Fetal and Neonatal Physiology

for the Advanced Practice Nurse

Amy J. Jnah, DNP, APRN, NNP-BC, is a veteran of the U.S. Navy Nurse Corps, as well as an alumna of the Marquette University School of Nursing (BSN), East Carolina University College of Nursing (MSN), and University of Alabama at Birmingham (DNP). Dr. Jnah holds the rank of clinical professor and is the director of the neonatal nurse practitioner program at the East Carolina University College of Nursing. She has received numerous awards and honors, which include the Reserve Officer Training Corps academic scholarship (1994–1998), distinguished graduate of the East Carolina University neonatal nurse practitioner program (2007–2008), and East Carolina University Scholar-Teacher of the Year (2017–2018) award.

Her clinical interests include hyperbilirubinemia, neonatal resuscitation, the transition to extrauterine life, and issues that affect late-preterm infants. Dr. Jnah is a master trainer for the American Academy of Pediatrics Helping Babies Breathe program, and an instructor-mentor for the Neonatal Resuscitation Program. Her academic interests include mentoring, role-modeling, and the integration of multisensory teaching innovations within distance education.

Amy J. Jnah, DNP, APRN, NNP-BC
EDITOR
Jacqui Hoffman, DNP, APRN, NNP-BC
Colleen R. Moss, DNP, APRN, NNP-BC
Jennifer Fitzgerald, DNP, APRN, NNP-BC
Amy Williford, MSN, APRN, NNP-BC
ASSOCIATE EDITORS

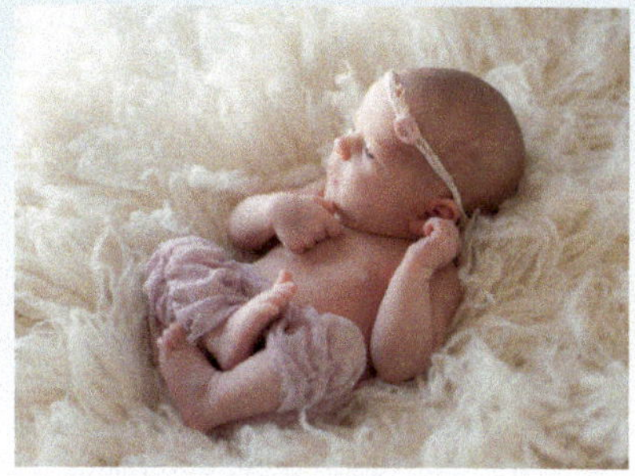

Fetal and Neonatal Physiology for the Advanced Practice Nurse

SECOND EDITION

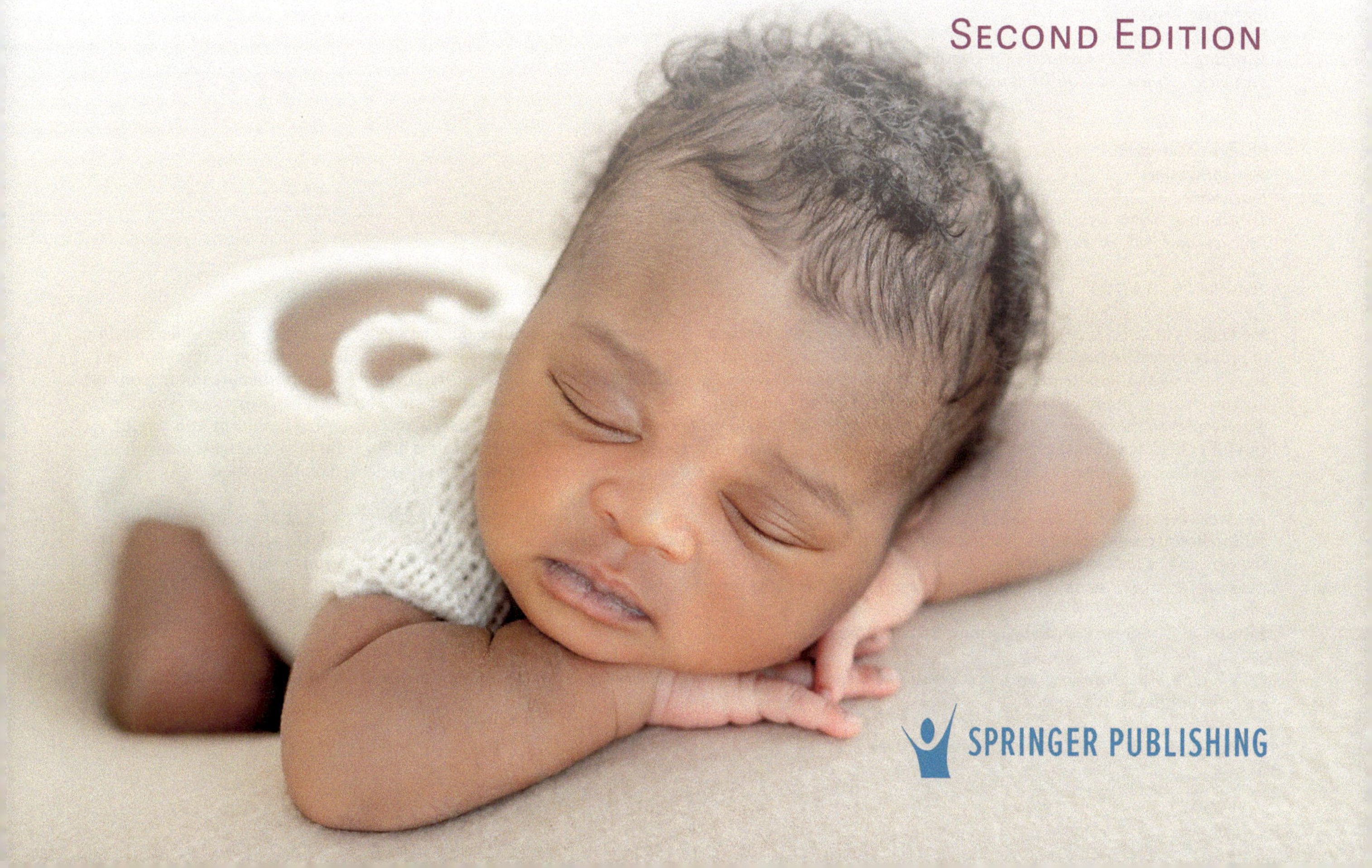

SPRINGER PUBLISHING

First Springer Publishing edition 978-0-8261-5731-7, 2018

Springer Publishing Company, LLC
902 Carnegie Center/Suite 140, Princeton, NJ 08540
www.springerpub.com
connect.springerpub.com

Acquisitions Editor: Joseph Morita
Development Editor: Brenna Croker
Production Editor: Diana Osborne
Compositor: Amnet

ISBN: 978-0-8261-7371-3
eBook ISBN: 978-0-8261-7372-0
DOI: 10.1891/9780826173720

SUPPLEMENTS:

A robust set of instructor resources designed to supplement this text is located at http://connect.springerpub.com/content/book/978-0-8261-7372-0. Qualifying instructors may request access by emailing textbook@springerpub.com.

Instructor Materials:
LMS Common Cartridge With All Instructor Resources
Instructor Test Bank
Instructor Image Bank
Mapping to AACN Essentials: Core Competencies for Professional Nursing Education
Transition Guide: First Edition to Second Edition

Student Materials:
Student Quizzes
Flashcards
Timelines of Organ Development
Podcasts and Podcast Transcripts

26 27 28 29 / 5 4 3 2 1

Library of Congress Control Number: 2025038207

Printed in the United States of America by Gasch Printing.

I would like to thank several special individuals who made this book possible:
To my family, Colonel Eric Jnah, Mya, and Ryan, thank you all for your grace, love, and support over the years and during the inception of both editions of this textbook. Thank you (again) for innovating drawings, teaching me to be a creative problem-solver who never gives up, and showing me that learning requires curiosity and engaging curiosity allows us to attain lasting knowledge.

To my co-editors (Jacqui, Colleen, Jen, and Amy), thank you for your hard work, dedication, and attention to detail in shaping this textbook. Your expertise and commitment have made it a valuable asset for neonatal nurse practitioner (NNP) students, and I truly appreciate the time and effort you put into refining the content.

To the talented East Carolina University NNP program student artists, thank you for role-modeling active learning behaviors. Your mind maps have helped you and will now be able to help future students for years to come!

To my dear colleagues Dr. Andrea N. Trembath and Dr. Lisa Mitchell, thank you for graciously peer-reviewing chapter content amid your hectic schedules, all while being steadfast voices of support and encouragement!

–AJ

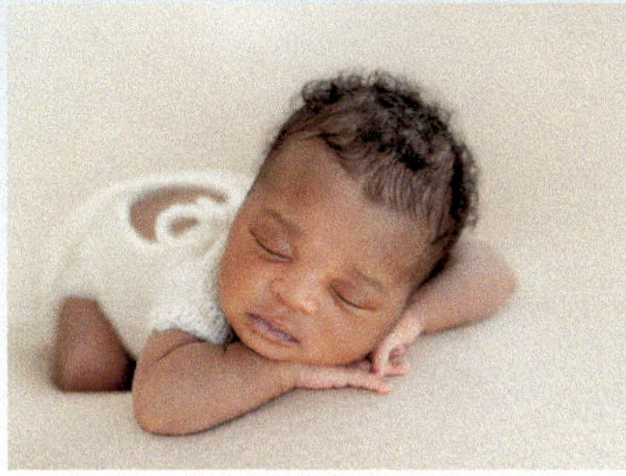 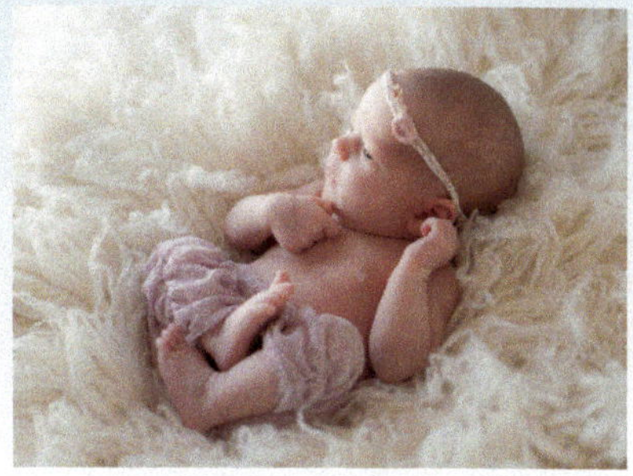

CONTENTS

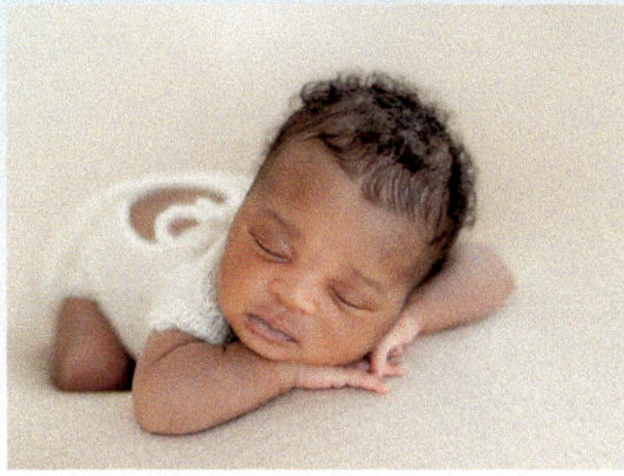 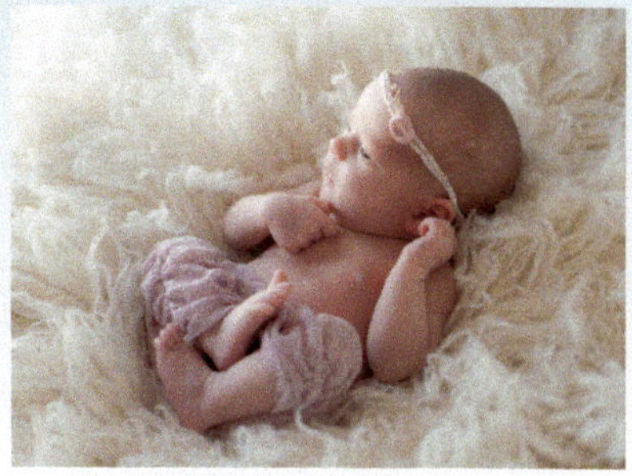

EDITORS

Amy J. Jnah, DNP, APRN, NNP-BC
Professor of Nursing (Clinical)
Director, Neonatal Nurse Practitioner Concentration
East Carolina University
College of Nursing
Greenville, North Carolina
Neonatal Nurse Practitioner
University of North Carolina at Chapel Hill
Chapel Hill, North Carolina

Jacqui Hoffman, DNP, APRN, NNP-BC
Assistant Professor, NNP Track–DNP Program
Rush University
College of Nursing
Chicago, Illinois

Colleen R. Moss, DNP, APRN, NNP-BC
Associate Professor
Director, Neonatal Nurse Practitioner Specialty
Vanderbilt University
School of Nursing
Nashville, Tennessee

Jennifer Fitzgerald, DNP, APRN, NNP-BC
Assistant Professor
Specialty Director, Neonatal Nurse Practitioner Program
University of Maryland Baltimore
School of Nursing
Baltimore, Maryland

Amy Williford, MSN, APRN, NNP-BC
Assistant Professor of Nursing (Clinical)
Neonatal Nurse Practitioner Concentration
East Carolina University
College of Nursing
Greenville, North Carolina

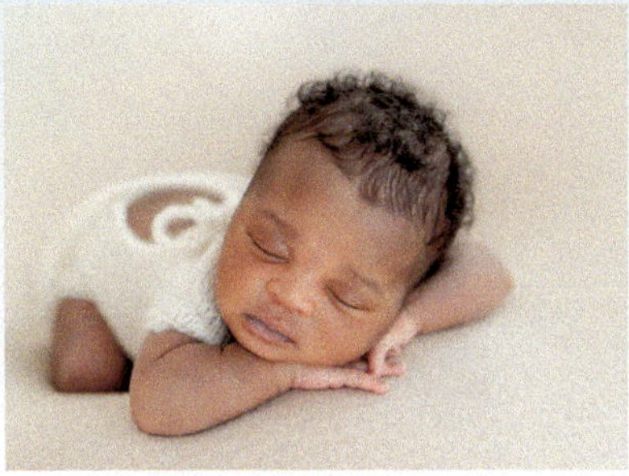

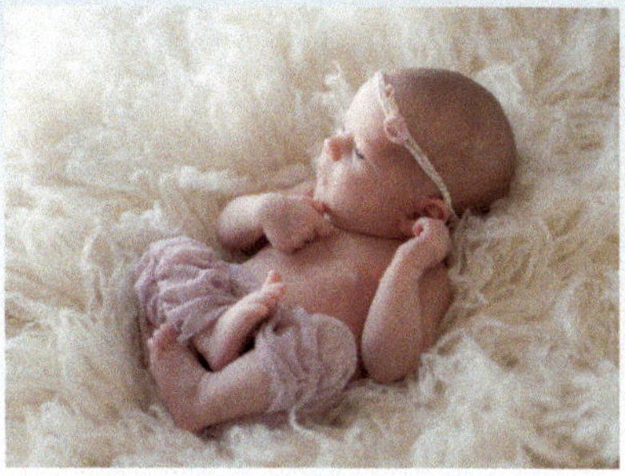

FOREWORD

Tell me and I forget, teach me and I may remember, involve me and I learn.

—Benjamin Franklin

In medicine, learning is a lifelong endeavor. Nowhere is that more apparent than in the NICU where the timely identification, diagnosis, and treatment of critically ill infants depends on our ability to rapidly translate information into knowledge. The second edition of this physiology textbook bridges that gap by providing the fundamental information and tools that neonatal APRNs need to navigate the rapidly advancing world of neonatal medicine. By emphasizing the importance of active learning through the creation of multisensory content, the editors inspire readers to become more engaged and advanced critical thinkers and learners.

The editors weave several successful teaching strategies into this edition of the textbook, which include case-based "clinical applications," drawings that visually enhance complex content, and podcasts written by expert neonatal clinicians. Dr. Jnah embedded this multisensory strategy within the East Carolina University neonatal nurse practitioner curricula over 10 years ago, and since that time, student outcomes and clinical performance have proven it works. Importantly, this type of high-stakes learning must occur within a supportive, trusting, and encouraging classroom environment for students to achieve a deeper understanding of content and long-term retention rather than passive receipt of information and short-term retention.

Learners tend to read much faster than they process information. Therefore, drawing out complex concepts in the form of "mind maps" forces them as learners to slow down and crystalize complex concepts, which enhances their critical thinking and problem-solving skills. Considering this information in the context of clinical scenarios encourages us to analyze, evaluate, and apply information to real-life scenarios, thus elevating the relevance of the content addressed in the textbook and the likelihood that learners will retain and recall that information. This also allows us as clinicians to discern the "why" behind how we manage and treat specific disease processes. Dr. Jnah uses clinical applications and visuals in this textbook for these reasons.

Last, let's not forget that collaboration and communication are critical in neonatal intensive care. For neonatal APRNs, collaboration begins in the graduate classroom. Faculty are called to lead this charge by creating engaging conversations with adult learners that help them translate complex concepts into understandable material. Students are called to help one another by discussing content, asking clarifying questions of one another and their faculty mentors, and seeking answers. This collaborative approach not only enhances retention but also prepares practitioners for working in multidisciplinary professional teams. Most importantly, active learning empowers learners to take ownership of their education—a process that should continue throughout their career.

Andrea N. Trembath, MD, MPH, FAAP
Professor of Pediatrics
University of North Carolina at Chapel Hill
Chapel Hill, North Carolina

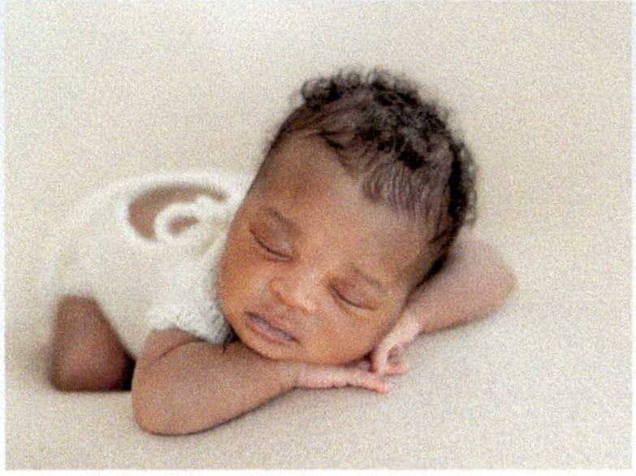 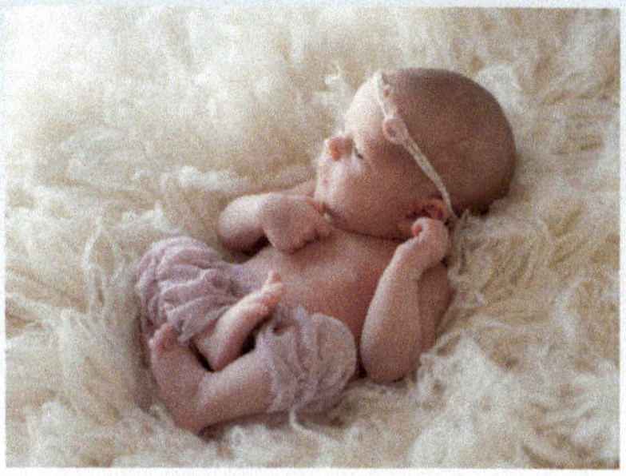

PREFACE

Fetal and Neonatal Physiology for the Advanced Practice Nurse offers a unique framework for the study of human physiology and common diseases that may afflict premature and term infants. The scope, sequence, and construct of each individual chapter is grounded in the Montessori method, which underpins My multisensory, active approach to didactic instruction and engaging, clinically relevant teaching methods.

This textbook provides APRNs with core concepts of fetal and neonatal physiology in a manner that promotes contemplative thinking, understanding, and retention. Therefore, this content is intended to precede the study of clinical diagnostics and management. Part I introduces core concepts, including fetal origins of disease, genetic inheritance patterns, and placental physiology. Part II investigates each major human body system. Part III offers an exploration into the transition to extrauterine life and common challenges facing perinatal and neonatal clinicians.

It is well known that teamwork, communication, and mentoring behaviors are associated with optimal outcomes for individuals and organizations. Therefore, each chapter reflects a purposeful, interprofessional integration of the knowledge of both junior and senior nursing and medical professionals. Most chapter mind maps and other select visuals are the work of aspiring neonatal nurse practitioners, who handpicked challenging concepts and, in consultation with academic faculty, created these graphic learning tools. Blank timelines are included to encourage active annotation during studying, self-directed learning, and the creation of feedback loops with academic or clinical mentors. Blank and completed timelines can be accessed at www.springerpub.com/courseconnect. See inside front cover and tear-out for CourseConnect details.

Audio podcasts offer learners a complementary method for studying common, core phenomena that affect the fetus and newborn. These podcasts, written by neonatal APRNs and physicians, mimic breakout teaching moments that occur during daily rounding at academic teaching hospitals. The podcasts are also available online by visiting www.springerpub.com/courseconnect.

Amy J. Jnah

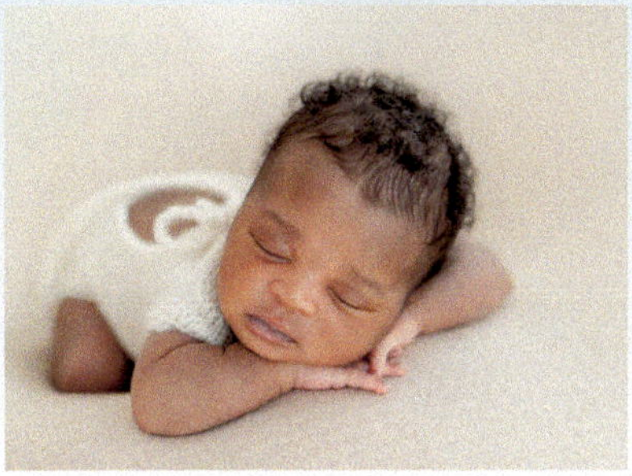 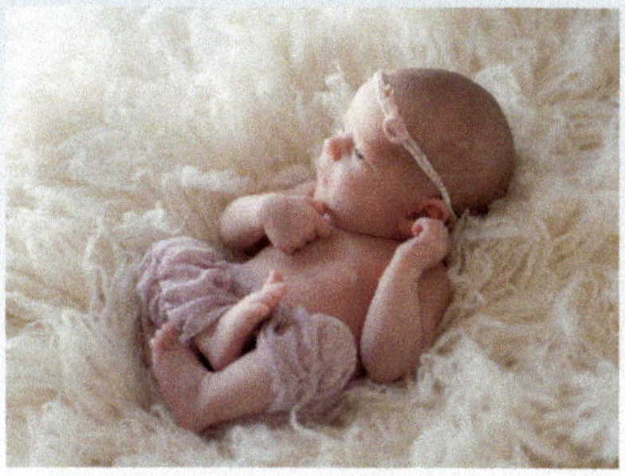

NOTE TO READERS

We recognize and support gender diversity among patients who seek obstetrical care and have optimized the use of the phrase "XX pregnant patient" as much as possible throughout this book in a sincere effort to be both scientifically accurate and inclusive of all persons. The use of the term "maternal" is used minimally and refers to pregnant individuals with biological characteristic XX assigned at birth.

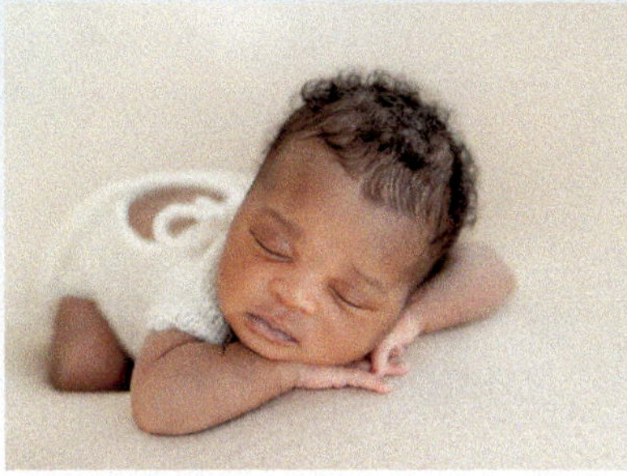 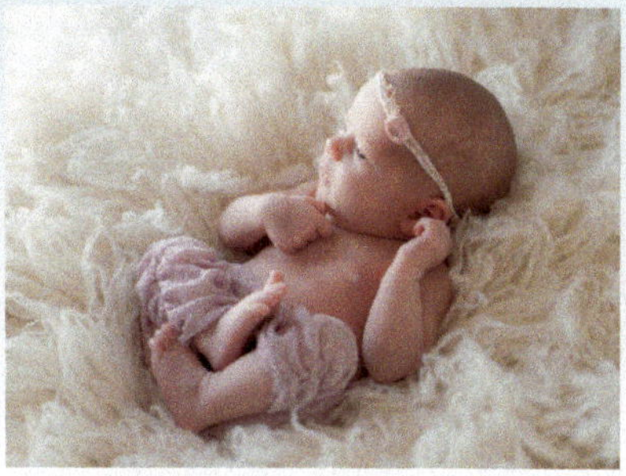

LIST OF PODCASTS

The supplemental audio podcasts listed below are provided as an adjunct to the content included within each chapter. Accessible anytime, the podcasts are an ideal complement to the written chapter content, and can reinforce learning through auditory engagement. Listen along to strengthen your grasp of concepts relevant to neonatal care. To access the podcasts and transcripts, visit www.springerpub.com/courseconnect. See inside front cover and tear-out card for CourseConnect details.

Chapter 2: Transplacental Gas Transfer
Mark Kadrofske

Chapter 3: Infant Sleep-Wake Pattern
Jenna Meredith and Amy J. Jnah

Chapter 4: Surfactant, Surface Tension, and LaPlace
Janice L. Wilson and Jennifer Fitzgerald

Chapter 5: Case-Based Learning: Patent Ductus Arteriosus
Jacqui Hoffman and Nicole Bowie

Chapter 6: Intestinal Immunity
Rani Delaney, Lauren Fraser, Maryellen Lane, and Melissa Bauserman

Chapter 7: Physiologic Hyperbilirubinemia
Christie del Castillo-Hegyi

Chapter 8: The Renin-Angiotensin-Aldosterone System
Amy J. Jnah

Chapter 9: Antibiotic Use in the NICU and the Role of the Neonatal Early-Onset Sepsis Calculator in Decreasing Antibiotic Consumption
Rani Delaney, Lauren Fraser, Maryellen Lane, and Melissa Bauserman

Chapter 10: Neonatal Dehydration and Hypoglycemia
Christie del Castillo-Hegyi

Chapter 11: Congenital Adrenal Hyperplasia/ 21-Hydroxylase Deficiency
Andrea N. Trembath

Chapter 12: Neonatal Skin and Innate Immunity: Differences Between the Term and Preterm Infant
Rani Delaney, Lauren Fraser, Maryellen Lane, and Melissa Bauserman

Chapter 13: #1—Visual Input; #2—Retinopathy of Prematurity; #3—The Red Reflux
Desi M. Newberry, Debbie Fraser, Sofia Aliaga, Bill Diehl-Jones, and Amy J. Jnah

Chapter 14: Transition to Extrauterine Life
Janice L. Wilson and Jennifer Fitzgerald

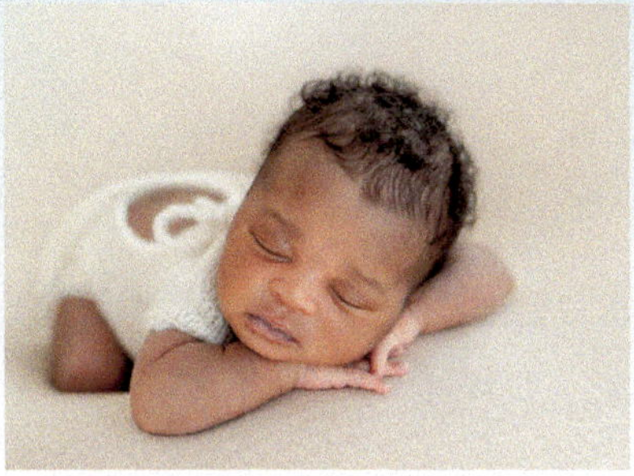 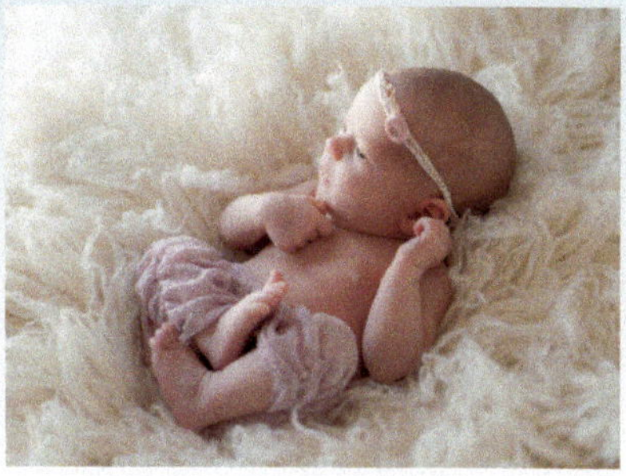

RESOURCES

STUDENT RESOURCES

To access self-assessment questions and interactive learning activities for this chapter, visit www.springerpub.com/courseconnect. See inside front cover and tear-out card for CourseConnect details.

- Student Quizzes
- Flashcards
- Timelines of Organ Development
- Podcasts with Transcripts

INSTRUCTOR RESOURCES

A robust set of resources designed to supplement this text is located at http://connect.springerpub.com. Qualifying instructors may request access by emailing textbook@springerpub.com. Available resources include:

- LMS Common Cartridge With All Instructor Resources
- Instructor Test Bank
- Instructor Image Bank
- Mapping to AACN Essentials: Core Competencies for Professional Nursing Education
- Transition Guide: First Edition to Second Edition

SPRINGER PUBLISHING

Visit https://connect.springerpub.com and look for the "**Show Additional Resources**" button on the **book homepage**.

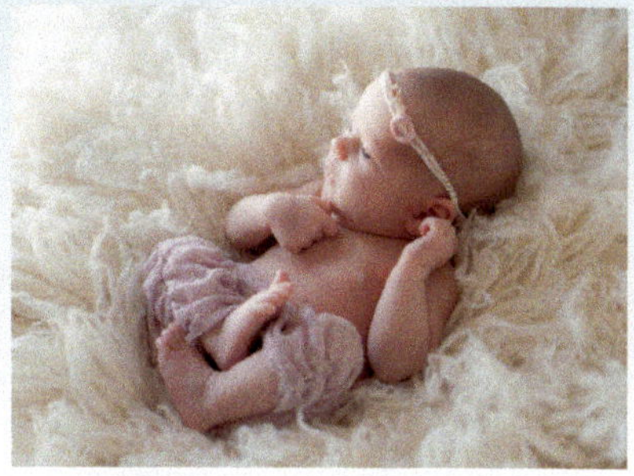

I

BASIC PRINCIPLES OF FETAL AND NEONATAL PHYSIOLOGY

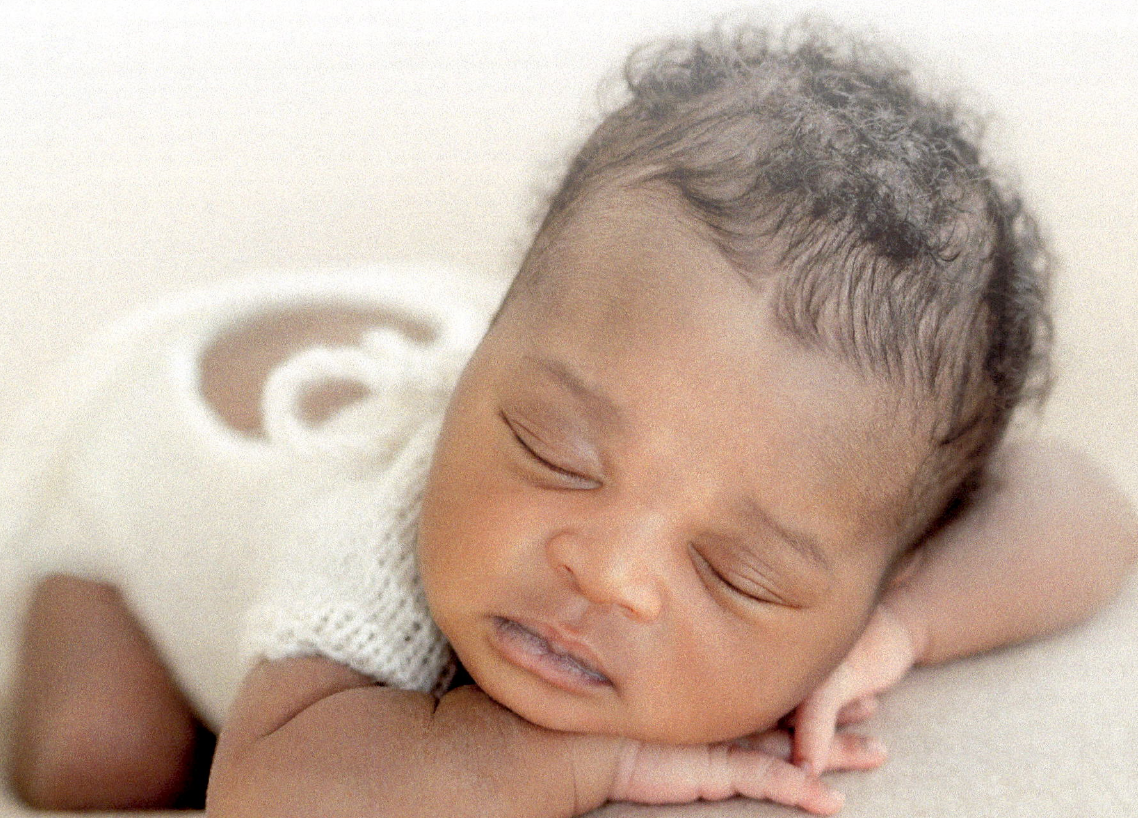

1

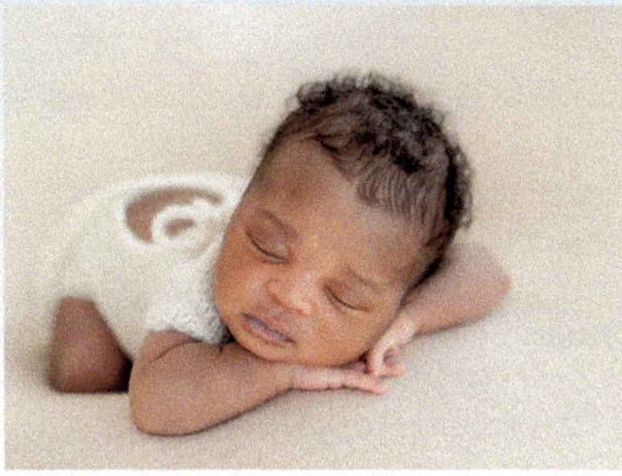

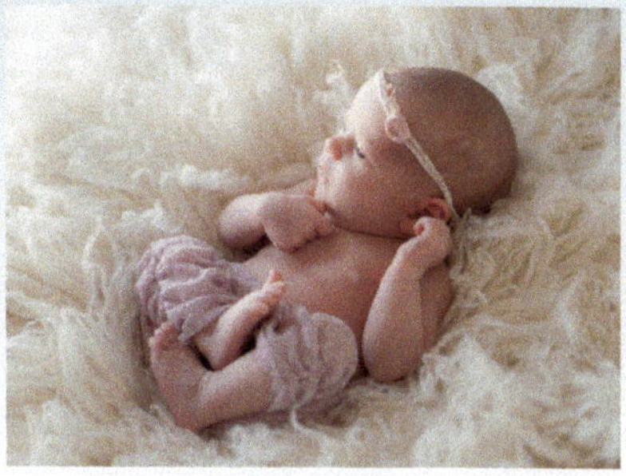

PRINCIPLES OF GENETICS

Amy J. Jnah and Jacqui Hoffman

LEARNING OBJECTIVES

After completing this chapter, the reader should be able to:

- Demonstrate a working understanding of common genetic terminology used in neonatal intensive care.
- Review basic principles of genetics, including DNA, genes and gene expression, and chromosomes.
- Apply existing knowledge of inheritance patterns to the investigation of Mendelian single-gene disorders.
- Evaluate common aneuploidies and chromosome structure disorders.
- Appraise disorders of metabolism and associated morbidity and mortality risks.
- Identify common genetic testing modalities used to evaluate for common and rare genetic disorders reported in neonates.

INTRODUCTION

The Human Genome Project was an international research project which spanned from 1990 to 2003. Scientists sought out to decode and sequence the entirety of the human genome. In total, upwards of 25,000 protein-coding genes and 3.2 billion base pairs in the human genome (Chail, 2008) were analyzed, and by 2003, more than 90% of the human genome was successfully sequenced. This project significantly enhanced our understanding of human sequence variation and the genetic basis for disease development in fetuses, newborns, infants, children, and adults. It also elucidated the key role for genomic medicine within perinatology and neonatology, flagging the importance of this topic of study for APRNs.

This chapter begins with a concise discussion of basic principles of genetics. Genetic terms are utilized throughout this chapter to begin to familiarize neonatal APRNs with terminology used in clinical practice (Table 1.1). Next, we investigate key genomic concepts, including common single-gene disorders and aneuploidies. From there, we analyze more complex concepts including translocation, mosaicism, uniparental disomy, and mitochondrial disorders. This information offers APRNs a foundational body of knowledge that can facilitate early identification of the newborn with a genetic disorder, multidisciplinary communications, diagnostics, and family counseling. We close the chapter with an overview of genetic testing modalities.

BASIC PRINCIPLES OF GENETICS

Deoxyribonucleic Acid

A eukaryote is a cell that contains a nucleus. The nucleus is the center of a eukaryotic cell where critical functions including DNA synthesis, RNA synthesis, DNA replication, and DNA transcription occur. DNA, first discovered by Watson and Crick in 1953, has two primary subtypes: nuclear and mitochondrial. *Nuclear DNA* is synthesized within the nucleus of eukaryotic cells. It modulates the

TABLE 1.1 Common Genetic Terms and Definitions

Term	Definition
Allele	Alternative form of a gene or sequence of DNA
Autosomes	22 pairs of "non-sex" chromosomes
Copy number variant	A sequence of the genome (base pairs) that is repeated or deleted in variable amounts
Deletion	Fracturing of a chromosome in two places with loss of the intervening portion
Exome	The portion of the genome which consists of protein-coding regions
Exome sequencing	The laboratory study of the order of nucleotides in the protein-coding regions of DNA
Fluorescence in situ hybridization (FISH)	The laboratory study of the location of one gene on a chromosome
Gene	Section of DNA that codes for biochemical molecules and proteins
Genome	The sum of all genetic material within a cell
Genome sequencing	The laboratory study of the order of nucleotides in the entire sequence of DNA
Genotype	The set of two inherited alleles found at a genetic locus
Human Genome Project	The title of a large study initiated in 1990 by the U.S. Department of Energy (US DOE) and National Institutes of Health (NIH) to create the first ordered set of human DNA and draft of the human genome. The project ended in 2003.
Karyotype	The laboratory study of chromosomes, which can detect abnormal numbers or structures
Mendelian disorder (single-gene disorder)	An inherited disease or trait that is identified by a gene at one specific locus
Microarray	The laboratory study of an ordered pattern of known nucleic acid sequences using fluorescent detection
Meiosis	The process of separation of somatic cells, as occurs during reproduction, such that the embryo gains half from each parent. Diploid cells (containing two sets of chromosomes) undergo two rounds of division to yield four haploid cells (gametes). The egg (gamete cell) and sperm (gamete cell) are therefore haploid cells (each containing 23 chromosomes) which can unite to form a zygote (a newly formed diploid cell known as the fertilized ovum).
Mitosis	The process by which embryonic cells replicate the chromosome complement. This produces two identical nuclei, or daughter cells. After fertilization, the zygote undergoes a series of several mitotic divisions, which in time gives rise to the human embryo.
Mosaicism	Abnormal germline (egg/sperm) or somatic (all cells except reproductive cells) cellular divisions resulting in two or more types of cells comprised of varying numbers of chromosomes
Mutation	The alteration of normal genetic material into a pathologic state and which leads to altered function
Phenotype	Observable physical features
Sex chromosomes	X (female) and Y (male)
Translocation	A segment of a chromosome that breaks from its original locus and is reinserted at a different location in the genome
Trisomy	Three copies of a chromosome within a somatic or germline cell

synthesis and function of specific genes (e.g., *POLG, TWNK, TK2, ANT1*) responsible for producing proteins which control the synthesis and replication of *mitochondrial DNA (mtDNA)*, found within the mitochondria. Mitochondria are organelles that use food (e.g., parenteral nutrition, formula, breast milk) to synthesize energy that cells can use to perform various functions. By way of oxidative phosphorylation, *mtDNA* modulate the production of adenosine triphosphate (ATP), energy which mitochondria depend upon to function properly.

DNA is inherited, and the process of inheritance is unique. At conception, sperm undergo meiotic cellular divisions and during this normal process, mtDNA in the sperm are degraded. In contrast, the oocyte (female germ cell, inherited from the mother, XX) contains a plethora of mtDNA that under normal circumstances remain intact. Proper inheritance of this genetic material requires normal mtDNA function during cellular mitosis (Podolak et al., 2022). mtDNA are known to be extremely fragile and vulnerable to mutations, which can disturb the production of ATP, reactive oxygen species, and free radical production. This can negatively affect embryogenesis and give rise to primary mitochondrial disorders (PMDs), which will be discussed later in this chapter.

Genes and Gene Expression

Recall that in the prior section of this chapter, we discussed that DNA modulates the synthesis and function of **genes**, which are nucleotide sequences of DNA that produce proteins. Gene sequences offer cells a transcript which guides the synthesis and secretion of protein molecules. Essentially, human cells extract gene sequences, then record and translate them, using the gene's "recipe," into biologically active proteins. These processes modulate human growth, development, and function. The process of "turning on" or "turning off" protein synthesis is referred to as *gene regulation*. When a gene is "turned on," a process called *gene expression* occurs. DNA will create RNA through a process called *transcription*. Next, the newly created messenger RNA (mRNA) couriers genetic information to the cytoplasm of the cell for processing. Mutations (germline/inherited or somatic/acquired) involving any of the transcription factors that regulate this process of DNA modification (e.g., methylation of cytosine) can give way for the development of genetic diseases that either affect a single nucleotide or an entire chromosome. Once transcription is complete, a process called mRNA *translation* occurs. Translation leads to the synthesis of a specific protein with a unique sequence of amino acids.

Clinical Application. The cystic fibrosis (CF) transmembrane conductance regulator gene, expressed on chromosome 7, is responsible for regulating the synthesis of a protein called cystic fibrosis transmembrane conductance regulator (*CFTR*). The *CFTR* protein is an amino acid glycoprotein and member of the ATP family. During periods of active *CFTR* gene expression, *CFTR* protein synthesis is regulated and synthesized. This *CFTR* protein allows for the proper transport of chloride out of epithelial cells, and regulates bicarbonate transport and epithelial sodium (ENaC) channel function. This facilitates water and salt balance in the airways, gastrointestinal system, pancreas, liver, gallbladder, and sweat glands, creating mucus that is of normal consistency. A mutation in this *CFTR* gene disrupts normal production of the *CFTR* protein and leads to the production of abnormally thick and sticky mucous within the airways and gastrointestinal system. Newborn screening can detect CF by measuring immunoreactive trypsinogen (IRT) in the dried blood spots. A substantially elevated IRT is significant for CF. Hallmark manifestations of this single-gene autosomal recessive inherited disorder include meconium ileus, distal intestinal obstruction, airway obstruction, and recurrent chronic bacterial infections or bronchiectasis. Given that individuals with CF have "salty sweat," the pilocarpine "sweat test" remains the gold standard test for diagnosing CF.

Chromosomes

Assuming that cell division is not deranged, the entire complement of genetic information is cloned every time cells replicate so that each daughter cell contains the same information. Genes are thereby arranged in an orderly, linear fashion on chromosomes. By definition, chromosomes are organized, long, thread-line strands that contain DNA, genes, proteins, and alleles and found within the nucleus of cells. Chromosomes are organized into pairs, with one chromosome from each pair donated from each parent. Normally, humans have 23 pairs of chromosomes, with 22 of those pairs considered homologous *autosomes* (non-sex chromosomes numbered 1–22 in order of decreasing size) and one pair considered *sex chromosomes* (i.e., XX, XY). The chromosomal pattern found within any human is regarded as their *karyotype* (e.g., 46, XY).

Chromosomes are made up of a short arm (*p*), long arm (*q*), and a centromere. The "p" originates from the French term "petit" (small) because the *p-arm* is normally the smaller end of a chromosome. The centromere is a constricted section of a chromosome, and while it may seem intuitive that a centromere would always be found in the center of a chromosome, in truth it can be found anywhere along the full length of a chromosome. For this reason, geneticists use different terms to denote where the centromere is found on a particular chromosome. Most chromosomes are *metacentric,* which means that the centromere is positioned in the middle of the chromosome, permitting equal-sized *p* and *q* arms. *Acrocentric* chromosomes (13, 14–15, 21, 22) have a centromere located at the end of a chromosome which leads to a *p-arm* of variable size (invisible to quite sizable). *Submetacentric* chromosomes (2, 4–12, 17, 18, X) also have a centromere off-set from the center of the chromosomes which leads to a shortened *p*-arm compared to the *q*-arm.

Alleles are specific variations of genes that are found within autosomes. Alleles are inherited in pairs (one from each parent) and these pairs might be homozygous (each allele in a pair is identical to the other) or heterozygous (different from the other). For example, consider a fetus who inherits heterozygous alleles for eye color (Figure 1.1). One parent donates a dominant allele for brown eye color and the other donates a recessive allele for blue eye color. The baby goes on to develop permanent brown eye color. (Note: Eye color is considered permanent between 6 and 9 months of age.) In this example, while both alleles coded for eye color, each parent donated one that was slightly unique from the other and ultimately the dominant allele controlled for eye color. This offers one example of how children inherit phenotypic characteristics from each parent, and in some ways their immediate ancestors.

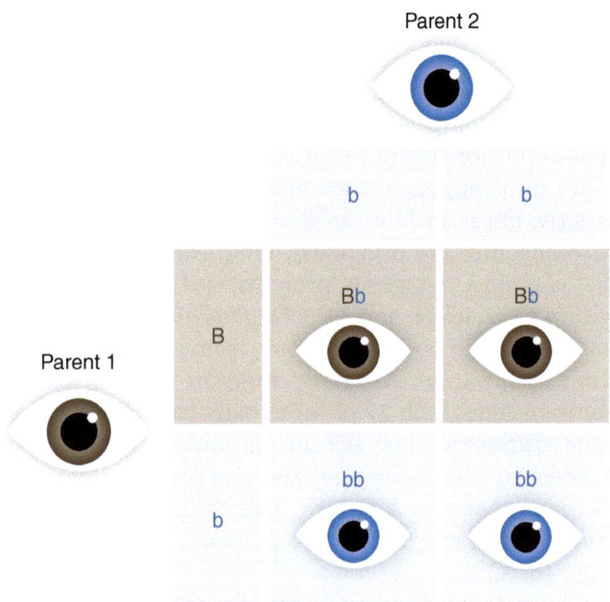

Figure 1.1 Punnett square of dominant and recessive alleles for eye color.

Note: "B" represents the dominant allele for brown eye color. "b" represents the recessive allele for blue eye color. Parent #1 is "Bb" and has brown eyes, meaning that parent can donate either the "B" or "b" at conception. Parent #2 is "bb" and has blue eyes, meaning this parent can only donate a "b" at conception. There is a 50% chance that an offspring will inherit the dominant "B" allele and develop "Bb" brown eyes, and a 50% chance that an offspring will inherit "bb" blue eyes.

SINGLE-GENE DISORDERS

To review, there are 46 chromosomes contained within every human cell. These chromosomes are organized into pairs; 50% of each pair is donated from each parent. Twenty-two of the chromosome pairs are numbered and considered "non-sex" alleles, or autosomes; autosomal genes usually produce similar outcomes in males and females. This leaves one pair to function under normal circumstances as the sex chromosomes; X-linked sex genes affect males and females differently. In females, despite the presence of two X chromosomes, only one is responsible for modulating gene product. The other X chromosome is subject to X-inactivation.

Phenotypes that occur as a result of variations in a single gene can be shared from parent to child by way of Mendelian inheritance patterns. Since the early 1960s, scientists have been cataloging Mendelian disorders and traits; as of October 2023, 7,430 phenotypes and 4,844 genes with phenotype-causing mutations are reported by the OMIM Online Catalog of Human Genes and Genetic Disorders scorecard (https://www.omim.org/statistics/geneMap). We investigate four common single-gene inheritance patterns in this section of the chapter: autosomal dominant, autosomal recessive, X-linked dominant, and X-linked recessive.

Autosomal Dominant

Dominant inheritance refers to the inheritance of one faulty, or mutated, dominant autosome (1–22) from either parent. In the case of autosomal dominance, the faulty gene copy *dominates* its working gene partner. Therefore, if one parent possesses an autosomal dominant gene defect, each child has a 50% chance of being affected by the disease. Children who do not inherit the abnormal gene will not develop or pass on the disease. In rare circumstances a child may inherit the same dominant faulty gene from both parents and display a severe manifestation of the trait or disease, which in some cases is fatal. Males and females are affected equally. Figure 1.2 describes outcomes based upon common parental carrier statuses.

Clinical Application. Achondroplasia is an autosomal dominant inherited genetic disorder characterized by short stature (rhizomelic shortening), large head size (narrow foramen magnum), and a characteristic facial appearance including a depressed nasal bridge. This means that individuals with achondroplasia incur a 50% chance of passing this condition to each offspring, regardless of the sex of the parent and child. Approximately 80% of children born with achondroplasia represent spontaneous new mutations in the *FGFR3* gene, meaning that

Parent 1 Unaffected and Parent 2 Affected

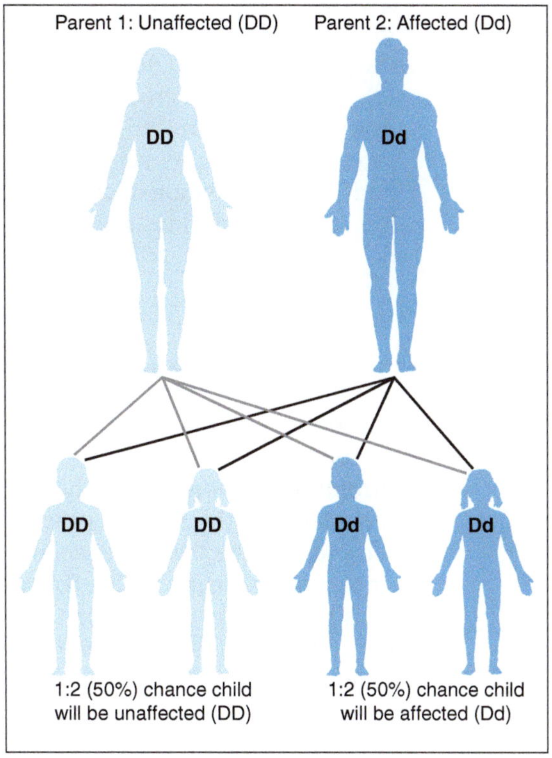

♂\♀	D	D
D	DD	DD
d	Dd	Dd

Parent 1 Affected and Parent 2 Affected

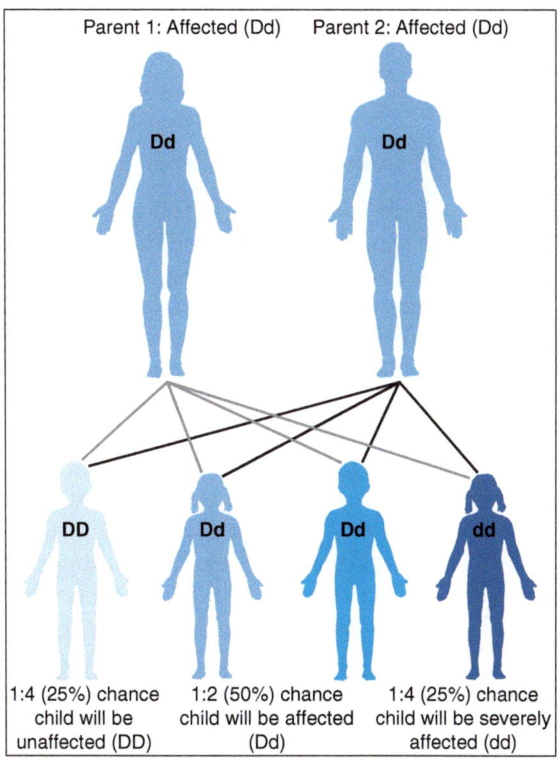

♂\♀	D	d
D	DD	Dd
d	Dd	dd

Figure 1.2 Autosomal dominant inheritance.

Note: Autosomal dominant inheritance. The working gene copy is represented as "D" and the faulty dominant gene copy is represented as "d" in all depictions in the figure. Autosomal dominant inheritance is presented in two different formats for student learners. The images on the left offer a visual representation of parents passing traits to offspring. The images on the right are Punnett squares, which can also be used to calculate the probability that male or female offspring will inherit a genetic disease. When neither parent is a carrier of a dominant faulty gene and they have a child affected by a condition known to be due to autosomal dominant inheritance, the condition is likely the result of a new (de novo) mutation in that gene during conception.

both parents are of normal stature yet the infant manifests with the genetic disorder due to the spontaneous mutation.

Germ-line mosaicism, also known as gonadal mosaicism, occurs when some germ cells are derived from a normal cell line, and some are derived from a cell line with a mutation. This has been reported in families with achondroplasia and means that two average-stature parents can have a child with achondroplasia. The recurrence risk of achondroplasia in sporadic cases by way of gonadal mosaicism is approximately 1%.

Many babies with achondroplasia reach their motor milestones later than normal because of hypotonia (low muscle tone) and large head size. A higher risk for central apnea within the first year of life is reported. Due to difficulties with head control, it is recommended that head support be provided at all times. Children with achondroplasia typically demonstrate normal intelligence and reach an average height of around 4 feet.

Autosomal Recessive

Recessive inheritance refers to the inheritance of a complete pair of faulty recessive autosomes (1–22), one from each parent. Unlike dominant inheritance, offspring must inherit a faulty gene pair to manifest an autosomal recessive disease or trait. Typically, both parents are unaffected carriers. For this reason, XX pregnant patients may choose to undergo prenatal screening for CF carrier status, a common autosomal recessive disease. When both parents are carriers, the offspring has a 25% chance of inheriting one faulty gene from each parent and becoming affected by the disease, or a 50% chance of carrying the trait. Males and females are affected equally. Figure 1.3 describes outcomes based upon common parental carrier statuses.

Clinical Application. Phenylketonuria (PKU), a single-gene disorder, is characterized by a deficiency of the phenylalanine hydroxylase (PAH) enzyme, which is necessary for the conversion of phenylalanine to tyrosine. The incidence of PKU in the United States is estimated to be 1:10,000 live births, whereas the incidence in Russia is 1:850 (Gundorova et al., 2018; Scriver, 2007). Newborn metabolic screening programs are credited with the rate of early identification, diagnosis, and treatment in U.S.-born infants.

Inheritance is autosomal recessive, meaning that parents who are both unaffected carriers of the PKU gene disorder incur a 25% chance of giving birth to a child affected by PKU, regardless of the sex of the parent and child. Prompt treatment with a low-Phe diet optimizes growth and neurodevelopment. Symptoms of untreated PKU in newborns include growth failure and seizures. Untreated infants and children demonstrate motor delays, ataxia, hypopigmented skin, and global developmental delay (Hillert et al., 2020).

X-Linked Dominant Inheritance

X-linked dominant inheritance refers to the inheritance of a faulty X chromosome. Among females, the faulty X chromosome "dominates" the normal, working copy of the gene and the disease process or trait manifests. Among males, the lack of a second X chromosome offers no recourse; males with a faulty X chromosome will express the disease process or trait. When the mother is affected by a condition caused by an X-linked dominant gene mutation, there is an equal (50%) chance that male and female offspring may, or may not, inherit the X-linked dominant gene mutation. When the father is affected by a condition caused by an X-linked dominant gene mutation, there is a 100% chance he will pass the faulty X chromosome to his female offspring; male offspring will be unaffected. Figure 1.4 describes outcomes based upon common parental carrier statuses.

X-Linked Recessive Inheritance

X-linked recessive inheritance commonly refers to the inheritance of one (in males) or a pair (in females) of faulty X chromosomes. Given that females inherit two X chromosomes, these X chromosomes can be homozygous for the diseased allele, homozygous for the normal allele, or heterozygous for the allele. In that way, X-linked recessive inheritance in females is very similar to autosomal recessive inheritance.

XX pregnant patients who carry one working copy and one faulty copy of the X chromosome are heterozygous unaffected (normal) carriers of the disease or trait. In these circumstances, the working copy of the X chromosome produces sufficient gene product and compensates for the faulty copy; the disease or trait does not manifest. Females who inherit a complete pair of faulty X chromosomes will be homozygous affected by the disease or trait. Rarely, females who possess one working and one faulty gene pair (heterozygous) express X-inactivation of the working copy of the X chromosome and manifest the disease or trait. On the other hand, males only inherit one X chromosome. Therefore, if a male inherits the faulty X chromosome, the disease or trait will be expressed. Figure 1.5 describes outcomes based upon common parental carrier statuses.

Parent 1 Carrier and Parent 2 Carrier

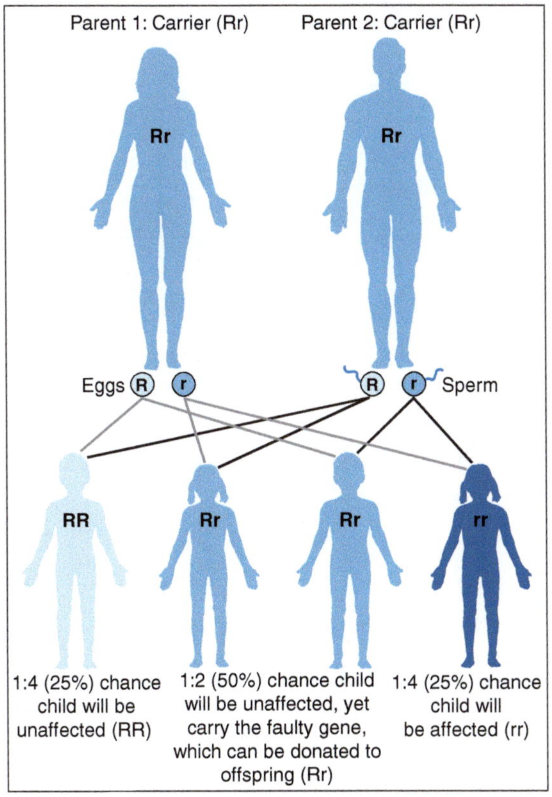

♂\♀	R	r
R	RR	Rr
r	Rr	rr

Parent 1 Affected and Parent 2 Carrier

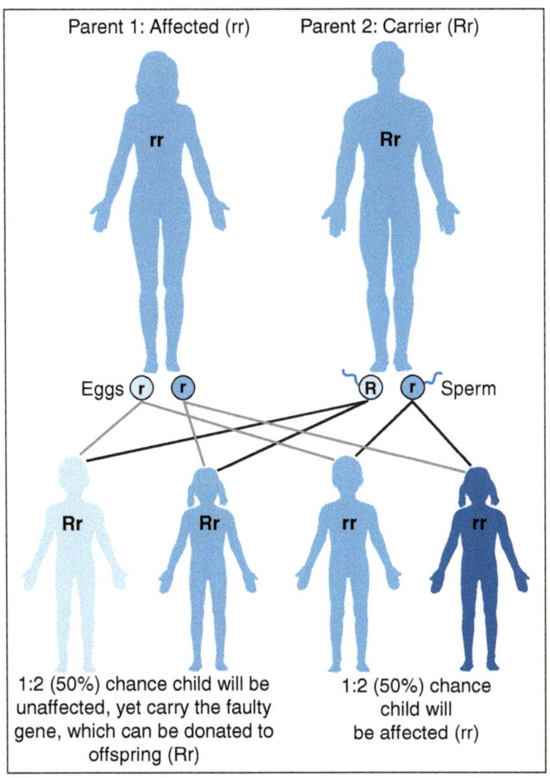

♂\♀	r	r
R	Rr	Rr
r	rr	rr

Figure 1.3 Autosomal recessive inheritance.

Note: Autosomal recessive inheritance. The working gene copy is represented as "R" and the faulty gene copy is represented as "r" in all depictions in the figure. The images on the left offer a visual representation of parents passing traits to offspring. The images on the right are Punnett squares, which can also be used to calculate the probability that male or female offspring will inherit a genetic disease. Of note, nearly 99% of all males with CF are infertile.

Mother Affected and Father Noncarrier

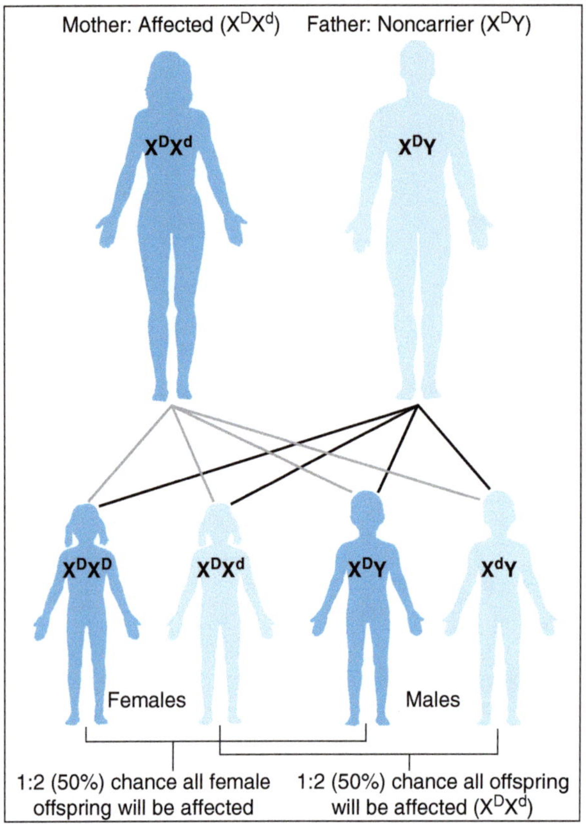

♂\♀	X^D	X^d
X^D	X^DX^D	X^DX^d
Y	X^DY	X^dY

Mother Noncarrier and Father Affected

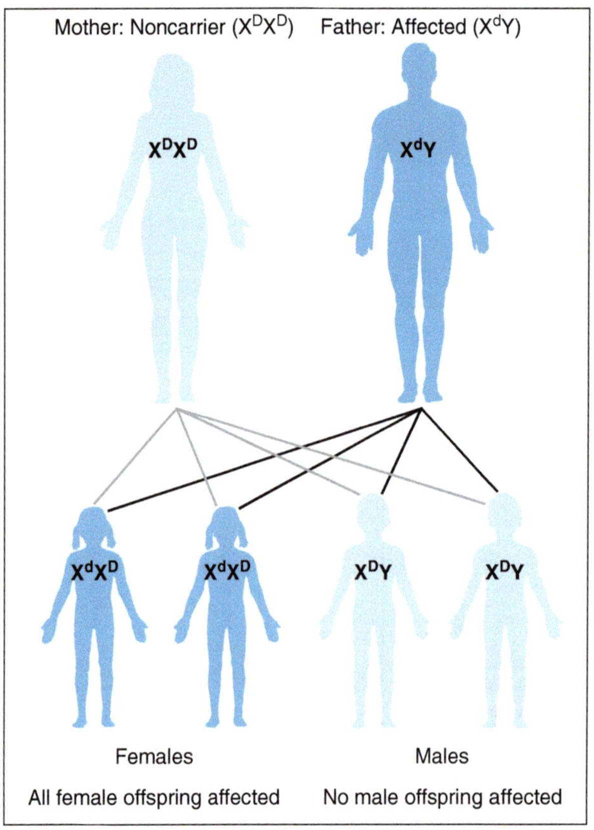

♂\♀	X^D	X^D
X^d	X^DX^d	X^DX^d
Y	X^DY	X^DY

Figure 1.4 X-linked dominant inheritance.

Note: X-linked dominant inheritance. The working gene copy is represented as "D" and the faulty gene copy is represented as "d."

Mother Carrier and Father Noncarrier

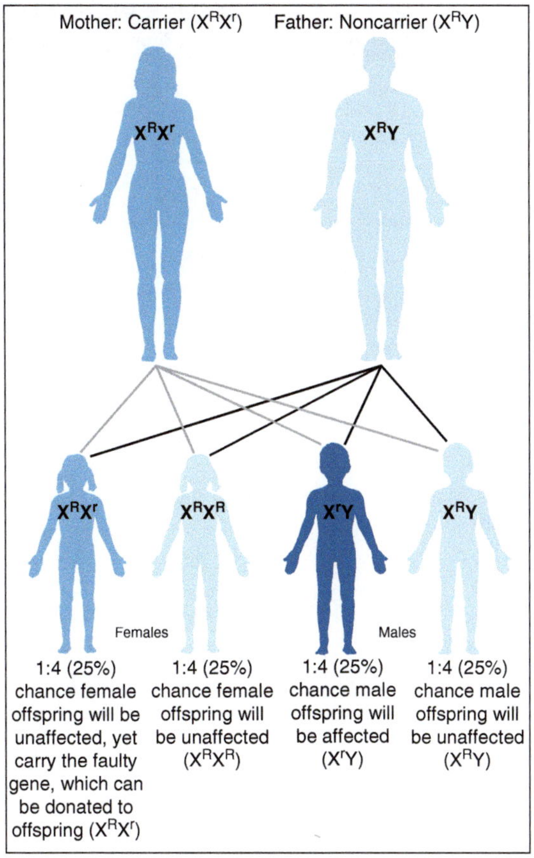

♂\♀	X^R	X^r
X^R	X^RX^R	X^RX^r
Y	X^RY	X^rY

Mother Noncarrier and Father Affected

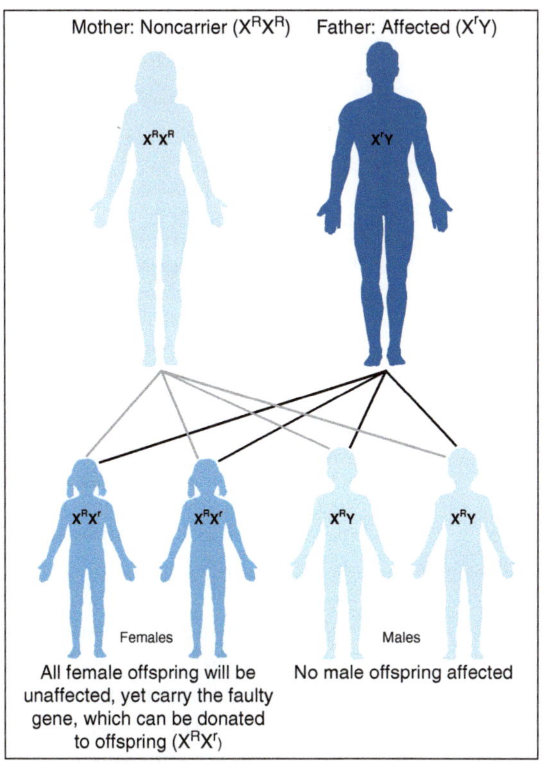

♂\♀	X^R	X^R
X^r	X^RX^r	X^RX^r
Y	X^RY	X^RY

Figure 1.5 X-linked recessive inheritance.

Note: X-linked recessive inheritance. The working gene copy is represented as "R" and the faulty gene copy is represented as "r." In rare circumstances, female offspring with *XRXr* inheritance may experience X-inactivation of the working gene copy and thereby manifest the disease or trait.

CHROMOSOME ANEUPLOIDIES

Under normal circumstances after conception, chromosomes separate, and human cells contain 46 chromosomes. *Nondisjunction* is the term used to describe a failed segregation of chromosomes, which will lead to an unequal distribution to the developing embryo, or an *aneuploidy*. The unequal distribution of chromosomes can result in a *monosomy*, where one copy of a chromosome is found in cells, leaving a total of 45 chromosomes in each cell within the body. Alternatively, a *trisomy* may occur, when three copies of a single chromosome are found in a cell. Nondisjunction that occurs during meiosis (when chromosomes are separated such that the embryo gains half from each parent) often leads to miscarriage. When nondisjunction occurs during mitosis (when embryonic cells exponentially divide and form the blastocyst, then morula, etc.), mosaicism is reported. A mosaic presentation of a disease may present as a milder phenotype. For example, with mosaic trisomy 21, newborns may lack visible dysmorphic features and this can precipitate a delay in diagnosis.

Advanced Maternal Age. The likelihood of chromosomal nondisjunction (e.g., trisomy 13, 18, and 21), congenital malformations, premature birth, and low birthweight increases with advancing maternal (XX) age, particularly among childbearing patients 35 years of age or older (Table 1.2; American College of of Obstetricians and Gynecologists' [ACOG] Committee on Clinical Consensus-Obstetrics et al., 2023). A linear relationship is reported; as maternal (XX) age (at the estimated date of delivery [EDD]) increases above age 35, this risk increases (relative risk [RR] 1.36; 95% CI; Sheen et al., 2018). ACOG makes the following recommendation related to genetic screening and diagnostic testing, which should alert neonatal providers to thoroughly inspect prenatal records for relevant test results:

> We recommend that prenatal genetic screening (serum screening with or without nuchal translucency ultrasonography or cell-free DNA screening) and diagnostic testing (chorionic villus sampling [CVS] or amniocentesis) options be discussed and offered to all pregnant individuals regardless of age or risk of chromosomal abnormality. After review and discussion, every patient has the right to pursue or decline prenatal genetic screening and diagnostic testing (GRADE 1A). (ACOG Committee on Clinical Consensus-Obstetrics et al., 2023)

TABLE 1.2 Risk of Chromosome Abnormalities Based on Age of the Pregnant Individual

Age at Estimated Due Date	Risk of Trisomy 13	Risk of Trisomy 18	Risk of Trisomy 21
35	1:4,000	1:1,060	1:272
36	1:3,333	1:800	1:205
37	1:2,857	1:600	1:153
38	1:2,000	1:444	1:114
39	1:1,667	1:333	1:85
40	1:1,250	1:255	1:65
41	1:1,000	1:200	1:51
42	1:800	1:162	1:42
43	1:606	1:136	1:35
44	1:465	1:117	1:30
45	1:357	1:104	1:27
46	1:278	1:94	1:24
47	1:215	1:87	1:22
48	1:167	1:82	1:21
49	1:128	1:79	1:20
50	Not reported	1:76	1:19

Note: These numbers represent population-specific risks, not individual risks, and are presented for teaching purposes only.

Sources: Hook, E. B. (1983). Chromosome abnormalities and spontaneous fetal death following amniocentesis: Further data and associations with maternal age. *American Journal of Human Genetics, 35*(1), 110–116; Hook, E. B., Cross, P. K., & Schreinemachers, D. M. (1983). Chromosomal abnormality rates at amniocentesis and in live-born infants. *JAMA, 249*(15), 2034–2038; Morris, J. K., Mutton, D. E., & Alberman, E. (2002). Revised estimates of the maternal age specific live birth prevalence of Down's syndrome. *Journal of Medical Screening, 9*(1), 2–6. https://doi.org/10.1136/jms.9.1.2

Patau Syndrome (Trisomy 13). Trisomy 13, also referred to as Patau syndrome, is the *third* most common aneuploidy. It is caused by an extra copy of chromosome 13, which can be present in all cells of the body or present within some cells of the body (mosaicism). Recall that chromosome 13 is considered an acrocentric chromosome. Acrocentric chromosomes can be subject to a Robertsonian translocation, where portions of two chromosomes (e.g., 13 and 14) become abnormally attached at a centromere, creating one chromosome with blended genetic material. Individuals can be unaffected carriers of a Robertsonian translocation and unknowingly pass this genetic material to offspring. In situations where one parent passes their intact chromosome 13 and the translocated chromosome 13/14 combination, and the other parent passes an intact chromosome 13, the offspring will inherit three copies of chromosome 13 and manifest with trisomy 13. Every cell in the fetus's body will contain the three copies of chromosome 13.

Classic fetal findings include CHDs (80%), holoprosencephaly (60%; hallmark neurologic finding), increased fetal neck thickness, nuchal translucency, intrauterine growth restriction, omphalocele (10%), cleft lip/palate, a two-vessel umbilical cord, and polydactyly (Descartes et al., 2018). Classic postnatal findings include ocular manifestations (microphthalmia, anophthalmia) and cutis aplasia (Table 1.3). CHDs often include ventricular and atrial septal defects (most common CHD), patent ductus arteriosus (PDA), double outlet right ventricle (DORV), and tetralogy of Fallot (Kosiv et al., 2023).

When concerns for aneuploidy are high, maternal fetal medicine experts often recommend cell-free DNA testing followed by CVS with fluorescence in situ hybridization (FISH). This test will analyze cells derived from the cytotrophoblast (inner layer of chorionic villus). In this case, if three hybridization signals are observed for chromosome 13 within 60% or more of cells that are sampled, the test is considered positive for trisomy 13 (46, XX, +13 or 46, XY, +13). Most pregnancies end in miscarriage or stillbirth. In-hospital mortality after delivery is estimated at 20% with an average survival time of 5 to 12.5 days (Glinianaia et al., 2023; Haghnazarian et al., 2019), particularly among newborns with cardiac defects (64.7%), respiratory issues (26.1%), or multiple organ failure (17.6%) and whose families prefer comfort care versus intensive care interventions (Peterson et al., 2017). Among infants who undergo a palliative cardiac procedure, in-hospital mortality decreases to 16%, with 5-year survival of 84% and 15-year survival of 70% (Kosiv et al., 2017; Peterson et al., 2017). Outcomes of a recent Western European study indicated that 55% of newborns survive the first week of life, 34% survive the first month of life, 17% survive to 1 year of age, and 11% survive to age 10 (Glinianaia et al., 2023).

Edwards Syndrome (Trisomy 18). Trisomy 18, also referred to as Edwards syndrome, is the *second* most common aneuploidy. It is caused by an extra copy of chromosome 18. Similar to Patau syndrome, trisomy 18 can present in all (complete trisomy) or some cells (mosaic) within the body. Common fetal markers include intrauterine growth restriction, CHDs (e.g., septal defects, poly-valvular disease), congenital diaphragmatic hernia, and horseshoe kidney. Other reported associated manifestations are summarized in Table 1.3. CHDs are reported in 90% of cases and include the same defects as with trisomy 13 (Kosiv et al., 2023). Outcomes of a recent Western European study indicated that 59% of newborns survive the first week of life, 38% survive the first month of life, 30% survive to age 1, and 8% survive to age 10 (Davisson et al., 2018; Glinianaia et al., 2023; Kosho et al., 2006). As mentioned in the prior section, in-hospital mortality risk is approximately 30% (vs. 55% in infants who do not undergo cardiac surgery, with 5-year survival identical to trisomy 13 at 84%, and 15-year survival of 70% (Kosiv et al., 2017; Peterson et al., 2017). Infants with complete trisomy 18 and who survive to childhood are not expected to use language to communicate or walk. Central apnea is reported and can lead to life-threatening hypoxia.

Down Syndrome (Trisomy 21). Trisomy 21, also referred to as Down syndrome, is the *most* common aneuploidy. This syndrome affects a total of one in 700 births, with a male prevalence. An incidence of one in 50 to 300 births involve XX pregnant patients classified as advanced maternal age (over age 35; Jones et al., 2022; NIH, 2020). It is caused by an extra copy of chromosome 21.

The overwhelming majority (95%) of cases are attributed to nondisjunction, with translocation and mosaicism accounting for the remainder of cases. In over 90% of cases, the additional chromosome is of maternal (XX) origin. Classic fetal findings include nuchal lucency, suggesting lymphedema. This state of congenital lymphedema carries into the postnatal period as lymphedema of the hands and feet (Table 1.4). CHDs are associated with 40% to 50% of trisomy 21 cases (Dimopoulos et al., 2023). Less known associations include Hirschsprung disease and congenital hypothyroidism. Ocular findings include epicanthal folds, upturned palpebral fissures, and Brushfield spots (see Chapter 13).

Clinical Application. Antepartum testing for chromosomal abnormalities is commonly offered to pregnant patients with advanced age at conception (35 years old or greater) and those with a history of chromosomal abnormalities with prior pregnancies. One particular noninvasive prenatal test is called the "MaterniT21 + ESS + SCA" test, which can determine fetal biological sex (male or female), and presence or absence of trisomies (13, 16, 18, 21, 22) and certain sex chromosome aneuploidies and microdeletions (45X, 47XXY, 47XXX, 47XYY, DiGeorge syndrome, Cri du chat syndrome, Prader-Willi syndrome [PWS], and 1p36 deletion syndrome). The positive predictive value for trisomy 21 is 97.9%. The negative predictive value for trisomy 13, 18, and 21 is greater than 99%. This test analyzes cell-free DNA in the maternal blood.

TABLE 1.3 Common Manifestations of Trisomy 13 and Trisomy 18 by Organ System

Organ System	Trisomy 13	Trisomy 18
Head/CNS	• Absent cerebellar vermis • Developmental delay • Enlarged cisterna magna • Facial nerve palsy • Holoprosencephaly • Meningomyelocele • Microcephaly with sloping forehead • Ventriculomegaly	• Choroid plexus cyst • Enlarged cisterna magna • Facial nerve palsy • Developmental delay • Meningomyelocele • Microcephaly • Seizures • Ventriculomegaly
Eyes	• Hypertelorism • Iris coloboma • Micropthalmia/anopthalmia	
Ears	• Low-set ears	• Hearing loss or deafness • Low-set ears
Nose/Mouth/Neck/ Throat	• Absent nasal bone • Cleft lip or palate • Retrognathia	• Absent nasal bone • Cleft lip or palate • Widely spaced nipples
Cardiac/Chest	• PDA • Septal defects • Tetralogy of Fallot	• PDA • Polyvalvular disease • Septal defects • Tetralogy of Fallot • Wharton's jelly cyst
Respiratory		• Pulmonary hypertension • Pulmonary vascular disease
Gastrointestinal	• Omphalocele	• Esophageal atresia and trachea-esophageal fistula • Malrotation • Meckel diverticulum • Omphalocele • Pyloric stenosis
Genitourinary	• Cryptorchidism • Fetal echogenic kidneys	• Bifid scrotum • Horseshoe kidney
Musculoskeletal	• Joint contractures • Postaxial polydactyly • Rounded appearance of the feet ("rocker bottom" feet)	• Clenched fists with overlapping second and fifth digits • Joint contractures, limb shortening (e.g., radial aplasia/hypoplasia/agenesis) • Rounded appearance of the feet ("rocker bottom" feet) • Sandal gap deformity • Scoliosis
Skin/Hair	• Cutis aplasia • Hair whorls	

Note: This table should not be considered inclusive of all manifestations of trisomy 13 and 18. Learners should spend time discerning manifestations unique to each trisomy in order to aid in the generation of a differential diagnosis. Additional manifestations may be presented in other chapters in this textbook.

CNS, central nervous system; PDA, patent ductus arteriosus.

TABLE 1.4 Common Manifestations of Trisomy 21 by Organ System

Organ System	Trisomy 21
Head/CNS	• Hypotonia
Eyes	• Epicanthal folds • Up-slanting palpebral fissures
Ears	• Low-set ears
Nose/Mouth/Neck/ Throat	• Flat nasal bridge • Flat faces • High-arched palate • Web neck
Cardiac/Chest	• Atrioventricular canal defect
Gastrointestinal	• Duodenal atresia
Musculoskeletal	• Fifth digit clinodactyly • Sandal gap deformity • Short fourth metacarpal bone • Short stature
Skin/Hair	• Nail dysplasia

CNS, central nervous system.

CHROMOSOME STRUCTURE DISORDERS

Under normal circumstances, newborns inherit a balanced karyotype. However, alterations to chromosome structure or complement, or a mosaicism, can occur. We review these concepts in this section of the chapter.

A chromosomal *translocation* occurs when genetic information "breaks off" of one chromosome and is transferred to a different chromosome. Translocations can be balanced, meaning a portion of two chromosomes "break off" and each broken portion is transferred to the other chromosome (e.g., balanced translocation of chromosomes 7 and 21 where a portion of chromosome 7 attaches to chromosome 21, and vice versa); a normal amount of genetic material is maintained in these situations. Newborns with balanced translocations demonstrate normal DNA protein synthesis. While rare, less than 0.1% of newborns are affected by unbalanced translocations, which can involve the *insertion* of additional DNA onto a chromosome (Jacobs et al., 1992). Unbalanced translocations typically lead to the development of congenital malformations (e.g., cardiac malformations, craniofacial malformations) that carry significant morbidity and mortality risk (Ishibashi et al., 2021).

Copy number variants (CNV) include chromosomal deletions and duplications. A chromosomal *deletion* occurs when a portion of a chromosome is deleted at conception. The loss of a portion of a chromosome leads to the loss of genes necessary for protein synthesis and often gives rise to congenital anomalies. A chromosomal *duplication* occurs when a portion of a chromosome is duplicated (two copies are created). This additional genetic material can derange normal development.

Clinical Application. Newborns affected by chromosomal deletions often manifest with obvious phenotypic malformations at birth. For example, consider Cri du chat (cat cry syndrome), a rare genetic disorder with an estimated incidence of 1:15,000 to 50,000 newborns (Cerruti-Mainardi, 2006). Cri du chat develops when the p-arm of chromosome 5 is deleted at conception. Newborns with Cri du chat are often of low birthweight. Common symptoms associated with the loss of genetic material at chromosome 5p include hypotonia, microcephaly, and a uniquely high-pitched cry. Children often develop expressive disorders associated with a reduced vocabulary as well as motor delays.

Alternatively, consider 22q11.2 deletion syndrome, also known as DiGeorge syndrome. In the majority of cases (90%), the deletion of the proximal long arm of chromosome 22 is de novo (a new mutation that is not inherited). Less often (10% of cases), DiGeorge syndrome is a result of autosomal dominant inheritance from a heterozygous parent. Newborns often present with congenital heart disease (e.g., tetralogy of Fallot, truncus arteriosus), palate deformities (e.g., cleft palate), thymic dysfunction (i.e., T-cell abnormality), parathyroid dysfunction (i.e., hypocalcemia), and phenotypic features (e.g., hypertelorism, short palpebral fissures, short philtrum, micrognathia, ear anomalies).

Mosaicism. Mosaicism occurs when two or more lines of cells contain different numbers of chromosomes. In this way, any cell line in the body (or the placenta) can be affected. Mosaicism can result from nondisjunction or even a de novo mutation. Mosaicism involving the placenta is termed *confined placental mosaicism*, and is associated with isolated fetal growth restriction without any other congenital phenotypic anomalies. In contrast, mosaicism that affects two or more cell lines in a fetus and newborn, termed a *somatic mosaicism*, will result in one or more observable phenotypic defects. Clinically, newborns with a mosaicism typically present with milder features. The most common genetic abnormality associated with mosaicism is Turner syndrome (Tuke et al., 2019).

Clinical Application. One of the most common X chromosome aneuploidies is Turner syndrome (45X), which on a global scale affects one in every 2,500 females. Turner syndrome results either from a monosomy (45%), chromosomal abnormality, or mosaicism. Of note, Turner syndrome is the most common genetic abnormality that presents as a mosaicism.

As a result of a spontaneous error, females have an absent or abnormal set of genes on the short arm of the X chromosome. This is associated with a very high (98%) risk for miscarriage.

Recall that with mosaicism, some cell lines demonstrate a normal 46,XX whereas others have one X chromosome that is missing (45,X). This means that affected newborns may present with a less severe presentation after birth. Common postnatal manifestations include undifferentiated gonads (hallmark manifestation), congenital renal anomalies (e.g., horseshoe kidney), CHDs (e.g., coarctation of the aorta, bicuspid aortic valve), and lymphedema which can be associated with cystic hygroma as well as edema of the hands and feet and wide-spaced nipples. In contrast, mosaic Turner syndrome is associated with fewer abnormalities. For example, female newborns with mosaic Turner syndrome may be healthy during the newborn period and infancy, and later develop short stature, primary amenorrhea, and ovarian failure leading to sterility. Given these rather late-onset findings, it is understandable that only 20% of cases are identified at birth with the rest diagnosed during childhood or puberty (Hemani et al., 2021; Jones et al., 2022; Levy et al., 2021; Sharma & Shankar Kikkeri, 2025).

Imprinting Disorders

We have established thus far that human genes are inherited from the mother (XX) and father. While it would seem logical that alleles inherited from both parents would cohesively function and remain active, this does not always occur. In some situations, one allele inherited from the mother (XX) might be inactivated while the other inherited allele remains active. This process of gene inactivation (or silencing) is termed *imprinting*. The affected gene(s) remain imprinted for life and can be isolated from nearly all human tissues. Three common imprinting disorders—PWS, Angelman syndrome, and Beckwith-Wiedemann syndrome (BWS)—will be reviewed.

PWS, or 15q11 deletion, is associated with a deletion of a portion of the long arm of chromosome 15, which occurs with gene silencing, or imprinting. PWS affects 1:5,000 to 1:10,000 newborns each year, with the majority of newborns inheriting a deletion of the paternal 15q11.2q13.1 region (Descartes et al., 2018). Common manifestations observed shortly after birth include characteristic facial features (e.g., decreased bifrontal diameter, facial depth, palpebral fissures), hypotonia, poor feeding, and small hands and feet (Dolci et al., 2022). Children with PWS often develop short stature (necessitating early diagnosis of the 15q11 deletion and intervention with growth hormone), hypogonadism, and mild to moderate neurocognitive impairment; in the absence of a strict dietary plan, morbid obesity can develop secondary to hyperphagia. In contrast, when the gene deletion is inherited from the mother (XX), a more severe condition known as Angelman syndrome develops. In this situation, the *UBE3A* gene, which is responsible for contributing to normal brain development and is only inherited from the mother (XX), is lost. Affected newborns manifest with seizures and go on to develop severe intellectual disability.

BWS is another common imprinting disorder affecting chromosome 11p. Unlike PWS, which can be elusive in the newborn period due to limited phenotypic findings, BWS is associated with more obvious findings. Altered expression of insulin growth factor (IGF) genes, as well as *CDKN1C, KCNQ1* genes responsible for growth-regulation results in a loss of growth inhibition, which explains many of the following common findings: macrosomia and large for gestational age (LGA) status, ear creases or pits, macroglossia, omphalocele, and hypoglycemia. BWS is associated with both Wilms tumor and hepatoblastoma.

DISORDERS OF METABOLISM

PMDs are often fatal and therefore require close involvement with pediatric metabolic and genetic specialists. It is important that APRNs understand the function of mitochondria and implications associated with mutations.

Primary Mitochondrial Disorders

Recall that mitochondria are regarded as the powerhouse of a cell because they produce ATP and moderate cellular proliferation, differentiation, and apoptosis, as well as calcium homeostasis. Other reactions, including urea cycle reactions, fatty acid oxidation, ketogenesis, and amino acid catabolism, occur within the mitochondria (Das et al., 2019; Gorman et al., 2016; Madeira, 2018; Wang et al., 2022). Disrupted mitochondrial function, due to a mutation incurred at conception, can give rise to PMDs.

PMDs customarily affect organs and tissues with high ATP demand (e.g., brain, heart). They affect 1:6,000 newborns, and are known to carry a high mortality risk (Gorman et al., 2016; Rahman & Rahman, 2018). Fetal and neonatal manifestations include severe growth restriction/low birthweight, hydrops fetalis, prematurity,

TABLE 1.5 Genetic Testing Methodologies Used in the NICU

	Karyotype	FISH	Chromosomal and Single-Nucleotide Microarray	Whole Exome Sequencing	Whole Genome Sequencing
Copy number variants (CNV)		X		X	X
Chromosomal deletions, duplications, translocations	X	X	X		X
Mosaicism	X[a]	X	X[a]		
Identification of new gene disorders			X	X	X

[a]High-resolution chromosomal microarray can scan the entire genome for gains/losses, detect mosaicisms, and novel disorders. Routine G-band karyotypes are tests that sample 5, 10, or 20-cells and cannot detect mosaicism. In contrast, an *extended* 30-cell karyotype can detect mosaicism.
FISH, fluorescence in situ hybridization.

worsening hypotonia, encephalopathy, seizures, apnea, feeding intolerance, lactic acidosis, cardiomyopathy or cardiorespiratory collapse, hypoglycemia, liver disease, and progressively worsening renal disease (Emmanuele et al., 2022). Of the previously listed symptoms, hypotonia (90%), lactic acidosis (87%), and apnea (69%) continue to be the most commonly reported manifestations, and likewise should increase the index of suspicion for a PMD (Honzik et al., 2012).

TABLE 1.6 Genetic Testing Methodologies for Specific Genetic Disorders

	First-line Test	Second-line Test	Reflex Test (as Indicated)
Trisomy 13, 18, 21	FISH	Confirmatory karyotype	Microarray
Turner syndrome	FISH	Confirmatory karyotype	Microarray
DiGeorge syndrome (22q11.2)	Microarray	n/a	n/a

FISH, fluorescence in situ hybridization; n/a, not applicable.
Source: Hopkins, M. K., Dugoff, L., & Kuller, J. A. (2019). Congenital heart disease: Prenatal diagnosis and genetic associations. *Obstetrical & Gynecological Survey, 74*(8), 497–503. https://doi.org/10.1097/OGX.0000000000000702

COMMON GENETIC TESTING MECHANISMS

Genetic diagnoses are always rendered in consultation with pediatric genetic specialists. Five common testing modalities are karyotyping, fluorescent FISH, microarray, whole exome sequencing, and whole genome sequencing. A summary of testing methods and associated utility is offered in Table 1.5. A summary of common genetic disorders and appropriate tests to consider is offered in Table 1.6.

Karyotype

The karyotype has been considered a gold standard genetic tool for detecting CNVs as well as chromosome deletions, duplications, and balanced and unbalanced translocations since the 1960s. Karyotyping uses a Giemsa stain (G-banding) technique and customarily analyzes 5, 10, or 20 metaphase-state cells. Extended cell (30-cell) karyotyping can detect high (more obvious) levels of mosaicism but may not detect very low levels of mosaicism.

A normal karyotype and trisomy 21 karyotype is shown in Figure 1.6; notice that this test involves organizing the chromosomes in an orderly fashion from 1 to 22, including the sex chromosomes. This makes for relatively simplistic interpretation by the clinical team and can be a helpful visual to share with families during genetic counseling. An important limitation is low test sensitivity compared to other modalities (e.g., FISH) due to low band resolution used with this test (3–5 million Mb). Turnaround time for results is approximately 24 to 48 hours.

Fluorescent In Situ Hybridization

FISH testing began to increase in the 1980s and often complements karyotyping. FISH can be used to detect duplications, deletions, balanced or unbalanced translocations, and mosaicisms. Two types of FISH testing are available: interphase FISH, which is typically ordered to evaluate for common aneuploidies, and metaphase FISH, which is used to evaluate for specific deletions

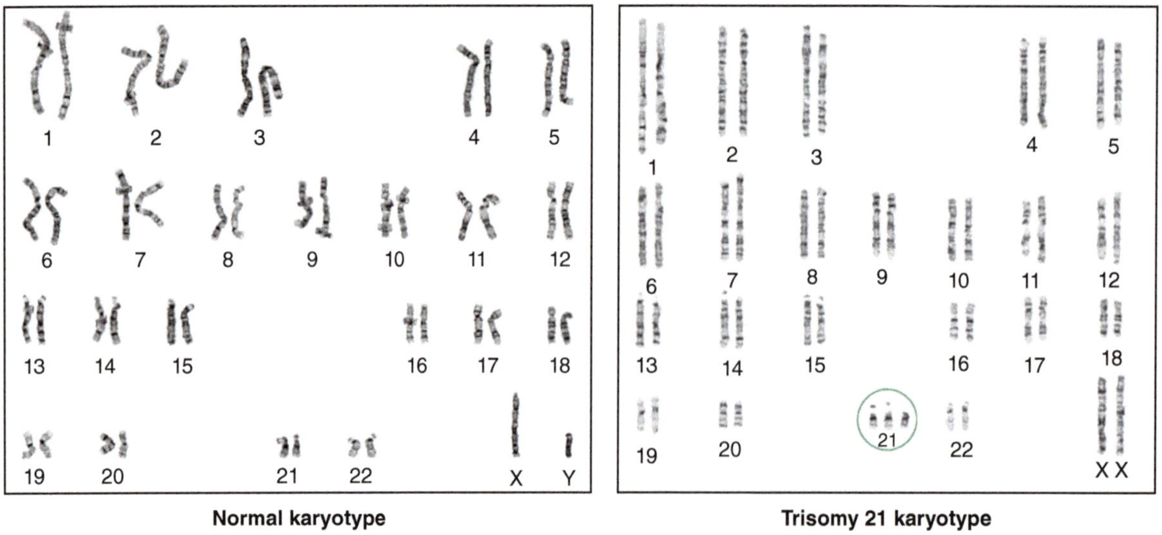

Figure 1.6 Normal karyotype compared to trisomy 21 karyotype.
Image Credit: Amy J. Jnah.

(e.g., PWS, 22q11 deletion syndrome; **Figure 1.7**). Fluorescent DNA probes are used to bind to regions of a chromosome that are complementary to the probe. Upon binding, the FISH probe emits a specific fluorescent color. This allows for detection of CNVs of chromosomes in cells when a trisomy is suspected. FISH is also used when clinicians are certain that a patient has a specific genetic abnormality and want to probe a specific chromosome, or as a "reflex" test when a karyotype is resulted as abnormal. The term "reflex" means the blood sample is held in the lab and secondary test (e.g., reflex microarray) is only pursued if the initial test (karyotype) in the series yields abnormal results.

There are some limitations to FISH testing. Interphase FISH is limited by the inability to rule out more complex trisomies (e.g., Robertsonian, partial trisomy), and analysis can be limited by the number of probes that can be used during a single test as well as the region that is being analyzed. Probes essentially analyze a specific segment of a chromosome and not the rest of the genome. For that reason, FISH may not detect a partial trisomy. Metaphase FISH offers condition-specific analysis, which makes this test appropriate only if the clinician highly suspects a particular deletion syndrome. Turnaround time for results is approximately 24 to 48 hours.

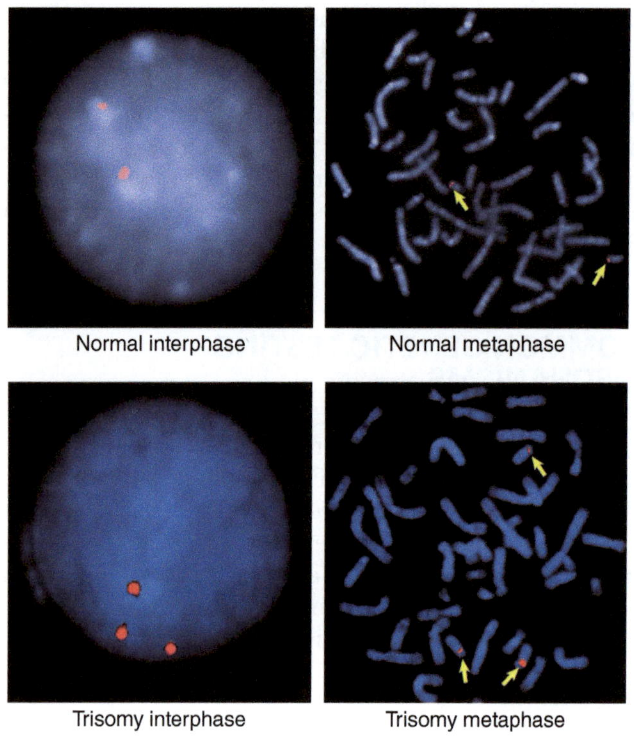

Figure 1.7 Interphase and metaphase FISH analysis for a trisomy.
Note: Fluorescent regions light up in a red coloration. The bottom images describe a trisomy, as three fluorescent regions are illuminated.
Image Credit: Amy J. Jnah.

Chromosomal Microarray

Readers may have experienced situations where genetics experts recommend obtaining a "DNA extract and hold" test. This is often because high resolution whole genome chromosomal microarray (CMA) is a reflex (second-tier) or third-tier genetic test. CMA is effective at detecting aneuploidy, *un*balanced translocations, and small deletions and duplications because this test scans the entire genome. The newborn's DNA and a control DNA are labeled with colored fluorescent dye (green for the patient, red for the control). The microarray slide is prepared with tiny spots of synthetically designed DNA, known as probes. Next, the newborn's DNA and control DNA are "washed" over the microarray slide. They will attempt to bind to a complementary probe. Next, the emission of colored fluorescent light is measured at each probe location. Typically, bright red regions represent a deletion (less newborn DNA compared to control DNA), and bright green regions represent a duplication (more newborn DNA compared to control DNA).

Whole Exome Sequencing and Whole Genome Sequencing

Whole exome sequencing (WES) and whole genome sequencing (WGS) may be used to diagnose PMDs (discussed earlier in this chapter) or other rare genetic disorders, and may be paired with mtDNA sequencing and deletion/duplication analysis. These tests customarily involve peripheral blood sampling, but can be expanded to include muscle tissues, urine, or even buccal cell testing. WES paired with mtDNA sequencing and deletion/duplication analysis is typically the first-line testing modality. WES amplifies and sequences protein-coding genes and, when paired with mtDNA sequencing and deletion/duplication, can successfully detect PMDs in up to 60% of cases (Ohtake et al., 2014; Tolomeo et al., 2021; Wortmann et al., 2015).

WGS offers an expanded analysis by sequencing both protein-coding and non–protein-coding regions of genes. WGS is considered more sensitive and specific compared to WES, as it can analyze for deletions and duplications (CNVs). Results for both WES and WGS options are typically obtained within 1 week, offering a relatively short turnaround time for families (Ouyang et al., 2021; Rius et al., 2021).

CONCLUSION

The future direction of genetics in neonatology should offer opportunities for earlier and precise diagnosis of genetic abnormalities. This will open the door for more timely and effective treatment, family counseling, and long-term outcomes. Interestingly, newborn screening programs may be enhanced in years to come, offering more than tandem mass spectrometry (Kavus & Chung, 2022). This could allow for enhanced screening for common genetic disorders.

LEARNING TOOLS AND RESOURCES

CourseConnect

To access self-assessment questions and interactive, competency-based learning activities for this chapter, visit www.springerpub.com/courseconnect. See inside front cover and tear-out card for CourseConnect details.

Discussion Prompts

1. Two parents are unaffected carriers of CF, which is detected during routine prenatal testing. What is the likelihood that a child will be affected by CF? Draw a Punnett square or pedigree chart to support your conclusion.
2. Discuss the common differences in phenotypic findings between trisomy 13 and 18 that would assist a novice clinician in distinguishing between the aneuploidies. What genetic testing should the neonatal APRN expect the genetics team to request?
3. A newborn is delivered by cesarean section at 33 weeks of gestation for fetal hydrops. The pregnancy was complicated by polyhydramnios over the third trimester. The newborn manifests with respiratory distress requiring positive pressure ventilation, endotracheal intubation, and high-frequency ventilation. Physical examination is significant for anasarca, macrosomia, a prominent tongue, and generalized hypotonia. Chest radiographs yield bilateral pleural effusions. Further testing reveals a normal head ultrasound, normal echocardiogram, and abdominal ascites with a large left kidney with a duplicated collecting system. Which genetic disorder, an imprinting disorder, is most likely associated with these findings? Discuss long-term risks, particularly associated with the renal findings, that apply to this case.

MIND MAP

Punnett squares describing X-linked inheritance

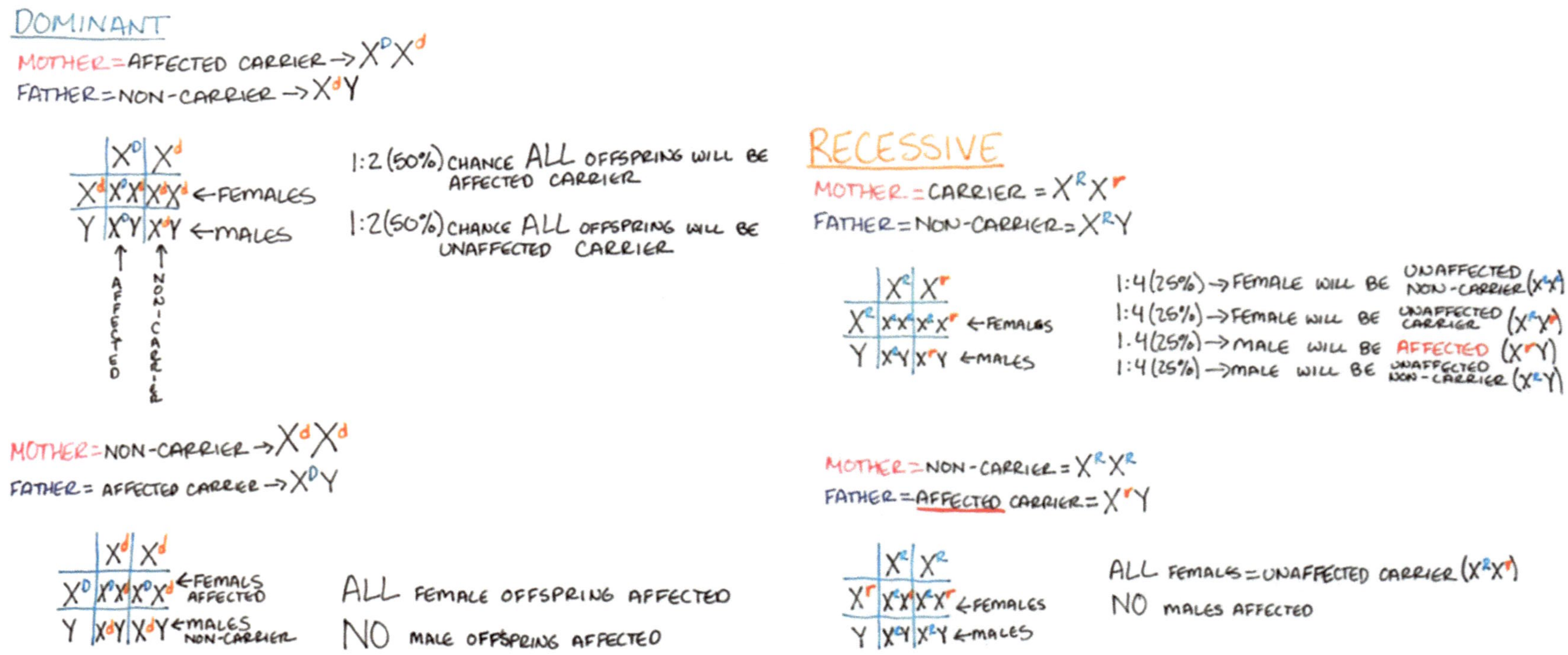

Note: *This mind map reflects one neonatal nurse practitioner student's interpretation of a concept addressed in this chapter. Readers should regard the mind maps woven throughout this textbook as examples of multisensory study tools that can be developed to aid conceptual understanding. Readers are encouraged to develop their own unique mind maps in consultation with academic faculty or clinical preceptors.*

Image Credit: Rhianon Brock, MSN, APRN, NNP-BC.

REFERENCES

American College of Obstetricians and Gynecologists' Committee on Clinical Consensus-Obstetrics, Gantt, A., Society for Maternal-Fetal Medicine, Metz, T. D., Kuller, J. A., Louis, J. M., Society for Maternal-Fetal Medicine, Cahill, A. G., Turrentine, M. A., & American College of Obstetricians and Gynecologists. (2023). Obstetric Care Consensus #11, Pregnancy at age 35 years or older. *American Journal of Obstetrics and Gynecology, 228*(3), B25–B40. https://doi.org/10.1016/j.ajog.2022.07.022

Cerruti-Mainardi, P. (2006). Cri du chat syndrome. *Orphanet Journal of Rare Diseases, 1*, 33. https://doi.org/10.1186/1750-1172-1-33

Chail, H. (2008). DNA sequencing technologies key to the Human Genome Project. *Nature Education, 1*(1), 219.

Das, M., Alzaid, F., & Bayry, J. (2019). Regulatory T cells under the mercy of mitochondria. *Cell Metabolism, 29*(2), 243–245. https://doi.org/10.1016/j.cmet.2019.01.012

Davisson, N. A., Clark, J. B., Chin, T. K., & Tunks, R. D. (2018). Trisomy 18 and congenital heart disease: Single-center review of outcomes and parental perspectives. *World Journal for Pediatric & Congenital Heart Surgery, 9*(5), 550–556. https://doi.org/10.1177/2150135118782145

Descartes, M., Korf, B. R., & Mikhail, F. M. (2018). Genetics and genetic abnormalities. In K. F. Swaiman, S. Ashwal, D. M. Ferriero, N. F. Schor, R. S. Finkel, A. L. Gropman, P. L. Pearl, & M. Shevell (Eds.), *Swaiman's pediatric neurology: Principles and practice* (6th ed., pp. 268–276). Elsevier.

Dimopoulos, K., Constantine, A., Clift, P., Condliffe, R., Moledina, S., Jansen, K., Inuzuka, R., Veldtman, G. R., Cua, C. L., Tay, E. L. W., Opotowsky, A. R., Giannakoulas, G., Alonso-Gonzalez, R., Cordina, R., Capone, G., Namuyonga, J., Scott, C. H., D'Alto, M., Gamero, F. J., ... for Down Syndrome International (DSi). (2023). Cardiovascular complications of Down syndrome: Scoping review and expert consensus. *Circulation, 147*(5), 425–441. https://doi.org/10.1161/CIRCULATIONAHA.122.059706

Dolci, C., Rigamonti, A. E., Cappella, A., Gibelli, D. M., Grugni, G., Caroli, D., Sforza, C., & Sartorio, A. (2022). Robustness of distinctive facial features in Prader-Willi syndrome: A stereophotogrammetric analysis and association with clinical and biochemical markers in adult individuals. *Biology, 11*(8), 1148. https://doi.org/10.3390/biology11081148

Emmanuele, V., Ganesh, J., Vladutiu, G., Haas, R., Kerr, D., Saneto, R. P., Cohen, B. H., Van Hove, J. L. K., Scaglia, F., Hoppel, C., Rosales, X. Q., Barca, E., Buchsbaum, R., Thompson, J. L., DiMauro, S., Hirano, M., & North American Mitochondrial Disease Consortium (NAMDC). (2022). Time to harmonize mitochondrial syndrome nomenclature and classification: A consensus from the North American Mitochondrial Disease Consortium (NAMDC). *Molecular Genetics and Metabolism, 136*(2), 125–131. https://doi.org/10.1016/j.ymgme.2022.05.001

Glinianaia, S. V., Rankin, J., Tan, J., Loane, M., Garne, E., Cavero-Carbonell, C., de Walle, H. E. K., Gatt, M., Gissler, M., Klungsøyr, K., Lelong, N., Neville, A., Pierini, A., Tucker, D. F., Urhoj, S. K., Wellesley, D. G., & Morris, J. K. (2023). Ten-year survival of children with trisomy 13 or trisomy 18: A multi-registry European cohort study. *Archives of Disease in Childhood, 108*(6), 461–467. https://doi.org/10.1136/archdischild-2022-325068

Gorman, G. S., Chinnery, P. F., DiMauro, S., Hirano, M., Koga, Y., McFarland, R., Suomalainen, A., Thorburn, D. R., Zeviani, M., & Turnbull, D. M. (2016). Mitochondrial diseases. *Nature Reviews. Disease Primers, 2*, 16080. https://doi.org/10.1038/nrdp.2016.80

Gundorova, P., Zinchenko, R. A., Kuznetsova, I. A., Bliznetz, E. A., Stepanova, A. A., & Polyakov, A. V. (2018). Molecular-genetic causes for the high frequency of phenylketonuria in the population from the North Caucasus. *PLoS One, 13*(8), e0201489. https://doi.org/10.1371/journal.pone.0201489

Haghnazarian, E., Hu, J., Song, A. Y., Friedlich, P. S., & Lakshmanan, A. (2019). The association of trisomy 13 and 18 and hospital discharge outcomes among neonates in California: A retrospective cohort study. *Pediatrics and Neonatology, 60*(6), 617–622. https://doi.org/10.1016/j.pedneo.2019.02.007

Hemani, F., Niaz, S., Kumar, V., Khan, S., Choudry, E., & Ali, S. R. (2021). A case of early diagnosis of Turner syndrome in a neonate. *Cureus, 13*(7), e16733. https://doi.org/10.7759/cureus.16733

Hillert, A., Anikster, Y., Belanger-Quintana, A., Burlina, A., Burton, B. K., Carducci, C., Chiesa, A. E., Christodoulou, J., Đorđević, M., Desviat, L. R., Eliyahu, A., Evers, R. A. F., Fajkusova, L., Feillet, F., Bonfim-Freitas, P. E., Giżewska, M., Gundorova, P., Karall, D., Kneller, K., ... Blau, N. (2020). The genetic landscape and epidemiology of phenylketonuria. *American Journal of Human Genetics, 107*(2), 234–250. https://doi.org/10.1016/j.ajhg.2020.06.006

Honzik, T., Tesarova, M., Magner, M., Mayr, J., Jesina, P., Vesela, K., Wenchich, L., Szentivanyi, K., Hansikova, H., Sperl, W., & Zeman, J. (2012). Neonatal onset of mitochondrial disorders in 129 patients: Clinical and laboratory characteristics and a new approach to diagnosis. *Journal of Inherited Metabolic Disease, 35*(5), 749–759. https://doi.org/10.1007/s10545-011-9440-3

Hopkins, M. K., Dugoff, L., & Kuller, J. A. (2019). Congenital heart disease: Prenatal diagnosis and genetic associations. *Obstetrical & Gynecological Survey, 74*(8), 497–503. https://doi.org/10.1097/OGX.0000000000000702

Ishibashi, M., Watanabe, T., Kyozuka, H., Yamaguchi, A., Sato, K., Sato, M., Go, H., & Fujimori, K. (2021). Perinatal diagnosis of a fetus with an unbalanced translocation 46,XY, der(10)t(6;10)(p22;q26.1) with multiple malformations: A case report and literature review. *Fukushima Journal of Medical Science, 67*(2), 83–88. https://doi.org/10.5387/fms.2020-28

Jacobs, P. A., Browne, C., Gregson, N., Joyce, C., & White, H. (1992). Estimates of the frequency of chromosome abnormalities detectable in unselected newborns using moderate levels of banding. *Journal of Medical Genetics, 29*(2), 103–108. https://doi.org/10.1136/jmg.29.2.103

Jones, K. L., Jones, M. C., & Del Campo, C. M. (2022). *Smith's recognizable patterns of human malformation* (8th ed.). Elsevier.

Kavus, H., & Chung, W. K. (2022). Basic genetic principles. In R. A. Polin, S. H. Abman, D. H. Rowitch, W. E. Benitz, & W. W. Fox (Eds.), *Fetal and neonatal physiology* (6th ed., pp. 1–11). Elsevier.

Kosho, T., Nakamura, T., Kawame, H., Baba, A., Tamura, M., & Fukushima, Y. (2006). Neonatal management of trisomy 18: Clinical details of 24 patients receiving intensive treatment. *American Journal of Medical Genetics. Part A, 140*(9), 937–944. https://doi.org/10.1002/ajmg.a.31175

Kosiv, K. A., Gossett, J. M., Bai, S., & Collins, R. T. (2017). Congenital heart surgery on in-hospital mortality in trisomy 13 and 18. *Pediatrics, 140*(5), e20170772. https://doi.org/10.1542/peds.2017-0772

Kosiv, K. A., Mercurio, M. R., & Carey, J. C. (2023). The common trisomy syndromes, their cardiac implications, and ethical considerations in care. *Current Opinion in Pediatrics, 35*(5), 531–537. https://doi.org/10.1097/MOP.0000000000001278

Levy, A. T., Berghella, V., & Al-Kouatly, H. B. (2021). Outcome of 45,X fetuses with cystic hygroma: A systematic review. *American Journal of Medical Genetics. Part A, 185*(1), 26–32. https://doi.org/10.1002/ajmg.a.61902

Madeira, V. M. C. (2018). Overview of mitochondrial bioenergetics. *Methods in Molecular Biology (Clifton, N.J.), 1782*, 1–6. https://doi.org/10.1007/978-1-4939-7831-1_1

National Institutes of Health. (2020). *Medline plus: Down syndrome*. https://medlineplus.gov/genetics/condition/down-syndrome/#statistics

Ohtake, A., Murayama, K., Mori, M., Harashima, H., Yamazaki, T., Tamaru, S., Yamashita, Y., Kishita, Y., Nakachi, Y., Kohda, M., Tokuzawa, Y., Mizuno, Y., Moriyama, Y., Kato, H., & Okazaki, Y. (2014). Diagnosis and molecular basis of mitochondrial respiratory chain disorders: Exome sequencing for disease gene identification. *Biochimica et Biophysica Acta, 1840*(4), 1355–1359. https://doi.org/10.1016/j.bbagen.2014.01.025

Ouyang, X., Zhang, Y., Zhang, L., Luo, J., Zhang, T., Hu, H., Liu, L., Zhong, L., Zeng, S., Xu, P., Bai, Z., Wong, L. J., Wang, J., Wang, C., Wang, B., & Zhang, V. W. (2021). Clinical utility of rapid exome sequencing combined with mitochondrial DNA sequencing in critically ill pediatric patients with suspected genetic disorders. *Frontiers in Genetics, 12*, 725259. https://doi.org/10.3389/fgene.2021.725259

Peterson, J. K., Kochilas, L. K., Catton, K. G., Moller, J. H., & Setty, S. P. (2017). Long-term outcomes of children with trisomy 13 and 18 after congenital heart disease interventions. *The Annals of Thoracic Surgery, 103*(6), 1941–1949. https://doi.org/10.1016/j.athoracsur.2017.02.068

Podolak, A., Woclawek-Potocka, I., & Lukaszuk, K. (2022). The role of mitochondria in human fertility and early embryo development: What can we learn for clinical application of assessing and improving mitochondrial DNA? *Cells, 11*(5), 797. https://doi.org/10.3390/cells11050797

Rahman, J., & Rahman, S. (2018). Mitochondrial medicine in the omics era. *Lancet (London, England), 391*(10139), 2560–2574. https://doi.org/10.1016/S0140-6736(18)30727-X

Rius, R., Compton, A. G., Baker, N. L., Welch, A. E., Coman, D., Kava, M. P., Minoche, A. E., Cowley, M. J., Thorburn, D. R., & Christodoulou, J. (2021). Application of genome sequencing from blood to diagnose mitochondrial diseases. *Genes, 12*(4), 607. https://doi.org/10.3390/genes12040607

Scriver, C. R. (2007). The *PAH* gene, phenylketonuria, and a paradigm shift. *Human Mutation, 28*(9), 831–845. https://doi.org/10.1002/humu.20526

Sharma, L., & Shankar Kikkeri, N. (2025). Turner syndrome [Updated 2025 Jun 22]. In: *StatPearls*. https://www.ncbi.nlm.nih.gov/books/NBK554621/

Sheen, J. J., Wright, J. D., Goffman, D., Kern-Goldberger, A. R., Booker, W., Siddiq, Z., D'Alton, M. E., & Friedman, A. M. (2018). Maternal age and risk for adverse outcomes. *American Journal of Obstetrics and Gynecology, 219*(4), 390.e1–390.e15. https://doi.org/10.1016/j.ajog.2018.08.034

Tolomeo, D., Orsucci, D., Nesti, C., Baldacci, J., Battini, R., Bruno, C., Bruno, G., Cassandrini, D., Doccini, S., Donati, M. A., Ferrari, A., Fiori, S., Fiorillo, C., Guerrini, R., Mari, F., Montomoli, M., Pochiero, F., Procopio, E., Ruggiero, L., ... Santorelli, F. M. (2021). The diagnostic approach to mitochondrial disorders in children in the era of next-generation sequencing: A 4-year cohort study. *Journal of Clinical Medicine, 10*(15), 3222. https://doi.org/10.3390/jcm10153222

Tuke, M. A., Ruth, K. S., Wood, A. R., Beaumont, R. N., Tyrrell, J., Jones, S. E., Yaghootkar, H., Turner, C. L. S., Donohoe, M. E., Brooke, A. M., Collinson, M. N., Freathy, R. M., Weedon, M. N., Frayling, T. M., & Murray, A. (2019). Mosaic Turner syndrome shows reduced penetrance in an adult population study. *Genetics in Medicine, 21*(4), 877–886. https://doi.org/10.1038/s41436-018-0271-6

Wang, H., Han, Y., Li, S., Chen, Y., Chen, Y., Wang, J., Zhang, Y., Zhang, Y., Wang, J., Xia, Y., & Yuan, J. (2022). Mitochondrial DNA depletion syndrome and its associated cardiac disease. *Frontiers in Cardiovascular Medicine, 8*, 808115. https://doi.org/10.3389/fcvm.2021.808115

Wortmann, S. B., Koolen, D. A., Smeitink, J. A., van den Heuvel, L., & Rodenburg, R. J. (2015). Whole exome sequencing of suspected mitochondrial patients in clinical practice. *Journal of Inherited Metabolic Disease, 38*(3), 437–443. https://doi.org/10.1007/s10545-015-9823-y

2

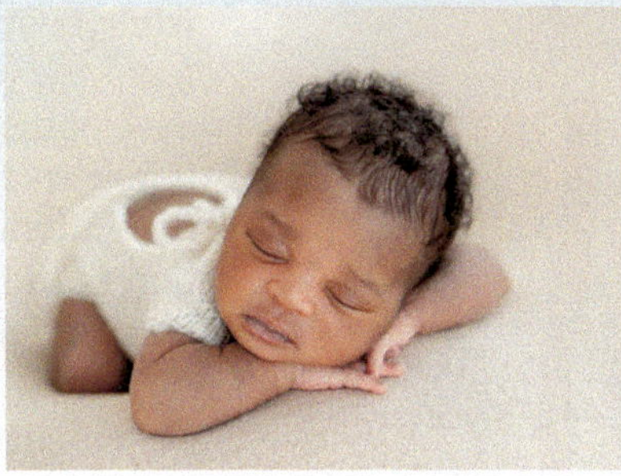

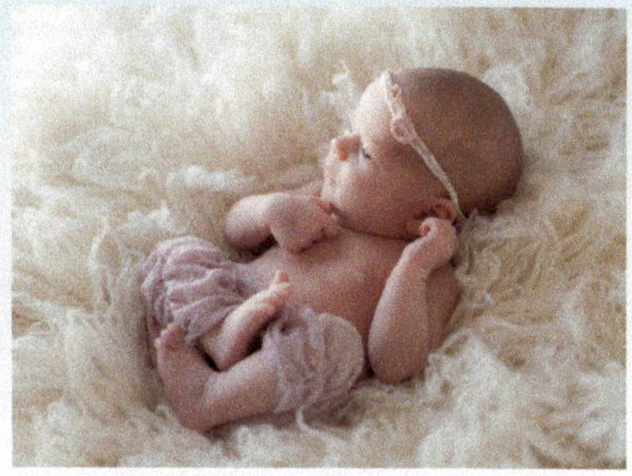

PLACENTAL DEVELOPMENT AND FUNCTION

Jennifer Fitzgerald, Amy Williford, and Amy J. Jnah

LEARNING OBJECTIVES

After completing this chapter, the reader should be able to:

- Discuss the development of individual structures of the placenta.
- Describe uteroplacental circulation from the XX pregnant patient to fetus through the placenta.
- Identify the major functions of the placenta.
- Analyze mechanisms involved in nutrient transfer to the fetus across the placenta.
- Relate altered placental development to abnormal fetal development.
- Discuss diseases diagnosed in pregnant individuals that result in altered placental and fetal development.

INTRODUCTION

During the menstrual cycle, follicle-stimulating hormone (FSH) and luteinizing hormone (LH) are released by the anterior pituitary. These hormones regulate ovarian follicle development and changes in the uterine mucosa. Next, the mature ovarian follicle ruptures and expels one (or more) oocyte (egg) into the fallopian tube, a process called *ovulation*. Subsequently, the remnant follicle becomes the corpus luteum and helps regulate ongoing changes to the uterine mucosa. These changes to the uterine mucosa, or endometrium, include growth with proliferation of spiral arteries and glands, all in anticipation of implantation of a fertilized oocyte (**Figure 2.1**). If fertilization occurs, changes in the architecture of the endometrium continue. The endometrium becomes the location for the development of the placenta, the feto–maternal organ that provides the life-sustaining connection between the developing fetus and maternal circulation. Then, after the birth of the infant, this organ ceases to function and is expelled.

This chapter focuses on placental development. In addition, alterations in fetal development and disease resulting from developmental abnormalities of the placenta, as well as diseases affecting the pregnant individual, will be discussed. Later chapters present the fetal phases of development specific to each body system.

TIMELINE OF PLACENTAL DEVELOPMENT

The timeline offered in **Figure 2.2** provides a high-level overview of the development of major structures of the placenta (*top*) and the fetal and neonatal problems potentially associated with a specific stage of placental development (*bottom*). The exact timing of events can vary and subtle differences are described in the literature.

DEVELOPMENTAL PHYSIOLOGY

The first week of human development begins at fertilization, as the oocyte is released into the fallopian tube and fertilized. This results in the formation of the first somatic cell, or zygote. Through the process of mitosis, the zygote grows into an aggregate of somatic cells,

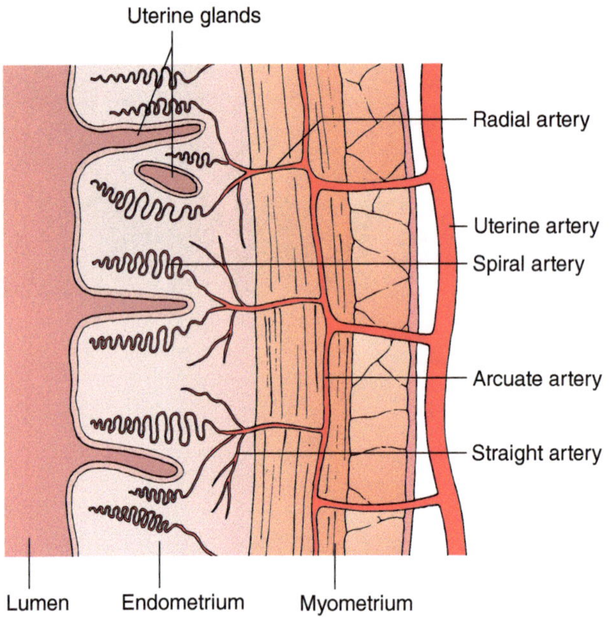

Figure 2.1 Uterine anatomy.

while being ushered through the fallopian tube and toward the uterus. Finally, by the end of the first week of development, the zygote matures into a blastocyst. Next, it reaches the uterine cavity and begins to implant within the endometrium (Torchia & Persaud, 2025). This section of the chapter will review key milestones related to fertilization, blastocyst formation, and implantation.

Fertilization

At the onset of ovulation, a spherical oocyte enters the distal end of a fallopian tube. Next, penetration of the ooctye by a spermatozoon induces fertilization. During fertilization, pronuclei from the oocyte and spermatozoon combine and form a zygote, which is now comprised of the genetic material necessary to create a unique human being (Sadler, 2024; Torchia & Persaud, 2025). Over the next 3 days, the zygote undergoes repeated, exponential cell divisions while being propelled through the fallopian tube (toward the uterus) by physiologic peristaltic movements and motile cilia lining the

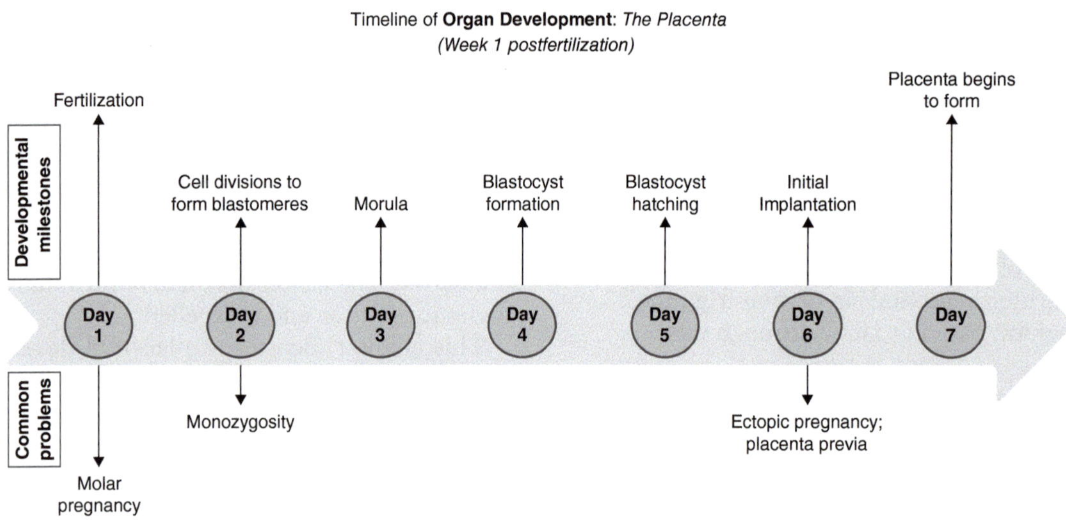

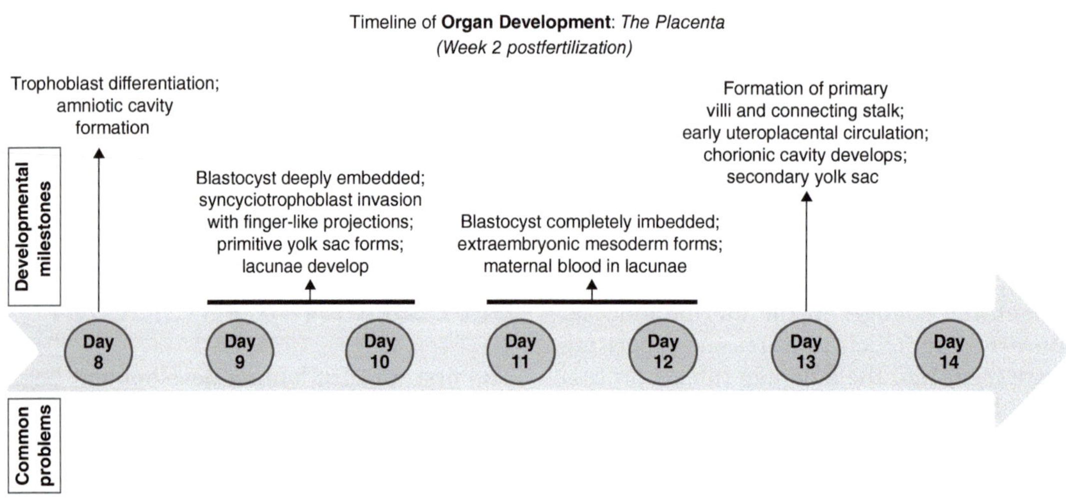

Figure 2.2 Visual timeline. *(continued)*

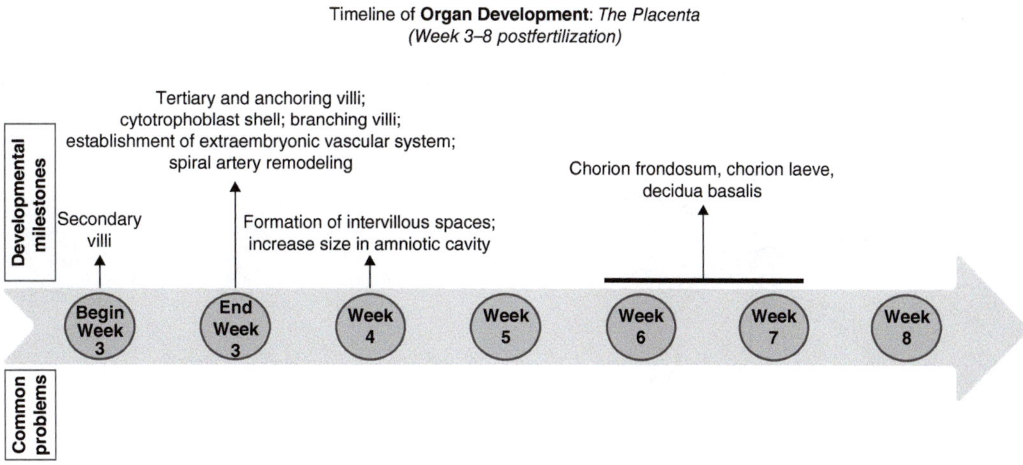

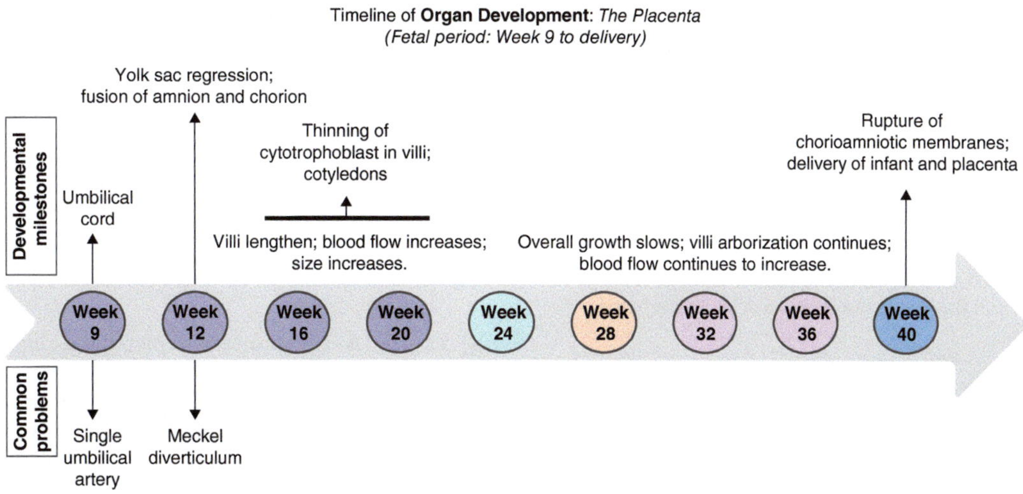

Figure 2.2 *(continued)*

Note: Placement of common problems is meant to offer visual/conceptual perspective on the timing of onset of these commonly reported malformations. Variation exists across the literature. Amniotic band disruption, intrauterine growth restriction, oligohydramnios, polyhydramnios, and abruptio placenta may arise at variable times.

fallopian tube. This process requires energy. Nutrients stored within the outer zona pellucida of the oocyte, a protective, shelllike glycoprotein matrix (comprised of glucose and protein), provide the necessary energy to nourish and support the zygote during this time as it migrates and proliferates into a blastocyst and is propelled toward the uterus (Sadler, 2024).

From Morula to Blastocyst

Throughout its migration, the zygote undergoes cleavage, or a series of cell exponential divisions (mitosis); the nomenclature changes as these cell divisions occur. This results in rapid doubling of genetically identical cells, and the zygote evolves into a *blastomere*. The blastomere undergoes compaction and realignment, and evolves into a tight cluster of eukaryotic cells, called a *morula*. The morula, a hollow 12- to 16-cell mass, finishes the journey through the fallopian tube and into the uterus (**Figure 2.3**). Next, the blastomeres begin to separate into an inner cell mass and an outer cell mass, or the future embryoblast and trophoblast, respectively (Torchia & Persaud, 2025). Fluid from the uterine cavity enters the morula, forming a cavity that will provide nutrients for continued development. At this point, the morula evolves into a *blastocyst* (**Figure 2.4A**).

Next, the outer zona pellucida of the blastocyst is shed, removing any mechanical constraints to future growth of the embryo (Sadler, 2024). This permits "hatching" of the blastocyst and implantation into the endometrium of the birthing parent (**Figure 2.4B**). The embryonic pole, which is the point of contact between the embryoblast and the trophoblast, is the first to implant.

Implantation

At the end of the first week of pregnancy, the outermost layer of cells that comprise the blastocyst, trophoblast

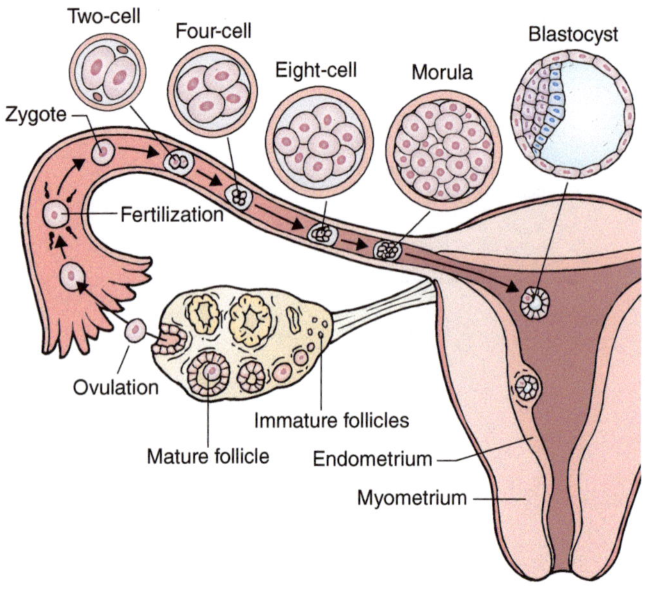

Figure 2.3 From ovulation to blastocyst formation: First, the two-cell embryo appears approximately 36 hours after fertilization. Twenty-four hours later, the embryo divides into a four-cell mass. Twelve hours later, the embryo divides into an eight-cell mass, and 6 hours afterward into a 16-cell morula ("mulberry"). Finally, approximately 4 hours after becoming a densely packed morula, the embryo changes into a hollow blastocyst.

Note: Failure of ciliated cells to propel the embryo through the fallopian tube and into the uterus results in an ectopic pregnancy.

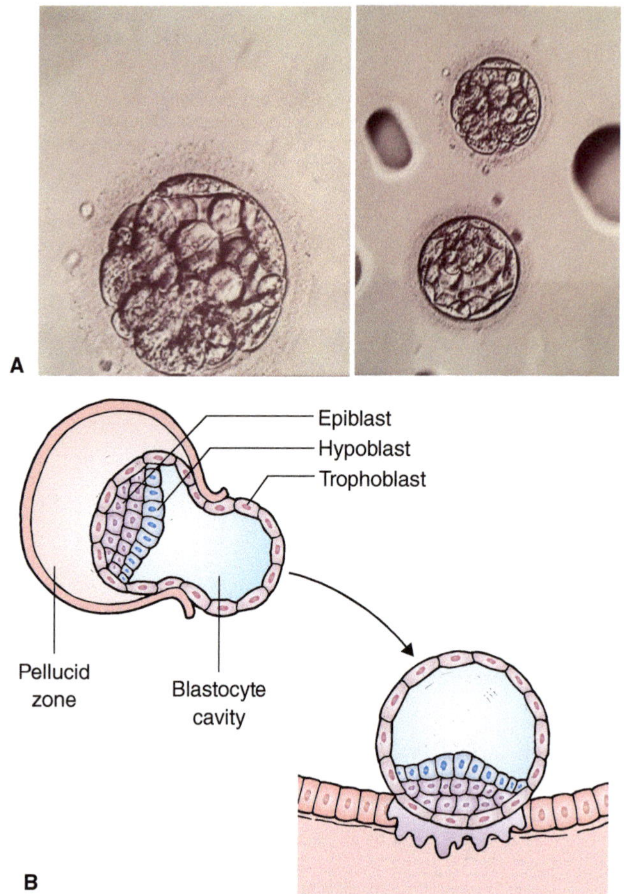

Figure 2.4 (**A**) Image on left depicts single blastocyst; image on right depicts splitting of the original blastocyst resulting in twin pregnancy. (**B**) The anatomic composition of the blastocyst is noteworthy, as its major components differentiate into the future embryo and placenta. The hollow inner portion will fill with fluid and become the embryoblast, or future embryo. The embryoblast will further differentiate into the hypoblast and the epiblast, the origin of all three germ layers of the fetus (endoderm, mesoderm, ectoderm; Torchia & Persaud, 2025). The one-cell thick outer layer, or trophoblast, will differentiate into placental structures including the chorionic villi, umbilical cord, and other critical structures such as the fetal membranes (Sadler, 2024).

Image Credit: Erin Broush, MSN, APRN, NNP-BC.

cells, invade the endometrial wall and begin the process of implantation (Figure 2.5). In a matter of days, trophoblast cells go on to differentiate into syncytiotrophoblast (the outer trophoblastic cell layer) and cytotrophoblast (the inner trophoblastic cell layer) cells (Park et al., 2022; Sadler, 2024). This differentiation sets the stage for the necessary changes in the endometrium and the development of the placental structures (e.g., umbilical cord) that will establish the feto–maternal circulation and support the growing embryo/fetus. By 11 to 12 days postfertilization, the blastocyst is fully implanted into the endometrium. A summary of the implantation process is provided in the following paragraphs.

Once trophoblast cells differentiate, newly formed cytotrophoblast undergo a series of critical tasks. The cells begin to penetrate the syncytiotrophoblast layer (syncytium) and facilitate its expansion. Then, cytotrophoblast cells migrate deeper into the endometrium and anchor the embryo to the uterine wall (anchoring villi; Sadler, 2024). Next, cytotrophoblast cells colonize the exterior surfaces of the spiral arteries to facilitate circulatory adaptation (a low-resistance system of flow) to support the rapidly growing fetus (Turco & Moffett, 2019). As the syncytium proliferates, lacunar (sunken) spaces appear. At the same time, the maternal capillaries found within the endometrium dilate and form sinusoids, allowing maternal blood to flow into the lacunar spaces (Torchia & Persaud, 2025). These lacunar spaces stop growing at about 12 days after fertilization and coalesce to form fused intervillous spaces. Once formed, the combined presence of intervillous spaces and chorionic villi give rise to the early feto–maternal circulation (Sadler, 2024).

Next, syncytiotrophoblasts secrete proteolytic enzymes which lyse (invade) the endometrium and permit the formation of chorionic villi. These villi go on to mature into structures composed of a bilayered epithelium (inner layer of cytotrophoblasts and an overlying layer of syncytiotrophoblast; Sadler, 2024; Turco & Moffett, 2019). During this process of implantation, the embryoblast moves toward the endometrial surface to accommodate correct placement of the future umbilical cord.

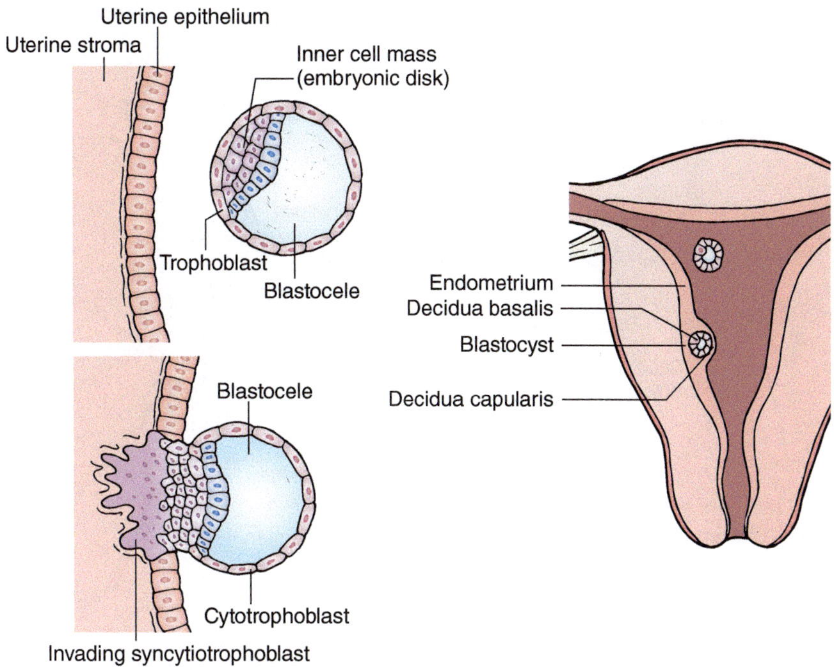

Figure 2.5 Implantation of the blastocyst.

Clinical Application. Syncytiotrophoblast cells (which comprise the syncytium) are detected early into pregnancy, given that they are a subdivision of trophoblast cells (the outermost layer of cells that comprise the blastocyst). Syncytiotrophoblasts begin to secrete two hormones, human chorionic gonadotropin (hCG) and progesterone, shortly after conception. The presence of adequate hCG prevents degradation of the corpus luteum, which makes hCG necessary for maintaining the pregnancy until the placenta can provide sufficient hormones (around week 8 of gestation). Progesterone maintains the thick endometrial lining of the uterus, an environment rich in blood vessels. Importantly, hCG is a hormone that can be detected in both urine and serum early pregnancy tests. Markedly elevated hCG levels have been associated with trisomy 21, whereas abnormally low hCG levels have been associated with trisomy 13 and 18. The syncytium is expected to expand and thin across pregnancy, as the nutrient demands of the fetus increase during advancing gestation. Altered rates of cell turnover and abnormal growth of the syncytium have been linked to fetal growth abnormalities.

Development of the Extraembryonic Membranes

During the second week after fertilization, the blastocyst differentiates into various layers that are vital to the embryo's survival. These extraembryonic membranes, which are required to support and protect the growing embryo, include the chorion, amnion, yolk sac, and the allantois.

The Chorion. The *chorion* represents the outermost layer of the fetal portion of the placenta and is derived from the trophoblast. As the extraembryonic mesoderm penetrates the core of the developing villi, the villi are contiguous with the chorionic plate. Blood vessels develop within the chorionic plate and connect to both the developing umbilical cord and developing blood vessels within the villi, forming the extraembryonic vascular system. The portion of the chorion that interfaces with the decidua capsularis undergoes atrophy and these villi disappear. The chorion fuses with the decidua parietalis and forms the membranous, nonvillus portion of the placenta (Sadler, 2024). This smooth area is called the chorionic laeve. The remaining portion of the chorion will form the villous portion of the placenta.

Chorionic Villi. Recall that the fingerlike projections of the *chorionic villi*, or chorionic frondosum, are created after the syncytiotrophoblast lyses the endometrial surface. At approximately 13 days after fertilization, primary chorionic villi are formed. These early villi are small and nonvascular, and branch outward from the chorionic plate toward the basal (or maternal) plate (Figure 2.6). Secondary villi develop during week 3 of gestation, increase in size, and contain a core of extraembryonic mesoderm surrounded by the cytotrophoblast; secondary villi cover the entirety of the chorionic sac (Torchia & Persaud, 2025). Shortly thereafter, the mesoderm differentiates into capillaries and venules that are regarded as vascular tertiary villi. The tertiary villi account for

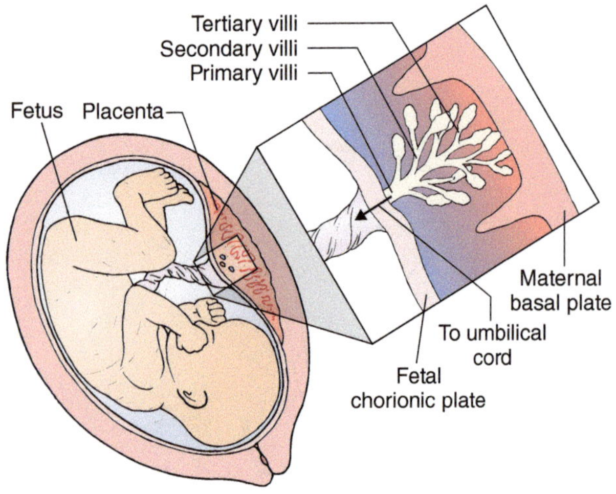

Figure 2.6 Chorionic villi. The chorion is the outermost layer of the fetal portion of the placenta. It arises from the cytotrophoblast layer of the blastocyst and the chorionic plate.

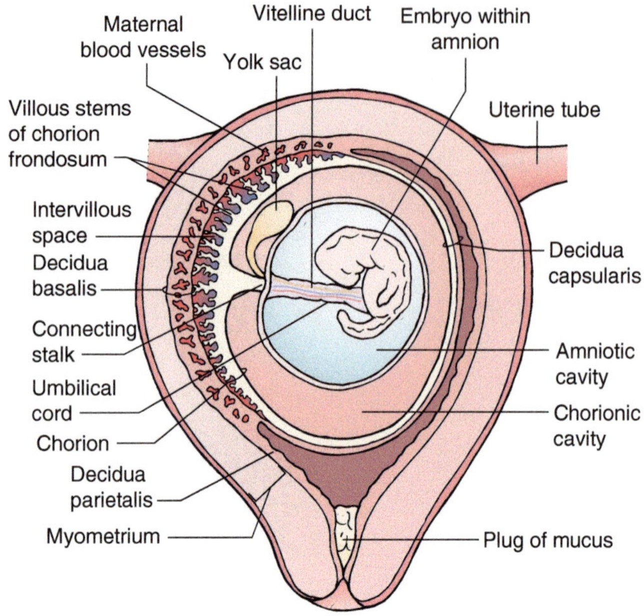

Figure 2.7 Orientation of chorionic structures within the uterus. The image represents the gravid uterus in the second month. The decidua basalis forms the maternal portion of the placenta. The decidua capsularis initially covers the growing embryo and disappears with development of the chorion. The decidua parietalis facilitates trophoblastic adhesion and migration.

the major site of nutrient and waste exchange between the XX pregnant patient and fetus (Cindrova-Davies & Sferruzzi-Perri, 2022; Moser et al., 2018; Sadler, 2024).

Maternal spiral arteries, which grow from the endometrium and extend into the decidua basalis, deliver pulsatile maternal blood to these intervillous spaces (Figure 2.7). Remodeling of the anatomic configuration of the maternal arteries, along with trophoblast-mediated pressure regulation, lowers resistance to flow into these intervillous spaces and increases volume capacity. This structural adaptation results from alteration of the endothelium and removal of the neurovascular control of the blood vessels (Cindrova-Davies & Sferruzzi-Perri, 2022). In instances where vascular regulation is imbalanced, there is an increased risk for vascularization abnormalities. Inadequate development of utero-placental blood vessels may give rise to conditions associated with poor placental perfusion (e.g., preeclampsia, fetal growth restriction, or placental abruption) whereas overgrowth and invasion of blood vessels into maternal organs may lead to disorders associated with placenta accreta (Cindrova-Davies & Sferruzzi-Perri, 2022).

The maternal endometrium, or inner layer of the uterine wall, also begins a process of structural change, or decidualization, which supports formation of the placenta and the developing future fetus. Three regions are formed as a result of the decidual process: the decidua basalis, decidua capsularis, and decidua parietalis. The decidua basalis provides a soft vascular bed on which the blastocyst rests, and along with uterine vessels and glands forms the maternal portion of the placenta (Torchia & Persaud, 2025). The decidua capsularis lies just above the area of trophoblastic proliferation, initially covers the growing embryo, and disappears with development of the chorion. The decidua parietalis (or vera) supports trophoblastic adhesion and migration (Cunningham et al., 2022; Sadler, 2024).

The decidua basalis (maternal portion of the placenta) extends septa between intervillous spaces resulting in about 15 to 20 subdivisions called *cotyledons* (Sadler, 2024). Each cotyledon is supplied by a maternal arteriole, contains a main stem of a chorionic villus and its branches, receives fetal blood, and contains all of the structures necessary for exchange of oxygen and nutrients between maternal blood and fetal capillaries (Torchia & Persaud, 2025). The decidua basalis and its cotyledons comprise the maternal circulation at the level of the placenta, located within the endometrial layer of the uterus. It is important to recognize that neither the maternal nor fetal circulations comingle or innervate one another, but rather communicate via diffusion.

The Amnion (and Amniotic Cavity). Early in week 2, a cavity is created in the embryoblast between the embryonic disc and the trophoblast, developing from the upper layer (epiblast) of the embryonic disc. The epiblasts form the floor of the cavity, which later becomes ectoderm, and gives rise to amnioblasts (Sadler, 2024). These amnion-forming cells create the amniotic membrane, which will cover the developing embryo. The *amnion* fills with fluid and expands to become the amniotic sac. The fluid volume increases over the next 3 to 4 weeks, and this volume expansion leads to adherence of the amnion to the inner surface of the chorion at about 12 to 14 weeks, forming the amniochorionic membrane (Cunningham et al., 2022; Gerson et al., 2019; Torchia & Persaud, 2025).

Composition of the amniotic fluid includes a filtrate of maternal plasma (early on) and then includes urine later once fetal kidney function is established. The function is to provide a neutral thermal environment, as well as a trauma-free environment that allows the fetus to move freely and initiate other acts, including breathing and swallowing. The amniotic fluid cushions the developing fetus, allows for symmetrical growth, and prevents adherence. In addition, amniotic fluid allows for movement of the fetus for development of skeletal structure and participates in development of the lungs and gastrointestinal (GI) system.

The Yolk Sac. While the placenta develops, the yolk sac plays an important role in supporting the developing embryo. During the first week after fertilization, the yolk sac develops and begins to provide nutrition via a primitive vitelline circulation, participates in blood development until approximately week 5 of gestation, and participates in development of the trachea, lungs, and bronchi, as well as GI, genitourinary, and reproductive systems (Schoenwolf et al., 2021). The vitelline circulation is characterized by the presence of a vitelline duct (conduit) that connects the yolk sac and midgut. This conduit allows for the early transfer of nutrients, until the placenta assumes the role of providing nutrition to the developing fetus. The yolk sac gradually shrinks in size over the course of the first weeks of embryonic development and usually disappears between weeks 10 and 20 of gestation (Clemente et al., 2021).

Clinical Application. The yolk sac should normally regress prior to birth. Failed regression of the yolk sac can leave persistent remnants of the urachus or vitelline duct (omphalomesenteric duct). These remnants may be partial or complete and may or may not connect to skin, bladder, or bowel. The presence of a partial remnant that is open to the skin at the region of the umbilicus is referred to as a urachal or umbilical sinus. The presence of a partial remnant that is open to the bladder or bowel is referred to as the Meckel diverticulum. In comparison, a partial remnant that is not open to the skin and does not connect to the bladder or bowel is referred to as a urachal or omphalomesenteric cyst. A complete remnant gives rise to a fistula that connects the bladder or bowel to the umbilicus; when the connection involves the bladder it is referred to as a patent urachus.

The Allantois (and Umbilical Cord). The umbilical cord provides a connection between the fetus and the placenta and quickly replaces the yolk sac as the source of nutrient delivery. Early in development, a primitive circulation via diffusion is established between the maternal spiral arteries and veins and the blood-filled lacunae. By the third week after fertilization, the umbilical cord develops from remnants of the yolk sac and the allantois. This primitive cord is composed of extraembryonic mesoderm extending from the chorionic plate to the developing embryo (Schoenwolf et al., 2021).

By week 5 of gestation, the primitive umbilical cord contains two umbilical veins, two umbilical arteries, the allantois, and other rudimentary elements such as the omphaloenteric duct and the umbilical coecum (Sadler, 2024). The second umbilical vein regresses by week 6 of gestation. The umbilical arteries arise initially from the dorsal aorta and, over time, the internal iliac arteries. The allantois arises from the yolk sac and develops into the urachus, which connects the yolk sac and fetal bladder and participates in the removal of waste from the fetal bladder (Torchia & Persaud, 2025). The allantois normally regresses by week 8 of gestation; failed regression can give rise to a patent urachus. The omphaloenteric duct (vitelline duct or yolk stalk) connects the yolk sac with the rudimentary intestinal tract and disappears by week 10 of gestation. The umbilical coelom, which connects both intraembryonic coelom (pleura, pericardial, and peritoneal spaces) and extraembryonic coelom (yolk sac, amniotic cavity, and chorionic cavity), disappears by week 12 of gestation (Schoenwolf et al., 2021).

The epithelium of the umbilical cord forms by week 12 of gestation and contains two arteries and one vein, both surrounded by Wharton's jelly. Wharton's jelly is formed from mucopolysaccharides, which produce a gelatinous material that protects the umbilical blood vessels (Cunningham et al., 2022). The umbilical vessels are longer than the cord and twist and spiral within the cord. Length of the umbilical cord depends on fetal movement, with more movement resulting in longer length and decreased movement shorter length. The cord is usually inserted in the center of the placenta and reaches maximal length by 30 weeks of gestation, with an average length of about 60 cm.

The Fetal Period: The Structurally Formed Placenta

The placenta is structurally mature by week 12 of gestation, though it continues to grow in size until term in order to meet the demands of the growing fetus (Sadler, 2024). The cytotrophoblast layer begins to thin out in order to decrease the distance for diffusion. The fetal part of the placenta, called the *chorionic plate*, contains the amnion, embryonic mesenchyme, and both cell layers (cytotrophoblast and syncytiotrophoblast). The maternal part of the placenta, the decidual plate, contains the decidua basalis, uterine vessels, and glands (Sadler, 2024). At term gestation, the placenta weighs about 500 grams with a diameter of approximately 18 to 25 cm, and 2 to 2.5 cm thickness (Cunningham et al., 2022; Sadler, 2024).

MATERNAL–FETAL CIRCULATION

Now that the structure of the placenta is described, blood flow can be followed from the maternal blood supply through the placenta to the fetus via the umbilical cord and then back to the mother (Figure 2.8). Oxygen-rich blood from the maternal uterine artery is delivered to the uterus, then to the maternal spiral arteries supplying the cotyledons. Maternal blood flows into the intervillous spaces in which the chorionic terminal villi extend. The fetal capillary system in the terminal villi take up contents of the maternal blood by diffusion and transport via the arteriovenous system, deliver it to the branching venules in the chorionic plate, and empty it into the single umbilical vein, which delivers oxygenated blood into the fetal circulation. Fetal circulation has a specialized architecture composed of fetal shunts (ductus venosus, foramen ovale, and ductus arteriosus [DA]) that allow the blood to circulate through the fetus within the context of the placenta, functioning as an organ of respiration, nutrition, and excretion.

The oxygenated blood enters the fetus via the umbilical vein, a portion of the blood enters the portal circulation, and the remaining blood (approximately 50%) flows through the ductus venosus into the inferior vena cava, joining deoxygenated blood returning from perfused organs. Minimal mixing occurs and the oxygenated blood is "preferentially streamed" into the right atrium, through the foramen ovale into the left atrium and ultimately to the aortic arch.

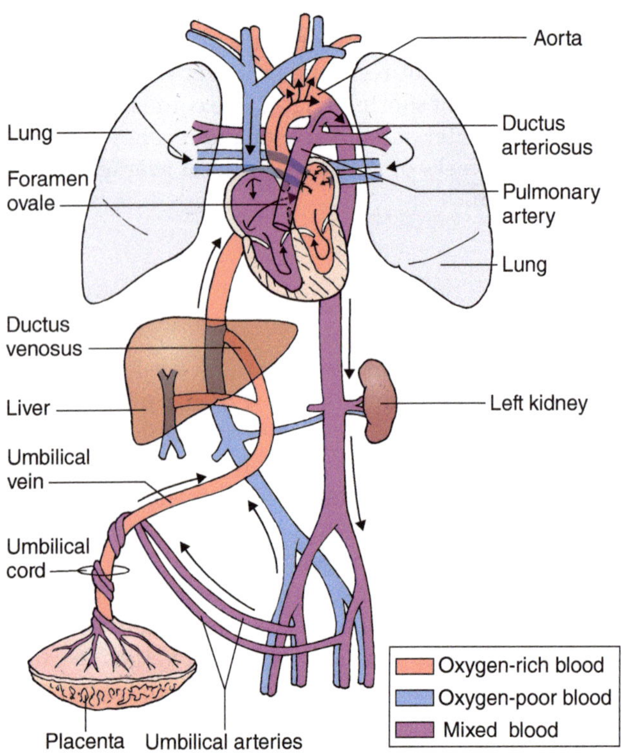

Figure 2.8 Maternal–fetal circulation.

Poorly oxygenated blood enters the right atrium from the superior vena cava and passes into the right ventricle and the pulmonary artery. Only about 10% of this blood flows to the lungs to nourish the proliferating pulmonary tissues; the majority of the blood volume is shunted through the DA, due to the high pulmonary vascular resistance, and into the descending aorta and returns to the placenta through the umbilical arteries.

Because only a small amount of blood is returning from the lungs via the pulmonary veins into the left atrium, the level of oxygenated blood sitting in the left atrium is minimally affected. This oxygenated blood in the left atrium flows into the left ventricle and the aorta and is delivered to the head and heart via the carotid and coronary arteries, with the remaining blood continuing down the aorta. This remaining blood is joined by the deoxygenated blood returning from the right ventricle that has shunted through the DA into the aorta. This mixed blood continues through the aorta, eventually drains into the umbilical arteries, and delivers waste products to the mother through the placenta via the chorionic villi to the maternal uterine vein.

In summary, fetal circulation occurs due to specific architecture:

1. The ductus venosus shunts blood from the placenta via the umbilical vein into the inferior vena cava.
2. This oxygenated blood from the umbilical vein enters the fetal cardiac circulation via preferential streaming and bypasses the lungs via the foramen ovale.
3. Poorly oxygenated blood from the right ventricle moves through the pulmonary artery, bypassing the lungs, and shunts into the descending aorta via the DA at a point distal to where the highest oxygenated blood has already been delivered to the heart and brain. This blood returns to the placenta through the umbilical arteries.

Other unique compensatory mechanisms that involve gas and nutrient delivery are discussed later in the chapter. The rate of fetal blood flow in the placenta is 500 mL/minute; it is dependent on fetal heart rate and regulated by interaction of blood pressure, fetal right to left shunts, and systemic and pulmonary vascular resistance. The placenta serves as a low-resistance circuit in the fetal circulatory system (Ali & Sawyer, 2024).

Placental Function

The placenta is an organ essential for transfer of nutrients and gases from the mother to the fetus and removal of fetal waste products from the fetus to the mother. The placenta performs four major functions to support growth and development of the fetus: (a) endocrine functions to facilitate a successful pregnancy, (b) fetal gas exchange, (c) nutrient delivery, and (d) waste product excretion (Cindrova-Davies & Sferruzzi-Perri, 2022). The transport of substances across the placenta increases during the course of gestation due to changes in placental structure (decreased distance between maternal and fetal blood), increased maternal and fetal blood flow, and greater demands of the growing fetus. The gas exchange, nutrition and excretion, immunologic, and endocrine functions will be described in detail later in the chapter.

Remember that the decidua basalis and chorionic villi are the site of communication between the mother and fetus. Maternal and fetal arteries and veins provide delivery of blood to and from mother and fetus. The actual exchange of nutrient uptake and waste exchange occurs via the fetal capillary bed in the terminal villi that are suspended in the intervillous spaces and bathed in maternal blood. How these nutrients are exchanged can be explained by different modes of placental transport.

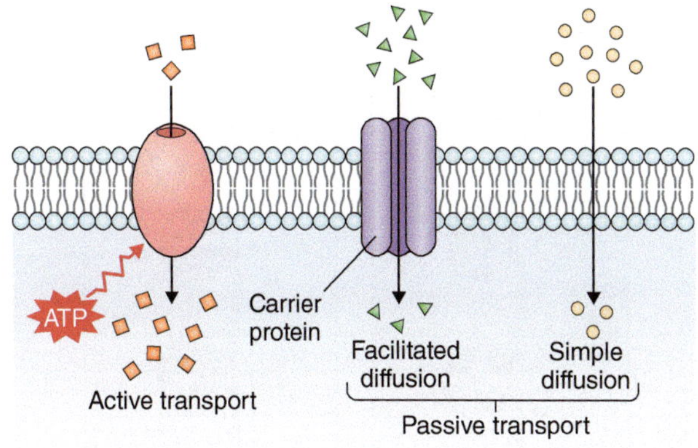

Figure 2.9 Simple diffusion, facilitated diffusion, and active transport. Simple diffusion allows substances to move from a higher to lower area of concentration. Facilitated diffusion requires the presence of a carrier protein in order for a particle to cross the desired membrane. Active transport requires the presence of energy (ATP) in addition to carrier proteins to facilitate transfer of substances between the maternal and fetal circulation.
ATP, adenosine triphosphate.

MODES OF PLACENTAL TRANSPORT

Fick's law of diffusion states that the rate of diffusion of a gas across a permeable membrane is determined by the chemical nature, density, and surface area of the membrane, and the partial pressure gradient of the gas (McNanley & Woods, 2008). There are five major processes involved in placental transfer, and each will be explored in this chapter.

Simple Diffusion

Simple diffusion, also called *passive diffusion*, is the simplest pathway across any membrane (Figure 2.9). Simple diffusion is concentration dependent and involves the movement of unbound substances across the lipid membrane of the cell or through channel proteins, from a higher to lower concentration. Diffusion is implicated by molecular size, membrane depth, and the water or fat solubility of the molecules. Not all substances diffuse with the same ease; some easily pass through the cell membranes (e.g., CO_2) whereas others are dependent on significant differences between the level of concentration on both sides of the membrane. In general, smaller, water-soluble molecules pass more readily with carbon dioxide transfer occurring faster than oxygen. Water, electrolytes, oxygen, carbon dioxide, urea, simple amines, creatinine, fatty acids, steroids, fat-soluble vitamins, narcotics, barbiturates, and anesthetics cross by the process of simple diffusion.

Given that the direction of movement is always from an area of higher concentration to an area of lower concentration, movement from mother to fetus is favored when a higher concentration of a substance (e.g., oxygen) is present in the maternal blood. Movement from fetus to mother is favored when the concentration of a substance (e.g., carbon dioxide) is present in the fetal blood.

Facilitated Diffusion

Facilitated diffusion requires the presence of specific "carrier" proteins that assist the transfer of the substance across a membrane. When a carrier protein is available, substances can move from a higher to lower concentration. Glucose, for example, is transferred via facilitated diffusion with the help of glucose transport proteins (GLUT transporters; Hufnagel et al., 2022).

Active Transport

Active transport is energy dependent as well as transfer protein specific, and results in the transfer of substances against concentration gradients with the assistance of adenosine triphosphate (ATP). This is the process used for transfer of most amino acids, potassium, water-soluble vitamins, calcium, phosphate, iron, and iodide. Active transport allows for concentrations of nutrients to be higher in the fetus (compared to mother) during critical growth periods.

Endocytosis and Exocytosis

The processes of endocytosis and exocytosis allow for substances to be enveloped or engulfed within a membrane for transport into the cell (endocytosis), or to be removed from a cell (exocytosis; Figure 2.10). These processes are used when substances are too large to be accommodated by simple or facilitated diffusion, or specific carrier proteins are not available. Iron and immunoglobulin G (IgG) antibodies are examples of substances that require endocytosis for transfer from maternal circulation to the fetal circulation (Cooke et al., 2021).

Bulk Flow

Bulk flow may result in large, rapid transfer of substances across the placental membrane resulting from changes in osmotic pressure and hydrostatic forces. When osmotic

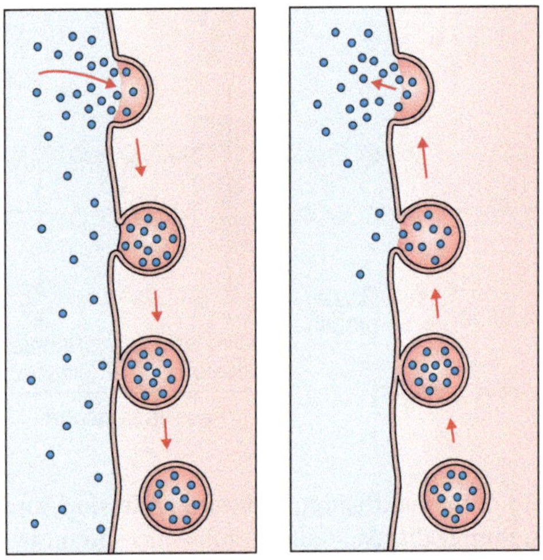

Figure 2.10 Endocytosis and exocytosis are reverse processes and involve fusion of substances (e.g., antibodies) within the plasma membrane for transport into and out of a cell.

pressure drops, the bulk movement of water will be from the higher to lower side of the maternal–fetal circuit. This movement results in concomitant electrolyte shifts, as certain electrolytes (e.g., sodium) follow water. This process may also include the use of special aqueous pores or water channels.

Clinical Application. During routine delivery or periods of maternal illness, hypotonic dextrose intravascular fluid delivery is a commonly used therapeutic intervention to ensure adequate maternal hydration, though instances of maternal fluid overload have been noted. Owing to the difference between maternal and fetal osmotic pressures and the principles of bulk flow, there is increased fluid transfer to the fetus. The result of this intervention on the neonate may present as increased birth weight (generalized edema) due to excess fluid transfer. Associated neonatal clinical features the APRN should be alerted to include hyponatremia, respiratory distress, and excessive weight loss following diuresis.

In addition to these processes for substance transfer, there may be transfer of fetal or maternal blood cells due to tiny capillary breaks within the villus covering, allowing small amounts of maternal blood to enter fetal circulation, and vice versa. Maternal leukocytes, some bacteria, and some viral organisms can also cross the placenta and infect the fetus, but the mechanisms by which these processes occur are unknown.

TRANSPLACENTAL GAS TRANSFER

Gas transfer is by simple diffusion across a 3.5-micron distance between the fetal and maternal circulations. In the case of oxygen, it is transferred down an average concentration gradient of 30 mmHg (Burton et al., 2021). Oxygen delivery to the uterus and placenta is from the maternal uterine artery and is delivered to the fetus via the umbilical vein. Fetal hemoglobin has a higher oxygen affinity (P50 = 18–20 mmHg) than adult hemoglobin (P50 = 26.6 mmHg), meaning that fetal hemoglobin is more saturated with oxygen at the same PaO_2. This optimizes fetal oxygen uptake. In addition, fetal hemoglobin lacks binding sites for 2,3-diphosphoglycerate (DPG), a key regulator of oxygen affinity. This also leads to a right shift (lower affinity) in the oxyhemoglobin dissociation curve (OHDC) and optimal delivery of oxygen to the fetal tissues. But, how does near perfect uptake and offloading of oxygen and carbon dioxide occur during pregnancy? This biochemical phenomenon which occurs in tandem is described as the Bohr and Haldane effects (or "double" Bohr and Haldane during pregnancy). Both the Bohr (role of CO_2 on the affinity of Hgb for oxygen) and Haldane (role of oxygen on the affinity of Hgb for CO_2) effects work synergistically on both the maternal and fetal sides to facilitate gas transfer and homeostasis within the fetus.

The *Bohr effect* refers to the role of carbon dioxide and pH on hemoglobin's affinity for oxygen, which implicates transplacental oxygen transfer. Increased pCO_2 (and lower pH) alters the structure of the hemoglobin molecule and results in lower oxygen affinity and a shift of the OHDC to the right, displacing oxygen molecules from hemoglobin. The net effect is an increase in the amount of oxygen dissolved in plasma, which is available for delivery to target tissues. Conversely, a low pCO_2 (and higher pH) results in higher oxygen affinity and a shift of the OHDC to the left. The net effect is a decrease in the amount of oxygen dissolved in the plasma. The "double" Bohr refers to this process occurring concurrently in both the maternal and fetal circulations (**Figure 2.11**). An increase in pCO_2 in the maternal intervillous sinuses of the placenta from uptake of displaced fetal CO_2 leads to unloading of oxygen by maternal adult hemoglobin. The subsequent decrease in the pCO_2 on the fetal side leads to an increase in oxygen uptake by the fetal hemoglobin. The double Bohr effect leads to a widening of the difference between the maternal and fetal hemoglobin OHDC for any given pO_2 (**Figure 2.12**).

The *Haldane effect* refers to the role of oxygen on hemoglobin affinity to carbon dioxide, which implicates transplacental CO_2 transfer. The higher pO_2 results in a lower capacity for hemoglobin to carry CO_2 (**Figure 2.13**). The "double" Haldane refers to this process occurring concurrently in both the maternal and fetal circulations. As fetal hemoglobin becomes saturated with oxygen, carbon dioxide is offloaded and

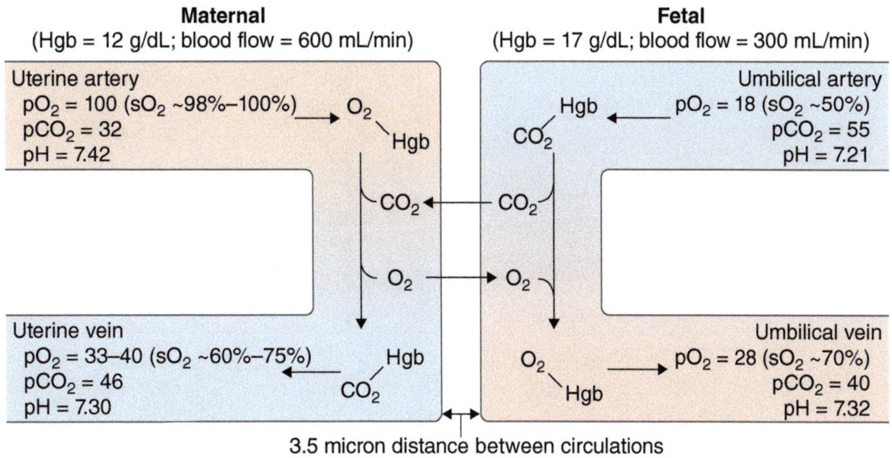

Figure 2.11 Double Bohr effect. *Right:* Carbon dioxide diffuses from fetal blood into the maternal blood more readily than oxygen due to solubility differences. As maternal hemoglobin absorbs more CO_2, the pH and affinity of maternal hemoglobin for oxygen decreases. This prompts displacement of oxygen from maternal hemoglobin (higher concentration), promoting uptake of the displaced oxygen by fetal hemoglobin (lower concentration). *Left:* As there is a decrease in carbon dioxide on fetal hemoglobin, the affinity of fetal hemoglobin for oxygen increases, strengthening oxygen binding to fetal hemoglobin.
Hgb, hemoglobin.

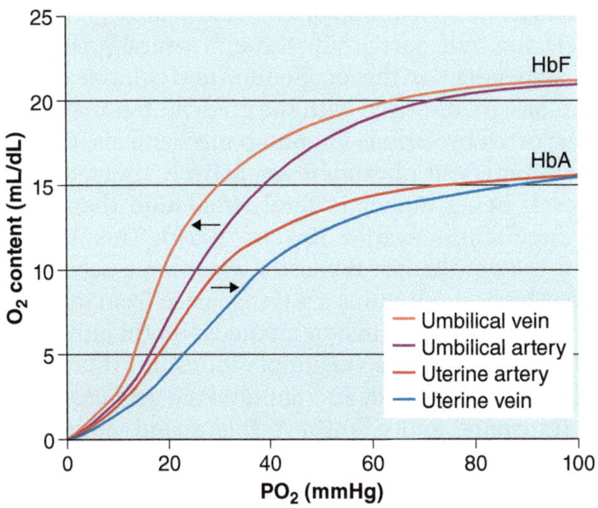

Figure 2.12 Oxyhemoglobin dissociation curve within the placenta.
HbA, adult hemoglobin; HbF, fetal hemoglobin.

returned by simple diffusion to the maternal circulation via the umbilical arteries and intervillous space. The comparatively lower maternal CO_2 levels (secondary to maternal hyperventilation) facilitates maternal uptake and expulsion.

Clinical Application. The APRN can apply the principles of the "double" Bohr and Haldane effects when considering the exchange of gases in the fetus experiencing impairments to placental blood flow. Consider the scenario of maternal hypertension or preeclampsia, where due to impaired vascular modeling in the placenta there is increased pressure in the placenta and a decrease in the volume of blood perfusing the placenta. The resultant placental hypoxia impairs both availability of oxygen delivery to the fetus (impaired Haldane effect) and CO_2 removal (impaired Bohr effect). This is exacerbated during labor, further impairing blood flow and gas exchange. Clinical features noted prior to and following delivery in the distressed fetus include poor HR variability, decelerations, fetal growth restriction, passage of meconium into the amniotic fluid, respiratory distress, delayed transition to extrauterine life, and acidosis noted on cord gases.

NUTRITION AND EXCRETION

Nutrients, waste products, and drugs are exchanged across the syncytiotrophoblast, passing in both directions—maternal to fetal and fetal to maternal circulation. This exchange occurs through various processes, including simple diffusion, facilitated diffusion, active transport, endocytosis and exocytosis, and bulk flow.

Glucose

The main source of carbohydrate is glucose; it is transported from maternal to fetal circulation by a protein-mediated, concentration-dependent, facilitated diffusion. There are several glucose transporters involved, each with a specific function. The fetus itself produces little glucose during gestation and relies on the concentration gradient to facilitate glucose transfer from the maternal circulation (higher concentration) to the fetal circulation

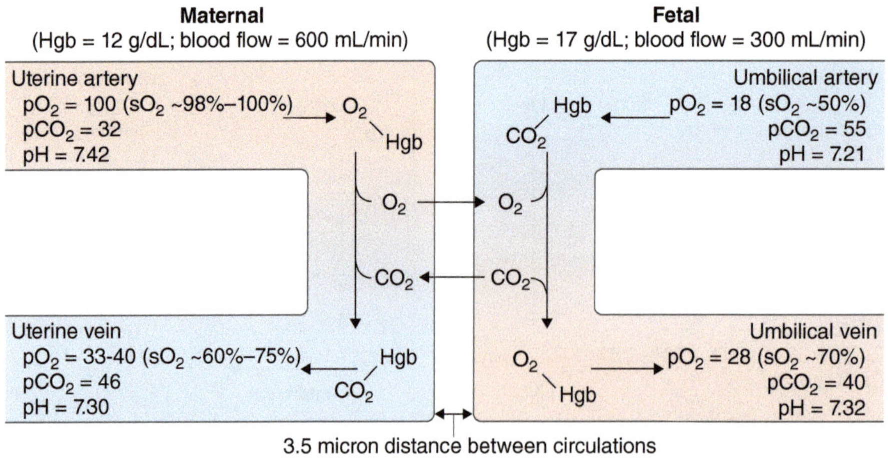

Figure 2.13 Double Haldane effect. *Left:* Oxygen is released from maternal hemoglobin (higher concentration) and is absorbed by fetal hemoglobin (lower concentration). In the presence of lower maternal hemoglobin oxygen saturation, there is an increase in carbon dioxide affinity by the maternal hemoglobin. *Right:* The oxygen that is absorbed by fetal hemoglobin results in a decrease in affinity for carbon dioxide.
Hgb, hemoglobin.

(lower concentration). Fetal glucose levels are approximately 70% to 80% of the maternal glucose levels (Fay et al., 2024). Elevated blood glucose in the mother causes elevated blood glucose in the fetus, with subsequent sequelae for the infants of diabetic mothers with poor glucose control (see Chapter 10 for further discussion on the impact of elevated maternal blood glucose levels on the fetus and neonate).

Amino Acids

Amino acids are transported across the placenta and can be metabolized by the fetus as well. Protein transfer across the placenta occurs via active transport (energy-requiring process that relies on amino acid transporters). Amino acid levels are higher in the fetal circulation than in maternal circulation.

Lipids

Lipids are present in many forms in both maternal and fetal circulation and transport varies based on the form. Free fatty acids and glycerol are transported via simple diffusion or facilitated through fatty acid binding proteins (Hirschmugl et al., 2021). The trophoblast itself can synthesize cholesterol and other fatty acids, but most cholesterol is transported across the placenta from the maternal circulation (Hirschmugl et al., 2021). Cholesterol is necessary during early development and is key in the function of Sonic Hedgehog (SHH), which is responsible for the control and development of the neurologic system and other organ systems (Cindrova-Davies & Sferruzzi-Perri, 2022).

Water, Ions, Vitamins, and Minerals

Water transport is thought to occur through several processes, including passive transport (osmosis) dependent on hydrostatic and osmotic pressure, and through water channels. Ion transport occurs through several processes as well, dependent on the ion. Sodium and chloride move through passive diffusion with the gradient but may also be transported by various ion pump mechanisms. Potassium, calcium, and phosphate are actively transported, with levels being higher in fetal circulation than maternal circulation (Ryan & Kovacs, 2020). This is particularly true in the last trimester when bone accretion activity is highest. Vitamins are transported from mother to fetus via multiple diffusion methods. Biotin and vitamins D, E, and K cross via simple diffusion; thiamine, riboflavin, nicotinic acid, and pantothenic acid cross via active transport; and vitamin A, folate, and vitamin C use facilitated transfer (McNanley & Woods, 2008).

In addition to the excretion of carbon dioxide, the placenta also excretes by-products of metabolism that would normally be excreted by the liver and kidneys. Ammonia is converted into uric acid and urea and passively diffuses across the placenta. For the most part, unconjugated bilirubin is thought to be diffused passively across the placenta.

IMMUNOLOGIC FUNCTION

One of the most significant immunologic functions of the placenta is its ability to permit implantation and maintenance of the pregnancy because the developing fetal tissue is semiallogeneic, having both maternal and paternal proteins. Several factors are involved in protecting the fetal tissues (which include the placenta) from being attacked by the maternal immune system. Human leukocyte antigen G (HLA-G) is a maternally derived antigen responsible for decreasing the maternal immune response to the fetal tissue. Fetal cells also contribute to this process by producing immunosuppressive cytokines, chemokines, and prostaglandins that limit T-lymphocyte proliferation and enhance progesterone production, which helps reduce immune response (Cindrova-Davies & Sferruzzi-Perri, 2022; Turco & Moffett, 2019). The syncytiotrophoblast and cytotrophoblast of the villi within the intervillous space do not produce tissue antigens. This prevents reactions between maternal and fetal blood that are in constant direct contact with the villi (fetal structures). The placenta itself also blocks maternal cytotoxic cells, further enhancing the antigenic mechanisms that promote human reproduction.

Passive immunity to many viruses is passed from mother to fetus by endocytosis. Maternal IgG antibodies developed in response to prior exposure to viruses, or through prior immunization, are taken up by membrane-bound vesicles and transported across the placenta into fetal circulation. IgG provides immunity for a limited period of time postnatally, until the neonate has adequate supply of innate or acquired immunity.

The placenta has several features that offer protection from many viruses and bacteria; however, this protection is limited. The first level of protection is provided by the syncytiotrophoblast itself. There are no intracellular junctions in the placenta, which limits the passage of most bloodborne pathogens. The decidual trophoblast has multiple cellular defenses in the form of macrophages and natural killer cells that enhance placental elimination of invading pathogens. The final layer of protection is afforded by the basement membrane of the placenta, separating the capillary endothelium and syncytiotrophoblast, which further limits transfer of infectious agents (Cunningham et al., 2022). There are, however, pathogens that are known to pass from mother to fetus, including syphilis, rubella, toxoplasmosis, cytomegalovirus (CMV), parvovirus B-19, herpes simplex, and mycobacterium tuberculosis, which cause devastating sequelae in the fetus.

Clinical Application. CMV infections affect up to 60% of adults in the United States, with approximately 0.64% of neonates born with congenital CMV, making it the most common congenital viral infection. Globally, the incidence of CMV is between 0.2% to 2.5% of all live births and may be implicated in up to 16% of the cases of fetal demise. Similar to other viral infections, the rate of vertical transmission is *highest* during the primary infection, with 30% to 50% of congenital infections as a result of a primary CMV infection. The CMV virus impacts the placenta by causing chronic inflammation and decreased vascularity of the villi. Though the CMV virus has a large size, inflammation within the placenta increases the possibility of viral exposure to the fetal bloodstream and subsequent fetal infection. The APRN should be highly suspicious of CMV infections in symptomatic neonates. Clinical symptoms of CMV infection include small for gestational age (SGA), hepatosplenomegaly, thrombocytopenia (with or without petechia), chorioretinitis, cerebral calcifications, hyperbilirubinemia, and abnormal liver enzymes. The majority of impacted neonates are asymptomatic at birth with the most common long-term sequelae being sensorineural hearing loss (SNHL). CMV infections are the most common non-genetic cause of SNHL in children.

The placenta does not offer protection to the fetus from drug transfer. Drugs that cross the placenta most readily are those with low molecular weight that are uncharged and lipophilic and have high levels of unbound drug in maternal circulation. Drugs that cross the placenta include most antibiotics, antivirals, anesthetics, analgesics, cardiovascular drugs, tobacco, caffeine, and alcohol. Very few drugs do not cross the placenta; this group includes heparin and insulin. The mechanisms of transfer follow the processes listed earlier: diffusion, facilitated diffusion, active transport, and endocytosis.

Drug safety in pregnancy is a complex issue, and a clear understanding of benefits and risks associated with the use of drugs during pregnancy is critical. In 2014, the U.S. Food and Drug Administration (FDA) overhauled its recommendations for drugs in pregnancy and lactation by enacting the Pregnancy and Lactation Labeling Rule (PLLR). The former alphabetical system (A, B, C, D, and X) was replaced with a summary of known and suspected risks in narrative form preceding each drug description, including the molecular weight of the drug (FDA, 2014). This new legislation holds pharmaceutical companies responsible for updating drug information as soon as information becomes outdated.

ENDOCRINE FUNCTION

The placenta produces hormones that are critical in maintenance of the pregnancy, preparation and coordination of the mother's body to sustain changes in function to support additional metabolic and circulation requirements of pregnancy and lactation, and regulation of fetal growth. This hormonal production begins during the blastocyst stage even before the placenta is formed and implantation has taken place (Cindrova-Davies & Sferruzzi-Perri, 2022; Turco & Moffett, 2019). The primary site of placental hormone synthesis is the syncytiotrophoblast. These hormones include, but are not limited to, estrogens, progesterone, oxytocin, hCG, human chorionic somatomammotropin (hCS), growth hormones, corticotropin-releasing hormone, human placental lactogen, and insulin-like growth factors. Some of the hormones initially produced in the placenta are also made in the fetal brain as gestation continues. Placental hormones may remain in the placenta, whereas others cross the placenta to maternal and/or fetal circulation (Cindrova-Davies & Sferruzzi-Perri, 2022).

Estrogen, progesterone, and oxytocin work to help maintain the endometrium, suppress gonadotropin secretion, trigger parturition, and have important roles in neuroendocrine processes. Estrogens also stimulate mammary gland development while progesterone stimulates the development of the alveolar tissue within the mammary glands. Lactogen is critical for maternal carbohydrate and lipid metabolism for nutrient availability for the fetus as well as milk production for the infant after birth. Chorionic gonadotropin is critical in maintenance of the corpus luteum, in synchrony with LH in the first few weeks of pregnancy, and also plays a role in suppressing the immune response, preventing rejection of the embryo. Somatomammotropin increases lipolysis in adipose tissue to provide placental energy, sparing glucose for use by the fetus.

GENETIC INFLUENCES ON PLACENTAL DEVELOPMENT

Currently, research on genetic and epigenetic defects that might have a direct effect on the developing placenta is ongoing. Investigation is warranted into the etiology of recurring early pregnancy loss to determine genetic mutations that may predispose a woman to early fetal demise as a direct result of abnormal placental development.

Chronic histiocytic intervillositis (CHIV) of the placenta occurs in less than 1% of pregnancies and is associated with fetal demise, premature delivery, and low birth weight/intrauterine growth restriction (IUGR; Moar et al., 2022). Histiocytic infiltration and lesions in the intervillous spaces of the placenta characterize CHIV (Moar et al., 2022). Resulting trophoblast degeneration and increased distance between maternal blood and the chorionic villi are suggested causes of fetal and neonatal sequelae (Moar et al., 2022).

XX pregnant patients with a mutation in methylenetetrahydrofolate reductase (MTFHR) suffer recurrent miscarriages, develop preeclampsia, and give birth to infants with congenital defects, for example, neural tube defects (Tabatabaei et al., 2022; Zhu et al., 2018). However, it is unclear whether these recurrent miscarriages are directly related to defective placental development. Current understanding of this genetic disease links high homocysteine levels to development of preeclampsia and failure of embryo implantation into the placenta (Zhu et al., 2018), but whether this is associated with faulty trophoblast invasion or defects in placental blood vessel development remains unclear. Development of neural tube defects appears to be related to altered folate metabolism as the MTHFR enzyme is necessary for folate metabolism and absent or decreased enzyme activity leads to hyperhomocysteinemia (Tabatabaei et al., 2022).

Simmons (2024) details the role in which maternal nutrient deprivation alters gene expression and ultimately the function of the placenta. These alterations in placental function focus on the impact of the maternal environment on adaptive gene expression and fetal brain development.

As scientific knowledge advances in genetic sequencing, epigenetics, and identification of biomarkers for diagnosis of maternal disease, and from examination of the placenta in early pregnancy losses, we may better understand the direct genetic influences on placental development. Currently, there are known placental developmental abnormalities and maternal illnesses that may not be genetic in nature, but affect fetal development, and these conditions are discussed in the following section.

COMMON DEVELOPMENTAL ABNORMALITIES OF THE PLACENTA AND THEIR EFFECT ON THE FETUS

During the development of the placenta, problems with site of implantation, individual placental structures, or development of placental vasculature can alter the normal structure and function of the placenta. These problems are presented as they occur from fertilization to later in fetal development. These can occur due to maternal illness and can impact the developing fetus or affect the future health of the human being.

Placental Structure: Zygosity and Abnormal Vasculature

The structure of the placenta is determined at the time of fertilization and depends on whether the pregnancy is single or multiple. A twin pregnancy is used here to illustrate differences in placental structure (Figure 2.14). Monozygotic (identical) twins account for a third of all twin pregnancies and arise from the division of a single ovum after fertilization. A twin pregnancy can result in a monochorionic or dichorionic placenta and the following possible placental structures: monochorionic–monoamniotic (same amniotic sac), monochorionic–diamniotic (separate amniotic sac), and dichorionic–diamniotic. Dizygotic (fraternal) twins account for two thirds of all twin pregnancies and arise when two ova enclosed within a single follicle are fertilized simultaneously, or when ovulation of two ova from one or both ovaries are independently fertilized. This results in two (dichorionic) placentas (separate or fused). There are instances when the placentas fuse

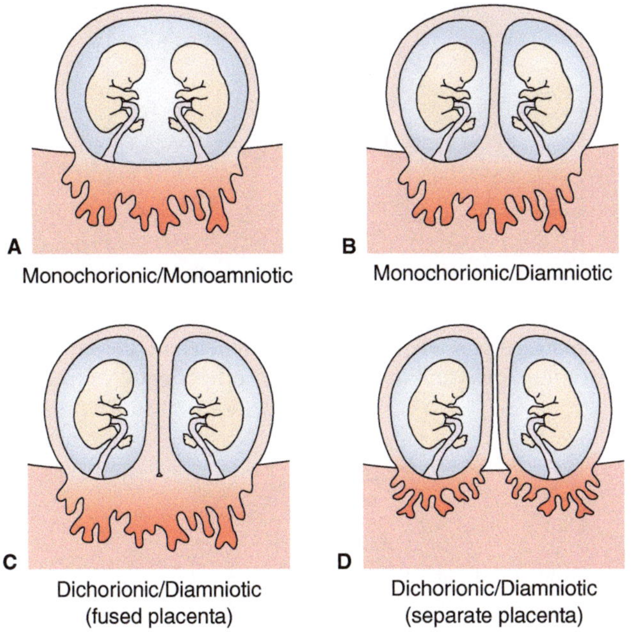

Figure 2.14 Zygosity. (**A**) Monochorionic/monoamniotic and (**B**) monochorionic/diamniotic resulting from division of a single ovum. (**C**) Dichorionic/diamniotic with a fused placenta may either be from division of a single ovum or as a result of fertilization of two ovum with placental implantation in close proximity. (**D**) Dichorionic/diamniotic with separate placentas result from fertilization of two ovum.

along a common border, making ultrasound distinction of monochorionic versus dichorionic difficult (Cunningham et al., 2022; Sadler, 2024).

Improper development of the vasculature in monozygotic twins can lead to placental vascular anastomoses that alter normal blood flow, decreasing blood flow to one fetus and increasing flow to the other fetus. In addition, given the high demands of a pregnancy with more than one fetus, insufficient blood flow may result in restricted growth and preterm delivery (Cunningham et al., 2022). Monochorionic/monoamniotic twins are at the highest risk for adverse pregnancy outcomes including maternal hypertension, preeclampsia, stroke, diabetes, and premature delivery. These twins are also at increased risk of conjoined twins, birth defects (cardiac), and abnormal vascular blood flow between the twins (Van Mieghem et al., 2022). Twin-to-twin transfusion syndrome is a disorder of monochorionic placentas in which the blood flow between each fetus is unequal and can occur in up to 15% of monochorionic twin pregnancies (Bamberg & Hecher, 2022). Owing to vascular anomalies within the placenta, blood flow is diverted from the "donor" twin and pumped to the larger "recipient" twin. The smaller, donor twin receives less blood flow, resulting in anemia, oliguria, and thus decreased amniotic fluid (oligohydramnios). This places the fetus at risk for abnormal organ development and compromises cushioning of the developing fetus. The larger, recipient twin receives an excess of blood flow, resulting in polycythemia and polyuria, and leads to a higher volume of amniotic fluid (polyhydramnios), risk for rupture of the sac, heart failure, and hydrops (Bamberg & Hecher, 2022).

Molar Pregnancy

A molar pregnancy, also called *gestational trophoblastic disease*, occurs in 0.1% of pregnancies and results from implantation of a fertilized egg that is not viable. The developing chorionic villi swell and form fluid-filled cysts in the placenta (Cunningham et al., 2022). Although most molar pregnancies are noncancerous growths and result in pregnancy loss, there are malignant forms.

Implantation Errors

Ectopic Pregnancy. An ectopic pregnancy occurs any time the fertilized egg implants in a location other than the uterine endometrium, although most often this occurs in the fallopian tubes (tubal pregnancy). Any conditions that affect the integrity of the tissue in the fallopian tubes, such as inflammation from infection or sexually transmitted infections, scar tissue, or abnormal tube shape, can lead to improper implantation of the fertilized egg in the tube, where the growing embryo cannot be supported. Ectopic pregnancies may occur in approximately 1% to 2% of first-trimester pregnancies, but can account for 6% to 10% of pregnancy-related deaths (Cunningham et al., 2022; Sadler, 2024). Early detection of a tubal pregnancy allows time for laparoscopic surgery and the prevention of tubal rupture, thereby reducing maternal morbidity risks. However, the risk remains for subsequent ectopic pregnancies and subsequent unsuccessful pregnancies (Cunningham et al., 2022).

Placenta Accreta. After a normal fertilization, the deep portion of the endometrium does not undergo decidualization and limits trophoblastic invasion beyond the endometrial layer into the maternal myometrium by secreting locally acting factors (Cunningham et al., 2022). However, in XX pregnant patients with previous cesarean deliveries or in conditions leading to endometrial damage or scarring, the placenta can invade the smooth muscle fibers and become inseparable from the uterine wall. Three types of abnormal attachment (accreta) are known. *Placenta accreta*, the most common type of abnormal attachment, occurs when the chorionic villi penetrate deep into the endometrium, but not the myometrium. *Placenta increta* occurs if the chorionic villi invade the myometrium, and *placenta percreta* occurs if the villi invade past the muscle layer into the serosal layer or even other organs such as the bladder (Cunningham et al., 2022). At delivery, these conditions create a risk for life-threatening maternal hemorrhage when the placenta does not appropriately separate from the uterine wall (**Figure 2.15**).

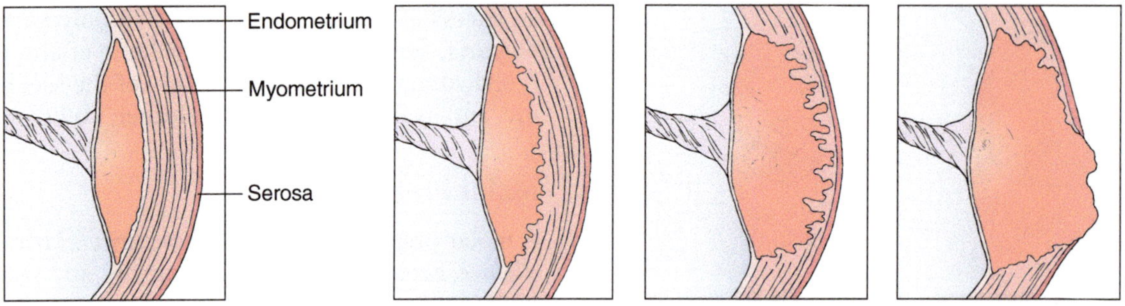

Figure 2.15 Diagram of degrees of abnormal placental infiltration. Placenta accreta is adherent to the myometrium. Placenta increta invades the myometrium. Placenta percreta extends beyond the uterine serosa and may invade any other organ.

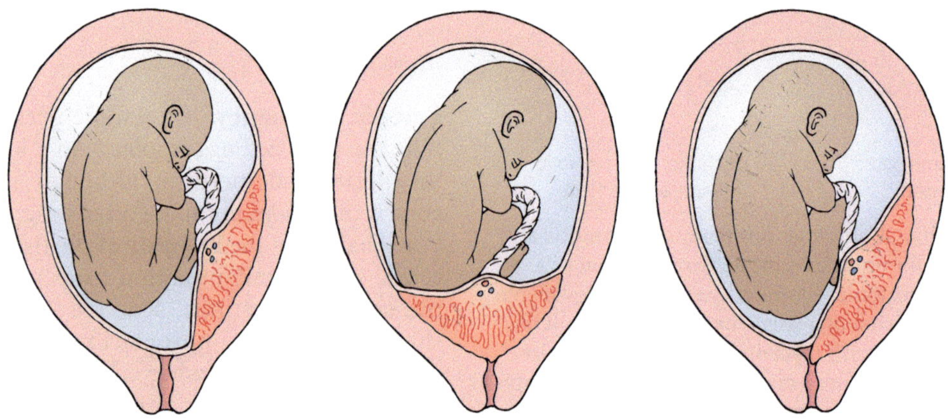

Figure 2.16 Placenta previa.

Placenta Previa. Placenta previa results from the improper implantation of the blastocyst close to or overlying the internal os of the uterus. At delivery, as the cervix dilates, risk of hemorrhage threatens the fetus and mother. The delivery route is determined by the severity of the previa and potential hemorrhage. In general, a complete previa describes two conditions: The cervical os is completely or partially covered by the placenta. In the low-lying placenta, the placenta extends to the edge of the cervix, but not over the os (Figure 2.16; Cunningham et al., 2022).

Velamentous Cord Insertion. Velamentous insertion of the cord occurs when the umbilical cord does not insert directly into the middle of the placenta, but instead attaches to the placental membrane between the amnion and the chorion. Abnormal cord placement may result from improper implantation of the blastocyst. The cord is not protected by Wharton's jelly and the vessels are vulnerable to compression and rupture leading to rapid fetal blood loss (Figure 2.17; Cunningham et al., 2022).

Vasa Previa. Vasa previa occurs when the umbilical vessels cross the cervical os. The vessels are vulnerable to tearing as the cervix dilates, which can lead to significant fetal blood loss and fetal mortality (Figure 2.18; Cunningham et al., 2022).

Abnormal Spiral Arteries

If the cytotrophoblast fails to correctly invade the uterus and its vasculature, transformation of the spiral arteries into low resistant circuits does not occur and can lead to decreased uteroplacental blood flow to the fetus. This developmental abnormality characterizes maternal preeclampsia and can lead to growth restriction of the fetus (Staff et al., 2022). Research continues into defining the mechanisms of vessel remodeling and altered hemodynamics and their relationship to preeclampsia and altered placental function.

Umbilical Cord Defects

Any compression or knotting of the umbilical cord can compromise normal blood flow to and from the placenta and affect normal function of the placenta. Umbilical cord compression during delivery, a knot in the cord, or a nuchal cord disrupts umbilical blood flow. Cord length can also cause problems; a longer cord may be prone to prolapse, knotting, or twisting; a short cord may limit sufficient blood volume delivery or tear during delivery (Cunningham et al., 2022).

Single Umbilical Artery. The normal umbilical cord contains one vein and two arteries. In most cases, there are no associated anomalies. However, in the 1% of

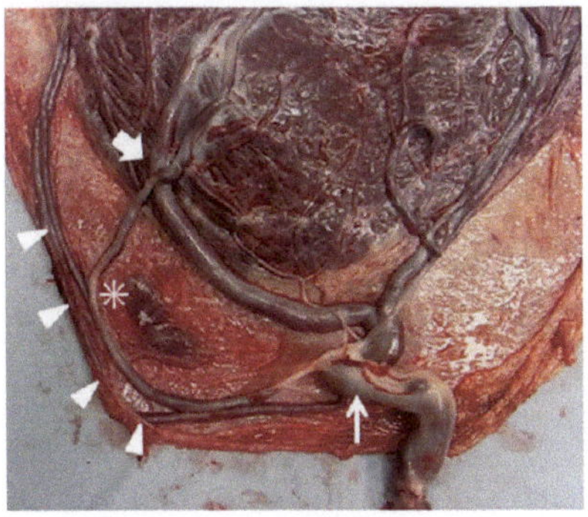

Figure 2.17 Velamentous cord insertion.
Source: Iwahashi, N., Ota, N., Shiro, M., Yagi, S., Minami, S., & Ino, K. (2016). Vasa previa evaluated by noncontrast time-of-flight magnetic resonance angiography. *Taiwanese Journal of Obstetrics & Gynecology, 55*(4), 585–587. doi:10.1016/j.tjog.2016.06.007

infants born with a single umbilical artery, there have been cases of associated cardiovascular and renal anomalies (Cunningham et al., 2022).

Fusion Failure of the Amnion and Chorion

During the first trimester of pregnancy, it is common to note separation of the amnion (inner layer) and the chorion (outer layer covering the placenta). Failure of the chorion and amnion to fuse by the end of week 12 of gestation, which is the beginning of the second trimester, is linked to increased rates of premature delivery, premature membrane rupture, fetal growth restriction, genetic abnormalities, or fetal demise. Invasive procedures, such as amniocentesis or fetal surgery, has been linked to disruption of the fetal membranes following initial fusion (Gerson et al., 2019).

Amnion (Amniotic Bands)

Rupture of the amniotic sac or accumulation of fluid in the space between the amnion and chorion leading to rupture of the amnion may lead to development of fibrous amniotic bands that can surround and constrict the umbilical cord or any area of the developing fetus, such as arms, legs, and forehead. Depending on the tightness of this banding, development of the affected fetal body area can be limited or totally impeded, leading to malformations or amputations (Sadler, 2024).

Abnormal Amniotic Fluid Volume

Oligohydramnios occurs when there is low volume of amniotic fluid for gestational age (less than 500 mL at term). This condition can result from placental insufficiency with diminished placental blood flow, premature rupture of amniochorionic membrane, or fetal renal anomalies (Taylor et al., 2025). Any of these conditions can lead to complications in fetal development (such as pulmonary hypoplasia) or defects from lack of protective cushioning and resulting compression (facial defects or structural limb defects).

Polyhydramnios occurs when there is a higher volume of amniotic fluid than normal, usually in excess of 2,000 mL. Etiology includes maternal factors, such as Rh isoimmunization or maternal diabetes, or fetal factors, such as esophageal atresia, which prevents swallowing of amniotic fluid (Taylor et al., 2025). Polyhydramnios can lead to premature rupture of membranes or abruptio placentae.

Placental Abruption

Premature separation of a normally implanted placenta prior to delivery characterizes placental abruption and is a common cause of antepartum bleeding (Lazebnik et al., 2025). With ensuing bleeding, the decidua basalis separates from the placenta and leads to disruption in normal uteroplacental exchange and therefore fetal compromise. Etiology of abruptio placentae includes abdominal trauma and maternal conditions that cause vasoconstriction, such as hypertension or use of tobacco or cocaine (Cunningham et al., 2022). Onset of hemorrhage may lead to preterm labor or, depending on the severity of the hemorrhage, may result in intrauterine fetal demise (Cunningham et al., 2022).

MATERNAL HEALTH INFLUENCES ON PLACENTAL DEVELOPMENT AND FUNCTION

Maternal conditions can alter normal placental implantation and development, disrupt placental blood flow, and affect placental function. As a result, normal growth of the fetus can be affected, or fetal diseases can develop. Specific diseases affecting the neonate will be discussed in detail in subsequent chapters specific to body systems.

Much has been learned about the many factors (growth and transcription) that impact the development of the placenta and which are necessary to sustain a healthy pregnancy. Particular focus has been placed upon the relationship between maternal growth factors, signaling molecules, and cytotrophoblastic proliferation necessary for placental growth and development. Any alteration in cytotrophoblast proliferation has the potential to impact normal fetal growth. For example, an increase in cell proliferation might lead to macrosomia, whereas a decrease in cell proliferation, and thus the failure to keep up with the expanding syncytium needed to support the growing fetus, could lead to fetal growth restriction (FGR; Cindrova-Davies & Sferruzzi-Perri, 2022). Progesterone is currently being utilized in XX pregnant patients with a history of pregnancy loss or failure to implant following in-vitro fertilization to optimize the decidua and increase the likelihood of successful implantation (Cindrova-Davies & Sferruzzi-Perri, 2022). Additional research is indicated to better understand these relationships.

Hypertension, which occurs in up to 10% of pregnancies (Cunningham et al., 2022), is characterized by

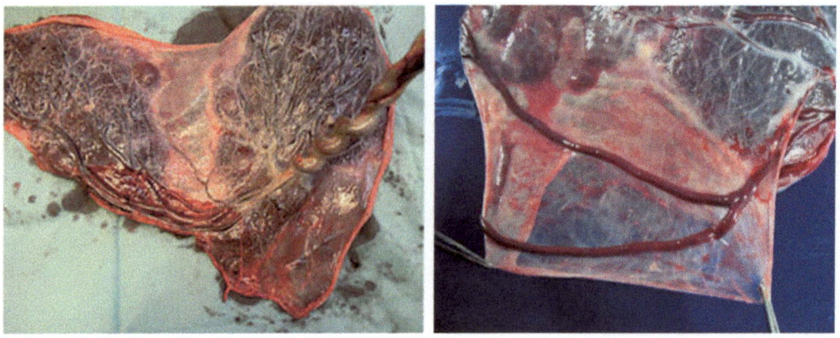

Figure 2.18 Vasa previa.

Sources: [Left] Rivera, M. J. C., Bachs, S. C., Vilarmau, M. G., Capdevila, J. P., & Pérez, F. O. (2009). Vasa previa: prenatal ultrasound diagnosis and obstetric management. *Advances in Obstetrics and Gynecology, 52*(11), 643–647. https://doi.org/10.1016/s0304-5013(09)72802-x; [Right] Iwahashi, N., Ota, N., Shiro, M., Yagi, S., Minami, S., & Ino, K. (2016). Vasa previa evaluated by noncontrast time-of-flight magnetic resonance angiography. *Taiwanese Journal of Obstetrics & Gynecology, 55*(4), 585–587. https://doi.org/10.1016/j.tjog.2016.06.007

constriction of blood vessels in the XX pregnant patient and can lead to uteroplacental insufficiency, which is the failure of the placenta to deliver sufficient nutrients to the fetus, often as a result of insufficient blood flow to the placenta. Chronic uteroplacental insufficiency is correlated with IUGR and preterm labor (Jeyabalan, 2025). The type and severity of the hypertensive disorder (gestational diabetes, preeclampsia, eclampsia, or preeclampsia with chronic hypertension) will determine the impact on mother's health, placental function, and fetal well-being (Cunningham et al., 2022). Investigation into the role of genetic variables that might be involved with the phenotypic expression of preeclampsia is ongoing.

Infection can alter tissue in the fallopian tubes and cause an implantation error. Any condition resulting in villitis, chorioamnionitis, or uterine inflammation can alter normal placental function, impede delivery of blood to the fetus, and result in growth restriction and preterm labor (Goldstein et al., 2020). Neonatal infection can occur as a result of transmission of infectious agents, such as bacteria and viruses, via the placenta and is discussed in detail in the chapter on neonatal infection.

Overall, diabetes mellitus (DM) affects about 8% to 9% of pregnancies and includes gestational DM or pregestational DM (Osterman et al., 2024). The severity of DM can impact the integrity of the vasculature, disrupt normal placental blood flow, and alter normal fetal growth. In mothers with pregestational DM who have a preexisting impairment to renal, ophthalmologic, or cardiac vasculature, perfusion to the placenta can be impacted leading to poor placental function and FGR. The placenta is sensitive to hyperglycemia, leading to villus immaturity and necrosis, which are associated with developmental abnormalities of the placenta (Ehlers et al., 2021). The surface area of the villi, the diffusion distance between maternal and fetal circulation, and placental metabolic and endocrine functions are affected by both types of DM (Ehlers et al., 2021). The type of diabetes, timing of diagnosis, and control of blood glucose levels in the XX pregnant patient will determine the effect on the fetus (Cunningham et al., 2022; Ehlers et al., 2021). However, pregestational DM is also associated with major congenital abnormalities of fetal organ systems, as poor glucose control present prior to pregnancy impacts organogenesis early in pregnancy. Neonatal hypoglycemia is a common postnatal problem in infants born to mothers with pregestational and gestational DM and is associated with glucose control (increased amounts of glucose crosses the placenta) and resulting fetal hyperinsulinism as insulin does not cross the placenta to the fetus. The degree of fetal hyperinsulinemia in response to poorly controlled glucose levels in the XX pregnant patient can lead to fetal macrosomia, as insulin is a growth factor. Macrosomia can lead to birth trauma during delivery and/or the need for cesarean delivery.

EFFECTS OF PLACENTAL FUNCTION ON DEVELOPMENT OF ADULT DISEASE

As the intrauterine environment should be a period of cell differentiation, organogenesis, and accelerated growth, alterations in placental development and function play a role in "fetal programming," including the development of chronic diseases in the adult. Fetal programming, or fetal adaptation to nutrient alteration across the placenta, occurs when a stimulus evokes an adaptive response in cell structure, tissue perfusion pattern, organ function, or metabolism in the fetus in an effort to minimize short-term deleterious outcomes; this may predispose the infant to the development of chronic disease in adult life (Simmons, 2024). Placental size is one factor that influences the overall efficiency of nutrient delivery to the fetus and there is evidence to support that infants whose placentas were either smaller or larger than normal are at increased risk for adult-onset diseases. In the fetus with reduced nutrient availability, whether due to poor nutrition or placental insufficiency, there is impaired nutrient and oxygen delivery which the fetus routes to systems necessary for survival. Poor nutrition in the XX pregnant patient impacts fetal growth due to deficiency in available nutrients for placental transfer.

In the fetus with IUGR resulting from placental insufficiency, there is a higher incidence of neurodevelopmental issues as well as increased rates of cardiovascular disease, obesity, and impairments in glucose metabolism. However, the studies that demonstrated these results were cohort studies which did not control for factors known to have an impact on epigenetics (Simmons, 2024). The mechanisms involved in this relationship continue to be investigated. However, at this time, the impact of fetal programming and gene expression on disease development is an area of rapid discovery and the APRN should continue to review the literature to ensure current management and anticipatory guidance for patients and families.

Anxiety and stress increase the level of circulating glucocorticoids. Glucocorticoids pass readily through the placenta and affect the regulation of nutrient delivery and subsequent growth in the fetus at many levels, including cell number and differentiation, organ structure, gene expression, and vascular response (McGowan & Matthews, 2018). High levels of stress in the XX pregnant patient, regardless of cause, have been linked to neurodevelopmental disorders, including increased risk for mental health disorders in childhood and adulthood (McGowan & Matthews, 2018).

CONCLUSION

A basic understanding of placental structure, development, and function provides the foundation for understanding the role of the placenta in normal fetal development. Examination of the placenta after birth may provide information on the etiology of abnormal fetal development and neonatal disease, though increased study is ongoing into gestational placental evaluation and early intervention. Assisted reproductive technology has improved due to an understanding of the blastocyst, leading to implantation techniques that limit the incidence of multiple embryos. Continued investigation into the impact of disease on abnormal placental development and function may lead to early therapeutic interventions that attenuate or eliminate placental abnormalities and ensure normal fetal development.

LEARNING TOOLS AND RESOURCES

CourseConnect

To access self-assessment questions and interactive, competency-based learning activities for this chapter, visit www.springerpub.com/courseconnect. See inside front cover and tear-out card for CourseConnect details.

Podcast

This podcast is available online by visiting www.springerpub.com/courseconnect. See inside front cover and tear-out card for CourseConnect details.

Transplacental Gas Transfer
Mark Kadrofske

Discussion Prompts

1. Describe how the exchange of nutrients and waste products occurs when there is no direct communication between the maternal and fetal vasculature.
2. Describe how the maternal–fetal environment facilitates gas exchange at the membrane level.
3. Identify three maternal factors that may be associated with implantation errors or placental insufficiency.
4. Discuss three transport mechanisms involved in the transfer of nutrients across the placenta.

MIND MAP

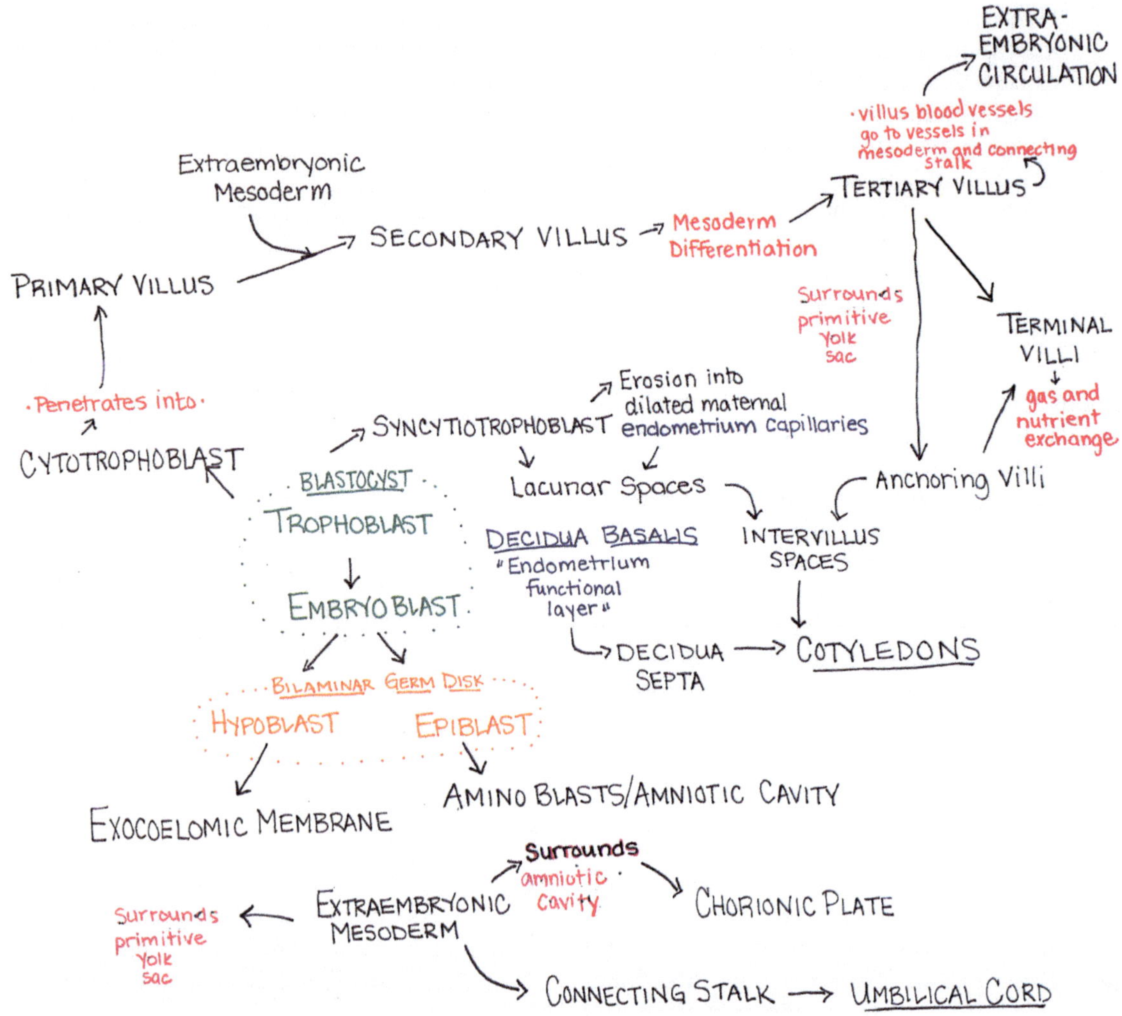

Note: *Readers should regard the mind maps woven throughout this textbook as examples of multisensory study tools that can be developed to encourage conceptual understanding. Readers are encouraged to develop their own unique mind maps in consultation with academic faculty or clinical preceptors.*

Image Credit: Leanne Nantais-Smith, PhD, RN, NNP-BC; Carolyn Herrington, PhD, RN, NNP-BC, CLC; and Mark Kadrofske, MD, PhD, FAAP.

REFERENCES

Ali, N., & Sawyer, T. (2024). Perinatal transition and newborn resuscitation. In C. A. Gleason & T. Sawyer (Eds.), *Avery's diseases of the newborn* (11th ed., pp. 159–171). Elsevier.

Bamberg, C., & Hecher, K. (2022). Twin-to-twin transfusion syndrome: Controversies in the diagnosis and management. *Best Practice & Research Clinical Obstetrics & Gynaecology, 84*, 143–154. https://doi.org/10.1016/j.bpobgyn.2022.03.013

Burton, G. J., Cindrova-Davies, T., Yung, H. W., & Jauniaux, E. (2021). Oxygen and development of the human placenta. *Reproduction, 161*, F53–F65. https://doi.org/10.1530/REP-20-0153

Cindrova-Davies, T., & Sferruzzi-Perri, A. N. (2022). Human placental development and function. *Seminars in Cell & Developmental Biology, 131*, 66–77. https://doi.org/10.1016/j.semcdb.2022.03.039

Clemente, E. J., Navarro, O. M., Irujo, M. N., Ladera, E., Columbo, C., Suñol, M., Sousa, P., & Martinez de la Torre, I. B. (2021). Omplahlomesenteric duct anomalies in children: A multimodality overview. *Radiographics, 41*(7), 1897–2192. https://doi.org/10.1148/rg.2021210048

Cooke, L. D. F., Tumbarello, D. A., Harvey, N. C., Sethi, J. K., Lewis, R. M., & Cleal, J. K. (2021). Endocytosis in the placenta: An undervalued mediator of placental transfer. *Placenta, 113*, 67–73. https://doi.org/10.1016/j.placenta.2021.04.014

Cunningham, F. G., Leveno, K. J., Dashe, J. S., Hoffman, B. L., Spong, C. Y., & Casey, B. M. (Eds.). (2022). *Williams obstetrics* (26th ed.). McGraw-Hill.

Ehlers, E., Talton, O. O., Schust, D. J., & Schulz, L. C. (2021). Placental structural abnormalities in gestational diabetes and when they develop: A scoping review. *Placenta, 116*, 58–66. https://doi.org/10.1016/j.placenta.2021.04.005

Fay, E., Simmons, L., & Brown, C. (2024). Maternal diabetes. In C. A. Gleason & T. Sawyer (Eds.), *Avery's diseases of the newborn* (11th ed., pp. 67–81). Elsevier.

Gerson, K. D., Modest, A. M., Hecht, J. L., & Young, B. C. (2019). Persistent amnion-chorion membrane separation. *Journal of Obstetrics and Gynaecology, 45*(2), 352–357. https://doi.org/10.1111/jog.13852

Goldstein, J. A., Gallagher, K., Beck, C., Kumar, R., & Gernand, A. D. (2020). Maternal-fetal inflammation in the placenta and the developmental origins of health and disease. *Frontiers in Immunology, 11*, 531–543. https://doi.org/10.3389/fimmu.2020.531543

Hirschmugl, B., Perazzolo, S., Sengers, B. G., Lewis, R. M., Gruber, M., Desoye, G., & Wadsack, C. (2021). Placental mobilization of free fatty acids contributes to altered materno-fetal transfer in obesity. *International Journal of Obesity (2005), 45*(5), 1114–1123. https://doi.org/10.1038/s41366-021-00781-x

Hufnagel, A., Grant, I. D., & Aiken, C. E. M. (2022). Glucose and oxygen in the early intrauterine environment and their role in developmental abnormalities. *Seminars in Cell and Developmental Biology, 131*, 25–34. https://doi.org/10.1016/j.semcdb.2022.03.041

Jeyabalan, A. (2025). Hypertensive disorders of pregnancy. In R. J. Martin & A. A. Fanaroff (Eds.), *Fanaroff and Martin's neonatal-perinatal medicine: Diseases of the fetus and infant* (12th ed., pp. 1068–1119). Elsevier.

Lazebnik, N., Ozcan, T., & Lazebnik, R. S. (2025). Perinatal ultrasound. In R. J. Martin & A. A. Fanaroff (Eds.), *Fanaroff and Martin's neonatal-perinatal medicine: Diseases of the fetus and infant* (12th ed., pp. 664–819). Elsevier.

McGowan, P. O., & Matthews, S. G. (2018). Prenatal stress, glucocorticoids, and developmental programming of the stress response. *Endocrinology, 159*(1), 69–82. https://doi.org/10.1210/en.2017-00896

McNanley, T., & Woods, J. (2008). Placental physiology. *Global Library of Women's Medicine, 10*(4). https://doi.org/10.3843/GLOWM.10195

Moar, L., Simela, C., Nanda, S., Marnerides, A., Al-Adnani, M., Nelson-Piercy, C., Nicolaides, K. H., & Shangaris, P. (2022). Chronic histiocytic intervillositis (CHI): Current treatments and perinatal outcomes, a systematic review and meta-analysis. *Frontiers in Endocrinology, 13*, 1–17. https://doi.org/10.3389/fendo.2022.945543

Moser, G., Windsperger, K., Pollheimer, J., Chuva de Sousa Lopes, S., & Huppertz, B. (2018). Human trophoblast invasion: New and unexpected routes and functions. *Histochemistry and Cell Biology, 150*, 361–370. https://doi.org/10.1007/s00418-018-1699-0

Osterman, M. J. K., Hamilton, B. E., Martin, J. A., Driscoll, A. K., & Valenzuela, C. P. (2024). Births: Final data for 2022. *National Vital Statistics Report, 73*(2), 1–56. https://www.cdc.gov/nchs/products/index.htm

Park, J. Y., Mani, S., Clair, G., Olson, H. M., Paurus, V. L., Ansong, C. K., Blundell, C., Young, R., Kanter, J., Gordon, S., Yi, A. Y., Mainigi, M., & Huh, D. D. (2022). A microphysiological model of human trophoblast invasion during implantation. *Nature Communications, 13*, 1252. https://doi.org/10.1038/s41467-022-28663-4

Ryan, B. A., & Kovacs, C. S. (2020). Calciotropic and phosphotropic hormones in fetal and neonatal bone development. *Seminars in Fetal and Neonatal Medicine, 25*(1), 1–8. https://doi.org/10.1016/j.siny.2019.101062

Sadler, T. W. (2024). *Langman's medical embryology* (15th ed.). Lipincott Williams & Wilkins.

Schoenwolf, G. C., Bleyl, S. B., Brauer, P. R., & Francis-West, P. H. (2021). *Larsen's human embryology* (6th ed.). Churchill Livingstone.

Simmons, R. A. (2024). Abnormalities of fetal growth. In C. A. Gleason & T. Sawyer (Eds.), *Avery's diseases of the newborn* (11th ed., pp. 33–41). Elsevier.

Staff, A. C., Fjeldstad, H. E., Fosheim, I. K., Turowski, G., Johnsen, G. M., Alnaes-Katjavivi, P., & Sugulle, M. (2022). Failure of physiological transformation and spiral artery atherosis: Their roles in preeclampsia. *American Journal of Obstetrics & Gynecology, 226*(Suppl 2), S895–S906. https://doi.org/10.1016/j.ajog.2020.09.026

Tabatabaei, R. S., Fatahi-Meibodi, N., Meibodi, B., Javaheri, A., Abbasi, H., Hadadan, A., Bahrami, R., Mirjalili, S. R., Karimi-Zarchi, M., & Neamatzadeh, H. (2022). Association of fetal MTHFR C677T polymorphism with susceptibility to neural tube defects: A systematic review and updated meta-analysis. *Fetal and Pediatric Pathology, 41*(2), 225–241. https://doi.org/10.1080/15513815.2020.1775734

Taylor, K. H., Simmons, P. M., & Magann, E. F. (2025). Amniotic fluid volume. In R. J. Martin & A. A. Fanaroff, *Fanaroff and Martin's neonatal-perinatal medicine: Diseases of the fetus and infant* (12th ed., pp. 1412–1479). Elsevier.

Torchia, M. G., & Persaud, T. V. N. (2025). *Before we are born: Essentials of embryology and birth defects* (11th ed.). Elsevier.

Turco, M. Y., & Moffett, A. (2019). Development of the human placenta. *Development (Cambridge, England), 146*(22), dev163428. https://doi.org/10.1242/dev.163428

U.S. Food and Drug Administration. (2014). *Content and format of labeling for human prescription drug and biological products; requirements for pregnancy and lactation labeling*. 21 CFR 201. https://www.federalregister.gov/documents/2014/12/04/2014-28241/content-and-format-of-labeling-for-human-prescription-drug-and-biological-products-requirements-for

Van Mieghem, T., Abbasi, N., Shinar, S., Keunen, J., Seaward, G., Windrim, R., & Ryan, G. (2022). Monochorionic monoamniotic twin pregnancies. *American Journal of Obstetrics & Gynecology Maternal Fetal Medicine, 4*(2), 1–6. https://doi.org/10.1016/j.ajogmf.2021.100520

Zhu, Y., Wu, T., Ye, L., Li, G., Zeng, Y., & Zhang, Y. (2018). Prevalent genotypes of methylenetetrahydrofolate reductase (MTHFR) in recurrent miscarriage and recurrent implantation failure. *Journal of Assisted Reproduction and Genetics, 35*, 1437–1442. https://doi.org/10.1007/s10815-018-1205-6

II

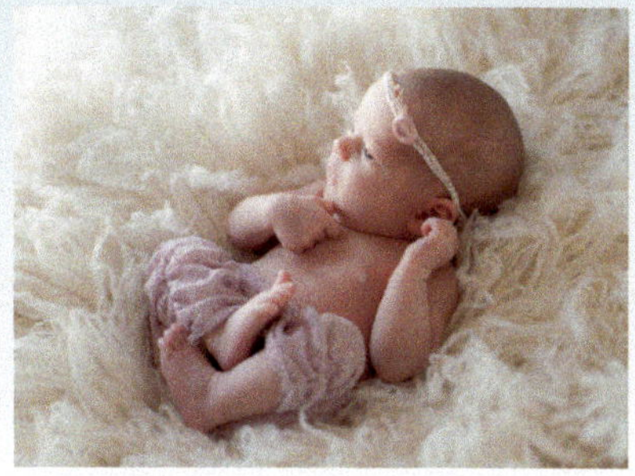

FETAL AND NEONATAL PHYSIOLOGY BY BODY SYSTEM

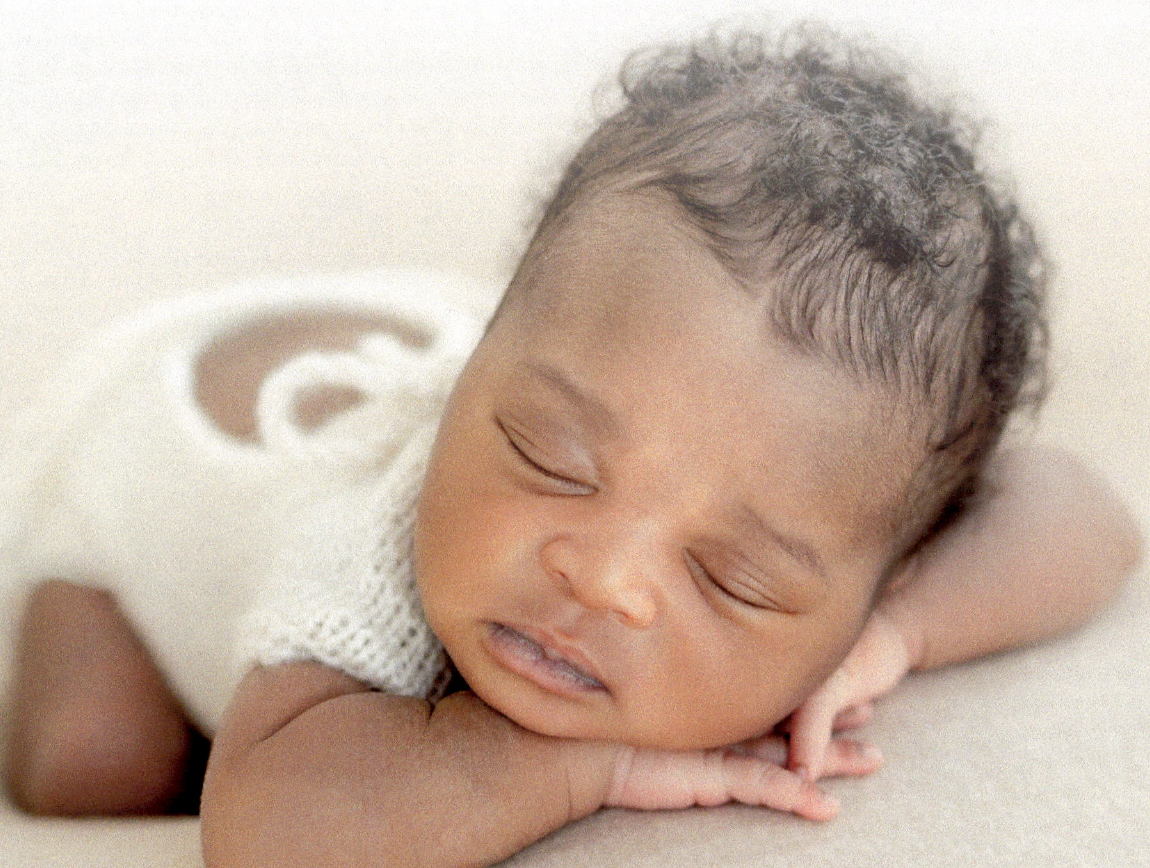

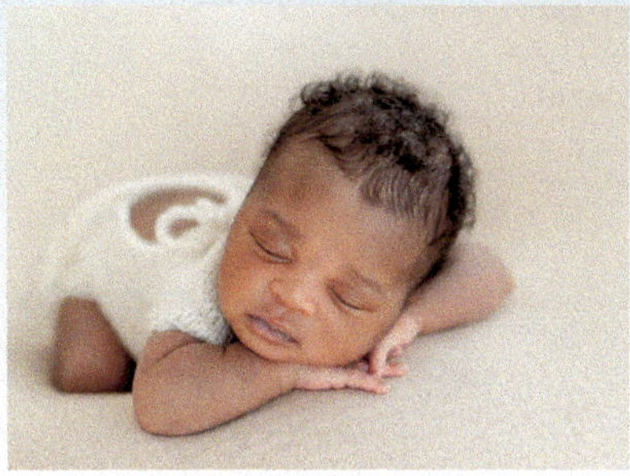

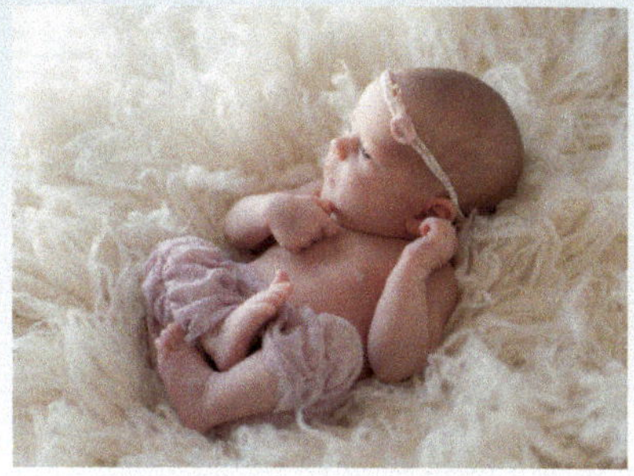

3

THE NERVOUS SYSTEM

Colleen R. Moss, Amy Williford, and Amy J. Jnah

LEARNING OBJECTIVES

After completing this chapter, the reader should be able to:

- Understand normal nervous system development.
- Analyze the physiologic function of the fetal and neonatal nervous system.
- Identify the impact of noxious stimuli on the developing brain.
- Discuss common inherited disorders and their effect on fetal and neonatal nervous system development and function.
- Identify health issues in the XX pregnant patient that have a potential impact on fetal and postnatal nervous system development and function.
- Evaluate common disorders that affect the nervous system and their implications across the life span.

INTRODUCTION

The greater nervous system is comprised of the central nervous system (CNS), peripheral nervous system (PNS), and the somatic and autonomic nervous systems (SNS and ANS, respectively; **Figure 3.1**). It is one of the most complex systems in the human body and communicates with other body systems to maintain physiologic homeostasis. A critical portion of the CNS is the human brain, a fragile and complicated organ with postnatal function dependent on normal embryologic and fetal development. Likewise, alterations in embryologic development, which may occur secondary to environmental factors, genetic factors, or diseases in the XX pregnant patient, can lead to the development of structural or functional pathologies affecting the spinal cord, motor neurons, or sensory neurons and impose lifelong neurologic consequences. We begin this chapter with a review of key milestones in normal CNS development and functional organization and progress to an exploration of inherited disorders and diseases in the XX pregnant patient that can affect nervous system function, and common congenital and acquired disorders that can affect the nervous system.

TIMELINE OF ORGAN DEVELOPMENT

Fetal neurologic development is dependent on a series of activities and progressions in specified sequencing. This process begins during week 3 of gestation, with the production of neurons. Numerous developmental processes follow and include gastrulation, neurulation, differentiation, proliferation and migration, organization, programmed cell death, synaptogenesis, and myelination. Some processes continue through childhood and even into late adolescence, with differentiation continuing across the life span. A summary of major developmental milestones and the time frame when development occurs is offered in **Table 3.1**.

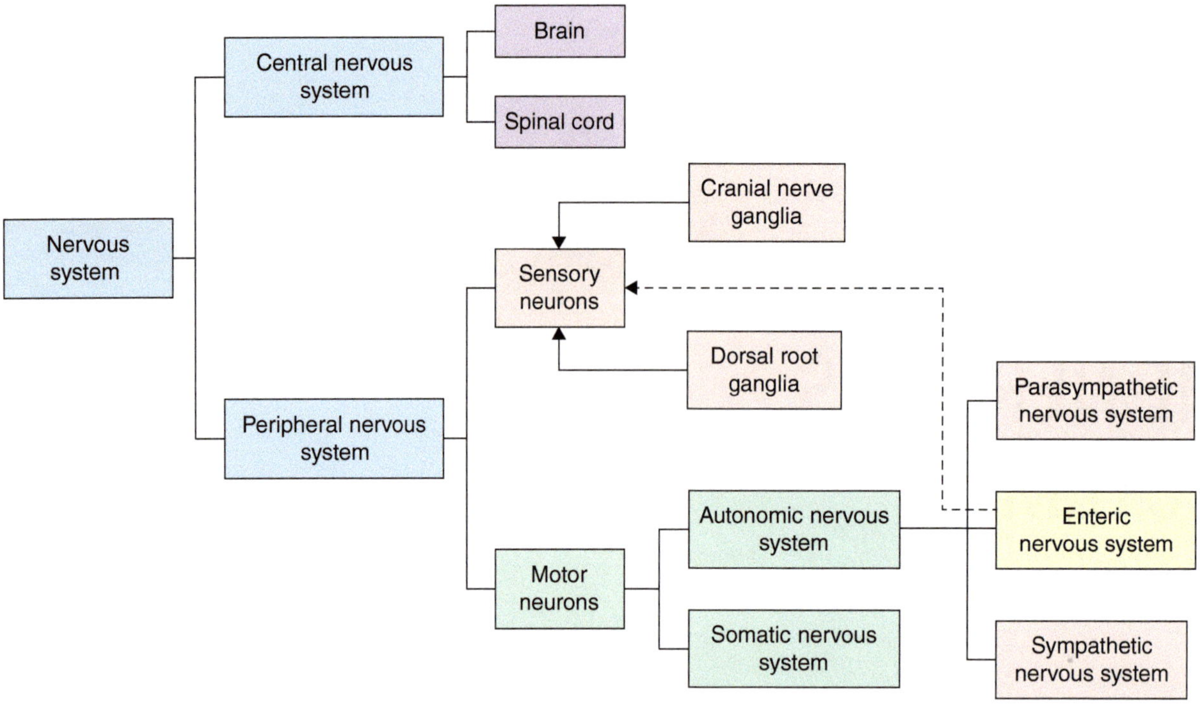

Figure 3.1 The nervous system.

TABLE 3.1 Major Developmental Milestones for the Developing Nervous System

Period of Neurologic Development	Peak Time Frame for Development (Weeks of Gestation)
Primary neurulation	3–4
Prosencephalic differentiation	8–12
Neuronal proliferation	12–16
Neuronal migration	12–20
Organization	20 to early childhood
Programmed cell death	28–41
Synaptogenesis	20 to early adolescence
Myelination	29–42[a]

[a]Myelination begins at the brainstem around 29 weeks and peaks at various time frames based upon the region of the brain that is developing, eventually reaching the centrum semiovale (base of the cerebral cortex) at 42 weeks.

Sources: Torchia, M. G., & Persaud, T. V. N. (2025). *The developing human: Clinically oriented embryology* (12th ed.). Elsevier; Volpe, J. J. (2025). *Volpe's neurology of the newborn* (7th ed.). Elsevier.

The Embryonic Period: Early Brain Development

Primary Neurulation. Primitive neurulation begins around day 18 of gestation and peaks between weeks 3 and 4 of gestation (Torchia & Persaud, 2025). This process involves cellular and structural differentiation, resulting in the formation of the neural plate and neural groove and, ultimately, the formation of the neural tube (**Figures 3.2** and **3.3**). The neural tube will then go on to differentiate into the brain and spinal cord.

Neurulation involves a four-step process: (a) formation of the neural plate; (b) morphogenic molding of the neural plate; (c) the formation of a groove within the neural plate; and (d) closure of the ends of the neural plate into a sealed neural tube. This process begins during the latter end of week 3 of gestation (days 18–22) with formation of the neural plate (Gressens & Hüppi, 2025). Next, two ridges flanked by neural progenitor cells form on either side of the neural plate (du Plessis & Volpe, 2025a). These ridges rise upward and begin to fold inward on themselves, forming a groove within the neural plate. The ridges continue to rise upward and toward one another, turning the neural plate into a tube-like structure. Finally, by day 22 of gestation, the ridges begin to fuse together (du Plessis & Volpe, 2025a). Fusion proceeds rostrally to form the anterior portion of the neural tube (the future brain) and then posteriorly. During this time frame, the three distinct pouches (primitive vessels)

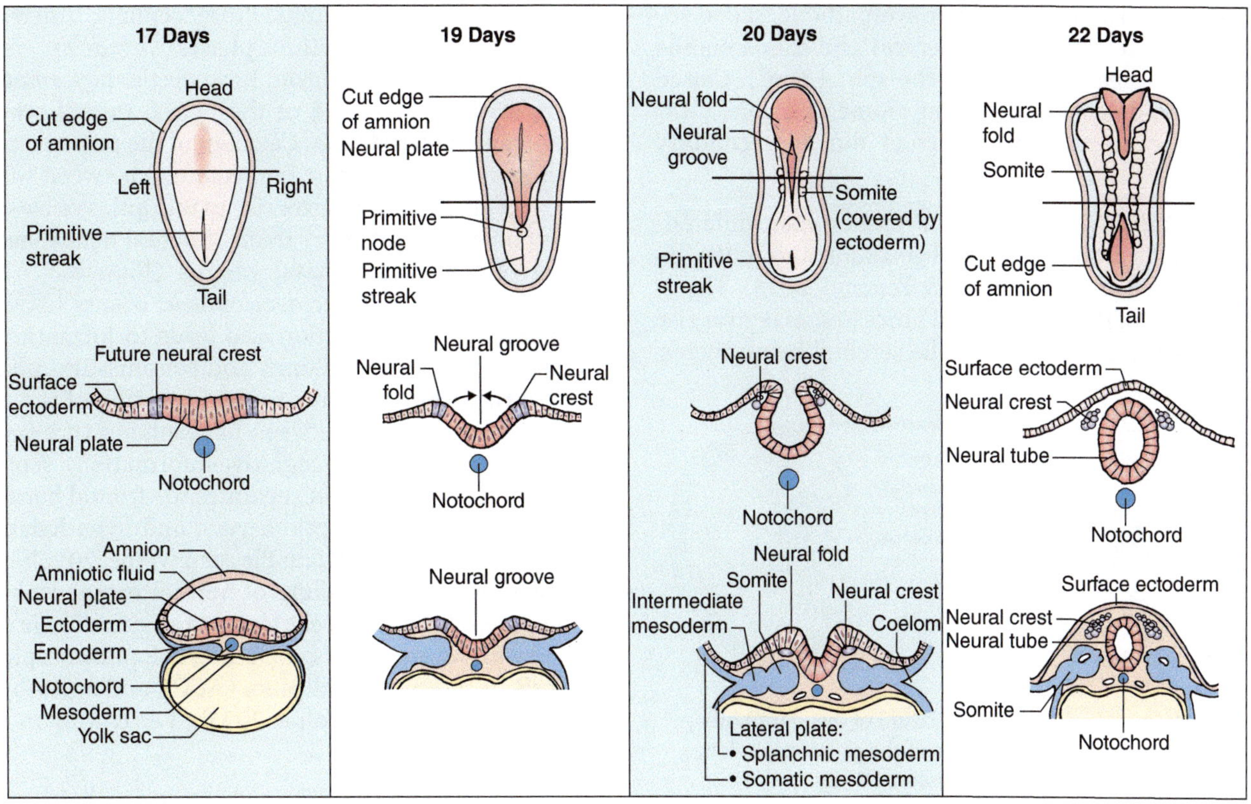

Figure 3.2 Neurulation.

appear. The first and most anterior of these pouches is the *prosencephalon*, which gives rise to the forebrain. Next is the *mesencephalon*, which gives rise to the midbrain. The third pouch is the *rhombencephalon*, precursor to the hindbrain (Table 3.2 and Figure 3.4). Anterior neural tube fusion is considered, is completed within a 48-hour period, by 24 days of gestation (du Plessis & Volpe, 2025a). At nearly the same time, fusion begins to occur in a caudal direction to form the posterior portion of the neural tube (future spinal cord). Posterior fusion is complete by 26 days of gestation (du Plessis & Volpe, 2025a).

In its most primitive form, the neural tube closely resembles a drinking straw. However, it quickly undergoes additional morphologic changes. Neural progenitor cells reorganize and cover the interior walls of the hollowed out neural tube (Cizmeci & deVries, 2025; du Plessis & Volpe, 2025a; Torchia & Persaud, 2025). Next, the cells separate and form a neural crest. The neural crest undergoes a unique process of differentiation which gives rise to facial bones and structures, sensory neurons, and cells located in the pia mater (innermost layer of the meninges) and arachnoid mater (middle layer of the meninges which offers a web-like protective covering for the brain and spinal cord).

Given the extremely early time frame in which primary neurulation occurs, errors can give rise to serious (and sometimes fatal) birth defects. Common defects associated with failed primary neurulation include anencephaly, encephalocele, myelomeningocele seen with

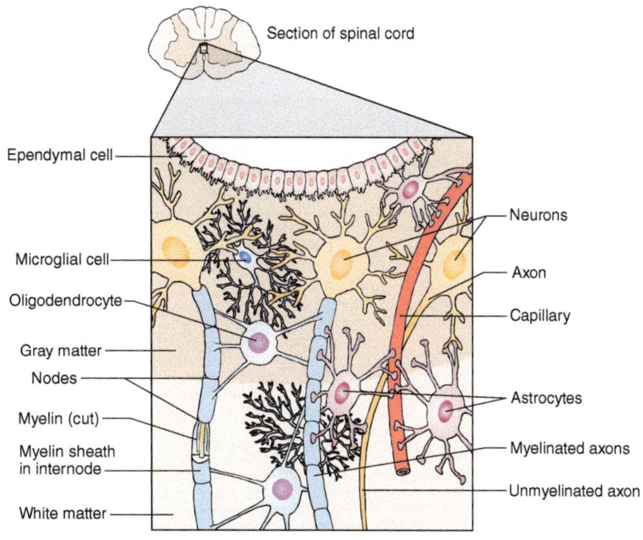

Figure 3.3 Glial cells hold nerve cells in place and assist with their function; examples include oligodendrocytes, astrocytes, microglia, and ependymal cells.

Chiari II malformation, and myeloschisis (du Plessis & Volpe, 2025a).

Secondary Neurulation. Secondary neurulation begins around day 26 of gestation and peaks during week 7 of gestation (du Plessis & Volpe, 2025a). This involves the formation of the caudal portion of the neural tube and structures including the conus medullaris (which gives rise to the lumbar sympathetic, sacral somatic, and parasympathetic nerves) and cauda equina (nerve roots near the base of the spinal cord). Closed neural tube defects (e.g., lipomyelomeningocele, tethered cord) can arise from errors during secondary neurulation.

Prosencephalic Differentiation. Prosencephalic differentiation begins around day 35 of gestation and peaks between weeks 8 and 12 (Torchia & Persaud, 2025). This is arguably one of the most critical processes, as it gives rise to major structures including the cerebral hemispheres, thalamus, and hypothalamus. Prosencephalic differentiation can be divided into three phases: *formation, cleavage,* and *midline development.* Prosencephalic *formation* occurs at the rostral end of the neural tube, between weeks 5 and 8 of gestation. *Cleavage* of the prosencephalon thereby begins (almost immediately) between weeks 5 and 6 of gestation and gives rise to the optic vesicles, olfactory bulbs and olfactory tracts, cerebral hemispheres, lateral ventricles, and basal ganglia (**Figure 3.5** and **Table 3.2**). Last, *midline development* occurs between weeks 8 and 12 of gestation and leads to formation of the chiasmatic, hypothalamic, and commissural plates. These structures contribute to the formation of the corpus callosum (conduit between hemispheres that transmits sensory, motor, and cognitive information), septum pellucidum (structure that separates the frontal horns of the lateral ventricles), optic nerves, and hypothalamus (Cizmeci & deVries, 2025; du Plessis & Volpe, 2025b; Lee & Mukundan, 2015). Failure of normal prosencephalic development between weeks 9 and 12 of gestation is correlated with severe defects, including holoprosencephaly, agenesis of the corpus callosum (ACC), and septo-optic dysplasia (du Plessis & Volpe, 2025b; Lee & Mukundan, 2015).

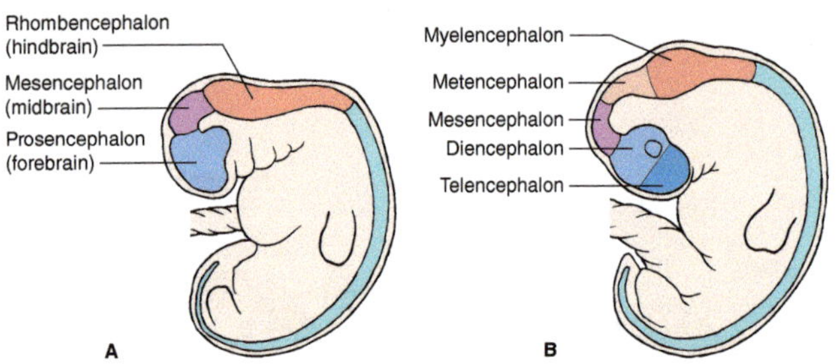

Figure 3.4 (**A**) Primitive differentiation of the neural tube, prior to fusion, includes the genesis of the prosencephalon, mesencephalon, and rhombencephalon. (**B**) By week 5 of gestation, the primitive neural tube begins a process of differentiation, which gives rise to five structures: telencephalon, diencephalon, mesencephalon, metencephalon, and myelencephalon.

Mesencephalic Differentiation. The mesencephalon gives rise to the midbrain, which is considered the communication center between the right and left hemispheres of the brain and is responsible for the integration of visual,

TABLE 3.2 Embryologic-to-Adult Brain Differentiation

Primary Structure	First Division	Second Division	Major Adult Structures & Vessels
Forebrain	Prosencephalon	Telencephalon	• Basal ganglia • Cerebrum • Lateral ventricles • Limbic system
		Diencephalon	• Hypothalamus • Thalamus • Third ventricle
Midbrain	Mesencephalon	Mesencephalon	• Cerebral aqueduct • Cerebral peduncles • Tectum • Tegmentum
Hindbrain	Rhombencephalon	Metencephalon	• Cerebellum • Fourth ventricle (upper portion) • Pons
		Myelencephalon	• Fourth ventricle (lower portion) • Medulla oblongata

Source: Fleiss, B., Stolp, H., Mezger, V., & Gressens, P. (2024). Central nervous system development. In C. A. Gleason & S. E. Juul (Eds.), *Avery's diseases of the newborn* (11th ed., pp. 781–786). Elsevier.

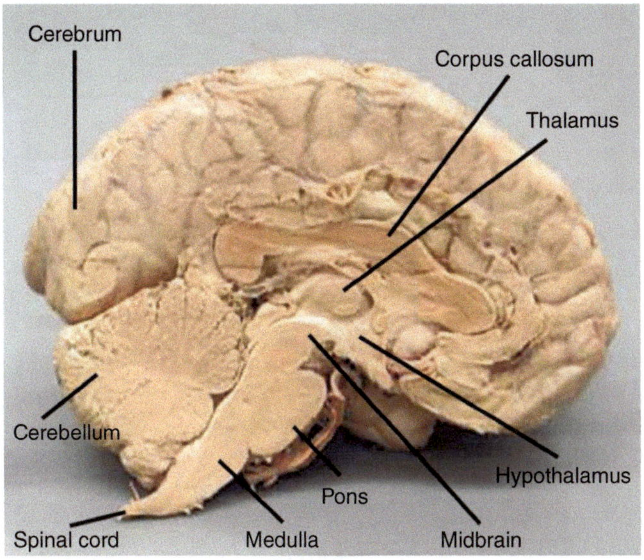

Figure 3.5 The limbic system.
Source: From Bryn Mawr College, 2017. Reprinted with permission.

auditory, and motor system information. Major midbrain structures that develop include the tectum, tegmentum, cerebral peduncles, and cerebral aqueduct, a channel that connects the third and fourth ventricles (du Plessis & Volpe, 2025b). Failure of normal mesencephalic development, which can be a consequence of prematurity or genetics, may result in aqueductal stenosis (narrowing of the cerebral aqueduct of Sylvius), hydrocephalus, or other obstructive disorders that impair the flow of cerebrospinal fluid (Patton et al., 2022; Torchia & Persaud, 2025).

Rhombencephalic Differentiation. The rhombencephalon gives rise to the hindbrain. Major hindbrain structures that develop include the pons, cerebellum, fourth ventricle, and medulla oblongata. Failed differentiation is associated with conditions including Dandy-Walker syndrome, a syndrome characterized by the following four major defects: (a) partial or complete cerebral agenesis, (b) cystic dilation of the fourth ventricle, (c) hydrocephalus, and (d) an enlarged posterior fossa (du Plessis & Volpe, 2025b; Torchia & Persaud, 2025; Yuskaitis & Pomeroy, 2022).

The Fetal Period: Major Milestones in Brain Development

The end of the embryonic period (week 8) and beginning of the fetal period (week 9) involves significant morphologic brain development. During week 8 of gestation, a longitudinal fissure arises within the prosencephalon and begins a process of subdividing the brain into two distinct and interconnected hemispheres. This fissure continues to proliferate and differentiate, until week 22 of gestation, when development is considered complete (Torchia & Persaud, 2025). As the fissure is developing, the circuitry inside the brain begins to emerge. This highly organized sequence of events includes the *proliferation* and *migration* of neurons, the *organization* of these neurons, and their encapsulation (*myelination*) by a myelin sheath.

Neuronal Proliferation. Neural progenitor cells situated just outside the lateral ventricles begin to divide (proliferate) toward the end of week 8 and peak between weeks 12 to 16 of gestation, producing neurons and radial glia. These newly synthesized neurons undergo *corticogenesis* and move outward toward the cortical region of the brain (outer layer of the brain), the "control center" of future behavior, thought, and intellectual capacity (D'Gama et al., 2025b; Torchia & Persaud, 2025). Radial glia are nonneuronal cells that assist with this migratory process and later differentiate into microglia and macroglia. Microglia function as primary immune defense cells in the CNS. Macroglia include astrocytes (funnel nutrients to neurons, repair nervous system tissues, regulate neuronal communications, and maintain the integrity of the blood-brain barrier [BBB]), oligodendrocytes (encapsulate neurons in the CNS with myelin), Schwann cells (encapsulate neurons in the PNS with myelin), and ependymal cells (located in the choroid plexus of lateral ventricles and produce cerebrospinal fluid as well as remove waste products). Glial proliferation continues after birth, as glia undergo a second phase of multiplication between 5 and 12 months of life (D'Gama et al., 2025b).

Clinical Application. Congenital viral infections (e.g., cytomegalovirus [CMV]) arising during the first trimester can disrupt normal neuronal proliferation. Aberrant proliferation is associated with fetal microcephaly.

Neuronal Migration. Neuronal migration to the cerebral cortex begins between weeks 8 and 9, and peaks between weeks 12 and 20 of gestation. Early migration involves radial and tangential movement of progenitor cells from the central ventricular zone and subventricular zones to specific locations in the CNS. Radial glia assist with early radial migration of neurons by providing the scaffolding for neurons to travel along. Radial migration in the cerebrum gives rise to the cerebral cortex and deep nuclear structures, including the basal ganglia, hypothalamus, thalamus, brainstem, cerebellum, and spinal cord (D'Gama et al., 2025a; Winn, 2017). Radial migration in the cerebellum gives rise to Purkinje cells and the dentate nucleus (regulator of voluntary movements). Tangential migration in the cerebellum gives rise to the inner portion of the cerebral cortex and in the cerebrum facilitates formation of the basal ganglia and gamma-aminobutyric acid (GABA) expressing neurons (D'Gama et al., 2025a; Q. Wu et al., 2014).

By week 20 of gestation, the cortex is fully affixed with excitatory and projection neurons, and by term the cortex has a full complement of GABA neurons (D'Gama et al., 2025a). At completion, a thin, 3- to 5-mm thick layer of approximately 85 to 100 billion neurons covers the cerebral cortex (J. E. Hall, 2020). These neurons serve an integral role in future postnatal processing of somatosensory stimuli (Brown et al., 2017; Rosenthal & Soto, 2016).

Clinical Application. Neuronal migration should provide the cortex with a substantial number of neurons, and this should prompt significant gains in cortical surface area. The rapid rate of cortical growth creates a state of compression, which somewhat forces the brain to create gyrations and sulcations. When neuronal migration fails, an inadequate complement of neurons reaches the cortical layers of the brain and gyri do not form. This is lissencephaly. Other disorders of migration include schizencephaly and ACC (normally found just below the cerebral cortex and above the thalamus).

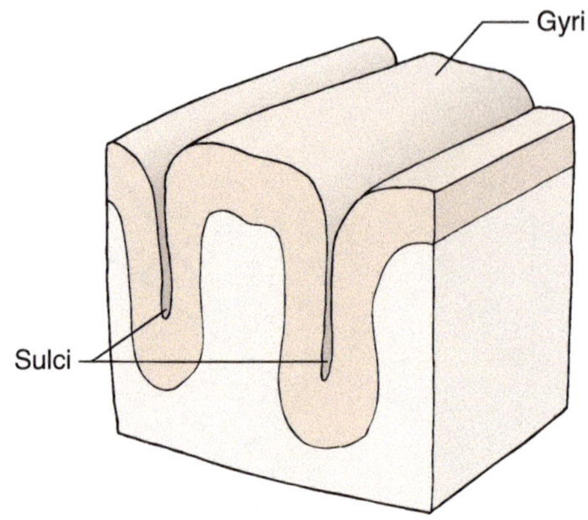

Figure 3.6 Gyri and sulci.

Clinical Application. Early cranial ultrasounds obtained in infants born less than 28 to 30 weeks of gestation demonstrate a relatively smooth brain surface. The smoothness of the brain is inversely proportional to gestational age; therefore, the *greatest period of gyrification occurs during the third trimester*. Under most circumstances, premature infants continue to develop gyri and sulci in the postnatal period, which can be seen on repeat cranial ultrasound at 36 to 40 weeks of gestation. Among infants born preterm, repeat cranial ultrasounds are often performed at term corrected gestational age to assess for periventricular leukomalacia (PVL). These images will also inform the extent of gyrations and sulcations present at this more mature gestational age.

Neuronal Organization. Peak timing for neuronal organization spans from week 20 to early childhood (Cizmeci & deVries, 2025). Events that occur during neuronal organization include (a) subplate neuron development and differentiation, (b) neuronal alignment and lamination, (c) the formation of neuronal synapses, (d) selective cell death and neuronal parsing, and (e) glial proliferation and differentiation (Haynes et al., 2025). Subplate neuron formation leads to the formation of neurons that contain important receptors for GABA, excitatory amino acids, neuropeptides, and growth factors, and the differentiation of grey and white brain matter (Haynes et al., 2025). Alignment describes the process of neurons becoming oriented and stacked on top of one another at the target locus. This results in a normal, evolving increase in cortical thickness, and by week 30 of gestation, the neocortex is impressively organized (Haynes et al., 2025).

Under normal circumstances (assuming migration was uninterrupted), cortical thickness increases during neuronal organization. This forces the brain tissue to begin a normal process of folding, which changes the landscape of the brain from smooth (lissencephalic) to an organ with elevations (gyri) and depressions (sulci; Figure 3.6). The process of creating gyrations and sulcations allows for significant gains in the volume of grey matter. The grey matter (which is actually gray-pink in color) is made up of dendrites, axon *terminals*, and other cell bodies. The expansion of the grey matter allows for more efficient electrical transmissions of information across the brain (Wandell, 2016).

Programmed Cell Death. Neuronal proliferation is an overzealous process resulting in the overproduction of neurons. The human brain mitigates this issue by eliciting a process of programmed cell death (apoptosis). Programmed cell death essentially prunes 10% to 50% of neurons and occurs between weeks 28 and 41 of gestation through the activation of genetic pathways and synthesis and secretion of proteolytic enzymes. These enzymes collapse and disassemble neurons, which leads to apoptosis and fragmentation of the nuclear DNA. Of note, apoptosis is a highly selective event that allows for targeted pruning, which averts damage to other nearby cells (Alberts, 2022; Cizmeci & deVries, 2025).

Although programmed cell death is an anticipated, normal physiologic process, it can be pathologically activated and exacerbated. For example, repetitious use of antenatal corticosteroids or antiepileptic drugs, or repetitive use of postnatal corticosteroids (e.g., dexamethasone to treat or prevent bronchopulmonary dysplasia) elicit pathophysiologic programmed neuronal cell death at the neocortex and basal ganglia (cortical grey matter). In fact, high-dose dexamethasone initiated within the first week of life is associated with an increased relative risk for acquired cognitive dysfunction and cerebral palsy, a key reason why this therapy is deferred for weeks after birth (Cizmeci & deVries, 2025).

Myelination. Myelination enables efficient transmission and communication of nerve impulses in both the CNS and PNS (Haynes et al., 2025). For myelination to occur, oligodendrocytes must have proliferated (beginning at around week 18 of gestation), migrated to target regions of the brain, differentiated, and matured. Assuming this occurs as described, myelin, a white, fatty substance composed primarily of lipids (80%) and water (20%), is synthesized during week 25 of gestation.

Beginning around week 29 of gestation, newly synthesized myelin proteins wrap around neuronal axon fibers (several times). This creates an insulating and all-encompassing protective sheath around the neurons (Haynes et al., 2025). Sensory neurons are first to become myelinated, and by term gestation, acoustic, vestibular, proprioceptive, and tactile neurons are covered in a myelin sheath. After the fetus or newborn reaches term gestation, myelination proceeds in the more peripheral regions within the hemispheres of the brain that are responsible for higher-level information processing and this continues all the way into adulthood (Torchia & Persaud, 2025).

Premature birth and certain diseases can interrupt normal oligodendrocyte development and function or interrupt normal axon function. Examples of diseases that can disrupt myelination include congenital viral infections (e.g., CMV), inborn errors of metabolism (e.g., amino and organic acidopathies), mitochondrial disorders, and PVL (Haynes et al., 2025). These diseases ultimately impede myelination and/or myelin production, which reduces white matter volume (detectable with MRI). In addition, neuromotor deficits are reported in infants who suffer hypoxia-related injury, secondary to abnormal myelin composition (Watzlawik et al., 2015).

Clinical Application. Human milk is the preferred form of enteral nutrition for premature infants. Human milk oligosaccharides (HMOs) are among the major constituents of human milk. Rajhans and colleagues (2023) report that HMOs positively influence postnatal myelination, motor function, cognition, language, and social-emotional well-being over the first 12 months of life.

Cerebrovascular Development

During week 3 of gestation, six paired aortic arches provide early blood supply to the developing brain. Shortly after, these primitive vessels undergo a series of modifications. The second pair of branch arteries fuse to form the pharyngeal artery (PA) and the third pair of primitive branch arteries fuse to form the internal carotid arteries (ICA). The ventral side of the PA and ICA fuse, giving rise to the common carotid artery (CCA) and the external carotid artery (ECA). The anterior end of the ICA differentiates into the anterior cerebral artery (ACA), middle cerebral artery (MCA), and the anterior choroidal artery (AChA). The posterior end of the ICA gives rise to the posterior cerebral artery (PCA) and posterior choroidal artery (PChA). These posterior vertebral arteries form the basilar artery, ultimately dividing to become two posterior cerebral arteries. The middle cerebral artery supplies the lateral surface of the cerebrum, the anterior artery supplies the midline of the cerebrum, and the posterior cerebral artery supplies the midtemporal region as well as a large portion of the brainstem. During week 8 of gestation, the left and right ACA join together and form the anterior communicating artery (ACOM), completing the circle of Willis. The circle of Willis provides a critical blood supply to the brain and eyes (Figure 3.7; Ruiz et al., 2021; Takakuwa et al., 2016).

Distal cerebral angiogenesis occurs concomitant with the development of the major structures of the brain. Arterial supply to the cerebrum, brainstem, and periventricular regions is established by week 24 of gestation. In the basal ganglia, diencephalon, and germinal matrix, arteriogenesis is complete by week 28 of gestation.

Vessels that form in the germinal matrix between 24 and 28 weeks of gestation are affixed with fewer structural support mechanisms (astrocyte end-feet and pericyte capillary coverage). It is evident that the timing of these developments places premature infants born at less than 28 weeks of gestation at increased risk for ischemic injury near the ventricles and within the white matter of the brain, as well as hemorrhage within the fragile germinal matrix (Brew et al., 2014; Fleiss et al., 2024).

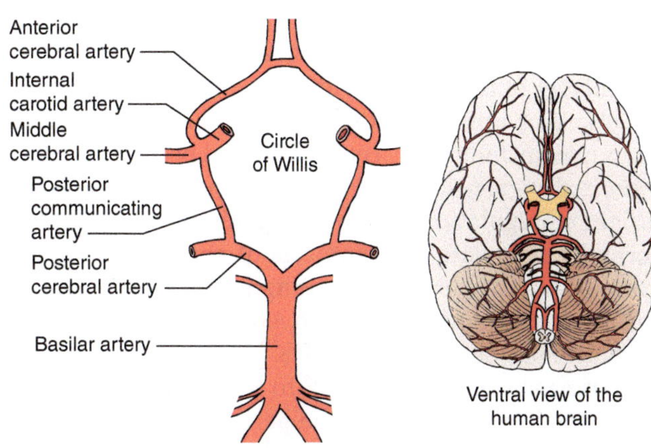

Figure 3.7 Circle of Willis.

DEVELOPMENTAL PHYSIOLOGY

Clearly, the nervous system is a complex network of vessels, structures, cells, and electrochemical impulses. The two major divisions of the nervous system are the PNS and CNS (brain and spinal cord), with the PNS further subdivided into the SNS, ANS, and enteric nervous system (ENS). These systems work collaboratively when activated by biochemical, electrical, or sensory inputs.

Principles of Cerebral Blood Flow and Autoregulation

Cerebral Blood Flow. The cerebral circulation consists of a complex network of intracranial and extracranial arteries and veins. Recall from basic anatomy coursework that all arteries have three layers: (a) an innermost endothelial layer; (b) a middle smooth muscle layer; and (c) an outer adventitia (fatty layer) comprised of collagen and nerve endings. Each layer uniquely influences vascular tone. The endothelial layer releases several mediators, including prostanoids (vasoconstrictor) and nitric oxide (vasodilator), to mediate the diameter of blood vessels (Brew et al., 2014; Takakuwa et al., 2016). The smooth muscle layer mediates vascular constriction and dilation by modulating intracellular calcium levels. For example, increased mechanical stretch or intraluminal pressure elicits an increase in intracellular calcium concentrations and resultant vasoconstriction. Perivascular nerves found in the adventitia can elicit both vascular constriction and vasodilation, whereas catecholamine release (e.g., epinephrine and norepinephrine) elicits only constriction (Brew et al., 2014; Takakuwa et al., 2016; Vutskits & Wolf, 2014).

Cerebral blood flow (CBF) can be affected by one or more of the following pathologies: (a) incomplete or dysregulaed angiogenesis, (b) diseases (e.g., asphyxia, sepsis) which affect cerebrovascular dynamics during birth, (c) poor vascular tone, or the (d) presence of cerebrovascular disorders including vein of Galen malformation, congenital heart diseases, and cerebral venous sinus thrombosis (Raybaud, 2010; Takakuwa et al., 2016). *Incomplete angiogenesis* may occur secondary to aplasia or hypoplasia of the ACOM, posterior communicating segment (P1), and posterior communicating artery (PCOM), or a merger of the right and left communicating arteries, vessels which normally supply blood and oxygen to major structures including the cerebellum and brainstem. *Dysregulated angiogenesis* may occur secondary to partial or variant upregulation of proangiogenic proteins, which normally stimulate the synthesis of new blood vessels from existing vessels, or following injuries that alter or obstruct blood flow, including hypoxia-ischemia and intraventricular hemorrhage (IVH).

A transient decrease in CBF to the cortical regions is understood to occur during the peripartum period, particularly among extremely low birthweight infants (lower gestational ages are associated with an increasingly lower cortical CBF nadir after birth). This is at least partially explained by the relative state of incomplete angiogenesis at birth, as this process is not fully complete until week 28 of gestation and vascular reactivity begins only a few weeks prior. This decrease in CBF can continue after birth when associated with a transient state of compensated shock; intrinsic neurohormonal responses are activated (e.g., adrenal activation) and blood flow is preferentially shunted to vital organs (heart, brainstem, adrenals). This preferential flow of blood to the heart helps maintain normal contractility and heart rate, thereby (at least temporarily) maintaining normal cardiac output while stroke volume and urinary output diminish after birth. These intrinsic compensatory mechanisms may produce a “normal” blood pressure reading after birth, but a normal systemic blood pressure does not always confer adequate CBF, especially to the cortical regions. Experts believe that the cortex is considered “nonvital” during the postnatal transition to extrauterine life and may experience a phase of vasoconstriction secondary to reduced cardiac output to these regions in the brain, including the periventricular white matter. Other disease states that can exacerbate abnormal CBF patterns after birth include perinatal asphyxia, acidosis, sepsis, microvascular dysfunction, cerebral edema, and hypercapnia or hypocapnia (Inder & Volpe, 2025; Sekhon et al., 2017).

Cerebrovascular Autoregulation. Cerebrovascular autoregulation is the mechanism which maintains homeostatic cerebral perfusion during changes in perfusion pressure. Healthy individuals experience physiologic oscillations (increases and decreases) in blood pressure, and an intact neurovascular autoregulatory system can recognize and modulate cerebral perfusion and avoid injury. This occurs with the assistance of autonomic, myogenic, and cellular mechanisms that are modulated by catecholamines, vasoactive peptides, nitric oxide, and the renin-angiotensin-aldosterone system. Among healthy individuals, when blood pressure oscillations (ebb and flow) occur, blood flow to the brain is autoregulated and the brain is protected from ischemia-reperfusion injuries.

Two conditions must be met for infants to autoregulate effectively: (a) *normal cerebral perfusion pressure (CPP)* and (b) *normal cerebrovascular reactivity* (resistance). CPP = mean arterial pressure (MAP) − intracranial pressure (ICP). MAP is influenced by gestational age and comorbid conditions and is calculated as $1/3 \times$ systolic blood pressure + $2/3 \times$ diastolic blood pressure. ICP remains low and stable under normal circumstances, so CPP is most dependent on MAP fluctuations. Thus, if MAP remains stable, so too will CPP. Cerebrovascular reactivity, or the ability of the cerebral blood vessels to react to changes in perfusion, is a more complex mechanism that only *begins* to develop during week 25 of gestation. This is a complex process that requires the help of metabolic response pathways, myogenic reflexes, and the sympathetic nervous system activity (Riera et al., 2014).

The metabolic hypothesis posits that either hypertensive states *or* reduced oxygen tension (a) activates a local reflex or (b) stimulates the release of adenosine and subsequent vasodilatory metabolites (nitric oxide and carbon monoxide) which are poorly developed in infancy (Austin, 2012; Brew et al., 2014). Myogenic (autonomic) responses are the primary autoregulatory response observed in preterm and term newborns. This involves changes in vascular wall tension. Vascular endothelial cells will elicit constriction and/or relaxation with the help of calcium-activated potassium channels to attenuate the effect of fluctuations in blood pressure. Last, activation of the sympathetic nervous system can modulate hypotensive states through the stimulation of perivascular nerves.

A basic, sigmoidal curve is used to visually depict the principles of cerebrovascular autoregulation. Essentially, use of this type of curve tells us that if blood pressure remains in the "stable" range (a rather ubiquitous term with the neonatal population), CBF will remain stable. Some experts posit that autoregulation can be maintained when the mean arterial blood pressure remains ~30 mmHg, but the gestational age range that coincides with this theory has yet to be agreed upon (Børch et al., 2010; Vesoulis & Mathur, 2017). If blood pressure falls below this threshold and the compensatory mechanisms discussed earlier in this section are insufficient, blood flow to areas of the brain, including the prefrontal cortex and white matter, can decrease and lead to ischemia. If the blood pressure subsequently increases significantly or rapidly, reperfusion injury or hemorrhage may occur next (particularly at the germinal matrices).

Not surprisingly, premature and critically ill term infants often exhibit neurovascular immaturity and ineffective autoregulation. In fact, experts believe that the autoregulatory range in preterm infants is far narrower than their term counterparts (Inder & Volpe, 2025). Furthermore, cortical blood vessels in extremely preterm infants are considered "nonvital." Therefore, during periods of compromised blood flow, the immature brain either cannot autoregulate CBF and it passively mimics arterial blood pressure (which can be significantly hypotensive), or blood flow is shifted away from the cortical vessels in an attempt to perfuse vital organs (Inder & Volpe, 2025). This is often a prolonged pathologic process in preterm infants and is associated with both cerebral hypoperfusion and overperfusion (Inder & Volpe, 2025). In other situations, autoregulation may be completely lost and the preterm brain becomes vulnerable to pressure passivity. These situations create conditions for ischemia-reperfusion brain injury.

Clinical Application. Continuous wave near-infrared spectroscopy (NIRS) is used to measure CBF and indirectly assess cerebral autoregulation. NIRS noninvasively measures the oxygen saturation of the brain using near-infrared light wavelengths, which can pass unskewed through skin, bones, and other tissues. Once the wavelength reaches hemoglobin, it can detect and quantify the difference between saturated and unsaturated hemoglobin molecules within the brain, in the same manner as pulse oximetry. When combined with transcutaneous carbon dioxide (TCOM) measurements, clinicians can assess for hypoxia and hypercarbia, both of which are strongly associated with altered cerebral autoregulation and pressure passivity.

The Sensory–Somatic System

Somatosensory function involves the receipt and neural processing of sensory information. Neurons within the cerebral cortex and other areas of the brain work collaboratively (in circuits) to transmit information received via afferent (input) pathways and respond via efferent (motor output) pathways. These pathways are either somatic or visceral and involve the cranial nerves. In addition, spinal nerves, which arise from the spinal cord, send sensory information via afferent pathways to the CNS for processing. Therefore, it is essential to digress briefly and recognize the spinal cord as a powerful modulator of somatosensory processing. We then discuss the cranial nerves and somatosensory response pathways.

The Spinal Cord and Nerves. Located in the vertebral canal, the spinal column extends from the brain to the lower portion of the first lumbar vertebrae and is supported and protected by the vertebral column. Brainstem–spinal cord sensory controls are postulated to be an influential feedback system for sensory processing as well as motor and autonomic function (Schwaller et al., 2017).

Recall that there are 31 pairs of spinal nerves connected to the spinal cord, numbered according to the vertebral column from which they emerge. Each spinal nerve (8 cervical, 12 thoracic, 5 lumbar, 5 sacral, and 1 coccygeal) innervates with skin, muscle, or bone. Therefore, the spinal nerves can be sensory, motor, or mixed. Each area of skin (dermatome), muscle, or bone typically innervates with only one spinal nerve (Figure 3.8; Ignatavicius et al., 2024; Vanderah & Gould, 2021).

Spinal nerves attach to the spinal cord by a ventral (anterior, motor) root and a dorsal (posterior, sensory) root. Once the nerves exit the intervertebral foramen, they branch out into several directions. This branching mechanism creates complex networks of interconnected nerves, which send electrochemical information to the CNS via afferent (input) pathways for processing and subsequent efferent (output) motor responses. For example, the *cervical plexus* is comprised

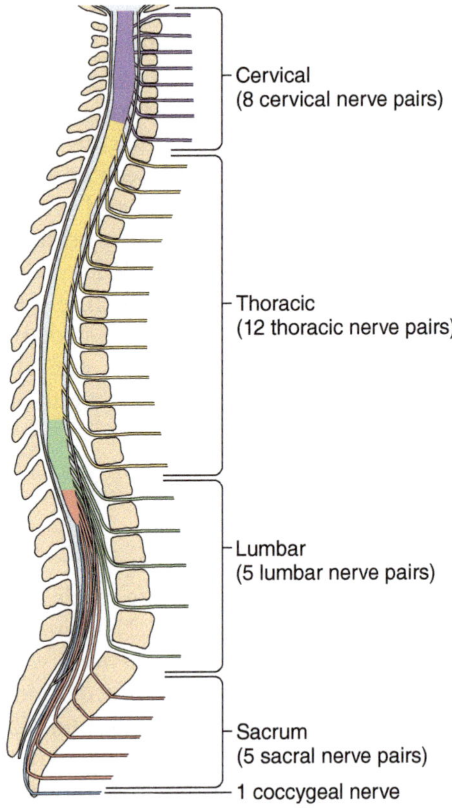

Figure 3.8 The spinal cord.

of a clustering of the anterior (motor) rami spinal nerves, C1 to C5. These nerves innervate the muscles of the neck, shoulders, and parts of the head (Patton et al., 2022). The *brachial plexus* is a clustering of anterior (motor) rami of the lower cervical nerves and first thoracic nerve, C5 to C8 and T1. This plexus innervates the shoulder and entire upper extremity (Schwaller et al., 2017; Vanderah & Gould, 2021).

For the developing fetus, any disruption in neural tube formation may negatively affect spinal cord development and spinal nerve function, causing later sensory processing dysfunction. For example, children with spina bifida often suffer urinary dysfunction, as the lowest spinal nerve modulates bowel and bladder control. Damage to the brachial plexus may be implicated in deliveries resulting in a shoulder dystocia (C5–C6 injury known as Erbs palsy; C8–T1 injury known as Klumpke palsy) and cause motor and respiratory dysfunction if injury to the phrenic nerve (C4) is involved (Ignatavicius et al., 2024; Patton et al., 2022; Vanderah & Gould, 2021).

The Cranial Nerves. No less important are the cranial nerves. These 12 nerves emerge from the brainstem through a small foramen in the cranial cavity (Figure 3.9). Typically, the cranial nerves are organized by their basic function or embryologic origin (Table 3.3). Most cranial nerves control a sensory or motor function. Similar to the spinal nerves, injury to any of the cranial nerves (CN V–VIII),

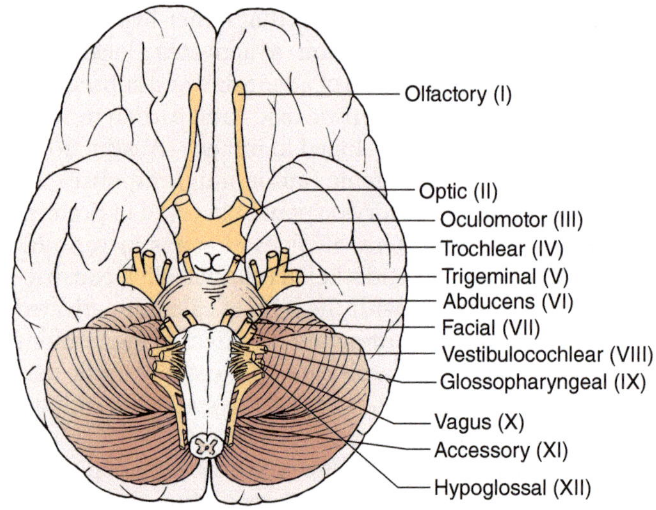

Figure 3.9 Anatomic location of the 12 cranial nerves.

as well as the first thoracic cranial nerve, may be associated with traumatic deliveries and shoulder dystocia.

Integrated Somatosensory Function: Input, Processing, and Response Systems

Sensory Inputting. Sensory inputs are external stimuli. In the presence of a sensory input, neurons direct electrochemical responses across axons to various areas of the cerebral neocortex and spinal cord for processing. For example, neurons in the spinal cord transmit information across afferent sensory axons secondary to sensory inputs from skin, muscle, or connective tissue receptors. Similarly, thalamic axons (axons residing on neurons located in the thalamus) transmit information about sensation, motor function, and internal physiologic state to the neocortex (Figure 3.10; Boron & Boulpaep, 2017).

Among premature and term infants, sensory inputs produce outputs primarily in the form of body movements (e.g., rooting, withdrawal from painful stimuli, startle reflex) and emotions to external stimuli (see Physiology of Pain). In children and adults, sensory inputs produce additional outputs, including awareness, cognition, and perception.

Sensory Processing. Sensory integration is an organizational process by which sensory neurons recognize sensory inputs and send appropriate responses across electrochemical circuits. This process involves identification, interpretation, modulation, and organization of stimuli.

Electrochemical Circuits. Electrochemical communications are critical for sensory processing. Communications primarily travel to and from (and within) the cerebrum. Recall that these communication pathways are established during neuronal migration and organization,

TABLE 3.3 Cranial Nerves

Number	Name	Innervation	Function	Associated Pathologies[a]
I	Olfactory	S	Olfaction	
II	Optic	S	Vision	Blindness
III	Oculomotor	M	Eye movement, pupillary constriction, and accommodation	Horner syndrome Infants with CN III palsy have a dilated, fixed pupil
IV	Trochlear	M	Eye movement	
V	Trigeminal	S, M	General sensation, mastication, tympanic membrane tension, rooting, sucking	Sturge Weber syndrome
VI	Abducens	M	Eye movement	Horner syndrome Mobius sequence
VII	Facial	S, M	Taste, facial movement, tension of ossicles, salivation, lacrimation	Asymmetric grimace and/or facial palsy following traumatic (or instrument-assisted) birth Differentiate from absence of depressor anguli oris muscle (DAOM) Mobius sequence
VIII	Vestibulocochlear	S	Hearing, proprioception, balance	Sensorineural hearing loss CHARGE syndrome
IX	Glossopharyngeal	S, M	General sensation, chemoreception/baroreception, taste, swallowing, salivation, gag reflex	CHARGE syndrome
X	Vagus	S, M	General sensation, chemoreception/ baroreception, visceral sensation, parasympathetic control of CVS, respiratory, and GI systems	Damage is manifested by hoarse cry, stridor, or aphonia CHARGE syndrome
XI	Accessory	M	Head and shoulder movement, sternocleidomastoid muscle function	
XII	Hypoglossal	M	Tongue movement	

[a]This list is not inclusive for all associated pathologies but highlights the most common pathologies.

CVS, cardiovascular system; GI, gastrointestinal; M, motor fiber innervation; S, sensory fiber innervation.

Sources: Lee, T. C., & Mukundan, S. (2015). Brainstem and cranial nerves. In T. C. Lee, S. Mukundan Jr., & F. H. Netter (Eds.), *Netter's correlative imaging: Neuroanatomy* (pp. 175–271). Elsevier Saunders; National Organization for Rare Disorders. (2023). *CHARGE syndrome.* https://rarediseases.org/rare-diseases/charge-syndrome

which spans the latter portion of fetal development into the postnatal period.

Once neurons migrate to their target areas of the brain, they must become functionally integrated. Functional integration (organization) involves morphologic change in the structure of the neuron. A single axon, the fibrous electrochemical signaling pathway, and hundreds of dendrites form at opposing ends of an individual neuron. With the help of a growth cone, the axon elongates (axonal outgrowth) makes contact with its target

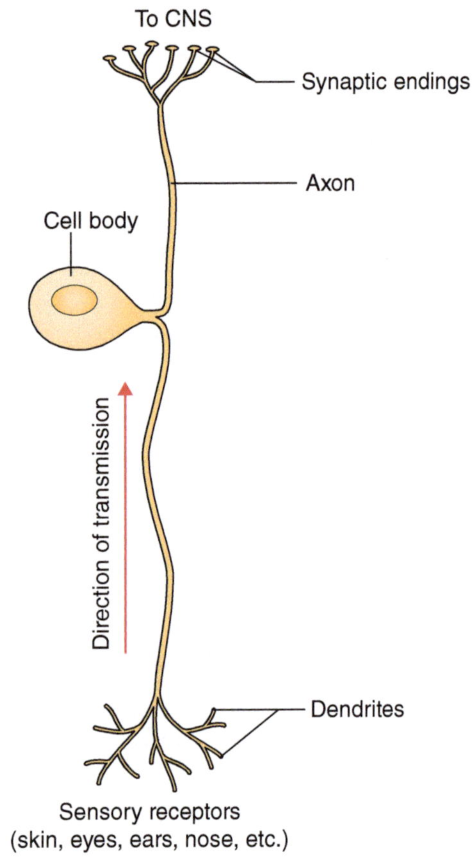

Figure 3.10 Sensory input transmission. CNS, central nervous system.
Image Credit: Mya Jnah.

cell, and creates a synapse. This establishes the electrochemical circuit, allowing transmission of information from the host neuron to the target cell. Dendrites (short, matrix-like pathways) extend off the neuron and receive electrochemical inputs from other neurons (**Figure 3.11**; D'Gama et al., 2025a; Rubenstein & Rakic, 2013).

These electrochemical communication tracts connect one part of the brain to another. Three types of communication tracts are known as *projection, association,* and *commissural tracts* (Patton et al., 2022). Projection tracts are part of the sensory spinothalamic and motor corticospinal tracts. The tracts extend vertically between higher and lower brain structures, transmitting information upward toward the cerebellum and cerebral cortex or downward toward motor neurons (**Figure 3.12**). Association tracts are axon fiber pathways connecting areas of the cerebrum, cerebral cortex, or gyri within the same hemisphere of the brain, linking memory and perception centers. Association tracts vary in length and shape, with some assuming a "U-shaped" appearance. Commissural tracts extend horizontally across hemispheres with many passing directly through the corpus callosum, a large mass of nerve fibers that integrates communication between the two cerebral hemispheres. Therefore, commissural tracts influence motor (e.g., hand–eye coordination), sensory, and cognitive function (Barbas, 2015; Patton et al., 2022).

Gestational age at birth (degree of prematurity), gender, and the education level of the XX pregnant patient are associated with reduced or sporadic sensory integration

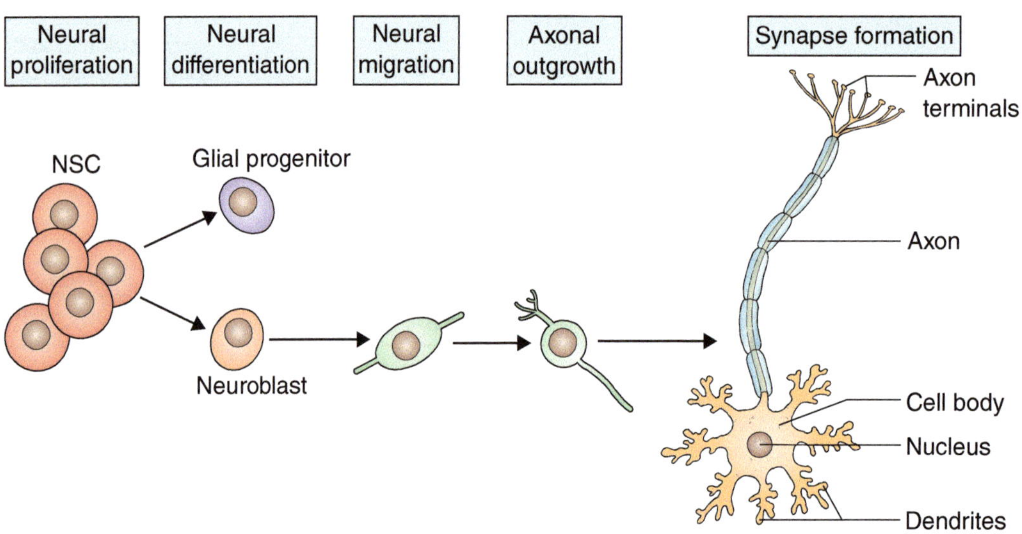

Figure 3.11 Genesis of the electrochemical communication pathway. NSC, neural stem cell.

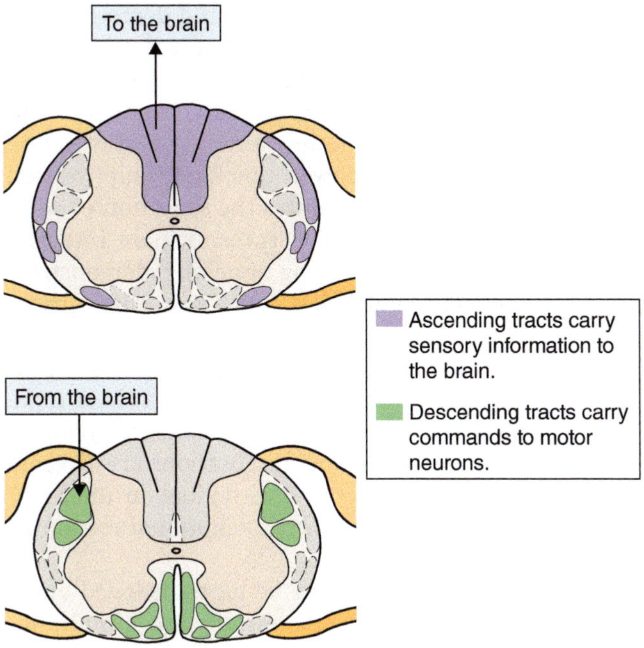

Figure 3.12 Projection electrochemical communication pathways.

(Pekçetin et al., 2016). This is attributed to the fact that sensory transmission pathways are present but immature by week 25 of gestation and progressively develop thereafter. More specifically, auditory, proprioceptive, and vestibular sensory hypoprocessing deficits are commonly reported among premature infants, with extremely low-birthweight (ELBW) infants at the highest risk for impairment (Pekçetin et al., 2016). As these pathways mature, additional sensory processing and higher order cognitive functioning emerge (Dumont et al., 2017). Disturbing the maturational aspect of sensory processing in the postnatal period, by way of sensory deprivation *or* sensory overload, can negatively impact the developmental physiology and later function of the somatosensory system. This is of great concern among infants born prematurely.

Motor Responses. Muscular maturation occurs in a caudocephalad direction and increases with advancing gestational age (Table 3.4). Motor responses are characterized as a physical response to a sensory stimulus. Motor responses regulated by the cerebral cortex (the frontal lobe specifically) by way of the motor cortex. Upper and lower motor neurons receive a sensory stimulus from sensory transmission pathways and translate the stimulus into a motor response. This creates a feedback system (feedback loop) which modulates muscle contractions, passive muscle tone, spinal control, and muscle stretch reflexes. The physiology of muscle contraction and relaxation will be discussed later in this chapter (see "Hypotonia").

TABLE 3.4 Timeline of Fetal Motor Development

Week of Gestation	Motor Function
7.5	Spontaneous flexion–extension of vertebral column and sideways bending
9	Spontaneous gross arm, leg, neck, and trunk movements (no patterning or sequencing)
10	Twitching movements
11	Harmonious leg movements
12	Hand-to-face movements Rotation of head and torso
13	Reciprocal and harmonious limb movements
14	Leg movements
15	Finger-sucking movements
16	Coordinated limb movements
24	Hand, face, respiratory movements

Note: Direction of motor function and tone follow a caudocephalad direction; onset of motor function and tone is approximate.
Sources: Piontelli, A. (2010). *Development of normal fetal movements: The first 25 weeks of gestation.* Springer Verlag; Torchia, M. G., & Persaud, T. V. N. (2025). *The developing human: Clinically oriented embryology* (12th ed.). Elsevier; van Merendonk, E. J. J. M., Brouwers, J. J. W. M., De Catte, L., Hasaerts, D., Nijhuis-van der Sanden, M. W. G., & Kerckhofs, E. (2017). Identification of prenatal behavioral patterns of the gross motor movements within the early stages of fetal development. *Infant and Child Development, 26*(5), e1–e15. https://doi.org/10.1002/icd.2012

Motor function responses to stimuli may be absent or immature among premature infants. In addition, infants who suffer hypoxia-related brain injury may display altered neurosensory and neuromotor responses to provocative events (Gulati et al., 2015).

Physiology of Pain

The human body contains an abundance of nerve endings commonly found in the eyes, gastrointestinal (GI) tract, connective tissues, and the skin. Most of these nerve endings are classified as *free nerve endings*, which are formed from sensory fibers in the skin. These free nerve endings (or cutaneous receptors) include mechanoreceptors, thermoreceptors, and nociceptive (pain) receptors. Nociceptors can be activated by mechanical stimulation (e.g., movement of an extremity, peristalsis), chemical stimulation (e.g., exposure to a noxious substance as with a peripheral intravenous catheter infiltration), cold, and heat. In other circumstances, nociceptors can remain dormant until activated by damage to surrounding tissues.

Free nerve endings, including nociceptors, first appear at the face during week 7 of gestation; the hands and feet by week 11; and the trunk, arms, and legs by week 15. It is understood that all components of pain processing are present by week 20 and they matriculate beyond the spinal horn and to the brain between weeks 22 to 24 of gestation. Maturation and development continue after birth and into infancy. Clearly, infants born at even the cusp of viability can experience pain. Furthermore, given that pain pathways continue to mature and develop after birth, postnatal illness can impair normal development and negatively alter an infant's perceptions and responses to pain (**Figure 3.13**; Ranger & Grunau, 2014).

Transmission of Pain. Nociceptors are stimulated when a noxious stimulus from the periphery (skin, viscera) activates free nerve endings. This creates action potentials that travel along one of several types of nociceptive nerve fibers (A-alpha, A-beta, A-delta, C-fibers) and toward to the spinal cord by way of *transduction*. Myelinated peripheral A-delta fibers sense acute pain (e.g., heel prick, sharp needle stick) and demonstrate a moderate conduction velocity (transmit the sensation quickly), yet are also *fast-adapting*. This means that the nerve endings demonstrate a burst-suppression tendency after the initial stimulus; a rapid burst of action potentials is released followed quickly by suppression of action potentials which mutes the sensation of pain. Unmyelinated C fibers, which transmit pain intensity as well as sensations of burning or aching, demonstrate slow and irregular conduction, and are *slow-adapting*; these nerve endings continuously fire action potentials, but at a much slower rate. This often leads to a prolonged or variable intensity of burning or aching pain. A-alpha and A-beta fibers sense touch, soft pressure, and even vibration. These touch sensations are directed to the spinothalamic tract and to regions in the brain like the amygdala, which control emotional responses (Tucker et al., 2023).

While action potentials are being transduced along afferent neurons, neurotransmitters are simultaneously (and endogenously) synthesized at the dorsal ganglion and dorsal horn. The neurotransmitters include glutamate (excitatory) and GABA (inhibitory), which can accentuate or mute the sensation of pain. In addition, endorphins and opioid peptides are synthesized to *modulate* the pain impulse. Opioids accomplish this by

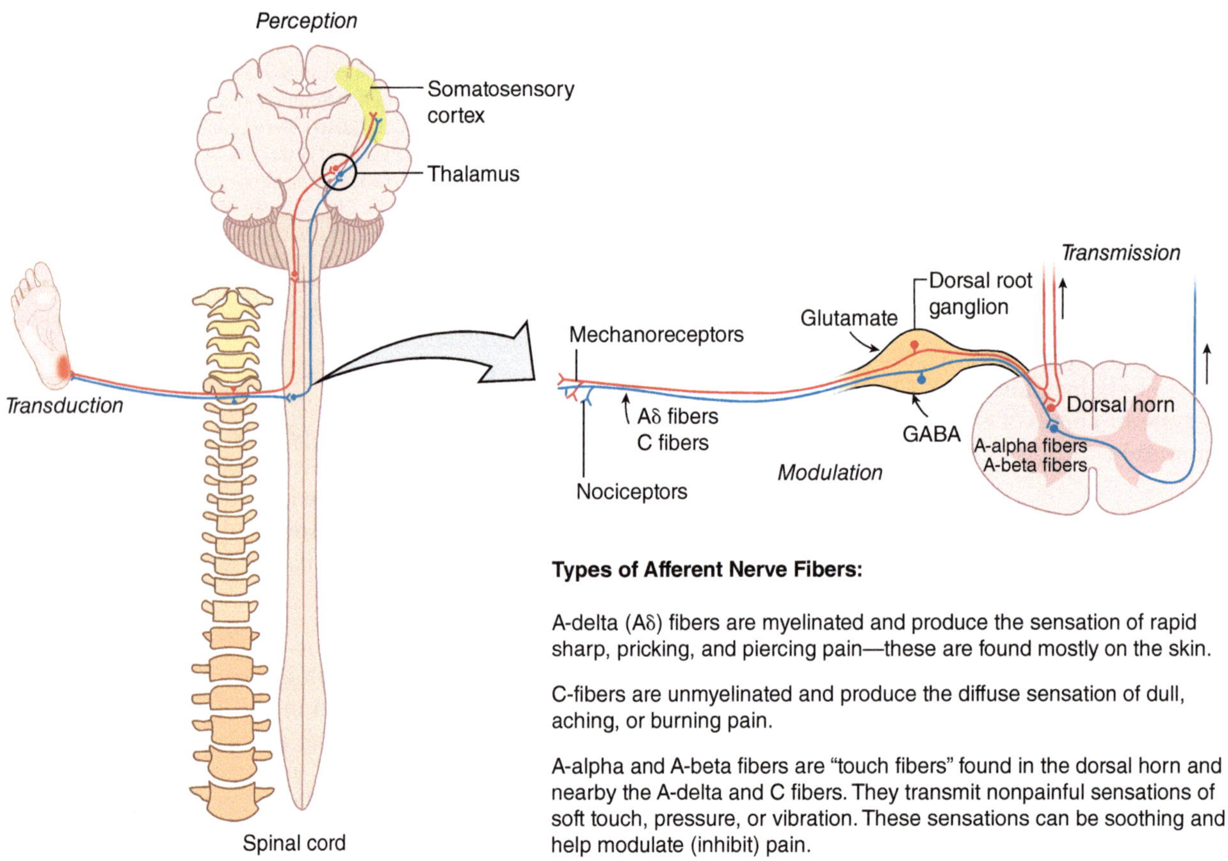

Types of Afferent Nerve Fibers:

A-delta (Aδ) fibers are myelinated and produce the sensation of rapid sharp, pricking, and piercing pain—these are found mostly on the skin.

C-fibers are unmyelinated and produce the diffuse sensation of dull, aching, or burning pain.

A-alpha and A-beta fibers are "touch fibers" found in the dorsal horn and nearby the A-delta and C fibers. They transmit nonpainful sensations of soft touch, pressure, or vibration. These sensations can be soothing and help modulate (inhibit) pain.

Figure 3.13 The pain pathway.
GABA, gamma-aminobutyric acid.
Image Credit: Amy J. Jnah.

binding at mu-receptors, which mutes pain sensation and intensity.

Next, the pain impulse is subject to *transmission*. The impulse migrates and ascends the spinothalamic tract toward the hypothalamus, brainstem, and thalamus, the major relay stations of sensory information. Neurons in the thalamus relay the information to the midbrain and cerebral cortex for processing and *perception*. In this instant, the infant perceives the pain and the clinician observes a visible and/or audible response to the stimulus. At the same time, the cortex attempts to mitigate that pain sensation by sending a message to the periphery to withdraw from the pain. Clinicians will notice the infant trying to pull away (e.g., pull arm away during a blood draw or peripheral IV insertion).

Pain and Preterm Infants. In the past, scientists believed that preterm infants were incapable of perceiving painful stimuli because some of the free nerve endings (e.g., C-fibers) were unmyelinated. More recent research has debunked this theory. First, we know that C-fibers remain unmyelinated or partially myelinated in adults, and yet adults can feel pain. Second, we know that the number of free nerve endings peaks by 24 weeks of gestation, meaning that preterm infants have the same complement of nerve endings as adults (Tucker et al., 2023). A key vulnerability for infants is their smaller body surface area compared to adults, which leads to a higher ratio of nerve fibers to surface area in infants. With more nerve fibers confined within a smaller surface area, and a shorter distance for impulses to travel (compared to adults), infants are far more responsive and reactive to sensory stimuli, both therapeutic and noxious (Brewer & Baccei, 2020; R. W. Hall & Anand, 2005). Last, studies have shown that injury to free nerve endings increases the risk for "excessive nerve sprouting" and hyperexcitability, or hyperalgesia (peripheral and/or visceral; Anand, 2000; Tucker et al., 2023).

Clinical Application. Both preterm and term infants with a history of GI disease (e.g., necrotizing enterocolitis, congenital diaphragmatic hernia) can experience a state of visceral hyperalgesia, or increased sensations of pain when the GI system is stimulated during or after feeding sessions. Common manifestations include irritability, increased tone, and arching or withdrawal during or after feeding that is not attributed to any other disease process. Emerging evidence suggests gabapentin may mitigate these symptoms and help facilitate oral feeding tolerance. Side effects to consider include nystagmus and bradycardia. Additional studies are needed before widespread adoption of this pharmacologic treatment strategy occurs.

The Peripheral Nervous System

The PNS, an integrated portion of the CNS and greater nervous system, is composed of sensory and motor neurons (spinal and cranial nerves) and is integral to somatosensory function. It is further subdivided into the SNS and ANS.

Somatic Nervous System. The SNS controls all *voluntary* motor responses as well as involuntary reflexes (see the "Motor Responses" section of this chapter).

Autonomic Nervous System. The ANS consists of both sensory and motor neurons and regulates *involuntary* responses, including heart rate, vascular tone, smooth muscle contraction, glandular secretion, and digestive motility (Carlson, 2024). The ANS is divided into *sympathetic* and *parasympathetic* pathways. Each pathway is composed of nerves, ganglia, and plexus that conduct impulses away from the brainstem or spinal cord and toward autonomic effectors (Patton et al., 2022; Powley, 2013).

The *sympathetic pathway* contains adrenergic neurons (axons) that transmit norepinephrine to target structures, including the sweat glands and blood vessels. This pathway is best known for its ability to activate the "fight or flight" response (see Chapter 10). Alternatively, the *parasympathetic pathway* consists of cholinergic neurons (axons). This pathway elicits "rest and digest" responses. Neurons project through certain cranial nerves (III, VIII, IX, and X) and target the brain, thorax, and abdomen. This allows the parasympathetic pathway to control the pupillary sphincter, ciliary muscles, salivary and lacrimal glands, mucus secretion, food ingestion and digestion, musculature of the heart and esophagus, and select structures of the conducting portion of the respiratory system (Powley, 2013).

Enteric Nervous System. The ENS is a complex network of nerves located within the intestinal wall (Patton et al., 2022). These nerves control visceral effectors, such as endocrine and exocrine cells and smooth muscles.

Neuroprotective Mechanisms

The Skull. The skull is a protective cavity for the brain. Cranial osteogenesis begins during week 4 of gestation. Mesenchyme, or loosely organized tissue, derived from the primitive streak, occipital sclerotomes, and the neural crest proliferate to cover the brain. The lower portion of mesenchyme gives rise to the base of the cranium and the upper portion gives rise to the calvaria (skullcap). Once the primitive skull is formed, it undergoes chondrification (conversion into cartilage). Portions of the skull convert into parachordal cartilage, which gives rise to the temporal bones. Hypophyseal cartilage forms the roof of the orbit, whereas trabecular cartilage gives rise to the ethmoid bone.

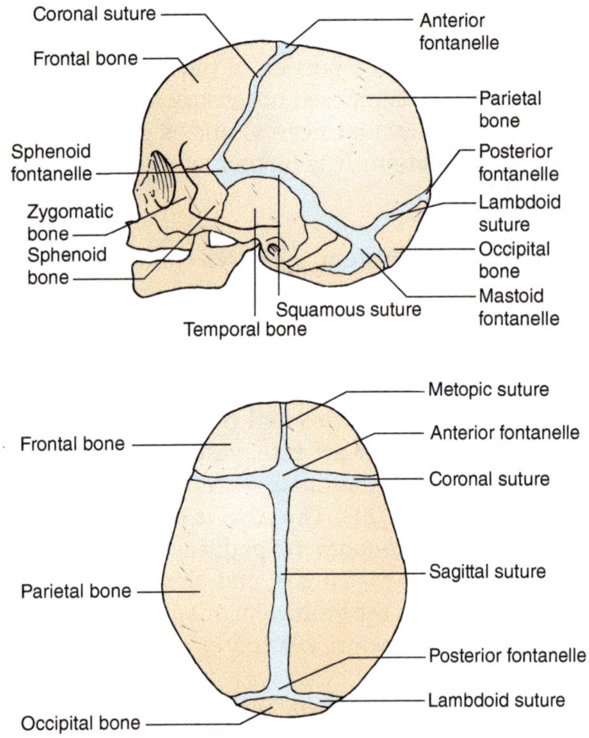

Figure 3.14 The cranial sutures.

TABLE 3.5 Cranial Sutures and Fontanelles

Suture	Closure or Fusion
Metopic	3 months–2 years of age
Lambdoid, sagittal, coronal	40 years of age
Squamosal	40–70 years of age
Fontanelle	**Closure or Fusion**
Posterior	2–3 months of age
Sphenoidal	6 months of age
Mastoid	6–18 months of age
Anterior	18 months–2 years of age

Source: Schoenwolf, G. C., Bleyl, S. B., Brauer, P. R., & Francis-West, P. H. (2022). *Larsen's human embryology* (6th ed.). Churchill Livingstone.

Ossification of the mesenchyme begins with week 13 of gestation (Duderstadt, 2019). Once formed, these bones remain independent of one another throughout fetal development and into infancy, permitting continued brain growth. Over time, the cranial bones approximate to form sutures and fontanelles. The cranial sutures include the metopic, lambdoid, coronal, and squamosal sutures (Figure 3.14). The anterior and posterior fontanelles are the two main fontanelles (Table 3.5). Ossification results in the formation of 45 bones; however, after fusion is complete, 22 bones remain (Som & Naidich, 2013). Craniosynostosis occurs due to premature closure and aberrant ossification of any one or more cranial sutures. Craniosynostosis is discussed in greater detail later in this chapter.

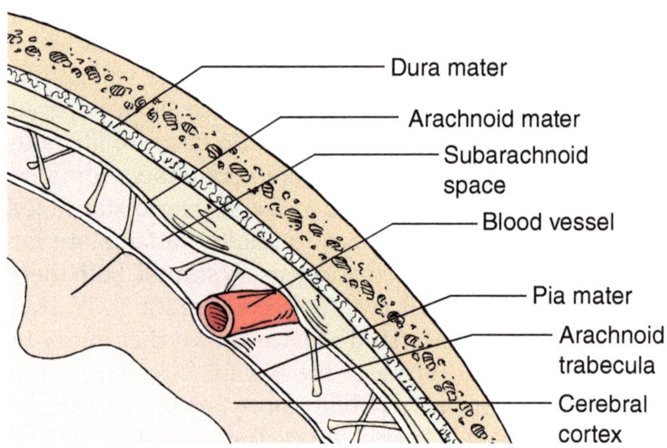

Figure 3.15 The meninges.

Meninges. The meninges are a three-layered protective covering around the brain and spinal cord. The outermost layer of the meninges is the dura mater. The arachnoid mater comprises the middle layer, and pia mater is the innermost layer (Figure 3.15).

Dura Mater. The dura mater is the thickest and most superior layer of the meninges. It is innervated by CN V, IX, X, and XII. The dura mater functions as a protective layer for the brain and spinal cord by forming several folds (structures) that separate the brain into various cavities. The *falx cerebri* divides the hemispheres of the brain, and the *falx cerebelli* separate the lobes of the cerebellum. The *tentorium cerebelli* divides the cerebrum and cerebellum. In addition to these protective and functional divisions, the dura mater also forms into several large pressure-dependent channels, or venous sinuses. These venous sinuses (superior sagittal, straight sinus, inferior sinus, and transverse sinus) drain blood from the brain and back to the heart, by way of the internal jugular veins.

APRNs should recognize that the anatomic location of the dura, its nerve innervations, and venous sinuses make it vulnerable to injury, in particular during traumatic operative vaginal deliveries (Vanderah & Gould, 2021). Hemorrhage may lead to blood sequestrations (accumulation and hematoma) within the (a) epidural space between the dura mater and the skull, or the (b) subdural space between the dura mater and arachnoid mater. This fluid accumulation can lead to increased ICP; subdural hemorrhage can be a life-threatening emergency for a newborn.

Arachnoid Mater, Subarachnoid Space, and Pia Mater. The middle layer of the meninges, which connects the dura and pia, is the *arachnoid mater*. Some projections of the arachnoid mater (known as the *arachnoid villi*) protrude into the venous sinuses of the dura. This innervation with the dura permits some cerebrospinal fluid (CSF) that normally travels through the arachnoid mater to traverse the arachnoid villi, enter the venous sinuses, and thereby enter the bloodstream.

Below the arachnoid mater is the *subarachnoid space*. This is regarded as a functionally significant portion of the brain for three important reasons: (a) It stores and circulates CSF, (b) it is innervated by the cranial nerves, and (c) it is generously supplied with blood vessels (Lee & Mukundan, 2015). In fact, the "arachnoid" is coined after the Greek term "arachne" (spider) because the arachnoid mater has a spiderweb-like vasculature.

The *pia* mater is the thinnest, innermost layer of the meninges. It adheres tightly to the surface of the brain and spinal cord (Lee & Mukundan, 2015). The pia merges with the membranous lining of the cerebral ventricles to form choroid plexuses. Recall that the choroid plexuses produce CSF. Disruptions during formation of these structures are associated with neural tube defects, whereas injuries to normally formed structures are often a result of a traumatic birth.

Choroid Plexus and Cerebrospinal Fluid. The choroid plexus produces 80% of CSF (Gomella et al., 2020). CSF protects the CNS while working as a barrier between the vasculature and the tissues of the brain.

The choroid plexus produces CSF in an energy-dependent active transport process; it is then reabsorbed by the arachnoid villi and directed into the superior sagittal sinus. CSF produced by the choroid sinuses in the lateral ventricles follows a pathway to the third ventricle and then passes through the cerebral aqueduct to the fourth ventricle. From the fourth ventricle, the CSF travels to the subarachnoid spaces. While in the subarachnoid spaces, CSF travels in a rostrocaudal direction toward the arachnoid villi (rostral) and central canal of the spinal cord (caudal; Figure 3.16; Brinker et al., 2014; Cizmeci & deVries, 2025). Structural defects, such as Chiari malformation, can interrupt normal movement of CSF.

Vertebral Column. The vertebral column is the bony structure that protects the spinal cord. Originally derived from the paraxial mesoderm, the vertebrae begin to form during week 4 of gestation. Sclerotome cells migrate around the spinal cord and notochord to combine with

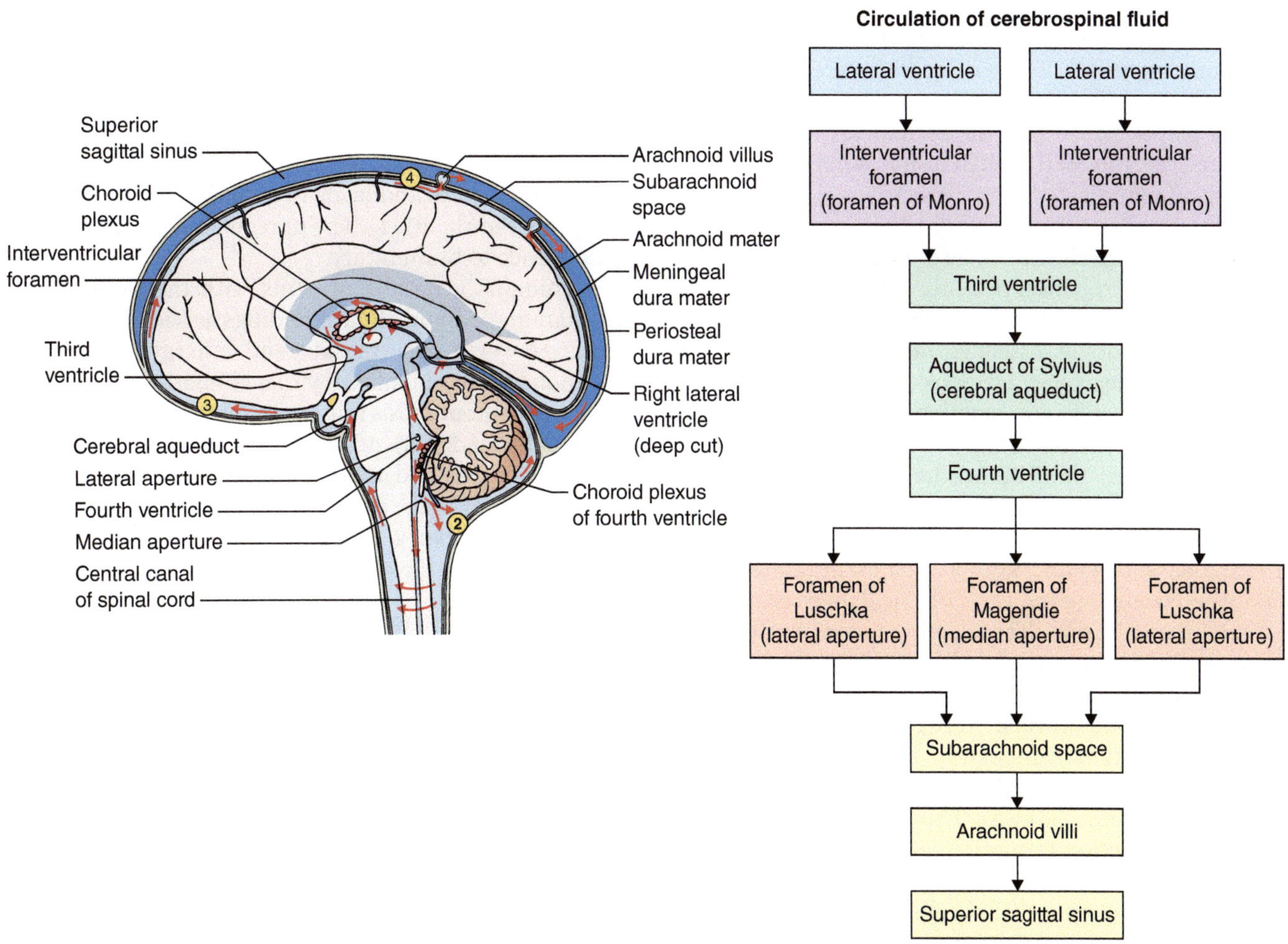

Figure 3.16 Cerebrospinal fluid circulation pathway. CSF is secreted by the choroid plexus (1) and travels through the lateral ventricles to the third and then fourth ventricles (2). When CSF reaches the subarachnoid spaces, it is directed caudally toward the spinal cord (3) and in a rostral direction toward the arachnoid villus (4), where it is absorbed into the venous sinuses of the dura.

cells on the opposing side of the neural tube. During development, resegmentation occurs when the caudal half of the sclerotome fuses with the cephalic half. This results in the formation of each individual vertebra (Schoenwolf et al., 2022). Once the vertebrae are fully formed, the vertebral column consists of 7 cervical, 12 thoracic, and 5 lumbar vertebrae, each separated by an intervertebral disc. The sacrum is comprised of 5 fused vertebrae and 2 coccygeal vertebrae. The 31 spinal nerves (8 cervical, 12 thoracic, 5 lumbar, 5 sacral, and 1 coccygeal), addressed earlier in this chapter, innervate accordingly. There are four curvatures that contribute to posture (Lee & Mukundan, 2015).

After early infancy, the vertebrae begin to ossify and grow. As such, the initial "C" shape of the spine begins to transition to an "S" shape (lateral view). The thoracic (T) to sacral (S) segment of vertebrae, denoted as T1-S1, is approximately 20 cm long at birth and 45 cm once mature. T1 to T12 is approximately 12 cm at birth and 27 cm once mature Finally, the lumbar (L) region spans L1 to L5 and is approximately 7.5 cm at birth and 16 cm once mature. Congenitally acquired, rare spinal deformities known to contribute to altered sitting height include scoliosis (lateral "S" curvature), kyphosis (abnormal outward "hunchback" curvature), and lordosis (abnormal inward "swayback" curvature; Canavese & Dimeglio, 2013; Lee & Mukundan, 2015). These deformities are the result of abnormal vertebral development and underdeveloped growth plates, which prevent normal vertical ascent of the spinal column. Early spinal fusion, before the age of 5 years, is often indicated.

Blood–Brain Barrier. BBB, also termed *neurovascular units*, function to inhibit potentially harmful substances in the bloodstream from entering the cerebral circulation and brain tissue. Although rarely discussed in fetal and neonatal physiology textbooks, five brain barrier interfaces exist as diffusion junctions to control ionic gradients between the blood and the CSF (Saunders et al., 2012). Therefore, the BBB is a neuroprotective mechanism for the developing fetus and neonate.

The BBB consists of endothelial cells, pericytes, microglia, astrocytes, and a basement membrane. Endothelial cells serve as a physical barrier against paracellular diffusion. These cells reduce permeability through the formation of tight junctions that restrict passage of small ions. Pericytes, microglia, astrocytes, and basement membrane strengthen endothelial cell junction formation. Although its intricacies are beyond the scope of this book, BBB function is influenced by the Wnt/β-catenin pathway. This pathway upregulates endothelial junction formation and modulates ongoing maintenance of the BBB.

The efficacy of endothelial cells as a barrier to diffusion in the fetus is complex and not well understood. Although previously regarded as "leaky" or "immature," more recent studies indicate the endothelial barrier in the fetus and premature infant is capable of resisting molecules as small as sucrose (Saunders et al., 2012). However, other properties of the BBB mechanism, including the cerebral vasculature and presence of protein transport mechanisms, may place the fetus and premature infant at risk for injury secondary to developmental and functional immaturity. Recent studies indicate endothelial cells located in the choroid plexus contain receptor/protein-binding molecules that hold a particular affinity for albumin. This mechanism may be associated with protein transfer and, in some cases, transfer of unconjugated bilirubin (bound to albumin) across the BBB and into the CSF. Other efflux transporters may contribute further to this pathology; however, additional investigation is necessary before the evidence can be reported with confidence (Saunders et al., 2014).

Meningitis may occur when bacteria enter the body through invasive procedures, such as umbilical vessel catheterization, endotracheal suctioning, or fetal scalp electrode placement. The bacteria attach to the mucosa and travel to other tissues in the body, leading to activation of the alternative complement pathway (discussed further in Chapter 9). When bacteria enter an infant's CSF, a large release of inflammatory mediators and increased permeability of the BBB results in meningitis. Host defense mechanisms, such as immunoglobulins, complement, and phagocytes, are unable to penetrate the BBB. The inability of the host defense mechanisms to penetrate the BBB allows the bacteria to replicate within the CSF. As bacteria die, they release lipopolysaccharides, which stimulate additional release of inflammatory mediators and leads to meningeal inflammation (Benitz & Smith, 2024). The unregulated bacterial replication leads to brain injury.

Meningitis generally presents with the same physical examination and clinical findings as seen in neonatal sepsis. However, hyperthermia and lethargy are the most common findings in infants with meningitis. Temperature elevation without sepsis is uncommon in the neonate (Edwards & Baker, 2023). Additional classic meningitic signs, such as seizures and a bulging anterior fontanelle, are often seen later in the course of meningitis among infants weighing more than 2,500 grams (Benitz & Smith, 2024).

GENETIC INFLUENCES

Genomic technologies, including linkage analysis, have been used in recent years to investigate the genome, transcriptome, and epigenome from a whole-genome perspective to better understand the genesis of certain neurologic defects. Several neurologic disorders are hereditary, commonly of Mendelian inheritance, and the result of errors during conception. Some present at birth, whereas others manifest during infancy, childhood, or later into adulthood. We present a discussion of several inherited disorders of the nervous system that manifest within the first 2 years of life. Additional disorders are provided in Box 3.1.

BOX 3.1 Other Inherited Disorders of the Nervous System

- Agenesis of corpus callosum (ACC)
- Anencephaly
- Apert syndrome (acrocephalosyndactyly)
- Congenital myotonic dystrophy
- Congenital neonatal myasthenia gravis
- Cri du chat
- Crouzon syndrome
- Dandy–Walker malformation
- Fragile X (Martin–Bell syndrome)
- Neurofibromatosis
- Prader–Willi syndrome
- Spina bifida
- Sturge–Weber syndrome
- Trisomy 21 (Down syndrome)
- Werdnig–Hoffman disease (spinal muscular atrophy [SMA] type 1)

Note: A more comprehensive list is provided by the National Institutes of Health, Genetic and Rare Diseases Information Center (GARD): https://rarediseases.info.nih.gov/diseases?category=Neurological%20 Diseases&page=1&letter=&search=

Autosomal Dominant Inherited Disorders

Neurofibromatosis. Neurofibromatosis (NF) is an autosomal dominant genetic disorder affecting the skin, nerves, brain, and spinal cord (Abramowicz & Gos, 2014). Neurofibromas (tumors) may grow along nerves throughout the body. NF is classified into two types, NF1 and NF2. NF1 is the most common form of NF and affects one in 3,000 to 4,000 births; no gender prevalence is reported (National Institutes of Health [NIH] 2025c). Mutations in the *NF1* gene are to blame for the development of NF1. *NF1* genes normally modulate the production of neurofibromin, which regulates cellular proliferation and acts as a tumor-suppressing gene. Infants with NF1 may present with café-au-lait spots (six or more), macrocephaly, or seizures. The importance of a comprehensive physical examination during the birth hospitalization, with astute recognition and classification of skin lesions, cannot be understated (see Chapter 12). Learning disabilities occur in up to 50% of children with NF1. NF2 typically presents with tumor-related symptoms around the age of 20 years.

Congenital Myotonic Dystrophy. Congenital myotonic dystrophy (CMD) affects one in every 47,000 births (Campbell et al., 2013). This is a multisystem genetic disease caused by expansions of a CTG trinucleotide repeat in the dystrophia myotonica protein kinase (DMPK) region (Rogers et al., 2022). Mutations in the *DMPK* gene alter normal cellular proliferation and function, which leads to muscular dystrophy (Muscular Dystrophy Association, 2025). CMD often manifests within the first hours of life. Typical clinical manifestations include persistent hypotonia, facial diplegia, areflexia, hyporeflexia, or muscle atrophy. Life-span implications include motor deficits, facial weakness, and developmental delays. Risk of death during the neonatal period is 30% to 40% (Ho et al., 2015).

Autosomal Recessive

Spinal Muscular Atrophy. SMA is a degenerative disorder that affects anterior horn cells and impacts lower motor neurons. The overall incidence of SMA is one in 8,000 to 10,000 births with Caucasian infants most commonly affected (National Library of Medicine, 2018; Ogino & Wilson, 2004). Mutations in the *SM1, UBA1, CYNC1H1,* and *VAPB* genes alter normal genetic modulation of the motor neurons in these patients, leading to failed nerve impulses and altered muscle control. SMA manifests with progressive muscle weakness and atrophy and is classified by type (0–IV; Nicolau et al., 2021). Type 0 and type I SMA present within the first 6 months of life. Common clinical manifestations include profound hypotonia and facial diplegia. Notable manifestations associated with type 1 SMA, or Werdnig–Hoffman disease, include "frog-leg" posturing, hyporeflexia, and areflexia. Life expectancy is less than 2 years (Nicolau et al., 2021).

Imprinting Disorders

Most human genes show equal expression of maternally and paternally derived alleles; however, a small percentage are expressed from only one parent without changing the fundamental genetic structure. This is called imprinting and typically occurs via DNA methylation (epigenetic modification). Imprinting disorders result from the loss of function of genes that are normally expressed from only one parental allele. Under ordinary circumstances, either the maternally or paternally derived allele is active, and the contribution from the other parent is silenced. In individuals with imprinting disorders, the allele that should be expressed is deleted or epigenetically silenced or there may instead be two copies of a chromosome from the wrong parent (uniparental disomy). Having no active copy of the relevant genes alters messenger ribonucleic acid (mRNA) function and production of proteins necessary for cellular function. This section discusses Prader–Willi and Angelman syndromes; other important examples of imprinting disorders include Beckwith-Wiedeman and Silver-Russell syndrome. Imprinting disorders are more common in pregnancies resulting from assisted reproductive technology for reasons that remain unclear (possibly due to subfertility or the technology itself; Hattori et al., 2019).

Prader-Willi. Prader-Willi syndrome (PWS) affects one in every 10,000 to 30,000 births and is the most common syndrome associated with obesity (NIH, 2021).

PWS results from the loss of expression of paternally expressed genes at 15q11-q13. Most cases (70%) occur from deletion of paternally inherited genes. Less frequently, the cause is maternal uniparental disomy; even less commonly, epimutations may occur (2%–4% of cases). There are numerous imprinted genes in this region that are implicated in the pathogenesis of PWS.

The pathogenesis of PWS involves hypothalamic dysfunction. An inadequate amount of growth hormone releasing hormone (GHRH) is released from the hypothalamus, which leads to deficient or absent production of growth hormone (GH) by the anterior pituitary gland. Biochemically, this results in deficient insulin-like growth factor 1 production (which modulates bone, cartilage, and muscle development), deficient gluconeogenesis, deficient lipolysis at the adipose tissue, and deficient amino acid uptake at the muscles. In addition, hypothalamic-pituitary-thyroid function can be disrupted, causing hypothyroidism.

Clinical manifestations observed during the fetal and neonatal period include decreased fetal movement, hypotonia (*the most common postnatal manifestation*), poor feeding, and failure to thrive. Later manifestations include hypogonadotropic hypogonadism, short stature, and obesity secondary to hyperphagia (excessive appetite), as well as cognitive and motor deficits (Carrel et al., 2022). Studies have also shown that prolonged GH deficiency can stunt the development of critical structures including the basal ganglia, corpus callosum, hippocampus, and thalamus, as well as the cerebellum (Carrel et al., 2022). Stunted development of these structures is associated with abnormal motor function and abnormal cognition (Martínez-Moreno et al., 2018). Prognosis varies due to the spectrum of neurodevelopmental involvement and consistency of outpatient continuing care, with an overall mortality risk of 2.7% (McCandless et al., 2020).

Clinical Application. PWS should be included in the differential diagnosis for an infant with hypotonia, poor feeding ability, and failure to thrive. Early diagnosis enables coordination of care and early initiation of growth hormone replacement therapy (GHRT), a U.S. Food and Drug Administration (FDA)–approved therapy since 2000. The effects of GHRT are noteworthy. Early GHRT can help normalize head growth and establish a normal head circumference (the head is often abnormally small at birth) and optimize muscle function, motor development, and body composition. Among children and adults, GHRT promotes increased linear growth (increased height velocity) as well as the size of hands and feet, and optimize lean body mass. GHRT can mitigate the effects of hypotonia by optimizing physical strength and mobility as well as respiratory function (minute ventilation). Last, GHRT has shown promise with optimizing cognitive function.

Angelman Syndrome. Angelman syndrome affects one in every 12,000 to 20,000 births (NIH, 2025a). Angelman involves loss of function inactivation in a different section of chromosome 15q11-13 than that seen in PWS. The characteristic features of this syndrome are caused by loss of function of the *UBE3A* gene. Although a copy of this gene is typically inherited from each parent, only the copy in the XX pregnant patient is active in normal neurons, with the paternal allele silenced by imprinting. When the copy in the XX pregnant patient is inactivated or deleted, AS occurs. Although this can be inherited, most cases arise as a de novo mutation in early embryonic development, conferring a low risk of recurrence in subsequent offspring from the same parents. A smaller percentage of cases involve paternal uniparental disomy of chromosome 15 or an imprinting defect. Common clinical manifestations include microcephaly and seizures, both of which manifest during early infancy (Lalande & Calciano, 2007; NIH, 2025a; Williams et al., 2010). Neurodevelopmental deficits are common and become apparent between 6 to 12 months of age.

Trisomies

Trisomy 18 (Edwards Syndrome). Trisomy 18 affects one in 5,000 live births; a female prevalence is reported (Chen, 2012). Nearly all (95%) infants are affected by a translocation of genetic material, which yields three copies of chromosome 18 within each cell in the body. Less often, infants may be affected by a mosaicism (partial trisomy) at the long arm of chromosome 18 (Senarante et al., 2024). Hallmark clinical manifestations include clenched hands and "rocker-bottom" feet, a small and narrow cranium, prominent occiput, and low-set ears. Midline defects may include **v**ertebral defects, **a**nal atresia, **c**ardiac defects (80%), **t**racheo**e**sophageal fistula, **r**enal anomalies, and other **l**imb abnormalities, including club feet (VACTERL). Long-term outcomes vary. Partial to severe forms of trisomy 18 are associated with moderate to severe neurologic deficits and hypotonia. Infants with a mosaicism may express fewer anomalies and have improved neurodevelopmental outcomes. Rarely, trisomy 18 is associated with fatal neural tube defects, such as anencephaly. This is usually the result of a somatic or unbalanced translocation.

Trisomy 21 (Down Syndrome). Trisomy 21 affects one in every 700 births. An increased incidence, estimated at one in 25 to 300 births, is reported among XX pregnant patients over 35 years of age (NIH, 2025b). Nearly all (94%) infants are affected by a translocation of genetic material, which yields three copies of chromosome 21 within each cell in the body. Less common, infants may be affected by a mosaicism and present with a milder form of the syndrome. Approximately 50% of fetuses with trisomy 21 are spontaneously aborted or stillborn. Hallmark clinical manifestations include microcephaly, congenital heart defects (atrioventricular canal defects, tetralogy of Fallot, and patent ductus arteriosus), brachycephaly, upward-slanted palpebral fissures, epicanthal folds, Brushfield spots, a flattened nasal bridge, prominent tongue, short neck, single palmar crease (suggestive of hypotonia in utero), and abnormal digits. Life-span implications include cognitive and intellectual deficits, including difficulty with reasoning, judgment, and emotional lability (NIH, 2025b).

Trisomy 13 (Patau Syndrome). Trisomy 13 affects an estimated one in 16,000 live births (Genetic and Rare Diseases Information Center, 2024). Most (80%) infants are affected by a translocation of genetic material, which yields three copies of chromosome 13 within each cell in the body. Mosaicism, associated with reduced disease severity, occurs in approximately 5% of all cases. Few fetuses affected by trisomy 13 survive to term; the majority of affected pregnancies result in spontaneous abortion or stillbirth. The hallmark clinical manifestations include holoprosencephaly (50% of patients), postaxial polydactyly, cardiac and renal anomalies, and microcephaly. Incomplete development of the forebrain, spinal cord abnormalities, hypotonia, and seizures are also reported. Infants affected by a mosaicism may express varying degrees of mental deficits and incur longer survival rates (National Organization for Rare Disorders [NORD], 2024a).

X-Linked Disorders

Agenesis of Corpus Callosum. ACC is a birth defect resulting from failed or partial development of fiber bundles connecting the cerebral hemispheres. ACC affects seven of every 1,000 births and may be an isolated defect or associated with brain malformations, including Chiari malformation, schizencephaly, holoprosencephaly, colpocephaly, Andermann syndrome, or Dandy–Walker malformation (NORD, 2024b; Volpe & Inder, 2025). Females may be concurrently affected by Aicardi syndrome, characterized by ACC, chorioretinal lacunae (punched out lesions in the pigmented layer of the retina), and seizures (Govil-Dalela et al., 2017; NORD, 2024b). Clinical manifestations include seizures, abnormalities of the spine, developmental delay, and congenital hydrocephalus. Life expectancy is related to extent and severity of associated disorders or abnormalities (NORD, 2024b).

Aqueductal Stenosis. Congenital stenosis of the aqueduct of Sylvius involves a narrowing of the passageway between the third and fourth ventricle, which slows the passage of CSF from the ventricles. This is an X-linked recessive disorder associated with 15% to 60% of all cases of congenital hydrocephalus (Cinalli et al., n.d., 2011). Hallmark clinical manifestations include congenital hydrocephalus with or without seizures, hypotonia, and weakness (Pina-Garza, 2013). Long-term outcomes are related to the underlying cause of aqueductal stenosis and associated disorders (Cinalli et al., n.d.).

Fragile X. Fragile X syndrome is the most common inherited cause for intellectual disability and affects one in every 4,000 to 8,000 births; a male prevalence (2:1) is reported (Raspa et al., 2017). Fragile X syndrome follows an X-linked dominant inheritance pattern and involves mutations in the Fragile X mRNA 1 gene (*FMR1*; Centers for Disease Control and Prevention [CDC], 2025a). Mutations effectively shut off transcription of the *FMR1* gene, which is normally responsible for modulating synapses between axons and target cells. Delayed speech and language development is common and typically identified by age 2. Therefore, common life-span implications include delayed neurocognitive development and behavioral problems. Seizure disorders and macrocephaly have also been reported (CDC, 2025a).

NOTEWORTHY DISEASES IN THE XX PREGNANT PATIENT AND KNOWN EFFECTS UPON CENTRAL NERVOUS SYSTEM DEVELOPMENT AND FUNCTION

Stability of the XX birthing parent–fetal dyad is critical for the developing fetus. Certain pharmacologic agents, infections, alterations in health status, and placental and delivery complications may impact neurologic system development.

Acute, Chronic, and Pregnancy-Associated Diseases

The health status of the XX pregnant patient is important to a stable fetal growth environment. Neurodevelopmental consequences of disease states, including malnutrition, may impose lifelong challenges for the affected child. Common disease states in XX pregnant patients that affect the fetal neurodevelopment are summarized in Table 3.6.

The presence of disease activates stress-response systems in the XX pregnant patient. For example, the hypothalamic–pituitary–adrenal (HPA) axis (see Chapter 10) may be activated to preserve homeostasis. Although this normal stress response is helpful to the XX pregnant patient, it can compromise the intrauterine environment and alter or interrupt normal fetal neurodevelopment. For example, placental blood flow may be reduced during the XX pregnant patient's stress responses. Recurrent activation of the HPA axis, or the hypothalamic–pituitary–thyroid axis in cases of thyroid disorders in XX pregnant patients, may impose long-lasting, deleterious effects on fetal neurodevelopment and across the life span. As such, the health and well-being of the XX pregnant patient are of critical importance throughout the entirety of the pregnancy (Vohr et al., 2017).

Pharmacologic Influences

Sufficient evidence exists related to the potential harmful effect of certain pharmacologic agents on the developing fetus. These substances may have a direct or indirect influence on developing fetal CNS. Direct impact may alter

TABLE 3.6 Summary of Common Diseases in XX Pregnant Patients and Risks to Fetal Neurodevelopment and Childhood Function

Disease States in XX Pregnant Patients	Risks
Infections (CMV,[a] chorioamnionitis)	*Fetal/neonatal:* Sensorineural hearing loss (CMV), impaired grey matter development (chorioamnionitis) *Childhood:* Cognitive deficits
Inflammatory diseases	*Fetal/neonatal*: Atypical brain development[b] *Childhood:* Cognitive deficits
Thyroid disorder	*Fetal/neonatal*: Craniosynostosis *Childhood:* Attention deficit disorder
Diabetes mellitus	*Fetal/neonatal*: Atypical brain development[b] *Childhood*: Language delay, impaired recognition, poor motor development, neuropsychologic impairment
Obesity	*Fetal/neonatal*: Inflammation-mediated atypical brain development[b] *Childhood*: Cognitive and language deficits
Micronutrient deficiencies (folate, B_{12}, choline, zinc, tryptophan, omega-3 fatty acids, iodine)	*Fetal/neonatal*: Neural tube defects, atypical brain development,[b] reduced myelination *Childhood*: Cognitive and language deficits; motor, socioemotional, and behavioral dysfunction[b]

[a]CMV is the most common congenital infection; however, the TORCH infections excluded from this table may cause similar neurologic consequences in the developing fetus.

[b]*Atypical brain development* refers to an interruption of normal embryologic and fetal brain development during neurogenesis (proliferation, migration, organization, or myelination). The correlation between maternal obesity and neurologic dysfunction in childhood may be confounded by sociodemographic factors.

CMV, cytomegalovirus; TORCH, *Toxoplasma gondii*, rubella, cytomegalovirus, and herpes simplex.

Source: Cizmeci, M. N., & deVries, L. (2025). Intracranial hemorrhage and stroke in the neonate. In R. J. Martin & A. A. Fanaroff (Eds.), *Fanaroff and Martin's neonatal-perinatal medicine: Diseases of the fetus and infant* (12th ed., pp. 1059–1084). Elsevier Mosby.

neuronal pathways, receptors, and structures resulting in potential short-term and long-term complications. Indirect impact includes alterations in health and nutrition, intrauterine growth restriction (IUGR), neonatal respiratory depression, hypotonia, apnea, and premature delivery. Clinicians must weigh the risks of pharmacologic exposures with the benefits of the intended medication on both the XX pregnant patient and the fetus. For patients using illicit substances, dosing and frequency are commonly inconsistent, providing a greater challenge for diagnosis and management of neonatal abstinence.

Any use of general or regional obstetric analgesia or narcotics should alert the clinician to potential adverse effects to the fetus (as well as the pregnant female). Opioid analgesics may precipitate hypotension and drowsiness, alter labor patterns, and arrest labor (Davidson et al., 2023). This may disrupt CBF patterns and fetal oxygen consumption. Fetal manifestations of obstetric analgesia may include decreased fetal heart rate variability and postnatal respiratory depression. General anesthesia may provoke hypotension, hypertension, tachycardia, vomiting (with possible aspiration), and laryngospasm in the XX pregnant patient (Davidson et al., 2023; Palanisamy, 2012). Fetal manifestations of general anesthesia include hypotonia and CNS depression. Regional spinal or epidural anesthesia risks include hypotension, allergic reaction, and prolonged second-stage labor. Potential fetal complications include toxic reaction to dosing, late decelerations, bradycardia, and variability (Tsen, 2011).

Antihypertensive agents are known to readily cross the placenta. These medications may precipitate IUGR, premature labor and delivery, hypoxia, and acidosis (Dekker, 2011; Sibai, 2012). Postnatal manifestations of antihypertensive use during the antepartum and intrapartum period include hypotonia, apnea, respiratory depression, and hypotension in the newborn (Dekker, 2011; Fitton et al., 2020; Sibai, 2012). High-dose antihypertensive therapy is associated with increased risk for neonatal neuromuscular and respiratory depression (Davidson et al., 2023).

Antiseizure medications readily cross the placental barrier and can lead to significant congenital malformations in the developing fetus. There is an approximate threefold increase in risk for major anomalies in the developing fetus when mothers use valproic acid (Valproate) for seizure management (Petersen et al., 2017). The most common risk to the fetus is the development of a neural tube defect.

Substance Abuse

Substance use disorders are a significant issue within the United States. The most abused substances include tobacco, alcohol, cannabinoids, opioids, and cocaine. Polysubstance abuse is common and, in certain cases, can exacerbate manifestations of neonatal opioid withdrawal syndrome (NOWS). The effects of drug abuse on fetal neurodevelopment include alterations to neurotransmitters and receptors, brain organization, and structural malformations. In addition, certain drugs disrupt the XX birthing parent–fetal placental interface, which can cause rapid shifts in fetal CBF and vascular resistance, thereby increasing the risk for brain injury.

Tobacco and Nicotine. Tobacco and nicotine products used during pregnancy include chewing tobacco, rolled cigarettes, e-cigarettes, and nicotine replacement therapies. From 2016 to 2021, the percentage of mothers who smoked cigarettes during pregnancy declined from 7% to 4% (Martin et al., 2023). Fetal neurodevelopmental consequences of tobacco or nicotine exposure include observed reductions in cortical grey matter. These findings are observed and reported using cohorts of children exposed to smoking during pregnancy (Chatterton et al., 2017). The pathophysiology of tobacco and nicotine exposure has been investigated using fetal rodent models. Abnormal development of cerebral dendrites and axon-mediated synapses within the cortex are observed. Epigenetic changes in DNA methylation are reported. Therefore, risk factors to the human fetus include cognitive impairment, behavioral issues, and reductions in executive function, which typically manifest in childhood (O'Keeffe et al., 2014). Of note, smoking during pregnancy is positively associated with antenatal anxiety and depression and a reduction in XX birthing parent–fetal bonding, as well as breast (or chest) feeding practices, in the postpartum period (Chatterton et al., 2017; Hernández-Martínez et al., 2017).

Alcohol. Approximately 10% of XX pregnant patients report current alcohol use, and nearly 5% of these patients report binge drinking (National Institute on Alcohol Abuse and Alcoholism [NIAAA], 2023). Alcohol consumption during pregnancy can be categorized as social consumption, moderate, binge, or heavy drinking. *Moderate drinking* is defined as up to one drink per day, *binge drinking* is defined as four or more drinks in about 2 hours, and *heavy drinking* refers to binge drinking on 5 or more days during a 30-day period (NIAAA, 2025). There is no safe range for alcohol consumption during pregnancy. The American College of Obstetricians and Gynecologists (ACOG) report even moderate drinking during early pregnancy can lead to neurodevelopment sequela (anxiety-like behavior) in offspring (ACOG, 2017; CDC, 2024a; NIAAA, 2025; Rouzer et al., 2017). Impaired oxidative and nonoxidative metabolism of ethanol is one proposed etiology for high circulating levels of ethanol within amniotic fluid (Heller & Burd, 2014). In addition, ethanol is known to impose placental and umbilical cord vasoconstriction and increase fetal–placental vascular resistance. Consequences of fetal exposure to alcohol include speech and language deficits, cognitive and behavior deficits, learning disabilities, hyperactivity, reduced executive functioning, and psychosocial dysfunction in adulthood (NIAAA, 2025).

Cannabis. Approximately 7% of individuals of child-bearing age use marijuana while pregnant (CDC, 2025c). The psychoactive component of cannabis is Δ9-tetrahydrocannabinol (THC). THC can cross the placenta as well as the BBB (CDC, 2025c). In doing so, it may function as a noxious stimulant to the endocannabinoid system, which can interfere with folic acid absorption, cerebral angiogenesis, neuronal proliferation, axon development, and synaptogenesis. In addition, fetal THC exposure disrupts fetal dopamine synthesis by impairing dopamine receptor cell maturation (Jaques et al., 2014; C. S. Wu et al., 2011). Prenatal exposure to THC is associated with neonatal tremors, irritability, and an exaggerated startle response. Life-span implications include learning disabilities, impaired higher order executive functions (impulse control, visual memory, and attention span) during school-age years, and neuropsychiatric disorders (drug addiction, schizophrenia, and depression) in older children and adults (Jaques et al., 2014; Volkow et al., 2017). Dose–response relationships between THC and fetal neurodevelopment have not been defined to date (Jaques et al., 2014).

Stimulants. Common reported stimulants ingested during pregnancy include cocaine, ecstasy, and methamphetamines. Prenatal stimulant use is more common than opioid use (Smid et al., 2019; Wouldes & Lester, 2023). Stimulants, such as amphetamine-dextroamphetamine and methylphenidate, are prescribed to treat attention deficit hyperactivity disorder (ADHD); approximately 1% of XX pregnant patients take these medications for ADHD during pregnancy (Anderson et al., 2018).

Mechanisms by which cocaine and methamphetamines complicate fetal neurodevelopment are poorly understood. Cocaine rapidly crosses the placenta by simple diffusion, causing generalized vasoconstriction of fetal blood vessels. Methamphetamine is also a vasoconstrictor, decreasing blood flow to the fetus which leads to hypoxia. Neonatal effects include lower birthweight, smaller head circumferences, and shorter length at birth (Wouldes & Lester, 2023). Neurologic manifestations of early cocaine use during pregnancy (first trimester) include impaired short-term memory and behavioral issues. Methamphetamines are neurotoxic, leading to impaired fetal brain development.

Opioids. Opioid use involves both prescription opioids as well as heroin and fentanyl. Rates of prenatal opioid use have stabilized in the past several years but remain at 7% (CDC, 2025b). Prenatal opioid exposure disrupts early cortical brain development, including neurogenesis, proliferation, and migration. These disruptions may negatively affect brain growth and basal ganglia development. Early consequences of opioid abuse include NOWS. NOWS manifests as crying, irritability, poor sleep, increased muscle tone, tremors, skin excoriation, hyperthermia, loose stools, yawning, sweating, nasal stuffiness, and sneezing (Patrick et al., 2020). Discussion of life-span implications for opioid abuse in the XX pregnant patient is confounded by the prevalence of polysubstance abuse. In addition, the severity of NOWS and pharmacologic treatment mechanisms, as well as environmental factors and parenting behaviors, may complicate infant developmental assessments in infancy and childhood (Benninger et al., 2023).

Xylazine, a nonopioid alpha-2 agonist, is an FDA-approved veterinary anesthetic that is now commonly added to illicitly manufactured fentanyl ("tranq dope") to hasten onset, extend the sedative effect, and possibly increase dependence and withdrawal (Perrone et al., 2024). It is therefore an increasingly frequent co-exposure for infants born to mothers who abuse fentanyl. Xylazine withdrawal in infants may extend or complicate opioid withdrawal symptoms. The specific details of a xylazine withdrawal syndrome in neonates remain murky primarily because of universal opioid co-exposure. Adults withdrawing from xylazine have reported increased anxiety, depressed mood, body aches, hypertension, and worsening of withdrawal symptoms from other substances that is not effectively treated by the medications for opioid use disorders (Spadaro et al., 2023). There are no studies of the symptoms or their treatment in infants and limited published information in adults. Clonidine, also an alpha-2 adrenergic agonist, has alleviated symptoms in adult sufferers (Ehrman-Dupre et al., 2022), has been studied in the pharmacologic management of NOWS (Bada et al., 2024), and may be helpful in symptomatic infants exposed to xylazine.

Acute and Chronic Infectious Diseases

Infections during pregnancy adversely affect the developing fetus in various ways. Complications may include alterations in fetal development (IUGR, microcephaly), premature delivery, alterations in cerebral tissue (intraventricular and intracerebral calcifications), seizures, or long-term neurodevelopmental complications. In many cases, the risk for adverse outcomes is inversely related to the infant's gestational age and age of infectious exposure during pregnancy. Of particular concern are those infectious agents capable of readily crossing the placenta (Neu et al., 2015). These infectious agents include **s**yphilis, **t**oxoplasmas, **o**thers (varicella-zoster, parvovirus B19), **r**ubella, CMV, and **h**erpes simplex virus (STORCH; Box 3.2). These infectious agents increase the risk for neonatal neurologic sequelae from prenatal infection. In some cases, the neurologic impact is related to the onset of infection during pregnancy.

BOX 3.2 Prenatal Infections

- (**S**) Congenital syphilis (Treponema pallidum)
- (**T**) Toxoplasmosis (*Toxoplasma gondii*)
- (**O**) Others (e.g., Varicella zoster virus, parvovirus B19)
- (**R**) Congenital rubella (German measles)
- (**C**) Congenital cytomegalovirus
- (**H**) Herpes simplex virus (HSV)

Sources: Elmore, S. A., Jones, J. L., Conrad, P. A., Patton, S., Lindsay, D. S., & Dubey, J. P. (2010). *Toxoplasma gondii*: Epidemiology, feline clinical aspects, and prevention. *Trends in Parasitology, 26*(4), 190–196. https://doi.org/10.1016/j.pt.2010.01.009; Neu, N., Duchon, J., & Zachariah, P. (2015). TORCH infections. *Clinical Perinatology, 42*(1), 77–103. https://doi.org/10.1016/j.clp.2014.11.001

COMMON PROBLEMS WITH IMPLICATIONS ACROSS THE LIFE SPAN

Disorders of Early Brain Development

Anencephaly. Anencephaly is a lethal disorder of early brain development resulting in incomplete or defective closure of the rostral end of the anterior neural tube. The incidence of anencephaly within the United States is one in every 4,600 births per year, with females more affected than males (CDC, 2025a). An increased prevalence of anencephaly among Hispanic infants has been reported (Dean & Doherty, 2024).

Risk factors for development of anencephaly include mineral deficits (such as deficiencies in folate, copper, and zinc), febrile illnesses during the first one third to one half of gestation, and diabetes in XX pregnant patients (Volpe & Inder, 2025). Recurrence risk ranges from 1.9% to 3% with subsequent pregnancies (Dean & Doherty, 2024; Jones et al., 2013). Causes of anencephaly are generally unknown (CDC, 2025a). Genetic and environmental influences appear to impact the development of this disorder (Volpe & Inder, 2025). Environmental factors may include toxins, certain medications, and folic acid deficiencies.

The pathogenesis of anencephaly involves closure of the cranial neuropore leading to incomplete brain and skull development. Direct exposure of the hemispheres of the brain to amniotic fluid, as well as prolonged trauma from fetal movement causing brain tissue to interface with the uterine wall, contributes to the development of this neural tube defect (Figure 3.17; Copel, 2018).

Anencephaly manifests as craniorachischisis totalis or myeloschosis. Large portions of the skull (and, in some cases, the scalp) are missing. Craniorachischisis totalis

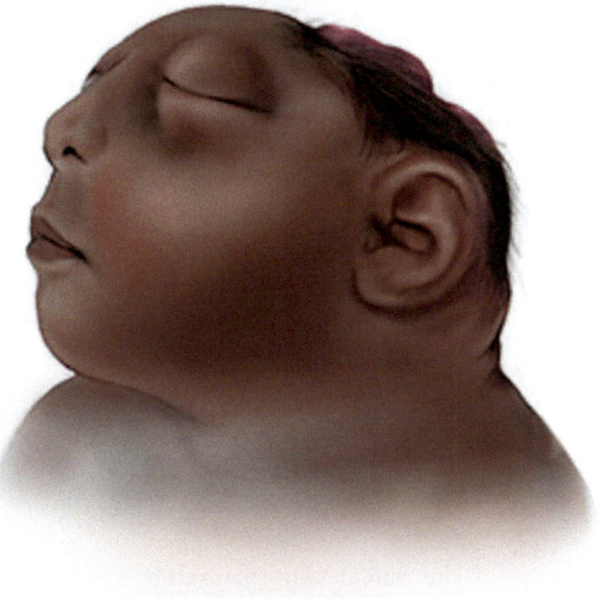

Figure 3.17 Anencephaly.
Source: Centers for Disease Control and Prevention. (2024, December 26). *Anencephaly*. https://www.cdc.gov/birth-defects/about/anencephaly.html?CDC_AAref_Val=https://www.cdc.gov/ncbddd/birthdefects/anencephaly.html

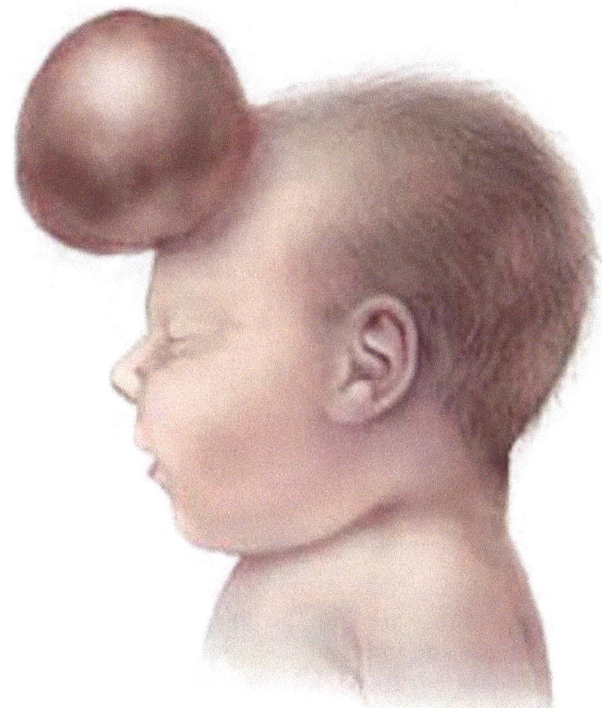

Figure 3.18 Encephalocele.
Source: Centers for Disease Control and Prevention. (2024c, November 21). *Encephalocele*. https://www.cdc.gov/birth-defects/about/anencephaly.html?CDC_AAref_Val=https://www.cdc.gov/ncbddd/birthdefects/anencephaly.html

involves absent dermal or skeletal coverage of the neural plate. Myeloschosis involves an open dermal layer, absent skeletal coverage, and exposed nerve tissue resulting in posterior exposure of the spinal cord. Prominent-appearing eyes, hypertonia, hyperactive reflexes, and myoclonus may be present. Life-span implications include fetal demise, stillbirth, or postnatal death within the first 2 months of life (Dean & Doherty, 2024).

Encephalocele. Encephalocele is a neural tube defect occurring from a failure of rostral neural tube closure during primary neurulation. Incidence rates for encephalocele in the United States are one in 10,500 live births (CDC, 2024b; Dean & Doherty, 2024). The majority of cases (80%) in the Western hemisphere involve occipital encephaloceles, whereas Eastern countries (Thailand, for example) report a higher incidence of frontal encephaloceles (Copel, 2018). Associated anomalies (microcephaly, cleft lip/palate, hydrocephalus, craniosynostosis, and spina bifida) are seen in 50% of all cases (Dean & Doherty, 2024). Risk factors include previous children with spina bifida or anencephaly, Meckel syndrome, Walker–Warburg syndrome, fetal exposure to teratogens or mineral deficits (such as deficiencies in folate, copper, and zinc), and febrile illnesses during early gestation in the XX pregnant patient (Dean & Doherty, 2024; Jones et al., 2013).

The pathogenesis of encephalocele involves one of two possible mechanisms: (a) failed anterior fusion of the neural folds, or (b) herniation of brain tissue outside of the cranial cavity and into a protuberant mass or fluid-filled saclike structure (Figure 3.18). Defects may also occur in the frontal, nasopharyngeal, or parietal regions (Volpe & Inder, 2025).

Life-span implications are related to location, size, and regional involvement. Cognitive deficits may occur in up to 50% of all cases (Dean & Doherty, 2024). Encephaloceles arising in the occiput are also associated with blindness (Ruge, 2023).

Spina Bifida. *Spina bifida* refers to incomplete formation, or absence, of the posterior vertebral arch, giving rise to a saclike protuberance at the base of the spinal column. Four forms of spina bifida are reported: (a) occulta (most common), (b) closed neural tube defects, (c) meningocele, and (d) myelomeningocele (Figure 3.19). Spina bifida affects between 1,500 to 2,000 infants each year in the United States. Rates are highest among the Hispanic population (3.8 per 10,000 live births), followed by Caucasian infants (3.09 per 10,000 live births) and African American infants (2.73 per 10,000 live births; CDC, 2025e). Risk factors include malnutrition (specifically folic acid deficiencies), diabetes, and the use of certain medications (e.g., valproic acid and carbamazepine) in XX pregnant patients (NIH, 2025d).

Clinical manifestations vary depending on the extent of tissue involvement and level of the defect. Increased neural tissue involvement and defects involving the cervical or upper thoracic spine are associated with

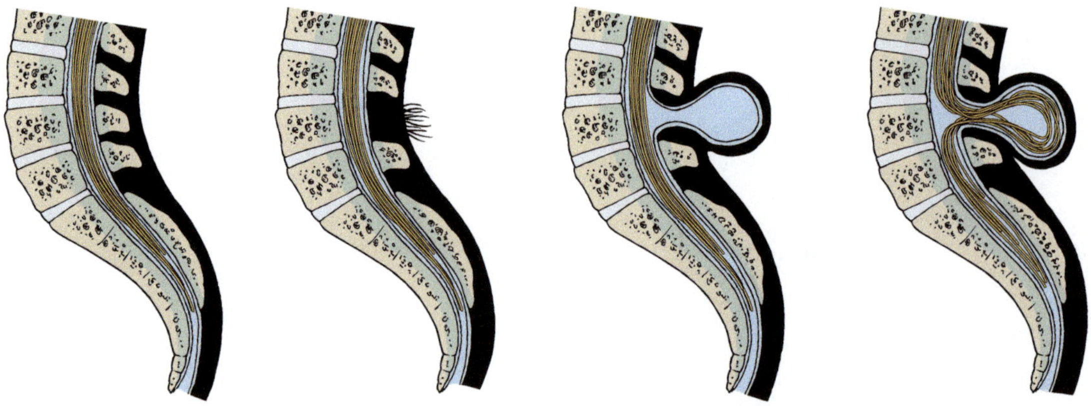

Figure 3.19 Normal spine and types of spina bifida.

increased morbidity risks. A tuft of hair, dimple, lipoma, or hemangioma located in the lower lumbar region should increase the index of suspicion for spina bifida (Cizmeci & deVries, 2025). Infants with an accompanying tethered cord and Chiari malformation may present with hydrocephalus, as 85% to 90% of cases involving thoracolumbar, lumbar, or lumbosacral lesions are associated with obstructed flow of CSF secondary to kinking of the fourth ventricle (Elgamal, 2012).

Clinical Application. The serum alpha-fetoprotein (AFP) test is performed early into pregnancy to evaluate for cases of *open* fetal spina bifida. AFP is a protein produced by the fetal liver as well as the yolk sac and can transfer (transplacentally) into the maternal blood. Maternal serum (MS) AFP testing can detect up to 80% of open fetal neural tube defects, and in these cases, the AFP level is abnormally high. However, closed neural tube defects may not be detected by this screening test. Amniocentesis is often the preferred method for measuring AFP levels in pregnant patients over the age of 35 years, per the ACOG.

Spina Bifida Occulta. Spina bifida occulta occurs in 12% of individuals and is referred to as "hidden" (occulta) because there is no obvious deformity and the spine and nerves are usually unaffected. Spina bifida occulta occurs secondary to failed closure of the posterior vertebral laminae, most often during week 4 of gestation, and results in failed fusion of one or more arches of the spine, which forms a small, spinal cleft. Most newborns are unaffected, and unless the condition is identified prenatally parents may be completely unaware of the defect. Approximately one in 1,000 affected individuals go on to develop complications including bowel and/or bladder dysfunction and neurologic deficits, which often trigger diagnostic evaluations and identification of the disorder (American Association of Neurological Surgeons, 2024).

Meningocele. A meningocele is a saclike dilation of the meninges that results in bulging below the skin. Meningoceles can be differentiated from myelomeningoceles based upon the position of the spinal cord. In this case, the spinal cord is contained within the spinal canal with the sac ("cele") containing only arachnoid mater, dura mater, and pia mater which herniates through open vertebrae (Schindelmann et al., 2021). Meningoceles occur equally along the cervical, thoracic, and lumbar spinal regions. The structures (meninges and spinal cord) are normally developed. No neurodevelopmental deficits are reported among infants and children.

Myelomeningocele. Myelomeningocele is a similar saclike dilation comprised of spinal fluid and neural tissue, spinal cord, nerves, or a combination of these neural structures. Myelomeningoceles can also be differentiated from meningoceles based upon the position of the spinal cord. In these cases, the spinal cord is not completely contained within the spinal canal. Rather, the sac contains the spinal cord and meninges (Schindelmann et al., 2021). Up to 80% of all myelomeningoceles occur in the lumbar and lumbosacral regions (Ruge, 2023; Volpe & Inder, 2025). Of those that do originate in these regions, nearly all are associated with Chiari II malformation (Ruge, 2023). Chiari II malformations involve the downward displacement of the brainstem, medulla, cerebellum, and fourth ventricle through the foramen magnum (**Figure 3.20**). Chiari II formations are associated with hydrocephalus secondary to obstruction of the fourth ventricle or to aqueductal stenosis (Volpe & Inder, 2025).

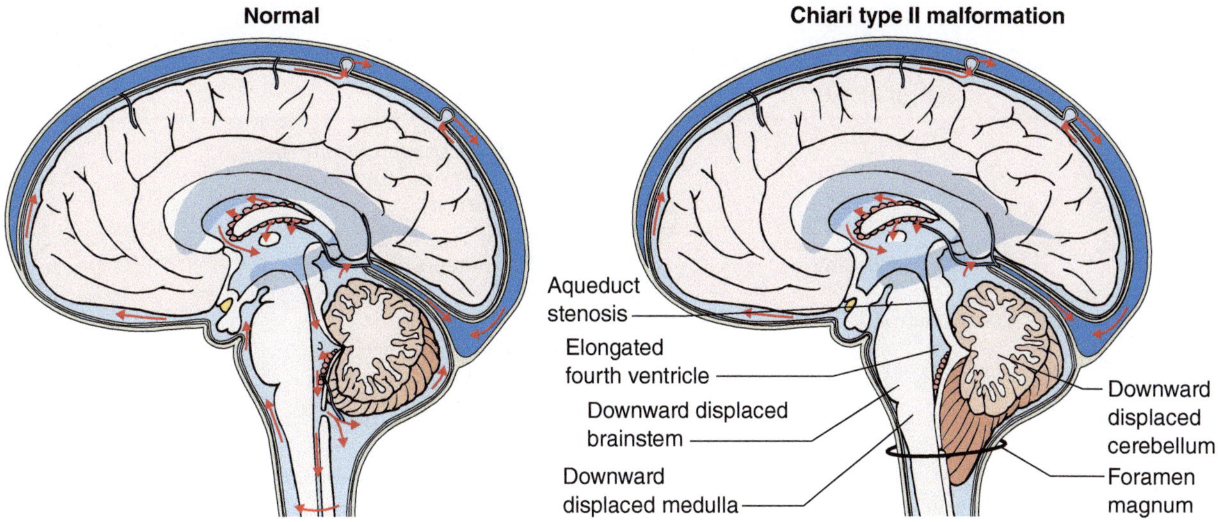

Figure 3.20 Chiari II malformation.

Life-span implications of these three variants of spina bifida include altered neurologic function below the level of the defect. Severity is related to the extent and location of the defect, integrity of associated structures, and comorbidities (Volpe & Inder, 2025). Closure of a meningocele may impose few, if any, long-term complications. Life-span implications of spina bifida occulta include altered gait, chronic back pain, bowel and bladder dysfunction, and alterations in spinal alignment (scoliosis; Volpe & Inder, 2025). Life-span implications of myelomeningocele include seizures (30% of all affected patients), issues with visual perception and astigmatism, talipes equinovarus (clubfoot), congenital hip dysplasia, and spinal alignment defects (kyphosis and scoliosis; Volpe & Inder, 2025). In particular, cognitive deficits are also common with the Chiari II malformation.

Congenital Hydrocephalus. Congenital hydrocephalus is known as *distention of the cerebral ventricles* (Table 3.7). The incidence of congenital hydrocephalus is approximately six per 10,000 live births (Pindrik et al., 2022). Congenital hydrocephalus is categorized as syndromic or nonsyndromic based on whether the hydrocephalus is part of an underlying genetic syndrome (Figure 3.21). Upwards of 70% of all cases of congenital hydrocephalus are associated with other congenital anomalies, including ACC, Dandy–Walker cysts, and aqueductal stenosis (Volpe & Inder, 2025).

Risk factors for the development of congenital hydrocephalus include Dandy–Walker malformation, exposure to excessive radiation, malnutrition and infections (such as toxoplasmosis and CMV) in XX pregnant patients, fetal aqueductal stenosis, congenital cerebral tumors, vein of Galen malformation, and intrauterine IVH (Garne et al., 2010; NORD, 2025b). Brain tumors, trauma, cysts, thrombi, spina bifida, and arteriovenous malformations are other causes of obstructive hydrocephalus.

The pathogenesis of congenital hydrocephalus relates to inhibition of flow of CSF from the cerebral ventricles (area of production) to the systemic circulation (area of absorption). This is a result of X-linked genetic aberrations or altered physiologic CSF function (McAllister, 2012). Ventriculomegaly and the resultant impedance or obstruction to normal flow of CSF alters the physiologic flow of CSF. In this case, ventriculomegaly creates a structural blockade that reduces flow of CSF through the ventricles, to the arachnoid space and cerebral microvasculature.

Congenital hydrocephalus manifests at birth as a constellation of physical findings. Typically, the anterior and posterior fontanelles are full, enlarged, and possibly bulging; cranial sutures are palpably separated. Frontal bossing may be observed. Scalp veins may be distended and bulging (Volpe & Inder, 2025). Ocular prominence (bulging) with a staring expression, with or without the sclera visible above the iris (sunset eyes), may be present. A high-pitched cry may accompany increasing ICP. Other manifestations include lethargy, irritability, poor feeding, and emesis.

Life-span implications correlate with the extent of the disease process, onset of treatment, and other comorbidities. With prompt and adequate neurosurgical evaluation and intervention, 5-year survival rates are more than 80% (Ruge, 2023). Following treatment, morbidities reported in the literature include epilepsy and impaired cognitive function (Persson et al., 2006; Smith & Buckley, 2012).

Microcephaly. Microcephaly is a disorder of neuronal proliferation involving an abnormal reduction in global brain growth. Cranial head circumference measurements are typically 2 to 3 SDs lower in affected infants compared to counterparts of similar gestational age, gender, and ethnicity (Volpe & Inder, 2025). The annual incidence within the United States is estimated to be one in every

TABLE 3.7 Categories of Hydrocephalus

Category	Subcategory	Etiology
Acquired	N/A	Intraventricular hemorrhage Infection/meningitis Tumor/cyst
Congenital	Nonsyndromic	Hydranencephaly
	Syndromic	Craniosynostosis Myelomeningocele Neural tube defect X-linked hydrocephalus

N/A, not applicable.
Source: Adapted from Flanders, T. M., Billinghurst, L., Flibotte, J., & Heuer, G. G. (2018). Neonatal hydrocephalus. *NeoReviews, 19*(8), e467–e477. https://doi.org/10.1542/neo.19-8-e467

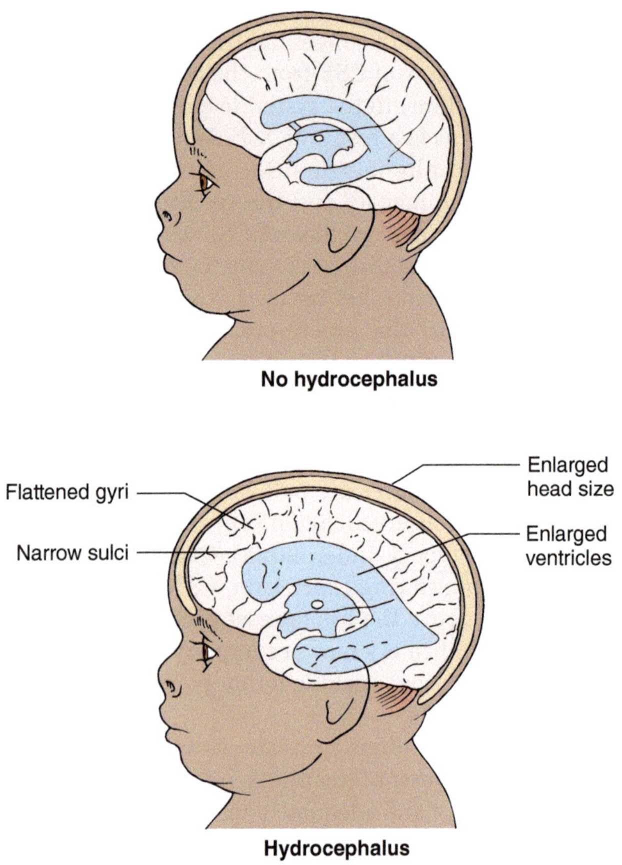

Figure 3.21 Normal infant brain and infant brain with hydrocephalus.

800 to 5,000 live births (CDC, 2025d). In the United States, microcephaly is attributed to infectious causes, such as rubella, toxoplasmosis, or CMV. Noninfectious causes of microcephaly include malnutrition, hypothyroidism, polysubstance abuse, and placental insufficiency in XX pregnant patients.

The pathophysiology of microcephaly involves increased apoptosis or reduced growth proliferation. Primary (true) microcephaly involves disruptions during primary neurulation, causing either dysfunction or death of neural progenitor cells. Secondary microcephaly develops during the postnatal period and involves disruptions to neuronal maturation (Devakumar et al., 2017). The cranial vault is within normal limits at birth but fails to grow and develop properly over time. Consideration of the delivery method is essential for an appropriate assessment of cranial size. Vaginal delivery may compress the skull, impose cranial molding, and cause a transient reduction in head circumference. In these cases, the transient cranial deformity resolves within a few days.

Life-span implications are related to underlying cause and comorbidities; the diagnosis does not automatically confer lifelong neurodevelopmental consequences. Infants with mild cases of microcephaly often exhibit minimal long-term neurodevelopmental complications. More severe forms of microcephaly result in moderate to severe long-term neurodevelopmental complications, including seizures, learning disabilities, and physical disabilities (CDC, 2025d).

Disorders of the Cerebral Vasculature Not Related to Birth Injury

Intraventricular Hemorrhage. Recall that germinal matrices are highly vascularized structures located at the fourth ventricle (subependymal region), cerebellum, and just below the pial surface of the cortex. Because of this, they are considered a preferentially low blood flow structure due to their fragility (Shafer et al., 2025). When reviewing imaging studies, the germinal matrix found around the fourth ventricle can be seen anterior to the choroid plexus, a location referred to as the *caudothalamic groove* (Riddle et al., 2024; Snyder et al., 2022).

This germinal matrix drains into the vein of Galen until it involutes around week 32 of gestation (Perlman, 2022).

IVH refers to a collection of blood within one or more ventricular spaces and often begins within the germinal matrix (GMH-IVH) or subependymal portions of the brain. Given the locus for IVH, it is a common hemorrhagic disorder that primarily affects premature infants. The incidence is inversely related to gestational age and birthweight. Approximately 25% of infants born at less than 32 weeks of gestation or weighing less than 1,500 grams at birth are diagnosed with GMH-IVH that may progress beyond the germinal matrix region (Shafer et al., 2025). Infants weighing less than 750 grams at birth have a 45% to 60% risk of acquiring IVH (Parsons et al., 2016; Volpe & Inder, 2025). In comparison, 3.5% to 4.6% of term infants develop IVH. Risk factors for IVH include gestational age, developmental fragility of germinal matrix vascularity, low birthweight, coagulation disturbances, delivery room resuscitation complications, illness severity, disturbances in CO_2 levels, respiratory distress syndrome, race, male sex, high-frequency ventilation, and fluctuating CBF (Inder et al., 2025; Shafer et al., 2025). The risk for IVH is also increased with multiple-gestation pregnancies because multiple-gestation pregnancies are more likely to result in preterm delivery.

The pathogenesis of IVH is well understood and reconciles the aforementioned risk stratifications. As eluded to earlier in this section, the hemorrhage typically begins with rupture of the thin-walled germinal matrix capillaries. These capillaries are susceptible to rupture because of their large diameter, which offers lesser resistance and resilience amid changes in intravascular pressure (Inder et al., 2025). Fluctuations in CBF (decreases and increases) can precipitate IVH and may occur secondary to hypoxia (or hyperoxia), hypercarbia, and coagulation disorders, as well as hypoglycemia, blood transfusions, rapid use of volume expanders, mechanical ventilation, and tracheal suctioning (Inder et al., 2025).

The majority of IVHs begin within the first 72 hours of life. Approximately 50% of IVH cases begin in the first 24 hours of life, 80% by 48 hours, and 90% by 72 hours of life (Shafer et al., 2025; Volpe & Inder, 2025). In 20% to 40% of cases, the hemorrhage progresses over the following 3 to 5 days. Clinical manifestations include lethargy, apnea, increase in ventilator support, hypotension, poor perfusion, thrombocytopenia, and anemia (Inder et al., 2025; Shafer et al., 2025).

Clinicians may opt to wait to obtain the first cranial ultrasound until day 7 to 10 of life to assess the extent of bleeding, as the hemorrhage is likely to have ceased by this point. Conditions that warrant earlier imaging include hemodynamic instability and severe anemia. The severity of IVH is defined with the use of either the Papile or Volpe grading system (Table 3.8). Using Volpe's classification system, risk thresholds for long-term neurodevelopmental impairment are as follows: Grade I

TABLE 3.8 Methods for Classifying Intraventricular Hemorrhage

Grade of IVH	Volpe	Papile
I	Site: Germinal matrix Degree of hemorrhage within ventricle: 0%–10% Ventricular distention? No	Site: Subependymal matrix Degree of hemorrhage within ventricle: N/A Ventricular distention? N/A
II	Site: Lateral ventricle Degree of hemorrhage within ventricle: 10%–50% Ventricular distention? No	Site: Lateral ventricle Degree of hemorrhage within ventricle: <50% Ventricular distention? No
III	Site: Lateral ventricle(s) Degree of hemorrhage within ventricle: >50% Ventricular distention? Yes	Site: Lateral ventricle(s) Degree of hemorrhage within ventricle: >50% Ventricular distention? Yes
IV	N/A	Site: Subependymal matrix or lateral ventricle(s) Degree of hemorrhage within ventricle: Any Ventricular distention? Absent or any degree of distention Other: Extension of hemorrhage into parenchyma

Note: Dr. Volpe's method states that bleeding into parenchymal tissue is multifactorial and not exclusive to IVH.
IVH, intraventricular hemorrhage.

Sources: Papile, L. A., Burstein, J., Burstein, R., & Koffler, H. (1978). Incidence and evolution of subependymal and intraventricular hemorrhage: A study of infants with birth weights less than 1,500 gm. *Journal of Pediatrics, 92*(4), 529–534. https://doi.org/10.1016/S0022-3476(78)80282-0; Volpe, J. J. (2025). *Volpe's neurology of the newborn* (7th ed.). Elsevier.

(15%), Grade II (25%), Grade III (50%), and Grade III with parenchymal injury (75%; Volpe & Inder, 2025). The implications of IVH across the life span are associated with the severity of IVH and associated comorbidities (Cizmeci & deVries, 2025; Inder et al., 2025; Shafer et al., 2025).

Intracerebellar Hemorrhage. Intracerebellar hemorrhage (ICH) involves bleeding within the cerebellum. Among fetuses, ICH most often occurs between 21 and 26 weeks of gestation; a known risk factor is anemia necessitating an in utero fetal blood transfusion (Limperopoulos et al., 2025). Postnatally, ICH may result from primary bleeding or be caused by the extension of a subarachnoid or GMH-IVH into cerebellar tissues. Approximately 19% of infants weighing less than 1,500 grams and being less than 32 weeks of gestation develop ICH, with infants weighing less than 750 grams at birth considered at highest risk for this type of bleed (Cizmeci & deVries, 2025; Limperopoulos et al., 2025). The prevalence of ICH in term infants is not reported in the literature.

Risk factors include respiratory distress, prematurity, hypoxic birth event, vitamin K deficiency, rapid fluid resuscitation, and complicated instrument-assisted deliveries. The majority of ICH in term infants is precipitated by birth trauma, hypoxic-ischemic injury, or coagulopathies. For preterm infants, risk factors predominantly mirror those of IVH (e.g., intubation, mechanical ventilation greater than 7 days, hypotension, use of volume expanders, high-dose caffeine, Grade III or IV IVH) and are implicated by the immaturity of the vasculature within the cerebellum (Limperopoulos et al., 2025).

The pathogenesis of ICH is not fully understood, but it is believed to be a result of intravascular, vascular, and extravascular insults. Intravascular factors include episodes of pressure-passive CBF, which can cause rupture of vessels in the cerebellum and resultant hemorrhage. Interestingly, the autoregulatory plateau in the cerebellum is narrower than the ventricles, making this region of the brain extremely vulnerable to bleeding (Limperopoulos et al., 2025). In addition, situations that lead to skull compression (e.g., aggressive downward force during bag-mask ventilation) can cause an increase in venous pressure at the back of the skull and lead to hemorrhage at the cerebellum. Vascular factors refer to the vulnerability of the cerebellar vasculature, which is inversely proportional to gestational age at birth. As germinal matrices involute, the vessels become even more fragile and at-risk for rupture. Extravascular factors focus upon the immature nature of the structures which contain the germinal matrix, which in this case is the cerebellum. Limperopoulos and colleagues (2025) characterize the immature cerebellum as "gelatinous," which emphasizes the lack of extravascular structural support and protection offered to the internal vessels.

Clinical manifestations of ICH include motor agitation, respiratory compromise, and apnea. These findings may be associated with brainstem compression (Whitelaw et al., 2016). Other general symptoms of ICH include bradycardia and lateral eye deviation. Life-span implications include possible long-term neurodevelopmental deficits (e.g., motor delays, cerebral palsy), which occur in approximately 30% to 100% of affected preterm infants (Limperopoulos et al., 2025).

Cerebral Artery Ischemic Stroke. The incidence of neonatal strokes is increasing, likely secondary to increased diagnostic testing methods. Formerly, one in 1,600 to 4,000 term neonates were affected per year, but more recent data suggests that one in 1,100 to 4,000 term births are affected (Bernson-Leung & Rivkin, 2016; Rivkin et al., 2025). Upwards of 80% of strokes are classified as ischemic and the balance are caused by a cerebral thrombosis or hemorrhage (Rivkin et al., 2025; Srivastava et al., 2022). The two major classifications for strokes include perinatal arterial ischemic strokes and sinovenous strokes. Perinatal strokes are most often a consequence of developmental vascular abnormalities, but can also be attributed to gene mutations or vasospasm (most commonly from cocaine use). Perinatal arterial ischemic strokes are classified as ischemic insults that lead to focal areas of necrosis within one or more major cerebral arteries. In contrast, sinovenous strokes are classified as ischemic insults that most often occur after birth and lead to focal areas of necrosis within the superior sagittal sinus (65% of cases), lateral sinus, or deep veins (e.g., vein of Galen).

Risk factors for the development of neonatal stroke are multifactorial and include infection, coagulation disorders, preeclampsia, and drug (cocaine) and tobacco use in XX pregnant patients (Bernson-Leung & Rivkin, 2016). Fetal risk factors include congenital heart disease, congenital infection, coagulation disorders, and difficult deliveries that require mechanical force or involve perinatal asphyxia (Rivkin et al., 2025). Postnatal risk factors include systemic or CNS-specific infections, dehydration, congenital heart disease, polycythemia, and coagulation disorders (disseminated intravascular coagulopathy, factor VIII or V deficiency, prothrombin abnormalities; Hielkema & Hadders-Algra, 2016; Sehgal, 2011).

The pathogenesis of cerebral artery infarcts correlates with risk factors. Vascular anomalies, emboli, arterial or venous thrombi, or impaired venous drainage within the periventricular white matter of the brain contribute to the formation of a thrombus and subsequent occlusion and infarct. Congenital heart defects, for example, are often associated with deranged vasculature, which may facilitate the formation of thrombi. Similarly, infections can trigger clotting mechanisms, which increase the risk for thrombi and resultant infarcts. Premature infants often suffer strokes secondary to impaired venous drainage within periventricular regions (Bernson-Leung & Rivkin, 2016; Hielkema & Hadders-Algra, 2016; Rivkin et al., 2025).

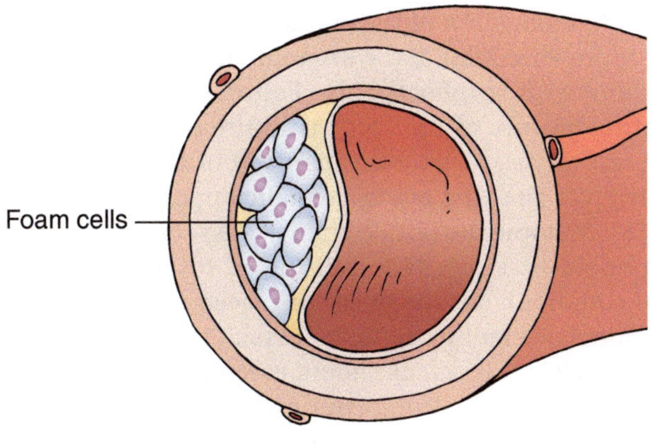

Figure 3.22 Foamy macrophages.

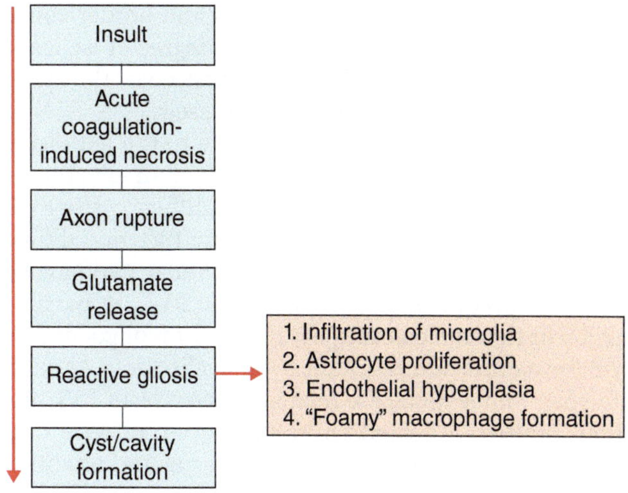

Figure 3.23 Pathogenesis of focal cystic periventricular leukomalacia.

Following the vascular injury, a period of oxidative stress and inflammation precedes necrosis of all affected cells. Within the next 24 hours, monocytes enter the affected space, wedge between vascular endothelial cells, and then migrate into subendothelial spaces. Over the next 24 to 48 hours, the monocytes transform into macrophages, ingest oxidized lipids, and transform into larger, "foamy"-looking cells (Figure 3.22). Release of glial fibrillary acidic protein is initiated, which causes astrocyte hypertrophy. Astroglial proliferation is elicited next as a reactive response to inflammation. This disorganized proliferation produces excessive glial fibrillary cells, which induce tissue reorganization, structural changes, and glial scar formation (Rivkin et al., 2025). In fact, astroglial proliferating cells only differentiate into astrocytes, which stunts the repair of injured tissue. Strategies to "loosen" the dense covering of glial fibrillary processes and promote neurulation and synthesis of oligodendrocytes are necessary to encourage healing (Kratzer et al., 2014).

The most common clinical manifestations of neonatal hemorrhagic stroke include seizures, hypotonia, focal weakness, apnea, encephalopathy, and poor feeding (Armstrong-Wells et al., 2009; Bruno et al., 2013; Cole et al., 2017). Life-span implications vary based on underlying pathology and comorbidities. More than 50% of infants affected by neonatal stroke display normal neurodevelopment in early childhood and beyond. Refractory seizures have been reported in some cases; however, the data is rather antiquated (Cizmeci & deVries, 2025). Cerebral palsy, cognitive disabilities, hemiparesis, hemisensory impairments, and cognitive dysfunction are other long-term complications (Westmacott et al., 2009). That said, approximately one in four premature infants and one in three term infants who suffer a stroke will develop a cognitive disability.

Periventricular Leukomalacia. PVL is a white-matter brain injury characterized by ischemic, necrotic periventricular white matter (Pierson & Volpe, 2025). The incidence of cystic and noncystic PVL is known to be inversely proportional to gestational age; however, sparse publications quantify this relationship. This is likely secondary to variable screening mechanisms and difficulty discerning microscopic lesions with noncystic PVL (Pierson & Volpe, 2025). Risk factors include prematurity, postnatal age greater than 3 days of life, cardiorespiratory disease, IVH, and infection/inflammation (e.g., maternal–placental infections; Pierson & Volpe, 2025; Shafer et al., 2025).

PVL typically affects regions of white matter dorsal and lateral to the lateral ventricles and around the foramen of Monro. The vessel most often implicated is the *middle cerebral artery*. The pathogenesis of PVL begins with necrosis (focal or diffuse) followed by gliosis and one of three possible end results: (a) diffuse white matter gliosis without the formation of cysts or scars; (b) cystic PVL (focal or diffuse), which includes the formation of cysts/cavities; or (c) noncystic PVL, which includes microscopic lesions. Cystic focal PVL is more severe when compared to cystic diffuse PVL (Pierson & Volpe, 2025). The progression pathway for focal cystic PVL is provided in Figure 3.23.

Vascular factors, specifically the anatomic state of the periventricular vessels, contribute to the pathogenesis of PVL. The brains of infants less than 32 weeks of gestation are completing the essential process of angiogenesis, proliferation, and branching of the cerebral vasculature throughout the brain and toward the deeper structures. Immature vessels, as previously described, contain a high number of vulnerable "end zones" and "border zones." These zones are particularly sensitive to changes in CBF and pressure; therefore, they are easily ruptured. From week 32 until term, the cerebral arteries (most notably, the middle cerebral artery) penetrate the brain. Long penetrations target deeper structures and short penetrations target subcortical white matter. This involves the establishment of connections (anastomoses) between vessels and elimination of end zones and border zones. Therefore, the relationship between degree of ischemia and permanent injury is directly influenced by the maturational state of the periventricular vessels.

Biochemical factors also contribute to the pathogenesis of PVL. Focal cystic PVL has less of an effect upon white matter volume as compared to diffuse cystic PVL. Diffuse cystic PVL as well as noncystic PVL and diffuse gliosis are associated with reduced cellular pathologies. Typical consequences of diffuse cystic PVL, in particular, include ventriculomegaly, reduced preoligodendrocyte formation, and resultant hypomyelination. As such, life-span implications are related to the type of PVL and comorbidities. Affected children may experience cognitive and visual impairment; behavioral and attention disorders; and motor deficits, including spastic diplegia. Motor deficits may improve with less severe cases of PVL (Pierson & Volpe, 2025; Shafer et al., 2025).

Disorders of the Cerebral Vasculature Related to Birth Injury

Hypoxic Ischemic Encephalopathy. See Chapter 14.

Disorders of Skull Development

Craniosynostosis. Craniosynostosis (craniostenosis) involves premature closure of one or more cranial sutures. More specifically, premature closure of a single suture line (nonsyndromic) or multiple (syndromic) closures may be observed. Although rare, syndromic craniosynostosis may present alongside birth defects and in the absence of a complementary syndrome (Fulton et al., 2024). Craniosynostosis occurs in one out of every 2,000 to 2,500 live births with a prevalence reported among males (Cornelissen et al., 2016). Risk factors include fetal tobacco and drug exposure, as well as rickets, idiopathic hypercalcemia, and hypophosphatemia.

Errors within gene-mediated signaling pathways, as well as environmental factors (intrinsic and extrinsic), are root causes for nonsyndromic cases of craniosynostosis (Katsianou et al., 2016). An intricate discussion of gene-mediated factors is beyond the scope of this textbook; however, mutations with the *EphrinA-4, FGFR*, and *TWIST-1* genes have been identified. Environmental factors include valproate ingestion, tobacco and drug use in XX pregnant patients, and compression of the developing skull during fetal growth. Regardless of the underlying pathobiology, premature fusion of a suture prevents growth of the affected cranial bones perpendicular to the fused site (Fulton et al., 2024). As a result, the brain compensates by growing in alternative directions. Over time, this distorts the shape of the skull and can lead to facial deformities, ocular and auditory malformations, and potential neurodevelopmental impairment (Twigg & Wilkie, 2015).

The most common form of craniosynostosis involves premature closure of the sagittal (midline) suture and is reported in 40% to 55% of all cases; a male prevalence is reported. This type of premature closure leads to elongation of the cranial contour in the anteroposterior direction and commonly manifests as frontal bossing with scaphocephaly (Fulton et al., 2024). Premature closure of the coronal suture occurs in 20% to 25% of all cases; lateral expansion of the cranial contour gives rise to a brachycephalic appearance (Figure 3.24). Metopic fusion accounts for 14% of cases. Finally, lambdoid fusion is reported in 3% to 5% of all cases and commonly results in ear displacement as well as an asymmetric skull base (Cornelissen et al., 2016; Fulton et al., 2024). Clinicians should carefully distinguish between benign skull deformities from pathologic skull deformities. Positional plagiocephaly is a benign form of cranial contour alteration that occurs secondary to supine positioning at rest (Ruge, 2023). Cranial contour may be flattened in the occipital or lateral regions of the skull.

Life-span implications are related to the number of sutures involved, onset of monitoring and treatment, genetic involvement, and additional comorbidities. Early surgical involvement reduces chronic increased ICP and reduces the risk for long-term neurologic damage. Custom-molded padded helmets are typically used to reshape the cranial contour of infants affected by positional plagiocephaly (benign). These infants often suffer no long-term neurologic dysfunction.

Neurologic Disorders

Hypotonia. Hypotonia, or "floppy baby syndrome," is the state of low muscle tone or reduced muscle strength. It is a manifestation of diseases or disorders that affect any level of the nervous system. The incidence of hypotonia varies based on the primary, underlying problem. Common etiologies are summarized in Table 3.9.

It is important to understand that hypotonia is not a primary problem—hypotonia is the result of an underlying disorder or disease process. Given the long list of primary problems manifested with hypotonia, and the range of subtle to severe weaknesses that can be observed among neonates, distinguishing the underlying pathology for the single manifestation of hypotonia (excluding all other manifestations of the primary problem) can be a daunting task.

Clinicians often find themselves asking, "What disruption in homeostasis is causing the baby to present with weakness?" Begin by recognizing that hypotonia occurs due to an injury *above* or *below* the lower motor neuron (Figure 3.25). Upper motor neurons synapse onto lower motor neurons located in the ventral horn of the spinal cord. Lower motor neurons project from their spinal origins onto muscles (at neuromuscular junctions) to create muscle contraction (motor responses). This gives rise to the sensory–motor feedback system, best explained as it applies to active muscle contraction.

Muscle contraction (active muscle tone) is modulated by way of a feedback loop between upper and lower

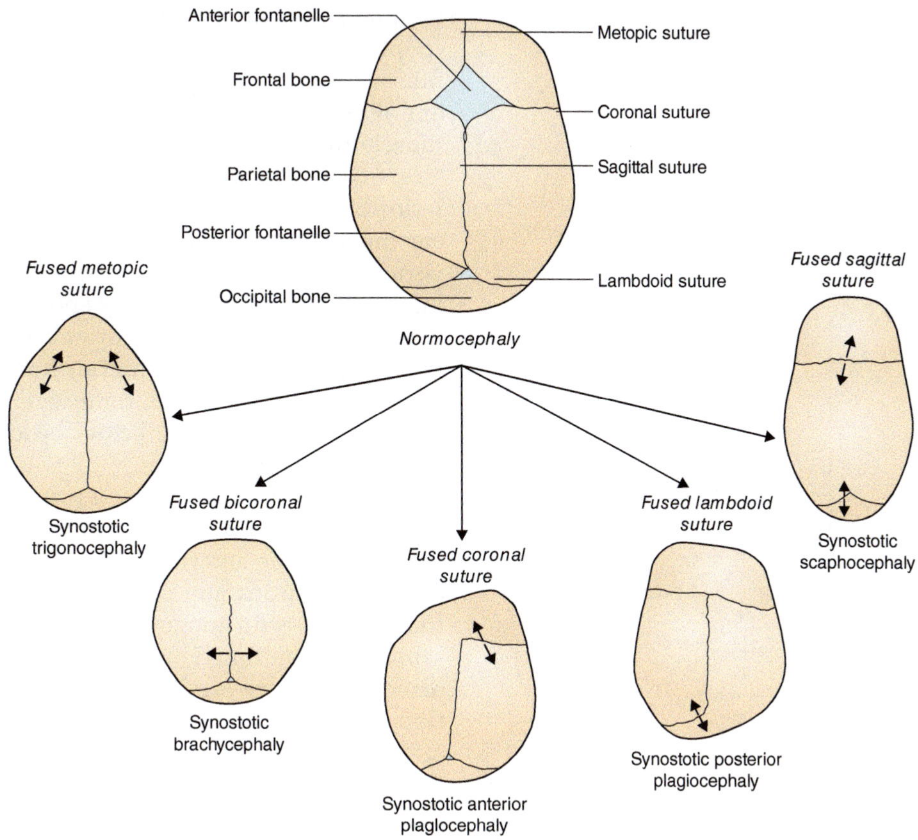

Figure 3.24 Different forms of craniosynostosis, indicating the premature fusion of one (or more) cranial sutures.
Source: Adapted from Shah, P. J. (2023). Craniosynostosis: A congenital anomaly. In U. Saha (Ed.), *Clinical anesthesia for the newborn and the neonate* (pp. 829–835). Springer International Publishing. https://link.springer.com/chapter/10.1007/978-981-19-5458-0_43

TABLE 3.9 Hypotonia as a Manifestation of Common Problems

System	Primary Disease Process
CNS	Hypoxic–ischemic encephalopathy, bilirubin-induced neurologic dysfunction, meningitis, encephalitis, motor neuron lesions, cerebellar lesions and palsies, spinal nerve and muscle disorders
Respiratory	Congenital hypothyroidism, cerebral palsy, teratogenesis
Gastrointestinal	Dehydration, hyperbilirubinemia
Metabolic/Endocrine	Hypoglycemia, hypermagnesemia, inborn errors of metabolism
Immune	Sepsis
Genetic	22q13 deletion syndrome, achondroplasia, CHARGE syndrome, Down syndrome (trisomy 21), trisomy 18, Fragile X syndrome, Marfan syndrome, myotonic dystrophy,[a] Noonan syndrome, Prader–Willi syndrome, Smith–Lemli Opitz syndrome, Williams syndrome, Zellweger syndrome
Other	Autoimmune disorders[a] in the XX pregnant patient

[a]Myotonic dystrophy is the most common inherited disorder associated with progressive muscle wasting and weakness. Myasthenia gravis is the most common maternal autoimmune disorder associated with neonatal hypotonia.
CHARGE, coloboma, heart defects, atresia choanae (choanal atresia), growth retardation, genital abnormalities, and ear abnormalities; CNS, central nervous system.
Sources: Bass, N. (2025). Hypotonia and neuromuscular disease in the neonate. In R. J. Martin & A. A. Fanaroff (Eds.), *Fanaroff and Martin's neonatal-perinatal medicine: Diseases of the fetus and infant* (12th ed., pp. 1117–1131). Elsevier Mosby; Natarajan, N., & Ionita, C. (2024). Neonatal neuromuscular disorders. In C. A. Gleason & S. E. Juul (Eds.), *Avery's diseases of the newborn* (11th ed., pp. 854–861). Elsevier; Sparks, E. S. (2015). Neonatal hypotonia. *Clinics in Perinatology, 42*(2), 363–371. https://doi.org/10.1016/j.clp.2015.02.008; Volpe, J. J. & Inder, T. E. (Eds). (2025). *Volpe's neurology of the newborn* (7th ed.). Elsevier.

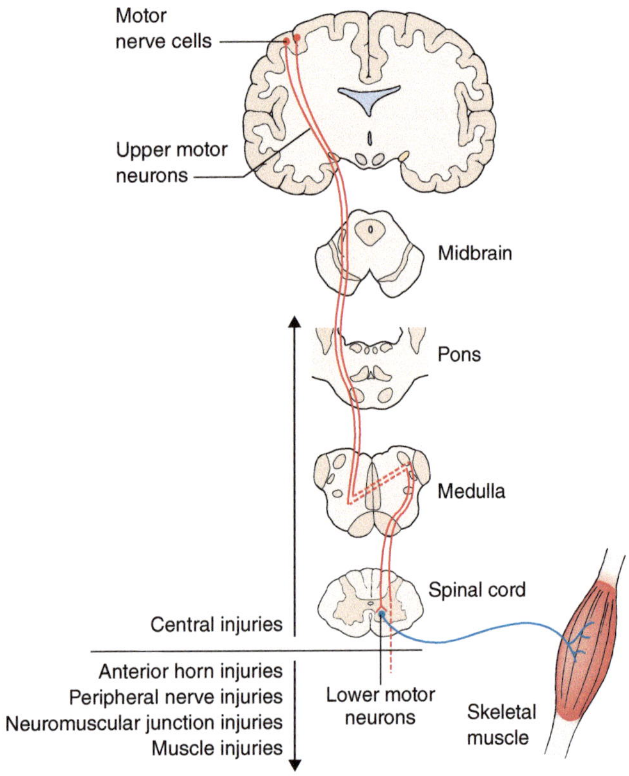

Figure 3.25 Upper and lower motor neurons.

motor neurons and begins with sensory inputs. Sensory inputs are sent via afferent pathways to the upper motor neurons. Upper motor neurons send efferent communications to alpha motor neurons in the ventral horn of the spinal cord, which elicit muscle contraction. Once adequate contraction is achieved, stretch reflexes become deactivated, completing this feedback loop. Active tone can be assessed with the pull-to-sit maneuver in infants. The infant is slowly pulled up to a sitting position. Under normal circumstances, the elbows will flex and the neck will raise the head (a normal feedback system with muscle contraction). In cases of hypotonia, the head will lag backward during the pull-to-sit, and once the infant is in a sitting position, the head will fall forward (altered feedback system with no muscle contraction). Postnatally, muscle cells increase in size, which correlates with progressively increasing muscle strength. Simultaneously, myelination of sensory (afferent) pathways modulates maturation of the motor cortex. The cumulative result is progressive maturation of neuromuscular feedback loops and muscle strength (Darras & Volpe, 2025; Volpe & El-Dib, 2025).

Passive tone refers to muscle resistance to passive movements during manipulation, and passive tone wanes as active tone increases. Passive motor tone is appraised during the birth hospitalization and remains evident during the first few months of life. Careful assessment of tone can alert the clinician to areas of weakness (hypotonia). Wrist (square window) and knee (popliteal angle) flexibility is an assessment of neuromuscular response to extensor stretch reflex responses and muscle tone of the arms and legs. Similarly, flexor muscle tone at the shoulder is assessed by way of the "scarf sign." Competency of stretch reflexes at the posterior hip flexor muscle are measured using the heel-to-ear maneuver. Facial muscle competency is appraised visually. Weakness in the arms, legs, and facial regions informs the location of injury and pathogenesis of neonatal hypotonia. Central injuries occur above the lower motor neuron, whereas anterior horn cell injuries, peripheral nerve injuries, neuromuscular junction injuries, and muscle injuries occur below the lower motor neuron (Darras & Volpe, 2025).

Central hypotonia implies a primary problem within the CNS and may manifest with seizures or hemiparesis. Disorders of the anterior horn cells involve dysfunction of motor neurons and commonly manifest with hypotonia paired with tongue fasciculations and areflexia; sensory system function is unaffected. Peripheral nerve disorders involve a reduction in motor nerve conduction, most often caused by reduced or absent myelination to peripheral nerves; sensory function is absent. Neuromuscular junction disorders involve altered communication (synapses) between motor neurons and skeletal muscle fibers. Muscle disorders impose muscle weakness, as the name suggests (Ahmed et al., 2016; Darras & Volpe, 2025).

Ultimately, in order to reverse or decrease muscle function, treatment must be directed toward correcting the primary, underlying problem. As such, life-span implications correlate with the primary problem. Hypotonia in tandem with central disorders is associated with neurodevelopmental impairment (Darras & Volpe, 2025).

Seizures. Neonatal seizures affect approximately 5 to 15 per 1,000 preterm infants of very-low-birthweight and 1 to 3.5 per 1,000 term infants; poor interrater reliability, reporting mechanisms, and hospital settings may affect these rates (Abend et al., 2025; Kayyal & Inder, 2025). Major risk factors are summarized in Box 3.3.

Recall that a seizure occurs when neurons located within the CNS depolarize in excess. Depolarization requires adenosine triphosphate (ATP), an influx of sodium ions, and resultant egress of potassium ions out of the neuron in the setting of an imbalance of excitatory and inhibitory neurotransmitters (Abend et al., 2025). Several mechanisms increase the likelihood for this to occur and include (a) failed ATP-pump activity, (b) an excess of excitatory neurotransmitters, (c) a deficiency of inhibitory neurotransmitters, or (d) an inherited inborn error of metabolism (Abend et al., 2025). Failed ATP-pump activity disrupts membrane potential. Excessive amounts of excitatory neurotransmitters provoke

BOX 3.3 Risk Factors for Onset of Neonatal Seizures

- Asphyxia
- Benign familial origin
- Congenital brain malformations
- Congenital infections
- Hypocalcemia
- Hypoglycemia
- Inborn errors of metabolism
- Neonatal abstinence syndrome
- Neonatal stroke

Sources: Kayyal, S., & Inder, T. E. (2025). Seizures in neonates. In R. J. Martin & A. A. Fanaroff (Eds.), *Fanaroff and Martin's neonatal-perinatal medicine: Diseases of the fetus and infant* (12th ed. pp. 1085–1116). Elsevier Mosby; Shafer, G. J. D. C., Vu Tran, J. S., & Inder, T. E. (2025). Neonatal brain disorders. In A. A. Fanaroff & J. M. Fanaroff (Eds.), *Klaus & Fanaroff's care of the high risk neonate* (8th ed., pp. 340-361). Elsevier Mosby; Volpe, J. J., Inder, T. E., Darras, B. T., de Vries, L. S., du Plessis, A. J., Neil, J. J., & Perlman, J. M. (2025). *Volpe's neurology of the newborn* (7th ed.). Elsevier.

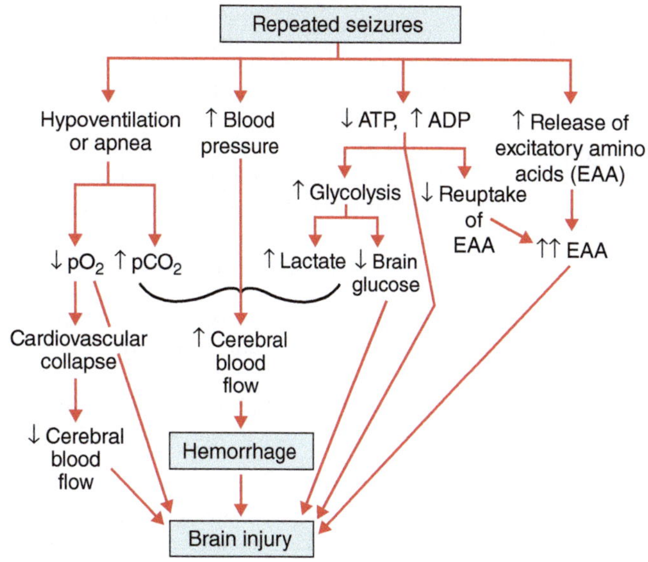

Figure 3.26 Energy metabolism.
ADP, adenosine diphosphate; ATP, adenosine triphosphate.
Source: Volpe, J. J., & Inder, T. E. (Eds.). (2025). *Volpe's neurology of the newborn* (7th ed.). Elsevier.

increased depolarization. GABA, which functions in an exclusive inhibitory capacity in the adult brain, functions in both capacities in the neonatal brain. Furthermore, levels of inhibitory GABA fall short of excitatory GABA levels in the neonatal brain; inhibitory GABA transmitters are also permeable to calcium (Abend et al., 2025; Kayyal & Inder, 2025).

The pathway evoked during a neonatal seizure, activated to metabolize energy to compensate for energy expenditure, is summarized in **Figure 3.26**. Upon review of the pathway, it is clear that glucose is an essential energy source during a seizure, and excessive glucose metabolism will increase the synthesis of lactate (a classic by-product of glucose metabolism). It is common for infants with prolonged and refractory seizures to consume available glucose and glycogen stores and develop a lactic acidosis secondary to the use of alternative energy sources. In situations where the available supply of energy does not match demand, insufficient energy metabolism becomes a mechanism for injury.

Other consequences of seizures that are correlated with injury include (a) hypoventilation, (b) hypertension, and (c) increased release of excitatory amino acids (Abend et al., 2025). Hypoventilation and apnea are commonly observed during prolonged seizures. This causes hypoxia and hypercarbia, which can decrease CBF and provoke injury. Alternatively, hypertension has also been observed, which can increase CBF and increase the risk for IVH with resulting seizures. Excessive release of amino acids (glutamate) serves as a noxious stimulant, similar to the noxious effect that GABA receptors impose preseizure, and may provoke injury.

Seizures may be visible yet undetectable on EEG (clinical only), visible and detectable on EEG (electroclinical), or not clinically visible yet detectable on EEG (subclinical; Hirsch et al., 2021). The types of seizures that may be observed among neonates include subtle (most common), clonic, myoclonic, and tonic seizures. These seizures may be focal, multifocal, or generalized (**Table 3.10**). Life-span implications of neonatal seizures are related to the underlying etiology. Commonly reported consequences include cognitive disability, cerebral palsy, motor deficits, and epilepsy (Abend et al., 2025; Kayyal & Inder, 2025).

Long-term consequences of seizure activity are stratified based upon if the seizures were intermittent and recurrent versus prolonged. Brief and recurrent seizures are associated with long-term cognitive deficits which occur because of developmental abnormalities of affected neurons primarily located within the hippocampus as well as an increased risk for epilepsy. The exact time frame that defines "prompt" treatment remains elusive. Prolonged seizures are associated with permanent cell loss, which occurs in part because the length of the seizure precipitates apnea, hypercapnia, and hypoxemia. Hypercapnia causes an initial increase in CBF (an adaptive response) but this increase in flow threatens the health of vascular matrices (e.g., germinal matrix) and can induce a hemorrhage. Over time, prolonged hypoxemia leads to ischemic injury and myocardial dysfunction, which decreases CBF and depletes energy sources (e.g., ATP), leading to additional brain injury. *Importantly, prompt treatment of seizure activity with supplemental glucose and antiepileptic medications (e.g., phenobarbital) can*

TABLE 3.10 Types of Seizures and Associated Clinical Manifestations

Type	Common Clinical Manifestations
Clonic[a]	*Focal:* Rhythmic jerking movements of face, upper/lower extremities (bilateral), or neck/trunk (unilateral) *Multifocal:* Rhythmic jerking movements of two or more body parts *Generalized:* Bilateral and symmetric synchronous movements
Myoclonic[a,b]	*Myoclonus:* Rapid, focal jerking of one or more muscle groups (commonly in upper extremities); may or may not be ictal *Multifocal:* Irregular twitching of several parts of the body *Generalized:* Bilateral jerking with flexion of upper limbs
Subtle[a,c]	Lip smacking, fluttering of one or both eyelids, horizontal eye deviation, excessive drooling, episodes of apnea or bradycardia, and abnormal extremity movements (such as stepping, leg rowing, and pedaling motions)
Tonic[a]	*Focal:* Prolonged posturing of one body part (arm, leg, neck, or trunk) *Generalized:* Extension of upper and lower limbs, flexion of upper limb with extension of lower limb

[a]clinically evident; [b]associated with epilepsy; [c]most common.
Source: Volpe, J. J., & Inder, T. E. (Eds.). (2025). *Volpe's neurology of the newborn* (7th ed.). Elsevier.

reduce the incidence of long-term deficits and epilepsy (Abend et al., 2025).

CONCLUSION

The nervous system is one of the most complex and integrated systems in the human body; it communicates with other body systems to maintain physiologic homeostasis. Postnatal neurologic function is largely dependent on a process of systematic and uncomplicated embryologic and fetal development. Environmental and genetic factors, along with myriad health influences in XX pregnant patients, may lead to alterations in embryologic development resulting in lifelong neurologic sequelae. Fetal neurologic development begins with primary neurulation (week 3 of gestation) and continues in sequence with prosencephalic differentiation, neuronal proliferation and migration (complete by 24 weeks), glial proliferation and migration, neuronal organization and migration (complete in early childhood), and neuronal myelination (complete in adulthood). The sequential process is most vulnerable during the first and second trimesters of fetal development; alterations may lead to disorders of early brain development (e.g., anencephaly, encephalocele, spina bifida, congenital hydrocephalus, and microcephaly). Cerebral vascular injuries (e.g., intraventricular and ICH, cerebral artery infarction, PVL) may result in a wide range of mild to severe neurodevelopmental short- and long-term complications. Other neurologic complications (e.g., seizures, hypotonia) may further affect long-term prognoses and prove a management challenge for families and healthcare providers following discharge from the NICU.

LEARNING TOOLS AND RESOURCES

CourseConnect

To access self-assessment questions and interactive, competency-based learning activities for this chapter, visit www.springerpub.com/courseconnect. See inside front cover and tear-out card for CourseConnect details.

Podcast

This podcast is available online by visiting www.springerpub.com/courseconnect. See inside front cover and tear-out card for CourseConnect details.

Infant Sleep-Wake Pattern
Jenna Meredith and Amy J. Jnah

Discussion Prompts

1. A former 24-week gestation infant, now 6 weeks old, receives a routine cranial ultrasound. Multiple periventricular cysts are noted on coronal view ultrasound imaging, consistent with PVL. Explain the relationship between PVL and spastic diplegia, the most common clinical sequela, and the effect upon the infant across the life span.
2. Recent research has shown that the environment in which the premature infant is exposed has influences on growth and development of the nervous system. The current standard of care for NICU design is the single family room; however, there are many open-bay style NICUs that still exist. Discuss the advantages of the single family room design, and which standard of care practices could be implemented into the open-bay style NICU in order to achieve best neurodevelopmental outcome.

MIND MAP

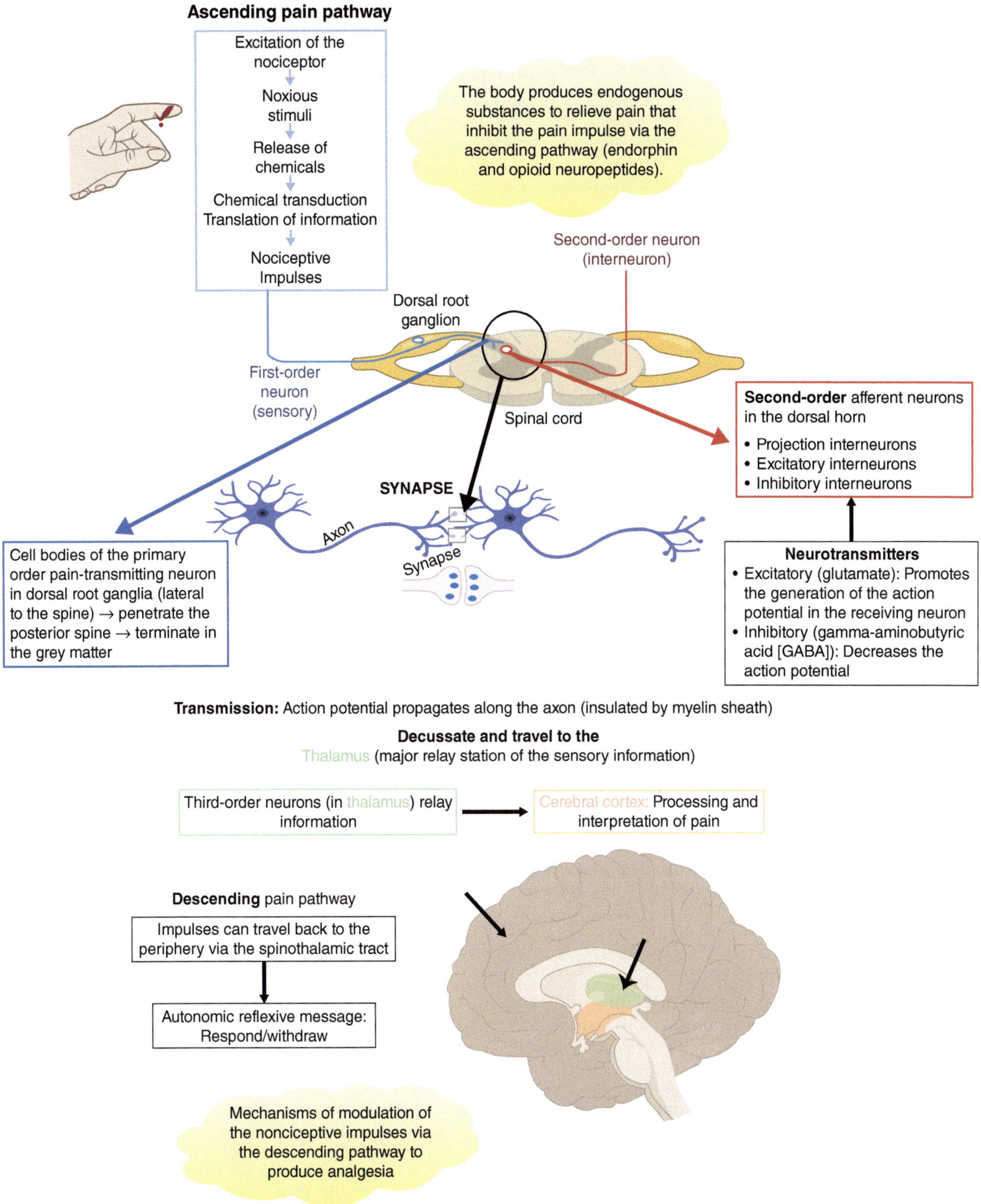

Note: *This mind map reflects one neonatal nurse practitioner student's interpretation of a concept addressed in this chapter. Readers should regard the mind maps woven throughout this textbook as examples of multisensory study tools that can be developed to aid conceptual understanding. Readers are encouraged to develop their own unique mind maps in consultation with academic faculty or clinical preceptors.*

Design Credit: Kerri Rassa, MSN, NNP, RNC-NIC, C-ELBW.

TIMELINE OF ORGAN DEVELOPMENT

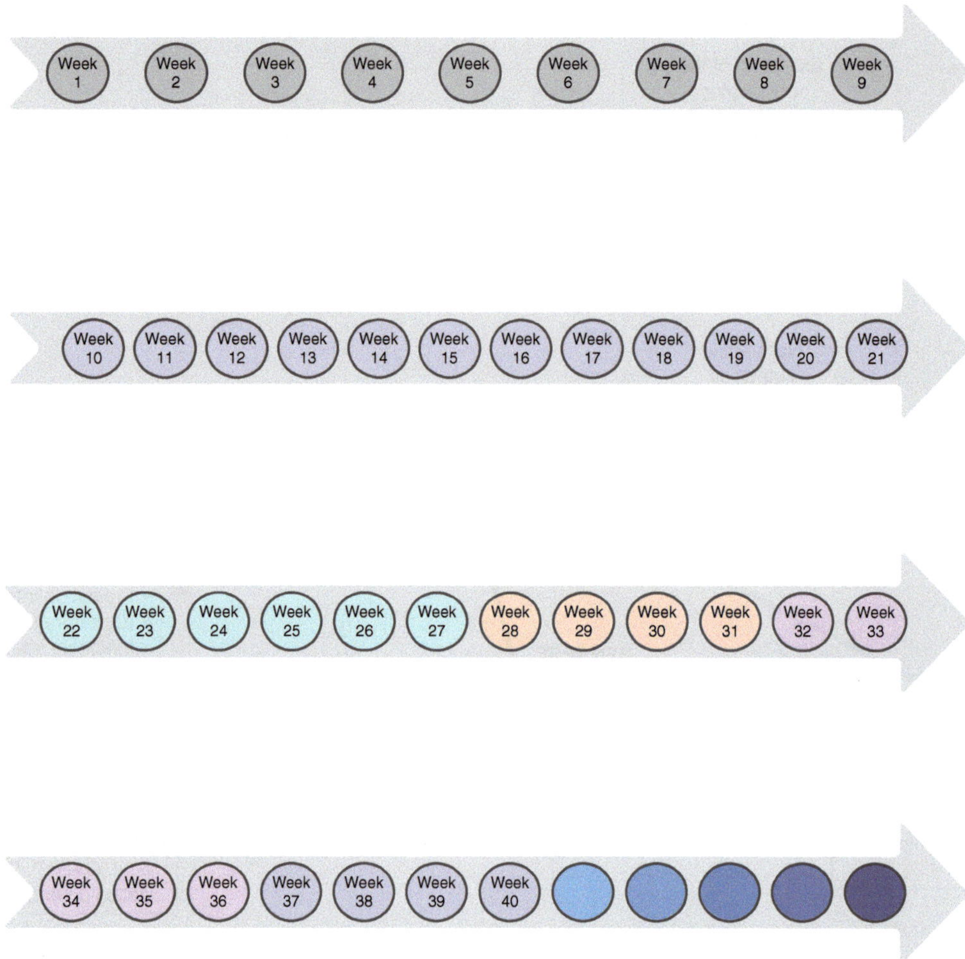

Note: Placement of common problems is meant to offer visual/ conceptual perspective on the timing of onset of these commonly reported malformations. Variation exists across the literature.	*Legend:* <22–27 6/7 weeks = extremely preterm 28–31 6/7 weeks = very preterm 32–36 6/7 weeks = late/moderate preterm 37–40 weeks = term

Note: Readers are encouraged to annotate the blank timeline during studying, self-directed learning, and with the help of mentors. To access the blank and completed timelines visit www.springerpub.com/courseconnect. See inside front cover and tear-out card for CourseConnect details.

REFERENCES

Abend N.S., Wusthoff, C.J., Jensen, F.E., Inder, T.E., & Volpe, J.J. (2025). Neonatal seizures. In J. J. Volpe & T. E. Inder (Eds.), *Volpe's neurology of the newborn* (7th ed., pp. 381–448). Elsevier.

Abramowicz, A., & Gos, M. (2014). Neurofibromin in neurofibromatosis type 1 mutations in *NF1* gene as a cause of disease. *Developmental Period Medicine, 18*(3), 297–306. https://www.ncbi.nlm.nih.gov/pubmed/25182393

Ahmed, M.I., Iqbal, M., & Hussain, N. (2016). A structured approach to the assessment of a floppy neonate. *Journal of Pediatric Neurosciences, 11*(2), 2-6. doi:10.4103/1817-1745.181250

Alberts, B. (2022). *Molecular biology of the cell* (7th ed.). W.W. Norton.

American Association of Neurological Surgeons. (2024). *Spina bifida*. https://www.aans.org/patients/conditions-treatments/spina-bifida

American College of Obstetricians and Gynecologists. (2017). *Neural tube defects* (ACOG Practice Bulletin No. 187). Author. https://www.acog.org/clinical/clinical-guidance/practice-bulletin/articles/2017/12/neural-tube-defects

Anand, K. J. (2000). Pain, plasticity, and premature birth: A prescription for permanent suffering? *Nature Medicine, 6*(9), 971–973. https://doi.org/10.1038/79658

Anderson, K.N., Ailes, E.C., Danielson, M., Lind, J.N., Farr, S.L., Broussard, C.S., & Tinker, S.C. (2018). Attention-Deficit/hyperactivity disorder mediation prescription claims among privately insured women aged 15–44 years - United States 2003–2015. *CDC Morbidity and Mortality Weekly Report, 67*(2). doi:10.15585/mmwr.mm6702a3

Armstrong-Wells, J., Johnston, S. C., Wu, Y. W., Sidney, S., & Fullerton, H. J. (2009). Prevalence and predictors of perinatal hemorrhagic stroke: Results from the Kaiser pediatric stroke study. *Pediatrics, 123*(3), 823–828. https://doi.org/10.1542/peds.2008-0874

Austin, T. (2012). 104 cerebral autoregulation in the newborn. *Archives of Disease in Childhood, 97*(Suppl. 2), A29. https://doi.org/10.1136/archdischild-2012-302724.0104

Bada, H. S., Westgate, P. M., Sithisarn, T., Yolton, K., Charnigo, R., Pourcyrous, M., Tang, F., Gibson, J., Shearer-Miller, J., Giannone, P., & Leggas, M. (2024). Clonidine as monotherapy for neonatal opioid withdrawal syndrome: A randomized trial. *Pediatrics, 154*(5), e2023065610. https://doi.org/10.1542/peds.2023-065610

Barbas, H. (2015). General cortical and special prefrontal connections: Principles from structure to function. *Annual Review of Neuroscience, 38*(1), 269–289. https://doi.org/10.1146/annurev-neuro-071714-033936

Benitz, W. E., & Smith, P. B. (2024). *Neonatology questions and controversies: Infectious disease, immunology, and pharmacology* (2nd ed.). Elsevier.

Benninger, K. L., McAllister, J. M., & Merhar, S. L. (2023). Neonatal opioid withdrawal syndrome: An update on developmental outcomes. *Clinics in Perinatology, 50*(1), 17–29. https://doi.org/10.1016/j.clp.2022.10.007

Bernson-Leung, M. E., & Rivkin, M. J. (2016). Stroke in neonates and children. *Pediatrics in Review, 37*(11), 463–477. https://doi.org/10.1542/pir.2016-0002

Børch, K., Lou, H. C., & Greisen, G. (2010). Cerebral white matter blood flow and arterial blood pressure in preterm infants. *Acta Paediatrica, 99*(10), 1489–1492. https://doi.org/10.1111/j.1651-2227.2010.01856.x

Boron, W. F., & Boulpaep, E. L. (2017). *Medical physiology* (3rd ed.). Elsevier.

Brew, N., Walker, D., & Wong, F. Y. (2014). Cerebral vascular regulation and brain injury in preterm infants. *American Journal of Physiology. Regulatory, Integrative and Comparative Physiology, 306*(11), R773–R786. https://doi.org/10.1152/ajpregu.00487.2013

Brewer, C. L., & Baccei, M. L. (2020). The development of pain circuits and unique effects of neonatal injury. *Journal of Neural Transmission, 127*(4), 467–479. https://doi.org/10.1007/s00702-019-02059-z

Brinker, T., Stopa, E., Morrison, J., & Klinge, P. (2014). A new look at cerebrospinal fluid circulation. *Fluids and Barriers of the CNS, 11*, 10. https://doi.org/10.1186/2045-8118-11-10

Brown, T. I., Uncapher, M. R., Chow, T. E., Eberhardt, J. L., & Wagner, A. D. (2017). Cognitive control, attention, and the other race effect in memory. *PLoS One, 12*(3), e0173579. https://doi.org/10.1371/journal.pone.0173579

Bruno, C. J., Beslow, L. A., Witmer, C. M., Vossough, A., Jordan, L. C., Zelonis, S., Licht, D. J., Ichord, R. N., & Smith, S. E. (2013). Haemorrhagic stroke in term and late preterm neonates. *Archives of Diseases in Childhood, Fetal and Neonatal Edition, 99*(1), F48–F53. https://doi.org/10.1136/archdischild-2013-304068

Campbell, C., Levin, S., Siu, V. M., Venance, S., & Jacob, P. (2013). Congenital myotonic dystrophy: Canadian population-based surveillance study. *Journal of Pediatrics, 163*(1), 120–125. https://doi.org/10.1016/j.jpeds.2012.12.070

Canavese, F., & Dimeglio, A. (2013). Normal and abnormal spine and thoracic cage development. *World Journal of Orthopedics, 4*(4), 167–174. https://doi.org/10.5312/wjo.v4.i4.167

Carlson, B. M. (2024). *Human embryology and developmental biology* (7th ed.). Elsevier/Saunders.

Carrel, A. L., Lee, P. D. K., & Mogul, H. R. (2022). Growth hormone and Prader-Willi syndrome. In M. G. Butler, P. D. K. Lee, & B. Y. Whitman (Eds.), *Management of Prader-Willi syndrome* (pp. 195–216). Springer International Publishing. https://doi.org/10.1007/978-3-030-98171-6_7

Centers for Disease Control and Prevention. (2024a). *About alcohol use during pregnancy.* https://www.cdc.gov/alcohol-pregnancy/about/index.html

Centers for Disease Control and Prevention. (2024b). *Facts about encephalocele.* https://www.cdc.gov/ncbddd/birthdefects/encephalocele.html#ref

Centers for Disease Control and Prevention. (2025a). *Fragile X syndrome (FXS).* https://www.cdc.gov/ncbddd/fxs/index.html

Centers for Disease Control and Prevention. (2025b). *About opioid use during pregnancy.* https://www.cdc.gov/overdose-prevention/hcp/clinical-care/opioid-use-and-pregnancy.html

Centers for Disease Control and Prevention. (2025c). *Cannabis and public health: Cannabis and pregnancy.* https://www.cdc.gov/cannabis/health-effects/pregnancy.html

Centers for Disease Control and Prevention. (2025d). *Microcephaly.* https://www.cdc.gov/birth-defects/about/microcephaly.html

Centers for Disease Control and Prevention. (2025e). *Spina bifida: Data and statistics.* https://www.cdc.gov/spina-bifida/data/index.html

Chatterton, Z., Hartley, B. J., Seok, M., Mendelev, N., Chen, S., Milekic, M., Rosoklija, G., Stankov, A., Trencevsja-Ivanovska, I., Brennand, K., Ge, Y., Dwork, A. J., & Haghighi, F. (2017). In utero exposure to maternal smoking is associated with DNA methylation alterations and reduced neuronal content in the developing fetal brain. *Epigenetics & Chromatin, 10*(1), e1–e11. https://doi.org/10.1186/s13072-017-0111-y

Chen, H. (2012). *Atlas of genetic diagnosis and counseling* (2nd ed.). Springer Verlag.

Cinalli, G., Mirone, G., Spennato, P., & Nastro, A. (n.d.). *Aqueductal stenosis in children.* https://www.ispn.guide/hydrocephalus-and-other-anomalies-of-csf-circulation-in-children/aqueductal-stenosis-in-children-homepage

Cinalli, G., Spennato, P., Nastro, A., Aliberti, F., Trischitta, V., Ruggiero, C., Mirone, G., & Cianciulli, E. (2011). Hydrocephalus in aqueductal stenosis. *Childs Nervous System, 27*(10), 1621–1642. https://doi.org/10.1007/s00381-011-1546-2

Cizmeci, M. N., & deVries, L. (2025). Intracranial hemorrhage and stroke in the neonate. In R. J. Martin & A. A. Fanaroff (Eds.), *Fanaroff and Martin's neonatal-perinatal medicine: Diseases of the fetus and infant* (12th ed., pp. 1059–1084). Elsevier Mosby.

Cole, L., Dewey, D., Letourneau, N., Kaplan, B. J., Chaput, K., Gallagher, C., Hodge, J., Floer, A., & Kirton, A. (2017). Clinical characteristics, risk factors, and outcomes associated with neonatal hemorrhagic stroke: A population-based case-control study. *JAMA Pediatrics, 171*(3), 230–238. https://doi.org/10.1001/jamapediatrics.2016.4151

Copel, J. (2018). *Obstetric imaging: Fetal diagnosis and care E-book* (2nd ed.). Elsevier.

Cornelissen, M., Ottelander, B., Rizopoulos, D., van der Hulst, R., Mink van der Molen, A. M., van der Horst, C., Delye, H., van Veelen, M-.L., Bonsel, G., & Mathijssen, I. (2016). Increase of prevalence of craniosynostosis. *Journal of Cranio-Maxillofacial Surgery, 44*(9), 1273–1279. https://doi.org/10.1016/j.jcms.2016.07.007

Darras, B. T., & Volpe, J. J. (2025). Evaluation, special studies. In J. J. Volpe & T. E. Inder (Eds.), *Volpe's neurology of the newborn* (7th ed., pp. 1011–1024). Elsevier.

Davidson, M. R., London, M. L., & Ladewig, P. A. (2023). *Olds' maternal-newborn nursing & women's health across the lifespan* (12th ed.). Pearson.

Dean, B., & Doherty, D. (2024). Congenital malformations of the central nervous system. In C. A. Gleason & T. Sawyer (Eds.), *Avery's diseases of the newborn* (pp. 787–808.e6). Elsevier. https://doi.org/10.1016/B978-0-323-82823-9.00053-2

Dekker, G. (2011). Hypertension. In D. James, P. Steer, C. Weiner, & B. Gonik (Eds.), *High risk pregnancy: Management options* (4th ed.). Elsevier.

Devakumar, D., Bamford, A., Ferreira, M. U., Broad, J. M., Rosch, R. E., Groce, N., Breuer, J., Cardoso, M. A., Copp, A. J., Alexandre, P., Rodrigues, L. C., & Abubakar, I. (2017). Infectious causes of microcephaly: Epidemiology, pathogenesis, diagnosis, and management. *Lancet Infectious Diseases, 18*(1), e1–e13. https://doi.org/10.1016/S1473-3099(17)30398-5

D'Gama, A. M., Poduri, A., & Volpe, J. J. (2025a). Neuronal migration. In J. J. Volpe & T. E. Inder (Eds.), *Volpe's neurology of the newborn* (7th ed., pp. 142–165). Elsevier.

D'Gama, A. M., Poduri, A., & Volpe, J. J. (2025b). Neuronal proliferation. In J. J. Volpe & T. E. Inder (Eds.), *Volpe's neurology of the newborn* (7th ed., pp. 122–141). Elsevier.

Duderstadt, K. (2019). *Pediatric physical examination* (3rd ed.). Elsevier.

Dumont, V., Bulla, J., Bessot, N., Gonidec, J., Zabalia, M., Guillois, B., & Roche-Labarbe, N. (2017). The manual orienting response habituation to repeated tactile stimuli in preterm neonates: Discrimination of stimulus locations and interstimulus intervals. *Developmental Psychobiology, 59*(5), 590–602. https://doi.org/10.1002/dev.21526

du Plessis, A. J., & Volpe, J. J. (2025a). Neural tube development. In J. J. Volpe & T. E. Inder (Eds.), *Volpe's neurology of the newborn* (7th ed., pp. 3–37). Elsevier.

du Plessis, A. J., & Volpe, J. J. (2025b). Prosencephalic development. In J. J. Volpe & T. E. Inder (Eds.), *Volpe's neurology of the newborn* (7th ed., pp. 3–37). Elsevier.

Edwards, M. S., & Baker, C. J. (2023). Bacterial infections in the neonate. In S. Long (Ed.), *Principles and practice of pediatric infectious diseases* (6th ed., pp. 566–572). Elsevier.

Ehrman-Dupre, R., Kaigh, C., Salzman, M., Haroz, R., Peterson, L. K., & Schmidt, R. (2022). Management of xylazine withdrawal in a hospitalized patient: A case report. *Journal of Addiction Medicine, 16*(5), 595–598. https://doi.org/10.1097/ADM.0000000000000955

Elgamal, E. A. (2012). Natural history of hydrocephalus in children with spinal open neural tube defect. *Surgical Neurology International, 3*, 112. https://doi.org/10.4103/2152-7806.101801

Fitton, C. A., Fleming, M., Steiner, M. F. C., Aucott, L., Pell, J. P., Mackay, D. F., & Mclay, J. S. (2020). In utero antihypertensive medication exposure and neonatal outcomes: A data linkage cohort study. *Hypertension, 75*(3), 628–633. https://doi.org/10.1161/HYPERTENSIONAHA.119.13802

Fleiss, B., Stolp, H., Mezger, V., & Gressens, P. (2024). Central nervous system development. In C. A. Gleason & S. E. Juul (Eds.), *Avery's diseases of the newborn* (11th ed., pp. 781–786). Elsevier.

Fulton, G. K., Blessing, M. S., & Evans, K. N. (2024). Craniofacial conditions. In C. A. Gleason & S. E. Juul (Eds.), *Avery's diseases of the newborn* (11th ed., pp. 1269–1293). Elsevier.

Garne, E., Loane, M., Addor, M. C., Boyd, P. A., Barisic, I., & Dolk, H. (2010). Congenital hydrocephalus—Prevalence, prenatal diagnosis and outcome of pregnancy in four European regions. *European Journal of Paediatric Neurology, 14*(2), 150–155. https://doi.org/10.1016/j.ejpn.2009.03.005

Genetic and Rare Diseases Information Center. (2024). *Trisomy 13*. https://rarediseases.info.nih.gov/diseases/7341/trisomy-13

Gomella, T.L., Eyal, F.G., & Bany-Mohammed, F. (2020). Gomella's Neonatology (8th edition). McGraw Hill.

Govil-Dalela, T., Kumar, A., Agarwal, R., & Chugani, H. T. (2017). Agenesis of the corpus callosum and Aicardi syndrome: A neuroimaging and clinical comparison. *Pediatric Neurology, 68*, 44–48. https://doi.org/10.1016/j.pediatrneurol.2016.12.002

Gressens, P., & Hüppi, P. S. (2025). Normal and abnormal brain development. In R. J. Martin & A. A. Fanaroff (Eds.), *Fanaroff and Martin's neonatal-perinatal medicine: Diseases of the fetus and infant* (12th ed., pp. 980–1010). Elsevier Mosby.

Gulati, I. K., Shubert, T. R., Sitaram, S., Wei, L., & Jadcherla, S. R. (2015). Effects of birth asphyxia on the modulation of pharyngeal provocation-induced adaptive reflexes. *American Journal of Physiology. Gastrointestinal and Liver Physiology, 309*(8), G662–G669. https://doi.org/10.1152/ajpgi.00204.2015

Hall, J. E. (2020). *Guyton and Hall textbook of medical physiology* (14th ed.). Elsevier.

Hall, R. W., & Anand, K. J. S. (2005). Physiology of pain and stress in the newborn. *Neoreviews, 6*(2), e61–e68. https://doi.org/10.1542/neo.6-2-e61

Hattori, H., Hiura, H., Kitamura, A., Miyauchi, N., Kobayashki, N., Takahashi, S., Okae, H., Kyono, K., Kagami, M., Ogata, T., & Arima, T. (2019). Association of four imprinting disorders and ART. *Clinical Epigenetics, 11*(1), 21. https://doi.org/10.1186/s13148-019-0623-3

Haynes, R. L., Kinney, H. C., & Volpe, J. J. (2025). Organizational events. In J. J. Volpe & T. E. Inder (Eds.), *Volpe's neurology of the newborn* (7th ed., pp. 166–198). Elsevier.

Heller, M., & Burd, L. (2014). Review of ethanol dispersion, distribution, and elimination from the fetal compartment. *Birth Defects Research Part A: Clinical and Molecular Teratology, 100*(4), 277–283. https://doi.org/10.1002/bdra.23232

Hernández-Martínez, C., Voltas Moreso, N., Ribot Serra, B., Arija Val, V., Escribano Macías, J., & Canals Sans, J. (2017). Effects of prenatal nicotine exposure on infant language development: A cohort follow up study. *Maternal and Child Health Journal, 21*(4), 734–744. https://doi.org/10.1007/s10995-016-2158-y

Hielkema, T., & Hadders-Algra, M. (2016). Motor and cognitive outcome after specific early lesions of the brain—A systematic review. *Developmental Medicine and Child Neurology, 58*(Suppl. 4), 46–52. https://doi.org/10.1111/dmcn.13047

Hirsch, L. J., Fong, M. W. K., Leitinger, M., LaRoche, S. M., Beniczky, S., Abend, N. S., Lee, J. W., Wusthoff, C. J., Hahn, C. D., Westover, M. B., Gerard, E. E., Herman, S. T., Haider, H. A., Osman, G., Rodriguez-Ruiz, A., Maciel, C. B., Gilmore,

E. J., Fernandez, A., Rosenthal, E. S., ... Gaspard, N. (2021). American Clinical Neurophysiology Society's Standardized Critical Care EEG Terminology: 2021 Version. *Journal of Clinical Neurophysiology: Official Publication of the American Electroencephalographic Society, 38*(1), 1–29. https://doi.org/10.1097/WNP.0000000000000806

Ho, G., Cardamone, M., & Farrar, M. (2015). Congenital and childhood myotonic dystrophy: Current aspects of disease and future directions. *World Journal of Clinical Pediatrics, 4*(4), 66–80. https://doi.org/10.5409/wjcp.v4.i4.66

Ignatavicius, D. D., Rebar, C. R., & Heimgartner, N. M. (2024). *Medical-surgical nursing: Concepts for clinical judgment and collaborative care* (11th ed.). Elsevier.

Inder, T. E., Perlman, J. M., & Volpe, J. J. (2025). Preterm intraventricular hemorrhage/posthemorrhagic hydrocephalus. In J. J. Volpe & T. E. Inder (Eds.), *Volpe's neurology of the newborn* (7th ed., pp. 777–846). Elsevier.

Inder, T. E., & Volpe, J. J. (2025). Encephalopathy of the preterm—Clinical aspects. In J. J. Volpe & T. E. Inder (Eds.), *Volpe's neurology of the newborn* (7th ed., pp. 547–591). Elsevier.

Jaques, S. C., Kingsbury, A., Henshcke, P., Chomchai, C., Clews, S., Falconer, J., Abdel-Latif, M. E., Feller, J. M., & Oei, J. L. (2014). Cannabis, the pregnant woman and her child: Weeding out the myths. *Journal of Perinatology, 34*(6), 417–424. https://doi.org/10.1038/jp.2013.180

Jones, K. L., Jones, M. C., & Casanelles, M. D. C. (2013). *Smith's recognizable patterns of human malformation* (7th ed.). Elsevier Saunders.

Katsianou, M. A., Adamopoulos, C., Vastardis, H., & Basdra, E. K. (2016). Signaling mechanisms implicated in cranial sutures pathophysiology: Craniosynostosis. *BBA Clinical, 6*, 165–176. https://doi.org/10.1016/j.bbacli.2016.04.006

Kayyal, S., & Inder, T. E. (2025). Seizures in neonates. In R. J. Martin & A. A. Fanaroff (Eds.), *Fanaroff and Martin's neonatal-perinatal medicine: Diseases of the fetus and infant* (12th ed. pp. 1085–1116). Elsevier Mosby.

Kratzer, I., Chip, S., & Vexler, Z. S. (2014). Barrier mechanisms in neonatal stroke. *Frontiers in Neuroscience, 8*, 359. https://doi.org/10.3389/fnins.2014.00359

Lalande, M., & Calciano, M. A. (2007). Molecular epigenetics of Angelman syndrome. *Cellular and Molecular Life Science, 64*(7–8), 947–960. https://doi.org/10.1007/s00018-007-6460-0

Lee, T. C., & Mukundan, S., Jr. (2015). Brainstem and cranial nerves. In T. C. Lee, S. Mukundan, Jr., & F. H. Netter (Eds.), *Netter's correlative imaging: Neuroanatomy* (pp. 175–271). Elsevier Saunders.

Limperopoulos, C., du Plessis, A. J., & Volpe, J. J. (2025). Cerebellar hemorrhage. In J. J. Volpe & T. E. Inder (Eds.), *Volpe's neurology of the newborn* (7th ed., pp. 760–776). Elsevier.

Martin, J. A., Osterman, M. J. K., & Driscoll, A. K. (2023). Declines in cigarette smoking during pregnancy in the United States, 2016–2021 (NCHS Data Brief, no. 458). National Center for Health Statistics. https://doi.org/10.15620/cdc:123360

Martínez-Moreno, C. G., Calderón-Vallejo, D., Harvey, S., Arámburo, C., & Quintanar, J. L. (2018). Growth hormone (GH) and gonadotropin-releasing hormone (GnRH) in the central nervous system: A potential neurological combinatory therapy? *International Journal of Molecular Sciences, 19*(2), 375. https://doi.org/10.3390/ijms19020375

McAllister, J. P. (2012). Pathophysiology of congenital and neonatal hydrocephalus. *Seminars in Fetal & Neonatal Medicine, 17*(5), 285. https://doi.org/10.1016/j.siny.2012.06.004

McCandless, S. E., Suh, M., Yin, D., Yeh, M., Czado, S., Aghsaei, S., Li, J. W., Francis, K., Hadker, N., & Stafford, D. E. J. (2020). SUN-604 U.S. prevalence & mortality of Prader-Willi syndrome: A population-based study of medical claims. *Journal of the Endocrine Society, 4*(Suppl. 1). https://doi.org/10.1210/jendso/bvaa046.993

Muscular Dystrophy Association. (2025). *Myotonic dystrophy*. https://www.mda.org/disease/myotonic-dystrophy

National Institute on Alcohol Abuse and Alcoholism. (2023). *Understanding fetal alcohol spectrum disorders*. https://www.niaaa.nih.gov/publications/brochures-and-fact-sheets/understanding-fetal-alcohol-spectrum-disorders#:~:text=About%201%20in%2010%20(9.8,10.5%25)%20reporting%20binge%20drinking

National Institute on Alcohol Abuse and Alcoholism. (2025). *Alcohol and pregnancy in the United States*. https://www.niaaa.nih.gov/alcohols-effects-health/alcohol-topics-z/alcohol-facts-and-statistics/alcohol-and-pregnancy-united-states

National Institutes of Health. (2021). *Prader Willi syndrome (PWS)*. https://www.nichd.nih.gov/health/topics/prader-willi

National Institutes of Health. (2025a). *Angelman syndrome*. https://www.ninds.nih.gov/health-information/disorders/angelman-syndrome

National Institutes of Health. (2025b). *Down syndrome*. https://www.nichd.nih.gov/health/topics/factsheets/downsyndrome

National Institutes of Health. (2025c). *Neurofibromatosis*. https://www.ninds.nih.gov/health-information/disorders/neurofibromatosis

National Institutes of Health. (2025d). *Spina bifida*. https://www.ninds.nih.gov/health-information/disorders/spina-bifida

National Library of Medicine. (2018). *Spinal muscular atrophy*. https://medlineplus.gov/genetics/condition/spinal-muscular-atrophy/

National Organization for Rare Disorders. (2024a). *Agenesis of corpus callosum*. https://rarediseases.org/rare-diseases/agenesis-of-corpus-callosu

National Organization for Rare Disorders. (2024b). *Dandy-Walker malformation*. https://medlineplus.gov/genetics/condition/dandy-walker-malformation

Neu, N., Duchon, J., & Zachariah, P. (2015). TORCH infections. *Clinical Perinatology, 42*(1), 77–103. https://doi.org/10.1016/j.clp.2014.11.001

Nicolau, S., Waldrop, M. A., Connolly, A. M., & Mendell, J. R. (2021). Spinal muscular atrophy. *Seminars in Pediatric Neurology, 37*, 100878. https://doi.org/10.1016/j.spen.2021.100878

Ogino, S., & Wilson, R. B. (2004). Spinal muscular atrophy: Molecular genetics and diagnostics. *Expert Review of Molecular Diagnostics, 4*(1), 15–29. https://doi.org/10.1586/14737159.4.1.15

O'Keeffe, L. M., Greene, R. A., & Kearney, P. M. (2014). The effect of moderate gestational alcohol consumption during pregnancy on speech and language outcomes in children: A systematic review. *Systematic Reviews, 3*(1), 1–11. https://doi.org/10.1186/2046-4053-3-1

Palanisamy, A. (2012). Maternal anesthesia and fetal neurodevelopment. *International Journal of Obstetric Anesthesia, 21*(2), 152–162. https://doi.org/10.1016/j.ijoa.2012.01.005

Parsons, J. A., Seay, A. R., & Jacobson, M. (2016). Neurologic disorders. In S. L. Gardner, B. S. Carter, M. Enzman-Hines, & J. A. Hernandez (Eds.), *Merenstein & Gardner's handbook of neonatal intensive care* (7th ed. pp. 727–762). Elsevier Saunders.

Patrick, S. W., Barfield, W. D., Poindexter, B. B., & Committee on Fetus and Newborn, Committee on Substance Use and Prevention. (2020). Neonatal opioid withdrawal syndrome. *Pediatrics, 146*(5), e2020029074. https://doi.org/10.1542/peds.2020-029074

Patton, K., Bell, F. B., Thompson, T., & Williamson, P. L. (2022). *Anatomy and physiology* (11th ed.). Elsevier.

Pekçetin, S., Aki, E., Üstünyurt, Z., & Kayihan, H. (2016). The efficiency of sensory integration interventions in preterm infants. *Perceptual and Motor Skills, 123*(2), 411–423. https://doi.org/10.1177/0031512516662895

Perlman, J. M. (2022). Periventricular-intraventricular hemorrhage in the premature infant—A historical perspective. *Seminars in Perinatology, 46*(5), 151591. https://doi.org/10.1016/j.semperi.2022.151591

Perrone, J., Haroz, R., D'Orazio, J., Gianotti, G., Love, J., Salzman, M., Lowenstein M., Thakrar, A., Klipp, S., Rae, L., Reed, M. K., Sisco, E., Wightman, R., & Nelson, L. S. (2024). National Institute on Drug Abuse Clinical Trials Network Meeting Report: Managing patients exposed to xylazine-adulterated opioids in emergency, hospital and addiction care settings. *Annals of Emergency Medicine, 84*(1), 20–28. https://doi.org/10.1016/j.annemergmed.2024.01.041

Persson, E.-K., Hagberg, G., & Uvebrant, P. (2006). Disabilities in children with hydrocephalus—A population-based study of children aged between four and twelve years. *Neuropediatrics, 37*(6), 330–336. https://doi.org/10.1055/s-2007-964868

Petersen, I., Collings, S. L., McCrea, R. L., Nazareth, I., Osborn, D. P., Cowen, P. J., & Sammon, C. J. (2017). Antiepileptic drugs prescribed in pregnancy and prevalence of major congenital malformations: Comparative prevalence studies. *Clinical Epidemiology, 9*, 95–103. https://doi.org/10.2147/CLEP.S118336

Pierson, C. R., & Volpe, J. J. (2025). Encephalopathy of prematurity: Neuropathology. In J. J. Volpe & T. E. Inder (Eds.), *Volpe's neurology of the newborn* (7th ed., pp. 506–522). Elsevier.

Pina-Garza, J. E. (2013). *Fenichel's clinical pediatric neurology* (7th ed.). Elsevier.

Pindrik, J., Schulz, L., & Drapeau, A. (2022). Diagnosis and surgical management of neonatal hydrocephalus. *Seminars in Pediatric Neurology, 42*, 100969. https://doi.org/10.1016/j.spen.2022.100969

Powley, T. L. (2013). Central control of autonomic functions: Organization of the autonomic nervous system. In L. R. Squire (Ed.), *Fundamental neuroscience* (4th ed., pp. 729–747). Elsevier/Academic Press.

Rajhans, P., Mainardi, F., Austin, S., Sprenger, N., Deoni, S., Hauser, J., & Schneider, N. (2023). The role of human milk oligosaccharides in myelination, socio-emotional and language development: Observational data from breast-fed infants in the United States of America. *Nutrients, 15*(21), 4624. https://doi.org/10.3390/nu15214624

Ranger, M., & Grunau, R. E. (2014). Early repetitive pain in preterm infants in relation to the developing brain. *Pain Management, 4*(1), 57–67. https://doi.org/10.2217/pmt.13.61

Raspa, M., Wheeler, A. C., & Riley, C. (2017). Public health literature review of Fragile X syndrome. *Pediatrics, 139* (Suppl. 3), S153–S171. https://doi.org/10.1542/peds.2016-1159C

Raybaud, C. (Ed.). (2010). Normal and abnormal embryology and development of the intracranial vascular system. *Neurosurgery Clinics of North America, 21*(3), 399–426. https://doi.org/10.1016/j.nec.2010.03.011

Riddle, A., Back, S. A., & Miller, S. P. (2024). Brain injury in the preterm infant. In C. A. Gleason & S. E. Juul (Eds.), *Avery's diseases of the newborn* (11th ed., pp. 809–826). Elsevier.

Riera, J., Cabañas, F., Serrano, J. J., Bravo, M. C., López-Ortego, P., Sánchez, L., Madero, R., & Pellicer, A. (2014). New time-frequency method for cerebral autoregulation in newborns: Predictive capacity for clinical outcomes. *Journal of Pediatrics, 165*(5), 897–902.e1. https://doi.org/10.1016/j.jpeds.2014.06.008

Rivkin, M. J., Inder, T. E., & Volpe, J. J. (2025). Stroke in the newborn. In J. J. Volpe & T. E. Inder (Eds.), *Volpe's neurology of the newborn* (7th ed., pp. 697–724). Elsevier.

Rogers, R., Moyer, K., & Moise, K. J. (2022). Congenital myotonic dystrophy: An overlooked diagnosis not amenable to detection by sequencing. *Prenatal Diagnosis, 42*(2), 233–235. https://doi.org/10.1002/pd.6105

Rosenthal, C. R., & Soto, D. (2016). The anatomy of non-conscious recognition memory. *Trends in Neurosciences, 39*(11), 707–711. https://doi.org/10.1016/j.tins.2016.09.005

Rouzer, S. K., Cole, J. M., Johnson, J. M., Varlinskaya, E. I., & Diaz, M. R. (2017). Moderate maternal alcohol exposure on gestational day 12 impacts anxiety-like behavior in offspring. *Frontiers in Behavioral Neuroscience, 11*(183), 1–13. https://doi.org/10.3389/fnbeh.2017.00183

Rubenstein, J., & Rakic, P. (Eds.). (2013). *Cellular migration and formation of neuronal connections: Comprehensive developmental neuroscience*. Academic Press.

Ruge, J. (2023). Alterations of neurologic function in children. In J. R. Rogers (Ed.), *McCance & Huether's pathophysiology: The biologic basis for disease in adults and children* (9th ed., pp. 640–660). Elsevier.

Ruiz, D. S. M., Barnett, B. P., & Gailloud, P. (2021). Craniocervical vascular anatomy. In M. A. Mauro (Ed.), *Image-guided interventions* (3rd ed., pp. 454–472). Elsevier Mosby.

Saunders, N. R., Dreifuss, J.-J., Dziegielewska, K. M., Johansson, P. A., Habgood, M. D., Møllgård, K., & Bauer, H.-C. (2014). The rights and wrongs of blood–brain barrier permeability studies: A walk through 100 years of history. *Frontiers in Neuroscience, 8*, 404. https://doi.org/10.3389/fnins.2014.00404

Saunders, N. R., Liddelow, S. A., & Dziegielewska, K. M. (2012). Barrier mechanisms in the developing brain. *Frontiers in Pharmacology, 3*, 46. https://doi.org/10.3389/fphar.2012.00046

Schindelmann, K. H., Paschereit, F., Steege, A., Stoltenburg-Didinger, G., & Kaindl, A. M. (2021). Systematic classification of spina bifida. *Journal of Neuropathology and Experimental Neurology, 80*(4), 294–305. https://doi.org/10.1093/jnen/nlab007

Schoenwolf, G. C., Bleyl, S. B., Brauer, P. R., & Francis-West, P. H. (2022). *Larsen's human embryology* (6th ed.). Churchill Livingstone.

Schwaller, F., Kanellopoulos, A. H., & Fitzgerald, M. (2017). The developmental emergence of differential brainstem serotonergic control of the sensory spinal cord. *Scientific Reports, 7*, 1. https://doi.org/10.1038/s41598-017-02509-2

Sehgal, A. (2011). Perinatal stroke: A case-based review. *European Journal of Pediatrics, 171*(2), 225–234. https://doi.org/10.1007/s00431-011-1509-3

Sekhon, M. S., Ainslie, P. N., & Griesdale, D. E. (2017). Clinical pathophysiology of hypoxic ischemic brain injury after cardiac arrest: A "two-hit" model. *Critical Care (London, England), 21*(1), 90. https://doi.org/10.1186/s13054-017-1670-9

Senarante, T. N., Zackai, E. H., & Saitta, S. C., (2024). Chromosome disorders. In C. A. Gleason & S. E. Juul (Eds.), *Avery's diseases of the newborn* (11th ed., pp. 347–361). Elsevier.

Shafer, G. J. D. C, Vu Tran, J. S., & Inder, T. E. (2025). Neonatal brain disorders. In A. A. Fanaroff & J. M. Fanaroff (Eds.), Klaus & Fanaroff's care of the high risk neonate (8th ed., pp. 340–361). Elsevier Mosby.

Sibai, B. M. (2012). Hypertension. In S. G. Gabbe, J. R. Niebyl, & J. L. Simpson (Eds.), *Obstetrics: Normal and problem pregnancies* (6th ed., pp. 661–705). Elsevier.

Smid, M. C., Metz, T. D., & Gordon, A. J. (2019). Stimulant use in pregnancy: An under-recognized epidemic among pregnant women. *Clinical Obstetrics and Gynecology, 62*(1), 168–184. https://doi.org/10.1097/GRF.0000000000000418

Smith, A. D., & Buckley, M. G. (2012). Spatial navigational impairments in hydrocephalus. *Cognitive Process, 13*(Suppl. 1), 329–332. https://doi.org/10.1007/s10339-0120505-5

Snyder, E. J., Pruthi, S., & Hernanz-Schulman, M. (2022). Characterization of germinal matrix hemorrhage in extremely premature infants: Recognition of posterior location and diagnostic pitfalls. *Pediatric Radiology, 52*(1), 75–84. https://doi.org/10.1007/s00247-021-05189-3

Som, P. M., & Naidich, T. P. (2013). Development of the skull base and calvarium: An overview of the progression from mesenchyme to chondrification to ossification. *Neurographics, 3*(4), 169–184. https://doi.org/10.3174/ng.4130069

Spadaro, A., O'Connor, K., Lakamana, S., Sarker, A., Wightman, R., Love, J. S., & Perrone, J. (2023). Self-reported xylazine experiences: A mixed-methods study of reddit subscribers. *Journal of Addiction Medicine, 17*(6), 691–694. https://doi.org/10.1097/ADM.0000000000001216

Srivastava, R., Mailo, J., & Dunbar, M. (2022). Perinatal stroke in fetuses, preterm and term infants. *Seminars in Pediatric Neurology, 43*, 100988. https://doi.org/10.1016/j.spen.2022.100988

Takakuwa, T., Koike, T., Muranaka, T., Uwabe, C., & Yamada, S. (2016). Formation of the circle of Willis during human embryonic development. *Congenital Anomalies, 56*(5), 233. https://doi.org/10.1111/cga.12165

Torchia, M. G., & Persaud, T. V. N. (2025). *The developing human: Clinically oriented embryology* (12th ed.). Elsevier.

Tsen, L. R. (2011). Neuraxial analgesia and anesthesia in obstetrics. In D. James, P. Steer, C. Weiner, & B. Gonik (Eds.), *High risk pregnancy: Management options* (4th ed., pp. 1211–1229). Elsevier Saunders.

Tucker, M. H., Tiwari, P., & Carter, B. S. (2023). The physiology, assessment, and treatment of neonatal pain. *Seminars in Fetal & Neonatal Medicine, 28*(4), 101465. https://doi.org/10.1016/j.siny.2023.101465

Twigg, S. R. F., & Wilkie, A. O. M. (2015). A genetic-pathophysiological framework for craniosynostosis. *American Journal of Human Genetics, 97*(3), 359–377. https://doi.org/10.1016/j.ajhg.2015.07.006

Vanderah, T. W., & Gould, D. J. (2021). *Nolte's the human brain: An introduction to its functional anatomy* (8th ed.). Elsevier.

Vesoulis, Z. A., & Mathur, A. M. (2017). Cerebral autoregulation, brain injury, and the transitioning premature infant. *Frontiers in Pediatrics, 5*, 64. https://doi.org/10.3389/fped.2017.00064

Vohr, B. R., Davis, E. P., Wanke, C. A., & Krebs, N. F. (2017). Neurodevelopment: The impact of nutrition and inflammation during preconception and pregnancy in low-resource settings. *Pediatrics, 139*(Suppl. 1), S38–S49. https://doi.org/10.1542/peds.2016-2828F

Volkow, N. D., Compton, W. M., & Wargo, E. M. (2017). The risks of marijuana use during pregnancy. *Journal of the American Medical Association, 317*(2), 129–130. https://doi.org/10.1001/jama.2016.18612

Volpe, J. J., & El-Dib, M. (2025). Neurological examination: Normal and abnormal features. In J. J. Volpe & T. E. Inder (Eds.), *Volpe's neurology of the newborn* (7th ed., pp. 293–323). Elsevier.

Volpe, J. J., & Inder, T. E. (Eds.). (2025). *Volpe's neurology of the newborn* (7th ed.). Elsevier.

Vutskits, L., & Wolf, A. (2014). Cerebral blood flow in the neonate. *Pediatric Anesthesia, 24*(1), 22–29. https://doi.org/10.1111/pan.12307

Wandell, B. A. (2016). Clarifying human white matter. *Annual Review of Neuroscience, 39*(1), 103–128. https://doi.org/10.1146/annurev-neuro-070815-013815

Watzlawik, J. O., Kahoud, R. J., O'Toole, R. J., White, K. A. M., Ogden, A. R., Painter, M. M., Wootla, B., Papke, L. M., Denic, A., Weimer, J. M., Carey, W. A., & Rodriguez, M. (2015). Abbreviated exposure to hypoxia is sufficient to induce CNS dysmyelination, modulate spinal motor neuron composition, and impair motor development in neonatal mice. *PLoS One, 10*(5), 1–24. https://doi.org/10.1371/journal.pone.0128007

Westmacott, R., MacGregor, D., Askalan, R., & deVeber, G. (2009). Late emergence of cognitive deficits after unilateral neonatal stroke. *Stroke, 40*(6), 2012–2019. https://doi.org/10.1161/STROKEAHA.108.533976

Whitelaw, A., Osredkar, D., & Thoresen, M. (2016). Neurological and neuromuscular disorders. In M. G. MacDonald & M. M. K. Seshia (Eds.), *Neonatology: Pathophysiology and management of the newborn* (6th ed.). Lippincott Williams & Wilkins.

Williams, C. A., Driscoll, D. J., & Dagli, A. I. (2010). Clinical and genetic aspects of Angelman syndrome. *Genetics in Medicine, 12*(7), 385–395. https://doi.org/10.1097/GIM.0b013e3181def138

Winn, H. R. (2017). *Youmans and Winn neurological surgery* (7th ed.). Elsevier.

Wouldes, T. A., & Lester, B. M. (2023). Opioid, methamphetamine, and polysubstance use: Perinatal outcomes for the mother and infant. *Frontiers in Pediatrics, 11*, 1305508. https://doi.org/10.3389/fped.2023.1305508

Wu, C. S., Jew, C. P., & Lu, H. C. (2011). Lasting impacts of prenatal cannabis exposure and the role of endogenous cannabinoids in the developing brain. *Future Neurology, 6*(4), 459–480. https://doi.org/10.2217/fnl.11.27

Wu, Q., Liu, J., Fang, A., Li, R., Bai, Y., Kriegstein, A. R., & Wang, S. (2014). The dynamics of neuronal migration. *Advances in Experimental Medicine and Biology, 800*, 25–36. https://doi.org/10.1007/978-94-007-7667-6_2

Yuskaitis, C. J., & Pomeroy, S. L. (2022). Development of the nervous system. In R. J. Polin, S. H. Abman, D. H. Rowtich, W. E. Benitz, & W. W. Fox (Eds.), *Fetal and neonatal physiology* (6th ed., pp. 1297–1318).Elsevier.

4

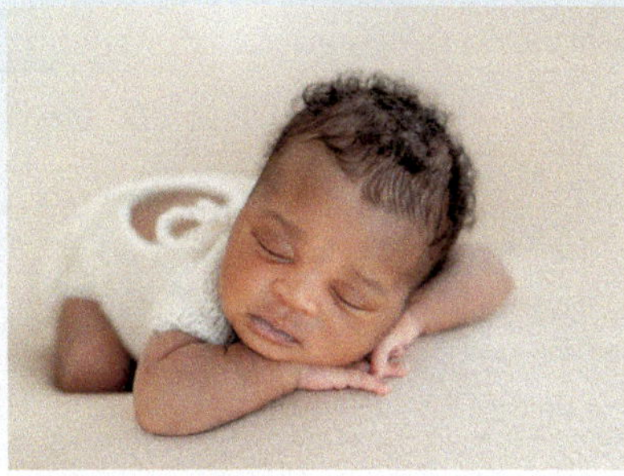

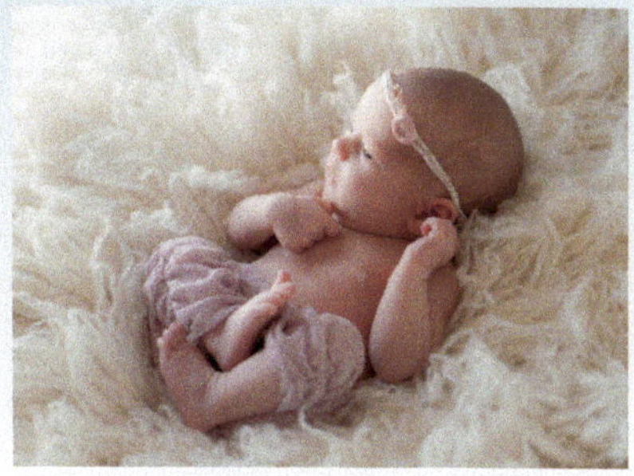

THE RESPIRATORY SYSTEM

Amy J. Jnah and Amy Williford

LEARNING OBJECTIVES

After completing this chapter, the reader should be able to:

- Understand normal respiratory organ development.
- Analyze the physiologic function of the fetal and postnatal respiratory systems.
- Discuss common inherited disorders and their effect on fetal and neonatal respiratory system development and function.
- Identify health conditions in XX pregnant patients that have a potential impact on fetal and postnatal respiratory system development and function.
- Evaluate common disorders that affect the respiratory system and their implications across the life span.

INTRODUCTION

Respiratory morbidities are some of the most common challenges facing neonatal healthcare providers, and they can have a lasting impact beyond infancy into childhood and adult life. This chapter discusses lung morphogenesis, the genetic drivers of lung development, fetal and neonatal lung function, common neonatal lung disorders, and long-term sequelae of neonatal lung disease.

TIMELINE OF ORGAN DEVELOPMENT

The respiratory system is one of the most complex of all organ systems. It is anatomically divided into separate entities: the upper respiratory tract (nose and nasal cavity, pharynx, and larynx) and the lower respiratory tract (trachea, bronchi, and lungs). While a review of embryologic development could progress in an anatomically minded fashion, organized by each supporting structure, the respiratory system does not develop in this manner. Rather, development occurs across gestation, from the early embryonic period through early adulthood. This normal progression is described using five phases of sequential development: the embryonic, pseudoglandular, canalicular, saccular, and alveolar phases (**Figure 4.1** and **Table 4.1**). Therefore, our review of the developing respiratory system will use this approach, which offers rising clinicians an opportunity to make connections between the timing of normal and aberrant development from early embryologic development to birth and identify the effect of interrupted development (premature birth) on postnatal respiratory function.

Phases of Lung Maturation

Embryonic Phase. The embryonic phase of respiratory development spans from week 4 to week 7 of gestation (**Table 4.1**; Cotton, 2017). During this time frame, the major airways, lung pleura, and early lung vasculature form. First, the *laryngotracheal groove* forms at the caudal end of the anterior foregut, during week 4 of gestation. The inner lining of the laryngotracheal groove gives rise to lung epithelium and glands that comprise the future larynx, trachea, and bronchi. By the end of week 4 of

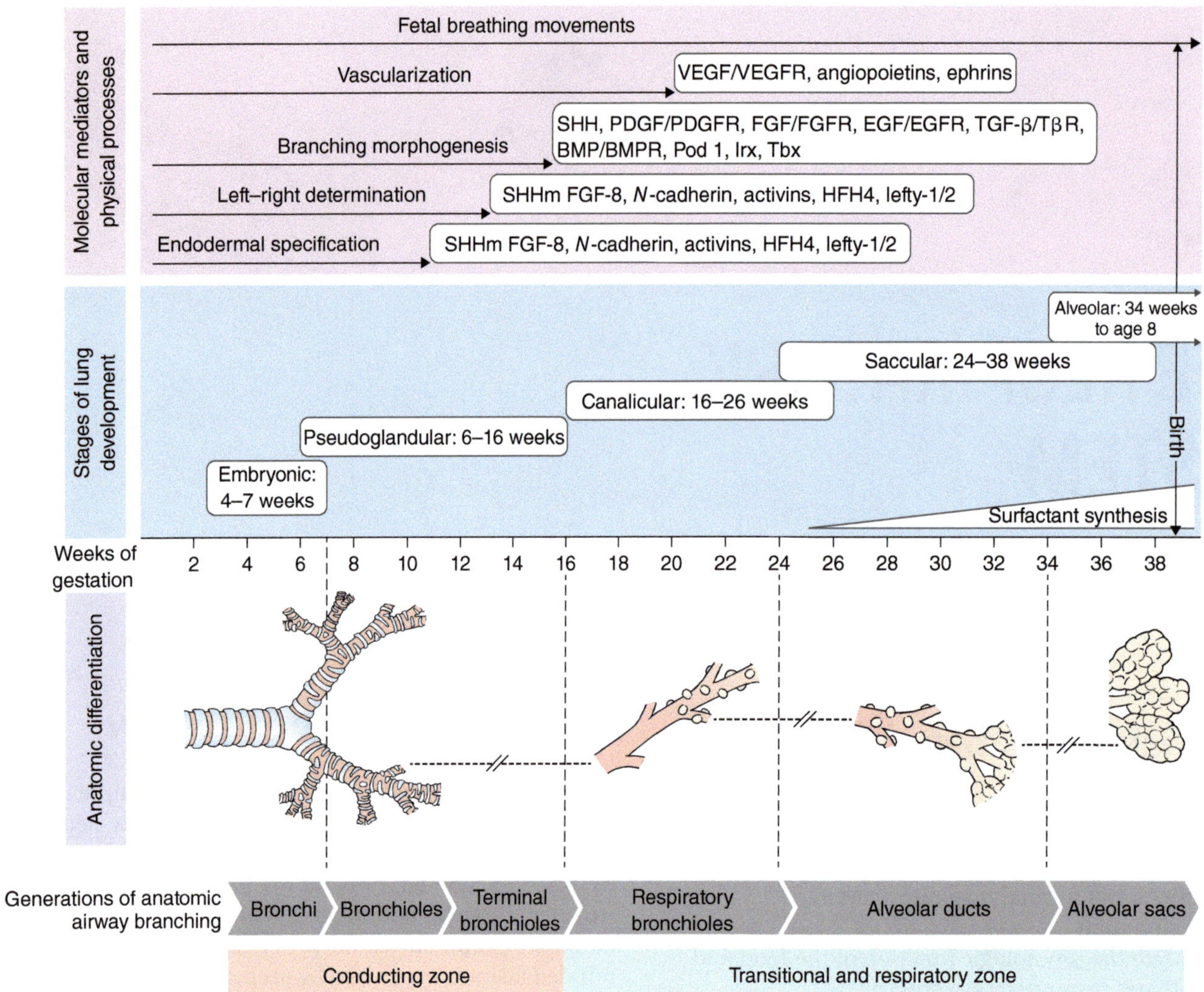

Figure 4.1 Five phases of pulmonary development. Morphogenic development is mediated by molecular mediators (transcription factors, polypeptides) and physical processes (FBMs). Like the systemic and pulmonary circulations, as the lungs progress through generations of branching, the number of branches increases yet their diameter and length progressively decrease. Airflow velocity decreases as air reaches the most distal bronchioles. Respiratory function is possible beginning at 22 to 23 weeks of gestation.
BMP, bone morphogenetic proteins; BMPR, bone morphogenetic protein receptor; EGF, epidermal growth factor; EGFR, epidermal growth factor receptor; FGF, fibroblast growth factor; FGFR, fibroblast growth factor receptor; HFH4, forkhead homologue hepatocyte nuclear family protein; Irx, Iroquois-complex homeobox family members; lefty-1/2, genes that help determine left-right determination; PDGF, platelet-derived growth factor; PDGFR, platelet-derived growth factor receptor; Pod 1, basic helix-loop-helix proteins; SHH, sonic hedgehog; Tbx, Tbox family proteins; TGF-β, transforming growth factor-β; TβR, transforming growth factor-β activating receptor; TGF-β receptor; VEGF, vascular endothelial growth factor; VEGFR,vascular endothelial growth factor receptor

Sources: Adapted from Bancalari, E., Keszler, M., Davis. P. G., & Polin. R. A. (2024). *The newborn lung: Neonatology questions and controversies* (4th ed.). Elsevier/Saunders; Copland, I., & Post, M. (2004). Lung development and fetal lung growth. *Paediatric Respiratory Reviews, 5,* (Suppl. 1), S259–S264. https://doi.org/10.1016/S1526-0542(04)90049-8

gestation, the laryngotracheal groove begins to protrude outward and quickly conforms into a pouchlike structure named the *laryngotracheal (respiratory) diverticulum* (Torchia & Persaud, 2025).

Next, the laryngotracheal (respiratory) diverticulum begins to morphologically change shape. It elongates and invaginates into a network of embryonic connective tissue (splanchnic mesenchyme) within the mesoderm (Sadler, 2024; Sun, 2022; Whitsett & Xu, 2016). During this process of elongation, the distal end of the laryngotracheal diverticulum takes on a rounded, budlike appearance, termed the *respiratory bud* (lung bud). This marks the earliest sign of development of the future tracheobronchial tree. Then, the lung bud transforms from a single primitive bud into two outpouchings, or *primary bronchial buds*. The bud thereby grows laterally, into the pericardioperitoneal canals that will give rise to pleural cavities during later development (Torchia & Persaud, 2025). Now that invagination is complete, an intricate process of folding ensues, resulting in formation of the tracheoesophageal septum. This occurs during week 5 of gestation. As the septum proliferates, it divides the foregut into two separate entities: (a) the trachea and (b) the esophagus (Sun, 2022).

TABLE 4.1 Phases of Lung Development

Phase	Weeks of Gestation	Summary of Major Developments
Embryonic	4–7	• Formation of the major airways, lung pleura, and primitive pulmonary vasculature
Pseudoglandular	6–16	• Formation of bronchi, terminal bronchioles, and alveolar ducts • Early differentiation of lung epithelial cells • Formation of muscle cells at the proximal end of distal airways • Differentiation and maturation of the pulmonary vasculature • Onset of fetal breathing movements
Canalicular	16–26	• Proliferation of pulmonary capillaries • Differentiation of terminal bronchioles into respiratory bronchioles and alveolar ducts • Widening and lengthening of alveolar ducts • Differentiation of the epithelium into type I and II cells • Formation of measurable amounts of surfactant begins
Saccular	24–38	• Septation and matriculation of alveoli, leading to smaller sized alveoli and a larger aggregate number of alveoli • Significant increases in lung volume and surface area with the formation of airway septations • Continued maturation of the pulmonary vasculature • Formation of the immature dual layer alveolar-capillary membrane • Development of the lymphatic system (for future assistance with the egress of lung fluid)
Alveolar	34 weeks–age 8	• Continued proliferation of alveoli (50 million by term gestation, 300 million by age 8) • Additional airway septations • Formation of the mature single layer alveolar-capillary membrane

Clinical Application. Under normal circumstances, between weeks 3 and 5 of gestation, the primitive foregut develops from the lung bud and separates into the trachea and esophagus. This process of differentiation and maturation is influenced by growth factors (i.e., NODAL and FGF4) and transcription regulators (e.g., Foxf1, Sox2, Nkx2.1, HEX, DoxA2). Failed septation is associated with tracheoesophageal communications, or fistulas (TEF). A common clinical manifestation of TEF with esophageal atresia (EA) is excessive oral secretions with the inability to pass a suction catheter through the mouth and esophagus, and into the stomach. The suction catheter will meet resistance at the location of the atresia and appear "coiled" on chest radiograph.

Next, the trachea begins to lengthen in a cephalocaudal fashion along its vertical axis, forming rudimentary right and left bronchi. Over time, the right main bronchus will grow slightly longer than the left, a pragmatic development to accommodate the superior, middle, and inferior lobes on that right side (Sun, 2022; Torchia & Persaud, 2025). Lengthening continues, and the right and left primary bronchi give rise to secondary bronchi, which thereby give rise to lower lobar, segmental, and intrasegmental bronchi. These branches then further divide into rudimentary upper, middle, and lower lobes (right side), and upper and lower lobes (left side). These lobar bronchi and rudimentary lung branches continue an intricate process of subdivision and branching throughout the greater portion of fetal development.

Cartilaginous plates form from the surrounding splanchnic mesenchyme and become the bronchial smooth muscle and connective tissue, as well as the pulmonary connective tissue and capillaries. In addition, cartilaginous tracheal rings and lobar airways form between weeks 5 and 7 of gestation. In total, this early embryonic period of lung development establishes the anatomic framework, which enables myriad maturational developments seen across the remaining pseudoglandular, canalicular, saccular, and alveolar stages of development.

Pseudoglandular Phase. It is interesting to note that bronchi discussed in the prior section arise from epithelial buds that are surrounded by mesenchyme. Within a matter of 1 week, this gives the immature lung a "glandularlike" appearance and explains the label "pseudoglandular" for this phase of maturation (Torchia & Persaud, 2025). The pseudoglandular phase encompasses weeks 6 to 16 of gestation and involves continued, intricate airway branching (Torchia & Persaud, 2025).

The tips of the epithelial buds also give rise to all of the other diverse types of cells found in the developing bronchi and bronchioles. Cartilage appears during week 10 of gestation in the trachea and bronchi and by week 16 in the segmental bronchi (Sun, 2022). Ciliated cells (responsible for the development of cilia that move debris within the airways), goblet cells (responsible for mucus production), and basal cells (responsible for the formation of a barrier against environmental damage) arise during week 13 of gestation (Kallapur & Jobe, 2025; Universities of Fribourg, Lausanne, & Bern, Switzerland, 2006). Simple columnar cells begin to accumulate within the lining of the terminal bronchioles between weeks 12 and 13 of gestation. These cells will participate in respiration and gas exchange, once fully formed (Torchia & Persaud, 2025). By the end of the pseudoglandular period, all the major components of the lung are formed, with the exception of structures involved in gas exchange.

Canalicular Phase. The canalicular phase of development extends between weeks 16 and 26 of gestation (Torchia & Persaud, 2025; Sun, 2022). Between weeks 16 and 20 of gestation, the lumen of the bronchi and terminal bronchioles continue to enlarge, while the pulmonary vasculature begins to rapidly proliferate (Bancalari et al., 2024; Torchia & Persaud, 2025). By week 20, primitive type I pneumocytes, the primary structural cell of the alveolus, are observed. Concurrently, lamellar bodies (LBs), surfactant storage repositories, appear within primitive type II alveolar cells and tiny amounts of surfactant production is observed. By week 24 of gestation, two or more *acini*, berry-like cell clusters, appear at the distal ends of the terminal bronchioles, giving rise to respiratory bronchioles. The respiratory bronchioles subdivide into three to six primitive alveolar ducts and saccules. In addition, capillaries derived from the mesenchyme form and surround the primordial alveoli. This marks the establishment of the primitive air-fluid interface for future gas exchange. Even though gas exchange is possible at the end of this developmental period, endogenous pulmonary surfactant production remains critically low (Sun, 2022).

Saccular Phase. The saccular phase spans between weeks 24 and 38 of gestation (Torchia & Persaud, 2025; Sun, 2022). Additional saccules continue to appear at the ends of the distal respiratory bronchioles and form primitive alveoli. By week 26 of gestation, squamous epithelial type I pneumocytes and secretory type II pneumocytes increase in abundance within the distal airways (compared to the prior phase of maturation). Type I pneumocytes prepare to modulate gas exchange, whereas type II pneumocytes begin to synthesize and secrete tiny amounts of surfactant at the inner walls of the alveolar sacs (Torchia & Persaud, 2025). As a result, surfactant begins to accumulate along these interior walls and reduce alveolar surface tension (also known as collapsing pressure). As more alveolar sacs develop, the barrier between the epithelium and the endothelium stretches and thins, establishing the primitive blood-air interface. Now, oxygen and carbon dioxide can be exchanged at this alveolar-capillary network (Torchia & Persaud, 2025).

Clinical Application. Extremely premature infants born before 26 to 28 weeks of gestation are known to have insufficient endogenous surfactant production and consequently high alveolar surface tension at birth. This means that collapsing pressure exceeds opening pressure at the alveoli and encourages atelectasis (alveolar collapse). The administration of exogenous surfactant will be necessary to attempt to reduce alveolar surface tension enough to open the alveoli and allow for the exchange of oxygen and carbon dioxide.

Alveolar Phase. The alveolar phase of development begins around week 34 of gestation and extends to age 8 (Sun, 2022; Torchia & Persaud, 2025). This stage marks a shift in lung capability from secretory organ to one capable of gas exchange. Saccular septation, or secondary septation, begins at the end of each respiratory bronchiole. This process of septation permits the formation of larger clusters of primordial alveolar sacs. Throughout the third trimester, these sacs produce increasing amounts of surfactant and transitions the fetal lungs away from exclusive dependence upon the placenta, to a state of readiness for independent postnatal gas exchange.

At birth (term gestation), the majority of alveoli (95%) are immature (primordial; Torchia & Persaud, 2025). These primordial alveoli are uniquely capable of stimulating the production of additional primitive alveoli, which allow for continued alveolar expansion and maturation after birth and through early childhood. Children are considered fully affixed with mature alveoli, incapable of regeneration, by age 8; any pathologic issues incurred during fetal or postnatal life may alter alveolar development and increase the risk for chronic respiratory problems.

Pulmonary Vascular Maturation

Blood is circulated throughout the body by way of the cardiovascular system. Blood circulates through one of two pathways: the *systemic circulation* or the *pulmonary circulation*. While the vasculature within each circulation is very similar histologically, the location and physiologic function of each differs. We discuss the evolution of the pulmonary vasculature in this section of the chapter.

The pulmonary vasculature arises from the sixth aortic arch and initially appears within the splanchnic mesenchyme during the embryonic phase of development. Vessel proliferation occurs in a cephalocaudal direction, in tandem with proliferation of lung buds. In fact, the pulmonary vascular development progresses caudally toward the lung buds (Sadler, 2024). Shortly thereafter, circulatory networks arise, modulated by the processes of angiogenesis, vasculogenesis, and fusion. Angiogenesis prompts vascular proliferation, whereby new vessels form off of preexisting vessels. Vasculogenesis results in the formation of blood vessels from angioblasts and endothelial precursor cells, creating new blood vessels (Steinhorn, 2025). Next, distal and proximal vessels fuse and form a circulatory network. Though not definitive, it is likely that these angiogenic and vasculogenic processes are also responsible for blood vessel development distal to the heart and lungs (Bancalari et al., 2024).

Vasculogenesis is influenced by three families of growth factors: vascular endothelial growth factor (VEGF), angiopoietin, and Ephrin (Eph; Alvira, 2016; Baker & Abman, 2015; Le Cras & Rabinovitch, 2016). The VEGF signaling system has been implicated in the early stages of vasculogenesis and may play an important role in later angiogenesis, vascular maintenance, and survival during the adult years (Le Cras & Rabinovitch, 2016). The angiopoietin system appears to be critical for the successful remodeling and stabilization of embryonic vessels and may facilitate blood vessel responsiveness to VEGF (Alvira, 2016; Baker & Abman, 2015; Le Cras & Rabinovitch, 2016; Sadler, 2024). The Eph family of growth factors influence vascular proliferation in the latter stages of pulmonary vascular development (Le Cras & Rabinovitch, 2016). Additional factors involved in vascular development include factors found in the extracellular matrix (fibronectin laminin, type IV collagen) as well as platelet-derived growth factor (PDGF).

As the pulmonary vasculature expands, vessels differentiate into arteries, capillaries, and veins, each enveloped by a layer of perivascular cells that participate in maintaining vascular homeostasis, angiogenesis, and tissue repair. Maturation of the pulmonary arteries progresses in the same fashion as the developing airways, from the proximal to distal ends of the lungs. More proximally located pulmonary arteries are comprised of a thick lumen made up of an outer extracellular matrix, nerves and collagen, and vaso vasorum (smaller vessels that supply nutrients to this outer vascular wall); a middle smooth muscle layer; and a thin inner elastic layer. The diameter of the arterial lumen and arterial wall progressively narrows toward the distal sections of the lungs. The more distal arteries are considered vulnerable to shearing forces, particularly among infants born premature, as these vessels are comprised of a very thin smooth muscle layer and no inner elastic layer. Pulmonary capillaries are only comprised of a single layer of epithelial cells that are surrounded by perivascular cells. The structure of the proximal and distal pulmonary veins mimics the pulmonary arteries (Kool et al., 2014; Sadler, 2024).

Over time, as the blood vessels proliferate and fuse, two circulatory pathways, known as the *pulmonary circulation* and *bronchial circulation*, emerge. The pulmonary circulation transports deoxygenated blood toward the alveolar capillary network for oxygenation, and newly oxygenated blood is transported to the four pulmonary veins and left atrium. During fetal development, high resistance (increased pulmonary vascular resistance [PVR]) is noted through these vessels, and likewise, the pulmonary circulation remains low until after birth. The bronchial circulation traverses the bronchial tree and perihilar regions of the lungs. These vessels transport oxygen and nutrients to the conducting airways, or portions of the lungs not directly involved in gas exchange, and subsequently drain blood into the right atrium (Bancalari et al., 2024; Kool et al., 2014; Sadler, 2024).

> **Clinical Application.** Disrupted molecular signaling that occurs early into lung development can alter vascular development and predispose newborns to pathologies including pulmonary hypertension. Pulmonary hypertension can develop idiopathically or from several other causes. These include aberrant pulmonary artery development and function ("pulmonary arterial hypertension"), left-sided congenital heart disease, lung disease (e.g., congenital diaphragmatic hernia [CDH], alveolar-capillary dysplasia, pulmonary hypoplasia, bronchopulmonary dysplasia), or gene mutations, or may occur in association with a genetic disorder (e.g., trisomy 21, DiGeorge syndrome, VACTERL [**V**ertebral anomalies, **A**nal atresia, **C**ardiovascular anomalies, **T**racheoesophageal fistula, **E**sophageal atresia, **R**enal and/or radial anomalies, **L**imb defects] syndrome, CHARGE [**C**oloboma of the eye, **H**eart defects, **A**tresia of the nasal choanae, **R**estricted growth/development, **G**enital or urinary anomalies, **E**ar anomalies/deafness] syndrome, or Noonan syndrome). Among newborns, the majority of cases of pulmonary hypertension are idiopathic or attributed to congenital heart disease.

The Pharyngeal Apparatus

Pharyngeal Arches. Before discussing the development of the facial region, which is significant to both respiratory and gastrointestinal (GI) function (see Chapter 6), a review of their derivatives is necessary. The six pharyngeal arches, also known as branchial arches, arise during week 4 of gestation. Each arch is initially comprised of mesenchyme from two of the primitive germ layers, the endoderm and ectoderm. They remain relatively static until innervated by neural crest cells, after which the arches begin increasing in size. The six arches and their major skeletal derivatives are provided in Table 4.2.

Pharyngeal Pouches. While the pharyngeal gut proliferates, the aforementioned brachial and pharyngeal arches become separated by brachial and pharyngeal clefts and form four pharyngeal pouches (Sadler, 2024). The first pouch gives rise to the middle ear, tympanic membrane, and Eustachian tube. The second pouch forms tonsils and lymph nodes. The third pouch gives rise to the thymus and inferior parathyroid gland, whereas the fourth pouch develops into the superior parathyroid glands and the parafollicular cells of the thyroid (Schoenwolf et al., 2021).

Other Structures That Influence Respiratory Development and Function

Nose and Nasal Cavity. The earliest facial features appear during week 4 of gestation and under the influence of two genes, sonic hedgehog signaling (*SHH*) and fibroblast growth factor 8 (*FGF-8*; Torchia & Persaud, 2025). During week 4 of gestation, the first pair of pharygneal arches give rise to five facial prominences. The frontonasal prominence gives rise to the forehead, nasal bridge, and septum. The maxillary prominence gives rise to the cheeks and lateral portion of the upper lip. The medial nasal prominence forms the philtrum of the upper lip, crest, and tip of the nose, while the lateral nasal prominence forms the alae (sides of the nose). Finally, the mandibular prominence forms the lower lip (Sadler, 2024).

Specific to nasal development, nasal placodes (embryonic structures that give rise to the nose) appear during week 5 of gestation and invaginate, under the influence of platelet-derived growth factor (PDGF) alpha polypeptide, to form nasal pits. In doing so, the placodes create a ridge of tissue surrounding each nasal pit, which forms nasal prominences (similar to facial prominences). The nasal prominences fuse with the maxillary prominences to form the nose, while the nasal pits mature into nasal sinuses. Of note, as the maxillary and nasal prominences fuse, a groove forms on either side of the developing nose, into the nasolacrimal duct and nasolacrimal sac. As the nasal pits continue to develop, an oronasal membrane (primary choana) separates each nasal pit from the primitive oral cavity (Sadler, 2024). The choana resides on each side of midline, behind the primary palate. During week 7 of gestation, the oronasal membrane ruptures, bringing the nasal and oral cavities into communication. As development continues, the secondary palate forms and separates the oral and nasal cavities. With these developments, the choana

TABLE 4.2 The Pharyngeal Arches

Pharyngeal Arch	Cranial Nerve Innervation	Primary Muscular Function	Skeletal Derivatives
1	V	Mastication	• Incus • Mandible • Malleus of middle ear • Maxilla • Meckel's cartilage • Tympanic ring
2	VII	Facial expression	• Hyoid • Stapes • Temporal styloid process
3	IX	Swallowing, elevation of larynx and pharynx	• Inferior parathyroid glands • Thymus
4	X	Pharyngeal and laryngeal muscle function	• Epiglottis cartilage • Superior parathyroid glands
6	X	Pharyngeal and laryngeal muscle function	• Arytenoid cartilages • Comiculate cartilage • Cricoid cartilage • Cuneiform cartilages

Note: The fifth pharyngeal arch is considered a rudimentary structure and regresses early in fetal development. The stylopharyngeus muscle is an internal muscle of the pharynx.

shifts to a definitive position, at the junction of the nasal cavity and pharynx (nasopharynx).

Errors in nasal development, in particular those which encourage anatomical closure of the posterior choanae, can lead to choanal atresia. Impaired RA down-regulation of FGF-8 may explain the emergence of this relatively rare disease (Kwong, 2015). In addition, failed development of the secondary palate may give rise to cleft palate, offering a continuous communication between the nasal and oral passages.

The Larynx. Just prior to the formation of the larynx, during week 5 of gestation, the tracheoesophageal septum forms (discussed earlier in this chapter). The formation of this septum divides the foregut into the ventral laryngotracheal tube and the dorsal primordial oropharynx and esophagus. The epithelium of the larynx arises from this laryngotracheal tube, while the cartilages develop from the fourth and sixth pairs of pharyngeal pouches and are innervated by the vagus nerve (cranial nerve X). Rapid cellular proliferation and differentiation between weeks 4 and 9 of gestation initially occludes the larynx; however, later organization during week 10 of gestation allows for recanalization and room for vocal cord development (Torchia & Persaud, 2025).

> **Clinical Application.** In some circumstances, as the vocal cords are developing, a mucous membrane can form and cover the vocal cords. This is referred to as a laryngeal web. Newborns will present with a hoarse cry at birth. A pediatric ear nose and throat (ENT) consult will be necessary, and treatment involves dilating the area affected by the web.

Meanwhile, the epiglottis begins to form from the third and fourth pharyngeal pouches. In order to make room for the formation of the epiglottis, the larynx assumes a high anatomic position and maintains this position through the first year of life. This allows the epiglottis to establish contact with the soft palate and create a functional separation between the respiratory and digestive tracts. Normal descent of the larynx (and vagus nerve) to its adult position is complete by 2 years of age, whereby children are able to switch from exclusive nasal to nasal and/or oral breathing.

> **Clinical Application.** Functional separation of the respiratory and digestive tracts encourages postnatal oral feeding proficiency (coordination) by deterring aspiration but also obligates the newborn to breathe exclusively from the nares (not the mouth). This is why we refer to newborns as “obligatory nasal breathers.”

Pleural Development. As the lungs develop within the mesenchyme, they develop two layers of pleura, or serous membranes (Torchia & Persaud, 2025). This begins during week 5 of gestation, with both layers of pleura (parietal and visceral) established by week 6 of gestation (Torchia & Persaud, 2025). The parietal pleura develops as a single layer of mesothelial cells supported by connective tissue and lines the thoracic wall and diaphragm. This serves as the outer membrane and, as a result, maintains direct communication with intercostal arteries and lymphatic vessels, as well as the intercostal and phrenic nerves. The visceral pleura covers the lungs and extends into each fissure while maintaining direct communication with the bronchial circulation. The pleural cavity is a space that forms between the two pleurae described earlier. This space is separated from the peritoneal cavity by a pleuroperitoneal membrane (Universities of Fribourg, Lausanne, & Bern, Switzerland, 2006). The pleural cavity is a hollowed out, yet narrow space composed of pleural fluid. During respiration, the pleurae should smoothly glide along each other’s exterior surface. Any accumulation of air into the pleural space, which may occur due to changes in the elasticity of the thoracic wall or lungs, may cause a pneumothorax.

Diaphragm. Diaphragm development in rodent models suggests multiple gene involvement, but that process is not as clear in humans. Many of the genes implicated play a critical role in lung morphogenesis, and studies in humans suggest an abnormality in the retinoic acid (RA) pathway (Ameis et al., 2017).

The diaphragm develops from four separate embryonic structures: the septum transversum, the pleuroperitoneal membranes, the dorsal esophageal mesentery, and the body wall. The septum transversum first appears as a thick mesodermal layer and develops into an incomplete wall that forms between the thoracic and abdominal cavities (Torchia & Persaud, 2025). The septum transversum most likely supplies the scaffolding for the continued development of the diaphragm (Ameis et al., 2017). Large openings in the septum on both sides of the esophagus remain and become the pericardioperitoneal canals. The septum fuses with the dorsal mesentery of the esophagus and the pleuroperitoneal membranes. This process of fusion creates the primitive diaphragm. As the lungs and pleural cavities grow, they extend into the body walls, and the body wall tissue separates into an internal and an external layer. The internal layer becomes the peripheral parts of the diaphragm, and the external layer becomes part of the abdominal wall (Torchia & Persaud, 2025).

Surfactant Development

Surfactant is first seen in measurable amounts at the end of the canalicular phase of development (around week 25 of gestation) and increases significantly across the last

2 weeks of gestation. Surfactant, produced from alveolar epithelial cells, is critical to normal alveolar stabilization and function. Its synthesis and secretion are modulated by type II pneumocytes and involves the breakdown, clearance, reuptake, and reprocessing of its phospholipid and protein components (Kallapur & Jobe, 2025).

Surfactant is primarily composed of phospholipids (80%); fats (10%), namely cholesterol; and proteins (10%; Figure 4.2; Kallapur & Jobe, 2025; Whitsett & Kingma, 2022). Numerous different phospholipids account for the majority of surfactant's composition; however, we highlight three significant phospholipids in this discussion. Phosphatidylcholine (PC) is the major phospholipid in surfactant, accounting for 80% of all phosopholipids contained within surfactant molecules. The second most prevalent phospholipid is phosphatidylglycerol (PG). PG contributes to maintaining the stability of the alveolar membrane, reducing alveolar surface tension, and holds a role in the immune response. Dipalmitoylphosphatidylcholine (DPPC) is the primary surface-active phospholipid and is directly responsible for reducing surface tension (Kallapur & Jobe, 2025). Unsaturated phospholipids and cholesterol help to maintain the fluidity of surfactant.

Surfactant proteins (SP) A, B, C, and D (SP-A, SP-B, SP-C, SP-D), contribute to surfactant function and host defenses (Table 4.3). SP-B and SP-C are hydrophobic proteins that modulate the movement of surfactant from myelin and toward the surface monolayer, as well as the spreading of surfactant along the alveolar membrane. More specific, SP-B is critical for the formation of the LBs within the type II pneumocyte, and because of this, deficiencies in SP-B synthesis and secretion will lead to abnormal SP-C processing. The remaining two SPs, SP-A and SP-D, are important for the function of the host defense immune system. In aggregate, both SP-A and SP-D function as opsonins that increase membrane permeability and facilitate the binding of phagocytes to pathogens. More specific, SP-A activates macrophages within the alveolus. SP-D binds to specific lipid and carbohydrate structures on the cell wall of invading bacteria, virus, fungi, and protozoa (Plosa & Sucre, 2024; Whitsett & Kingma, 2022). Of note, neonates with gene mutations affecting SP-B production manifest with severe respiratory distress syndrome (RDS) that often progresses to death unless lung transplantation is performed (this will be discussed later in the chapter; Whitsett & Kingma, 2022). This type of surfactant deficiency is extremely rare.

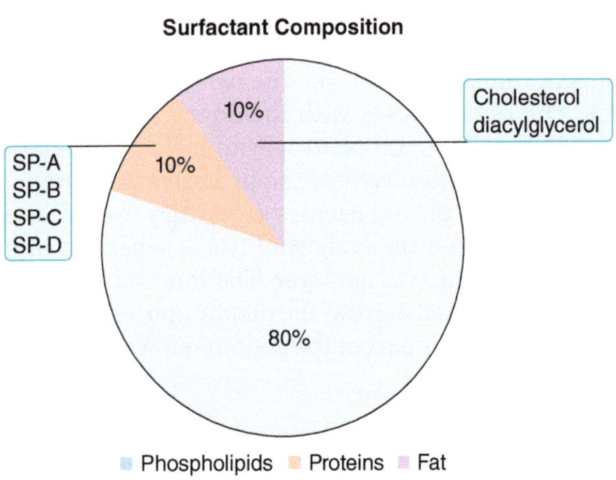

Figure 4.2 Surfactant composition. Percentages are approximations; minor differences are reported in the literature. SP, surfactant protein.

The synthesis, secretion, metabolism, and recycling of surfactant is slower in newborns, especially preterm neonates, given the decreased number and relative immaturity of alveoli and type II pneumocytes (Figure 4.3). Nearly all components that comprise surfactant are synthesized and secreted from LBs, small vesicles found within the type II pneumocytes that produce and store surfactant before secreting surfactant into the alveolar space. Surfactant secretion occurs by way of several biochemical and mechanical signaling pathways, the most common being mechanical stretch. Stretching of the type II pneumocytes activates the migration of phospholipids, SP-B, and SP-C into the LBs, which are packaged with surfactant phospholipids, and subsequently excreted into the alveoli, forming the tension-reducing bioactive film. The surfactant molecules are thereby metabolized and degraded by alveolar macrophages or taken up by the type II cell for recycling (Akella & Desphande, 2013; Jobe & Kallapur, 2022; Kallapur & Jobe, 2025; Plosa & Sucre, 2024).

Surfactant Function

Surfactant functions by (a) lowering surface tension at the air–liquid interface, (b) disrupting the biological lipid membrane and serving as antimicrobial agents, and (c) modulating the innate immune response (see Chapter 9). Surfactant synthesis, secretion, and metabolism, as well as the recycling of surfactant, are slower in newborns compared to older children and adults. A low surface tension is critical to prevent alveolar collapse during expiration. Yet, attractive forces found at the air–liquid interface favor increased surface tension, also known as increased collapsing pressure. Further complicating matters is the fact that alveoli have a natural tendency to collapse because of their spherical shape and small size. Fortunately, the chemical composition of surfactant, specifically its high concentration of DPPC, works to resist (and even lower) the surface tension to zero (Plosa & Sucre, 2024).

DPPC is a saturated phospholipid that forms a cohesive bioactive film within the alveoli. One end of the DPPC molecule is hydrophilic, allowing it to dissolve in water and attach in a perpendicular fashion to the alveolar wall. The opposite or hydrophobic end protrudes into the alveolus. The hydrophobic ends of the DPPC molecules crowd together during expiration, which opposes

TABLE 4.3 Surfactant Proteins: Overview and Availability

Surfactant Protein Type	Overview of Function	Available in Commercial Surfactant Preparations
SP-A	Regulator of lung inflammation; binds to bacterial and viral pathogens; facilitates phagocytosis and clearance of surfactant	No
SP-B	Secretory protein that facilitates surfactant homeostasis; participates in LB formation; facilitates lipid absorption and reduction in surface tension along with SP-C; complete SP-B deficiency leads to respiratory failure and death	Yes
SP-C	Works in conjunction with SP-B to facilitate lipid absorption and decreasing surface tension	Yes
SP-D	Regulator of lung inflammation; binds to bacterial and viral pathogens; facilitates phagocytosis and clearance of pathogens	No

LB, lamellar body; SP, surfactant protein.

surface tension and holds the alveoli open (Han & Mallampalli, 2015).

While SP-B and SP-C consistently lower surface tension, SP-A and SP-D participate in host defenses, immunomodulation, and the clearance and metabolism of surfactant. SP-A and SP-D modulate and degrade bacteria (e.g., *Escherichia coli*) and clear them from the distal airways. Last, surfactant plays a role in the innate immune response. In this capacity, surfactant protects infants from pathogens prior to a directed immune response and then participates in the directed immune response. Upregulation of SP-A and SP-D by alveolar epithelial type II pneumocytes is observed when foreign agents, such as dust or pollen, enter the airways. This upregulation functions to stunt allergic reactions by inhibiting the proliferation of lymphocytes and decreasing the allergic histamine response. Children with asthma commonly suffer from deficient SP-A– and SP-D–modulated immune responses (Han & Mallampalli, 2015).

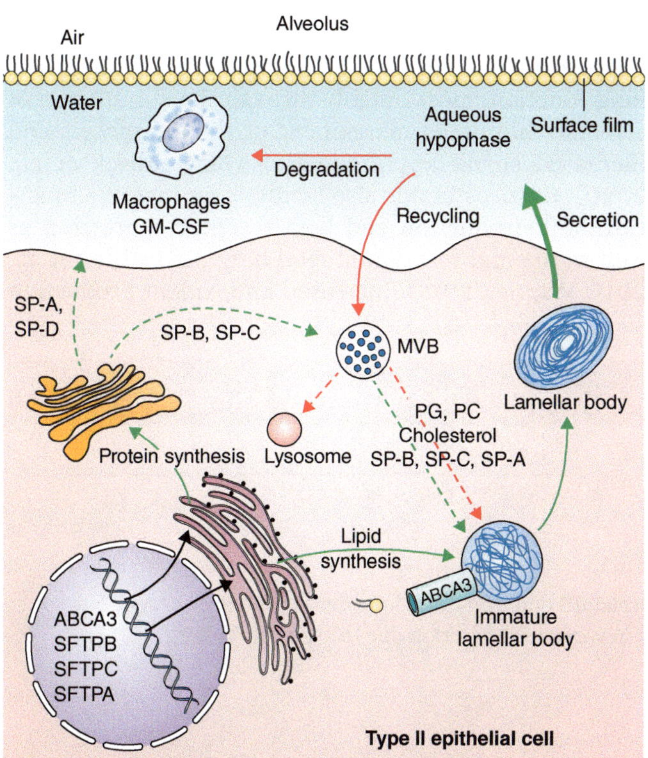

Figure 4.3 Synthesis, secretion, metabolism, and recycling of surfactant.

GM-CSF, granulocyte-macrophage colony-stimulating factor; MVB, multivesicular bodies; PC, phosphatidylcholine; PG, phosphatidylglycerol; SP, surfactant protein.

Fetal Lung Mechanics

Fetal Breathing Movements. Fetal breathing movements (FBMs) are essential to pulmonary growth and development and begin during the second trimester, toward the latter end of the pseudoglandular phase. FBMs strengthen the diaphragm and respiratory accessory muscles, facilitate lung growth and differentiation, and facilitate development of the neural control of the respiratory center (Malleske, 2015). Observed episodes of FBM are cyclical and typically occur over a 20- to 30-minute period. They alternate with apnea and appear to coincide with sleep cycles (Malleske, 2015). Peripheral chemoreceptors facilitate FBM in the normal lung through the response to oxygen and carbon dioxide levels. This mimics their function after birth.

With each breathing movement, the glottis opens, yet the presence of fetal lung fluid deters the influx of amniotic fluid into the airways. These breathing movements encourage the peristaltic migration of fetal lung fluid from proximal to more distal airspaces and facilitates necessary stretching and growth of distal airways. Mechanical stretching elicits the synthesis of growth factors which, in turn, encourage the proliferation of additional epithelial cells and the synthesis of surfactant (Cotton, 2017).

Extremely preterm infants are considered at high risk for pulmonary hypoplasia because limited epithelial cells are present and capable of producing fetal lung fluid, FBM have not been well established, and limited growth factor production has ensued prior to birth; this hinders postnatal lung maturation. Similarly, oligohydramnios and lung masses (e.g., congenital pulmonary airway malformation) restrict available space for respiratory stretching and proliferation, and precipitate reduced FBMs and pulmonary hypoplasia. Injury to the vagus nerve is associated with congenital hypoventilation syndrome ("Ondine curse") and is linked to pulmonary hypoplasia given the absence of FBMs. In addition, fetal exposure(s) to central nervous system depressants and stimulants negatively affect fetal lung development and breathing movements (Table 4.4; Malleske, 2015).

The Role of Antenatal Steroids. Discussions focused on antenatal and postnatal diagnosis and treatment mechanisms are largely beyond the scope of this textbook. However, antenatal steroids exert a significant effect on fetal lung development and postnatal physiologic function. These factors elevate the significance of this topic and warrant its inclusion in this chapter.

The administration of antenatal corticosteroids is one of the most significant prenatal therapies used in light of threatened premature labor and delivery to improve neonatal outcomes. Based on extensive research and meta-analyses, the American College of Obstetricians and Gynecologists (ACOG, 2024) makes certain recommendations regarding definitive administration versus the consideration for antenatal steroid administration. More specific, ACOG recommends that pregnant patients between 24 0/7 weeks and 33 6/7 weeks' gestation with threatened preterm delivery definitively receive a single course (2 doses) of antenatal steroids ("steroid complete" status is achieved 24-hours after the second dose is administered). ACOG suggests that clinicians consider antenatal steroid administration in pregnant patients who are 23 0/7 and 23 6/7 weeks as well as 34 0/7 and 36 6/7 weeks of gestation (ACOG, 2024). The provision of at least one complete course of antenatal steroids has been associated with significant reductions in RDS, necrotizing enterocolitis, intraventricular hemorrhage, and death (ACOG, 2024). A repeat 2-dose course of steroids should be considered for pregnant patients who are less than 34 0/7 weeks of gestation, with threatened preterm labor, and who previously received steroids at least 14 days prior. Rescue corticosteroid dosing can be considered by obstetric experts when the prior course of steroids occurred at least 7 days prior (ACOG, 2024).

Corticosteroids can be categorized as glucocorticoids or mineralocorticoids. Among healthy infants, children, and adults, glucocorticoids are hormones released by the adrenal glands in response to stimulation of the hypothalamic–pituitary–adrenal (HPA) axis, as a means to respond to a stressor and reestablish homeostasis (see Chapter 10; Oakley & Cidlowski, 2013). The ligand-dependent family of transcription factors, known as *glucocorticoid receptors (GR)*, are present on target cells throughout the body and mediate the effects of glucocorticoids. Among pregnant patients and fetuses, antenatally administered glucocorticoids (betamethasone or dexamethasone) can accelerate fetal lung maturity because of their anti-inflammatory properties. Glucocorticoids impart a pleiotropic effect on neonatal lung function, most notably through the stimulation of alveolar thinning, enlargement of the air spaces, and increased surfactant production (McGoldrick et al., 2020). Corticosteroids also facilitate an increase in antioxidant production and beta-receptor expression as well as the reabsorption of fetal lung fluid (Riley et al., 2011; Wapner, 2013). Increased antioxidant production

TABLE 4.4 Effects of Licit and Illicit Drug Use on Fetal Lung Development and Function

Drug Category	Risks to Lung Development and Function
Depressant	↑ Fetal growth restriction ↑ Teratogenic effects
Opioid	↑ Risk of premature birth: insufficient surfactant and immature lung development ↑ Risk of placental abruption: alterations in surfactant function due to asphyxia ↑ Fetal growth restriction
Stimulant	↑ Risk of premature birth ↑ Risk of placental abruption ↑ Fetal growth restriction ↓ Alveolarization

Note: Premature birth is associated with immature lung development and insufficient surfactant production. Placental abruption is associated with alterations in surfactant function due to hypoxia. Fetal growth restriction may negatively restrict lung development.

is important in countering the effects associated with increased oxidative stress commonly seen with the transition to an oxygen-rich environment. An increase in beta-receptor expression leads to bronchial smooth muscle relaxation and increased surfactant production.

Fetal Lung Fluid Production and Clearance

Fetal lung fluid is an important factor in structural and functional development of the respiratory system. Beginning as early as week 6 of gestation, fetal lung fluid develops from active chloride (Cl^-) secretion by epithelial cells, which fills the alveolar lumen and encourages spatial expansion. The composition of fetal lung fluid is uniquely different than amniotic fluid, with the most notable difference being the disproportionately higher concentration of chloride in fetal lung fluid (Table 4.5).

The volume of fetal lung fluid increases throughout the first half of pregnancy, from approximately 4 mL/kg to 6 mL/kg of body weight at 20 weeks of gestation to approximately 30 mL/kg at term, before it progressively decreases in preparation for birth (Plosa & Sucre, 2024). Fetal lung fluid prepares the lungs for extrauterine life. It accomplishes this by creating a distending end-expiratory pressure within the lungs of approximately 2 to 4 cmH_2O. This "trains" the fetal lungs to resist the natural recoil of the chest wall. The lung fluid moves up the respiratory tract with a small amount escaping the trachea during FBM; this is either swallowed or expelled into the amniotic fluid volume (Gao & Raj, 2010; te Pas & Hooper, 2016).

Fetal lung fluid production slows as the neonate approaches term. This is a logical transition, as the neonatal lungs need to quickly shift from a fluid-filled to air-filled cavity. By term gestation and prior to birth, the lungs contain approximately 100 mL of lung fluid (Alhassen et al., 2021). In preparation for life outside of the womb, the lungs transition from active fluid (Cl^-) secretion to fluid (Na^+) absorption (Katz et al., 2011). Just prior to the onset of labor (in term fetuses), glucocorticoid and thyroid hormone synthesis is upregulated, which activates Na+ channels. Once labor ensues, fetal synthesis of catecholamines significantly increases. This activates epithelial Na^+ channels (ENaC) and upregulates the transition from Cl^- secretion to Na^+ absorption by way of ENaC. Type I cells modulate the bulk of water transport and Type II cells modulate the active transport of Na^+ across the epithelium of alveoli, where both are functionally reabsorbed (Alhassen et al., 2021; Hillman et al., 2012). This reabsorption is a two-step process: (a) Na^+ is passively absorbed into the cellular membrane through ENaC, and (b) Na^+ is actively excreted into the interstitial space, where it can be absorbed by the pulmonary vasculature and lymphatic systems (Figure 4.4; Hillman et al., 2012). With vaginal births, mechanical forces imposed during fetal descent into the pelvis assist (to a small degree) with additional fluid evacuation from the lungs. After birth and within 2 to 6 hours of life, catecholamine levels have decreased to insignificant levels, and in most circumstances lung fluid has evacuated the airspaces. Failed reabsorption of fetal lung fluid increases the risk for transiently obstructive lung disease known as transient tachypnea of the newborn (TTN).

Cardiopulmonary Changes at Birth

With advancing gestational age, fetal pulmonary vascular tone increases. This encourages high PVR and low pulmonary blood flow; recall that less than 20% of cardiac output reaches the lungs during fetal development (Gao & Raj, 2010; Hooper et al., 2019). Explanations for this phenomenon include the active (in utero) secretion of fluid into the alveolar spaces combined with increased hydrostatic pressure, which promotes lung distention and compression of the pulmonary vasculature (Gao & Raj, 2010; Hillman et al., 2012; Hooper et al., 2019). As the fetus approaches term, vasomotor tone becomes more reactive, a necessary adaptation in preparation for extrauterine life.

In the meantime, the placenta continues to modulate gas exchange until birth occurs. Recall that oxygenated blood leaves the placenta and travels to the fetus via the umbilical vein, with most of the blood shunting past the hepatic circulation via the ductus venosus and into the right atrium. This oxygenated blood mixes with blood returning to the right atrium and shunts across the foramen ovale into the left atrium, where it mixes with the small volume of blood returning from the lungs via the pulmonary veins, into the left ventricle, then out the

TABLE 4.5 Comparison of Fetal Lung Fluid and Amniotic Fluid Composition

	pH	Bicarbonate (mEq/L)	Sodium (mEq/L)	Potassium (mEq/L)	Chloride (mEq/L)	Protein (g/dL)
Fetal lung fluid	6.27	3	150	6.3	157	0.03
Amniotic fluid	7.02	19	113	7.6	87	0.10

Source: Plosa, E., & Sucre, J. (2024). Lung development. In C. A. Gleason & T. Sawyer (Eds.), *Avery's diseases of the newborn* (11th ed.; pp. 535–547). Elsevier/Saunders.

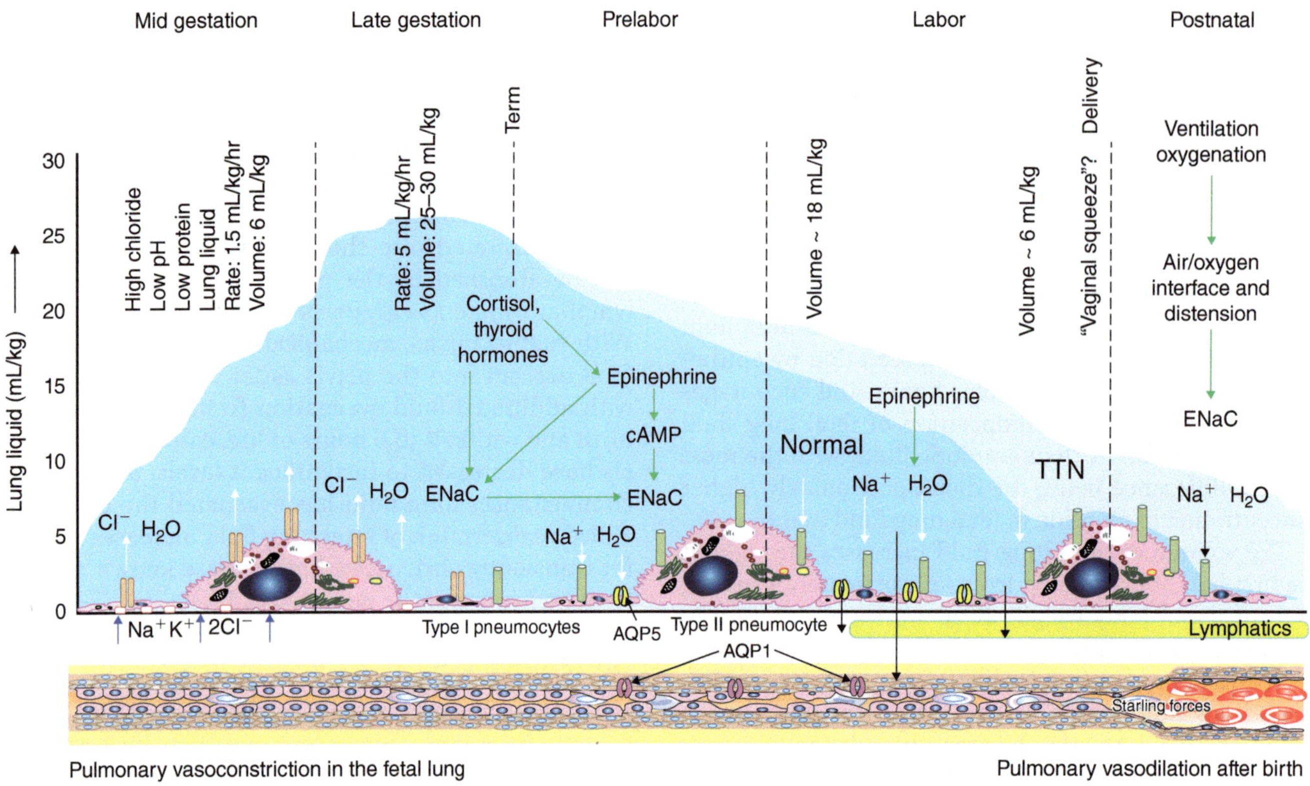

Figure 4.4 Fetal and neonatal lung fluid secretion and absorption.

AQP1, aquaporin-1 channels; AQP5, aquaporin-5; ENaC, epithelial sodium channel; NKCC, Na+-K+-Cl– cotransporter, TTN, transient tachypnea of the newborn.

Source: Alhassen, Z., Vali, P., Guglani, L., Lakshminrusimha, S., & Ryan, R. M. (2021). Recent advances in pathophysiology and management of transient tachypnea of newborn. *Journal of Perinatology: Official Journal of the California Perinatal Association, 41*(1), 6–16. https://doi.org/10.1038/s41372-020-0757-3. Copyright Satyan Lakshminrusimha, MD. Used with permission.

aorta to the body. Blood returning to the right atrium via the superior vena cava travels primarily to the right ventricle, then out the pulmonary artery and either shunts across the ductus arteriosus (DA), rejoining the blood flow in the aorta, or travels on to the lungs providing nutrients to the developing lung tissue (**Figure 4.5**). The transition to extrauterine life requires prompt changes within a narrow time frame. Blood flow must change from the aforementioned parallel circulation to one that flows in series (right heart side flowing into the left heart side following a series of steps). In addition, fetal lung fluid secretion must slow.

Fortunately, catecholamines and glucocorticoid release during labor stimulates the opening of epithelial Na^+ channels in late preterm and term newborns, and this action prompts the egress of lung fluid from the alveoli and into lung tissues (Gao & Raj, 2010; Guglani et al., 2008; Hillman et al., 2012). Importantly, the mode of delivery (cesarean versus vaginal) does *not* influence adrenaline production nor the rate of lung fluid clearance into lung interstitium before it is reabsorbed into the lymphatics or pulmonary capillary network (Hooper et al., 2019). Of note, preterm newborns do not benefit from the effect of increased circulating adrenaline because increased synthesis during labor does not occur until near term gestation.

Clamping of the umbilical cord and the first postnatal breath promote the neonatal lung to primary modulator of oxygenation. The alveoli expand with each subsequent breath and the distending pressure that once compressed the pulmonary vasculature abates. PVR begins to fall, and systemic vascular resistance (SVR) increases (see Chapters 5 and 14; Van Woudenberg et al., 2012). These processes activate the critical air–fluid interface, which under normal circumstances causes a temporary increase in surface tension and elastic recoil (Hooper et al., 2019; te Pas & Hooper, 2016). Surfactant secretion is critical in these moments, and is essential to the continuation of a normal extrauterine transition; deficiencies are associated with respiratory distress. Synthesis and secretion of surfactant modulate alveolar stability, or functional residual capacity (FRC), and decrease surface tension (collapsing pressure). Over time, chest wall rigidity increases in opposition to lung recoil, allowing the neonatal lung to tolerate greater negative intrapleural pressures while maintaining lung inflation (te Pas & Hooper, 2016; Truog & Manimtim, 2024).

With the rising postnatal SVR and falling PVR, functional fetal shunts are no longer necessary and the foramen ovale closes. Blood flow returning from the body to the heart is directed from the right ventricle into the pulmonary artery to the lungs. With the postnatal decline

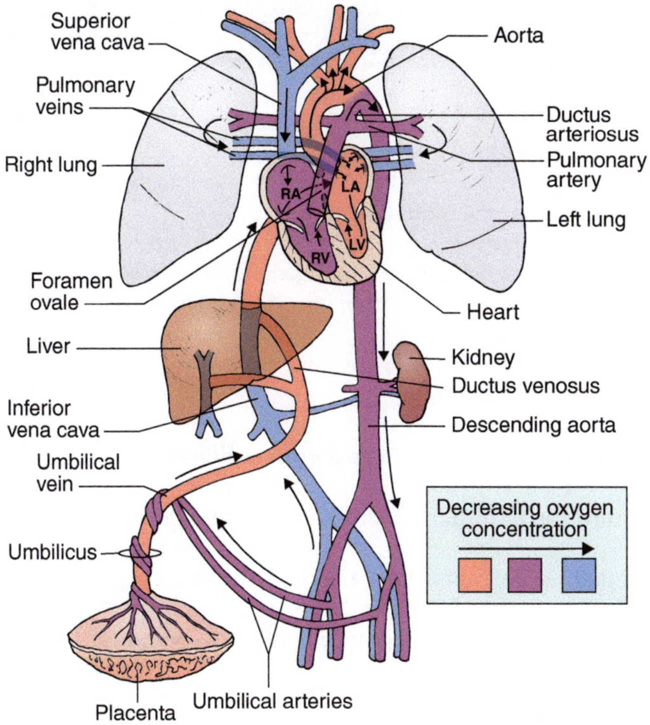

Figure 4.5 Newborn transition to extrauterine life.
LA, left atrium; LV, left ventricle; RA, right atrium; RV, right ventricle.

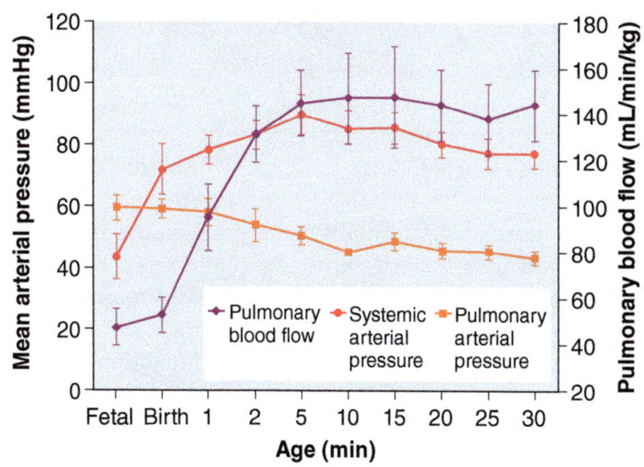

Figure 4.6 Changes in pulmonary blood flow through transition to neonatal life.
Source: Adapted from Nair, J., & Lakshminrusimha, S. (2014). Update on PPHN: Mechanisms and treatment. *Seminars in Perinatology, 38*, 78–91. https://doi.org/10.1053/j.semperi.2013.11.004

of circulating prostaglandins (PGE2), increased elimination of PGE2 by the lungs, increased arterial oxygenation, and decreased vascular tone in the ductus, the DA constricts; this marks the process of functional closure of the DA (Ali & Sawyer, 2024).

Vasoactive properties, activated by the shearing stress of pulmonary vasodilatation, lead to further reductions in PVR. These properties, synthesized in the endothelium of the pulmonary vasculature, include endogenous nitric oxide (EDNO), prostacyclin (PGI2), PGE2, endothelin-1 (ET-1), and platelet-activating factor (PAF). EDNO, mediated by cyclic guanosine monophosphate (cGMP), stimulates pulmonary vasodilatation. The prostanoids (PGI2 and PGE2) provide control of vasodilatation, a process modulated by the cAMP pathway (Gao & Raj, 2010). Postnatal ET-1 activity at ET_B receptors promotes vasodilation (Gao & Raj, 2010). Due to increased oxygen levels, PAF levels decrease following delivery and contribute to vasodilation of the pulmonary blood vessels postdelivery (Figure 4.6; Gao & Raj, 2010). In the healthy newborn adapting to extrauterine life, these changes happen rather seamlessly. Failed transition may manifest as respiratory diseases or persistent pulmonary hypertension of the newborn (PPHN).

Postnatal Lung Mechanics

The biochemical changes noted previously are critical to postnatal survival. In addition, mechanical changes, albeit more gradual, must occur. Recall that the anatomy and mechanics of the neonatal thorax differ from that of the adult and older child. The neonatal chest is more cylindrical than the elliptical shape of the adult thorax. The ribs have a more horizontal orientation in comparison to the oblique orientation seen in adults; this results in a relative shortening of the intercostal muscles (Keszler & Abubakar, 2022). As a result, neonates are less able to elevate their rib cage during inspiration and increase intrathoracic volume. The combination of the horizontal nature of the newborn diaphragm and the compliant chest wall results in an inward movement of the lower ribs during inspiration and lungs that are more prone to collapse. Maturation of the intercostal muscles and establishment of mature lung compliance progresses across infancy, childhood, and into adulthood. See Table 4.6 for additional definitions of neonatal pulmonary mechanics.

Clinical Application. The newborn's chest wall is primarily comprised of highly elastic cartilage. This makes the chest wall very compliant and prone to collapse during exhalation. Newborns will attempt to avoid collapse (and maintain FRC) by exhibiting any of the following maneuvers:

- laryngeal adduction with narrowing of the glottis; and
- maintaining the contractile state of inspiratory muscles during exhalation (creating a stiff chest wall); and/or
- increasing the respiratory rate to retain gas and limit the available time for exhalation.

While these maneuvers may help maintain FRC and therefore overcome the elastic and resistive forces complicating normal respiratory movements, they are fatiguing and often are accompanied by signs of increased work of breathing (audible grunting, nasal flaring, and retractions).

TABLE 4.6 Pulmonary Mechanics/Lung Measurement Definitions

Mechanic	Definition
Tidal volume (TV or VT)	Amount of gas moved during one normal inspiration and expiration
Functional residual capacity (FRC)	Volume of gas left in lung after a normal expiration
Residual volume	Minimum lung volume possible—air left in lung after maximum expiration
Vital capacity	Maximum amount of air that can be moved
Total lung capacity	Total amount of volume present in the lung
Inspiratory capacity	Maximum volume of air that can be inspired after a normal expiration
Inspiratory reserve volume	Additional amount of air that can be inspired after a normal inspiration
Expiratory reserve volume	Additional amount of air that can be expired after a normal expiration
Lung compliance	The change in lung volume divided by the change in lung pressure, which is influenced by the elastic recoil of the lungs
Minute volume	Combination of tidal volume and respiratory rate
Anatomic dead space	Part of airway where no gas exchange occurs (trachea, bronchi, etc.)
Physiologic dead space	Alveoli that is ventilated but under- or not perfused

Postnatal Gas Exchange. Following birth, the neonate transitions, over the first 3 to 6 months of life, to the production of adult hemoglobin (HgA); concurrent increases in 2,3-DPG production are also observed. Recall that HgA has a decreased affinity for oxygen, meaning that less oxygen will remain bound to hemoglobin in the lungs as more is released to the tissues. As such, this gradual postnatal transition from HgF to HgA is associated with reduced oxygen affinity and rightward shift of the oxyhemoglobin dissociation curve (ODC). Hemoglobin readily releases oxygen in an effort to ensure adequate tissue oxygenation, as oxygen demand is increased after birth. Postnatal blood transfusions can cause shifts in the ODC (right shift secondary to loss of HgF and increased acquisition of HgA), as well as alterations in pH, 2,3 DPG levels, and body temperature (Juul & Christensen, 2024; Rios et al., 2022). Refer to Figure 4.7 (and Chapter 7) to associate increases or decreases in these factors with corresponding shifts in oxygen affinity.

Ventilation and Perfusion. Gas exchange is dependent on matching of ventilation and perfusion, referred to as *V (ventilation)/Q (perfusion) matching* (V/Q ratio). The V/Q ratio is a description of the balance between ventilation (airflow at the alveoli) and perfusion (blood flow entering the lungs). In that sense, the V/Q is a reflection of alveolar ventilation divided by cardiac output. If part of the lung is ventilated but not perfused, or perfused but not ventilated, a V/Q mismatch occurs. This leads to either hypoxemia or hypercarbia.

Acid–Base Status. Blood gas evaluation is used to assess ventilation and oxygenation status, the severity of lung disease, the effectiveness of treatment modalities, and acid–base status. Arterial blood gas sampling is the gold standard; venous and capillary gas sampling are clinically useful methodologies and often associated with less invasive and noxious stimuli. The elements of blood gas analysis include pH, pO_2 (partial pressure of oxygen), pCO_2 (partial pressure of carbon dioxide), HCO_3^- (bicarbonate), base excess or base deficit, and oxygen saturation. The pH, pO_2, and pCO_2 are directly measured. The HCO_3^- and base deficit/base excess values are calculated and not directly measured. Depending on the blood gas analyzer used, the oxygen saturation can be directly measured or calculated. Table 4.7 presents normal ranges for blood gas components.

Neonatal Pulmonary Function. Pulmonary function can be assessed, in part, through visual observation. Although a discussion of the pulmonary examination is beyond the scope of this textbook, clinicians should understand that respiratory rate, retractions, nasal flaring, grunting, and cyanosis are invaluable in the identification of abnormal pulmonary function or pulmonary mechanics. Hypoventilation leads to decreases in alveolar

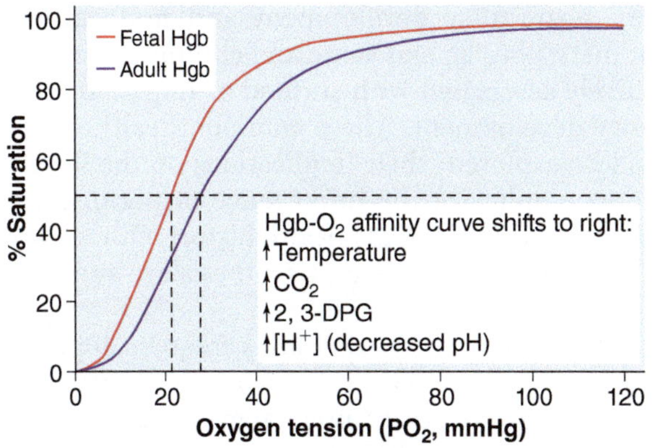

Figure 4.7 Postnatal oxygen dissociation curve.
Hgb, hemoglobin; PO_2, partial pressure of oxygen; DPG, disphosohoglyceric acid.
Source: Adapted from Ohls, R. K. (2011). Core concepts: The biology of hemoglobin. *NeoReviews, 12*(1), e29–e38. https://doi.org/10.1542/neo.12-1-e29

TABLE 4.7 Blood Gas Components

Value	Normal Range
pH	7.35–7.45
pO_2	60–95 mmHg
pCO_2	35–45 mmHg
HCO_3^-	22–26 mmol/L
BD/BE	−5/+5

BD, base deficit; BE, base excess; HCO_3^-, bicarbonate; pCO_2, partial pressure of carbon dioxide; pO_2, partial pressure of oxygen.

minute ventilation, whereas tachypnea yields low tidal volume. Retractions may suggest low lung compliance, obstruction, or atelectasis. Nasal flaring is a compensatory mechanism used to reduce airway resistance and total lung resistance. Grunting is a compensatory attempt to maintain FRC and maximize the partial pressure of oxygen; infants exhale against a closed or partially closed glottis. Central cyanosis, detected by the examination of the lips, tongue, and oral mucosa, suggests hypoxia. The value of the integrated physical assessment, as a critical component of identifying and diagnosing pulmonary dysfunction, cannot be understated.

GENETIC INFLUENCES

A myriad of genetically linked respiratory disorders can manifest in the neonatal period, or later into childhood and early adulthood. Although a discussion of all genetically linked respiratory disorders is beyond the scope of this textbook, we present two rare surfactant deficiencies that manifest within the first 2 years of life. In addition, we discuss cystic fibrosis (CF), a common genetic disorder that affects respiratory function. Additional inherited disorders affecting the respiratory system are provided in Box 4.1.

Hereditary Surfactant Protein Deficiencies

Recall that SP-B stimulates the formation of LBs within the type II pneumocytes and the synthesis and secretion of surfactant. SP-B formation is modulated by the SP-B gene (*SFPTB*), which is found on chromosome 2. Hereditary SP-B deficiency, a rare autosomal recessive disorder, develops in the presence of *SFPTB* mutations. At present, more than 40 mutations have been identified (Fleury et al., 2025). The deficiency of SP-B deficiency alters the composition of surfactant molecules, and this leads to widespread increased alveolar surface tension, alveolar collapse, and respiratory distress or failure. This disease is associated with a high mortality risk; most infants do not survive beyond the first 3 to 6 months of life (Fleury et al., 2025; Marinicak & Lomas, 2017).

In contrast, SP-C facilitates lipid recruitment and spreading of the surfactant film within the alveoli. SP-C deficiency is an autosomal dominant disorder caused by mutations in the SP-C gene (*SFTPC*), which is found on chromosome 8 (8p21). At present, more than 50 mutations have been identified and upwards of 55% of cases involve de novo mutations (Singh et al., 2021). The most severe *SFTPC* mutations manifest with severe respiratory failure, usually within the first few days of life. Less severe mutations have been associated with progressive interstitial lung disease, which manifests in infancy, as well as idiopathic pulmonary fibrosis in adults.

Cystic Fibrosis

Recall from Chapter 1 that CF is the most common autosomal recessive disorder diagnosed during infancy. The

BOX 4.1 Other Inherited Disorders That Affect the Respiratory System

- ABCA3 transporter disorder
- Apert syndrome
- Congenital hypoventilation syndrome
- Crouzon disease
- Gaucher disease
- Neurofibromatosis (NF1)/von Recklinghausen's disease
- Smith–Lemli–Opitz disorder
- Tuberous sclerosis

Note: A more comprehensive list is provided by the National Institutes of Health, Genetic and Rare Diseases Information Center (https://rarediseases.info.nih.gov/).

incidence is one in every 5,130 live births in the United States and one in every 3,848 live births in Canada, a decreasing trend (Stanojevic et al., 2022). CF occurs due to mutations in the cystic fibrosis transmembrane conductance regulator (*CFTR*) gene (Marinicak & Lomas, 2017). The *CFTR* gene, located on the long arm of chromosome 7, is responsible for the production of the CFTR protein (Marinicak & Lomas, 2017). CFTR protein regulates ion and water balance at the epithelial membrane located in the lung, GI tract, pancreas, sweat glands, and genitourinary system (Terlizzi et al., 2018). Deficient protein concentrations permit the formation of abnormally thick mucosal secretions, which impairs respiratory function.

Meconium ileus is the hallmark clinical manifestation of cystic fibrosis, occurring in approximately 71% of affected newborns younger than 2 weeks of age, with a slight male predominance noted in the literature (Huang et al., 2021). The incidence of MI in older children with CF is 10% (Dingeldein, 2025; Huang et al., 2021). Manifestations during infancy and childhood include varying degrees of cough and respiratory disease. Older infants commonly develop a chronic cough, copious thick sputum production, and are considered at risk for pneumonia. In the most severe of cases, respiratory failure secondary to bronchiectasis and lung scarring occurs (Spoonhower & Davis, 2016).

Due to state-mandated newborn metabolic screening programs, CF is typically identified during the newborn period. Most states offer combined blood spot analysis and reflexive screening for *CFTR* gene mutations. Blood spot analysis can detect elevated levels of immunoreactive trypsin (IRT), which is a substance normally released from the pancreas and which aids in the digestion of enteral proteins. In newborns with CF, mucus plugs can block the release of trypsin into the intestinal tract and lead to abnormally high serum IRT levels.

Newborns with elevated IRT levels or confirmed mutations reported on the newborn metabolic screening test will require "gold standard" sweat chloride testing once they weigh greater than 2.5 kg. This test assesses *CTFR* function in the sweat glands located in the skin. An elevated sweat chloride result greater than 60 mmol/L is consistent with CF (Terlizzi & Dolce, 2023). Among individuals with CF, the median life expectancy is currently 65 years, which is a significant improvement from 39 years in 2010 and near immediate death in the late 1930s (Cystic Fibrosis Foundation, 2021).

NOTEWORTHY DISEASES IN THE XX PREGNANT PATIENT THAT INFLUENCE FETAL RESPIRATORY DEVELOPMENT AND FUNCTION

The health status of the XX pregnant patient impacts all aspects of fetal and neonatal growth and development, including respiratory development and maturation. High-fat diets, obesity, and acute and chronic infections are positively associated with stunted or impaired fetal respiratory development. These common health influences will be explored; their implications on the developing fetus emphasize the importance of performing comprehensive analysis of the health history. Other conditions that implicate surfactant synthesis are summarized in Table 4.8.

Components of a healthy diet are a frequent topic of conversation between the obstetrician and pregnant patient during all stages of pregnancy. Research into the composition of a healthy diet has included a focus on avoiding high-fat diets and prioritizing daily vitamin intake, docosahexaenoic acid (DHA), and folic acid supplementation. Among pregnant smokers, vitamin C supplementation appears to optimize respiratory function and reduce wheezing associated with asthma in exposed newborns (McEvoy et al., 2023). A high-fat diet during pregnancy has been linked to impaired respiratory system development, obesity, metabolic disease, anxiety, depression, and attention deficit disorder in offspring (Calco et al., 2023; Gawlińska et al., 2021). High-fat diets also predispose the pregnant patient to obesity. Approximately 75% of individuals of childbearing age (20–39) are overweight (body mass index [BMI] 25–30) with 40% considered obese BMI greater than 30; Britt et al., 2013; Dingeldein, 2025; March of Dimes, 2020). Metabolic syndrome (visceral obesity, dyslipidemia, hypertension, and hyperglycemia) among pregnant patients has been linked to elevations in proinflammatory cytokines and an increase in wheezing/asthma of their offspring (Britt et al., 2013). Diabetes or hyperglycemia in the XX pregnant patient encourages fetal hyperinsulinemia,

TABLE 4.8 Other Conditions in XX Pregnant Patients Which Affect Surfactant Production

Disease Process	Increased	Decreased
Cardiovascular disease	X	
Cesarean section		X
Cholestasis		X
Chorioamnionitis	X	
Chronic hypertension	X	
Diabetes		X
Pregnancy-induced hypertension	X	
Prolonged rupture of membranes	X	

which in turn delays the functional maturation of the lungs and prolongs the time in which a neonate is at risk for RDS (Britt et al., 2013). Macrosomia in the fetus born to a pregnant patient with diabetes increases the risk for birth trauma, asphyxia, delayed reabsorption of fetal lung fluid, and respiratory distress.

Intrauterine growth restriction (IUGR), which is associated with impaired nutrient and oxygen delivery to the fetus, has also been linked to aberrant fetal pulmonary development. IUGR is defined as an estimated fetal weight (EFW) that is less than the tenth percentile expected for the gestational age and is reported in 3% to 7% of pregnancies that are often complicated by chronic hypertension, preeclampsia, and diabetes (Briana & Malamitsi-Puchner, 2020). Developmental problems include the development of fewer alveoli, thickened alveolar septation, and abnormal vascular development (Pike et al., 2012). Postnatal problems can include RDS and pulmonary hypertension (Devaskar et al., 2025). Late-onset problems can include asthma and chronic obstructive pulmonary disease (COPD; Briana & Malamitsi-Puchner, 2020).

COMMON PROBLEMS WITH IMPLICATIONS ACROSS THE LIFE SPAN

Multiple etiologies and overlapping factors contribute to neonatal respiratory distress. For learning purposes, we present two categories of respiratory diseases: (a) congenital or development problems and (b) acquired diseases. The incidence, manifestations, pathophysiology, and life-span implications of the more common disease processes will be discussed next.

Congenital and Developmental Problems

Many lung abnormalities occur early in fetal life and are related to genetic causes, whereas others may be related to in utero events that impact the developing lung. Prenatal fetal imaging is critical to the early identification of these lesions to counsel parents adequately and to guide appropriate management strategies. Although many of these disorders can be diagnosed prenatally, some do present later in childhood or adulthood.

Pulmonary Hypoplasia. Pulmonary hypoplasia is a rare disorder estimated to occur in 12.9% of pregnancies affected by premature prelabor rupture of membranes (PPROM), which occurs between 15 and 28 weeks of gestation (Winn et al., 2000). This disease is one part of a triad of pulmonary abnormalities known as *pulmonary underdevelopment complex*, with the triad also including pulmonary aplasia and pulmonary atresia. With pulmonary hypoplasia, the lung is incompletely developed. This results in the development of fewer lung cells, airways, alveoli, and corresponding pulmonary vasculature, which severely limits gas exchange (Crowley, 2025; Triebwasser & Treadwell, 2017).

Pulmonary hypoplasia is classified as primary or secondary. Primary hypoplasia is most likely due to inappropriate lung-bud development as a result of abnormal expression of growth factors and transcription factors (Crowley, 2025; Hsu et al., 2012). Secondary pulmonary hypoplasia is more common and results from processes that impede normal lung development. Common pathologic processes that contribute to secondary pulmonary hypoplasia include:

- *Oligohydramnios:* Lung fluid and lung fluid exchange facilitate fetal lung expansion. With diminished fluid, adequate lung growth does not occur. Renal anomalies (decreased urine production), early amniotic fluid loss as with early membrane rupture, placental abnormalities, and IUGR can all contribute to decreased lung fluid.
- *Lung compression from space-occupying lesions:* Lung compression and inadequate thoracic space for lung growth can result in hypoplasia (Triebwasser & Treadwell, 2017). CDH, cystic lung lesions, congenital heart disease with cardiomegaly, and decreased pulmonary blood flow can contribute to lung compression.
- *Decreased fetal breathing movements:* Normal diaphragm movement is essential for normal lung growth. Central or peripheral nervous system disorders or lesions, as well as musculoskeletal disorders, can contribute to decreased fetal breathing (Crowley, 2025; Hsu et al., 2012).

At birth, infants with hypoplasia often present with respiratory failure, severe respiratory distress, hypoxia, and reduced lung volume by x-ray, and they can require significant amounts of respiratory support. Respiratory distress is further complicated by the presence of PPHN and the development of pneumothoraces.

Survival and prognosis are dependent on the severity, extent, and cause of the hypoplasia. The timing of the disruption of lung growth and development predict the severity of the disease. The earlier the disruption, the more severe the disease. Mortality is high, and those who survive often develop chronic lung disease or bronchopulmonary dysplasia (BPD), which will be discussed later in the chapter. Patients with chronic lung disease have a higher incidence of both upper and lower respiratory tract infections (Crowley, 2025; Hsu et al., 2012). It is not uncommon for those children who survive the early newborn period to require oxygen therapy and/or prolonged ventilatory support.

Congenital Diaphragmatic Hernia. CDH is a developmental defect of the diaphragm that permits the abnormal migration of abdominal contents into the thoracic cavity. CDH is estimated to occur in one of every 2,000 to 3,000 live births (Crowley, 2025). Herniation can occur on the left or right side of the diaphragm, as well as centrally. The most common location for the herniation is the posterior and lateral (left side) region of the diaphragm, and it is titled a Bochdalek hernia. Bochdalek hernias account for 70% of all cases of CDH (Keijzer & Puri, 2010). Anterior (right side) defects, titled Morgagni hernias, account for 25% to 30% of all cases, and central hernias are rare (Chandrasekharan et al., 2017; Keijzer & Puri, 2010). Bilateral hernias and diaphragmatic agenesis are usually fatal.

The defect can occur in isolation, or in conjunction with other congenital anomalies—heart, genitourinary, chromosomal, GI, and musculoskeletal (Chandrasekharan et al., 2017; Crowley, 2025; Kumar, 2015)—as well as in conjunction with trisomy syndromes (Stark et al., 2015). Abdominal contents compress the lung, which affects normal growth and results in pulmonary hypoplasia. Pulmonary hypoplasia can be unilateral or bilateral but is most severe on the side of the hernia (ipsilatera).

The pathogenesis of CDH is complex and not exclusively associated with the herniation of abdominal contents and subsequent reduction in space for lung growth and development. CDH is most likely a multifactorial disease and results from some of the same genetic factors that drive lung and diaphragm development, meaning that this defect arises even before the diaphragm begins to form. Once the diaphragm begins to develop (around week 4 of gestation), disrupted migration of mesenchymal cells (which differentiate into various types of connective tissues) impedes the normal formation of the muscular wall of the diaphragm and gives rise to the herniation. Then, later migration of abdominal contents into the chest cavity compresses the available space for lung development and further contributes to lung hypoplasia. Therefore, the size of the herniation, severity of the pulmonary hypoplasia, severity of the PPHN, presence (or absence) of liver in the thoracic cavity, and the presence of other anomalies influence the severity of the CDH and associated mortality risk (Chandrasekharan et al., 2017; Crowley, 2025; Kumar, 2015; Reed-McCullough & Jnah, 2021).

In the most severe cases, infants present at birth with significant respiratory distress and respiratory insufficiency. Most develop persistent pulmonary hypertension a short time after birth. Less severe forms may present with mild respiratory symptoms, or with symptoms that develop later within the newborn period or even later in life (Reed-McCullough & Jnah, 2021). Among affected neonates, breath sounds are often diminished on the affected side with a shift in prominence of heart sounds to the opposite (contralateral) side. Chest radiographs will demonstrate bowel contents in the thoracic cavity on the ipsilateral side with mediastinal shift to the contralateral side.

Pulmonary function in CDH patients may remain abnormal through childhood and into adult life. Pulmonary function is predictably worse in those patients with significant pulmonary hypoplasia and prolonged ventilatory support (Danzer et al., 2012; Pantich et al., 2014). Obstructive airway disease, bronchospasm, pulmonary hypertension, and pneumonia are common reasons for hospital readmission within the first few years of life (Danzer et al., 2012; Reed-McCullough & Jnah, 2021; Register et al., 2016). The anatomy of the CDH defect, particularly if the defect is large, contributes to gastroesophageal reflux (GER) that can persist into adulthood. GER, feeding difficulties, and oral aversions contribute to poor growth, which can require gastrostomy placement to ensure adequate nutritional intake (Danzer et al., 2012). The incidence of hearing loss and neurodevelopmental delays is higher in this population, and they impact patients across the life span. Overall, CDH outcomes are improved when infants are delivered at tertiary care centers with access to multidisciplinary collaborative expertise.

Congenital Cystic Lung Lesions. Cystic lung malformations are a collection of developmental lung lesions that include congenital pulmonary airway malformation (CPAM), bronchopulmonary sequestration (BPS), bronchogenic cyst (BC), and congenital lobar emphysema (CLE; **Table 4.9**; Chowdhury & Chakraborty, 2015; Crowley, 2025; Durell & Lakhoo, 2014). These lesions are estimated to develop in one in 2,500 to 8,000 live births (Zobel et al., 2019). They are usually identified during the antenatal period and are assumed to have a common embryonic/fetal origin; many regress before birth. Some more rarely present during infancy, childhood, or adulthood and are commonly associated with other congenital anomalies.

The pathogenesis for this family of lung lesions is poorly understood. The onset of aberrant development seems to occur during the pseudoglandular period of lung development (Sfakianaki & Copel, 2012). Pathogenic theories include failed lung-bud and branching morphogenesis, triggered by abnormal gene expression (e.g., sonic hedgehog, bone morphogenic protein) and abnormal transcription factor expression (e.g., thyroid transcription factor), airway obstruction, and metaplasia and dysplasia of otherwise normal tissues (Chowdhury & Chakraborty, 2015; Correia-Pinta et al., 2010; David et al., 2016; Fowler & Gould, 2015; Lamberti et al., 2023).

Congenital Pulmonary Airway Malformation. CPAM, formerly known as congenital cystic adenomatoid malformation (CCAM), is the most commonly diagnosed congenital cystic lung lesion. CPAM accounts for the majority (95%) of all congenital cystic lung lesions (Sun, 2022). CPAM is classified into one of five types (0–4), based on Stocker's classification system (**Table 4.10**; Stocker, 2009).

The specific pathogenesis of CPAM is poorly understood. It appears that the cysts arise within the bronchiolar region. Therefore, CPAM likely involves malformations of the distal pulmonary bronchioles and

TABLE 4.9 Congenital Cystic Lung Lesions

Disease Process	Systemic Blood Supply?	Tracheobronchial Connection?	Malignancy Risk
Bronchogenic cyst	No	No[a]	Yes
Bronchopulmonary sequestration—ELS	Yes[b] (aorta)	No	No
Bronchopulmonary sequestration—ILS	Yes[b] (aorta)	No	Yes
Congenital lobar emphysema	No	No	No
Congenital pulmonary airway malformation	No (pulmonary vessels)	Yes	Yes (Type 1 & 4)

[a]Most bronchogenic cysts do not communicate with the airway. Rarely, a patent connection exists that increases the likelihood for infection.
[b]Systemic blood supply to bronchopulmonary sequestrations is derived from anomalous vessels originating from the aorta.
ELS, extralobar sequestration; ILS, intralobar sequestration.

TABLE 4.10 Stocker Classification System for Congenital Pulmonary Airway Malformations

Type	Location of Malformation	Notes
0	Tracheobronchial region	Rarest and most severe (dense) cystic lesions that frequently involve all lobes of the lung. Defects are associated with other anomalies (cardiovascular, renal) and pulmonary hypoplasia.
1	Bronchial area; bronchioles	*Most common* type of CPAM that affects one lobe of a lung. These cystic lesions are often large and can lead to pulmonary hypoplasia and hydrops. This type of lesion may regress as pregnancy advances. There is an increased risk of bronchioalveolar carcinoma with these lesions in children and adults.
2	Bronchioles	Cystic lesions that are small (compared to type 1) and often associated with other congenital extrapulmonary anomalies (renal, cardiovascular, diaphragmatic hernia, and extrapulmonary sequestration). If the associated congenital anomalies are severe, the outcome will be poor.
3	Bronchioles; alveoli	Lesions are considered noncystic and involve glandular tissues. These cysts do not regress during pregnancy and are associated with an increased risk of developing fetal hydrops and postnatal pulmonary hypertension.
4	Acini	Cystic lesions located at the distal acini that are large, air-filled, and usually covered by type 1 and 2 pneumocytes

CPAM; congenital pulmonary airway malformation.
Sources: Crowley, A. (2025). Spectrum of neonatal respiratory disorders. In A. A. Fanaroff & R. J. Martin (Eds.), *Fanaroff and Martin's neonatal-perinatal medicine: Diseases of the fetus and infant* (11th ed., pp. 1271–1303). Elsevier/Saunders; Stocker, J. T. (2009). Cystic lung disease in infants and children. *Fetal and Pediatric Pathology, 28*(4), 155–184. https://doi.org/10.1080/15513810902984095

lung parenchyma. More specific, type I to III CPAM is associated with failed branching during the pseudoglandular stage of pulmonary development, whereas type IV CPAM is associated with malformations that arise during the canalicular and saccular stages (Sun, 2022).

Up to 50% of all neonates with CPAM present as well-appearing newborns. Respiratory distress, when present, can range from mild to severe and can manifest any time from birth to adulthood. The most common comorbidity associated with CPAM is pulmonary hypoplasia (Crowley, 2025).

Life-span implications include postsurgical complications as well as cough, fever, and recurrent infections in later childhood. There is an increased risk for postoperative complications with emergency surgery when compared to elective surgery (Sfakianaki & Copel, 2012). Few long-term follow-up reports are available, but there is a small risk of malignancy later in life, most notable with type I and type IV lesions (Casagrande & Pederiva, 2016; Plosa & Sucre, 2024).

Bronchopulmonary Sequestration. BPS are masses of nonfunctional dysplastic pulmonary tissue that do not connect to the tracheobronchial tree and include a blood supply, making these lesions distinctly different from CPAM and CLE (which have no blood supply). The anomalous systemic arterial supply typically originates at the thoracic aorta (Hong et al., 2017; Plosa & Sucre, 2024). Two types of BPS are reported, intralobar sequestrations (ILS) or extralobar sequestrations (ELS). ILS lesions are 4 times more common than ELS lesions; 98% of all ILS occur within the lower lobes and most often within the left lung. ILS malformations are enveloped by and connected to normal lung tissue, whereas ELS lesions are completely separate from the lung and covered in their own pleura. ELS lesions may also be extrathoracic (Biyyam et al., 2010; Sfakianaki & Copel, 2012).

The pathogenesis of BPS remains unclear. The most widely accepted explanation dates back to Pryce's (1946) seminal work. Nonfunctioning lung tissue is thought to arise from the primitive foregut. During week 4 of gestation, capillaries formerly connecting the dorsal aorta and lung bud normally regress, separate, and are absorbed. Failed absorption results in the formation of an anomalous vasculature, which over time disrupts normal lung development and displaces the embryonic lung tissue into separate parts. This results in the formation of either an ILS or ELS (Hong et al., 2017).

Clinical manifestations in the immediate postnatal period include respiratory distress and congestive heart failure. Large lesions are associated with pulmonary hypoplasia. BPS may be associated with CDH, which also manifests as severe respiratory distress in the immediate postnatal period. More common, this lesion goes unnoticed in infancy and is discovered later into childhood secondary to cough, fever, dyspnea, hemoptysis, or congestive heart failure. Due to their location, an ELS lesion may be mistaken for an adrenal mass.

Life-span implications of BPS include high-output cardiac failure, hemoptysis, blood loss, or hemothorax. Patients with ILS lesions are at higher risk for malignancy risk later in childhood and adulthood (Casagrande & Pederiva, 2016). Latent ILS is associated with obstruction of the lower, posterior basal segments of the bronchus secondary to repetitive episodes of necrotizing pneumonia (Hong et al., 2017).

Bronchogenic Cyst. BCs, also known as duplications of the foregut, are cysts coated with cartilage and smooth muscle cells from the tracheobronchial tree (Crowley, 2025). The majority (67%) are found in the mediastinal area near the carina, followed by the lung parenchyma (33%), pleura, and the diaphragm (Chowdhury & Chakraborty, 2015; Sun, 2022). A paucity of recent literature exists that presents current epidemiologic trends, likely due to the rare status of this type of lung lesion.

Similar to other cystic lung lesions, the pathogenesis of BCs is poorly understood. The paucity of literature specific to this diagnosis adds to the mystery surrounding its genesis during early development. Experts posit that BCs are derived from the primitive foregut and occur secondary to abnormal ventral budding of the tracheobronchial tree between day 26 and 40 of gestation (Crowley, 2025).

These single-chambered cysts commonly present as smooth-appearing, spherical, and noncalcified masses containing clear fluid or, less often, blood or air (Sarper et al., 2003). Most newborns are asymptomatic at birth and the diagnosis is incidentally conferred when a radiograph (for other indications) is obtained. When the cysts exert a compressive effect on the trachea, bronchi, or esophagus, newborns can manifest with stridor, wheezing, dysphagia, and dyspnea, prompting further investigation. Older children whose cysts are undetected during infancy often develop recurrent cough, dyspnea, pneumonia, hemoptysis, or dysphagia, and these findings prompt a more focused diagnostic workup leading to detection of the cysts. Chest pain and dysphagia are the most common complaints reported among newly diagnosed adults.

Surgical excision is the only definitive treatment for BCs and significantly reduces the risk for malignancy. Lesions may regenerate if incompletely resected. Symptomatic infants may be subject to palliative aspiration for the first few months of life, to allow for growth and development until surgery is deemed feasible. Prognosis is excellent after surgical excision; no long-term sequelae are currently reported (Casagrande & Pederiva, 2016; Chowdhury & Chakraborty, 2015; Crowley, 2025).

Congenital Lobar Emphysema/Congenital Lobar Overinflation. CLE, also known as lobar overinflation, involves hyperinflation of one or more of the pulmonary lobes with corresponding marked distention of the alveoli. The left upper lobe and right middle lobes are more commonly implicated (Plosa & Sucre, 2024).

The etiology of CLE is thought to be due to disruptions in bronchopulmonary development secondary to abnormal interactions between embryonic endodermal and mesodermal lung components. These disruptions allow for the formation of an abnormal pathway that permits progressive hyperinflation of one or more lobes of the lung and mediastinal displacement (Kravitz, 1994). Intrinsic causes include dysplastic bronchial cartilage, thick plug-like mucus, extensive mucosal proliferation, bronchial torsion, and bronchial atresia. Extrinsic causes include compression of the bronchi, abnormal cardiopulmonary vasculature, and infection (Olutoye et al., 2000). If the lesion is large enough, mediastinal shift and compression of surrounding structures may occur (Chowdhury & Chakraborty, 2015; Durell & Lakhoo, 2014; Plosa & Sucre, 2024).

Infants typically present with varying symptoms of respiratory distress; larger lesions are associated with acute respiratory distress (Durell & Lakhoo, 2014). Sparse outcome data on the life-long sequelae of CLE exists. When grouped with other congenital pulmonary malformations, wheezing and increased infection rates persist through early childhood, but improve with age (Calzolari et al., 2016). Therefore, outcomes and prognosis appear to be good with excision of the abnormality.

Tracheoesophageal Fistula. Tracheoesophageal fistula (TEF), although not exclusively a disorder of pulmonary origin, is an abnormality that can result in significant respiratory distress and is presented in this chapter for that reason. EA is often part of the TEF, and therefore the defect is often labeled as EA/TEF. EA/TEF is an anomaly of the foregut that arises during week 4 of gestation due to an abnormal connection between the trachea and the esophagus. The incidence of EA is estimated at one in 2,500 to 4,000 live births and one in 3,000 to 4,500 with TEF (Wolfe & Jnah, 2024). Upwards of 50% of all infants with EA/TEF also present with other midline anomalies, with 14% to 29% of EA/TEF cases linked with vertebral anomalies, anal atresia/anorectal malformations, or renal and/or limb abnormalities (VACTERL association; Wolfe & Jnah, 2024). Other genetic associations include CHARGE spectrum, Feingold syndrome, and Opitz syndrome. EA/TEF is also reported among infants diagnosed with trisomy 18 and 21 (Sadreameli & McGrath-Morrow, 2016).

The pathogenesis of EA/TEF is thought to be multifactorial. Genetically induced abnormalities in branching of the primitive lung bud and poorly understood environmental and epigenetic influences are likely to blame (Sadreameli & McGrath-Morrow, 2016). Interrupted gene signaling disrupts the function of transcription factors (*NKX2-1*, a respiratory marker, and *SOX2*, a GI marker). This interrupts normal foregut separation during weeks 3 to 5 of gestation. Normally, the foregut develops from the lung bud and separates into the trachea and esophagus. However, interrupted gene signaling and transcription leads to abnormal separation of the foregut and development of EA/TEF (Wolfe & Jnah, 2024).

The five major types of EA/TEF and common associated clinical manifestations are provided in Table 4.11. A focused look at common manifestations and associated pathology is provided in Table 4.12. Rarely, esophageal stenosis is observed. In these cases, no EA or fistulous connection to the trachea exists (Sadreameli & McGrath-Morrow, 2016; Sun, 2022).

Life-span implications are optimal with isolated defects and overall survival with EA/TEF exceeds 90% (Wolfe & Jnah, 2024). Infants with low birthweight, genetic associations, and cardiac defects incur increased mortality risk (Dingeldein, 2025; Javia et al., 2016; Wolfe & Jnah, 2024). Long-term respiratory complications include wheezing, asthma, pneumonia, and abnormal pulmonary function tests (Sadreameli & McGrath-Morrow, 2016). Esophageal dysfunction, esophageal strictures, fistula recurrence, dysphagia, and reflux are reported after surgical correction. Dysphagia may persist into adulthood (Dingeldein, 2025; Sadreameli & McGrath-Morrow, 2016; Wolfe & Jnah, 2024).

Clinical Application. Currently, prenatal screening for EA/TEF is not mandated and most cases are diagnosed postnatally after hallmark symptoms present. Other cases may go undetected for weeks or months after birth, particularly when symptoms are subtle because the fistula is narrow in diameter. Prenatally, MRI tends to be more sensitive and specific compared to ultrasonography. Postnatally, the swallow study, esophagogram, and/or bronchoscopy can be helpful when symptoms suggest TEF/EA and radiographs are inconclusive. Currently, experts are investigating routine use of proton pump inhibitors (PPI) in the postoperative period, as the efficacy of use in preventing postoperative anastomotic strictures has not been proven.

Acquired Respiratory Problems

As previously discussed in this chapter, the stages of lung development and maturation impact the severity and type of respiratory distress that a neonate can experience following delivery. The following sections discuss some of the respiratory challenges a neonate may experience after birth as they begin to transition to extrauterine life.

Respiratory Distress Syndrome. Survival among premature neonates has improved with the advancements made in neonatal care and the understanding of disease processes affecting them. Over the past 50 years, our knowledge of physiologic changes that lead to RDS has grown, resulting in developments that have improved neonatal outcomes, leading to new challenges and opportunities for continued research and advancement. Gestational age at the time of delivery is inversely related to survival, with the highest morbidity and mortality rates noted for those neonates born at extremely preterm gestational ages (22–24 weeks of gestation), with RDS listed as the leading cause of mortality and morbidity among premature neonates (Lagoski et al., 2025; Stevens et al., 2007). Risk factors for RDS are summarized in Box 4.2.

Gestational age at the time of delivery impacts the severity of RDS and response to treatments, both antenatal and neonatal. Confounding variables, such as chorioamnionitis, prolonged rupture of membranes, need

TABLE 4.11 Five Classifications of Esophageal Atresia/ Tracheoesophageal Fistula

Incidence	Types	Clinical Manifestations	Image
8%	"A": Isolated esophageal atresia with no tracheal communication	• Scaphoid abdomen • Hypersalivation	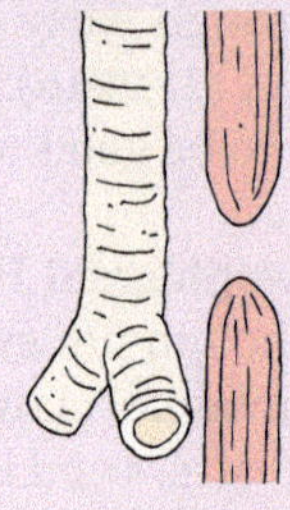
1%	"B": Esophageal atresia (upper pouch) with proximal TEF	• Scaphoid abdomen • Hypersalivation with possible entry into lungs	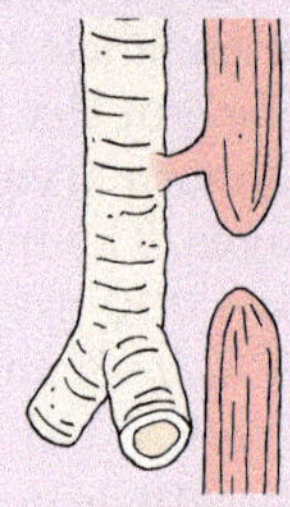
85%	"C": Esophageal atresia (upper pouch) with distal TEF just above carina	• Distended abdomen • Hypersalivation • Reflux of gastric secretions into lungs	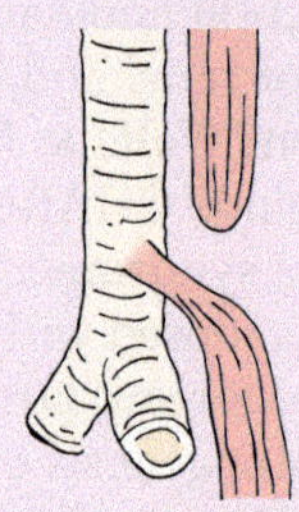
1%	"D": Esophageal atresia (upper pouch) with double TEF; note separate attachments with the upper and lower esophagus to the trachea	• Distended abdomen • Hypersalivation into lungs • Reflux of gastric secretions into lungs	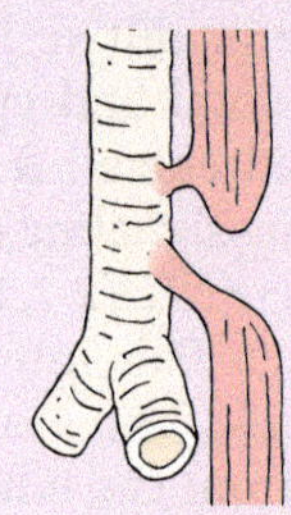
4%	"E": Isolated TEF ("H" type)	• Asymptomatic • Coughing with feedings • Aspiration pneumonia	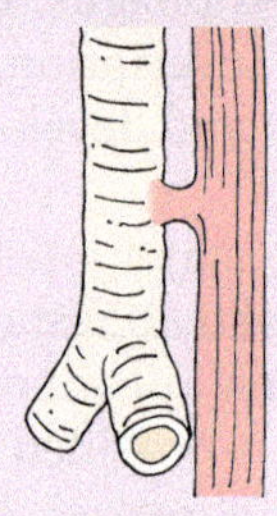

TEF, tracheoesophageal fistula.

for resuscitation at delivery, and early mechanical ventilation impacts recovery from RDS. Extremely preterm neonates born between 22 and 25 weeks of gestation are subject to interrupted canalicular development, and because of this, primitive gas exchange units do not resemble or function as mature alveoli.

The pathogenesis of RDS involves surfactant deficiency which discourages alveolar opening and gas exchange, leaving the lungs relatively airless and significantly atelectatic. Initially, the epithelial lining of the terminal bronchioles and alveolar ducts becomes injured, fibrous, and cluttered with cellular debris. The surfactant deficiency permits the persistence of high surface tension and decreased FRC as well as ventilation to perfusion mismatch. This leads to cyanosis, impaired O_2/CO_2 exchange, acidosis, and increased pulmonary

TABLE 4.12 Common Manifestations of EA/TEF With Associated Pathophysiology

Manifestation	Pathophysiology—Why Does the Symptom Develop?
Increased oral secretions with coughing or choking	Loss of cilia and narrowing of the airway lead to a decrease in clearing oral secretions and coughing, choking, and/or accumulation of oral secretions and predispose the infant to bacterial growth/ infection.
Emesis/regurgitation	Distention of the stomach paired with delayed motility of the esophagus and delayed clearance may cause regurgitation of gastric contents into the esophagus, which can lead to aspiration.
Respiratory distress with cyanosis	The connection of the airway and the esophagus can cause a large accumulation of air in the stomach, causing respiratory distress. Cyanosis occurs more frequently during crying episodes that collapse the trachea because of increased pressure.
Dysphagia	The connection between the airway and the stomach may cause gastric contents to be aspirated into the lungs through the fistula; breast milk or formula during feedings may be aspirated as well.
Gastric distention	The connection of the airway and esophagus can cause air to become trapped in the stomach, leading to distention.

EA, esophageal atresia; TEF, tracheoesophageal fistula.

BOX 4.2 Risk Factors for RDS

- Prematurity
- Prematurity without antenatal steroid administration
- Elective cesarean section without trial of labor
- European descent
- Infant of a diabetic mother
- Male gender
- Perinatal asphyxia

RDS, respiratory distress syndrome.

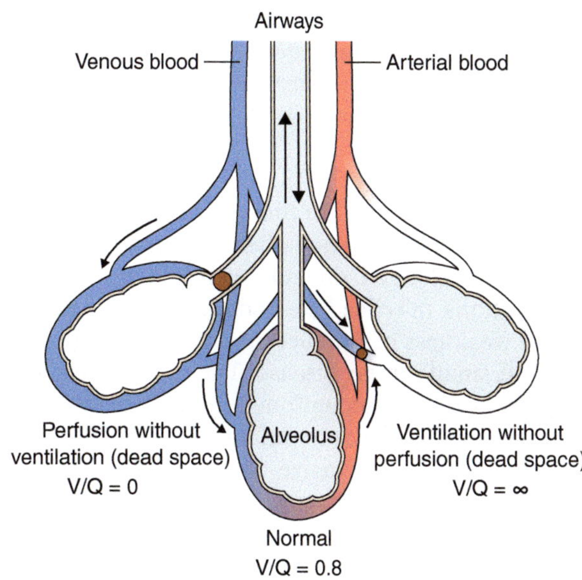

Figure 4.8 Ventilation-perfusion mismatching.
V/Q, ventilation-perfusion ratio.

pressures, which delays the normal adaptation to extrauterine life (Figure 4.8). In fact, persistent hypothermia, acidosis, hypovolemia, and/or hypoxemia suppresses endogenous surfactant production after birth, encouraging persistence of the disease process. Life-saving therapies including assisted mechanical ventilation and supplemental inspired oxygen risk injury to the respiratory epithelium, through volutrauma, and summon the infiltration of inflammatory cytokines, further suppressing surfactant production and function. Worsening inflammation can precipitate additional injury and the leakage of blood products (e.g., fibrin) into the alveolar spaces, which also suppresses surfactant production (Lagoski et al., 2025).

Hallmark clinical manifestations of RDS include increased work of breathing (nasal flaring, grunting, retractions), cyanosis, an increasing oxygen requirement, and apnea. In these circumstances, the neonate has a limited ability to combat alveolar collapse. Nasal flaring (inspiratory volume) and grunting (end-expiratory volume) are compensatory mechanisms aimed to increase lung volume, stabilize FRC, and improve gas exchange. Due to the relative compliance of the chest wall in premature infants, retractions (intercostal, subcostal, and sternal) are seen with increased exertion leading to exhaustion, hypercarbia, and apnea. Repeated efforts by the neonate to reestablish lung inflation, or ventilation efforts that lead to alveolar overdistension, cause repeated shearing stress on the alveoli.

Radiographic findings and laboratory findings are noteworthy. A reticulogranular ("ground-glass") appearance and air bronchograms of the larger branching airways with low lung volumes are typically noted on radiographic images. This classic appearance is a result of atelectatic alveoli alternating with alveolar distension in addition to alveolar and interstitial edema (Figure 4.9). Early laboratory manifestations of RDS

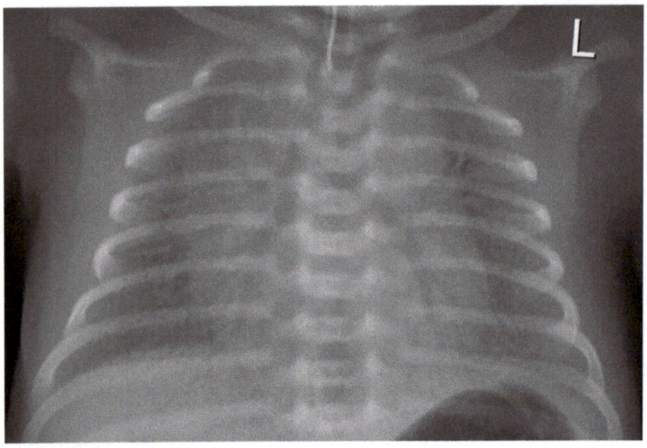

Figure 4.9 This is a 33-week preterm infant who is intubated with respiratory distress syndrome. Radiographic findings include symmetric granular opacifications with air bronchograms.

Source: van Schuppen, J., Kox, L., Onland, W., Smithuis, R., & van Rijn, R. (n.d.). *Neonatal chest x-ray.* https://radiologyassistant.nl/pediatrics/pediatric-chest-ct/neonatal-chest#respiratory-distress-syndrome-rds

include uncompensated respiratory acidosis with hypoxemia. With worsening RDS, the respiratory acidosis can become mixed with metabolic acidosis due to the accumulation of lactic acid.

Life-span implications of RDS are often determined by the severity of the disease, the timing of disease presentation, existing congenital anomalies, and any additional comorbidities. Prolonged, difficult, or repeated endotracheal intubations may lead to tracheobronchomalacia (congenital weakness of conducting airways), subglottic stenosis, and small airway disease. The relative risk for accruing any of the aforementioned upper airway traumas increases with each day an infant is intubated, most notably after *7 days* of invasive therapy (Zhang et al., 2016). High levels of oxygen and significant respiratory support may be required to sustain adequate ventilation and oxygenation for some neonates. Exposure to positive-pressure ventilation and inspired oxygen has been demonstrated to result in the presence of inflammatory cytokines resulting in an abnormal repair of the epithelium, persistent inflammation, and remodeling of the lung endothelium, all of which are seen in BPD. Affected infants will most likely require multiple hospital readmissions and a higher utilization of healthcare services, both of which are costly (Noritz et al., 2017). Families of these children are challenged financially as well as emotionally in managing their care.

Bronchopulmonary Dysplasia. Following the first description of BPD by Dr. Northway and colleagues in 1967, much has changed in the definition, development, and treatment of this most common form of pediatric chronic lung disease. The first patients with a diagnosis of BPD were premature neonates with a birthweight greater than 1,000 grams who underwent prolonged positive-pressure ventilation with high concentrations of inspired oxygen culminating in respiratory failure with radiographic and histopathologic changes (Bancalari et al., 2024). The damage seen in the lungs of these neonates included smooth muscle hypertrophy, neutrophilic inflammation, parenchymal fibrosis, and airway damage (Trembath & Laughon, 2012).

Since the original description of BPD, many advancements (antenatal steroids, improved ventilation techniques, surfactant replacement therapy) have improved outcomes and survival of neonates once thought to be born at the cusp of viability (Abman et al., 2017; Bancalari et al., 2024; Cohen & Cotten, 2022; Trembath & Laughon, 2012). Currently, between 10,000 and 15,000 infants are diagnosed with BPD every year in the United States, with 40% of these patients weighing less than 1,000 grams at birth (Bancalari et al., 2024; Gao & Raj, 2010; Higgins et al., 2018; Schmidt & Bancalari, 2025).

The etiology is multifactorial, encompassing antenatal and postnatal risk factors which disrupt lung development (Table 4.13). Prenatal risk factors for BPD include prematurity and chorioamnionitis in the pregnant patient. In the context of relative risk for postnatal BPD development, prematurity is defined as birth less than 28 weeks of gestation, which aligns with birth occurring during the canalicular or early saccular phase of lung development. Chorioamnionitis is associated with an increased risk for premature birth, as well as postnatal respiratory distress, BPD, and even perinatal death. This unequivocally increases the risk for altered anatomic and physiologic pulmonary development and chronic disease. Postnatal risk factors for BPD include

TABLE 4.13 Common Risk Factors for BPD

Antenatal Risks	Postnatal Risks
• Chorioamnionitis • Epigenetics • Intrauterine growth restriction • Maternal drug use • Maternal hypertension and/or preeclampsia • Maternal smoking • Placental insufficiency	• Lung parenchymal disease • Nutritional deficits • Oxygen toxicity • Patent ductus arteriosus • Prematurity • Pulmonary vascular disease • Respiratory failure • Sepsis • Volutrauma (ventilator-induced)

BPD, bronchopulmonary dysplasia.

Sources: Higgins, R. D., Jobe, A. H., Koso-Thomas, M., Bancalari, E., Viscardi, R. M., Hartert, T. V., Ryan, R. M., Kallapur, S. G., Steinhorn, R. H., Konduri, G. G., Davis, S. D., Thebaud, B., Clyman, R. I., Collaco, J. M., Martin, C. R., Woods, J. C., Finer, N. N., & Raju, T. N. K. (2018). Bronchopulmonary dysplasia: Executive summary of a workshop. *The Journal of Pediatrics, 197*, 300–308. https://doi.org/10.1016/j.jpeds.2018.01.043; Jensen, E. A., Dysart, K., Gantz, M. G., McDonald, S., Bamat, N. A., Keszler, M., Kirpalani, H., Laughon, M. M., Poindexter, B. B., Duncan, A. F., Yoder, B. A., Eichenwald, E. C., & DeMauro, S. B. (2019). The diagnosis of bronchopulmonary dysplasia in very preterm infants: An evidence-based approach. *American Journal of Respiratory and Critical Care Medicine, 200*(6), 751–759. https://doi.org/10.1164/rccm.201812-2348OC

prolonged ventilation, oxidative stress, and nosocomial infections (Bancalari et al., 2024; Metcalfe et al., 2017; Rook et al., 2014; Schmidt & Bancalari, 2025; Trembath & Laughon, 2012). Oxidative damage occurs with exposure to high oxygen concentrations as well as with fluctuations between hyperoxia and hypoxia and arrested alveolarization and vascular development (Bancalari et al., 2024; Madurga et al., 2013; Schmidt & Bancalari, 2025).

The definition of BPD has changed over the years and the most recent revisions offer succinct classifications for disease severity (**Table 4.14**). These modifications seek to inch closer toward a definition that appropriately classifies the disease state, guides management, and accurately characterizes pulmonary outcomes across the life span. In addition, newer definitions are inclusive of modern modes of respiratory support. Susceptible infants are those born prematurely and who possess a genetic predisposition to altered lung development or function, or fetuses subject to asphyxia or infection.

The pathogenesis of the "new" BPD is attributed to alveolar hypoplasia and dysmorphic pulmonary circulation which emerges from injuries incurred after birth. These injuries include sepsis, volutrauma, and mechanotrauma from the provision of positive-pressure ventilation, pulmonary edema, and oxygen toxicity. The occurrence of these injuries during a time frame when the lungs are continuously developing and maturing, and subsequently attempting to repair postinjury, give rise to BPD (Abman et al., 2017; Bancalari et al., 2024; Keller & Steinhorn, 2024; Schmidt & Bancalari, 2025; Trembath & Laughon, 2012).

Four stages summarize the development of BPD (**Figure 4.10**). The first stage involves selection of a vulnerable host. Second, acute lung injury occurs, often secondary to surfactant deficiency, barotrauma, inflammation, or infection, or exposure to the other antepartum and postnatal risk factors summarized earlier in this section. Acute lung injury involves an interruption of the normal anatomic canalicular and saccular (alveolar) development. An influx of chemotactic and chemokinetic factors into respiratory secretions is noted, which recruit inflammatory cells (including neutrophils, macrophages,

TABLE 4.14 Current NICHD Definitions of BPD in Premature Infants

	Mild BPD (Grade I)	Moderate BPD (Grade II)	Severe BPD (Grade III)
Higgins et al., 2018 Among infants born <32 weeks of gestation, who are 36 weeks PMA, there is persistent and radiographically confirmed parenchymal lung disease *and* the infant requires one of the following respiratory support modalities and ranges of supplemental oxygen to maintain an arterial oxygenation saturation between 90%–95%.	N-CPAP, NIPPV, or NC <3 LPM + FiO_2 0.21 **—or—** NC 1–3 LPM + FiO_2 0.22–0.29 **—or—** Oxyhood + FiO_2 ≥0.3 **—or—** NC <1 LPM + FiO_2 0.22–0.7	Invasive IPPV + FiO_2 0.21 **—or—** N-CPAP, NIPPV, or NC <3 LPM + FiO_2 0.22–0.29 **—or—** NC 1–3 LPM + FiO_2 ≥0.3 **—or—** Oxyhood + FiO_2 ≥0.3 **—or—** NC <1 LPM + FiO_2 >0.7	Invasive IPPV + FiO_2 >0.21 **—or—** N-CPAP, NIPPV, or NC <3 LPM + FiO_2 0.21
Jensen et al., 2019 Among infants born <27 weeks of gestation, who are 36 weeks PMA, the infant requires one of the following respiratory support modalities.	NC <2 LPM	Noninvasive PPV **—or—** NC >2 LPM	Invasive PPV

BPD, bronchopulmonary dysplasia; IPPV, intermittent positive-pressure ventilation; LPM, liters per minute; NC, nasal cannula; N-CPAP, nasal continuous positive airway pressure; NICHD, National Institute of Child Health and Human Development; NIPPV, nasal intermittent positive-pressure ventilation; PMA, postmenstrual age; PPV, positive-pressure ventilation.

Sources: Higgins, R. D., Jobe, A. H., Koso-Thomas, M., Bancalari, E., Viscardi, R. M., Hartert, T. V., Ryan, R. M., Kallapur, S. G., Steinhorn, R. H., Konduri, G. G., Davis, S. D., Thebaud, B., Clyman, R. I., Collaco, J. M., Martin, C. R., Woods, J. C., Finer, N. N., & Raju, T. N. K. (2018). Bronchopulmonary dysplasia: Executive summary of a workshop. *The Journal of Pediatrics, 197*, 300–308. https://doi.org/10.1016/j.jpeds.2018.01.043; Jensen, E. A., Dysart, K., Gantz, M. G., McDonald, S., Bamat, N. A., Keszler, M., Kirpalani, H., Laughon, M. M., Poindexter, B. B., Duncan, A. F., Yoder, B. A., Eichenwald, E. C., & DeMauro, S. B. (2019). The diagnosis of bronchopulmonary dysplasia in very preterm infants: An evidence-based approach. *American Journal of Respiratory and Critical Care Medicine, 200*(6), 751–759. https://doi.org/10.1164/rccm.201812-2348OC

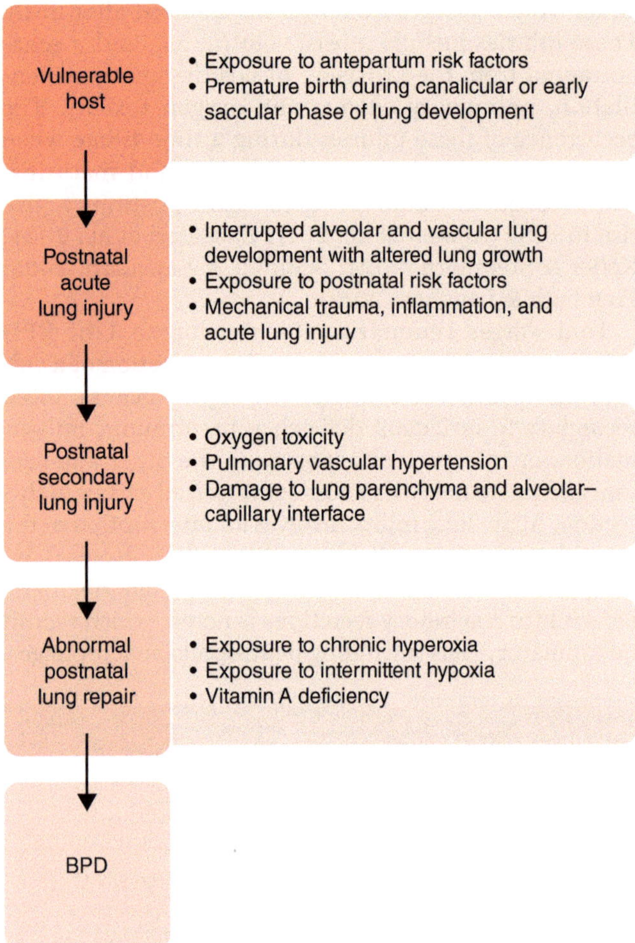

Figure 4.10 Pathogenesis of BPD.
BPD, bronchopulmonary dysplasia.

and proinflammatory cytokines) into the pulmonary tissues. Neutrophil invasion occurs often after just minutes of artificial respiratory therapy. Neutrophils adhere to the pulmonary tissues and vascular system and release various proteolytic enzymes as well as oxygen metabolites and radicals. This marks the second stage of lung injury, which permits deranged architectural changes at the alveolar–capillary interface and parenchymal damage. Thickening of what should be a very thin, easily accessed alveolar–capillary interface disrupts gas exchange. Once parenchymal and vascular damage has occurred, further exposure to hyperoxic or hypoxic states allows for insufficient, abnormal healing. This often occurs concurrent with a vitamin A deficiency, which further reduces healing capacity. Upregulation of genes that modulate fetal lung development and surfactant formation is reduced, resulting in stunted growth (Schmidt & Bancalari, 2025).

The histopathologic characteristics of BPD are noteworthy (Table 4.15). A milder form of BPD has been observed with the onset of gentler forms of positive-pressure support. Infants with mild BPD demonstrate diffuse injury without fibrosis or emphysema, dysmorphic pulmonary capillaries, and a reduced complement of alveoli and

TABLE 4.15 Characteristics of "New" Bronchopulmonary Dysplasia

Contemporary Clinical Management Strategies
• Antenatal steroid exposure • Exogenous surfactant administration • Reduced exposure to positive-pressure ventilation • Reduced exposure to supplemental oxygen
Contemporary Histologic Changes[a]
• Diffuse disease • Reduced hyperinflation • Reduced alveoli and capillaries • Minimal fibrosis

[a]Histologic changes observed among animal models.
Source: Trembath, A. N., & Laughon, M. M. (2012). Predictors of bronchopulmonary dysplasia. *Clinics in Perinatology, 39*(3), 585–601. https://doi.org/10.1016/j.clp.2012.06.014

surface area for gas exchange. Infants who require long-term invasive positive-pressure ventilatory support as well as supplemental oxygen may manifest with the more classic and severe form of BPD. Common features include diffuse injury with fibrosis and areas of emphysema and cysts surrounded by atelectasis, interstitial edema, and bronchiolar hyperplasia. Right ventricular hypertrophy is often present (Schmidt & Bancalari, 2025).

Life-span implications of BPD include abnormal pulmonary function, asthma with increased bronchodilator use, persistent wheezing, airflow obstruction, COPD, lower respiratory tract infections, and altered neurodevelopment (Islam et al., 2015; Schmidt & Bancalari, 2025). Altered neurodevelopment may include cerebral palsy, developmental delay, or cognitive and behavioral disorders, with an increase in the need for learning disability support services when compared to infants born at a similar gestational age and without BPD. Hearing and vision deficits are also reported. Among adults, consequences of BPD include wheezing and COPD with radiologic evidence of emphysema (correlated with moderate to severe BPD diagnosis); these individuals often require long-term subspecialty follow-up for pulmonary dysfunction (Islam et al., 2015; Li et al., 2023).

Neonatal Pneumonia. Pneumonia is the primary cause for infectious disease-related deaths among children across the globe, particularly in developing countries. Neonatal pneumonia is classified as early-onset and late-onset. As discussed in Chapter 9 ("The Immune System"), early-onset infections occur within the first 72 hours of life and late-onset infections occur after 72 hours of life. Specific to early-onset pneumonia, there are three routes of infection: transplacental (congenital), intrauterine, and intrapartum (Moujaes et al., 2025;

Mukherjee & Ryan, 2024). A summary of associated pathogens by timing and mode of infection is provided in Table 4.16. The fetus and neonate are particularly vulnerable to pneumonia. Risk factors include prematurity, immature innate and adaptive immune function, injury to the respiratory epithelium, and GI reflux.

The pathogenesis of pneumonia varies based on timing of infection. Asphyxia, intrauterine infection, or a combination of both factors are responsible for congenitally acquired pneumonia. Pathogens colonizing the vaginal canal vertically ascend the birth canal and, once rupture of membranes occurs, traverse the cervix, infiltrate the chorioamniotic membrane, and enter and contaminate the amniotic fluid (Figure 4.11). Once the fetus aspirates this amniotic fluid that is contaminated with birth parent leukocytes, amniotic debris, and pathogens, infection ensues. Similarly, pneumonia acquired during the intrapartum period involves aspiration of pathogens colonizing the vaginal canal. Postnatal infection typically stems from infiltration of pathogens, often at injured regions of the respiratory tract, from sources that include contaminated equipment or caregivers.

Clinical manifestations of pneumonia overlap with RDS and meconium aspiration syndrome (MAS), making the process of clinical, laboratory, and radiographic correlation necessary to distinguish among these disease processes. Pneumonia may manifest with temperature instability, apnea, tachycardia or bradycardia, increased and potentially discolored respiratory secretions, oxygen desaturations, and escalating demand for respiratory support. Laboratory derangements commonly include neutropenia with bandemia. Common radiographic evidence of pneumonia includes pleural effusion, reticulonodular densities (similar to reticulogranular densities observed with RDS), or patchy and asymmetric infiltrates with areas of hyperaeration (similar to MAS).

TABLE 4.16 Types of Pneumonia That Affect the Fetus and Neonate

Classification of Infection	Mode of Infection	Mechanism of Infection	Onset of Symptoms	Common Pathogens
Early onset	Transplacental (Congenital)	• Ascending (vertical) infection of chorioamniotic membrane **or** • Transplacental (blood-borne) maternal–fetal infection	• During fetal development, at birth, or within the first 48 hours of life	• Cytomegalovirus • Herpes simplex virus • *Listeria monocytogenes* • *Treponema gondii* • *Treponema pallidum*
	Intrauterine	• Fetal aspiration of infected amniotic fluid	• At birth or during first 3 days of postnatal life	• Group B *Streptococcus* • *Escherichia coli* • *Klebsiella* • *Chlamydia trachomatis*
	Intrapartum	• Fetal aspiration of vaginal pathogens	• At birth or during first 3 days of postnatal life	• Group B *Streptococcus* • *Escherichia coli* • *Klebsiella* • *Chlamydia trachomatis*
Late onset	N/A	• Infection acquired from human-to-human contact or exposure to contaminated equipment	• After first 72 hours of postnatal life	• Group B Streptococcus • *Escherichia coli* • *Klebsiella* • *Pseudomonas*

Note: List of pathogens limited to common exemplars and is therefore not all inclusive.

Sources: Hooven, T. A., & Polin, R. A. (2017). Pneumonia. *Seminars in Fetal and Neonatal Medicine, 22*(4), 206–213. https://doi.org/10.1016/j.siny.2017.03.002; Moujaes, L., Barnett, E. D., & Malley, R. (2025). Bacterial infections of the respiratory tract. *Remington and Klein's infectious diseases of the fetus and newborn infant* (8th ed., pp. 225–262). Elsevier/Saunders; Mukherjee, D., & Ryan, R. M. (2024). Postnatal bacterial infections. In A. A. Fanaroff, & R. J. Martin (Eds.), *Fanaroff and Martin's neonatal-perinatal medicine: Diseases of the fetus and infant* (11th ed., pp. 857–880). Elsevier/Saunders.

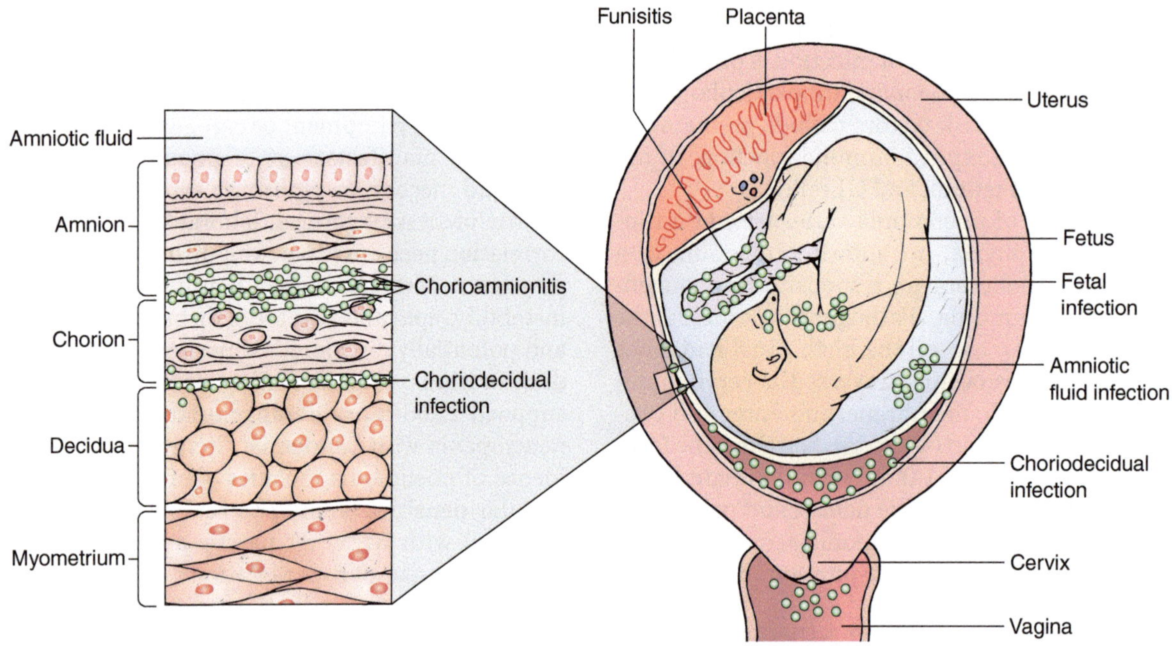

Figure 4.11 Vertical transmission of pathogens from birth canal to fetus (transplacental route).

Life-span implications vary depending on the pathogen, severity of illness, and recurrence. Prolonged exposure to broad-spectrum antibiotics increases the risk for chronic drug resistance, alteration of the GI microbiome, as well as hearing deficits.

Transient Tachypnea of the Newborn. TTN is a common physiologic problem associated with incomplete reabsorption of fetal lung fluid prior to birth. TTN affects approximately six of every 1,000 liveborn infants (Alhassen et al., 2021). Risk factors include diabetes in the XX pregnant patient, male gender, prematurity, fetal macrosomia, twin gestation, small for gestational age status at birth, and birth by cesarean section without a trial of labor (Alhassen et al., 2021; Dyess et al., 2024; Kassab et al., 2015).

The pathogenesis of TTN begins during the transition to extrauterine life. As described earlier in this chapter, successful transition involves the clearance of fetal lung fluid from the pulmonary bed. The reabsorption of fetal lung fluid normally occurs via transport of Na^+ through epithelial sodium channels (ENaCs). Failed reabsorption of fetal lung fluid leads to tachypnea and delayed transition to extrauterine life (Crowley, 2025; Dyess et al., 2024). Elective cesarean delivery is associated with reduced endogenous catecholamine secretion and stunted resorption of fetal lung fluid.

Clinical manifestations of TTN include respiratory rates higher than 60 breaths per minute often accompanied by cyanosis, retractions, and grunting. Radiographic findings include mild hyperinflation with increased perihilar markings and fluid trapped within fissures of one or both lungs. Significant laboratory findings may include elevated inflammatory markers.

TTN is considered a diagnosis of exclusion, as the manifestations described previously overlap with other respiratory diseases. The neonatal clinician must rule out more significant causes for tachypnea before settling on the diagnosis of TTN, as delays in treatment of congenital cardiac or pulmonary disease processes may confer deleterious consequences for the newborn and family unit. Life-span implications are associated with any associated defects or disease process; TTN is self-limiting and typically resolves within the first 72 to 96 hours of life.

Meconium Aspiration Syndrome. Meconium, a complex mixture of bile acids, vernix, hair, epithelial cells, mucus, and blood, is first seen in the fetal ileum between 10 to 16 weeks of gestation. Meconium is not normally excreted during fetal development and the birth process but can be released in response to hypoxic/ischemic stress or from increased synthesis of motilin (Dyess et al., 2024; Gien & Kinsella, 2022). Approximately 13% of all liveborn infants pass meconium in utero and approximately 5% of those infants go on to aspirate meconium and develop signs of respiratory distress (Crowley, 2025; Dyess et al., 2024; Gien & Kinsella, 2022). The frequency of neonates born through meconium-stained amniotic fluid (MSAF) increases with advancing gestational age.

The pathogenesis of MAS is attributed to one of two mechanisms. First, fetal hypoxic/ischemic stress can increase parasympathetic activity (increased peristalsis, anal sphincter relaxation) and cause the evacuation of stool into the amniotic fluid. Any mechanism which reduces blood flow through the umbilical cord stresses the fetus and induces vagal stimulation. Increased parasympathetic tone increases intestinal peristalsis and relaxation of the anal sphincter, which permits the passage of meconium in utero. Second, and particularly with postterm fetuses, increased synthesis of motilin within the GI tract upregulates peristalsis and can encourage the evacuation of stool into the amniotic fluid.

When meconium is prematurely evacuated prior to birth, aspiration into the trachea and lungs can occur and induce several pathologic changes to the lung parenchyma. Meconium elicits a ball-valve obstructive effect within the distal airways of the lung. In addition, it inactivates surfactant and encourages the development of pneumonitis. Alveolar overdistension and gas trapping caused by meconium particles blocking the distal airways during expiration increases the risk of air leaks and may result in an increased anterior-to-posterior diameter, or barrel-chest appearance. Cholesterol and bile acids found in meconium have been demonstrated to inactivate pulmonary surfactant in the lung and impair its performance (Lopez-Rodriguez et al., 2011; Perez-Gil & Weaver, 2010). Damage to the type II pneumocyte can lead to further dysfunctions in the production, recycling, and secretion of surfactant (Crowley, 2025; Stenson & Smith, 2012). A chemical pneumonitis, or inflammatory response, further causes damage to the lung epithelium resulting in pulmonary vasoconstriction, alveolar edema, and imbalances of the vasoactive properties (ET-1, NO, PGI2) needed to establish a successful transition to extrauterine life (Lee et al., 2016). Pulmonary vasoconstriction raises PVR over SVR, which encourages a postnatal right to left shunting across the foramen ovale and clinically observed hypoxemia (**Figure 4.12**).

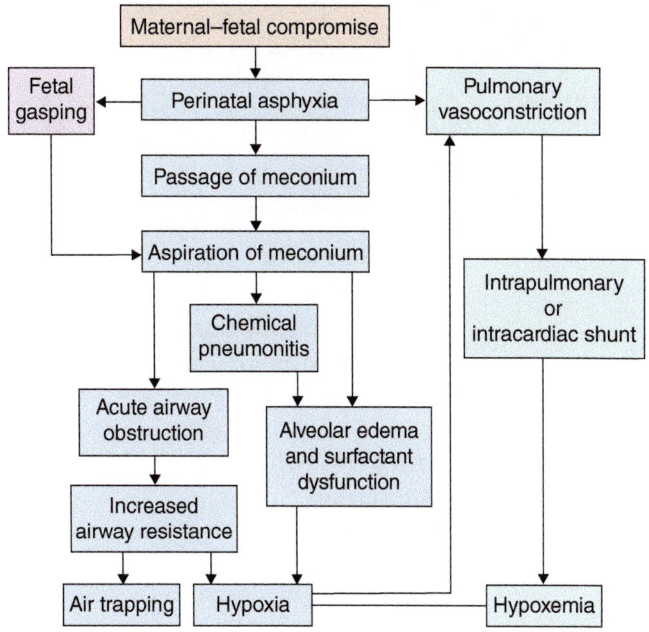

Figure 4.12 Pathogenesis of meconium aspiration syndrome.
Source: Adapted from MacDonald, M. G., Mullett, M. D., & Seshia, M. M. K. (Eds.). (2005). *Avery's neonatology: Pathophysiology and management of the newborn* (6th ed.). Lippincott Williams & Wilkins.

The clinical presentation of a neonate with MAS is variable but frequently includes worsening respiratory distress with cyanosis (Crowley, 2025; Stenson & Smith, 2012). Respiratory symptoms include cyanosis, tachypnea, grunting, and a prolonged expiratory phase. Severely affected neonates may manifest with air leak syndrome or persistent pulmonary hypertension. Meconium staining to the skin, umbilical cord, or nail beds may be evident. Radiographic findings of neonates with MAS include course, diffuse, and heterogeneous infiltrates with areas of hyperaeration (similar to TTN). Overinflation often displaces the left and right diaphragm to the 10th and 11th ribs.

There is a wide range of possible long-term outcomes which are contingent upon the severity of injury incurred during the disease process and recovery phase; outcomes include progression to BPD. Pharmacologic adjuncts used during management of the disease process may increase the risk for abstinence and other neurodevelopmental consequences.

Pulmonary Hemorrhage. Considered a life-threatening emergency, pulmonary hemorrhage (PH) involves an acute hemorrhage of blood into the trachea which causes cardiorespiratory decompensation. Approximately one to 12 per 1,000 liveborn infants are affected each year, with the risk inversely proportional to gestational age at birth (Welde et al., 2021). Other risk factors are summarized in **Table 4.17**. PH most often occurs within the first 72 to 96 hours of life.

The pathogenesis of PH is complex and incompletely understood. Experts believe that certain exposures or disease states lead to increased pulmonary blood flow increases with insufficient drainage into the pulmonary veins and left heart; this is exacerbated in situations where left ventricular preload is concurrently elevated and cardiac contractility is poor. The increase in pulmonary blood flow increases mechanical pressure within the pulmonary capillaries and imposes potentially devastating shearing forces upon vulnerable and relatively immature vessels (particularly among neonates who weigh less than 1 kg at birth). Fluid shifts into the interstitium may lead to pulmonary edema (which can be appreciated on chest radiographs), rupture of the vessels and alveoli, resulting in a mild, moderate, or severe PH.

Common prenatal etiologies for PH include cocaine use, hypertension, placental abruption, and antibiotic exposure during the intrapartum period. Common postnatal etiologies include a large patent ductus arteriosus (PDA) with left-to-right shunting, respiratory distress, sepsis, and asphyxia. With a large PDA (left-to-right shunting), pulmonary overcirculation develops, and this increases pressure within the pulmonary capillaries, which can lead to edema, shearing, and hemorrhage. Respiratory distress in preterm infants is associated with the risk for alveolar edema and leakage, inflammatory responses, and damage to the alveolar membrane leading to rupture and hemorrhage. Sepsis, specifically gram-negative sepsis, is associated with upregulation of proinflammatory cytokines and

TABLE 4.17 Pulmonary Hemorrhage Risk Factors

Birth parent	• Cocaine exposure • Hypertension • Intrapartum antibiotic use • Placental abruption
Neonatal	• Asphyxia • Coagulopathy • Congenital heart disease • Disseminated intravascular coagulation • **Extreme prematurity** • **Hemodynamically significant PDA with left-to-right shunt** • Hypothermia • Intrauterine growth restriction • Intubation and positive-pressure ventilation in the delivery room • Low Apgar scores • Low birthweight • Male gender • Mechanical ventilation • Meconium aspiration • Multiple birth • Neutrophil activation in cord blood in the setting of RDS • Polycythemia • Sepsis • **Surfactant administration** • Urea cycle defects with hyperammonemia

Note: Bold font indicates primary risk factors.
PDA, patent ductus arteriosus; RDS, respiratory distress syndrome.
Source: Data from Welde, M. A., Sanford, C. B., Mangum, M., Paschal, C., & Jnah, A. J. (2021). Pulmonary hemorrhage in the neonate. *Neonatal Network*, *40*(5), 295–304. https://doi.org/10.1891/11-T-696

other inflammatory mediators, increased vascular permeability, and the risk for hemorrhage. Finally, asphyxia is associated with cardiopulmonary failure. As the left-side heart failure worsens and blood is insufficiently ejected from the left ventricle, pulmonary capillary pressure increases, fluid accumulates, edema develops, and shearing forces can lead to hemorrhage.

Manifestations are linked to the severity of the hemorrhage. Mild PH may be subclinical as bleeding is often limited to the intra-alveolar spaces or lung interstitium. Moderate PH is associated with bleeding that reaches conducting airways and symptoms including respiratory distress (retractions, grunting, gasping breaths), cyanosis, and frothy, blood-tinged secretions in suction tubing or in the mouth or nares. Severe PH will include symptoms of moderate PH as well as bradycardia, pallor, hypotension, shock, and a larger volume of frothy, blood-tinged secretions in suction tubing, the mouth, or the nares.

The mortality risk is estimated between 38% to 65% (Welde et al., 2021). Limited outcomes data are reported. One study reported an increased risk for periventricular leukomalacia, seizures, and cerebral palsy through 18 months of age (Alfaleh et al., 2008). Other studies did not report an increased risk for neurodevelopmental deficits among infants who suffered PH (Crowley, 2025).

Persistent Pulmonary Hypertension of the Newborn. PPHN involves circulatory maladaptation or maldevelopment, which leads to a failed intrauterine to extrauterine transition and pulmonary arterial hypertension. As many as two of every 1,000 infants develop PPHN. Of infants who present with primary respiratory failure, mild PPHN is associated with 10% of all cases, while moderate to severe PPHN is associated with 2% to 6% of all cases (Lakshminrusimha & Steinhorn, 2022; Steinhorn, 2025). Common risk factors for primary, or *maladaptive PPHN* include MAS, RDS, sepsis, pneumonia, and perinatal asphyxia (Lakshminrusimha & Steinhorn, 2022). Common risk factors for *maldevelopmental PPHN* include congenital heart disease, CDH, and pulmonary hypoplasia.

The pathogenesis of primary PPHN focuses on deranged pulmonary vascular structure, reactivity, and right ventricular responses to high afterload. Less frequently, PPHN is the result of increased pulmonary blood flow or left ventricular dysfunction, causing an increase in capillary wedge pressures. Physiologically, increased pulmonary vasoconstriction raises PVR above that of SVR. This elevated PVR discourages blood flow through the right ventricle and pulmonary system, shunting the blood in a right-to-left direction across the foramen ovale and through the DA. The ventilation-perfusion mismatch (V/Q) leads to hypoxemia. In these situations, a discordance in pulse oximetry readings, with elevated preductal oxygen saturations compared to those obtained at a postductal location, is common.

Chronic pulmonary hypertension, also known as pulmonary hypertension of infancy, is commonly considered a comorbidity of other primary pulmonary diseases and manifests as altered pulmonary vascular development. New evidence also suggests that this pulmonary vascular maldevelopment may occur during early angiogenesis, secondary to interactions between environmental (in utero), epigenetic factors, and disrupted signaling pathways. These dysfunctional interactions lead to abnormal pulmonary vascular growth, which in turn contributes to narrowing of pulmonary vessel diameter, reduced compliance, and a noted reduction in available alveolar surface area for gas exchange (Abman et al., 2014; Lakshminrusimha & Steinhorn, 2022; Steinhorn, 2025).

Chronic PPHN is associated with increased mortality as well as increased healthcare costs during infancy. Among children, exercise intolerance, respiratory infections, and respiratory compromise are reported. Pulmonary arterial hypertension is common among affected adults (Lakshminrusimha & Steinhorn, 2022; Mourani & Abman, 2013; Naumberg et al., 2015).

Pulmonary Air Leaks. Air leaks include a spectrum of disorders that involve alveolar rupture and collapse with subsequent air leak into the interstitium or pleural spaces (Table 4.18). Pneumothorax is the most commonly identified air leak and primarily affects premature infants less than 1,000 grams or less than 28 weeks of gestation (Figure 4.13; Crowley, 2025; Oh et al., 2023). The most common etiology for air leak syndrome is supraphysiologic respiratory support by way of mechanical respiratory support devices. Additional risk factors for air leaks are summarized in Table 4.19.

Secondary to the pressures needed to establish pulmonary function following delivery, air leaks occur more often in the neonatal period than at any other time of life. The pathogenesis involves leakage of air from an overdistended and subsequently ruptured alveolus into the perivascular and tracheobronchial tree (Figure 4.14). The air either may remain trapped in the interstitium or track into the mediastinal spaces or pleural space.

TABLE 4.18 Common Types of Pulmonary Air Leak

Type	Location of Air Accumulation
Pneumothorax	Thorax
Pneumomediastinum	Mediastinum
Pneumopericardium	Pericardial space
Pneumoperitoneum	Peritoneum
Pulmonary interstitial emphysema	Interstitium
Subcutaneous emphysema	Subcutaneous tissue

Source: Data from Whitsett, J. A., Rice, W. R., Pryhuber, G. S., & Wert, S. E. (2016). Acute respiratory disorders. In M. G. MacDonald & M. M. K. Seshia (Eds.), *Avery's neonatology: Pathophysiology and management of the newborn* (7th ed., pp. 397–415). Wolters Kluwer.

Clinical manifestations may include respiratory distress, grunting, tachypnea, retractions, and cyanosis with increased severity of symptoms noted when large air leaks result in lung collapse and mediastinal shift. Tension pneumothoraces are associated with decreased breath sounds on the affected side, an increased anterior–posterior diameter on the affected side, and the potential for acute hypotension and cardiovascular collapse if left uncorrected. Like tension pneumothoraces, a significant pneumopericardium may impose excessive pressure upon the heart and manifest with acute hemodynamic decompensation and cardiac tamponade (Figure 4.15). Radiographic findings aid in the differentiation of air leaks. For example, radiographic evidence of a pneumothorax includes an area of hyperlucency without superimposed pulmonary vascular markings. Radiographic evidence of a pneumomediastinum yields elevation of the thymic lobes, often called a *spinnaker sail sign* (Jeng et al., 2012).

Neonates who develop air leaks are at an increased risk of death and disability, with mortality rates greater than 50% for premature neonates who develop pulmonary interstitial emphysema. Mortality risk is 20% to 38.6% higher when air leaks occur at nontertiary medical centers (Kastein & Coe, 2023).

Congenital Chylothorax. Congenital chylothorax is the most common cause for the accumulation of pleural lymph fluid (pleural effusion) in the fetus and neonate. The estimated incidence is one in 10,000 live births (Al-Tawi et al., 2000). Chylothorax can present as an isolated disorder or be associated with genetic disorders including Down syndrome, Noonan syndrome, and Turner syndrome.

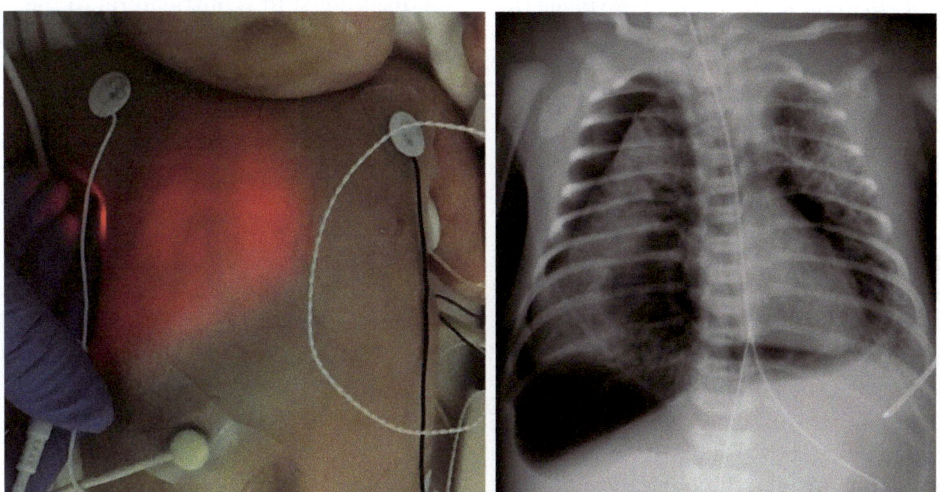

Figure 4.13 Right pneumothorax as illustrated by transillumination on image on the left and confirmed by chest radiograph on the right.

TABLE 4.19 Common Risk Factors for Air Leak

Disease Processes	Procedural	Management
• Prematurity (<28 weeks) • Pulmonary hypoplasia • Respiratory distress syndrome • Amniotic fluid aspiration • Infection	• Endotracheal intubation • Endotracheal suctioning • Needle thoracentesis	• ↑ Peak inspiratory pressures • ↑ Peak end-expiratory pressure • ↑ Tidal volume • ↑ Mean arterial pressures • Prolonged inspiratory time (>0.5 seconds)

Source: Duong, H. H., Mirea, L., Shah, P. S., Yange, J., Lee, S. K., & Sankaran, K. (2014). Pneumothorax in neonates: Trends, predictors, and outcomes. *Journal of Neonatal and Perinatal Medicine, 7*, 29–38. https://doi.org/10.3233/NPM-1473813

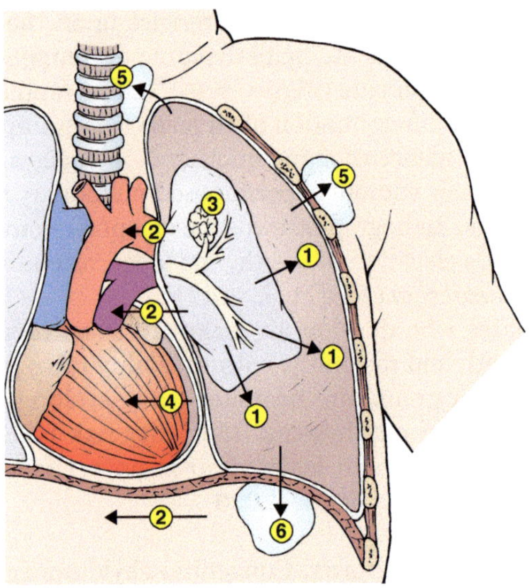

Figure 4.14 Air accumulation by type of air leak. **1,** pneumothorax; **2,** pneumomediastinum; **3,** pulmonary interstitial emphysema; **4,** pneumopericardium; **5,** subcutaneous emphysema; **6,** pneumoperitoneum. Arrows indicate directions of air leaks.

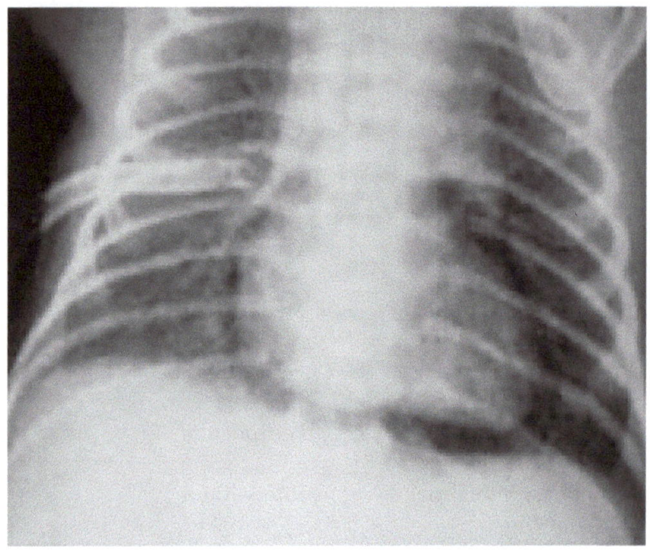

Figure 4.15 Pneumopericardium.
Note: The band of air completely surrounding the heart creates a radiolucent "halo."

The pathology of congenital chylothorax involves (a) direct leakage of lymph fluid from the thoracic duct, (b) obstructed drainage of lymph fluid, or (c) overproduction of lymph fluid. The ever-accumulating effusion increases intrathoracic pressure and suppresses fetal swallowing behaviors. This leads to the development of polyhydramnios, and in some cases, hydrops fetalis. Further, the accumulation of lymph in the pleural space impedes pulmonary development and explains why chylothorax is associated with pulmonary hypoplasia and impaired cardiovascular and pulmonary vascular function. Prenatal mitigation can involve transabdominal thoracentesis, pleurodesis, and dietary changes of the pregnant patient involving the intake of low-fat and high medium-chain-triglyceride foods. While these interventions may not completely resolve the chylothorax, they can stave off the reaccumulation of lymph fluid.

Common postnatal clinical manifestations in newborns include respiratory distress, which is often severe when chylothorax is associated with hydrops fetalis. A mediastinal shift (contralateral to the side with fluid accumulation) is likely to be seen on chest radiograph, both with unilateral or bilateral effusions. When sampled, chylous fluid will initially appear straw-colored and then change to milky-white after the newborn begins to ingest enteral feedings (due to the fat content of the feedings). These infants will require specialized formula that is low in long-chain fats.

The mortality risk ranges from 20% to 98% (Resch et al., 2022). Less favorable outcomes are associated with bilateral effusions and hydrops fetalis. The prognosis is more favorable when treatment leads to resolution of the effusion without reaccumulation.

CONCLUSION

One of the most common reasons for admission to the NICU is respiratory dysfunction. The test of successful mastery of the understanding of respiratory development and function is the ability of providers to explain the complex concepts to the parents and families of infants under their care.

LEARNING TOOLS AND RESOURCES

CourseConnect

To access self-assessment questions and interactive, competency-based learning activities for this chapter, visit www.springerpub.com/courseconnect. See inside front cover and tear-out card for CourseConnect details.

Podcast

This podcast is available online by visiting www.springerpub.com/courseconnect. See inside front cover and tear-out card for CourseConnect details.

Surfactant, Surface Tension, and LaPlace
Janice L. Wilson and Jennifer Fitzgerald

Discussion Prompts

1. Identify the major developmental milestones that occur during the major stages of lung development. At which stage is the lung considered viable and how might diseases in the XX pregnant patient implicate normal lung development?
2. Discuss the short-term and long-term complications associated with pneumothorax, persistent pulmonary hypertension, and chronic lung disease.
3. Discuss the role of the neonatal nurse practitioner in counseling the family of an extremely low birthweight infant, now 32 weeks postnatal age, who requires more than 30% oxygen by nasal cannula. What resources are available that offer predictive ability for risk for bronchopulmonary dysplasia?

MIND MAP

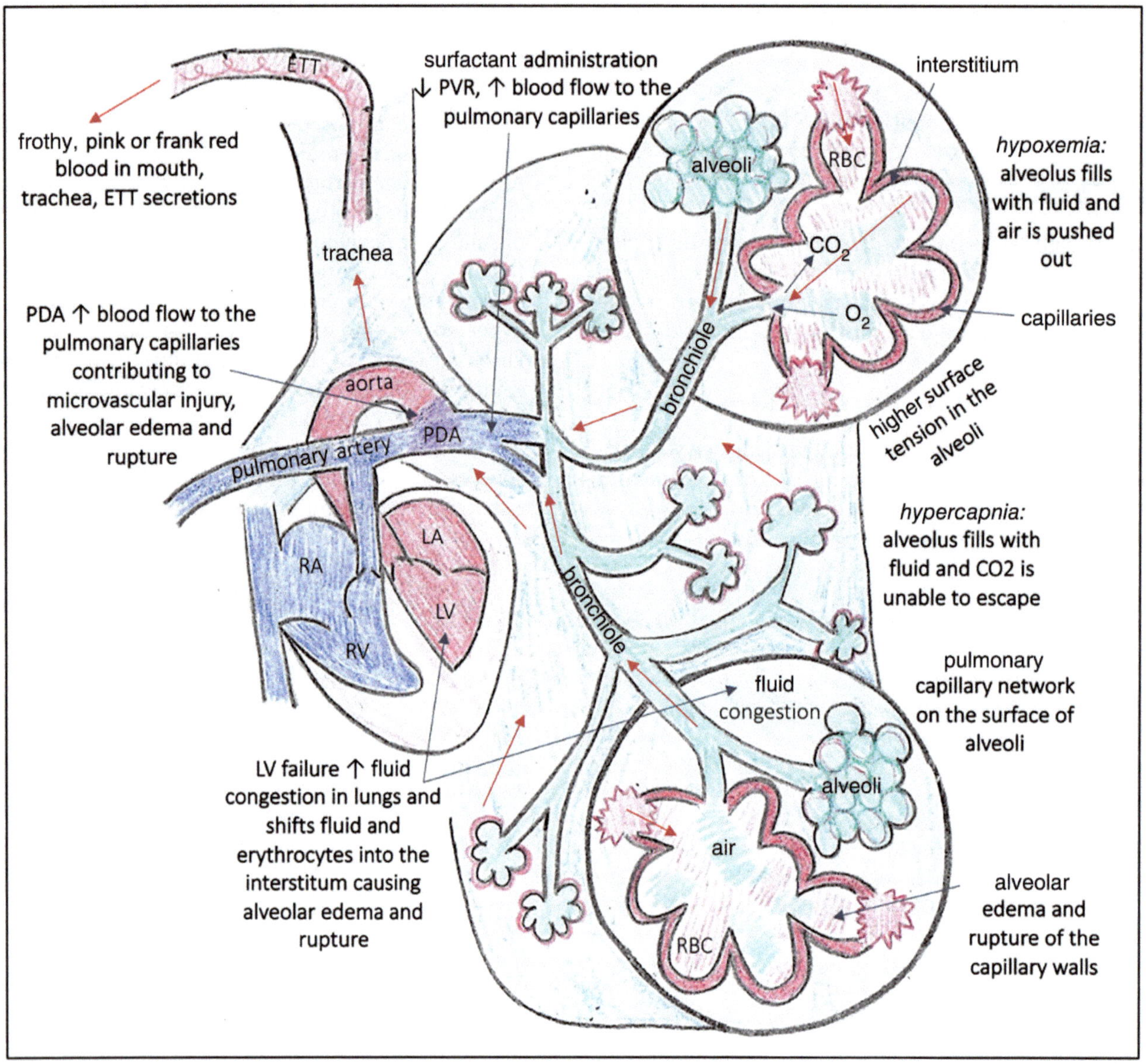

Note: This mind map reflects one neonatal APRN's interpretation of a portion of one or more concepts addressed in this chapter. Readers should regard the mind maps woven throughout this textbook as examples of multisensory study tools that can be developed to encourage conceptual understanding. Readers are encouraged to develop their own unique mind maps in consultation with academic faculty or clinical preceptors.
ETT, endotracheal tube; LA, left artery; LV, left ventricle; PDA, patent ductus arteriosus; ETT, endotracheal tube; PVR, pulmonary vascular resistance; RA, right artery; RBC, red blood cells; RLV, right left ventricle.
Image Credit: Cassidy Sanford, MSN, APRN, NNP-BC.

TIMELINE OF ORGAN DEVELOPMENT

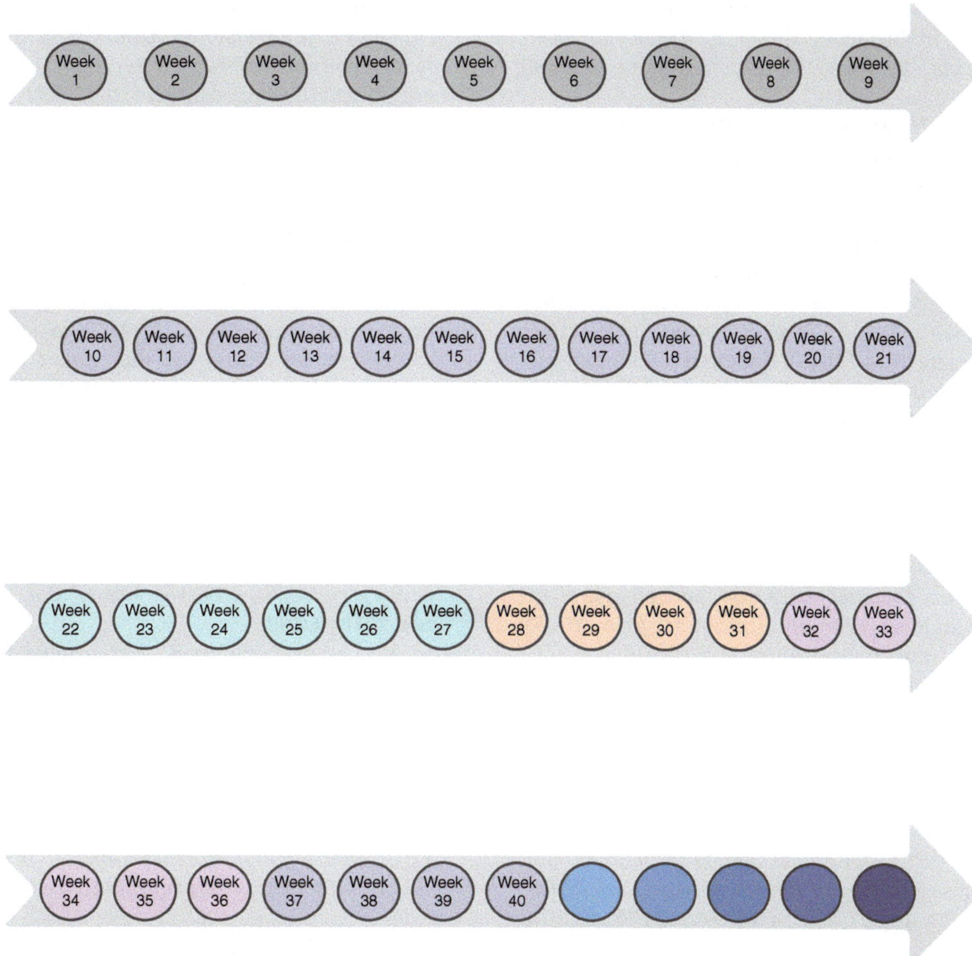

Note: Placement of common problems is meant to offer visual/ conceptual perspective on the timing of onset of these commonly reported malformations. Variation exists across the literature.	***Legend:*** <22–27 6/7 weeks = extremely preterm 28–31 6/7 weeks = very preterm 32–36 6/7 weeks = late/moderate preterm 37–40 weeks = term

Note: Readers are encouraged to annotate the blank timeline during studying, self-directed learning, and with the help of mentors. To access the blank and completed timelines, visit www.springerpub.com/courseconnect. See inside front cover and tear-out card for CourseConnect details.

REFERENCES

Abman, S. H., Baker, C., Gien, J., Mourani, P., & Galambos, P. (2014). The Robyn Barst Memorial lecture: Differences between the fetal, newborn, and adult pulmonary circulations: Relevance for age-specific therapies. *Pulmonary Circulation, 4*(3), 424–440. https://doi.org/10.1086/677371

Abman, S. H., Bancalari, E., & Jobe, A. (2017). The evolution of bronchopulmonary dysplasia after 50 years. *American Journal of Respiratory and Critical Care Medicine, 195*(4), 421–424. https://doi.org/10.1164/rccm.201611-2386ED

Akella, A., & Desphande, S. B. (2013). Pulmonary surfactants and their role in pathophysiology of lung disorders. *Indian Journal of Experimental Biology, 51*(1), 5–22. PMID: 23441475.

Alfaleh, K., Smyth, J. A., Roberts, R. S., Solimano, A., Asztalos, E. V., Schmidt, B., & Trial of Indomethacin Prophylaxis in Preterms Investigators. (2008). Prevention and 18-month outcomes of serious pulmonary hemorrhage in extremely low birth weight infants: Results from the trial of indomethacin prophylaxis in preterms. *Pediatrics, 121*(2), e233–e238. https://doi.org/10.1542/peds.2007-0028

Alhassen, Z., Vali, P., Guglani, L., Lakshminrusimha, S., & Ryan, R. M. (2021). Recent advances in pathophysiology and management of transient tachypnea of newborn. *Journal of Perinatology: Official Journal of the California Perinatal Association, 41*(1), 6–16. https://doi.org/10.1038/s41372-020-0757-3

Ali, N., & Sawyer, T. (2024). Perinatal transition and newborn resuscitation. In C. A. Gleason & S. E. Juul (Eds.), *Avery's diseases of the newborn* (11th ed., pp. 159–171). Elsevier.

Al-Tawi, K., Ahmed, G., Al-Hathal, M., Al-Jarallah, Y., & Campbell, N. (2000). Congenital chylothorax. *American*

Journal of Perinatology, 17(3), 121–126. https://doi.org/10.1055/s-2000-9281

Alvira, C. M. (2016). Aberrant pulmonary vascular growth and remodeling in bronchopulmonary dysplasia. *Frontiers in Medicine, 3*(21), 1–14. https://doi.org/10.3389/fmed.2016.00021

Ameis, S., Khoshgoo, H., & Keijzer, R. (2017). Abnormal lung development in congenital diaphragmatic hernia. *Seminars in Pediatric Surgery, 26*, 123–128. https://doi.org/10.1053/j.sempedsurg.2017.04.011

American College of Obstetricians and Gynecologists. (2024). Committee opinion no. 677: Antenatal corticosteroid therapy for lung maturity. *Obstetrics and Gynecology, 128*, e187–e194. https://doi.org/10.1097/AOG.0000000000001715

Baker, C. D., & Abman, S. H. (2015). Impaired pulmonary vascular development in bronchopulmonary dysplasia. *Neonatology, 107*(4), 344–351. https://doi.org/10.1159/000381129

Bancalari, E., Keszler, M., Davis. P. G., & Polin. R. A. (2024). *The newborn lung: Neonatology questions and controversies* (4th ed.). Elsevier/Saunders.

Biyyam, D. R., Chapman, T., Ferguson, M. R., Deutsch, G., & Dighe, M. K. (2010). Congenital lung abnormalities: Embryologic features, prenatal diagnosis, and postnatal radiologic–pathologic correlation. *RadioGraphics, 30*(6), 1721–1739. https://doi.org/10.1148/rg.306105508

Briana, D. D., & Malamitsi-Puchner, A. (2020). Perinatal biomarkers implying 'Developmental origins of health and disease' consequences in intrauterine growth restriction. *Acta Paediatrica, 109*(7), 1317–1322. https://doi.org/10.1111/apa.15022

Britt, R. D., Faksh, A., Vogel, E., Martin, R. J., Pabelick, C. M., & Prakash, Y. S. (2013). Perinatal factors in neonatal and pediatric lung diseases. *Expert Review of Respiratory Medicine, 7*(5), 515–531. https://doi.org/10.1586/17476348.2013.838020

Calco, G. N., Alharithi, Y. J., Williams, K. R., Jacoby, D. B., Fryer, A. D., Maloyan, A., & Nie, Z. (2023). Maternal high-fat diet increases airway sensory innervation and reflex bronchoconstriction in adult offspring. *American Journal of Physiology-Lung Cellular and Molecular Physiology, 325*(1), L66–L73. https://doi.org/10.1152/ajplung.00115.2023

Calzolari, F., Braguglia, A., Valfrè, L., Dotta, A., Bagolan, P., & Morini, F. (2016). Outcome of infants operated on for congenital pulmonary malformations. *Pediatric Pulmonology, 51*, 1367–1372. https://doi.org/10.1002/ppul.23472

Casagrande, A., & Pederiva, F. (2016). Association between congenital lung malformations and lung tumors in children and adults: A systemic review. *Journal of Thoracic Oncology, 11*(11), 1837–1845. https://doi.org/10.1016/j.jtho.2016.06.023

Chandrasekharan, P. K., Rawat, M., Madappa, R., Rothstein, D. H., & Lakshminrusimha, S. (2017). Congenital diaphragmatic hernia: A review. *Maternal Health, Neonatology and Perinatology, 3*(6), 1–16. https://doi.org/10.1186/s40748-017-0045-1

Chowdhury, M. M., & Chakraborty, S. (2015). Imaging of congenital lung malformations. *Seminars in Pediatric Surgery, 24*, 168–175. https://doi.org/10.1053/j.sempedsurg.2015.02.001

Cohen, J. L., & Cotton, M. (2022). Genetic variants and neonatal disease. In R. A. Polin, D. H. Rowitch, S. H. Abman, W. E. Benitz, & W. W. Fox (Eds.), *Fetal and neonatal physiology* (6th ed., pp. 1846–1854). Elsevier/Saunders.

Correia-Pinta, J., Gonzaga, S., Huang, Y., & Rottier, R. (2010). Congenital lung lesions—Underlying molecular mechanisms. *Seminars in Pediatric Surgery, 19*, 171–179. https://doi.org/10.1053/j.sempedsurg.2010.03.003

Cotton, M. C. (2017). Pulmonary hypoplasia. *Seminars in Fetal and Neonatal Medicine, 22*, 250–255. https://doi.org/10.1016/j.siny.2017.06.004

Crowley, A. (2025). Spectrum of neonatal respiratory disorders. In A. A. Fanaroff & R. J. Martin (Eds.), *Fanaroff and Martin's neonatal-perinatal medicine: Diseases of the fetus and infant* (11th ed., pp. 1271–1303). Elsevier/Saunders.

Cystic Fibrosis Foundation. (2021). *Cystic Fibrosis Foundation patient registry annual data report.* https://www.cff.org/sites/default/files/2021-11/Patient-Registry-Annual-Data-Report.pdf

Danzer, E., Zarnow, D., Gerdes, M., D'Agostino, J. A., Siegle, J., Bebbington, M. W., Flake, A. W., Adzick, S. N., & Hedrick, H. L. (2012). Abnormal brain development and maturation on magnetic resonance imaging in survivors of severe congenital diaphragmatic hernia. *Journal of Pediatric Surgery, 47*(3), 453–461. https://doi.org/10.1016/j.jpedsurg.2011.10.002

David, M., Lamas-Pinheiro, R., & Henriques-Coelho, T. (2016). Prenatal and postnatal management of congenital pulmonary airway malformation. *Neonatology, 110*, 101–115. https://doi.org/10.1159/000044894

Devaskar, S. U., Jazen, C., & Calkins, K. L. (2025). Fetal growth restriction: A complex interplay between the intrauterine and maternal environment. In R. J. Martin & A. A. Fanaroff (Eds.), *Fanaroff and Martin's neonatal-perinatal medicine: Diseases of the fetus and infant* (11th ed., pp. 259-273). Elsevier

Dingeldein, R. L. (2025). Selected gastrointestinal anomalies in neonates. In R. J. Martin & A. A. Fanaroff (Eds.), *Fanaroff and Martin's neonatal-perinatal medicine: Diseases of the fetus and infant* (11th ed., pp. 1626–1652). Elsevier/Saunders.

Durell, J., & Lakhoo, K. (2014). Congenital cystic lesions of the lung. *Early Human Development, 90*, 935–939. https://doi.org/10.1016/j.earlhumdev.2014.09.014

Dyess, N., Kinsella, J. P., & Parker, T. A. (2024). Acute neonatal respiratory disorders. In C. A. Gleason & T. Sawyer (Eds.), *Avery's diseases of the newborn* (11th ed., pp. 594–613). Elsevier.

Fleury, M., Delestrain, C., Roditis, L., Perisson, C., Renoux, M., Thumerelle, C., Epaud, R., Fletcher, C., Jedidi, N., Coulomb L'Hermine, A., Corvol, H., Ducou le Pointe, H., Fanen, P., Sileo, C., Louvrier, C., de Becdelievre, A., Legendre, M., & Nathan, N. (2025). Surfactant protein B deficiency: The RespiRare cohort. *Thorax, 80*(2), 109–112. https://doi.org/10.1136/thorax-2024-221947

Fowler, D. J., & Gould, S. J. (2015). The pathology of congenital lung lesions. *Seminars in Pediatric Surgery, 24*(4), 176–182. https://doi.org/10.1053/j.sempedsurg.2015.02.002

Gao, Y., & Raj, J. U. (2010). Regulation of the pulmonary circulation in the fetus and newborn. *Physiology Review, 90*, 1291–1335. https://doi.org/10.1152/physrev.00032.2009

Gawlińska, K., Gawliński, D., Filip, M., & Przegaliński, E. (2021). Relationship of maternal high-fat diet during pregnancy and lactation to offspring health. *Nutrition*

Reviews, 79(6), 709–725. https://doi.org/10.1093/nutrit/nuaa020

Gien, J., & Kinsella, J. P. (2022). Pathophysiology of meconium aspiration syndrome. In R. A. Polin, S. H. Abman, D. H. Rowitch, W. E. Benitz, & W. W. Fox (Eds.), *Fetal and neonatal physiology* (6th ed., pp. 1696–1703). Elsevier/Saunders.

Guglani, L., Lakshminrusimha, S., & Ryan, R. M. (2008). Transient tachypnea of the newborn. *Pediatrics in Review, 29*, e59–e65. https://doi.org/10.1542/pir.29-11-e59

Han, S., & Mallampalli, R. K. (2015). The acute respiratory distress syndrome: From mechanism to translation. *Journal of Immunology, 194*(3), 855–860. https://doi.org/10.4049/jimmunol.1402513

Higgins, R. D., Jobe, A. H., Koso-Thomas, M., Bancalari, E., Viscardi, R. M., Hartert, T. V., Ryan, R. M., Kallapur, S. G., Steinhorn, R. H., Konduri, G. G., Davis, S. D., Thebaud, B., Clyman, R. I., Collaco, J. M., Martin, C. R., Woods, J. C., Finer, N. N., & Raju, T. N. K. (2018). Bronchopulmonary dysplasia: Executive summary of a workshop. *The Journal of Pediatrics, 197*, 300–308. https://doi.org/10.1016/j.jpeds.2018.01.043

Hillman, N., Kallapur, S. G., & Jobe, A. (2012). Physiology of transition from intrauterine to extrauterine life. *Clinics in Perinatology, 39*(4), 769–783. https://doi.org/10.1016/j.clp.2012.09.009

Hong, C., Yu, G., Tang, J., Liu, Q., & Xia, B. (2017). Risk analysis and outcomes of bronchopulmonary sequestrations. *Pediatric Surgery International, 33*(9), 971–975. https://doi.org/10.1007/s00383-017-4097-0

Hooper, S. B., Roberts, C., Dekker, J., & te Pas, A. B. (2019). Issues in cardiopulmonary transition at birth. *Seminars in Fetal & Neonatal Medicine, 24*(6), 101033. https://doi.org/10.1016/j.siny.2019.101033

Hsu, J., Lee, Y., Lin, C., Li, F., Jeng, M., Soong, W., Chen, S. J., & Tang, R. (2012). Primary congenital pulmonary hypoplasia of a neonate. *Journal of the Chinese Medical Association, 75*, 87–90. https://doi.org/10.1016/j.jcma.2011.12.004

Huang, E. N., Quach, H., Lee, J. A., Dierolf, J., Moraes, T. J., & Wong, A. P. (2021). A developmental role of the cystic fibrosis transmembrane conductance regulator in cystic fibrosis lung disease pathogenesis. *Frontiers in Cell and Developmental Biology, 9*, 742891. https://doi.org/10.3389/fcell.2021.742891

Islam, J. Y., Keller, R. L., Aschner, J. L., Hartet, T. V., & Moore, P. E. (2015). Understanding the short- and long-term respiratory outcomes of prematurity and bronchopulmonary dysplasia. *American Journal of Respiratory and Critical Care Medicine, 192*(2), 134–156. https://doi.org/10.1164/rccm.201412-2142PP

Javia, L., Harris, M. A., & Fuller, S. (2016). Rings, slings, and other tracheal disorders in the neonate. *Seminars in Fetal & Neonatal Medicine, 21*, 277–284. https://doi.org/10.1016/j.siny.2016.03.005

Jeng, M., Lee, Y., Tsao, P., & Soong, W. (2012). Neonatal air leak syndrome and the role of high-frequency ventilation in its prevention. *Journal of the Chinese Medical Association, 75*, 551–559. https://doi.org/10.1016/j.jcma.2012.08.001

Jobe, A. H., & Kallapur, S. G. (2022). Surfactant treatment. In R. Polin, S. H. Abman, D. H. Rowtich, & W. Benitz (Eds.), *Fetal and neonatal physiology* (6th ed., pp. 813–825). Elsevier/Saunders.

Juul, S. E., & Christensen, R. D. (2024). Developmental hematology. In C. A. Gleason & T. Sawyer (Eds.). *Avery's diseases of the newborn* (11th ed., pp. 957–964). Elsevier.

Kallapur, S. G., & Jobe, A. H. (2025). Lung development and maturation. In R. J. Martin & A. A. Fanaroff (Eds.), *Fanaroff and Martin's neonatal-perinatal medicine: Diseases of the fetus and infant* (12th ed., pp. 1190–1209). Elsevier.

Kassab, M., Khriesat, W. M., & Anabrees, J. (2015). Diuretics for transient tachypnoea of the newborn. *Cochrane Database of Systematic Reviews, 2015*(11), CD003064. https://doi.org/10.1002/14651858.CD003064.pub3

Kastein, K., & Coe, K. (2023). Management of air leaks in the newborn. *Advances in Neonatal Care, 23*(2), 160–166. https://doi.org/10.1097/ANC.0000000000001040

Katz, C., Bentur, L., & Elias, N. (2011). Clinical implication of fetal lung fluid balance in the perinatal period. *Journal of Perinatology, 31*, 230–235. https://doi.org/10.1038/jp.2010.134

Keijzer, R., & Puri, P. (2010). Congenital diaphragmatic hernia. *Seminars in Pediatric Surgery, 19*(3), 180–185. https://doi.org/10.1053/j.sempedsurg.2010.03.001

Keller, R. L., & Steinhorn, R. H. (2024). Chronic respiratory disorders. In C. A. Gleason & T. Sawyer (Eds.). *Avery's diseases of the newborn* (11th ed., pp. 614–625). Elsevier.

Keszler, M., & Abubakar, K. (2022). Physiologic principles. In M. Keszler & K. S. Gautham (Eds.), *Goldsmith's assisted ventilation of the neonate* (7th ed., pp. 11–32.e3). Elsevier.

Kool, H., Mous, D., Tibboel, D., de Klein, A., & Rottier, R. J. (2014). Pulmonary vascular development goes awry in congenital lung abnormalities. *Birth Defects Research. Part C. Embryo Today, 102*(4), 343–358. https://doi.org/10.1002/bdrc.21085

Kravitz, R. M. (1994). Congenital malformations of the lung. *Pediatric Clinics of North America, 41*(3), 453–472. https://doi.org/10.1016/s0031-3955(16)38765-x

Kumar, V. H. S. (2015). Current concepts in the management of congenital diaphragmatic hernia in infants. *Indian Journal of Surgery, 77*(4), 313–321. https://doi.org/10.1007/s12262-015-1286-8

Kwong, K. W. (2015). Current updates on choanal atresia. *Frontiers in Pediatrics, 3*(52), 1–7. https://doi.org/10.3389/fped.2015.0052

Lagoski, M., Hamvas, A., & Wambach, J. A. (2025). Respiratory distress syndrome in the neonate. In A. A. Fanaroff & R. J. Martin (Eds.), *Fanaroff and Martin's neonatal-perinatal medicine: Diseases of the fetus and infant* (11th ed., pp. 1226–1239). Elsevier/Saunders.

Lakshminrusimha, S., & Steinhorn, R. H. (2022). Pathophysiology of persistent pulmonary hypertension of the newborn. In R. A. Polin, S. H. Abman, D. H. Rowtich, W. E. Benitz, & W. W. Fox. (Eds.), *Fetal and neonatal physiology* (6th ed., pp. 1648–1662). Elsevier.

Lamberti, R., Canali, G., Romero, A., Ghezzi, M., Vincenzo-Zuccotti, G., & D'Auria, E. (2023). Congenital pulmonary airways malformation: State of the art review. *Pediatric Respiratory Journal, 1*(3), 120–126. https://doi.org/10.56164/PediatrRespirJ.2023.26

Le Cras, T. D., & Rabinovitch, M. (2016). Pulmonary vascular development. In A. Jobe, J. Whitsett, & S. Abman (Eds.), *Fetal and neonatal lung development: Clinical correlates and technologies for the future* (pp. 34–57). Cambridge University Press.

Lee, J., Romero, R., Lee, K. A., Kim, E. N., Korzeniewski, S. J., Chaemsaithong, P., & Yoon, B. Y. (2016). Meconium aspiration syndrome: A role for fetal systemic inflammation. *American Journal of Obstetrics and Gynecology, 214*(3), 366.e1–366.e9. https://doi.org/10.1016/j.ajog.2015.10.009

Li, W., Wang, Y., Song, J., Zhang, C., Xu, Y., Xu, F., Wang, X., & Zhu, C. (2023). Association between bronchopulmonary dysplasia and death or neurodevelopmental impairment at 3 years in preterm infants without severe brain injury. *Frontiers in Neurology, 14*, 1292372. https://doi.org/10.3389/fneur.2023.1292372

Lopez-Rodriguez, E., Echaide, M., Cruz, A., Taeusch, W., & Perez-Gil, J. (2011). Meconium impairs pulmonary surfactant by a combined action of cholesterol and bile acids. *Biophysical Journal, 100*, 646–655. https://doi.org/10.1016/j.bpj.2010.12.3715

Madurga, A., Mizíková, I., Ruiz-Camp, J., & Morty, R. E. (2013). Recent advances in late lung development and the pathogenesis of bronchopulmonary dysplasia. *American Journal of Physiology—Lung Cellular and Molecular Physiology, 305*(12), L893–L905. https://doi.org/10.1152/ajplung.00267.2013

Malleske, D. (2015). Book review: *Advances in fetal and neonatal physiology. American Journal of Human Biology, 27*(5), 739–740. https://doi.org/10.1002/ajhb.22768

March of Dimes. (2020). *Being overweight during pregnancy.* https://www.marchofdimes.org/find-support/topics/pregnancy/being-overweight-during-pregnancy

Marinicak, S. J., & Lomas, D. A. (2017). Inherited pulmonary disorders. *Encyclopedia of Life Sciences.* John Wiley. https://doi.org/10.1002/9780470015902.a0005517.pub3

McEvoy, C. T., Shorey-Kendrick, L. E., Milner, K., Harris, J., Vuylsteke, B., Cunningham, M., Tiller, C., Stewart, J., Schilling, D., Brownsberger, J., Titus, H., MacDonald, K. D., Gonzales, D., Vu, A., Park, B. S., Spindel, E. R., Morris, C. D., & Tepper, R. S. (2023). Effect of vitamin C supplementation for pregnant smokers on offspring airway function and wheeze at age 5 years: Follow-up of a randomized clinical trial. *JAMA Pediatrics, 177*(1), 16–24. https://doi.org/10.1001/jamapediatrics.2022.4401

McGoldrick, E., Stewart, F., Parker, R., & Dalziel, S. R. (2020). Antenatal corticosteroids for accelerating fetal lung maturation for women at risk of preterm birth. *Cochrane Database of Systematic Reviews, 12*(12), CD004454. https://doi.org/10.1002/14651858.CD004454.pub4

Metcalfe, A., Lisonkova, S., Sabr, Y., Stritzke, A., & Joseph, K. (2017). Neonatal respiratory morbidity following exposure to chorioamnionitis. *BMC Pediatrics, 17*(1), 1–7. https://doi.org/10.1186/s12887-017-0878-9

Moujaes, L., Barnett, E. D., & Malley, R. (2025). Bacterial infections of the respiratory tract. In Y. Maldonado, V. Nizet, E. D. Barnett, K M. Edwards, & R. Malley (Eds.), *Remington and Klein's infectious diseases of the fetus and newborn infant* (9th ed., pp. 255–262). Elsevier.

Mourani, P., & Abman, S. H. (2013). Pulmonary vascular disease in bronchopulmonary dysplasia: Pulmonary hypertension and beyond. *Pulmonology, 25*, 329–337. https://doi.org/10.1097/MOP.0b013e328360a3f6

Mukherjee, D., & Ryan, R. M. (2025). Postnatal bacterial infections. In A. A. Fanaroff, & R. J. Martin (Eds.), *Fanaroff and Martin's neonatal-perinatal medicine: Diseases of the fetus and infant* (11th ed., pp. 857–880). Elsevier.

Naumberg, E., Axelson, I., Huber, D., & Soderstrom, L. (2015). Some neonatal risk factors for adult pulmonary arterial hypertension remain unknown. *Foundation Acta Paediatrica, 104*, 1104–1108. https://doi.org/10.1111/apa.13205

Noritz, G., Madden, M., Roldan, D., Wheeler, T. A., Conkol, K, Brilli, R. J., Barnard, J., & Gleeson, S. (2017). A population intervention to improve outcomes in children with medical complexity. *Pediatrics, 139*(1), e20153076. https://doi.org/10.1542/peds.2015-3076

Oakley, R. H., & Cidlowski, J. A. (2013). The biology of the glucocorticoid receptor: New signaling mechanisms in health and disease. *Journal of Allergy and Clinical Immunology, 132*(5), 1033–1044. https://doi.org/10.1016/j.jaci.2013.09.007

Oh, S. H., Jin, H., & Park, C. (2023). Risk factors and neonatal outcomes of pulmonary air leak syndrome in extremely preterm infants: A nationwide descriptive study. *Medicine, 102*(34), e34759. https://doi.org/10.1097/md.0000000000034759

Olutoye, O., Coleman, B., Hubbard, A. M., & Adzick, N. S. (2000). Prenatal diagnosis and management of congenital lobar emphysema. *Journal of Pediatric Surgery, 35*, 792–795. https://doi.org/10.1053/jpsu.2000.6084

Pantich, H. B., Weiner, D. J., Feng, R., Perez, M. R., Healy, F., McDonough, J. M., Rintoul, N., & Hedrick, H. L. (2014). Lung function over the first 3 years of life in children with congenital diaphragmatic hernia. *Pediatric Pulmonology, 50*(9), 896–907. https://doi.org/10.1002/ppul.23082

Perez-Gil, J., & Weaver, T. E. (2010). Pulmonary surfactant pathophysiology: Current models and open questions. *Physiology, 25*, 132–141. https://doi.org/10.1152/physiol.00006.2010

Pike, K., Pillow, J., & Lucas, J. S. (2012). Long term respiratory consequences of intrauterine growth restriction. *Seminars in Fetal and Neonatal Medicine, 17*(2), 92–98. https://doi.org/10.1016/j siny.2012.01.003

Plosa, E., & Sucre, J. (2024). Lung development. In C. A. Gleason & T. Sawyer (Eds.), *Avery's diseases of the newborn* (11th ed., pp. 535–547). Elsevier/Saunders.

Pryce, D. M. (1946). Lower accessory pulmonary artery with intralobar sequestration of lung: A report of seven cases. *Journal of Pathology and Bacteriology, 58*(3), 457–467. https://doi.org/10.1002/path.1700580316

Reed-McCullough, S., & Jnah, A. J. (2021). Congenital diaphragmatic hernia: Core review and novel updates. *Neonatal Network, 40*(5), 305–312. https://doi.org/10.1891/11-T-701

Register, C. H., Jnah, A. J., & Newberry, D. (2016). Congenital diaphragmatic hernia: Interprofessional care of the neonate and family grounded in Swanson's theory of caring. *Neonatal Network, 35*(6), 381–390. https://doi.org/10.1891/0730-0832.35.6.381

Resch, B., Sever Yildiz, G., & Reiterer, F. (2022). Congenital chylothorax of the newborn: A systematic analysis of published cases between 1990 and 2018. *Respiration: International Review of Thoracic Diseases, 101*(1), 84–96. https://doi.org/10.1159/000518217

Riley, C. A., Boozer, K., & King, T. L. (2011). Antenatal corticosteroids at the beginning of the 21st century. *Journal of*

Midwifery and Women's Health, 56, 591–597. https://doi.org/10.1111/j.1542-2011.2011.00119.x

Rios, D. R., El-Khuffash, A. F., & McNamara, P. J. (2022). Oxygen transport and delivery. In R. A. Polin, S. H. Abman, D. H. Rowtich, W. E. Benitz, & W. W. Fox. (Eds.), *Fetal and neonatal physiology* (6th ed., pp. 684–696). Elsevier.

Rook, D., Schierbeek, H., Vento, M., Vlaardingerbroek, H., van der Eijk, A. C., Longini, M., Giuseppe Buonocore, G., Escobar, J., van Goudoever, J. B., & Vermeulen, M. J. (2014). Resuscitation of preterm infants with different inspired oxygen fractions. *Journal of Pediatrics, 164*(6), 1322–1326.e3. https://doi.org/10.1016/j.jpeds.2014.02.019

Sadler, T. W. (2024). *Langman's medical embryology* (15th ed.). Wolters Kluwer.

Sadreameli, S. C., & McGrath-Morrow, S. A. (2016). Respiratory care of infants and children with congenital trachea-oesophageal fistula and oesophageal atresia. *Paediatric Respiratory Reviews, 17*, 16–23. https://doi.org/10.1016/j.prrv.2015.02.005

Sarper, A., Ayten, A., Golbasi, I., Demircan, A., & Isin, E. (2003). Bronchogenic cyst. *Texas Heart Institute Journal, 30*(2), 105–108. PMID: 12809250; PMCID: PMC161894.

Schmidt, A. F., & Bancalari, E. H. (2025). Bronchopulmonary dysplasia in the neonate. In R. J. Martin & A. A. Fanaroff (Eds.), *Fanaroff and Martin's neonatal-perinatal medicine: Diseases of the fetus and infant* (11th ed., pp. 1330–1345). Elsevier.

Schoenwolf, G. C., Bleyl, S. B., Brauer, P. R., & Francis-West, P. H. (2021). *Larsen's human embryology* (6th ed.). Elsevier.

Sfakianaki, A. K., & Copel, J. A. (2012). Congenital cystic lesions of the lung: Congenital cystic adenomatoid malformation and bronchopulmonary sequestration. *Reviews in Obstetrics & Gynecology, 5*(2), 85–93. https://doi.org/10.3909/riog0183a

Singh, J., Jaffe, A., Schultz, A., & Selvadurai, H. (2021). Surfactant protein disorders in childhood interstitial lung disease. *European Journal of Pediatrics, 180*(9), 2711–2721. https://doi.org/10.1007/s00431-021-04066-3

Spoonhower, K. A., & Davis, P. B. (2016). Epidemiology of cystic fibrosis. *Clinics in Chest Medicine, 37*(1), 1–8. https://doi.org/10.1016/j.ccm.2015.10.002

Stanojevic, S., Swaleh, S., Sykes, J., Ma, X., Desai, S., Quon, B. S., Faro, A., Marshall, B., Ramos, K., Ostrenga, J., Elbert, A., Cromwell, E., Goss, C. H., & Stephenson, A. L. (2022). WS08.02 contemporary incidence of cystic fibrosis in Canada and the United States. *Journal of Cystic Fibrosis, 21*, S15–S16. https://doi.org/10.1016/S1569-1993(22)00196-5

Stark, Z., Behrsin, J., Burgess, T., Ritchie, A., Yeung, A., Tan, T. Y., Brown, N. J., Savarirayan, R., & Patel, N. (2015). SNP microarray abnormalities in a cohort of 28 infants with congenital diaphragmatic hernia. *American Journal of Medical Genetics, Part A, 167A*(10), 2319–2326. https://doi.org/10.1002/ajmg.a.37177

Steinhorn, R. H. (2025). Pulmonary vascular development. In R. J. Martin & A. A. Fanaroff (Eds.), *Fanaroff and Martin's neonatal-perinatal medicine: Diseases of the fetus and infant* (11th ed., pp. 1372–1386). Elsevier.

Stenson, B. J., & Smith, C. L. (2012). Management of meconium aspiration syndrome. *Paediatric Child Health, 22*(12), 532–535. https://doi.org/10.1016/j.jnn.2015.05.002

Stevens, T. P., Blennow, M., Meyers, E. H., & Soll, R. (2007). Early surfactant administration with brief ventilation vs. selective surfactant and continued mechanical ventilation for preterm infants with or at risk for respiratory distress syndrome (Review). *Cochrane Database of Systematic Reviews, 2007*(4), 1–32. https://doi.org/10.1002/14651858.CD003063.pub3

Stocker, J. T. (2009). Cystic lung disease in infants and children. *Fetal and Pediatric Pathology, 28*(4), 155–184. https://doi.org/10.1080/15513810902984095

Sun, X. (2022). Normal and abnormal structural development of the lung. In R. A. Polin, S. H. Abman, D. H. Rowitch, W. E. Benitz, & W. W. Fox (Eds.), *Fetal and neonatal physiology* (pp. 586–599). Elsevier.

te Pas, A. B., & Hooper, S. (2016). Initiation of breathing at birth. In A. Jobe, J. Whitsett, & S. Abman (Eds.), *Fetal and neonatal lung development: Clinical correlates and technologies for the future* (pp. 164–186). Cambridge University Press.

Terlizzi, V., DiLullo, A. M., Comegna, M., Centrone, C., Pelo, E., Castaldo, G., Raia, V., & Braggion, C. (2018). S737F is a new *CFTR* mutation typical of patients originally from Tuscany region in Italy. *Italian Journal of Pediatrics, 44*(2), 1–7. https://doi.org/10.1186/s13052-017-0443-z

Terlizzi, V., & Dolce, D. (2023). Variability of the sweat test in children with cystic fibrosis previously CRMS/CFSPID: A retrospective monocenter experience. *Journal of Cystic Fibrosis, 22*(3), 496–498. https://doi.org/10.1016/j.jcf.2023.04.018

Torchia, M. G., & Persaud, T. V. N. (2025). *The developing human: Clinically oriented embryology* (12th ed.). Elsevier.

Trembath, A., & Laughon, M. M. (2012). Predictors of bronchopulmonary dysplasia. *Clinics in Perinatology, 39*(3), 585–601. https://doi.org/10.1016/j.clp.2012.06.014

Triebwasser, J. E., & Treadwell, M. C. (2017). Prenatal prediction of pulmonary hypoplasia. *Seminars in Fetal and Neonatal Medicine, 22*, 245–249. https://doi.org/10.1016/j.siny.2017.03.001

Truog, W. E., & Manimtim, W. M. (2024). Neonatal pulmonary physiology. In C. A. Gleason & T. Sawyer (Eds.), *Avery's diseases of the newborn* (11th ed., pp. 548–558). Elsevier.

Universities of Fribourg, Lausanne, & Bern, Switzerland, (2006). *Module 18: Respiration tract*. https://embryology.ch/en/organogenesis/respiration-tract/

Van Woudenberg, C. D., Willis, C. A., & Rubarth, L. B. (2012). Newborn transition to extrauterine life. *Neonatal Network, 31*(5), 317–322. https://doi.org/10.1891/0730-0832.31.5.317

Wapner, R. J. (2013). Antenatal corticosteroids for periviable birth. *Seminars in Perinatology, 37*, 410–413. https://doi.org/10.1053/j.semperi.2013.06.024

Welde, M. A., Sanford, C. B., Mangum, M., Paschal, C., & Jnah, A. J. (2021). Pulmonary hemorrhage in the neonate. *Neonatal Network, 40*(5), 295–304. https://doi.org/10.1891/11-T-696

Whitsett, J. A., & Kingma, P. S. (2022). Surfactant homeostasis: Composition and function of pulmonary surfactant lipids and proteins. In R. Polin, S. H. Abman, D. H. Rowtich, & W. Benitz (Eds.), *Fetal and neonatal physiology* (6th ed., pp. 776–787). Elsevier/Saunders.

Whitsett, J. A., & Xu, Y. (2016). Transcriptional mechanisms regulating pulmonary epithelial maturation: A systems biology approach. In A. Jobe, J. Whitsett, & S. Abman (Eds.), *Fetal and neonatal lung development: Clinical correlates and technologies for the future* (pp. 58–76). Cambridge University Press.

Winn, H. N., Chen, M., Amon, E., Leet, T. L., Shumway, J. B., & Mostello, D. (2000). Neonatal pulmonary hypoplasia and perinatal mortality in patients with mid-trimester rupture of amniotic membranes--a critical analysis. *American Journal of Obstetrics and Gynecology, 182*(6), 1638–1644. https://doi.org/10.1067/mob.2000.107435

Wolfe, C., & Jnah, A. (2024). Tracheoesophageal fistula with esophageal atresia: A case series. *Neonatal Network, 43*(2), 65–75. https://doi.org/10.1891/NN-2023-0051

Zhang, H., Zhang, J., & Zhao, S. (2016). Airway damage of prematurity: The impact of prolonged intubation, ventilation, and chronic lung disease. *Seminars in Fetal & Neonatal Medicine, 21*, 246–253. https://doi.org/10.1016/j.siny.2016.04.001

Zobel, M., Gologorsky, R., Lee, H., & Vu, L. (2019). Congenital lung lesions. *Seminars in Pediatric Surgery, 28*(4), 150821. https://doi.org/10.1053/j.sempedsurg.2019.07.004

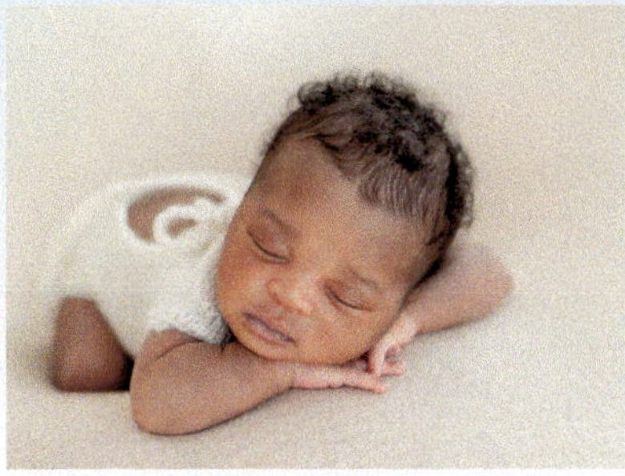

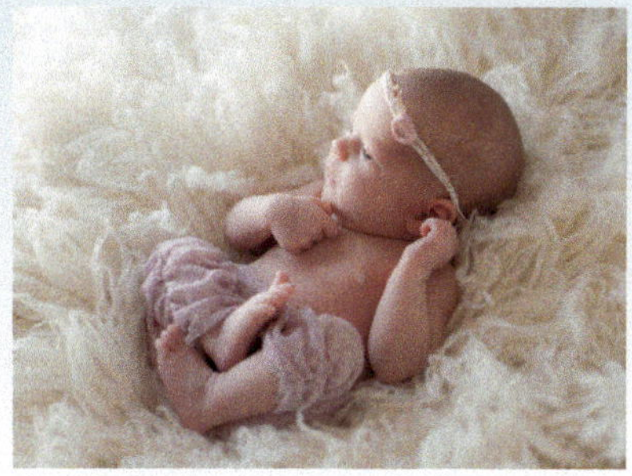

5 THE CARDIOVASCULAR SYSTEM

Amy Williford, Jennifer Fitzgerald, and Amy J. Jnah

LEARNING OBJECTIVES

After completing this chapter, the reader should be able to:

- Understand normal cardiovascular system development.
- Analyze the physiologic function of the fetal and neonatal cardiovascular system.
- Discuss common inherited disorders and their effect on fetal and neonatal cardiovascular system development and function.
- Identify health issues in XX pregnant patients that have a potential impact on fetal and postnatal cardiovascular system development and function.
- Evaluate common disorders that affect the cardiovascular system and their implications across the life span.

INTRODUCTION

Congenital heart defects (CHDs) are defined as cardiovascular malformations of the structure of the heart or great vessels that are present at birth (Bouma & Mulder, 2017). CHDs are the most common type of congenital anomaly observed among neonates and affect approximately 1% of all live-born infants in the United States, with an increasing prevalence in milder types of CHDs (Centers for Disease Control and Prevention [CDC], 2024a; Duca et al., 2020). Despite significant surgical and medical advancements, globally, CHDs remain a major cause of infant mortality due to birth defects (Wu et al., 2020).

Any deviations in the normal development of the heart which may result from genetic, environmental, or multifactorial influences during embryologic and fetal development can cause a CHD. CHDs lead to acyanotic, cyanotic, or obstructive blood flow patterns. Although over 120 different types of CHD are reported, ranging from mild to major malformations, the more common defects that implicate the fetus and neonate are discussed in this chapter (**Figure 5.1**).

Clinicians must be adept at differentiating between benign and life-threatening CHDs. Certain CHDs are associated with significant morbidity and mortality risks, substantial healthcare costs, and the need for lifelong care, especially when left undiagnosed during the early postnatal period. These factors may impose substantial emotional and socioeconomic challenges on patients and families (Bakker et al., 2019). Graduate-level and continuing nursing and medical education, as well as ongoing quality-improvement efforts, have improved prenatal and postnatal recognition of CHDs narrowing the gap in the identification, diagnosis, and initiation of medical care. As a result of these ongoing and concerted efforts among clinicians, approximately 85% to 90% of all U.S.-born infants with a CHD will celebrate their 18th birthday (Bouma & Mulder, 2017; Congenital Heart Public Health Consortium [CHPHC], 2024).

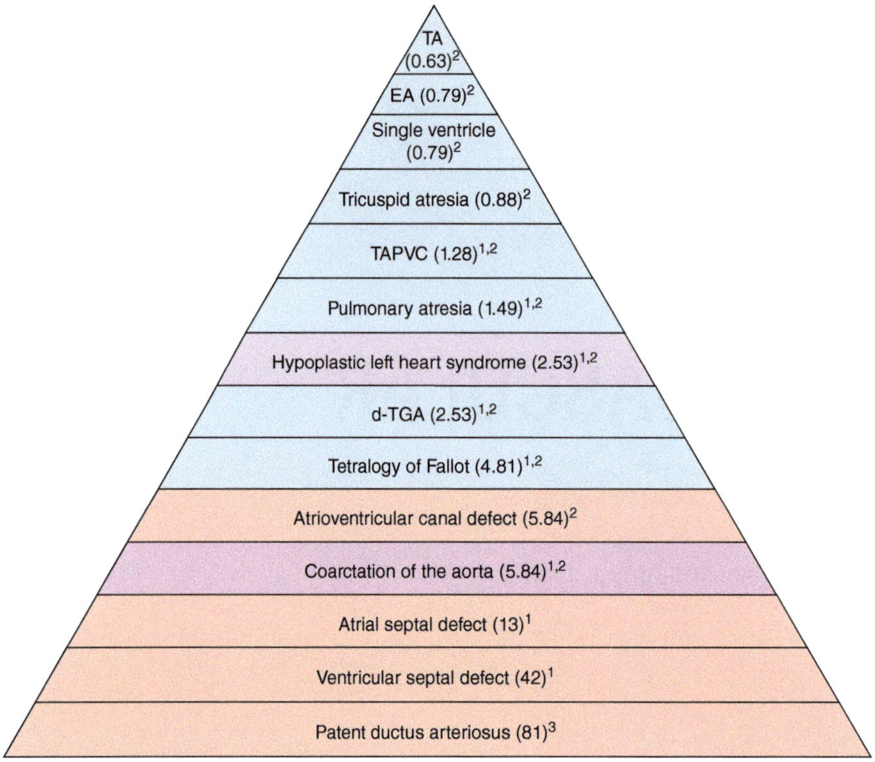

Figure 5.1 Incidence of various congenital heart defects.

Notes: The number in parentheses reflects the number of affected liveborn infants per 10,000 live births. Orange signifies acyanotic CHDs; blue signifies cyanotic CHDs; and purple signifies obstructive CHDs.

CHD, congenital heart defect; d-TGA, dextro-transposition of the great arteries; EA, Ebstein anomaly; TA, truncus arteriosus; TAPVC, total anomalous pulmonary venous connection.

[1]Centers for Disease Control and Prevention. (2024, October 21). *About tricuspid atresia.* https://www.cdc.gov/heart-defects/about/tricuspid-atresia.html

[2]Stallings, E. B., Isenberg, J. L. Rutkowsk, R. E., Kirby, R. S., Nembhard, W. N., Sandidge, T., Villavicencio, S., Nguyen, H. H., McMahon, D. M., Nestoridi, E., Pabst, L. J., & National Birth Defects Prevention Network. (2024). National population-based estimates for major birth defects, 2016-2020. *Birth Defects Review, 116*(1), e2301. https://doi.10.1002/bdr2.2301

[3]Park, J., Yoon, S. J., Han, J., Song, I. G., Lim, J., Shin, J. E., Eun, H. S., Park, K. I., Park, M. S., & Lee, S. M. (2021). Patent ductus arteriosus treatment trends and associated morbidities in neonates. *Scientific Reports, 11*(1), 10689. https://doi.org/10.1038/s41598-021-89868-z

TIMELINE OF ORGAN DEVELOPMENT

The heart is the first organ to reach functional status within the developing fetus. This is necessary, as simple diffusion of oxygen and nutrients across the placenta cannot singlehandedly and adequately nourish the rapidly proliferating embryo (Torchia & Persaud, 2025). In fact, early heart function is a stimulus for maturation of other organ systems, namely the hematologic system, by way of the movement of primitive and definitive red blood cells throughout the body (see Chapter 7).

From the early period of gastrulation through week 8 of gestation, the heart undergoes complex morphogenetic changes and differentiates into three distinct portions: the mesothelium (outer lining), endothelium (inner lining), and myocardium (muscle layer). First, a linear heart, or "primary" myocardium, forms. Second, a specialized ventricular chamber myocardium develops at the ventral surface of the linear heart tube. Concurrently, the left and right atrial myocardium form more caudally on the laterodorsal surfaces. Heart looping thereby occurs, aligning these primordial chambers. As a result, five distinct regions form: (a) truncus arteriosus, (b) bulbus cordis, (c) primitive ventricle, (d) primitive atrium, and (e) sinus venosus. Blood cells cluster to form blood islands (see Chapter 7), which form the vasculature. These and other significant changes in cardiac development continue up to the end of the embryonic period, at 10 weeks of gestation. In the text that follows, we describe the major phases of embryologic development as separate events; however, it is important to understand that most morphologic changes overlap.

Primordial Heart Tube

The primordial heart and vascular system begin to form during the period of gastrulation, between days 16 to 18 of gestation (Torchia & Persaud, 2025). Progenitor cells migrate from the endoderm, specifically tasked with forming a cardiogenic crest within the splanchnic mesoderm. The primary heart tube arises from this splanchnic mesoderm as a crescent-shaped formation at the cranial border of the mesoderm (Torchia & Persaud, 2025). This region becomes the cardiogenic region of the developing embryo.

By day 19, angiogenic cells cluster and form two primitive endocardial tubes. Each individual tube develops synchronously on either side of the cardiogenic region. During week 3 of gestation, both tubes begin migrating toward one another and merge in a cranial–caudal fashion. By day 22 of gestation, the tubes fuse and form one primordial heart tube (**Figure 5.2**; Gittenberger-de Groot et al., 2013; Goble et al., 2016). The inner aspect of the tube forms the endocardium. The outer aspect of the tube forms the myocardium, or muscular wall of the heart (England, 1996; Fineman & Clyman, 2004). Both the endocardium and myocardium become separated by *cardiac jelly*, an extracellular matrix. At this point in development, the heart tube is bilaterally symmetrical, appearing as an inverted Y, anchored in place by arterial trunks (cranial end) and venous channels (caudal end). By day 23 of gestation, the heart can beat and pump blood (Torchia & Persaud, 2025). Now, the heart is ready for looping and further differentiation.

Cardiac Looping

Soon after cardiac contractions (heartbeats) begin, asymmetric dextral looping of the primitive heart ensues. This process precedes the transformation of the single heart tube into a four-chamber heart (Ford & Watanabe, 2025). Growth at the cranial and caudal ends of the primitive heart tube encourages stretching or elongation of the tube. Concurrently, the dorsal mesocardium bends ventrally and to the right; this process is known as *cardiac looping* (dextro- or D-looping; **Figure 5.3**). Looping enables the initial positioning of the primitive heart, formation and alignment of cardiac chambers, development of accurate septation, alignment of the outflow tracts, and valvular morphogenesis (Robbins & Arruda, 2025). Once cardiac looping is complete, the primitive circulatory pattern is established.

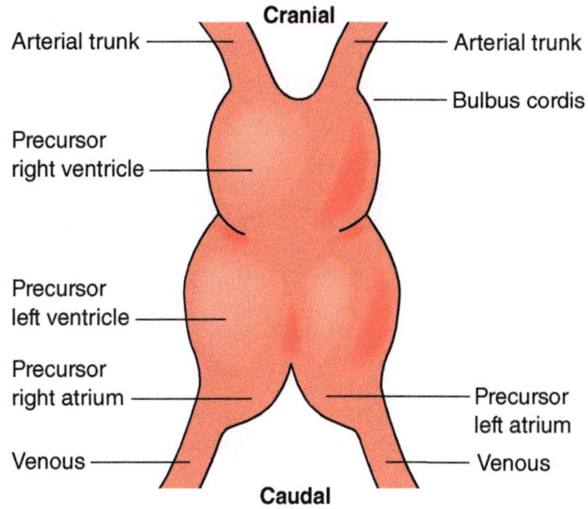

Figure 5.2 The primordial heart tube.

Clinical Application. Conotruncal defects are a specific group of CHDs that occur from abnormal migration of cardiac neural crest cells. This impairs normal elongation of the outflow tract and leads to abnormal primordial heart tube formation and septation, as well as cardiac looping. For example, defective arterial septation leads to truncus arteriosus and defective arterial rotation leads to transposition of the great vessels. The table that follows synthesizes common conotruncal defects, rotation, and clinical "pearls" to be aware of. Clinicians must be prepared to obtain a chest radiograph and arterial blood gas, and establish IV access for a prostaglandin E (PGE) infusion, while awaiting an echocardiogram (gold standard

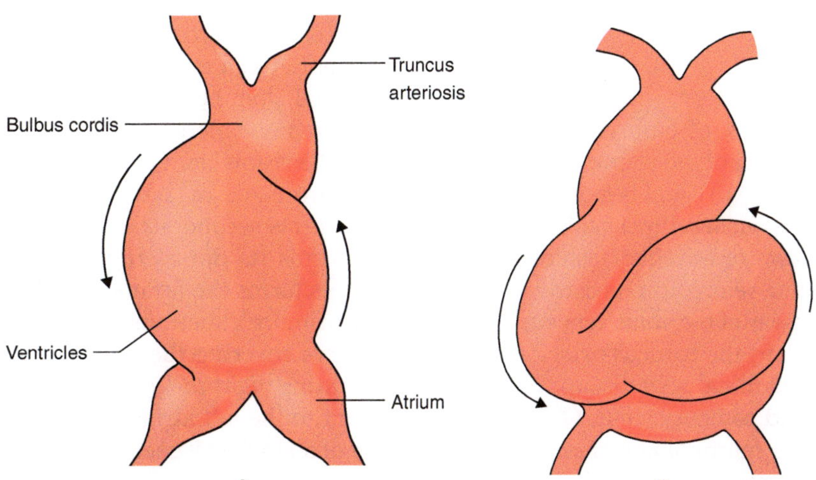

Figure 5.3 Cardiac looping. (**A**) Initial phase of cardiac looping. Note that the right side of the heart rotates in a leftward direction, while the left side of the heart twists in a rightward direction. (**B**) Continued cardiac looping. Note that the ventricles begin to take shape at the caudal end of the tube (ventral plane), while the atria form at the cranial end of the tube (dorsal plane).

diagnostic test). Hyperthermia and apnea are the two most common side effects of PGE exposure.

Conotruncal Defect	Degree of OFT Rotation	Clinical Presentation	PGE Infusion Needed
Transposition of the great arteries	Absent	Cyanosis	Yes for PBF
Double outlet right ventricle	Absent to incomplete	Cyanosis depends on location of VSD	No
Truncus arteriosus	Incomplete	Cyanosis	No
Tetralogy of Fallot with or without pulmonary atresia	Incomplete	Cyanosis depends on degree of pulmonary OFT obstruction	Yes for PBF
Pulmonary atresia with or without ventricular septal defect	Incomplete	Cyanosis	Yes for PBF
Interrupted aortic arch type B	Excessive	Signs of shock	Yes for SBF

OFT, outflow tract; PBF, pulmonary blood flow; PGE, prostaglandin E; SBF, systemic blood flow; VSD, ventricular septal defect.

Source: Data from Houyel, L., & Meilhac, S. M. (2021). Heart development and congenital structural heart defects. *Annual Review of Genomics and Human Genetics, 22*(1), 257–284. https://doi.org/10.1146/annurev-genom-083118-015012

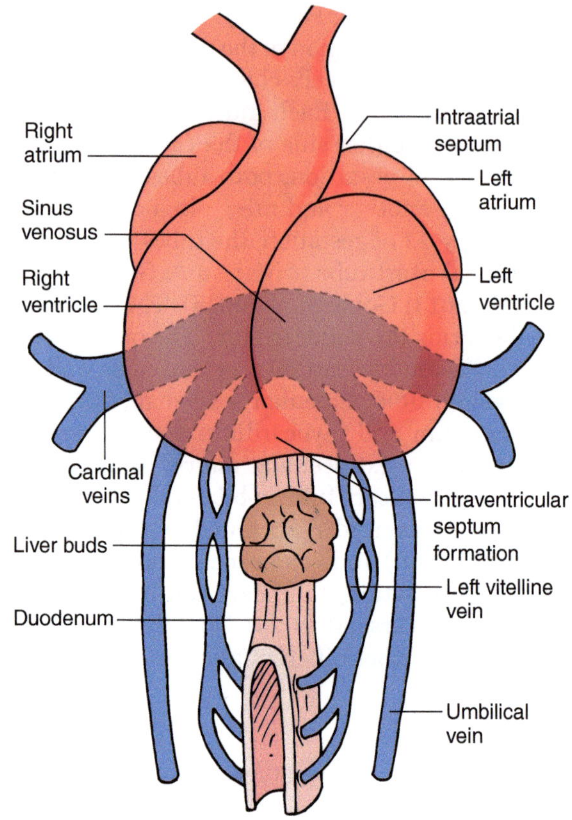

Figure 5.4 Chamber formation.

Chamber Formation

Around the middle of week 4 of embryonic development, septation or partitioning of the primitive ventricle, atrium, and atrioventricular (AV) canal begins. Throughout this process, the heart is remarkably capable of pumping blood in an ebb and flow (or wavelike) fashion. Blood is received from the vitelline vein, common cardinal vein, and the umbilical vein by way of the sinus venosus which is propelled cranially toward the truncus arteriosus. By week 10 of gestation, the cardinal vein disappears, leaving only the left atrium and coronary sinus. Quickly, the primitive heart undergoes morphologic changes (dilations) along its anteroposterior axis, facilitating unidirectional blood flow through the evolving heart chambers. The right and left ventricles emerge simultaneously, partitioned by the AV canal (AVC; Figure 5.4).

Atrial Partitioning. Toward the end of week 4 of gestation, the endocardium proliferates, producing dorsal and ventral bulges in the wall of the AV aperture. These bulges are invaded by mesenchymal cells, causing inward proliferation of the endocardial cushions. During week 5 of gestation, the endocardial cushions approach each other and fuse, dividing the atrium and ventricle into two separate cavities (van den Hoff & Wessels, 2022). Simultaneously, a rapidly proliferating muscular ridge grows from the intraventricular septum toward the base of the heart, and the intraatrial septum grows toward the fused endocardial cushions. This proliferation works to constrict and eventually close a foramen left between the atrial chambers, known as the *foramen primum*. A new foramen emerges as the foramen primum closes toward the cranial end of the intraatrial septum. A fold of atrial myocardium (*septum secundum*) begins migrating toward this second atrial foramen (*foramen secundum*) and forms its dorsal roof. This series of morphologic changes forms the foramen ovale (Figure 5.5). The septum primum functions as a type of membranous flutter valve covering the dorsal end of the *foramen ovale*, permitting *right-to-left* shunting of blood from the right atrium to the left atrium, throughout fetal development (van den Hoff & Wessels, 2022).

Ventricular Partitioning. Consider that the stem (caudal end) of the formerly Y-shaped primitive heart tube served as the primary site for the ventricular cavity. As

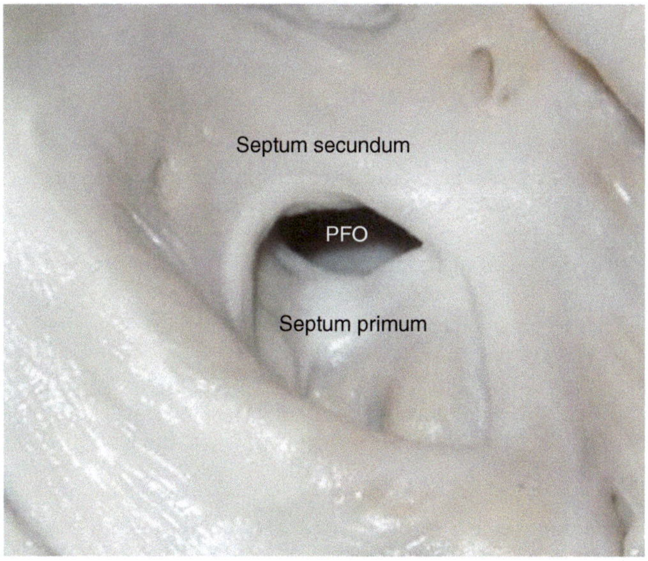

Figure 5.5 Patent foramen ovale (PFO). The caudal membranous septum primum approaches the cranial muscular septum secundum, thereby closing the PFO. The PFO accounts for up to 95% of all right-to-left shunts.
Source: Meier, B., Frank, B., Wahl, A., & Diener, H. C. (2012). Secondary stroke prevention: Patent foramen ovale, aortic plaque, and carotid stenosis. *European Heart Journal, 33*(6), 705–713. https://doi.org/10.1093/eurheartj/ehr443

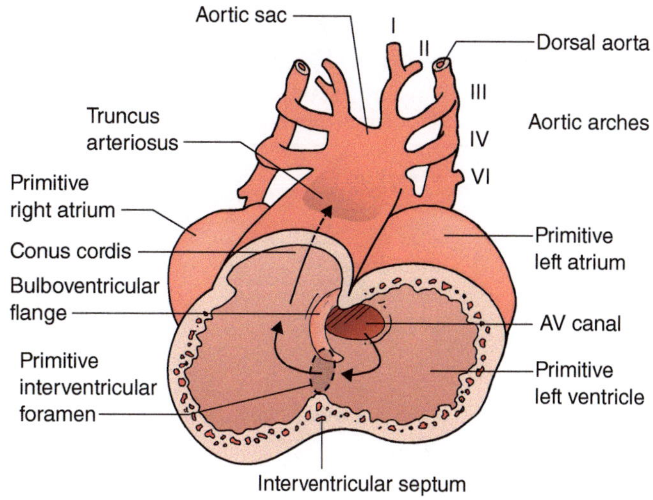

Figure 5.6 Ventricular bulging and partitioning. AV, atrioventricular.

mentioned previously, blood entered this cavity and traveled cranially toward the outflow tract. This changes during the fourth week of gestation, when looping begins and the early ventricular cavity shifts to the right of midline. Next, the ventricular cavity is pulled to a midline position, and bulging occurs at the point of D-looping. Bulging gives rise to each ventricle. The left ventricle arises to the left of the intraventricular groove, whereas the right ventricle, or bulbar cordis region, arises to the right of the interventricular foramen (Figure 5.6). In its primitive form, the conjoined left and right ventricles share a communication channel with the primitive truncus arteriosus (van den Hoff & Wessels, 2022).

Formation of the Aortic Arches

During week 4 of gestation, the superior end of the primitive truncus arteriosus gives rise to the aortic arches. Aortic arches I and II regress, whereas III, IV, and VI go on to form functional anatomic structures. However, if the right dorsal arch persists instead of the left, a right-sided aortic arch results. If the right dorsal aorta involutes proximal to the seventh intersegmented artery, an aberrant right subclavian artery results. If both dorsal aortae persist, a double aortic arch results.

Between weeks 6 and 8 of gestational development, the aortic arches are transformed into the adult arterial arrangement of the carotid, subclavian, and pulmonary arteries. A summary of the aortic arches and their primary function during embryogenesis is provided in Table 5.1. (See also Figure 5.7.)

Partitioning of the Truncus Arteriosus

Beginning during week 4 of gestation, a miraculous spiraling process occurs that bifurcates the truncus arteriosus and gives rise to the pulmonary artery (PA) and aorta. What once was a one-directional, single caudocranial heart tube becomes a bifurcated tunnel, capable of funneling deoxygenated blood to the lungs (PA) and oxygenated blood back to the heart and out to the body (aorta). Spiraling begins with the formation of tissue ridges at the cranial end of the truncus arteriosus. The ridges matriculate into endocardial tissue and complete a 180-degree spiral down the truncus arteriosus toward the superior end of the intraventricular septum. Fusion of the ridges results in formation of the *aortic-pulmonary septum*, which bifurcates the truncus arteriosus into two separate pathways (Figure 5.8).

If mesenchymal tissue fails to properly deposit on endocardial cushions during this period of cardiac development, a partial or complete failure of fusion of the AV canal can occur. A complete lack of septation allows blood to mix between all four chambers of the heart and results in one abnormal common AV valve. A partial defect typically has both a tricuspid and mitral valve (although usually less competent) and a cleft between either the atria or ventricles (CDC, 2023c).

DEVELOPMENTAL PHYSIOLOGY

Even in its most immature, primitive form, the heart supplies other developing body systems with enough blood flow to nourish growing tissues. Several events are required for the initiation of blood flow. The formation of the initial vascular network, blood vessel endothelial lumen development, initiation of heart contractions, and entry of red blood cells (erythrocytes) into the circulation are major events (Jones, 2011). The maturation of cardiac muscle cells, ion channels, and action

TABLE 5.1 Embryologic Timeline and Function of the Aortic Arches

Aortic Arches (Pairs)	Week of Gestation When Structure Appears	Regression	Function
I	4 (early)	Yes	Give rise to the maxillary artery; contributes to formation of external carotid artery.
II	4 (midweek)	Yes	Give rise to stapedial and hyoid arteries.
III	4 (end of week)	No	Give rise to common carotid and proximal portions of internal carotid arteries.
IV	4 (end of week)	No	Right side: Proximal portion of right subclavian artery. Left side: Persists as arch of aorta, giving rise to the left subclavian artery.
V	5 (early)	Yes	Rudimentary vessels; no derivatives; does not develop in 50% of embryos.
VI	5 (midweek)	Partial	Give rise to right and left pulmonary arteries. Right side: Complete regression after formation of right pulmonary artery. Left side: Proximal portion persists as proximal segment of left pulmonary artery; distal portion paired with dorsal aorta to form *ductus arteriosus*. After birth, functional closure of ductus arteriosus leaves *ligamentum arteriosum*.

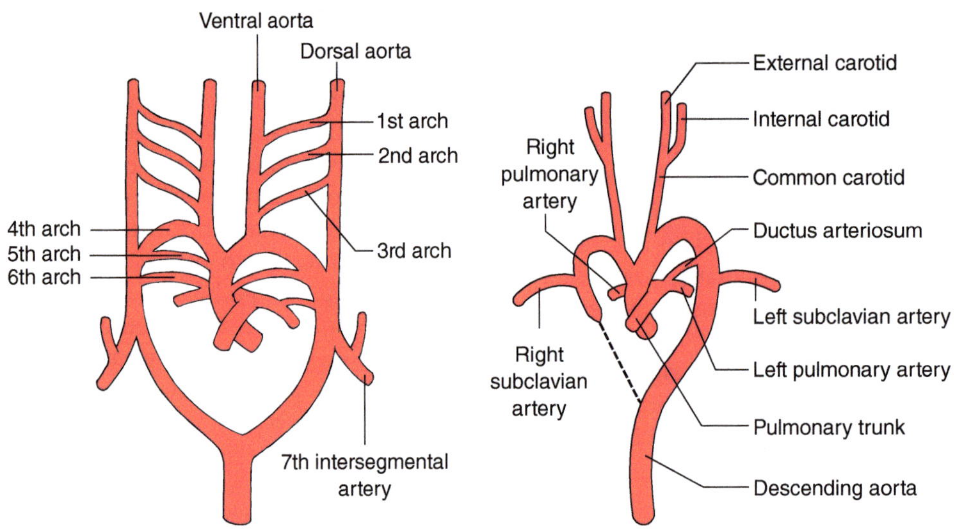

Figure 5.7 The aortic arches.

potentials occurs in cadence, which enables the heart to mature into a competent organ capable of generating the necessary stroke volume (SV) and cardiac output (CO) to support life outside the womb. This section of the textbook begins with a review of the core principles of cardiovascular function.

Cardiac Muscle Tissue

The cardiac conduction system develops from the myocardium and transforms into a specialized electrical wiring network responsible for initiating and coordinating the heartbeat (Jongbloed et al., 2012). In that sense, it is important to recognize the major role of the myocardium with regard to cardiac conduction. We begin with a focused review of the anatomy of the cardiac muscle cell, or cardiomyocyte. This is followed by a review of noteworthy ion channels and exchanges. These conversations are an appropriate predecessor to a later investigation into the cardiomyopathies. Next, we will review action potentials and associated relevant ion channels.

Cardiac Muscle Cells. *Cardiomyocytes* are muscle cells located within the heart. These cells are covered by a thin cytoskeleton of sarcoplasmic reticulum (the sarco-

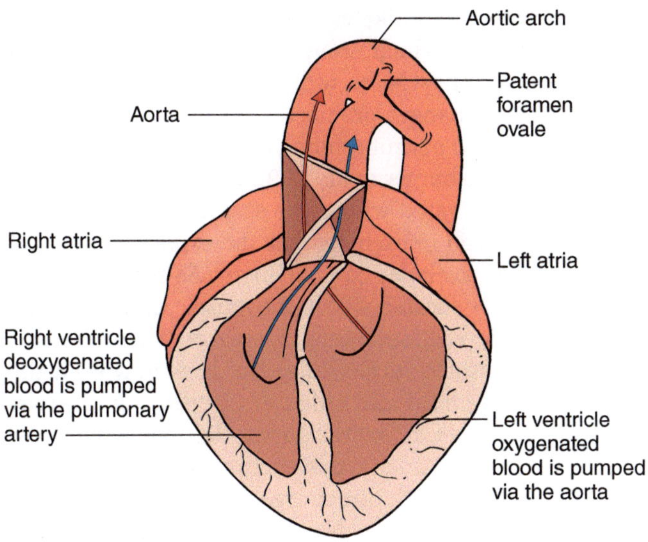

Figure 5.8 Partitioning of the truncus arteriosus.

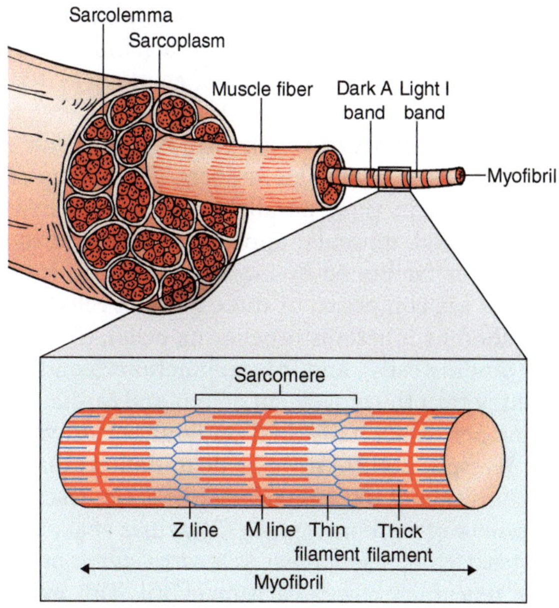

Figure 5.9 The myofibril.

Note: The I-band contains the thin filaments. The A-band marks the center area of overlap between the thin and thick filaments. The Z-line denotes the attachment zone of two neighboring sarcomeres. Thin filaments attach to each side of the Z-line.

lemma). This cytoskeleton offers structural support as well as a means for mechanical and chemical signaling within and between cardiomyocytes. The interior of the cardiomyocyte is comprised of *sarcomeres*, repeating and interconnected functional units of striated muscle (Figure 5.9). Sarcomeres are comprised of actin (thin) and myosin (thick) filaments, which yield the striated appearance of these cardiac muscle cells. The actin filaments contain regulatory proteins, namely cardiac troponins and α-tropomyosin, which regulate the interaction between the contractile proteins (actin and myosin) that enable depolarization. The myosin filaments contain myosin-binding proteins (van den Hoff & Wessels, 2022).

Clinical Application. Cardiac biomarkers, such as troponins and brain natriuretic peptides (BNPs), are commonly used for clinical decision-making in the adult population. Cardiac troponins are regulatory proteins that mediate the interaction between actin and myosin. This is important in order to ensure adequate depolarization (contraction) and repolarization (relaxation). Normally, troponin is found within the cells and is barely detectable in the bloodstream (0.02 ng/mL or less). Elevated levels of cardiac troponins are generally indicative of myocardial injury (e.g., secondary to intrapartum asphyxia), and a 10-fold increase (0.2 ng/mL) in circulating troponin might be observed (Bohn et al., 2021).

BNP are hormones that are triggered when the ventricles experience "stress" (e.g., pressure overload or volume expansion). The prohormone, proBNP, is released in response to ventricular stress, which leads to the splitting of the active hormone, BNP, and the inactive N-terminal fragment (NT-proBNP). Both BNP and NT-proBNP levels are elevated in the setting of cardiac disease due to myocardial stress and volume overload. However, other clinical pathologies affecting blood volume may cause increased levels as well (e.g., anemia, sepsis, renal dysfunction; Novack & Zubair, 2025).

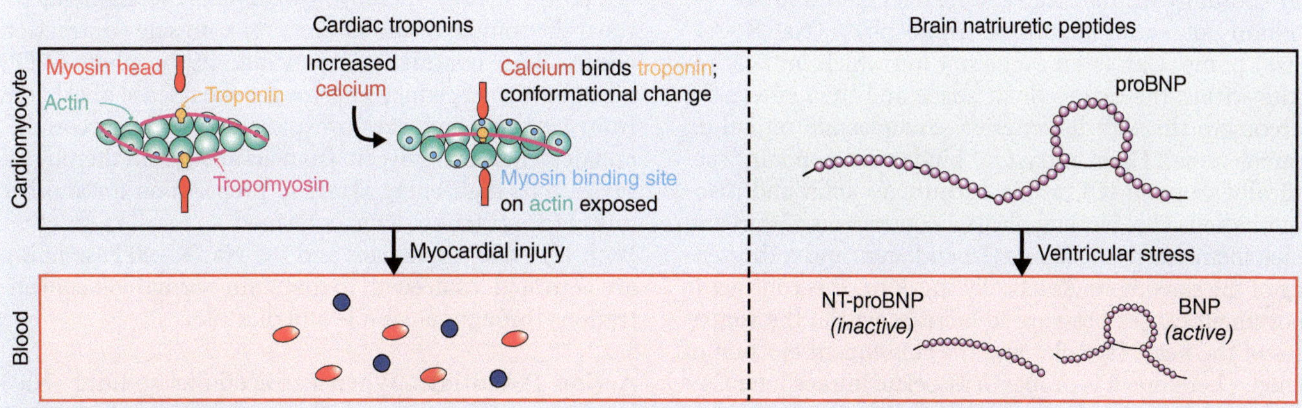

The healthy human heart contains more than two to three billion cardiomyocytes. Within each individual cardiomyocyte are repeating chains of as many as 10,000 3-micrometer-long sarcomeres. These sarcomeres form end-to-end attachments, which yield *myofibrils* or contractile threads of myofilament fibers. The arrangement of these fibers, in their parallel orientation, gives the heart its striated, muscular appearance. The end-to-end attachment is facilitated by *intercalated disks*. Intercalated disks are comprised of three types of cells, known as (a) adherens junctions (anchoring cells), (b) desmosomes (binding cells), and (c) gap junctions (conducting cells that permit the movement of ions and cardiac depolarization across the individual cardiomyocytes; van den Hoff & Wessels, 2022). Any genetic mutations that alter the composition of the intercalated disks can lead to the development of cardiomyopathy (Martinez et al., 2022).

A cytoskeleton, also known as a *sarcolemma* or *sarcoplasmic reticulum*, covers each myofibril. This cytoskeleton is comprised of numerous filaments, which directly influence both mechanical and chemical signaling that occurs within heart muscle. A discussion of each type of filament is beyond the scope of this chapter; however, a few influential filaments will be summarized. Desmin is one filament located at the Z-line. Desmin links adjacent Z-lines of sarcomeres to one another. In addition, γ-actin, another noteworthy microfilament, links sarcomeres to costameres. *Costameres* are the perpendicularly oriented structural components that connect myofibrils to the sarcolemma at the Z-line and within the I-Band and transmit force. In that manner, costameres serve a mechanical role by transducing force from one myofibril to another, mainly in a perpendicular direction. To a lesser extent, costameres transduce force longitudinally across sarcomeres until the end of a myofibril is reached. Therefore, genetic mutations that alter the proteins that comprise costameres increase the likelihood of altered mechanical signaling and the development of cardiomyopathy (Martinez et al., 2022; Peter et al., 2011).

Cardiac Electrophysiology

Ion Channels. Chemical signaling between cardiomyocytes, also known as *excitation-contraction coupling*, occurs by way of three ion channels: (a) Ca^{2+}-ATPase pump, (b) sodium-calcium (Na^{+}-Ca^{2+}) exchanger, and the (c) sodium-potassium-adenosine triphosphate (Na^{+}-K^{+}-ATPase) pump. Ca^{2+} is an excitatory ion which initially resides within the extracellular space and then enters the sarcomere through its exterior sarcoplasmic reticulum (sarcolemma). Upon entry, Ca^{2+} binds with troponin (specifically, troponin-C), which encourages actin and myosin binding. This binding elicits a contraction of thin and thick filaments at the Z-line (I-band area) and a shortening of the sarcomere. Practically speaking, this contractile movement causes pressure to increase within the ventricles of the heart (systole) and the subsequent ejection of blood. Therefore, it is proper to associate intracellular Ca^{2+} levels and the strength of calcium binding with contractile force during systole. Likewise, appropriate levels of ATP and tropomyosin, which unbind Ca^{2+} from troponin and relax the heart muscle, as well as sodium ions through the Na^{+}-Ca^{2+} exchanger, are necessary to lower Ca^{2+} levels during diastole to permit refilling of the ventricles (Eisner et al., 2017; Strasburger et al., 2022). When the Na^{+}- Ca^{2+} exchanger is activated within the sarcolemma, three Na^{+} ions enter the cell in exchange for the export of one Ca^{2+} back to the extracellular compartment. As such, intracellular Na^{+} (or Na^{+} located within the muscle, skin, subcutaneous tissue, or red blood cells) increases. Therefore, any preexisting, elevated intracellular Na^{+} level may limit the efficacy of this pump and efflux of Ca^{2+} during diastole. This may increase Ca^{2+} sparks during diastole, which over time can lead to contractile dysfunction or a cardiomyopathy (Ottolia et al., 2013; Strasburger et al., 2022).

Last, let's consider the Na^{+}-K^{+}-ATPase pump. Recall that electrochemical forces normally push K^{+} into the extracellular space and Na^{+} into the intracellular compartment during resting conditions. Action potentials exaggerate this process. In order to maintain normal intracellular concentrations of Na^{+} and K^{+}, the Na^{+}-K^{+}-ATPase pump is utilized. Similar to the aforementioned ion channels, this pump is also located within the sarcolemma. When the Na^{+}-K^{+}-ATPase pump is activated, three Na^{+} ions are removed from the cell and pushed to the extracellular compartment, while two K^{+} ions are pushed into the cell. Therefore, infants subject to potassium losses secondary to diuretic therapy (i.e., aldosterone antagonists) may exhibit reduced Na^{+}-K^{+}-ATPase pump activity. On the contrary, infants receiving angiotensin-converting enzyme (ACE) inhibitors may exhibit increased Na^{+}-K^{+}-ATPase pump activity and resultant biochemical imbalances, which negatively affect cardiovascular function. Clearly, a functional disturbance of these ion channels could explain arrhythmias commonly observed with cardiomyopathies, primarily a dilated cardiomyopathy (DCM).

In summary, all components needed for muscle contraction are contained within the sarcomere. Once a muscle is excited by a neuron, calcium (Ca^{2+}) is released from the sarcoplasmic reticulum. Calcium binds with troponin at the I-band. This causes the sarcomere to shorten, which likewise shortens the I-band. A high-energy attachment occurs between actin and myosin proteins. The end result is a power stroke, whereby myosin pulls the filaments toward the middle of the sarcomere; a muscle contraction occurs. After contraction, adenosine triphosphate (ATP) binds to myosin, which encourages the release of calcium from troponin, relaxation/expansion of the sarcomere, and detachment of myosin from actin. Myosin thereby returns to its high-energy state in preparation for another muscle contraction. This is termed a *cross-bridge cycle*. Both Na^{+}/ Ca^{2+} exchanges and the Na^{+}-K^{+}-ATPase pump are activated, as needed, to maintain normal ion concentrations throughout systole and diastole.

Action Potentials. When extracellular sodium (Na^{+}) levels are within a normal range (approximately 135–145 mEq/L) and intracellular K^+ levels are within a normal range (approximately 3.5–5 mEq/L), the voltage within the atrial and ventricular myocytes (intracellular voltage), as well as Purkinje fibers, is considered to be at equilibrium, at approximately -90 millivolts (mV). A cardiac action potential occurs when the intracellular voltage becomes less negative (changes from -90 mV to +10 mV), causing ion fluctuations (chemical and electrical potentials) across channels in the sarcolemma of the cardiomyocyte and, ultimately, atrial-to-ventricular contraction. Chemical potentials explain the movement of an ion across its selective concentration gradient. Electrical potentials explain the movement of ions away from those with a similar electrical charge. This process is best described as a series of five phases.

The action potential begins with *phase 0* within the sarcolemma, or sarcoplasmic reticulum. Cell membrane permeability to potassium decreases, and sodium channels open. This causes the intracellular voltage to become less negative (i.e., -90 mV to +10 mV), which elicits rapid cellular depolarization. Fast Na^+ channels open, permitting the influx of Na^+ into the cell. Once the voltage increases from -90 mV to -40 mV, calcium (Ca^{2+}) channels open, and a small amount of Ca^{2+} travels across its concentration gradient. Once the voltage reaches 0 mV, the time-dependent, fast Na^+ channels close. *Phase 1* marks a state of partial repolarization, secondary to the closure of the sodium ion channels, a subsequent decrease in sodium ion exchanges across the cell membrane, and a temporary reversal of voltage change back toward the negative. This also causes the voltage to change from a negative to a positive charge to approximately +10 to +30 mV (Strasburger et al., 2022). As a result, K^+ channels open, and K^+ is permitted to leave the cell. As extracellular K^+ levels increase, the intracellular voltage decreases in a negative direction. This drives the voltage back to approximately 0 mV. This marks the beginning of *Phase 2*—a plateau phase. Ca^{2+} and K^+ continue to enter and leave the cell, respectively, yet in a balanced state (electrical potential). The voltage is maintained close to 0 mV. Thereafter, a period of repolarization occurs. *Phase 3* marks this period of repolarization. Ca^{2+} channels close while K^+ continues to exit the cell. This creates an imbalanced exchange of ions and drives the voltage in a negative direction, back toward its resting state of -90 mV. In order to prevent excessive ionic shifts, which could occur during phase 3, three ion pumps (which will be further described later in this chapter) are activated. These are the Na^+-Ca^{2+} exchanger, Ca^{2+}-ATPase, and Na^+-K^+-ATPase pump. *Phase 4* thereby begins with this resting state, as ion pumps and exchangers are closed while a slow, persistent leak of K^+ out of the cell occurs. This helps maintain the voltage of -90 mV as the cell waits for the next stimulus (action potential; Figure 5.10).

Cardiac Conduction Pathways

The three main components of the cardiac conduction system are (a) the sinoatrial (SA) node, (b) the AV node, and (c) the bundle of His (Figure 5.11). These three major parts work collaboratively as the electrical switchboard that modulates the movement of action potentials and coordination of ventricular contractions (Strasburger et al., 2022). In order to recognize and understand the genesis of abnormal electrical conduction, one must understand the anatomic arrangement of the conduction system in a healthy heart. Therefore, this section of the chapter reviews the normal transmission of electrical currents from the SA node to the AV node and His–Purkinje system.

Sinoatrial Node. In the early developing heart, the atrium and ventricle muscle layers are continuous. The primordial pacemaker is initially located in the caudal portion of the left heart tube. After development of the sinus venosus myocardium, which occurs during week 5 of development, the SA node is recognizable as a tadpole-shaped structure. The “head” of the SA node is located at the border of the superior caval vein and the right atrium, and the “tail” is located along the terminal crest (Jongbloed et al., 2012; Strasburger et al., 2022).

Once mature, the SA node functions as the pacemaker for the heart. Cardiac action potential is initiated here and follows a pathway ending in contraction of heart muscle (also known as a heartbeat). Current research supports that the electrical activity initiated in the SA node results from the expression of ion channels, gap junction proteins responsible for electrical coupling between myocytes, and calcium-handling proteins (Strasburger et al., 2022).

Atrioventricular Node. Cells from the left wall of the sinus venosus are incorporated into the interatrial septum; these cells are combined with cells from the AVC region, forming the AV node and the bundle of His. The AV node is located at the right side of the base of the atrial septum in the triangle of Koch, superior to the tricuspid valve, and acts as the electrical bridge from the atria to the ventricles.

The AV node innervates the ventricular septum. It permits a frequency-dependent delay or refractory period in the cardiac action potential (initiated at the SA node). This normal delay allows atrial systole to take place and permits complete filling of the ventricles prior to ventricular systole. This highly coordinated series of events offers protection from atrial tachycardia by limiting the number of action potentials sent from the SA node to the AV node (ventricles; Jongbloed et al., 2012; Strasburger et al., 2022). In some cases, the SA node may fail to initiate an electrical impulse. In these circumstances, the AV node can take over as a secondary pacemaker, although the pacemaker activity of the AV node is slower than the SA node (Hund et al., 2014; Strasburger et al., 2022). Maturation of the AV node continues into early childhood.

His–Purkinje System. The bundle of His is comprised of right and left bundle branches and the

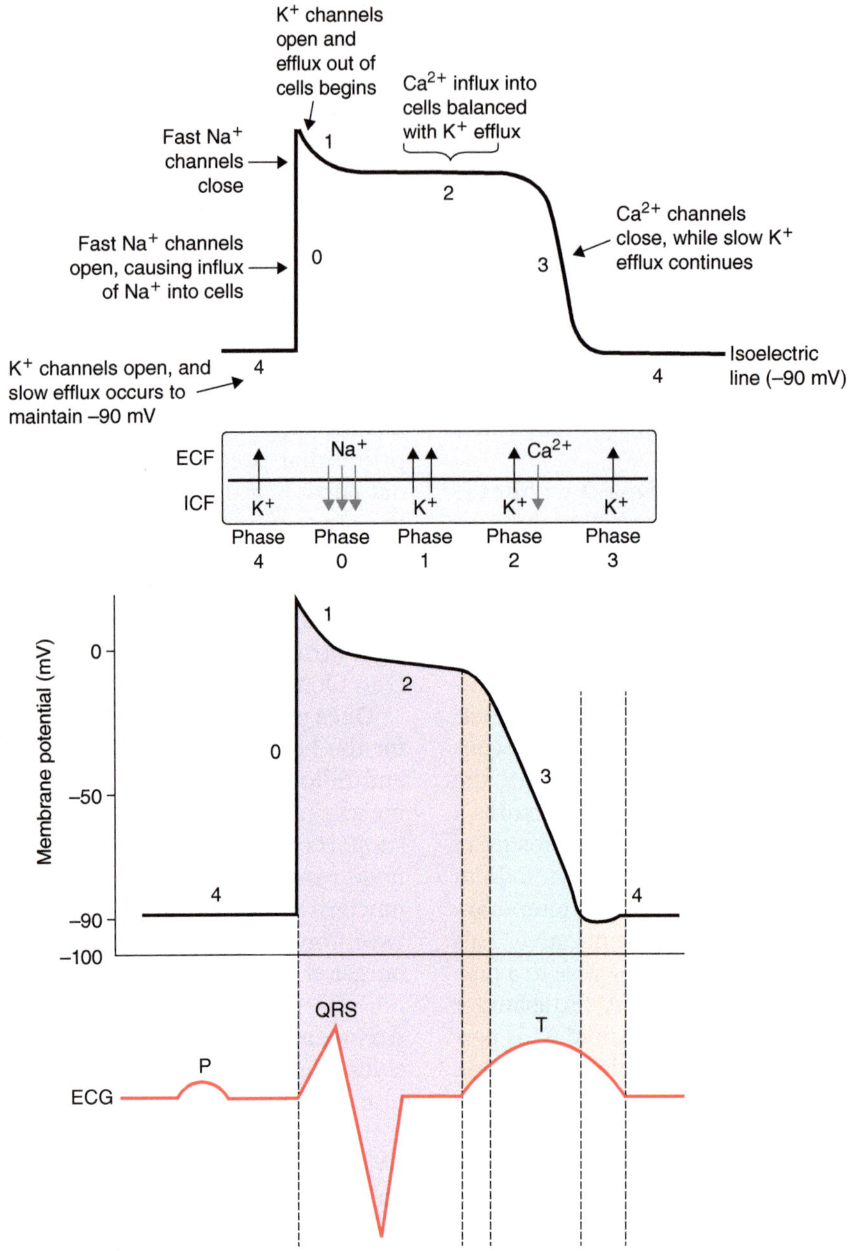

Figure 5.10 Typical action potential of a ventricular myocyte with associated ion currents.

Note: This figure is limited to a visual depiction of the status of electrical conduction during the ventricular action potential. During this time, the atria are refilling. More broadly, learners should recognize that the P wave reflects the start of the cardiac action potential cycle and atrial depolarization (not depicted here). Isoelectric conduction occurs as the action potential moves from the SA node to the AV node. The QRS interval reflects the time needed for ventricular depolarization (depicted here; phases 0–2), and the QT interval represents the time needed for ventricular repolarization (depicted here; phases 3–4).

AV, atrioventricular; ECF, extracellular fluid; ICF, intracellular fluid; SA, sinoatrial; TMP, transmembrane potential.

Purkinje fibers; this network is commonly referred to as the His–Purkinje system. An electrical impulse from the AV node continues down the thin myocardial fibers arising from a common bundle (the bundle of His) located on top of the ventricular septum. In contrast to the SA and AV nodes, the His–Purkinje system is derived from working cardiomyocytes that differentiate early in gestation (Strasburger et al., 2022). The fibers of the bundle split into right and left bundle branches that are distributed throughout the ventricular myocardium. The bundle branches terminate into the Purkinje fibers, a complex network of cardiac muscle cells extending from the bundle branches that are specialized for conduction and are responsible for synchronous activation of the ventricular myocardium to ensure that the ventricular muscles simultaneously contract (Jongbloed et al., 2012). In the event of heart block, the His–Purkinje system acts as a secondary ventricular pacemaker, once again at an even slower and less robust rate (Strasburger et al., 2022).

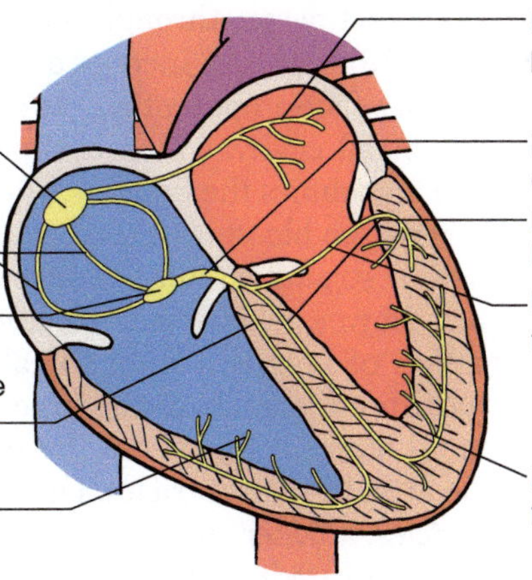

Figure 5.11 The conduction system. The SA node is the pacemaker that initiates electrical activity. The electrical activity is then transmitted to the AV node and onto the His–Purkinje system. The end result is a ventricular contraction (heartbeat).
AV, atrioventricular; SA, sinoatrial.

Indeed, alterations in the normal development of the heart may increase the risk of disturbed electrical conduction. For infants, this may range from benign occurrences, such as isolated premature atrial contractions, to life-threatening rhythms, including supraventricular tachycardia (SVT) or atrial fibrillation (Table 5.2). This aberrant electrical activity may be the result of fluid and electrolyte imbalances or malpositioned central venous catheters, a risk associated with prematurity and critical illness.

TABLE 5.2 Cardiac Conduction System Abnormalities

Electrical Conduction Abnormality	Clinical Significance
SA node dysfunction or "sick sinus syndrome"	• Sinus bradycardia • Sinus arrest/sinus pause • Sinus node exit block • Alternating atrial bradyarrhythmias/tachyarrhythmias
AV node dysfunction	• AV node reentrant tachycardia (e.g., type of SVT) • Atrial fibrillation • Heart block (first, second, and third degree)
His–Purkinje system dysfunction	• Bundle branch reentry ventricular tachycardia • Bundle branch block • Fascicular tachycardia • Torsade de pointes arrhythmia • Ventricular tachycardia

AV, atrioventricular; SA, sinoatrial; SVT, supraventricular tachycardia.

Primordial Cardiovascular Physiology

In the human embryo, the presence of primordial cardiac contractions has been detected as early as week 5 of gestation at an average rate of 100 beats per minute (BPM). This heartbeat increases as fetal development progresses (Hagen-Ansert & Guthrie, 2023; van den Hoff & Wessels, 2022). Cardiac systolic and diastolic function, blood flow, SV, and CO also increase over time. This early function is essential to normal structural cardiovascular development; alterations in these processes will lead to abnormal functional or structural defects. It is important to understand the differences between fetal blood flow patterns and postnatal circulation. Neonatal APRNs are often challenged to identify and stabilize infants with CHD during the peripartum period, in particular, those that depend upon ductal patency.

The Embryonic Period. While anatomic development begins during week 2 of gestation, physiologic function begins between weeks 5 and 6 of gestation. This begins on approximately day 23 of gestation, as a series of "ebb and flow" peristaltic movements, and over time changes to a one-directional blood flow (Acharya et al., 2016; Ford & Watanabe, 2025). Recall that three major paired veins communicate with the primitive heart during the embryonic period and supply the heart with blood flow. These veins are the (a) two umbilical veins, (b) vitelline veins, and (c) common cardinal veins. They drain blood into the heart through the sinus venosus, a cavity that communicates with the primitive atrial cavity. A brief digression to review pertinent anatomy is an appropriate predecessor to a review of primordial blood flow.

Two umbilical veins deliver oxygenated blood from the chorionic villi to the sinus venosus and into the heart. However, shortly after primitive blood flow begins, the right umbilical vein becomes obliterated, atrophies, and disappears. The left umbilical vein anastomoses with the ductus venosus in the liver, enabling incoming blood from the placenta to proceed directly to the heart without traversing the vascular networks of the liver. This facilitates the "first pass" effect observed when medications ingested by the XX pregnant patient cross the placenta and enter the fetal circulation, only to bypass the metabolic center (liver) and travel directly to the heart and onto the systemic circulation.

Deoxygenated blood (from the peripheral tissues) enters the sinus venosus through the vitelline veins and cardinal veins. By approximately week 6 of gestation, the vitelline veins (and duct) regress, leaving the paired cardinal veins to continue transporting venous return from the periphery back to the sinus venosus and into the heart. As the heart matures, the left cardinal vein and leftmost portion of the sinus venosus form the coronary sinus. The coronary sinus receives venous return from the coronary system. The right cardinal vein and the rightmost portion of the sinus venosus merge and form the superior vena cava (SVC). The SVC receives venous return from the head, neck, arms, and chest. By week 8 of gestation, the SVC drains blood as in the adult. A summary of the embryonic function of the primitive vessels and their final adult structure is provided in Table 5.3.

Recall that as blood enters the sinus venosus, the blood flows through the primordial heart in an "ebb and flow" peristaltic pattern. Blood flows forward, down the vessels, during systole and flows backward, up the vessels, during diastole. As cardiac looping ensues, the atria assume the role of interim pacemaker, and the early function of the conduction system can be appreciated. Thereafter, the sinus venosus takes on a dual role of blood reservoir and pacemaker; increasingly coordinated conduction and blood flow patterns are observed. However, since smooth muscles within the sinus venosus have not differentiated, the myocardium cannot dynamically regulate the diameter of vessel lumens to maintain equilibrium.

Let's consider the pattern of blood flow through the primordial heart once the primitive conduction system is established. As blood passes through the sinus venosus, it enters the atrial cavity. An increased propagation of electrical impulses (action potentials) is observed as blood enters this atrial cavity, which encourages conduction velocity. This mimics the function of the mature SA node. From here, the blood is pushed to the AVC, a region comprised of strong, circular connective fibers, yet a significantly slower conduction velocity. This delays the conduction of impulses from the atria to the ventricular myocardium, similar to the function of the mature AV node. Likewise, this slows the conduction velocity from the atria to the ventricles. Once the blood reaches the ventricles, a faster electrical impulse propagation is observed. This mimics the function of the mature His–Purkinje system. In fact, during embryologic development, cardiomyocytes within the ventricles are rapidly differentiating to offer optimal contractility, electrical conduction (ion channel maturation), and energy metabolism. This prepares the ventricles for the role of primary pumping chamber. Contractions within the ventricles move the blood into the conotruncal region (outflow tract) and out to the body.

TABLE 5.3 Blood Vessels' Embryonic Function and Final Mature Structure

Vein	Primitive Function	Final Adult Structure
Right vitelline vein	Returns poorly oxygenated blood from the umbilical vein	Terminal part of the inferior vena cava
Left vitelline vein	Returns poorly oxygenated blood from the umbilical vein	Regresses
Right anterior *and* common cardinal veins	Drainage system	Superior vena cava
Left common cardinal vein	Drainage system	Tributary of the coronary sinus
Right umbilical vein	Carries oxygenated blood from the chorionic sac (placenta) to the sinus venosus (embryo)	Regresses
Left umbilical vein	Carries oxygenated blood from the chorionic sac (placenta) to the sinus venosus (embryo)	Ligamentum venosum

The Fetal Period. The fetal period of development marks the maturation of the conduction system, which is generally reported as fully mature by week 12 of gestation. Action potentials predictably arise within the SA node and travel to the AV node and His–Purkinje system. This elicits a pattern of serial, rapid atrial and ventricular contractions that facilitate blood flow through the heart. At this point, the electrocardiogram begins to resemble that of a mature heart (Acharya et al., 2016; Boulgakoff et al., 2024).

The following content incorporates content from Chapters 2 and 4 and offers readers an intentional spiraling of core curricular concepts. Here, we describe the parallel cardiovascular circuits present during fetal development. Essentially, the right and left ventricles supply the fetal organ systems through combined ventricular output. This differs from postnatal and adult function due to structural (anatomic) differences as well as mechanisms by which the fetus increases CO.

The fetal circulation is characterized by two parallel circuits that permit the mixing of oxygenated and deoxygenated blood at the atrial and great vessel levels via three intracardiac and extracardiac shunts. These shunts, which allow fetal survival despite the presence of a complex CHD, include the ductus arteriosus (extracardiac), foramen ovale (intracardiac), and ductus venosus (extracardiac). Blood flow is influenced by the high-resistance pulmonary circuit and the low-resistance systemic circuit.

Recall that during fetal development, the placenta serves as the major site for the exchange of oxygen, carbon dioxide, nutrients, and waste materials with the placenta receiving approximately 40% of fetal CO (Goldsmith, 2025). The two umbilical arteries bring the fetal blood to the placenta. This blood circulates through the capillaries of the chorionic villi, where gas exchange takes place. Blood rich in oxygen and nutrients leaves the placenta, returning via a single umbilical vein to the fetus. This blood traverses the portal circulation; an average of 30% to 70% of blood bypasses the portal veins and is shunted across the ductus venosus and to the inferior vena cava (Strainic, 2025). Normally, flow across the ductus venosus is phasic and anterograde (forward flowing); abnormal flow patterns may suggest possible fetal stress as the fetus attempts to ensure oxygenation of the heart and the brain (Braga et al., 2019; Kiserud, 2005).

The oxygenated blood traveling via the inferior vena cava enters the right atrium, where it is divided into two streams by the crista dividens; the majority of flow travels across the foramen ovale and into the left atrium, where it mixes with blood returning from the pulmonary venous system. This oxygen-rich blood passes through the mitral valve, enters the left ventricle, and is thereby pumped out of the ascending aorta and toward the developing brain and upper extremities (Figure 5.12). Normally, flow across the aortic isthmus is both systolic and diastolic as well as anterograde; retrograde flow reflects fetal distress and is a mechanism for preserving cerebral perfusion (F. T. Lee et al., 2021). The remainder of the blood flow moves down the descending aorta (systemic circulation); delivers oxygen to the systemic circulation, becoming progressively deoxygenated in the process; and then enters either of two umbilical arteries that branch from the internal iliac arteries in order to return to the placenta (Figure 5.11). This poorly oxygenated blood (now highly saturated with carbon dioxide) travels back to the placenta for disposal (see Chapter 2, Haldane & Bohr effect).

Deoxygenated blood from the IVC and hepatic vein mix with venous return from the SVC (Dyer & Ikemba, 2012). This mixed blood is directed toward the tricuspid valve and right ventricle. Blood flowing to the right ventricle enters the pulmonary trunk, with 90% to 95%

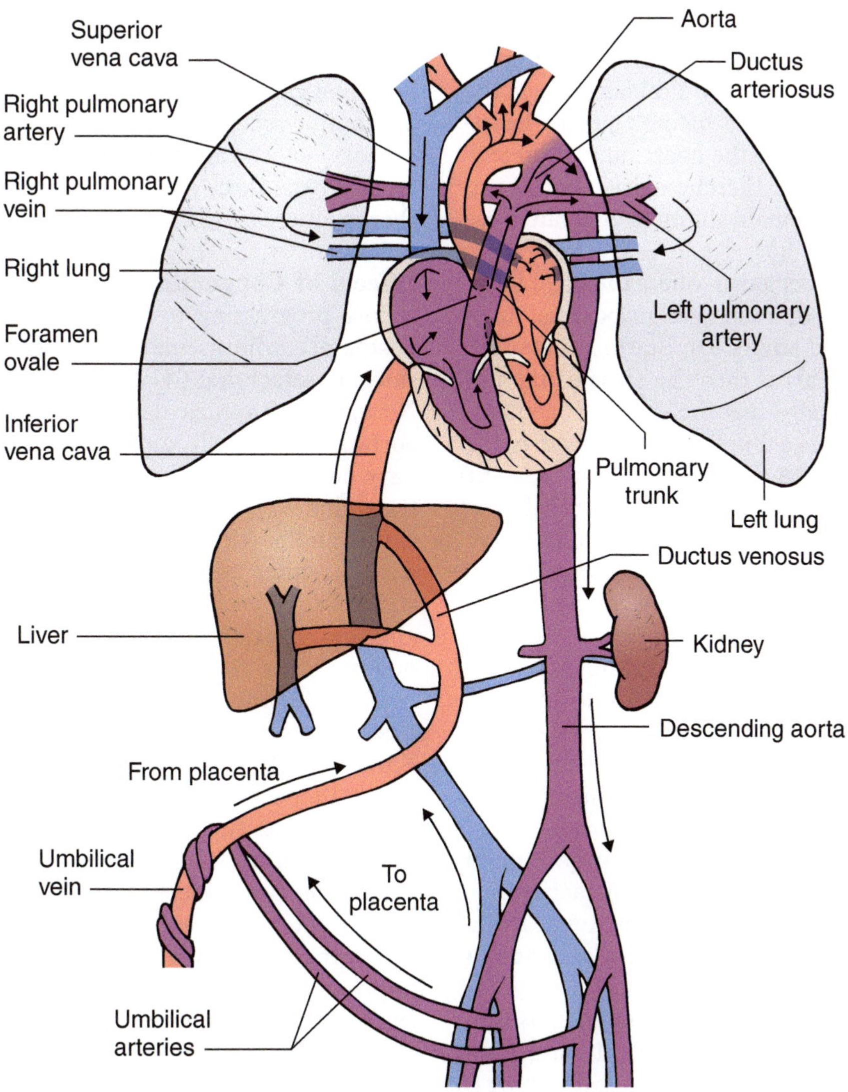

Figure 5.12 Fetal circulation.

shunted across the patent ductus arteriosus (PDA), thereby bypassing the pulmonary circulation; this is due to high pulmonary vascular resistance (PVR; Goldsmith, 2025). The ductus arteriosus is a wide, muscular vessel connecting the pulmonary arterial trunk to the descending aorta; the ductus is approximately the same size as the PA and the descending aorta in the fetus. Blood flow shunted across the PDA goes out the descending aorta to the systemic circulation and then returns to the placenta.

Fetal Cardiovascular Physiology

Fetal cardiovascular physiology involves the coordinated activities of two parallel circuits. Essentially, the right and left ventricles supply the fetal organ systems through combined ventricular output. This differs from postnatal and adult function due to structural (anatomic) differences as well as mechanisms by which the fetus increases CO.

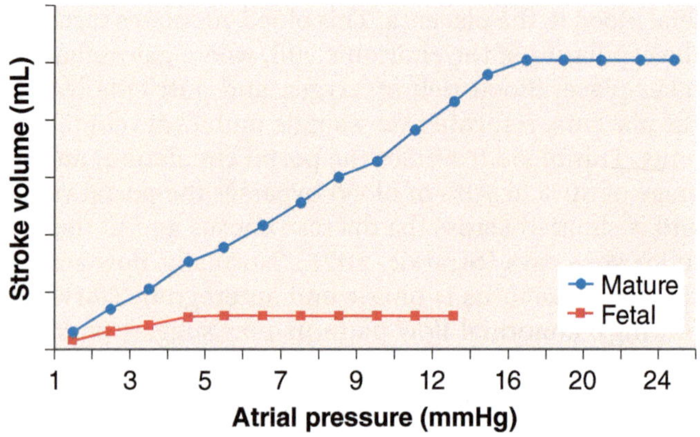

Figure 5.13 Frank–Starling mechanism (fetal vs. adult stroke volume capacity). Fetal stroke volume has little response despite increasing atrial pressure, unlike the adult, which rapidly increases following the Frank–Starling law. *Source:* Adapted from Rychik, J. (2004). Fetal cardiovascular physiology. *Pediatric Cardiology, 25*(3), 201-209. https://doi.org/10.1007/s00246-003-0586-0

Myocardial Function. Recall that CO equals the heart rate multiplied by the SV (HR × SV = CO). SV is the amount of blood squeezed from the heart with each heartbeat, and this volume is contingent upon preload, afterload, and cardiac contractility. Preload reflects the amount of blood in the ventricles before ("pre") a heartbeat. Afterload is the pressure the heart must overcome *after* filling to contract and thereby eject blood. Last, contractility is the heart's innate ability to generate force to contract.

The Frank–Starling mechanism offers the ideal foundation for distinguishing differences in myocardial function between fetuses and adults. Dr. Starling stated (in 1915), "the law of the heart is thus the same as the law of muscular tissue generally, that the energy of contraction, however measured, is a function of the length of the muscle fibre" (Starling, 1918, p. 43). In other words, the increase in pressure within the atria or ventricles during filling (preload) causes heart muscle fibers to lengthen. This lengthening is associated with an increase in the force of contraction (SV), increase in atrial or ventricular output, and increase in venous pressure.

While the Frank–Starling mechanism holds true in adults, the fetus has a narrower capacity to increase SV in the face of increased preload. In fact, the fetus typically reaches a peak SV of 4 to 5 mmHg compared to adults, who may compensate by increasing SV to 16 to 18 mmHg in the face of increased preload (Figure 5.13; Han et al., 2022). Several factors may explain this functional immaturity. Decreased contractile proteins within the myocardium, inefficient myocardial calcium uptake, as well as limited passive ventricular filling capacity during diastole help explain why the fetus is seemingly incapable of modulating increases in CO in light of increasing atrial pressure. In addition, spatial constraints imposed by nearby organs (lungs) may limit the heart's ability to contract effectively. Last, cholinergic nerves derived from the vagus nerve (not adrenergic receptors) primarily drive changes in the fetal heart rate. Therefore, the heart rate changes based on vagal stimuli. Later in infancy and adulthood, adrenergic receptors (specifically, beta-1-adrenergic receptors) exert a meaningful effect on the heart by increasing the force and rate of myocardial contraction, thereby increasing CO.

Effects of Congenital Heart Defects on the Fetus. Before progressing to a discussion of transitional and postnatal cardiovascular physiology, it is prudent to consider the effect that CHDs exert on the developing fetus. Normally, left ventricular output traverses the ascending aorta and primarily supplies the head and brain, coronary circulation, and upper extremities. Blood exiting the pulmonary vessels passes through the ductus arteriosus and aortic isthmus and through the descending aorta in order to supply the lower extremities. Certain structural defects derange this flow pattern, which may alter oxygenation to various organs as well as alter venous pressure (Strainic, 2025).

Consider the implications with pulmonary atresia (PA), tricuspid atresia, and tetralogy of Fallot (TOF). These structural defects alter blood flow patterns in utero. Blood flow through the PA is obliterated or reduced, and as such, blood is primarily diverted across the foramen ovale and into the left ventricle. Left ventricular output is increased, which, over time, stretches the diameter of the ascending aorta and aortic isthmus. In contrast, hypoplastic left heart syndrome (HLHS) imposes an increased workload on the right heart. Right ventricular pressure increases as this ventricle assumes full responsibility for providing ventricular output. Blood flows through the PA to the engorged pulmonary vasculature, ductus arteriosus, and across the aortic isthmus; little (if any) flow is ejected from the left heart. Retrograde flow patterns across the aortic isthmus are required to redirect output to the brain, coronary circulation, and upper extremities (Strainic, 2025).

Although the fetus can compensate for aberrant structural development in utero, prolonged intrauterine cardiopulmonary compensation, in combination with removal of the placental circuit, can provoke rapid postnatal decompensation. An understanding of normal transitional cardiovascular physiology is essential to develop fluency in linking fetal cardiovascular physiology and postnatal manifestations of CHDs.

Transitional Cardiovascular Physiology at Birth

The cardiac and pulmonary systems undergo drastic changes at birth in response to respirations and loss of the placenta, from parallel circuits to one circuit that operates in series. The abrupt cessation of placental blood flow leads to an accumulation of carbon dioxide and a decrease in oxygen saturation, which stimulates the onset of postnatal breathing. The first postnatal breath inflates the lungs and increases partial pressures of oxygen in the arterial blood (PaO_2). This modulates the postnatal decrease in PVR and a more than 20-fold increase in pulmonary blood flow and reversal of the left-to-right shunting across the PDA (Estévez & Ansah, 2024). At this time, 90% of blood flow is redirected to the lungs and the lungs assume the primary role of gas exchange. In addition, the release of vasodilators and endothelial-derived releasing factors occurs, further decreasing PVR and aiding in the redirection of blood flow through the pulmonary circuit.

Closure of the Fetal Shunts. Postnatal cardiovascular function does not depend on fetal shunts. In fact, these shunts must functionally close during the immediate postnatal period in order for the cardiopulmonary circuit to properly transition to extrauterine life; permanent anatomic closure can occur later without inducing pathologic problems. To summarize this key concept, functional closure of the intracardiac and extracardiac shunts precedes anatomic closure. On occasion, shunts may functionally close and later reopen; shunts have the ability to intermittently close and reopen before anatomic closure occurs. This may result in transient, functional, and, occasionally, hemodynamically significant murmurs, which are more common among premature infants.

As placental circulation ceases, there is a drop in pressure within the inferior vena cava and right atrium. Pulmonary venous return increases, and left atrial pressure exceeds right atrial pressure. These changes lead to the functional closure of the foramen ovale (Strainic, 2025). On the contrary, a patent foramen ovale (PFO) may persist among neonates with pulmonary stenosis or other defects associated with increased right atrial pressure. Permanent anatomic closure of the foramen ovale is typically achieved by 2.5 years of age.

Among term infants, functional closure of the PDA is usually noted within the first 3 to 4 days after birth (Benitz & Bhombal, 2025). Closure occurs as a result of increasing arterial oxygenation saturations amid decreasing PVR, as well as decreased responsiveness to naturally synthesized prostaglandins (see Chapter 4). In fact, functional closure occurs in approximately 50% of term infants by 24 hours of life and 90% by 48 hours of life (Clyman et al., 2012). Respiratory distress syndrome, septicemia, excessive fluid administration, furosemide therapy, phototherapy, and prematurity encourage delayed functional closure of the PDA. Anatomic closure is typically noted by 2 to 3 months of life; the PDA remnant is labeled the *ligamentum arteriosum* (Benitz & Bhombal, 2025; Clyman et al., 2012).

Within the first minute of life, umbilical blood flow drops to less than 20% of fetal values. During this time, the diameter of the umbilical arteries and veins decreases significantly. This leads to functional closure of the umbilical vessels. Fibrous proliferation occurs within 2 to 3 months, which completely obliterates both vessels.

Next, functional closure of the ductus venosus occurs shortly after birth. This occurs once the parallel circuitry disappears; blood flow from the placenta through the umbilical vein and ductus venosus ceases. Anatomic closure is completed by 2 months of age. The remnant of the ductus venosus is thereby labeled the *ligamentum venosum*. Spasms with prompt closure of the ductus venosus can be particularly problematic when postnatal umbilical venous access is necessary, especially in cases of CHD that require IV prostaglandin administration to maintain ductal integrity. Prompt closure may prevent cannulation with umbilical venous catheters.

Clinical Application. It is important to maintain awareness of when functional closure of the PDA occurs. Many well newborns are discharged home before the ductus arteriosus closes. Although rare (0.2%), a critical congenital heart defect (CCHD) that is dependent upon a PDA for either systemic or pulmonary blood flow is life-threatening and requires urgent intervention (American Academy of Pediatrics [AAP], 2024). Screening using pulse oximetry monitoring can pick up lower oxygen saturations associated with ductal-dependent CCHDs. Screening should be done after 24 hours of life to reduce the likelihood of false positive results (0.06%; AAP, 2025; Sneeringer et al., 2022). Other considerations, like high altitude, may impact CCHD screening, leading to false positives and the need for repeat testing. The AAP suggests areas with high elevation may need to modify the recommended algorithm to account for this factor. A recent study of infants at an elevation greater than 6,000 feet found that reducing the CCHD screen pass threshold from ≥95% to ≥93% significantly increased the number of infants passing their first CCHD screen (p<.001) and safely reduced false positive screenings (Sneeringer et al., 2022).

Postnatal Cardiovascular Physiology

Postnatal Blood Flow. Here, we offer intentional cycling of curriculum from Chapter 4, with a particular focus on blood flow patterns after birth. After birth, blood flows in series through the heart and lungs as an organized pattern of flow distinctly different from the parallel pattern observed during fetal development. Deoxygenated blood from the lower body and upper body is returned to the heart via the inferior vena cava and SVC. Blood enters the right atrium and is directed through the trileaflet tricuspid valve and into the right ventricle. From the right ventricle, blood flows through the trileaflet semilunar pulmonary valve and into the main PA. The main PA thereby splits into the right and left pulmonary arteries and blood is diverted to either side for oxygenation within either lung.

Oxygenated blood leaves the lungs by way of four pulmonary veins. These four pulmonary veins innervate with the left atrium. Blood thereby flows from the left atrium, through the bileaflet mitral valve, and into the left ventricle, the cavity solely responsible for generating postnatal CO. The left ventricle thrusts the blood through the aortic valve, where some of the CO enters the ascending aorta and is distributed through the three branches of the aorta and to the brain; the remaining CO is diverted in a downward direction through the descending aorta and to the distal organs and tissues.

Postnatal Cardiovascular Function. The normal postnatal decrease in pulmonary arterial pressure, in combination with the expected rise in systemic arterial pressure, exerts a major impact on myocardial function (Bensley et al., 2016). Similar to fetal myocardial function, ventricular preload and afterload, myocardial contractility, and heart rate all influence CO after birth and across the life span. The major difference between fetal and postnatal myocardial function is the ability to increase CO with increasing atrial pressures (preload).

Ventricular Preload. Recall that ventricular preload is a measure of end-diastolic volume in the neonate and is influenced by many factors, including circulating blood volume, myocardial relaxation and compliance, contractility, and afterload (Noori et al., 2022). After birth, left ventricular filling and SV improve once PVR decreases below systemic vascular resistance (SVR). In addition, increased end-diastolic pressure leads to increased myocardial fiber length and improved contractility. This results in increased SV and a resultant increase in CO.

Ventricular Afterload. Recall that ventricular afterload is the myocardial force that pumps blood out of the ventricles during the ejection period (Noori et al., 2022). It is inversely proportional to contractility and, as such, as afterload increases, contractility decreases. The normal postnatal fall in PVR causes a decrease in right ventricular afterload. Over time, right ventricular end-diastolic pressures decrease as ventricular filling is optimized. The end result is improved cardiac compliance and ventricular ejection (Artman et al., 2017).

Myocardial Contractility. Myocardial contractility is dependent on the force of the cardiac contraction, preload, inotropy, and afterload. It is immature among fetuses and neonates; reduced cellular and structural organization and decreased compliance are noted, leaving the heart less responsive to volume demands. The lack of noncontractile proteins leaves the myocardium stiff and less compliant, with little reserve to increase contractility. Therefore, in order to increase CO, the heart rate increases (Artman et al., 2017; Hines, 2013; Noori et al., 2022).

Immediately after birth, clamping of the umbilical cord removes the low resistance placenta, and SVR increases. This abrupt increase in SVR can stress the immature myocardium and lead to transient dysfunction, which manifests as (transient) tricuspid regurgitation. The result is decreased left ventricular CO and reduced systemic blood flow. The resultant low systemic blood flow usually resolves within 24 to 36 hours after birth (Noori et al., 2022). In addition, decreased myocardial contractility may be observed in the presence of acidosis, hypercarbia, and hypoxia. These conditions alter cellular permeability and the effectiveness of the sodium–potassium (Na^+-K^+) pump.

Heart Rate. With maturation of the parasympathetic system, resting heart rate in the neonate decreases. Any event that provokes catecholamine release, parasympathetic stimulation, or parasympathetic withdrawal will manifest with tachycardia. In the preterm infant, tachycardia is related to sympathetic nervous system control of cardiac function.

GENETIC INFLUENCES

Genetic (syndromic) and environmental influences are capable of altering structural and functional development of the heart. Although 80% of CHDs are not associated with genetic syndromes and occur sporadically, the remaining 20% of cases are positively associated with Mendelian and chromosomal syndromes and can manifest with CCHDs (Chung et al., 2012; Miller et al., 2011). Changes in chromosome number (aneuploidy), or rearrangement of chromosomal material from one chromosome to another (translocation), or loss of chromosomal material (deletions) may be at fault for altering embryonic development of the heart. Here, we present common chromosomal aneuploidy, associations, and sporadic genetic malformations that involve aberrant heart development or function. In addition, a summary of rare single gene disorders, which involve the formation of common CHDs, are summarized in Table 5.4.

Chromosomal Aneuploidy Influences

Chromosomal aneuploidy was the first reported genetic basis for syndromic CHDs and currently accounts for the largest percentage of identifiable, syndromic CHDs (Kosiv et al., 2023; Williams et al., 2019). The most common aneuploidy disorders with associated CHDs include trisomy 13, 18, and 21, as well as Turner syndrome (Table 5.5; Bouma & Mulder, 2017).

Trisomy 13. Trisomy 13 (Patau syndrome) results from a translocation of genetic material, resulting in the presence of three copies of chromosome 13 in each cell in the body. It affects an estimated one in 16,000 live births (National Organization for Rare Disorders [NORD], 2007). Nearly 80% of infants with trisomy 13 have three complete copies of chromosome 13. Less than 3% of fetuses affected by trisomy 13 survive to term; the majority of affected pregnancies result in spontaneous abortion or stillbirth (Senartne et al., 2024). Complex CHDs are noted in 25% to 100% of live-born neonates; hallmark defects include conotruncal defects, septal defects, and valvular anomalies (Kosiv et al., 2023; Williams et al., 2019).

Trisomy 18. Trisomy 18 (Edwards syndrome) commonly results from a translocation of genetic material, causing three copies of chromosome 18 in each cell in the body. Nearly 95% of infants with trisomy 18 have three complete copies of chromosome 18, and 5% are affected by a mosaicism (partial trisomy) of most of the long arm of chromosome 18 (National Organization for Rare Disorders, 2024). The incidence of Edwards syndrome is one in 5,000 live births; a female prevalence is reported (H. Chen, 2012; National Institutes of Health [NIH], 2021b). CHD is noted in up to 26% to 100% of live-born neonates with this chromosomal disorder; hallmark defects include septal and polyvalvular dysplasia (Kosiv et al., 2023; Williams et al., 2019).

Trisomy 21. Trisomy 21 (Down syndrome) commonly results from placement of three copies of chromosome 21 on each cell; the majority (94%) of infants with trisomy 21 have three complete copies of chromosome 21, whereas 2% may present with mosaicism (Haldeman-Englert et al., 2018). This syndrome affects one in 700 births; an increased incidence, estimated at one in 25 to 300 births, is reported among pregnant patients over the age of 35 years of age (NIH, 2020; Torchia & Persaud, 2025). Approximately 23% to 58% of infants with trisomy 21 are affected by a CHD; hallmark defects include AV and ventricular septal defects (VSDs). AV defects are more common among females and those of Caucasian race (Kosiv et al., 2023; Williams et al., 2019).

TABLE 5.4 Single-Gene Mutation Syndromes Associated With Congenital Heart Defects

Gene Mutation Syndromes	Common Associated Congenital Heart Defects
Noonan syndrome (AD)	• Septal defects (e.g., ASD) • **Valvular anomalies** (e.g., PS) • Cardiomyopathy
Alagille syndrome (AD)	• Right-sided heart defects (e.g., peripheral or valvular pulmonary stenosis, TOF) • Coarctation of the aorta
Holt–Oram syndrome (AD)	• **Septal defects** (e.g., ASD, VSD) • **PDA** • **Left ventricular outflow tract defects** (e.g., HLHS) • Atrioventricular conduction delays
CHARGE syndrome (AD)	• Conotruncal defects (e.g., TOF, DORV) • Aortic arch anomalies
Smith–Lemli–Opitz syndrome (AR)	• **Septal defects** (e.g., ASD, VSD) • **Left ventricular outflow tract defects** (i.e., HLHS) • PDA

Note: Defects in bold type denote common CHD associations reported in the literature.

AD, autosomal dominant; AR, autosomal recessive; ASD, atrial septal defect; CHD, congenital heart defect; DORV, double outlet right ventricle; HLHS, hypoplastic left heart syndrome; PDA, patent ductus arteriosus; PS, pulmonary stenosis; TOF, tetralogy of Fallot; VSD, ventricular septal defect.

Sources: Chung, W., Boskovski, M. T., Brueckner, M., Anyane-Yeboa, K., & Gupta, P. (2012). The genetics of fetal and neonatal cardiovascular disease. In C. S. Kleinman & I. Seri (Eds.), *Hemodynamics and cardiology: Neonatology questions and controversies* (2nd ed., pp. 343–376). Elsevier Saunders; Corrigan, N., Brazil, D., & McAuliffe, F. (2009). Fetal cardiac effects of maternal hyperglycemia during pregnancy. *Birth Defects Research (Part A): Clinical and Molecular Teratology, 85*, 523–530. https://doi.org/10.1002/bdra.20567; Ornoy, A., Reece, E., Pavlinkova, G., Kappen, C., & Miller, R. (2015). Effect of maternal diabetes on the embryo, fetus, and children: Congenital anomalies, genetic and epigenetic changes and developmental outcomes. *Birth Defects Research. Part C, Embryo Today, 105*(1), 53–72. https://doi.org/10.1002/bdrc.21090; Williams, K., Carson, J., & Lo, C. (2019). Genetics of congenital heart disease. *Biomolecules, 9(12)*, 879. https://doi.org/10.3390/biom9120879

TABLE 5.5 Chromosomal Aneuploidy Syndrome Associated With Congenital Heart Defects

Chromosomal Abnormality	Common Associated Congenital Heart Defects
Trisomy 13	• **Septal defects** (e.g., VSD, ASD) • Conotruncal defects (e.g., TOF, DORV) • PDA • Valvular anomalies
Trisomy 18	• Septal defects (e.g., VSD, ASD) • Conotruncal defects • Polyvalvular dysplasia
Trisomy 21	• **Septal defects** (e.g., VSD) • **Atrioventricular** (e.g., complete AVSD, partial AVSD) • Conotruncal defects (e.g., TOF, DORV) • PDA
Turner syndrome	• **Valvular anomalies** (e.g., bicuspid aortic valve, aortic stenosis, mitral valve defect) • **Coarctation of the aorta** • Left ventricular outflow tract defects (e.g., HLHS) • Aortic dissection

Note: Defects in bold type denote common CHD associations reported in the literature.

ASD, atrial septal defect; AVSD, atrioventricular septal defect; CHD, congenital heart defect; DORV, double outlet right ventricle; HLHS, hypoplastic left heart syndrome; PDA, patent ductus arteriosus; TOF, tetralogy of Fallot; VSD, ventricular septal defect.

Sources: Chung, W., Boskovski, M. T., Brueckner, M., Anyane-Yeboa, K., & Gupta, P. (2012). The genetics of fetal and neonatal cardiovascular disease. In C. S. Kleinman & I. Seri (Eds.), *Hemodynamics and cardiology: Neonatology questions and controversies* (2nd ed., pp. 343–376). Elsevier Saunders; Corrigan, N., Brazil, D., & McAuliffe, F. (2009). Fetal cardiac effects of maternal hyperglycemia during pregnancy. *Birth Defects Research (Part A): Clinical and Molecular Teratology, 85,* 523–530. https://doi.org/10.1002/bdra.20567; Ornoy, A., Reece, E., Pavlinkova, G., Kappen, C., & Miller, R. (2015). Effect of maternal diabetes on the embryo, fetus, and children: Congenital anomalies, genetic and epigenetic changes and developmental outcomes. *Birth Defects Research. Part C, Embryo Today, 105*(1), 53–72. https://doi.org/10.1002/bdrc.21090; Williams, K., Carson, J., & Lo, C. (2019). Genetics of congenital heart disease. *Biomolecules, 9(12),* 879. https://doi.org/10.3390/biom9120879

Turner Syndrome. Turner syndrome is a result of the loss of one X chromosome (most common) or structural abnormalities to one X chromosome (i.e., monosomy) affecting the normal course of development before and after birth only in females. A large number of affected fetuses spontaneously abort or are stillborn. Incidence in live-born neonates is about one per 2,000 (NIH, 2023b). CHDs are noted in about 38% of 45, XO live-born neonates. The most common associated CHDs involve left-sided cardiac structures; most notable are aortic arch and valve abnormalities (Williams et al., 2019).

Chromosomal Deletion Influences

Deletion of a small, discrete chromosomal region may yield a CHD. The most common deletion syndromes are 22q11.2 (DiGeorge), 11q23 (Jacobsen syndrome), or 7p11.23 microdeletion (Williams syndrome; Table 5.6).

TABLE 5.6 Chromosomal Deletion Syndromes Associated With Congenital Heart Defects

Chromosomal Deletion Syndromes	Common Associated Congenital Heart Defects
DiGeorge (22q11.2)	• **Conotruncal defects** (e.g., interrupted aortic arch type B, truncus arteriosus, TOF, TGA) • Septal defects (e.g., perimembranous VSD)
Jacobsen syndrome (11q23)	• Left ventricular outflow tract defects (e.g., **HLHS**) • Septal defects (e.g., VSD) • Coarctation of the aorta
Williams syndrome (7p11.23 microdeletion)	• Valvular anomalies (e.g., **supravalvular aortic stenosis,** supravalvular pulmonary stenosis) • **Peripheral pulmonary stenosis**

Note: Defects in bold type denote common CHD associations reported in the literature.

CHD, congenital heart disease; HLHS, hypoplastic left heart syndrome; TGA, transposition of the great arteries; TOF, tetralogy of Fallot; VSD, ventricular septal defect.

Sources: Chung, W., Boskovski, M. T., Brueckner, M., Anyane-Yeboa, K., & Gupta, P. (2012). The genetics of fetal and neonatal cardiovascular disease. In C. S. Kleinman & I. Seri (Eds.), *Hemodynamics and cardiology: Neonatology questions and controversies* (2nd ed., pp. 343–376). Elsevier Saunders; Corrigan, N., Brazil, D., & McAuliffe, F. (2009). Fetal cardiac effects of maternal hyperglycemia during pregnancy. *Birth Defects Research (Part A): Clinical and Molecular Teratology, 85,* 523–530. https://doi.org/10.1002/bdra.20567; Kosiv, K. A., Mercurio, M. R., & Carey, J. C. (2023). The common trisomy syndromes, their cardiac implications, and ethical considerations in care. *Current Opinion in Pediatrics, 35*(5), 531–537. https://doi.org/10.1097/MOP.0000000000001278; Ornoy, A., Reece, E., Pavlinkova, G., Kappen, C., & Miller, R. (2015). Effect of maternal diabetes on the embryo, fetus, and children: Congenital anomalies, genetic and epigenetic changes and developmental outcomes. *Birth Defects Research. Part C, Embryo Today, 105*(1), 53–72. https://doi.org/10.1002/bdrc.21090; Williams, K., Carson, J., & Lo, C. (2019). Genetics of congenital heart disease. *Biomolecules, 9(12),* 879. https://doi.org/10.3390/biom9120879

DiGeorge Syndrome. DiGeorge syndrome is the most frequent deletion syndrome and involves the loss of chromosomal material on the long arm of chromosome 22 (22q11.2). This syndrome affects one in every 4,000 live births (Goldmuntz, 2020). CHDs are noted in up to 80% of liveborn infants; conotruncal anomalies are the most commonly reported CHDs (Williams et al., 2019).

Jacobsen Syndrome. Jacobsen syndrome is a rare disorder characterized by deletions at the end of the long arm of chromosome 11 (11q23). Jacobsen syndrome occurs in approximately one in every 100,000 live-born neonates (NIH, 2023a). Normal function of 11q23 is critical for the development of the brain, face, and heart (Williams et al., 2019). VSD, left heart obstructive malformations, valvular defects, coarctation of the aorta, or HLHS are reported in up to 56% of all affected infants. The most common CHDs are VSD and left heart obstructive defects (Williams et al., 2019).

Williams Syndrome. Williams syndrome is a microdeletion syndrome involving the loss of genetic material from the short arm of chromosome 7. This syndrome affects roughly one in every 7,500 to 10,000 infants (NIH, 2022). The loss of the chromosomal material results in marked variability of clinical presentation, including facial, skeletal, renal, and heart anomalies. CHDs are reported in up to 82% of all affected infants; supravalvular aortic stenosis and pulmonary stenosis are the two most commonly reported CHDs (Williams et al., 2019).

Sporadic Malformation Syndromes

Many cardiac malformations occur as part of a constellation, or association, of defects. Two common associations that manifest with multiple anomalies are the VACTERL association and Beckwith–Wiedemann syndrome (BWS).

VACTERL Association. VACTERL association is a combination of multiple anomalies involving **V**ertebral defects, **A**nal atresia, **C**ongenital heart defects, **Tr**acheo**e**sophageal fistulas (TEF), **R**enal abnormalities, and **L**imb defects. The incidence has been estimated to be between one in 10,000 to 40,000 live births (NIH, 2011; NORD, 2020). The majority of cases occur sporadically (Brosens et al., 2013). Cardiac malformations are reported in approximately 40% to 80% of neonates affected by the VACTERL association (NORD, 2020). Commonly reported malformations range from clinically insignificant CHDs, including VSDs and atrial septal defects (ASDs), to clinically significant, complex congenital heart malformations requiring surgical interventions and continuing care across the life span (Brosens et al., 2013; Y. Chen et al., 2016; Cunningham et al., 2013; Solomon et al., 2014).

Beckwith–Wiedemann Syndrome. BWS is one of the most commonly described overgrowth disorders. BWS affects one in 10,500 to 13,700 infants (worldwide). Over time, these infants exhibit abnormally accelerated and often asymmetrical tissue growth (NIH, 2021a). Although classic manifestations include macroglossia and abdominal wall defects, cardiac anomalies are reported in approximately 20% of confirmed cases of BWS (Mussa et al., 2016). Hallmark manifestations include mild cardiomegaly, PDA, and PFO. Rare findings include long QT syndrome (Mussa et al., 2016; Shuman et al., 2016). Continuing care across the life span is indicated. Affected children are at risk for developing cancerous and noncancerous tumors, including hepatoblastoma, nephroblastoma (Wilms tumor), and pancreatoblastoma, which typically manifest during early to late childhood (Edmondson & Kalish, 2015).

NOTEWORTHY DISEASES IN THE XX PREGNANT PATIENT THAT INFLUENCE FETAL CARDIOVASCULAR DEVELOPMENT AND FUNCTION

Exposures of the pregnant patient to environmental toxins, such as pesticides, certain medications (sodium valproate, retinoic acid, lithium), or substances, including ethanol, cocaine, and other licit and illicit drugs, can exert a teratogenic effect on fetal cardiovascular development (Table 5.7; Bouma & Mulder, 2017; Fahed et al., 2013; Mone et al., 2004; Rolfo et al., 2020; Zeliger, 2023). Fetal myocytes are particularly vulnerable to injury among cocaine and alcohol exposed fetuses (Muralidharan et al., 2013; Yang et al., 2015; Zeliger, 2023).

Other influences associated with an increased risk of CHDs include advanced age at conception, viral infections during the first trimester of pregnancy (rubella, cytomegalovirus, coxsackie virus), a history of previous spontaneous abortions or stillbirths, diabetes, and other illness, such as systemic lupus erythematosus (SLE; Abqari et al., 2016; Bouma & Mulder, 2017; Gomersall et al., 2024; Yazigi et al., 2017).

Advanced Age at Conception

A 20% increased risk of CHD is conferred upon offspring born to XX pregnant patients 35 years of age or older, which defines advanced age at conception (or advanced maternal age). More specific, conotruncal defects, left ventricular outflow track obstructions, right ventricular outflow tract defects, AV septal defects (AVSDs), and VSDs are commonly associated with advanced age at conception and pregnancy (Miller et al., 2011).

Systemic Lupus Erythematosus in the Pregnant Patient

Presence of anti-Ro or anti-La antibodies resulting from SLE places the fetus at risk for heart block. There is

TABLE 5.7 Congenital Heart Defects Associated With Toxic In-Utero Exposures

Exposure	Common Associated Congenital Heart Defects
Rubella infection (in the pregnant patient)	• Septal defects (e.g., VSD, ASD) • **PDA** • Persistent pulmonary stenosis
Lupus (in the pregnant patient)	• **Heart block** • Cardiomyopathy
Diabetes mellitus (in the pregnant patient)	• Septal defects (e.g., VSD) • Conotruncal defects (e.g., TGA, TOF) • HLHS • Cardiomyopathy • Dextrocardia
Fetal alcohol exposure	• **Septal defects** (e.g., VSD, ASD) • PDA • Conotruncal defects
Fetal amphetamine exposure	• Septal defects (e.g., VSD, ASD) • PDA • TGA
Fetal cocaine exposure	• **Septal defects (e.g., VSD)** • Intracardiac conduction abnormalities
Fetal indomethacin exposure	• Premature closure of PDA
Fetal lithium exposure	• Septal defects (e.g., ASD) • **Ebstein anomaly** • RVOT • TA
Fetal progesterone exposure	• Septal defects (e.g., VSD) • Conotruncal defects (e.g., TGA, TOF)
Fetal hydantoin syndrome	• Septal defect • PDA • Valve stenosis
Fetal warfarin syndrome	• PDA • PPS

Note: Defects in bold type denote common CHD associations reported in the literature.

ASD, atrial septal defect; HLHS, hypoplastic left heart syndrome; PDA, patent ductus arteriosus; PPS, peripheral pulmonic stenosis; RVOT, right ventricular outflow tract; TA, truncus arteriosus; TGA, transposition of the great arteries; TOF, tetralogy of Fallot; VSD, ventricular septal defect.

Sources: Mone, S., Gillman, M., Miller, T., Herman, E., & Lipshultz, S. (2004). Effects of environmental exposures on the cardiovascular system: Prenatal period through adolescence. *Pediatrics, 113*(Suppl. 3), 1058–1069. http://pediatrics.aappublications.org/content/113/Supplement_3/1058..info; Patorno, E., Huybrechts, K. F., Bateman, B. T., Cohen, J. M., Desai, R. J., Mogun, H., Cohen, L. S., & Hernandez-Diaz, S. (2017). Lithium use in pregnancy and the risk of cardiac malformations. *New England Journal of Medicine, 376*(23), 2245–2254. https://doi.org/10.1056/NEJMoa1612222; Yazigi, A., De Pecoulas, A., Vauloup-Fellous, C., Grangeot-Keros, L., Ayoubi, J.-M., & Picone, O. (2017). Fetal and neonatal abnormalities due to congenital rubella syndrome: A review of literature. *Journal of Maternal-Fetal & Neonatal Medicine, 30*(3), 274–278. https://doi.org/10.3109/14767058.2016.1169526

transplacental passage of the antibodies associated with SLE, with resultant antibody and complement deposition in the fetal myocardium, leading to inflammation, calcification, necrosis, and fibrosis of the conducting tissue (Biron-Shental & Hershkovich-Shporen, 2025). Cardiovascular damage secondary to heart block is evident between 16 and 30 weeks of gestation, and as gestation advances, fetal conduction defects often worsen and increase the risk for hydrops fetalis and congestive heart failure (CHF; Mone et al., 2004; Society for Maternal-Fetal Medicine et al., 2023).

Diabetes Mellitus in the Pregnant Patient

Type 1 or type 2 diabetes mellitus before pregnancy (pregestational), with poorly controlled hyperglycemia before conception and during the first trimester, is associated with a fivefold higher risk for congenital cardiovascular malformations compared to the general population. Cardiac defects occur in roughly 8.5% of cases of pregestational diabetes, which is approximately tenfold higher than the incidence of CHDs in the general population (Corrigan et al., 2009; Ornoy et al., 2015). High glycosylated hemoglobin (HbA1c) levels and hyperglycemia during the critical early embryonic development periods appear teratogenic (Corrigan et al., 2009). Abnormal migration of cardiac neural crest cells occurs, leading to conotruncal malformations (Nakano et al., 2021). Additionally, interruption of secondary heart field cell proliferation may contribute to septal defects and malpositioning of the great vessels. The developing endocardial cushion cells are also highly sensitive to the effects of hyperglycemia. The most common CHDs associated with pregestational diabetes include AVC defects, dextro-transposition of the great arteries (D-TGA), aortic stenosis, PA, dextrocardia, and conotruncal defects (Ornoy et al., 2015). The fetal heart is also at risk for the development of hypertrophic cardiomyopathy (HCM), most commonly seen during the second and third trimesters. It has been suggested that hypertrophy results from fetal hyperinsulinism, leading to the proliferation and hypertrophy of cardiac myocytes triggered by increased proteins and fat synthesis. Hyperglycemia can also alter the embryonic epigenome and impact latent gene expression and regulation among offspring; a higher incidence of latent diabetes and cardiovascular disease is reported among exposed fetuses (Ornoy et al., 2015).

COMMON PROBLEMS WITH IMPLICATIONS ACROSS THE LIFE SPAN

Before beginning a conversation focused on the abnormal, it is always beneficial to establish a firm understanding of the normal. As such, Figure 5.14 provides a visual summary of normal heart anatomy and blood flow. This can be used to compare with the following

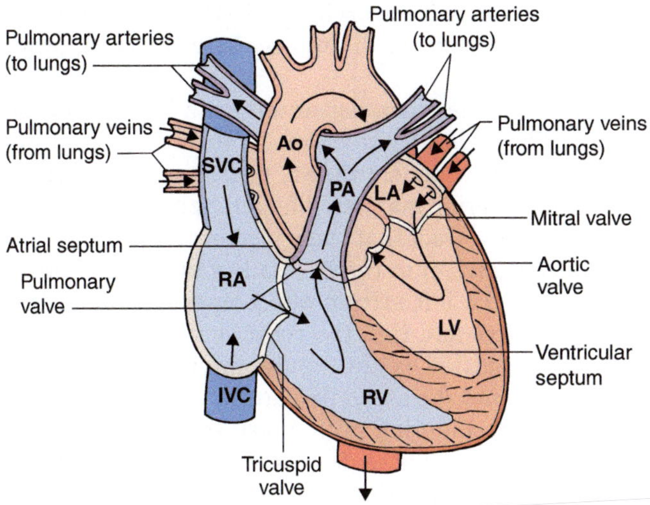

Figure 5.14 Normal heart anatomy. Arrows reflect blood flow pattern.

Ao, aorta; IVC, inferior vena cava; LA, left atrium; LV, left ventricle; PA, pulmonary artery; RA, right atrium; RV, right ventricle; SVC, superior vena cava.

common congenital heart lesions. The global incidence of all CHDs is 17.9 per 1,000 liveborn infants, with a slightly increased prevalence among males; the incidence in the United States is estimated at 10.1 to 15 per 1,000 liveborn infants (Wu et al., 2020). We explore cyanotic and acyanotic heart lesions in the following sections of this chapter.

Cyanotic Heart Defects

Cyanotic heart defects are a group of congenital malformations that lead to low circulating blood oxygen levels. These types of defects involve the systemic recirculation of desaturated venous blood, which occurs by one of two common mechanisms: (a) mixing of deoxygenated and oxygenated blood at the atrial, ventricular, or ductal level; or (b) a structural diversion redirecting deoxygenated blood returning to the heart away from the lungs and back to the systemic circulation. This shunting of blood from right to left results in hypoxemia, low arterial saturations, and cyanosis.

Transposition of the Great Arteries. Transposition of the great arteries (TGA) is the most common cyanotic heart defect that manifests during the neonatal period. The prevalence of TGA in the United States is estimated to be one in every 3,957 live births (CDC, 2024e). Within the United States, TGA accounts for 3% of all CHDs, and further accounts for 20% of all cyanotic heart defects. A 1.8:1 male-to-female preponderance is reported, and fetuses exposed to pregestational diabetes mellitus are considered at higher risk for developing TGA (Estévez & Ansah, 2024). TGA most likely occurs secondary to an abnormality in conotruncal development that happens between weeks 4 and 5 of gestation (Kirby, 2002). Two types of TGA are known: (a) dextro-transposition (D-TGA) and (b) levo-transposition (L-TGA). D-TGA is the most common type of TGA.

Dextro-Transposition. With D-TGA, the heart tube loops to the right during organogenesis, yielding normal ventricular orientation and great vessel formation, but the aorta and PA fail to rotate, resulting in the reversal of these two vessels (see previous discussion regarding the development of conotruncal defects). The aorta ultimately arises from the right ventricle, and the PA arises from the left ventricle (CDC, 2024e; Robbins & Arruda, 2025). This transposition of the two great vessels results in two independent and parallel circulations (Figure 5.15).

The first circuit involves the persistent recirculation of deoxygenated blood from the right atrium to the right ventricle through the aorta and out to the systemic circulation. The second circuit involves the recirculation of oxygenated blood from the pulmonary veins to the left atrium, left ventricle, and PA; blood enters this circuit by way of the PDA (Robbins & Arruda, 2025; Torchia & Persaud, 2025). This type of circulation is incompatible with life; therefore, early identification is critical to establishing an open communication between the two parallel circuits by way of an ASD, VSD, or PDA (Torchia & Persaud, 2025).

Affected neonates manifest with cyanosis at or within a few hours after birth. Due to increased right ventricular pressure and close proximity of the mitral valve, bowing of the ventricular septum occurs, which causes an outflow obstruction at the aortic inlet. Infants require a PDA to perfuse the pulmonary circuit and

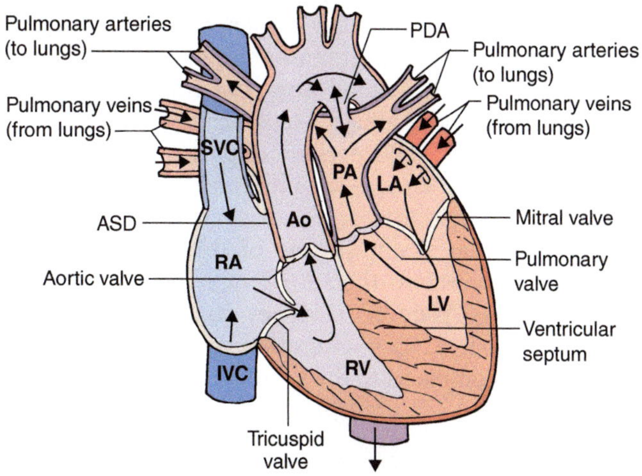

Figure 5.15 Dextro-transposition of the great arteries. Arrows reflect the parallel blood flow pattern. When the PDA is open, this allows the shunting of pulmonary blood flow from the PA to the Ao during systole, and the blood flow reverses direction from the Ao to the PA during diastole.

Ao, aorta; ASD, atrial septal defect; IVC, inferior vena cava; LA, left atrium; LV, left ventricle; PA, pulmonary artery; PDA, patent ductus arteriosus; RA, right atrium; RV, right ventricle; SVC, superior vena cava.

facilitate the uptake of oxygen. This blood is returned to the heart by way of a left-to-right shunting across the foramen ovale. Infants with a patent ventricular septum (a VSD) benefit from a greater opportunity for mixing of deoxygenated and oxygenated blood, which often results in better arterial oxygenation. However, a large VSD may increase the risk of pulmonary overcirculation and the risk of CHF.

Life-span implications include a 95% survival rate at 15 to 25 years following discharge status after the arterial switch procedure (Khairy et al., 2013). Children with repaired D-TGA often have functional limitations on exercise capacities. Neurodevelopmental delays have also been reported. Continuing care across the life span is indicated.

Clinical Application. The initial assessment of an infant with a suspected CCHD includes continuous pulse oximetry monitoring, specifically evaluating potential differences between preductal and postductal oxygen saturations (Karlsen & Cowley, 2021). This helps assess the right-to-left shunt of blood flow at the level of the PDA with the right hand/wrist (preductal saturation) greater than the left upper or lower extremities (postductal saturation). This is known as *differential cyanosis*. It may be seen with coarctation of the aorta, interrupted aortic arch, or persistent pulmonary hypertension of the newborn. *Reverse differential cyanosis* occurs when the preductal saturation is abnormally lower than the postductal saturation. This suggests TGA (the most common cyanotic CHD to manifest during the newborn period). Recall that when the PDA is open, and pulmonary vascular resistance remains high after birth, the deoxygenated blood flow first travels up the abnormally positioned aorta arising from the right ventricle. The earliest opportunity to mix deoxygenated and oxygenated blood does not occur until the blood travels past the PDA, where shunting may occur in one of three directions (from the aorta to the PA or vice versa, or in a bidirectional fashion). This results in blood flow with a lower oxygen saturation in the preductal vessels as compared to the postductal vessels.

Levo-Transposition. L-TGA is also referred to as *congenitally corrected TGA* because the systemic deoxygenated venous blood returns to the pulmonary circulation, and oxygenated pulmonary venous blood returns to the systemic circulation, yet the heart tube is abnormally rotated to the left. Isolated L-TGA is extremely rare; this defect usually presents with other cardiac malformations. Despite the rarity of this CHD, we present a concise overview of L-TGA such that clinicians can discern the differences between both forms of transposition.

In L-TGA, the aorta lies anterior and to the left of the PA. The right atrium connects through the mitral valve to a left ventricle that is positioned in a rightward and anterior manner. The left ventricle empties into an outflow tract that leads posteriorly through the pulmonary valve, into the PA, and to the lungs. Blood then enters the left atrium and empties through the tricuspid valve and into the right ventricle; the right ventricular outflow is anterior, emptying through the aortic valve into the ascending aorta, which is anterior and leftward, pumping pulmonary venous blood outward to the body. These defects lead to misplacement of the cardiac conduction system, which increases the risk of varying degrees of heart block. In addition, the positioning of coronary arteries is reversed, with the right coronary artery supplying the anterior descending branch.

L-transposition rarely exists without other major cardiac anomalies, which determine the outcome. The physiologic problems seen with L-transposition are directly related to the associated defects. The neonate may be asymptomatic after birth. In some cases, significant tricuspid insufficiency and systemic ventricular dysfunction can occur. Cyanosis can be present if there is an accompanying VSD and pulmonary stenosis (Bernstein, 2025).

Long-term sequelae for patients with L-TGA are dependent on the other cardiac malformations associated with it. Mortality risk after early surgical correction is low; however, the long-term prognosis is poor. Overall 15-year survival without need for a heart transplant in patients who received a Fontan repair or biventricular repair is estimated at 90%; however, the likelihood for surgical reintervention increases as patients age (71% likelihood for surgical reintervention at 15 years post initial procedure; Sun et al., 2019).

Tetralogy of Fallot. TOF, first described by Étienne Fallot in 1888, is *the most common congenital cyanotic defect that manifests during infancy.* TOF is associated with a prevalence of approximately four to five per every 10,000 live births within the United States (CDC, 2024e, 2024h). This defect accounts for about 7% to 10% of cases of CHD and is one of the most common congenital heart lesions that requires surgical intervention within the first year of life (Kulik & Levy, 2022; Robbins & Arruda, 2025). TOF occurs equally in males and females. Approximately 80% of cases are sporadic; the remaining 20% of cases of TOF have associated risk factors, including pregestational diabetes mellitus; advanced age at conception; family history of CHD; fetal exposure to medications, including valproate, amantadine, and Coumadin; trisomy 21; prune belly syndrome; CHARGE (**C**oloboma of the eye, **H**eart defects, **A**tresia of the choanae, **R**etardation of **G**rowth and development, and **E**ar abnormalities and deafness) syndrome; as well as pyloric stenosis; renal agenesis; hypospadias; and polydactyly (Nies & Brenner, 2013; Simeone et al., 2016).

TOF involves a constellation of four anatomic findings: (a) PA stenosis, (b) VSD, (c) overriding aorta, and (d) right ventricular hypertrophy (Figure 5.16; Swamy et al., 2015). The major defect is the right ventricular outflow obstruction, which limits pulmonary blood flow and impedes adequate oxygenation. Pulmonary stenosis results in right ventricular outflow obstruction, which leads to right ventricular hypertrophy. This leads to increased ventricular pressure and causes the perimembranous portion of the ventricular septum to rupture, yielding the large VSD of the conal septum. Furthermore, the aorta is enlarged and displaced to the right, straddling the ventricular septum, which permits aortic uptake of blood from both ventricles. The resultant right ventricular hypertrophy and upward tilting of the left ventricular axis yields the classic "boot-shaped" cardiac silhouette on radiographic studies.

Infants will manifest with either "blue" or "pink" TOF; few cases involve TOF with balanced pulmonary stenosis. Severe pulmonary stenosis is associated with *blue* TOF and is responsible for the audible murmur heard during early disease states. Blood is preferentially shunted in a right-to-left direction across the VSD; patients will present with varying degrees of cyanosis, which is contingent upon the severity of the outflow tract obstruction and patency of the ductus arteriosus.

Pink tetralogy involves minimal ventricular outflow obstruction, no significant directional shunt across the VSD, and, likewise, no cyanosis. The disease process may remain subclinical for years, even into adulthood. In between the aforementioned blue and pink extremes are cases of TOF with *balanced pulmonary stenosis*. In these circumstances, equivocal pressures protect the pulmonary arteries from overcirculation and reactive pulmonary hypertension. The main and central pulmonary arteries are typically small or hypoplastic in contrast to the aorta, which is comparatively larger. The amount of right ventricular outflow obstruction is proportionate to the degree to which the aorta overrides the ventricular septum.

Infants with blue TOF may manifest with paroxysmal hypercyanotic episodes, also known as *tet spells*. This leads to increased pulmonary stenosis and reduced blood flow to the PA. As a result, increased right-to-left shunting occurs with an acute reduction in the oxygen content of the blood. With severe hypoxemia, a switch from aerobic to anaerobic metabolism occurs and leads to lactic and metabolic acidosis. These hypercyanotic episodes can be fatal if left untreated. Parents must receive ongoing education on mechanisms to reverse tet spells.

Survival is estimated at greater than 97% among patients who undergo corrective procedures; uncorrected TOF is associated with 50% mortality risk in early childhood (Romeo et al., 2020; Ye et al., 2023). Continuing care is needed for patients with TOF. Lifespan implications include a risk for atrial reentrant

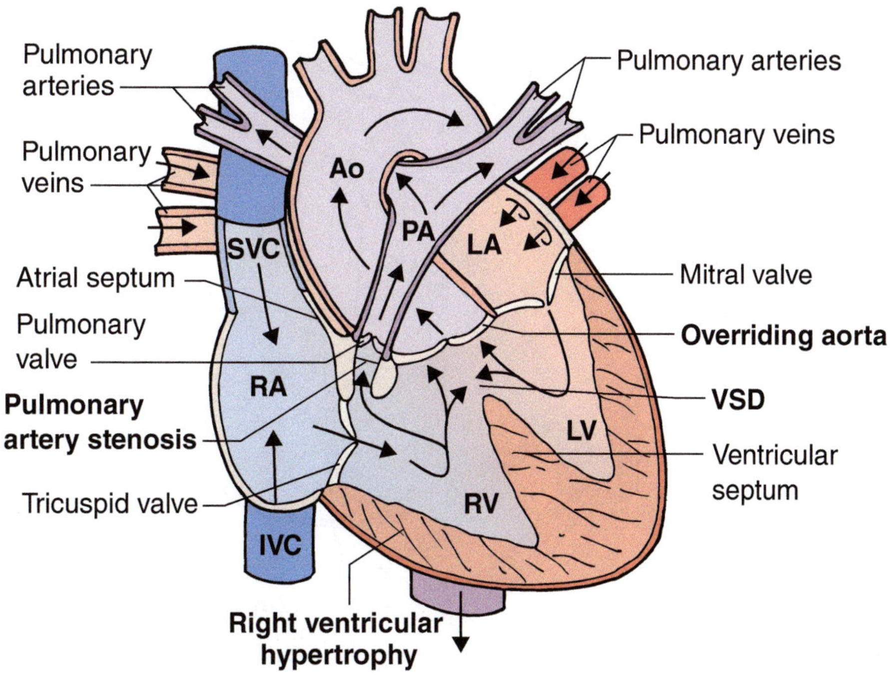

Figure 5.16 Tetralogy of Fallot. Arrows reflect the abnormal blood flow pattern.
Ao, aorta; IVC, inferior vena cava; LA, left atrium; LV, left ventricle; PA, pulmonary artery; RA, right atrium; RV, right ventricle; SVC, superior vena cava; VSD, ventricular septal defect.

tachycardia (30%), ventricular arrhythmias (10%), and sudden cardiac death (0.2%) as a result of scarring at the right ventricular incision site (Hoffman, 2017; Villafañe et al., 2013). Pulmonary valve regurgitation predisposes patients to ventricular dilatation. As the right ventricular dilatation progresses, tricuspid valve regurgitation occurs, which encourages right atrial enlargement. The constellation of these factors increases the risk for the ventricular and atrial arrhythmias described earlier. Affected adults are at increased risk for aortic dilation, likely related to increased aortic blood flow observed prior to surgical correction (McRae, 2015a). Reports indicate that affected individuals of childbearing age who undergo surgical correction can safely tolerate pregnancy and the birth process (Wijesekera, 2024).

Total Anomalous Pulmonary Venous Connection. Total anomalous pulmonary venous connection (TAPVC), also known as total anomalous pulmonary venous return (TAPVR), involves abnormal drainage of all pulmonary venous blood into the systemic venous system (Cruz-Lemini et al., 2026; Karlsen & Cowley, 2021). TAPVC is the fifth most common cause of cyanotic CHD, with an estimated incidence of one per every 10,000 live births (CDC, 2024i). Risk factors include heterotaxy syndromes, which include asplenia and polysplenia.

Four types of TAPVC are known: supracardiac, cardiac, mixed, and infracardiac (Figure 5.17). Supracardiac TAPVC is the most common type, accounting for 44% of all cases of TAPVC (Jaramillo et al., 2017). Recall that in normal anatomy, two pulmonary veins from each lung drain oxygenated blood into the left atrium. Supracardiac TAPVC involves the movement of pulmonary venous drainage (oxygenated blood returning from the lungs) to a common pulmonary venous channel located behind the left atrium. This pulmonary venous channel drains into the brachiocephalic vein, then the SVC, and into the right atrium, where it mixes with deoxygenated blood (Jaramillo et al., 2017; Martin et al., 2016).

Cardiac TAPVC accounts for 21% of all reported cases (Jaramillo et al., 2017). In these cases, all pulmonary veins drain into a common pulmonary venous channel, which then drains into the right atrium, or more commonly into the coronary sinus (Jaramillo et al., 2017; Martin et al., 2016).

The mixed type of TAPVC accounts for 9% of all cases (Jaramillo et al., 2017). Mixed TAPVC involves situations in which the pulmonary venous system drains

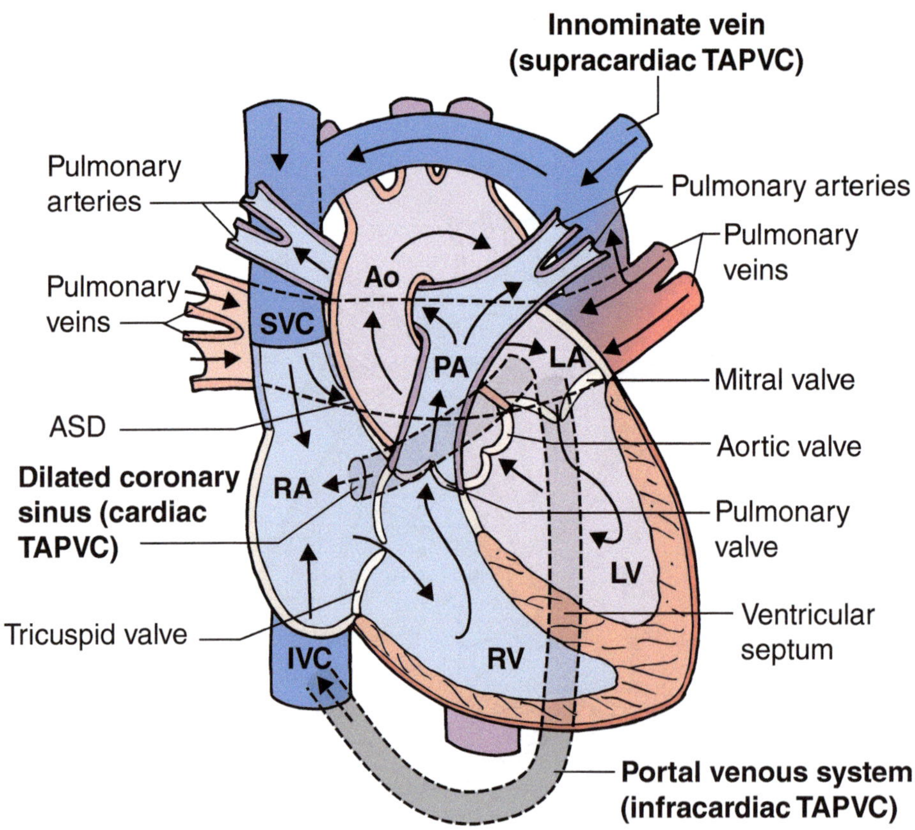

Figure 5.17 Total anomalous pulmonary venous connection. Image depicts anatomy with supracardiac, cardiac, and infracardiac TAPVC. Arrows reflect the abnormal blood flow pattern.

Ao, aorta; ASD, atrial septal defect; IVC, inferior vena cava; LA, left atrium; LV, left ventricle; PA, pulmonary artery; RA, right atrium; RV, right ventricle; SVC, superior vena cava; TAPVC, total anomalous pulmonary venous connection.

into two or more locations. For example, left pulmonary veins may pass through the innominate vein, by way of a supracardiac route, whereas the right pulmonary veins drain directly into the right atrium by way of an infracardiac route.

Infracardiac TAPVC accounts for 26% of all cases (Jaramillo et al., 2017). All pulmonary veins drain into a common pulmonary vein behind the left atrium, where the pulmonary venous blood passes inferiorly through the diaphragm and into the inferior vena cava, the portal venous system, or hepatic veins (Martin et al., 2016). In order to reenter the heart, this blood must pass through the portal vein and ductus venosus to the inferior vena cava and back to the right atrium. Infracardiac TAPVC is often associated with obstruction to flow at the diaphragm or ductus venosus; the portal system is often unable to tolerate CO, which often leads to significant pulmonary venous congestion. Other important consequences seen include pulmonary edema and PA hypertension (Karlsen & Cowley, 2021).

All types of TAPVC involve a degree of obstruction to blood flow at certain anatomic locations; obstruction is most common with infracardiac TAPVC (78%; Jaramillo et al., 2017). Obstruction may occur secondary to compression from adjacent structures or occur within the pulmonary venous system. Severe obstruction is associated with respiratory distress and cyanosis during the neonatal period and is considered a surgical emergency (Martin et al., 2016).

The most significant risk factor that associates with increased mortality risk is weight less than 2 to 6 kg at the time of surgery, followed by the infracardiac and mixed subtype (Nahle et al., 2024; Sakamoto et al., 2018). Surgical correction is associated with 5-year survivability of 97% and 88% survivability among adolescents; pulmonary vein stenosis (5%–19%), pulmonary hypertension, and pulmonary venous obstruction are the most common postsurgical complications (Jaramillo et al., 2017). Life-span implications may include neurocognitive delays and cardiac arrhythmias (Sakamoto et al., 2018). Continuing care is warranted. Patients who progress into adulthood often develop pulmonary vascular disease.

Ebstein Anomaly. While uncommon, occurring in less than 1% of infants with CHD, Ebstein anomaly (EA) can be a particularly challenging neonatal lesion depending upon its severity (Karlsen & Cowley, 2021; Mille & Ravishankar, 2023). The tricuspid valve located between the two right chambers of the heart is abnormally displaced in a more apical position within the right ventricle. The malposition of the tricuspid valve prevents its leaflets from closing properly, leading to valve regurgitation and enlargement of the right atrium. The area of the right ventricle above the tricuspid valve melds into the right atrium, becoming "atrialized," leaving the remaining right ventricle hypoplastic (varying degrees of this can occur) and less able to contribute pulmonary blood flow through the pulmonary valve into the PA and lungs. This can create a functional pulmonary outflow tract obstruction because of the right ventricle's poor contractility. Blood flow preferentially flows right-to-left across the PFO or ASD, mixing deoxygenated blood from the right side of the heart with oxygenated blood in the left atrium. In severe cases, there can be profound cyanosis. Cardiomegaly from right atrial dilation may impact fetal lung development as the heart crowds the chest cavity, leading to pulmonary hypoplasia.

EA is associated with other cardiac defects including the aforementioned ASD, pulmonary valve stenosis or atresia (anatomical), VSD, and, more rarely, coarctation of the aorta (Karlsen & Cowley, 2021; Kumar, 2021). A PDA is necessary for pulmonary blood flow if PA is present. SVT, specifically Wolff-Parkinson-White syndrome, occurs in 10% to 20% of cases (Karlsen & Cowley, 2021; Kumar, 2021; Mille & Ravishankar, 2023). Fetal exposure to lithium early in gestation is linked to EA (see Table 5.7).

The clinical presentation of EA varies based on its severity, with those infants with extreme tricuspid valve displacement and regurgitation, with resulting cardiomegaly, typically producing the most acute symptoms (Karlsen & Cowley, 2021; Kumar, 2021). Infants with large right-to-left shunting at the atrial level and poor pulmonary blood flow, either due to functional or anatomical pulmonary outflow tract obstruction, will be severely cyanotic. Elevated PVR after birth contributes to the impediment of pulmonary blood flow, which may be compounded by hypoxemia and acidosis (Mille & Ravishankar, 2023). The chest x-ray reveals a massive heart in severe cases, which can appear "wall-to-wall."

The management of EA depends upon its presentation. For neonates presenting early with signs of cyanosis and poor heart function, initial stabilization should be focused on efforts to lower the PVR and improve pulmonary blood flow. Inhaled nitric oxide may be considered to treat pulmonary hypertension. Prostaglandin E_1 is used to maintain ductal patency in the setting of pulmonary valve atresia. Inotropes may be needed to ameliorate heart function, namely, to assist the right ventricle in antegrade flow across the pulmonary valve. SVT should be treated without delay as it may be poorly tolerated.

Those with milder forms of EA may be managed medically and may not even be diagnosed until later in life. The prognosis for EA is poorer for those developing symptoms earlier, with fetal demise rates at 20% and overall perinatal mortality rates at 45% (Kumar, 2021). Surgical repair and its timing depend upon the stability of the infant, current ventilatory and pharmacologic support, and any additional CHDs present (see Figure 5.18).

Truncus Arteriosus. Truncus arteriosus is a less common condition, representing 1% to 3% of neonatal CHDs, and approximately 250 cases per year in the United States (CDC, 2024j; Karlsen & Cowley, 2021). Truncus

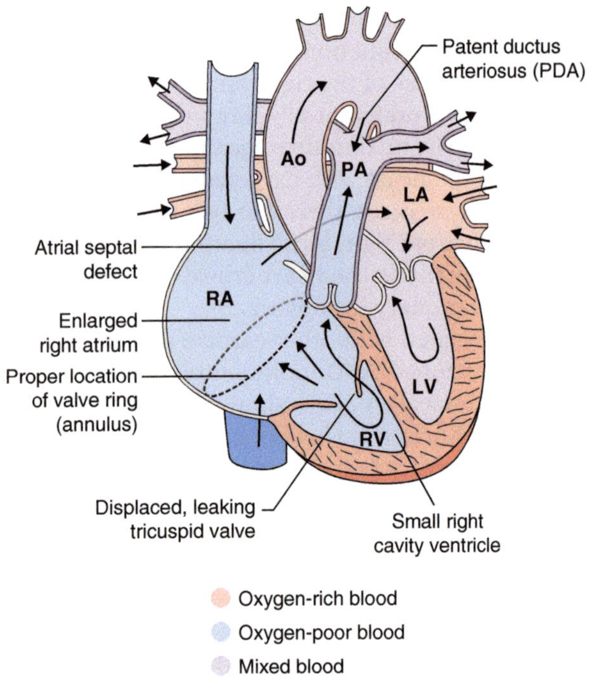

Figure 5.18 Ebstein anomaly.
Ao, aorta; LA, left atrium; LV, left ventricle; PA, pulmonary artery; RA, right atrium; RV, right ventricle.

arteriosus is a conotruncal defect that develops as a result of the incomplete rotation of the outflow tract during early heart development. The great vessels fail to separate, leaving one single vessel situated over the right and left ventricles as the origin of the aorta, pulmonary, and coronary arteries. A VSD is present in more than 98% of cases (Mille & Ravishankar, 2023). The truncus has a single valve, which is usually abnormal, with a variable number of leaflets that may be stenotic or regurgitant (Karlsen & Cowley, 2021). The large VSD allows mixing of deoxygenated blood from the right ventricle with oxygenated blood from the left ventricle. The blood travels via the truncus to the aorta, pulmonary, and coronary arteries.

The literature describes three types of truncus arteriosus depending on the location where the pulmonary arteries insert into the truncal root. Type I and type II are the most common (combined 85% of cases). Other associated anomalies include a right aortic arch, interrupted aortic arch, and coarctation (Mille & Ravishankar, 2023). Chromosome 22q11 deletion is present in more than 25% of patients with truncus arteriosus (see Table 5.6).

Clinical manifestations appear early in the neonatal period as the PVR fall and cyanosis becomes more apparent. As PVR drops, pulmonary blood flow is enhanced. The insufficient truncal valve combined with increased diastolic runoff in the pulmonary circulation leads to signs of pulmonary overcirculation and CHF (e.g., tachypnea, tachycardia, diaphoresis, increased work of breathing, and poor feeding; Karlsen & Cowley, 2021). Chest x-ray may show modest cardiomegaly with increased pulmonary markings due to overcirculation.

The initial management of truncus arteriosus includes avoiding supplemental oxygen if possible while maintaining oxygen saturations within a range of 75% to 85% to avoid excessive pulmonary blood flow. Prostaglandin E_1 is not necessary unless an interrupted aortic arch is also present. Surgical repair includes closing the VSD, creating a channel or conduit from the right ventricle to the PA, and maintaining the existing single truncus as the aorta (CDC, 2024j; see Figure 5.19).

Tricuspid Atresia. Tricuspid atresia affects about 3% of neonates with CHDs, with approximately 325 cases per year in the United States (CDC, 2024k; Karlsen & Cowley, 2021). There are three classifications of tricuspid atresia: (a) tricuspid atresia with normally related great arteries (70%–80%), (b) tricuspid atresia with D-TGA (10%–25%), and (c) tricuspid atresia with L-TGA (3%–6%; Karlsen & Cowley, 2021). The first classification is discussed here. There is congenital absence of the tricuspid valve with no direct communication between the right chambers of the heart. The right ventricle is hypoplastic due to limited blood flow in utero. Most all have a VSD (greater than 90%), allowing blood flow from the left ventricle to the right ventricle and into the PA. The size of the VSD, however, determines the pulmonary blood flow. Blood arriving from the right atrium is dependent upon an atrial level communication reach to the

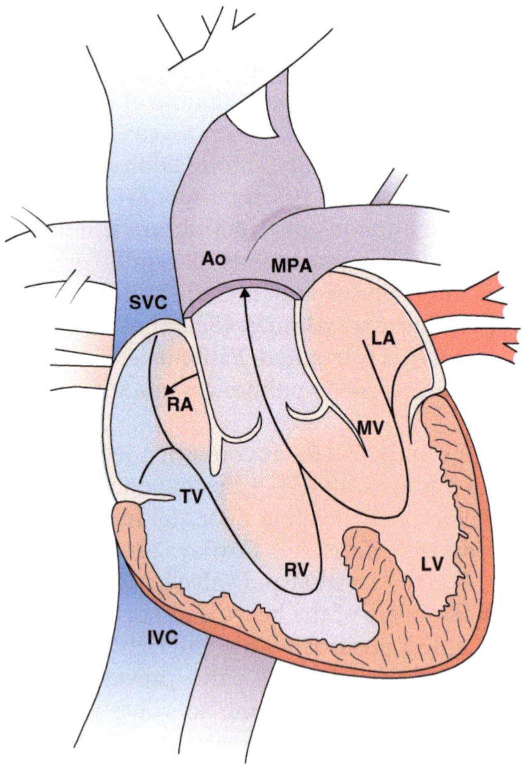

Figure 5.19 Truncus arteriosus.
Ao, aorta; IVC, inferior vena cava; LA, left atrium; LV, left ventricle; MPA, main pulmonary artery; MV, mitral valve; RA, right atrium; RV, right ventricle; SVC, superior vena cava; TV, tricuspid valve.

pulmonary and systemic circuits (see Figure 5.20 for blood flow pattern). Pulmonary valve stenosis is present in as many as 50% of cases.

The clinical presentation of tricuspid atresia can vary depending on the adequacy of pulmonary blood flow. If the VSD is restrictive or pulmonary valve stenosis (or atresia) is present, then cyanosis may be moderate to severe. If pulmonary blood flow is sufficient, there may be little cyanosis. In the setting of a known tricuspid atresia, this infant should be monitored closely for any signs of progressing hypoxemia. On chest x-ray, the heart appears normal or moderately increased if unrestricted pulmonary blood flow is present.

Medical management strategies for tricuspid atresia with normally related great arteries include providing supplemental oxygen to reduce hypoxemia and PVR. While most infants with tricuspid atresia are not PDA-dependent, oxygen saturations should be monitored closely during the first days of life to ensure adequate pulmonary blood flow. Infants with unrestricted pulmonary blood flow should be closely followed for signs of pulmonary edema and CHF. Surgical repair depends upon the presence and severity of accompanying heart defects (CDC, 2024k). Palliative techniques may be necessary with definitive correction later. Typically, a septostomy is performed early on to enlarge the ASD. If pulmonary blood flow is restrictive, a Blalock-Taussig shunt is created from the aorta to the PA to increase flow. If pulmonary blood flow is excessive, banding of the PA may be necessary to reduce flow.

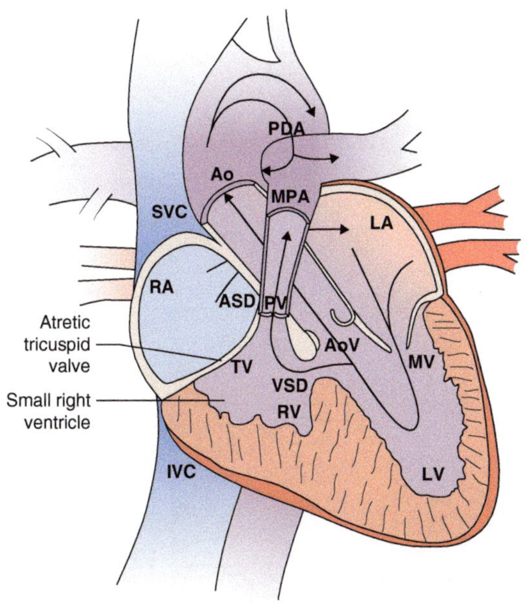

Figure 5.20 Tricuspid atresia.
Ao, aorta; AoV, aortic valve; ASD, atrial septal defect; IVC, inferior vena cava; LA, left atrium; LV, left ventricle; MV, mitral valve; MPA, main pulmonary artery; PDA, patent ductus arteriosus; PV, pulmonary valve; RA, right atrium; RV, right ventricle; SVC, superior vena cava; TV, tricuspid valve; VSD, ventricular septal defect.

The Single Ventricle. Single-ventricle defects involve the presence of one ventricular chamber or one large and functionally dominant ventricle with a rudimentary or hypoplastic opposing ventricle. Common single-ventricle defects include tricuspid atresia, HLHS, double outlet left ventricle, and double outlet right ventricle. Less frequent, AVC defects and PA may manifest as single-ventricle defects.

Recall that during early embryonic development, the AVC opens into the ventricular portion of the primitive heart tube and later becomes the left ventricle. Blood passes to the bulbus cordis from the ventricular portion of the primitive heart tube, contributing to right ventricle development. The arterial trunk arises from the bulbus cordis, later becoming the aorta and main PA. With an interventricular septation defect or arrest in development, a double-inlet single left ventricle with a rudimentary right ventricle forms.

The most common type of single ventricle is a single left ventricle with L-transposition of the great arteries. In these circumstances, the aorta arises from a very small, leftward-leaning right ventricle. The PA arises posteriorly, and the mitral valve is located on the right side of the heart, whereas the tricuspid valve is located to the left. The degree of pulmonary stenosis or amount of PVR determines the amount of pulmonary blood flow and the clinical presentation after delivery. If there is no pulmonary stenosis and pulmonary venous resistance decreases, CHF will develop. When PA is present, the neonate is dependent on a right-to-left shunt through the PDA in order to maintain systemic CO. The degree of cyanosis is thereby determined by the amount of pulmonary blood flow supplied by the collateral circulation.

Life-span implications are associated with venous hypertension and include esophageal varices, liver fibrosis or cirrhosis, protein-losing enteropathy from the intestine, leg varicosities, and pleural effusions. Sinus node dysfunction, intraatrial reentry tachycardia, and ventricular tachycardia are arrhythmias reported among patients treated with the Fontan procedure. The right atrium to PA Fontan connection increases the risk for postsurgical right atrial thrombi as well as pulmonary emboli, which is due to passive blood flow and subsequent right atrial enlargement (McRae, 2015b).

Acyanotic Heart Defects

Unlike cyanotic heart defects, which present with clinical symptoms in the first day of life, acyanotic defects may go undetected. Acyanotic heart defects may become clinically apparent days to weeks after birth. As PVR decreases during the postnatal period, increased left-to-right shunting occurs, resulting in increased pulmonary blood flow. Shunting at the atrial level results in right ventricular overload, whereas shunting at the ventricular or great vessel level results in left ventricular overload (Backer et al., 2016). Common acyanotic congenital cardiac defects described here include VSD, ASD, AVC, and PDA.

Ventricular Septal Defect. VSDs are the most common CHD diagnosed during the first year of life and occur in approximately 50% to 60% of infants affected by CHDs (Puri et al., 2017). VSD often presents as an isolated defect, or may occur in combination with other CHDs, including AVC, TOF, and occasionally D-TGA.

The anatomical defect is caused by abnormal ventricular septation. Single or multiple openings at various locations within the ventricular septum result (Torchia & Persaud, 2025). As a consequence, oxygenated blood mixes with deoxygenated blood during fetal and postnatal development. Postnatally, as the left side of the heart becomes dominant, blood flow via the abnormal ventricular opening(s) permits persistent left-to-right shunting and pulmonary overcirculation, which may increase the risk for CHF.

VSDs are classified into four major types with the embryological basis varying depending on the septal defect location. The four classifications are (a) perimembranous, (b) juxta-arterial (subarterial), (c) muscular, and (d) inlet VSD (atrioventricular canal; Figure 5.21). Perimembranous VSDs, the most common type of VSD, are reported in approximately 75% to 80% of all cases (Backer et al., 2016; McRae, 2015a; Puri et al., 2017). This type of VSD occurs in the upper, thinner, membrane-like portion of the ventricular septum as a result of fibrous deficiencies (McRae, 2015a; Puri et al., 2017). Juxta-arterial VSDs arise between the pulmonic and aortic valves, at the infundibular septum. Muscular VSDs are located in the lower, thicker trabecular portion of the ventricular septum (McRae, 2015a). These are understood to occur secondarily due to excessive excavation of myocardial tissue during ventricular growth (Torchia & Persaud, 2025). Inlet VSDs arise inferior to the perimembranous region and slightly below the tricuspid and mitral valves.

Clinical manifestations are contingent on the size and severity of the defect. Small to moderate defects that do not encourage significant pulmonary overcirculation are associated with a harsh pan-systolic murmur best heard over the left lower sternal border. Large VSDs are often hemodynamically significant and present with signs of pulmonary overcirculation with or without CHF.

Life-span implications depend on the type and severity of the VSD. Perimembranous and muscular VSDs may close over time; muscular VSDs close as the septum grows. Closure of a perimembranous VSD may be the result of aortic valve prolapse and therefore must be carefully followed. Hemodynamically significant VSDs often require diuretic therapy to treat pulmonary overcirculation. As such, these infants incur increased risk for nutritional deficits and poor linear growth (Puri et al., 2017).

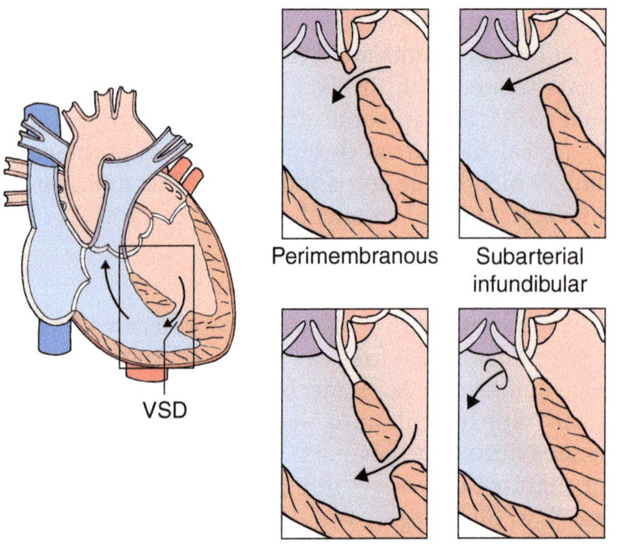

Figure 5.21 Ventricular septal defects.
VSD, ventricular septal defect.

Atrial Septal Defect. An ASD is an opening or series of openings anywhere within the atrial septum. In the United States, approximately 1,966 babies are born each year with an ASD, either as an isolated defect or part of a more complex CHD. A female-to-male prevalence (2:1) is reported (CDC, 2024b).

ASDs are classified into four major types: (a) ostium secundum defects, (b) ostium primum defects (common atrium or atrioventricular septal defect are broader categories), (c) sinus venosus defects, and (d) coronary septal defects (unroofed coronary sinus; Figure 5.22). The ostium secundum is the most common form, constituting about 75% of ASDs; in this type of defect the atrial opening is located in the center of the

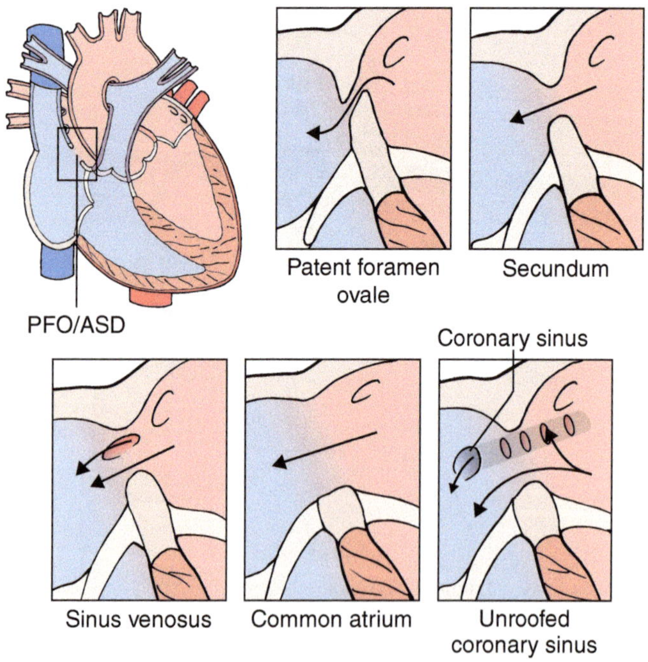

Figure 5.22 Atrial septal defects.
ASD, atrial septal defect; PFO, patent foramen ovale (a temporary opening in the atrium).

atrial septum in the area of the foramen ovale (McRae, 2015a). This defect arises secondary to defective development of the septum primum. Ostium primum defects arise secondary to failed proliferation of the endocardial cushion. Sinus venosus defects are seen at the level of the superior vena or pulmonary veins, and rare coronary defects occur near the coronary sinus (Puri et al., 2017).

After delivery, the amount of shunting is determined by the size of the defect and compliance of both ventricles (Backer et al., 2016). Initially, left-to-right shunting is minimal as the right ventricle is not very compliant. As the right ventricle becomes more compliant with age, left-to-right shunting increases, sending increased blood flow across the pulmonic valve. This increases the risk for right atrial and right ventricular dilatation (Backer et al., 2016).

Clinical manifestations, commonly identified during infancy, include tachypnea, decreased activity levels, and poor linear growth with failure to thrive. A focused cardiovascular examination will typically yield a split murmur heard over the pulmonic region secondary to the aforementioned increased blood flow across the pulmonic valve, as well as potential for a diastolic murmur heard over the left lower sternal border (Puri et al., 2017). Patients who require surgical repair during childhood usually endure uncomplicated postoperative courses and are generally free of latent complications and activity restrictions.

Atrioventricular Septal Defect. An AVSD results from failed fusion of the endocardial cushion (Figure 5.23). This acyanotic heart lesion leaves a hole in the center of the heart between the AV septums and is associated with a myriad of valvular anomalies. In the United States, approximately 2,000 infants are born each year with an AVSD. Complete AVSD is present in up to 75% of fetuses with trisomy 21 (Backer et al., 2016; Puri et al., 2017). AVSDs may be associated with a heterotaxy syndrome confirmed by the presence of asplenia or polysplenia. Diabetes mellitus has been associated with increased risk for the development of AVSDs among exposed offspring.

Recall from the review of cardiovascular embryology that the left ventricle connects to the atria by way of the primitive AVC. Ridges of mesenchymal tissue comprise the circumference of the canal and naturally divide during development into four distinct endocardial cushions: the (a) inferior (upper part of the ventricular septum), (b) superior (lower part of the atrial septum), (c) left (anterior leaflet of the mitral valve), and (d) right (septal leaflet of the tricuspid valve) endocardial

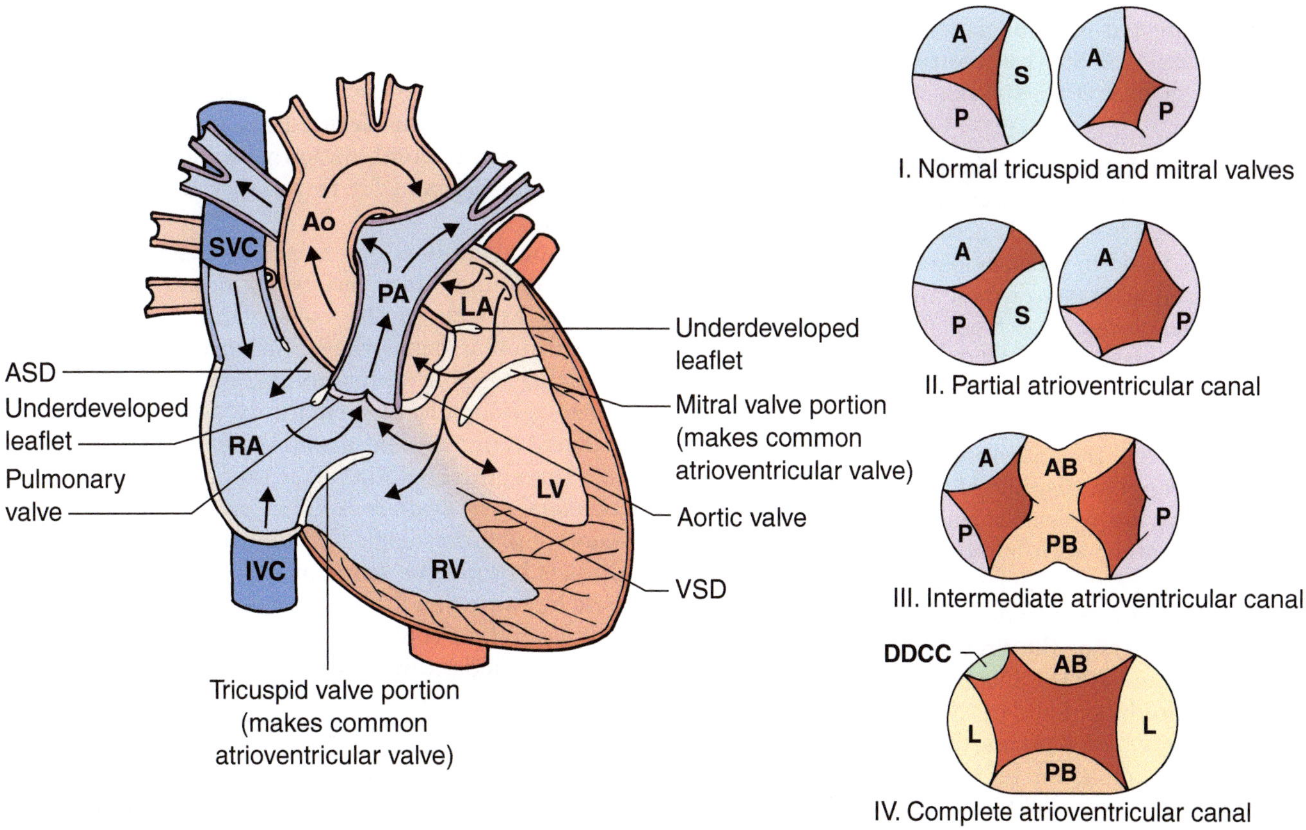

Figure 5.23 Atrioventricular canal defect. Arrows reflect the abnormal blood flow pattern.

A, anterior leaflet; AB, anterior bridging leaflet; Ao, aorta; ASD, atrial septal defect; DDCC, dextrodorsal conus cushion; IVC, inferior vena cava; L, lateral leaflet; LA, left atrium; LV, left ventricle; P, posterior leaflet; PA, pulmonary artery; PB, posterior bridging leaflet; RA, right atrium; RV, right ventricle; S, septal leaflet; SVC, superior vena cava; VSD, ventricular septal defect.

cushions. Abnormal development of the endocardial cushions gives rise to AVSD malformations.

AVC defects are commonly categorized as either *complete* or *partial*. A complete AVSD is characterized by an AVSD that is contiguous with an inlet VSD and a common AV valve with five leaflets. A partial AVSD is limited to an ASD with cleft anterior mitral leaflet; no inlet VSD is observed (Robbins & Arruda, 2025). Both variations of the defect cause mixing of blood in the centralized areas of the heart, but the flow is usually left to right due to the left heart dominance and low pulmonary pressures. Two additional subtypes, *intermediate* and *transitional* AVSDs, are also reported. The intermediate AVSD is a variant of the complete AVSD and involves an ASD, inlet VSD, and common AV valve annulus bifurcated into anterior and posterior segments by a thin flap of septal tissue. The transitional AVSD is considered a variant of the partial AVSD and involves an ASD, inlet VSD, and two annular cavities separated by a cleft anterior mitral leaflet (Puri et al., 2017).

Postnatal clinical manifestations include left-to-right shunting at both the atrial and ventricular levels, as well as mitral valve regurgitation, resulting in pulmonary overcirculation and CHF. Latent consequences of AVSD commonly include arrhythmias, subaortic stenosis, and pulmonary vascular disease. Continuing care involves monitoring for unbalanced pulmonary and systemic circulations with worsening mitral valve regurgitation; 10% to 20% of affected individuals will require additional corrective surgeries. Survival postrepair is estimated at 97.5% (Schumacher et al., 2023).

Patent Ductus Arteriosus. The PDA is a normal fetal intracardiac shunt that connects the main PA to the descending aorta. This cannula permits shunting of right-sided venous blood to the systemic circulation; elevated fetal PVR facilitates this purposeful pulmonary bypass and functional movement of blood flow (Benitz & Bhombal, 2025; Torchia & Persaud, 2025).

The pathogenesis of postnatal PDA closure is well understood. Ductal constriction appears to be stimulated by increasing arterial oxygen tension, increasing blood pH, and the increased availability of vasoactive substances. Removal of the low resistance placental circuit, onset of crying and spontaneous respirations, and uptake of oxygen initiate the progressive constriction and functional closure of the PDA. During this time, SVR increases and exceeds PVR, reversing the direction of flow through the intracardiac shunt (PDA). Blood flow entering the PDA is redirected to the pulmonary system through the left-to-right shunt, which temporarily increases demand on the pulmonary circulation. In the full-term infant, ductal closure typically begins within the first 24 hours of life and the ligament is functionally closed by day 4 of postnatal life (Robbins & Arruda, 2025). Of note, infants of more than 28 weeks' gestation and weighing more than 1 kg at birth, who do not manifest with respiratory distress, are also likely to experience normal and unassisted postnatal functional closure of the PDA (Benitz & Bhombal, 2025).

Failed closure of the PDA results in persistent and increasing left-to-right blood flow to the pulmonary circuit and, likewise, risks atrial and ventricular distension and pulmonary overcirculation. A consistent diversion of systemic blood flow away from the descending aorta and back across the PDA in a left-to-right direction is commonly referred to as the *diastolic steal phenomenon*. This type of flow pattern can lead to inadequate oxygen delivery to the cerebral arteries, mesentery, and renal system and risks associated ischemic damage (Benitz & Bhombal, 2025). Factors that favor the postnatal persistence of the PDA include hypoxemia, acidosis, prostaglandin administration, and postnatal glucocorticoid exposure, in addition to other factors associated with prematurity and critical illness.

Common clinical manifestations of PDA include bounding pulses, widened pulse pressures, and increased left ventricular SV with hyperdynamic precordial activity. A holosystolic or "machinery-like" murmur is typically heard over the right upper sternal border; large and even hemodynamically significant defects may offer such low resistance to flow that no murmur may be heard. As excessive blood flow continues, enlargement occurs and additional left-to-right shunting across the foramen ovale occurs, leading to further volume overload and the development of CHF (Backer et al., 2016). In these circumstances, worsening hypercapnia as well as an elevated alveolar-arterial (A-a) gradient, often in combination with increased work of breathing or demand for respiratory support, may be observed.

Life-span implications relate to the direct consequences of pulmonary recirculation and cardiac dysfunction, as well as the consequences of ischemia. Intraventricular hemorrhage, bronchopulmonary dysplasia, necrotizing enterocolitis, renal parenchymal damage, retinopathy of prematurity, and later neurodevelopmental impairment are all associated with cases of treated and untreated PDA. Due to substantial advances in neonatal care, death is rarely reported. Although a discussion of pharmacologic and surgical treatment mechanisms is beyond the scope of this textbook, clinicians should be aware that the management of pathologic PDA continues to be a contentious topic and wide variations in clinical practices are observed.

Obstructive Congenital Heart Defects

Obstructive lesions are CHDs that result in obstructed blood flow involving either the left or right side of the heart. The majority of clinical manifestations are a result of ventricular hypertrophy and diminished blood flow to the area distal to the obstruction.

Hypoplastic Left Heart Syndrome. HLHS is a spectrum resulting from underdevelopment of the left heart–aorta complex that involves the atresia, stenosis, or hypoplasia of the mitral and aortic valves, and hypoplasia of the left ventricle, preductal aorta, and aortic arch (**Figure 5.24**; Kulik & Levy, 2022; Robbins & Arruda, 2025). In the United States, approximately 929 infants are born each year with HLHS; this is equivalent to an incidence of one in every 3,955 live births (CDC, 2024f). A male prevalence (1.5:1) is reported and sibling recurrence risk is 0.5% (Robbins & Arruda, 2025).

The pathophysiology of HLHS relates to the severity of obstruction caused by the constellation of anatomic defects and associated hypoplasia. HLHS involves parallel pulmonary and systemic circulations, both modulated by the right ventricle. Several factors may implicate left ventricular hypoplasia and predispose the right ventricle to its dueling role. One such factor is incompetence of the aortic valve. An atretic, stenosed, or hypoplastic aortic valve inhibits evacuation of blood from the left ventricle and into the ascending aorta. This leads to increased afterload (pressure) within the left ventricle, which over time leads to left ventricular hypertrophy. The constant distending pressure created by increased afterload inhibits normal flow into the left ventricle, which over time inhibits growth and leads to ventricular hypoplasia.

A second root cause for left ventricular hypoplasia relates to aberrant development of the mitral valve. This leads to reduced preload into the left ventricle. Blood aggregates within the left atrium, which increases afterload within this locale and encourages blood flow to divert across the PFO (if present). Over time, this permits ongoing reductions in blood flow into the left ventricle, thereby encouraging hypoplasia.

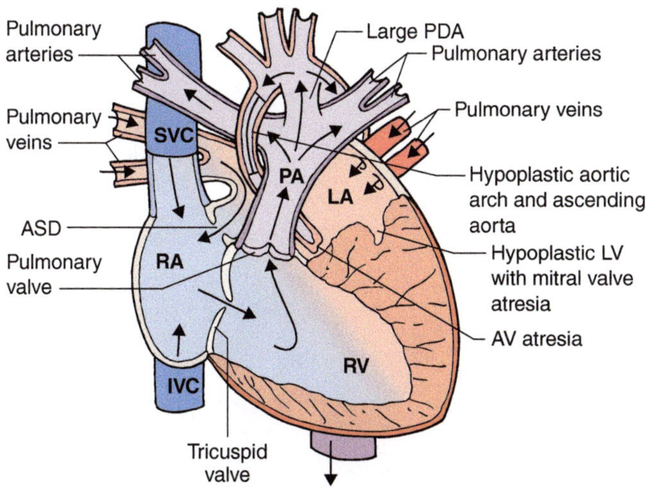

Figure 5.24 Hypoplastic left heart syndrome. Arrows reflect the abnormal blood flow pattern.

ASD, atrial septal defect; AV, atrioventricular valve; IVC, inferior vena cava; LA, left atrium; LV, left ventricle; PA, pulmonary artery; PDA, patent ductus arteriosus; RA, right atrium; RV, right ventricle; SVC, superior vena cava.

Third, right-sided compensation leads to enlargement and inhibits normal development of the left side of the heart. In cases of mitral valve stenosis or atresia, increased left atrial afterload encourages left-to-right movement of blood flow across the foramen ovale and back into the right side of the heart. This results in compensatory expansion of the right heart. Over time, right-sided enlargement competes spatially with the left side of the heart and contributes to left-sided hypoplasia.

It is important that clinicians understand the need for ductal patency during the postnatal period; early identification and diagnosis is absolutely critical to maintaining function of the PDA after birth. In the immediate postnatal period, PVR exceeds SVR and blood is redirected across the foramen ovale and, most significantly, the PDA. As PVR begins to decrease, blood flow is preferentially directed across the PDA and toward the pulmonary circulation. The PDA is the only mechanism by which gas exchange may occur. This directional flow across the PDA leads to "diastolic stealing," pulmonary overcirculation, edema, and systemic hypoperfusion. As a result, systemic blood flow decreases. SV and heart rate increase in an attempt to preserve systemic CO, but in doing so limit right ventricular output. This predisposes the infant to CHF, given that the right ventricle modulates both pulmonary and systemic circulation. Should the PDA begin to close, pressure will accumulate within the right ventricle, and perfusion to the systemic circulation, most notable in the coronary arteries, will be further compromised. The right ventricle will dilate and hypertrophy, tricuspid regurgitation may develop, and vital organs, including the kidneys, risk ischemic damage from poor systemic perfusion (Pigula & Mettler, 2017).

Term infants with HLHS who maintain a PFO and do not develop severely restricted disease during fetal development usually present as well-appearing infants after birth. However, the pathogenesis of the disease process quickly leads to pulmonary edema, restricted pulmonary blood flow, and increased work of breathing, tachypnea, cyanosis, and acidosis (Pigula & Mettler, 2017; Robbins & Arruda, 2025). The increased pulmonary blood flow and obstructed outflow from the left atrium leads to increased pulmonary venous pressure, which often causes the neonate to manifest with a "gasping" respiratory effort. This may precede or present alongside cardiogenic shock. Auscultation typically yields a single or third heart sound and any regurgitation across the valves will yield a murmur. Uneven upper and lower extremity pulses are common among infants affected by significant aortic narrowing or coarctation; peripheral pulses become increasingly difficult to palpate after functional closure of the PDA (Robbins & Arruda, 2025).

HLHS is responsible for 25% to 40% of all cardiac-related deaths among neonates (Simeone et al., 2016).

Advances in surgical palliation, involving the Norwood, Glenn, and Fontan procedures, have optimized survivability; survival to age 12 without a heart transplant is estimated between 54% and 63% (Goldberg et al., 2023). Cardiac transplantation is required in certain cases; organ rejection remains a potential contributor to mortality. Commonly reported (postsurgical) life-span implications for infants and children include an increased risk for intracranial hemorrhage, protein-losing enteropathy, arrhythmia, thrombotic stroke, neurodevelopmental impairment, and reduced exercise capacity (Gobergs et al., 2016).

Coarctation of the Aorta. Coarctation of the aorta is a narrowing or constriction of varying lengths of the aortic arch, distal to the aortic root. In the United States, four of every 10,000 infants are diagnosed with coarctation of the aorta (CDC, 2024d). A male-to-female prevalence is reported. Risk factors include chromosomal abnormalities such as Turner syndrome and DiGeorge syndrome and preexisting diabetes mellitus in the XX pregnant patient (Strainic, 2025).

The most common type of coarctation is the juxtaductal coarctation, which arises where the ductus arteriosus invaginates with the aorta (Choi et al., 2024). The ductus arteriosus is composed of smooth muscle in addition to elastic tissue. Some of this tissue extends into the wall of the aorta, comingling the ductal tissue with a section of the wall of the aorta. After birth, when the ductal smooth muscle begins its normal process of constriction, the tissue that innervated within the wall of the aorta also constricts. This gives rise to the juxtaductal coarctation.

Alternatively, coarctations may arise at a more proximal (preductal) or distal (postductal) segment of the aorta (**Figure 5.25**). The embryologic basis for this is poorly understood; however, postductal coarctations typically manifest in partnership with other complex heart lesions, including HLHS. Regardless of the etiology, the aortic constriction causes a mechanical outflow tract obstruction.

The pathogenesis of coarctation involves an increase in left ventricular afterload. This results in left ventricular failure, left atrial hypertension, and left-to-right shunting across the foramen ovale. Increasing pulmonary flow encourages a right-to-left shunt across the ductus arteriosus, as pulmonary vascular pressure exceeds systemic vascular pressure. Once the ductus arteriosus closes, CO to the descending aorta and distal organs is interrupted.

Clinical manifestations depend on the location and severity of the coarctation. Approximately 50% of patients will manifest symptoms during the neonatal period (first 28 days of life) and the majority of these cases involve a coarctation at a location on the aortic arch that occurs before innervation with the ductus arteriosus (preductal coarctation; Choi et al., 2024). Affected infants may exhibit normal perfusion to the upper extremities and decreased perfusion to the lower extremities, as well as feeding difficulties, lethargy, and decreased urine output (Puri et al., 2017). Coarctations that arise proximal to both subclavian arteries will manifest with diminished blood pressures and pulses to all four extremities. Severe narrowing typically manifests as discordant upper versus lower extremity blood pressures, pulses and oxygen saturations, hypoperfusion, metabolic acidosis, and heart failure (HF). Mild cases may remain subclinical through childhood or even into adulthood and manifest as chest pain or involve recurrent headaches. Older children and adults seem to develop collateral circulations over time, which circumvent the coarctation and distribute blood to the distal organs (Choi et al., 2024; Puri et al., 2017).

Life-span implications relate to operative mortality risk, survivability, and recurrence risk. Operative

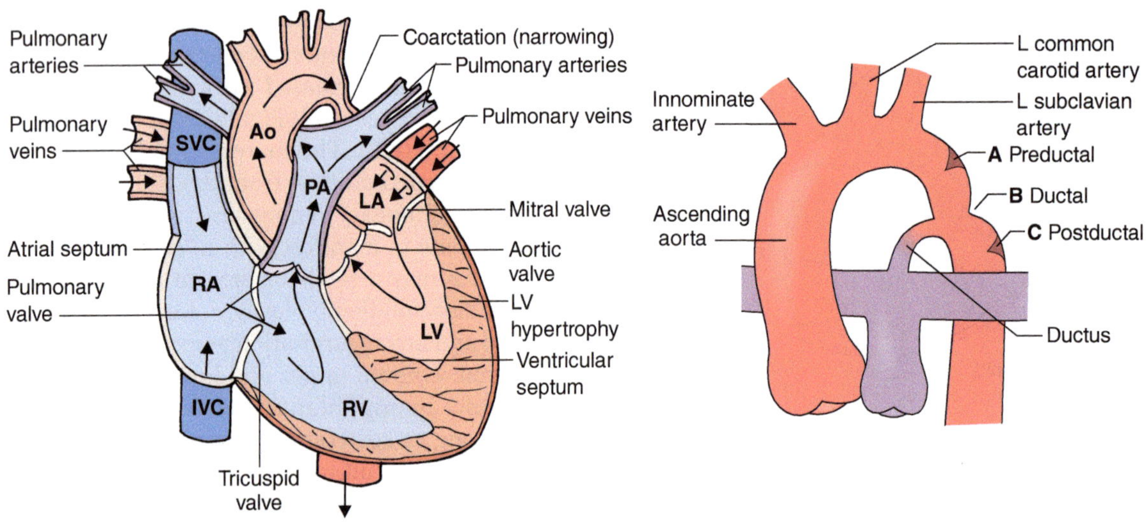

Figure 5.25 Coarctation of the aorta (postductal type). Arrows reflect the abnormal blood flow pattern.
Ao, aorta; IVC, inferior vena cava; L, left; LA, left atrium; LV, left ventricle; PA, pulmonary artery; RA, right atrium; RV, right ventricle; SVC, superior vena cava.

mortality is estimated at 1% to 5% (Choi et al., 2024). Survivability at 10 years postcorrection is 90%, whereas 70% of individuals survive for an additional three decades after surgical repair. Recurrence risk is higher among younger children, who may require additional corrective surgeries if the narrowing reappears. Hypertension is common among affected children.

Pulmonary Atresia (With Stenosis and an Intact Ventricular Septum). PA is a right-sided obstructive lesion. The pulmonary valve is completely fused, which obstructs the egress of blood from the right ventricle and into the lungs. PA affects one in every 10,000 liveborn infants within the United States (CDC, 2024g). The atresia may accompany an intact ventricular septum, or present with a VSD and a degree of PA stenosis (Figure 5.26).

The pathogenesis of PA with an intact ventricular septum is well understood. Blood enters the right atrium, traverses the tricuspid valve, and travels into the right ventricle. Blood is thereby unable to enter the PA, due to the atretic pulmonary valve, and is redirected toward the right atrium. Regurgitation across the tricuspid valve occurs, right atrial preload increases, and blood is preferentially shunted in a right-to-left direction across the foramen ovale. Once within the left atrium, the blood mixes with oxygenated blood exiting the pulmonary system and is routed to the left ventricle and through the aorta. A portion of this blood is redirected across the PDA, which is the only mechanism by which blood reaches the pulmonary system. Once the PDA closes, the conduit to the pulmonary system is removed and infants quickly manifest cyanosis and respiratory distress. Auscultation of the heart yields a single (not split) second heart sound with or without a murmur. Once surgically corrected, the prognosis is promising. Aerobic and exercise capacity are typically decreased among older adults (Karamlou et al., 2013). In rare circumstances, affected infants require cardiac transplantation.

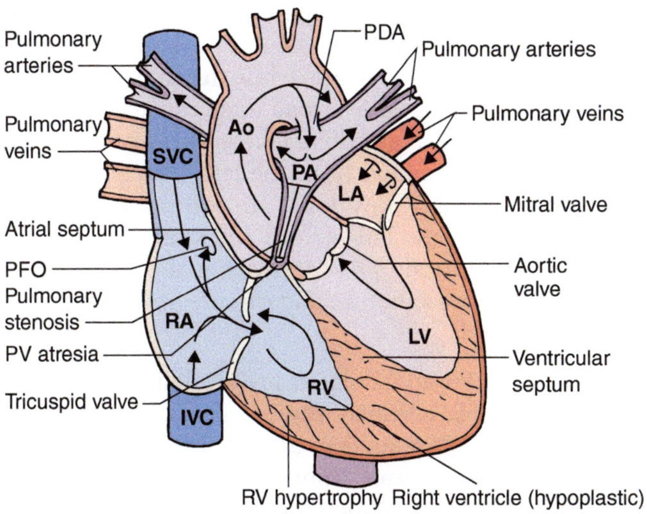

Figure 5.26 Pulmonary valve atresia with stenosis and intact ventricular septum. Arrows reflect the abnormal blood flow pattern.

Ao, aorta; IVC, inferior vena cava; LA, left atrium; LV, left ventricle; PA, pulmonary artery; PDA, patent ductus arteriosus; PFO, patent foramen ovale; PV, pulmonary valve; RA, right atrium; RV, right ventricle; SVC, superior vena cava.

Aortic Stenosis. Aortic stenosis is the most common valvular disease. It is a left-sided obstructive cardiac defect that results in decreased systemic perfusion to the body. The global incidence of all forms of congenital aortic stenosis is estimated at 1% to 2%, with a male-to-female (3:1) prevalence (Bonow & Greenland, 2015; Mordi & Tzemos, 2012). Narrowing of the valve orifice leads to the left-sided outflow obstruction. We focus this discussion upon bicuspid aortic valve disease, the most common congenital form of aortic stenosis. A male-to-female prevalence of bicuspid (dual-leaflet) aortic stenosis, as well as recurrence risk within families, is reported. Genetic influences, specifically related to mutations in the *NOTCH1* gene, may predispose the fetus to developing a bicuspid aortic valve (Irtyuga et al., 2017).

Normally, heart valves have three fleshy flaps, or cusps, which open with each beat of the heart. Stenotic valves, however, have less leaflet mobility due to thickening or fusion of one or both of the leaflets. This prevents the valve from opening up widely, resulting in obstruction to left ventricular outflow (Figure 5.27).

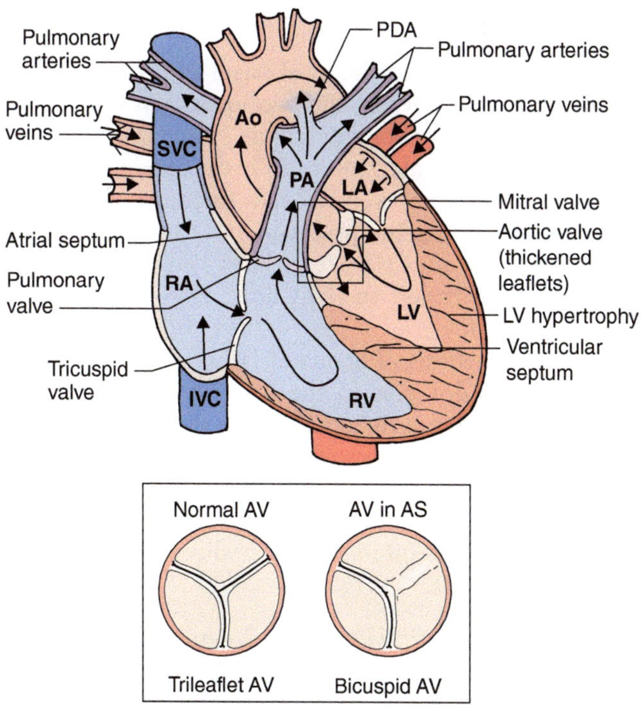

Figure 5.27 Aortic stenosis. Arrows reflect the abnormal blood flow pattern.

Ao, aorta; AS, aortic stenosis; AV, atrioventricular; IVC, inferior vena cava; LA, left atrium; LV, left ventricle; PA, pulmonary artery; PDA, patent ductus arteriosus; RA, right atrium; RV, right ventricle; SVC, superior vena cava.

As previously reviewed, aortic stenosis creates an obstruction to flow out of the left ventricle. As the stenosis progresses, increased afterload is noted within the left ventricle. This leads to endocardial ischemia and hypertrophy, scarring (endocardial fibroelastosis), ventricular failure, and decreased systemic CO. As left ventricular incompetence progresses, blood is diverted in a left-to-right direction across the foramen ovale, which increases pulmonary recirculation and magnifies the ensuing CHF. Once the PDA closes (the only significant conduit to the pulmonary system and systemic circulation), systemic CO significantly decreases (Estévez & Ansah, 2024).

The pathogenesis described here may escalate to a severe level, referred to as *critical aortic stenosis.* In these cases, the aortic pressure gradient increases from 30 mmHg (mild stenosis) to 60 mmHg (severe stenosis), further compromising systemic CO (Estévez & Ansah, 2024). Although manifestations of milder forms of aortic stenosis may be delayed, critical aortic stenosis typically manifests in the immediate postnatal period. Indices of cardiogenic shock, including diminished peripheral pulses with prolonged capillary refill time, are typically observed. Auscultation yields a harsh ejection murmur over the aortic region. Early identification is critical to reestablish ductal patency. Life-span implications extend across the life span. Valvular replacement therapy is not considered curative, and patients often require exercise restrictions.

Other Cardiovascular Disease Processes

Heart Failure. HF, in the most basic terms, can be defined as the inability of the cardiovascular system to meet systemic metabolic demands (Mille & Ravishankar, 2023; Ryan et al., 2018). While the incidence of HF in the neonate is not well-defined, the most commonly reported etiology is the presence of a cardiomyopathy, followed by certain CHDs (e.g., large ventricular septal defect, PDA with left-to-right flow; Levy et al., 2018; Ryan et al., 2018).

The pathogenesis of neonatal HF is described using myriad methodologies in the literature. We encourage APRN students to consider the three root causes for HF: (a) pulmonary over-perfusion, (b) pressure overload, and (c) pump failure, and explore applicable cause-and-effect relationships (McGinn et al., 2023). The following text offers a concise discussion of these root causes for HF.

Pulmonary Overperfusion. From a cardiovascular lens, "overperfusion" refers to a state of high pressure and flow through the vasculature, and most notably the heart and pulmonary vasculature. Under normal circumstances, the first breaths after birth inflate the lungs, establish transpulmonary pressure, and encourage the egress of fetal lung fluid. Transepithelial fluid is typically cleared within a few hours of birth and fetal lung fluid moves from the interstitium to the pulmonary microcirculation by 6 hours of life. This process increases pulmonary blood flow and decreases hydrostatic pressure in the pulmonary circulation. However, certain pathologies (e.g., congenital heart lesions) can impede normal process, causing overperfusion, increased hydrostatic pressure, and HF. Examples include a large and unrestricted VSD, AVC defect, truncus arteriosus, aortopulmonary window, and PDA (Ryan et al., 2018). Extracardiac shunts, such as arteriovenous malformations, can also lead to cardiomyopathy-inducing HF (Mille & Ravishankar, 2023; Ryan et al., 2018).

The pathogenesis of pulmonary overcirculation is complex. As PVR decreases after birth, blood flow into the pulmonary microvasculature is increased. Over time, this increases the normal workload of the left ventricle, ultimately leading to dilation of the left ventricle and atria. Under normal conditions in a healthy heart, stretching the heart muscle encourages improved CO via the Frank–Starling mechanism (see prior discussion). However, the immature heart is less responsive and unable to compensate for this additional preload, leading to decreased CO and increased myocardial oxygen consumption (Sahni et al., 2015). Hepatomegaly and pulmonary venous congestion develop secondary to the volume overload manifesting clinically as tachypnea, tachycardia, feeding intolerance, and failure to thrive (McGinn et al., 2023; Ryan et al., 2018).

Pressure Overload. Left-sided obstructive heart lesions, such as aortic stenosis, coarctation of the aorta, and HLHS, result in left-heart pressure overload, reduced CO, and precipitate HF (McGinn et al., 2023; Mille & Ravishankar, 2023; Ryan et al., 2018). Given the presence of a left-side obstruction, blood flowing from the four pulmonary veins into the left heart creates a state of pressure overload. This forces ventricular remodeling (changes in the size, shape, structure, and function of the left heart) while the consistently elevated state of pressure overload upon the left ventricle forces an increase in afterload (the amount of pressure necessary to eject blood from the left ventricle). Over time, left-sided HF develops. In addition, elevated pressures within the left atrium and ventricle lead to increased hydrostatic pressure within the pulmonary veins and microvasculature and can precipitate pulmonary edema.

Pump Failure. Pump failure, or myocardial dysfunction, may be further subdivided into primary and secondary causes (Mille & Ravishankar, 2023). Primary causes of cardiomyopathies result from inherited disorders including inborn errors of metabolism, genetic conditions, or myocarditis linked to an inflammatory or infectious etiology. Common secondary causes include prolonged tachyarrhythmias (e.g., reentrant tachyarrythmias, SVT), perinatal asphyxia, sepsis, and abnormalities of the coronary arteries (e.g., anomalous left coronary artery from the pulmonary artery [ALCAPA]). Sustained tachycardia in utero may result in hydrops fetalis if ventricular dysfunction is profound (Ryan et al., 2018). Whatever the antecedent cause, ventricular dysfunction leads to reduced CO and reduced systemic (and pulmonary) blood flow, giving way for the onset of HF (McGinn et al., 2023).

Clinical Manifestations. The timing of the presentation of manifestations of HF depends upon the underlying cause for the disease process. Fetal HF (as well as hydrops and death) is often linked to refractory arrhythmias (that do not respond to transplacental cardioversion, fetal cardioversion, or combination pharmacotherapies including digoxin and flecainide), a CHD like Ebstein anomaly, or even the result of high CO states like anemia or twin-to-twin transfusion (Sahni et al., 2015). Early HF in the first days of life is typically attributed to causes that disrupt myocardial function (e.g., perinatal asphyxia, sepsis, persistent pulmonary hypertension). HF beyond the second week of life is often related to a pulmonary overcirculation and pressure overload etiology.

Characteristic signs of HF include edema (although this is less common in neonates), respiratory distress (e.g., tachypnea, increased work of breathing, rales on auscultation), tachycardia, delayed capillary refill, hepatomegaly, diaphoresis, growth failure, and inability to tolerate activity (Mille & Ravishankar, 2023; Ryan et al., 2018; Sahni et al., 2015).

Life-span implications are determined by the underlying cause. While HF due to congenital heart disease is the most frequent cause in neonates, the overall mortality for these patients is lower compared to HF due to other causes (Hinton & Ware, 2017). HF is an associated morbidity in the adult living with CHD, developing in approximately 25% by age 30 and increasing with advancing age.

Cardiomyopathies. Cardiomyopathies are defined as abnormalities of the ventricular myocardium resulting in mechanical or electrical cardiac dysfunction. Five types of cardiomyopathies are recognized: (a) DCM, (b) HCM, (c) restrictive cardiomyopathy (RCM), (d) arrhythmogenic ventricular cardiomyopathy (AVCM), and (e) left ventricular noncompaction cardiomyopathy (LVNC). These diseases are classified as inherited or acquired. Cardiomyopathies affect one in every 100,000 children; children less than 1 year of age are considered at highest risk (Lipshultz et al., 2013). With the exception of AVCM, most cardiomyopathies present at birth or during early infancy. If not previously recognized, infants may present with life-threatening decompensation associated with an unrelated minor illness such as viral infection. Cardiomyopathy is the primary reason for heart transplantation in infants and children. This discussion will focus on the two most common cardiomyopathies that implicate infants: DCM and HCM (see Table 5.8). An understanding of these types of cardiomyopathy will allow the practitioner to determine the most appropriate diagnostic workup. A final diagnosis

TABLE 5.8 Cardiomyopathies and Associated Conditions

Diseases Associated With Dilated Cardiomyopathy	Diseases Associated With Hypertrophic Cardiomyopathy
Idiopathic in approximately 75% of cases	Idiopathic in >60% of cases
Myocarditis • Viral: parvovirus B19, coxsackievirus, adenovirus, echovirus, cytomegalovirus	Malformation syndromes • Noonan syndrome (autosomal dominant mutation on the *PTPN11* gene) • Beckwith-Wiedemann syndrome • Costello syndrome • Eagle Barrett (prune belly) syndrome
Neuromuscular disorders • Duchenne or Becker muscular dystrophy (X-linked)	Metabolic disorders • Pompe disease (autosomal recessive glycogen storage type II) Fatty acid oxidation disorders • Carnitine deficiency • Medium-chain acyl-coenzyme A (CoA) dehydrogenase deficiency
Familial DCM (majority are autosomal dominant)	Mitochondrial defects • Disorders of oxidative phosphorylation including Complex I, III, and IV deficiency • MELAS syndrome (**M**itochondrial myopathy, **E**ncephalopathy, **L**actic **A**cidosis, and **S**troke-like episodes)
Mitochondrial defects • Barth syndrome • Kearns-Sayre syndrome tRNA(Leu(UUR))-3242 mutation most common)	Hyperinsulinism • IDMs • Congenital hyperinsulinism

DCM, dilated cardiomyopathy; IDMs, infants of diabetic mothers.

Sources: Mallavarapu, A., & Taksande, A. (2022). Dilated cardiomyopathy in children: Early detection and treatment. *Cureus, 14*(11), e31111. https://doi.org/10.7759/cureus.31111; Wallis, G., & Fricker, F. J. (2012). Neonatal cardiomyopathy. *NeoReviews, 13*(12), e711–e723. https://doi.org/10.1542/neo.13-12-e711; Wilkinson, J. D., Westphal, J. A., Bansal, N., Czachor, J. D., Razoky, H., & Lipshultz, S. E. (2015). Lessons learned from the Pediatric Cardiomyopathy Registry (PCMR) Study Group. *Cardiology in the Young, 25*(Suppl. 2), 140–153. https://doi.org/10.1017/S1047951115000943

may lead to optimal therapy but more importantly may facilitate the genetic evaluation of other family members if indicated.

Dilated Cardiomyopathy. DCM is the most prevalent type of cardiomyopathy in children. DCM affects 0.57 per 100,000 children and accounts for approximately 50% or more of all cases of pediatric cardiomyopathy (Lipshultz et al., 2003). Various etiologies for DCM are reported across the literature. Acquired causes include placental insufficiency, nonimmune hydrops, renal or hepatic failure, acute stress (i.e., hypoxia), myocarditis, and chemotherapy-induced DCM. Alternatively, DCM can develop secondary to genetic mutations, within all of the known genes that code the actin (thin) filament, and, to a lesser extent, thick (myosin) filament. In addition, gene mutations in the Z-line, cytoskeleton, and desmosome are reported. Inherited and metabolic forms of the disease include carnitine deficiency and glycogen storage disease (Kulik & Levy, 2022; T. M. Lee et al., 2017).

Acquired or genetic causes give rise to abnormal shortening of the sarcomere during contraction and depressed ventricular function. Thinning of the wall of the left ventricle occurs. This leads to progressive myocardial incompetence and enlargement of the left ventricle, with resultant systolic and diastolic dysfunction.

After delivery in the infant with significant DCM, there is impairment of the ventricles to contract, leading to decreased CO. The infant attempts to respond initially by increasing the heart rate to improve CO. Left atrial filling pressure is elevated due to diastolic dysfunction of the dilated left ventricle, especially if there is mitral insufficiency (Martinez et al., 2022). The clinical presentation ranges from asymptomatic to acute HF and shock. Findings reported among neonates include irritability, feeding difficulties, poor distal perfusion, and poor growth velocity. Atrial or ventricular arrhythmias, sinus tachycardia, mitral valve regurgitation, and gallop rhythms are common. Radiographic evidence includes cardiomegaly, pulmonary edema, and pleural effusions as a result of left ventricular dysfunction, increased left atrial pressures, and pulmonary venous congestion. An elevated B-type natriuretic peptide is present as a result of worsening CO. Progressive worsening of myocardial function may manifest with hepatomegaly. Flattening of the T waves and ST segment depression can be seen on EKG; with carnitine deficiency, a giant T wave is seen. Survivability among patients who do not receive cardiac transplantation is between 60% and 75%, and of those patients, merely 20% to 45% recapture normal cardiovascular function (Kulik & Levy, 2022; T. M. Lee et al., 2017).

Hypertrophic Cardiomyopathy. HCM is the second most prevalent type of cardiomyopathy in children. The incidence is 0.47 per 100,000 children, and this disease implicates approximately 40% of the pediatric population (Martinez et al., 2022). HCM can occur in isolation but it is most commonly a consequence of autosomal dominant genetic inheritance. Genetic etiologies include gene mutations that code the thin (actin) and thick (myosin) filaments in the sarcomere, RASopathies, and neurodegenerative and mitochondrial disorders (T. M. Lee et al., 2017). In addition, HCM is a commonly recognized complication in infants of diabetic mothers (IDM), as well as infants with congenital hyperinsulinism. It has been suggested that the hypertrophy in IDMs is a result of fetal hyperinsulinism, leading to proliferation and hypertrophy of cardiac myocytes triggered by increased proteins and fat synthesis. Few cases have been reported that link transient HCM with perinatal stress.

The pathogenesis of HCM involves symmetrical or asymmetrical hypertrophy, or thickening, of the walls and interventricular septum of the left ventricle, resulting in left ventricular outflow tract obstruction. Some affected infants develop hypertrophy of both the left and right ventricles. Hypertrophy of cardiomyocytes occurs. This leads to aberrant cardiac depolarization and contraction, which gives rise to myofibrillar disarray and interstitial fibrosis (Kulik & Levy, 2022). With significant left ventricular hypertrophy, there is diastolic dysfunction with an increase in the end-diastolic pressure. Coronary insufficiency and ischemia can occur as a result of decreased coronary perfusion pressure from the increased end-diastolic pressure and the increased myocardial oxygen demand (Martinez et al., 2022).

Specific to the IDM, fetal hyperinsulinism in response to hyperglycemia in the XX pregnant patient results in this pathologic, yet reversible, hypertrophy of the ventricular wall and septum. The immediate neonatal course may be complicated by diastolic dysfunction and LVOT obstruction resulting in significant CHF (Yeh & Berger, 2015). In cases of congenital hyperinsulinism, gene mutations to ion channels, including the highly sensitive β-cell ATP-sensitive potassium (K_{ATP}) channel, lead to hypersecretion of insulin by β-cells in either a focal or diffuse manner. Unlike HCM associated with the IDM, that which is associated with congenital hyperinsulinism is not reversible and is often refractory to K_{ATP} channel agonists and diazoxide (Huang et al., 2013).

The clinical presentation ranges from asymptomatic to HF. Left ventricular outflow tract obstruction and dysfunction, and ventricular arrhythmias, are common. Outflow tract obstructions resulting in an increased afterload on the heart may give rise to mitral valve regurgitation and manifest with an audible murmur. Diastolic dysfunction resulting in elevated pulmonary venous pressure is associated with a pathologic gallop rhythm. Radiographic evidence includes cardiomegaly. Twenty-five percent will have normal EKGs; if there is not left ventricular outflow tract obstruction, the remaining will have ST- and T-wave changes. Mortality risk is 30% among infants diagnosed with HCM as a result of progressive CHF. Five-year survivability is estimated at 97%

and 10-year survivability is at 94% (Kulik & Levy, 2022; T. M. Lee et al., 2017). Of infants who develop HCM secondary to congenital hyperinsulinism, pancreatectomy is often required.

CONCLUSION

Heart defects are the single most common congenital defects reported in the literature. As such, it is critical that APRNs establish core understanding of normal and abnormal fetal and postnatal cardiovascular physiology. APRNs are encouraged to adopt active and multisensory learning methods; connecting core content with a clinical vignette adds meaning to the mundane. Rehearsing the creation of simple sketches of heart lesions during the learning process conditions clinicians to provide parents with a concrete look at their child's anatomy during difficult conversations. Parents are often overwhelmed and anxious to blame themselves for their infant's diagnosis. Long-term risks vary; however, cognitive and social impairment are common among children affected by CHDs (Figure 5.28). Therefore, the ability to clearly communicate complex information and evidence-based prognostics, balanced with sentiments of support and hope for the future, is essential. This allows parents to understand the relationship between current medical management plans and health promotion (Brosig et al., 2017).

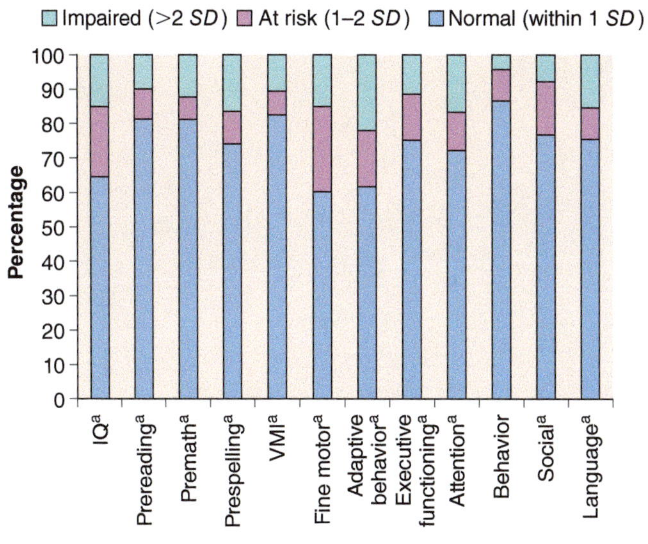

Figure 5.28 Percentage of children with congenital heart disease tested at 4 to 5 years in the normal, at risk, and impaired ranges on neurodevelopmental measures.

[a]More delays than normal, adjusted $p < .05$.

VMI, visual motor integration.

Source: Adapted from Brosig, C. L., Bear, L., Allen, S., Hoffmann, R. G., Pan, A., Frommelt, M., & Mussatto, K. A. (2017). Preschool neurodevelopmental outcomes in children with congenital heart disease. *The Journal of Pediatrics, 183*, 80–86. https://doi.org/10.1016/j.jpeds.2016.12.044

This Chapter Is Dedicated to the Memory of Dhillon Shah

A message from Dhillon's family:

Dhillon Jordan Shah was diagnosed with complex single ventricle, a variant of HLHS, in the first few days of life, but despite numerous surgeries and setbacks lived a life of joy, hope, and courage. Sadly, he passed away at the age of 12½ during a long-awaited heart transplant. His family and friends provided him unconditional support during those years, and the skill of his healthcare providers was critical.

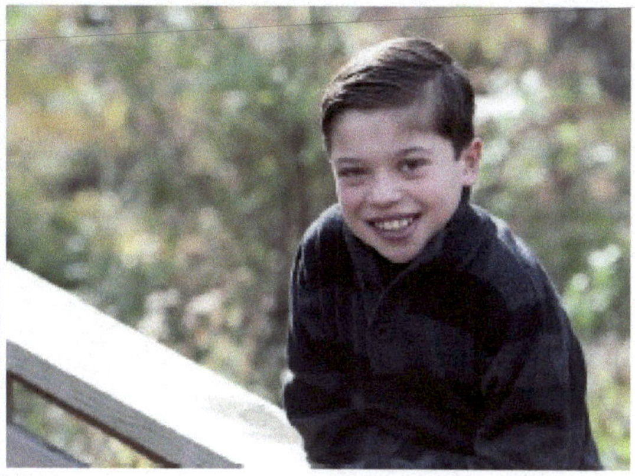

What are the attributes of those caregivers, mostly nurses, that we remember most, that prompted us to take photos of them, that produced big hugs and smiles when they were at the bedside? They conveyed caring in so many small things they did: a smile, the appreciation of a joke, a shared board game, the attempt to do treatments just the way he wanted, the tolerance of favorite foods, the offering of respite time for Mom so she could get a shower, their support of his family. They conveyed hope and positive energy along with the technical expertise that we trusted. They communicated effectively, listening carefully and letting us know they were with us every step of the way. They provided information we could hang on to and later read. They listened to our family, respected our needs and rules, and took the time to understand Dhillon's unique journey, anticipating next steps so we were prepared. They were hypervigilant, always advocating for Dhillon's care. They were our lifeline to other valued members of the health team, our allies, our partners, and some of Dhillon's best friends. When we sadly celebrated his short life in a memorial gathering, they supported us there as well and even beyond as we grieved. Many thanks to those who traveled with Dhillon on his journey, and to all who will have the privilege to do so with other children. You are very special!

LEARNING TOOLS AND RESOURCES

CourseConnect

To access self-assessment questions and interactive, competency-based learning activities for this chapter, visit www.springerpub.com/courseconnect. See inside front cover and tear-out card for CourseConnect details.

Podcast

This podcast is available online by visiting www.springerpub.com/courseconnect. See inside front cover and tear-out card for CourseConnect details.

Case-Based Learning: Patent Ductus Arteriosus

Jacqui Hoffman and Nicole Bowie

Discussion Prompts

1. Explain expected cardiovascular embryologic development and defects that may occur as a result of abnormal development.
2. Compare and contrast fetal circulation, transitional circulation after delivery, and neonatal circulation.
3. Sinus bradycardia may be a normal finding in hospitalized infants. Discuss the physiology of sinus bradycardia and how it typically manifests in the newborn.
4. The cardiovascular physical examination aids in the development of a differential diagnosis list with a suspected congenital heart infant. Correlate the pearls of the cardiovascular exam with your understanding of cardiac anatomy and physiology.

Advice From the Editors

The cardiovascular system, at first glance, may seem like a daunting body system to learn. However, I suggest approaching this content in a multisensory manner. If you thrive by listening to content, rely on podcasts and create your own mini-lectures. If you are a visual learner, take the time to draw out the normal heart and common defects, mapping out the blood flow and any mixing that may occur. And last, test yourself by explaining these concepts to others in your workplace. The more senses you incorporate into your learning process, and the more iterations you weave into the learning process, the more likely you are to retain the information and be able to apply it in practice.

MIND MAP

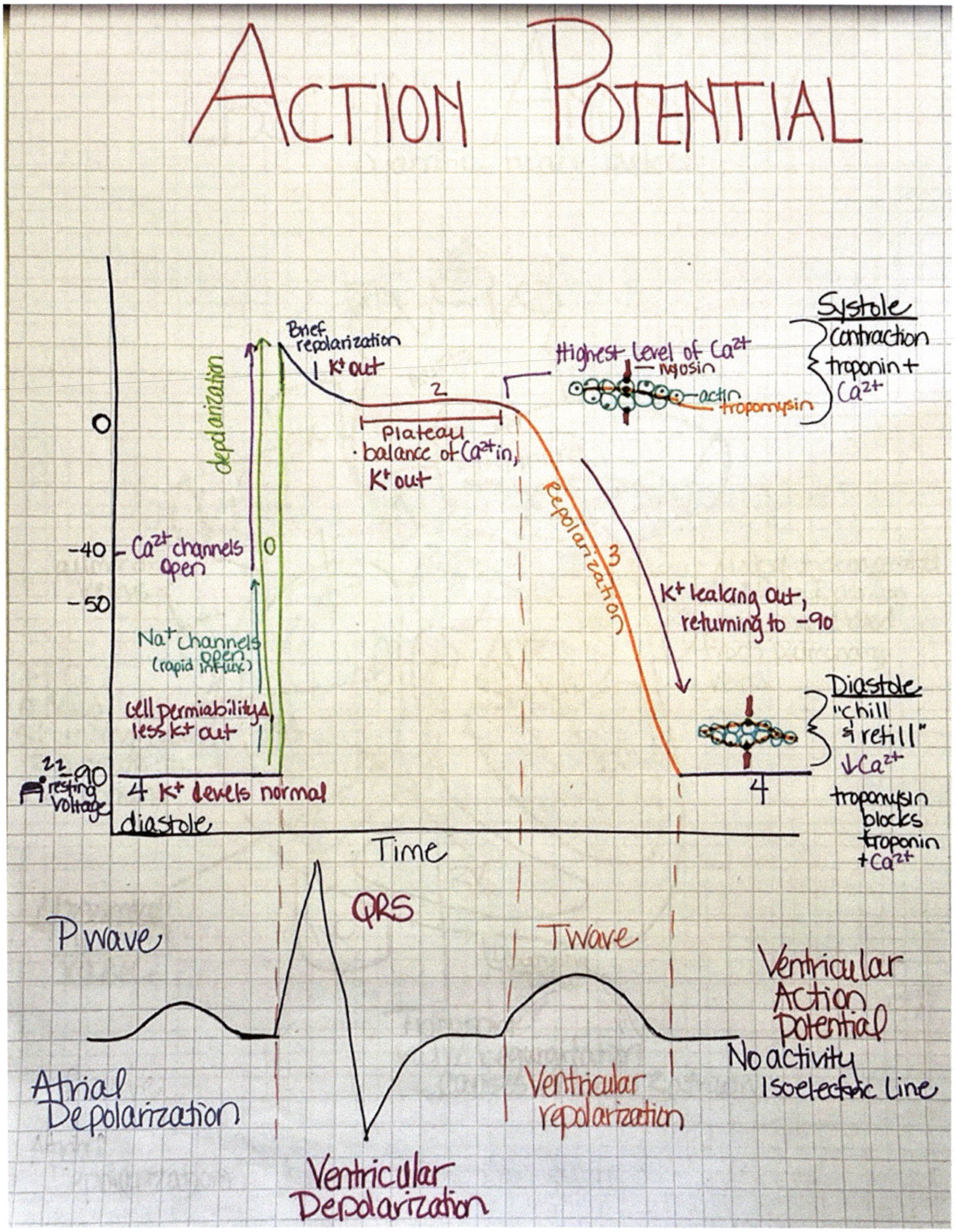

Note. *This mind map reflects one neonatal nurse practitioner student's interpretation of a concept addressed in this chapter. Readers should regard the mind maps woven throughout this textbook as examples of multisensory study tools that can be developed to aid conceptual understanding. Readers are encouraged to develop their own unique mind maps in consultation with academic faculty or clinical preceptors.*

Image credit: Lauren McCotter, MSN, APRN, NNP.

TIMELINE OF ORGAN DEVELOPMENT

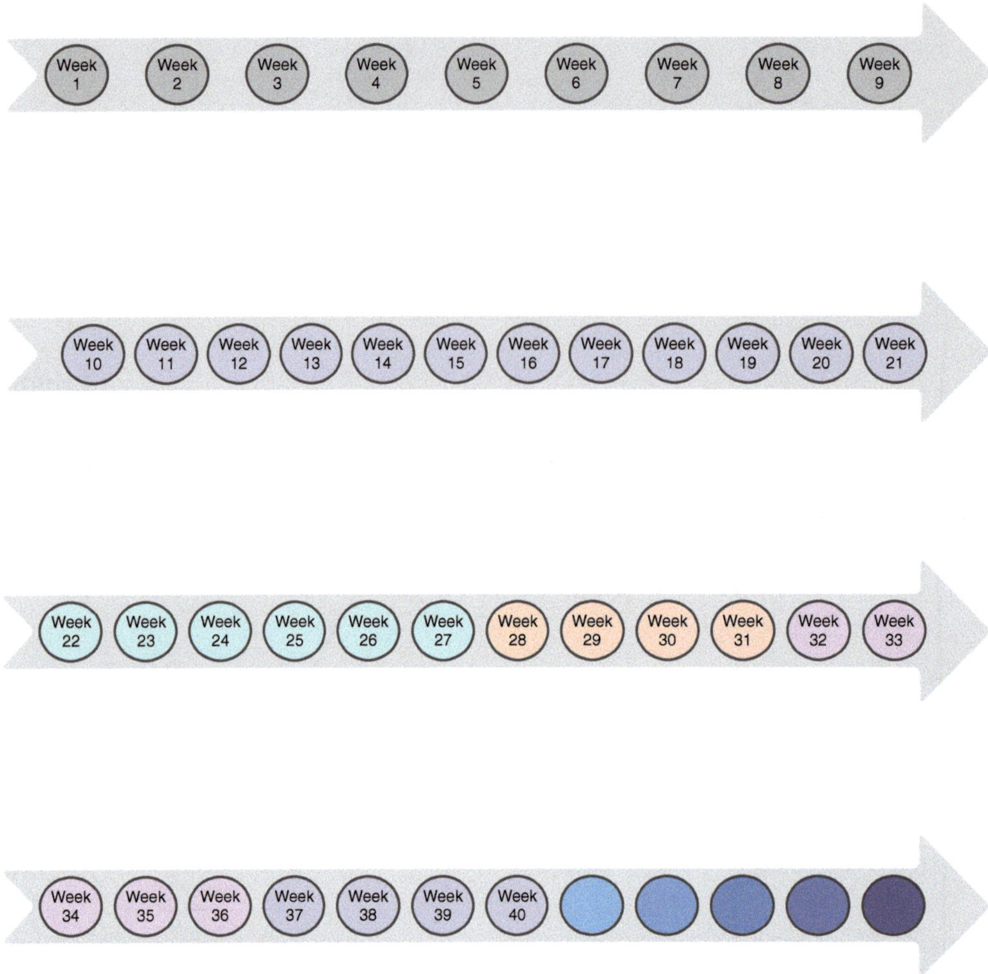

Note: Placement of common problems is meant to offer visual/ conceptual perspective on the timing of onset of these commonly reported malformations. Variation exists across the literature.	***Legend:*** <22 – 27 6/7 weeks = extremely preterm 28 – 31 6/7 weeks = very preterm 32 – 36 6/7 weeks = late/moderate preterm 37 – 40 weeks = term

Note: Readers should annotate the blank timeline during studying, self-directed learning, and creation of feedback loops with mentors. To access the blank and completed timelines visit www.springerpub.com/courseconnect. See inside front cover and tear-out card for CourseConnect details.

REFERENCES

Abqari, S., Gupta, A., Shahab, T., Rabbami, M. U., Ali, S. M., & Firdaus, U. (2016). Profile and risk factors for congenital heart defects: A study in a tertiary care hospital. *Annals of Pediatric Cardiology, 9*(3), 216–221. doi:10.4103/0974-2069.189119

Acharya, G., Gui, Y., Cnota, W., Huhta, J., & Wloch, A. (2016). Human embryonic cardiovascular function. *Acta Obstetricia et Gynecologica Scandinavia, 95*(6), 621–628. https://doi.org/10.1111/aogs.12860

Artman, M., Mahoney, L., & Teitel, D. (2017). *Neonatal cardiology* (3rd ed.). McGraw-Hill.

Backer, C., Eltayeb, O., Mongé, M., Mazwi, M., & Costello, J. (2016). Shunt lesions part I: Patent ductus arteriosus, atrial septal defect, ventricular septal defect, and atrioventricular septal defect. *Pediatric Critical Care Medicine, 17*(8 Suppl.), S302–309. https://doi.org/10.1097/PCC.0000000000000786

Bakker, M. K., Bergman, J. E. H., Krikov, S., Amar, E., Cocchi, G., Cragan, J., de Walle, H. E. K., Gatt, M., Groisman, B., Liu, S., Nembhard, W. N., Pierini, A., Rissmann, A., Chidambarathanu, S., Sipek Jr, A., Szabova, E., Tagliabue, G., Tucker, D., Mastroiacovo, P., & Botto, L. D. (2019). Prenatal diagnosis and prevalence of critical congenital heart defects: An international retrospective cohort study. *BMJ Open, 9*(7), e028139–e028139. https://doi.org/10.1136/bmjopen-2018-028139

Benitz, W. E., & Bhombal, S. (2025). Patent ductus arteriosus. In R. J. Martin & A. A. Fanaroff (Eds.), *Fanaroff and Martin's neonatal-perinatal medicine: Diseases of the fetus and infant* (12th ed., pp. 1401–1410). Elsevier.

Bensley, J., De Matteo, R., Harding, R., & Black, M. (2016). The effects of preterm birth and its antecedents on the cardiovascular system. *Acta Obstetricia et Gynecologica Scandinavica, 95*(6), 652–663. https://doi.org/10.1111/aogs.12880

Bernstein, D. (2025). Cyanotic congenital heart disease: Lesions associated with increased pulmonary blood flow. In R. M. Kliegman, J. W. St Geme, N. J. Blum, R. C. Tasker, K. M. Wilson, A. M. Schuh, & C. L. Mack (Eds.), *Nelson textbook of pediatrics* (pp. 2811–2826.e2). Elsevier.

Biron-Shental, T., & Hershkovich-Shporen, C. (2025). Fetal effects of autoimmune disease. In R. J. Martin & A. A. Fanaroff (Eds.), *Fanaroff and Martin's neonatal-perinatal medicine: Diseases of the fetus and infant* (12th ed., pp. 352–360). Elsevier.

Bohn, M. K., Steele, S., Hall, A., Poonia, J., Jung, B., & Adeli, K. (2021). Cardiac biomarkers in pediatrics: An undervalued resource. *Clinical Chemistry, 67*(7), 947–958. https://doi.org/10.1093/clinchem/hvab063

Bonow, R. O., & Greenland, P. (2015). Population-wide trends in aortic stenosis incidence and outcomes. *Circulation, 131*(11), 969–971. https://doi.org/10.1161/CIRCULATIONAHA.115.014846

Boulgakoff, L., D'Amato, G., & Miquerol, L. (2024). Molecular regulation of cardiac conduction system development. *Current Cardiology Reports, 26*(9), 943–952. https://doi.org/10.1007/s11886-024-02094-7

Bouma, B., & Mulder, B. (2017). Changing landscape of congenital heart disease. *Circulation Research, 120*, 908–922. https://doi.org/10.1161/CIRCRESAHA.116.309302

Braga, M., Moleiro, M. L., & Guedes-Martins, L. (2019). Clinical significance of ductus venosus waveform as generated by pressure-volume changes in the fetal heart. *Current Cardiology Reviews, 15*(3), 167–176. https://doi.org/10.2174/1573403X15666190115142303

Brosens, E., Eussen, H., van Bever, Y., van der Helm, R. M., Ijsselstijn, H., Zaveri, H. P., Wijnen, R., Scott, D. A., Tibboel, D., & de Klein, A. (2013). VACTERL association etiology: The impact of de novo and rare copy number variations. *Molecular Syndromology, 4*, 20–26. https://doi.org/10.1159/000345577

Brosig, C., Bear, L., Allen, S., Hoffmann, R., Pan, A., Frommelt, M., & Mussatto, K. (2017). Preschool neurodevelopmental outcomes in children with congenital heart disease. *Journal of Pediatrics, 183*, 80–86.e1. https://doi.org/10.1016/j.jpeds.2016.12.044

Centers for Disease Control and Prevention. (2024a, October 11). Specific congenital heart defects. CDC website. https://www.cdc.gov/heart-defects/about/specific-heart-defects.html

Centers for Disease Control and Prevention. (2024b, October 21). *About atrial septal defect.* https://www.cdc.gov/heart-defects/about/atrial-septal-defect.html

Centers for Disease Control and Prevention. (2024c, October 11). *About atrioventricular septal defect.* https://www.cdc.gov/heart-defects/about/atrioventricular-septal-defect.html

Centers for Disease Control and Prevention. (2024d, October 19). *About coarctation of the aorta.* https://www.cdc.gov/heart-defects/about/coarctation-of-the-aorta.html

Centers for Disease Control and Prevention. (2024e, May 15). *About dextro-transposition of the great arteries (d-TGA).* https://www.cdc.gov/heart-defects/about/d-tga.html

Centers for Disease Control and Prevention. (2024f, October 4). *About hypoplastic left heart syndrome.* https://www.cdc.gov/heart-defects/about/hypoplastic-left-heart-syndrome.html

Center for Disease Control and Prevention (2024g). About pulmonary atresia. CDC Website. https://www.cdc.gov/heart-defects/about/pulmonary-atresia.html

Centers for Disease Control and Prevention. (2024g, October 21). *About tetralogy of Fallot.* https://www.cdc.gov/heart-defects/about/tetralogy-of-fallot.html

Centers for Disease Control and Prevention. (2024h, October 21). *About total anomalous pulmonary venous return.* https://www.cdc.gov/heart-defects/about/tapvr.html

Centers for Disease Control and Prevention. (2024i, October 21). *About truncus arteriosus.* https://www.cdc.gov/heart-defects/about/truncus-arteriosus.html

Centers for Disease Control and Prevention. (2024j, October 21). *About tricuspid atresia.* https://www.cdc.gov/heart-defects/about/tricuspid-atresia.html

Centers for Disease Control and Prevention. (2024b, May 15). *Facts about ventricular septal defect.* U.S. Department of Health and Human Services. https://www.cdc.gov/heart-defects/about/ventricular-septal-defect.html

Chen, H. (2012). *Atlas of genetic diagnosis and counseling* (2nd ed.). Springer Verlag.

Chen, Y., Liu, Z., Chen, J., Zuo, Y., Liu, S., Chen, W., Liu, G., Qiu, G., Giampietro, P. F., Wu, N., & Wu, Z. (2016). The genetic landscape and clinical implications of vertebral anomalies in VACTERL association. *Journal of Medical Genetics, 53*, 431–437. https://doi.org/10.1136/jmedgenet-2015-103554

Choi, P. S., Baird, C. W., & Emani, S. M. (2024). Patent ductus arteriosus, coarctation of the aorta and vascular rings. In F. W. Sellke, P. J. del Nido & S. J. Swanson (Eds.), *Sabiston and Spencer surgery of the chest* (10th ed., pp. 2280–2302). Elsevier.

Chung, W., Boskovski, M. T., Brueckner, M., Anyane-Yeboa, K., & Gupta, P. (2012). The genetics of fetal and neonatal cardiovascular disease. In C. S. Kleinman & I. Seri (Eds.), *Hemodynamics and cardiology: Neonatology questions and controversies* (2nd ed., pp. 343–376). Elsevier Saunders.

Clyman, R. I., Couto, J., & Murphy, G. M. (2012). Patent ductus arteriosus: Are current neonatal treatment options better or worse than no treatment at all? *Seminars in Perinatology, 36*(2), 123–129. https://doi.org/10.1053/j.semperi.2011.09.022

Congenital Heart Public Health Consortium. (2024, March 29). *Health supervision for adolescents and young adults.* American Academy of Pediatrics. https://www.aap.org/en/patient-care/congenital-heart-defects/health-supervision-for-adolescents-and-young-adults

Corrigan, N., Brazil, D., & McAuliffe, F. (2009). Fetal cardiac effects of maternal hyperglycemia during pregnancy. *Birth Defects Research (Part A): Clinical and Molecular Teratology, 85*, 523–530. https://doi.org/10.1002/bdra.20567

Cruz-Lemini, M., Crispi, F., & Martinez Crespo, J. M. (2026). Anomalies of pulmonary venous return. In J. A. Copel, M. E. D'Alton, H. Feltvich, E. Gratacós, D. Krakow, A. O. Odibo, L. D. Platt, & B. Tutschek (Eds.), *Obstetric imaging: Fetal diagnosis and care* (3rd ed., pp. 284-286). Elsevier.

Cunningham, B. K., Hadley, D. W., Hannoush, H., Meltzer, A. C., Niforatos, N., Pineda-Alvarez, D., Sachdev, V., Warren-Mora , N., & Solomon, B. D. (2013). Analysis of cardiac anomalies in VACTERL association. *Birth Defects Research Part A: Clinical and Molecular Teratology, 97*(12), 792–797. https://doi.org/10.1002/bdra.23211

Duca, L. M., Pyle, L., Khanna, A. D., Ong, T., Kahn, M. G., DiGuiseppi, C., Scott, K., Daley, M. F., Costa, E., Davidson, A. J., & Crume, T. L. (2020). Estimating the prevalence of congenital heart disease among adolescents and adults in Colorado adjusted for incomplete case ascertainment. *The American Heart Journal, 221*, 95–105. https://doi.org/10.1016/j.ahj.2019.11.012

Dyer, A., & Ikemba, C. (2012). Core concepts: Fetal cardiac physiology. *NeoReviews, 13*(10), e583–e589. https://doi.org/10.1542/neo.13-10-e583

Edmondson, A. C., & Kalish, J. M. (2015). Overgrowth syndromes. *Journal of Pediatric Genetics, 4*(3), 136–143. https://doi.org/10.1055/s-0035-1564440

Estévez, N. G., & Ansah, D. A. (2024). Congenital heart disease. In C. A. Gleason & T. Sawyer (Eds.), *Avery's diseases of the newborn* (11th ed., pp. 743–771). Elsevier.

England, M. (1996). *Life before birth* (2nd ed.). Mosby-Wolfe.

Fineman, J., & Clyman, R. (2004). Fetal cardiovascular physiology. In R. Creasy, R. Resnik, & J. Iams (Eds.), *Maternal-fetal medicine: Principles and practice* (5th ed., pp. 160–163). Elsevier.

Ford, S. M., & Watanabe, M. (2025). Cardiac embryology. In R. J. Martin, A. A. Fanaroff, & M. C. Walsh (Eds.), *Fanaroff and Martin's neonatal-perinatal medicine: Diseases of the fetus and infant* (12th ed., pp. 1358–1371). Elsevier.

Gittenberger-de Groot, A. C., Bartelings, M. M., Poelmann, R. E., Haak, M. C., & Jongbloed, M. R. M. (2013). Embryology of the heart and its impact on understanding fetal and neonatal heart disease. *Seminars in Fetal and Neonatal Medicine, 18*(5), 237–244. https://doi.org/10.1016/j.siny.2013.04.008

Gobergs, R., Salputra, E., & Lubaua, I. (2016). Hypoplastic left heart syndrome: A review. *Acta Medica Lituanica, 23*(2), 86–98. https://doi.org/10.6001/actamedica.v23i2.3325

Goble, M. M., Yeh, J., von Alvensleben, J., & Panchangam, C. (2016). Cardiology and the newborn. *International Journal of Child Health and Human Development, 9*(1), 39. https://www.proquest.com/scholarly-journals/cardiology-newborn/docview/1781594869/se-2

Goldberg, C. S., Trachtenberg, F., William Gaynor, J., Mahle, W. T., Ravishankar, C., Schwartz, S. M., Cnota, J. F., Ohye, R. G., Gongwer, R., Taylor, M., Paridon, S., Frommelt, P. C., Afton, K., Atz, A. M., Burns, K. M., Detterich, J. A., Hill, K. D., Cabrera, A. G., Lewis, A. B., . . . on behalf of the Pediatric Heart Network Investigators. (2023). Longitudinal follow-up of children with HLHS and association between norwood shunt type and long-term outcomes: The SVR III study. *Circulation, 148*(17), 1330–1339. https://doi.org/10.1161/CIRCULATIONAHA.123.065192

Goldmuntz, E. (2020). 22q11.2 deletion syndrome and congenital heart disease. *American Journal of Medical Genetics. Part C, Seminars in Medical Genetics, 184*(1), 64–72. https://doi.org.10.1002/ajmg.c.31774

Goldsmith, J. P. (2025). Overview and initial management of delivery room resuscitation. In R. J. Martin & A. A. *Fanaroff (Eds.), Fanaroff and Martin's neonatal-perinatal medicine: Diseases of the fetus and infant* (12th ed., pp. 530–544). Elsevier.

Gomersall, J. C., Moore, V. M., Fernandez, R. C., Giles, L. C., Grzeskowiak, L. E., Davies, M. J., & Rumbold, A. R. (2024). Maternal modifiable factors and risk of congenital heart defects: Systematic review and causality assessment. *BMJ Open, 14*(8), e082961. https://doi.org/10.1136/bmjopen-2023-082961

Hagen-Ansert, S. J., & Guthrie, J. (2023). Fetal echocardiography: Beyond the four chambers. In S. J. Hagen-Ansert (Ed.), *Textbook of diagnostic sonography* (9th ed., pp. 1007-1030). Elsevier.

Han, J., Taberner, A. J., Loiselle, D. S., & Tran, K. (2022). Cardiac efficiency and Starling's law of the heart. *Journal of Physiology, 600*(19), 4265–4285. https://doi.org/10.1113/JP283632

Hines, M. (2013). Neonatal cardiovascular physiology. *Seminars in Pediatric Surgery, 22*, 174–178. https://doi.org/10.1053/j.sempedsurg.2013.10.004

Hinton, R. B., & Ware, S. M. (2017). Heart failure in pediatric patients with congenital heart disease. *Circulation Research, 120*, 978–994. https://doi.org/10.1161/CIRCRESAHA.116.308996

Hoffman, J. I. (2017). At what age should tetralogy of Fallot be corrected? *Cardiology in the Young, 27*(4), 625. https://doi.org/10.1017/S104795111600264X

Huang, T., Kelly, A., Becker, S. A., Cohen, M. S., & Stanley, C. A. (2013). Hypertrophic cardiomyopathy in neonates with congenital hyperinsulinism. *Archives of Disease in Childhood: Fetal and Neonatal Edition, 98*(4), F351–F354. https://doi.org/10.1136/archdischild-2012-302546

Hund, T. J., Smith, S. A., Makara, M. A., & Mohler, P. J. (2014). Cellular and molecular pathobiology of the cardiac conduction system. In M. S. Willis, J. W. Homeister, & J. R. Stone (Eds.), *Cellular and molecular pathobiology of cardiovascular disease* (pp. 121–134). Elsevier.

Irtyuga, O., Malashicheva, A., Zhiduleva, E., Freylikhman, O., Rotar, O., Bäck, M., Tarnovskaya, S., Kostareva, A., & Moiseeva, O. (2017). NOTCH1 mutations in aortic stenosis: Association with osteoprotegerin/RANK/RANKL. *BioMed Research International, 2017*, 6917907-10. https://doi.org/10.1155/2017/6917907

Jaramillo, F., Hernandez, C., Garzón, J. P., Sánchez Herrera, A. P., & Velasco Morales, M. L. (2017). Infracardiac type total anomalous pulmonary venous return with obstruction and dilatation of portal vein. *Radiology Case Reports, 12*(2), 229–232. https://doi.org/10.1016/j.radcr.2017.01.010

Jones, E. (2011). The initiation of blood flow and flow induced events in early vascular development. *Seminars in Cell & Developmental Biology, 22*, 1028–1035. https://doi.org/10.1016/j.semcdb.2011.09.020

Jongbloed, M. R. M., Steijn, R. V., Hahurij, N. D., Kelder, T. P., Schalij, M. J., Gittenberger-de Groot, A. C., & Blom, N. A. (2012). Normal and abnormal development of the cardiac conduction system; implications for conduction and rhythm disorders in the child and adult. *Differentiation, 84*(1), 131–148. https://doi.org/10.1016/j.diff.2012.04.006

Karamlou, T., Poynter, J. A., Walters, H. L., Rhodes, J., Bondarenko, I., Pasquali, S. K., Fuller, S. M., Lambert, L. M., Blackstone, E. H., Jacobs, M. L., Duncan, K., Caldarone, C. A., Williams, W. G., & McCrindle, B. W. (2013). Long-term functional health status and exercise test variables for patients with pulmonary atresia with intact ventricular septum: A Congenital Heart Surgeons Society study. *Journal of Thoracic and Cardiovascular Surgery, 145*(4), 1018–1027.e3 https://doi.org/10.1016/j.jtcvs.2012.11.092

Karlsen, K. A., & Cowley, C. G. (2021). *S.T.A.B.L.E.-cardiac module: Recognition and stabilization of neonates with severe CHD* (2nd ed.). S.T.A.B.L.E.

Khairy, P., Clair, M., Fernandes, S. M., Blume, E. D., Powell, A. J., Newburger, J. W., Landzberg, M. J., & Mayer, J. E. (2013).

Cardiovascular outcomes after the arterial switch operation for D-transposition of the great arteries. *Circulation, 127*(3), 331–339. https://doi.org/10.1161/circulationaha.112.135046

Kirby, M. L. (2002). Embryogenesis of transposition of the great arteries: A lesson from the heart. *Circulation Research, 91*(2), 87–89. https://doi.org/10.1161/01.RES.0000028301.40791.4F

Kiserud, T. (2005). Physiology of the fetal circulation. *Seminars in Fetal & Neonatal Medicine, 10*, 493–503. https://doi.org/10.1016/j.siny.2005.08.007

Kosiv, K. A., Mercurio, M. R., & Carey, J. C. (2023). The common trisomy syndromes, their cardiac implications, and ethical considerations in care. *Current Opinion in Pediatrics, 35*(5), 531–537. https://doi.org/10.1097/MOP.0000000000001278

Kulik, J. T., & Levy, P. T. (2022). Physiology of congenital heart disease in the neonate. In R. A. Polin, S. H. Abman., D. H. Rowitch, W. E. Benitz, & W. W. Fox (Eds.), *Fetal and neonatal physiology* (6th ed., pp. 521–534.e2). Elsevier.

Kumar, T. K. S. (2021). Ebstein's anomaly in the neonate. *Indian Journal of Thoracic and Cardiovascular Surgery, 37*(Suppl. 1), 17–25. https://doi.org/10.1007/s12055-020-00942-z

Lee, F. T., Seed, M., Sun, L., & Marini, D. (2021). Fetal brain issues in congenital heart disease. *Translational Pediatrics, 10*(8), 2182–2196. https://doi.org/10.21037/tp-20-224

Lee, T. M., Hsu, D. T., Kantor, P., Towbin, J. A., Ware, S. M., Colan, S. D., Chung, W. K., Jefferies, J. L., Rossano, J. W., Castleberry, C. D., Addonizio, L. J., Lal, A. K., Lamour, J. M., Miller, E. M., Thrush, P. T., Czachor, J. D., Razoky, H., Hill, A., & Lipshultz, S. E. (2017). Pediatric cardiomyopathies. *Circulation Research, 121*(7), 855–873. https://doi.org/10.1161/CIRCRESAHA.116.309386

Levy, P. T., Tissot, C., Horsberg Eriksen, B., Nestaas, E., Rogerson, S., McNamara, P. J., El-Khuffash, A., & de Boode, W. P. (2018). Application of neonatologist performed echocardiography in the assessment and management of neonatal heart failure unrelated to congenital heart disease. *Pediatric Research, 84*(Suppl. 1), 78–88. https://doi.org/10.1038/s41390-018-0075-z

Lipshultz, S. E., Orav, E. J., Wilkinson, J. D., Towbin, J. A., Messere, J. E., Lowe, A. M., Sleeper, L. A., Cox, G. F., Hsu, D. T., Canter, C. E., Hunter, J. A., Colan, S. D.; Pediatric cardiomyopathy registry study group. (2013). Risk stratification at diagnosis for children with hypertrophic cardiomyopathy: An analysis of data from the Pediatric Cardiomyopathy Registry. *Lancet, 382*(9908), 1889–1897. doi:10/1016/S0140-6736(13)61685-2

Mallavarapu, A., & Taksande, A. (2022). Dilated cardiomyopathy in children: Early detection and treatment. *Cureus, 14*(11), e31111. https://doi.org/10.7759/cureus.31111

Martin, B. J., Karamlou, T., & Tabbutt, S. (2016). Shunt lesions part II: Anomalous pulmonary venous connections and truncus arteriosus. *Pediatric Critical Care Medicine, 18*(Suppl. 8), S310–S314. https://doi.org/10.1097/PCC.0000000000000822

Martinez, H. R., Thomas, D. R., & Towbin, J. A. (2022). Pathophysiology of cardiomyopathies. In R. A. Polin, S. H. Abman., D. H. Rowitch, W. E. Benitz, & W. W. Fox (Eds.), *Fetal and neonatal physiology* (6th ed., pp. 1633–1648.e4). Elsevier.

McGinn, C., Casey, F. A., Watson, C., & Morrison, L. (2023). Paediatric heart failure–understanding the pathophysiology and the current role of cardiac biomarkers in clinical practice. *Cardiology in the Young, 33*, 503–513. https://doi.org/10.1017/S1047951123000331

McRae, M. (2015a). Long-term outcomes after repair of congenital heart defects: Part 1. *American Journal of Nursing, 115*(1), 24–35. https://doi.org/10.1097/01.NAJ.0000459628.07668.db

McRae, M. (2015b). Long-term outcomes after repair of congenital heart defects: Part 2. *American Journal of Nursing, 115*(2), 34–45. https://doi.org/10.1097/01.NAJ.0000460674.59200.1f

Meier, B., Frank, B., Wahl, A., & Diener, H. C. (2012). Secondary stroke prevention: Patent foramen ovale, aortic plaque, and carotid stenosis. *European Heart Journal, 33*(6), 705–713. https://doi.org/10.1093/eurheartj/ehr443

Mille, F. K., & Ravishankar, C. (2023). Cardiac disorders. In E. C. Eichenwald, A. R. Hansen, C. R. Martin, & A. R. Stark (Eds.), *Cloherty and Stark's manual of neonatal care* (9th ed., pp. 534–593). Wolters Kluwer.

Miller, A., Riehle-Colarusso, T., Siffel, C., Frias, J., & Correa, A. (2011). Maternal age and prevalence of isolated congenital heart defects in an urban area of the United States. *American Journal of Medical Genetics, Part A*, 155A, 2137–2145.

Mone, S., Gillman, M., Miller, T., Herman, E., & Lipshultz, S. (2004). Effects of environmental exposures on the cardiovascular system: Prenatal period through adolescence. *Pediatrics, 113*(Suppl. 3), 1058–1069. http://pediatrics.aappublications.org/content/113/Supplement_3/1058..info

Mordi, I., & Tzemos, N. (2012). Bicuspid aortic valve disease: A comprehensive review. *Cardiology Research and Practice, 2012*, 196037. https://doi.org/10.1155/2012/196037

Muralidharan, P., Sarmah, S., Zhou, F., & Marrs, J. (2013). Fetal alcohol spectrum disorder (FASD) associated neural defects: Complex mechanisms and potential therapeutic targets. *Brain Science, 3*, 964–991. https://doi.org/10.3390/brainsci3020964

Mussa, A., Di Candia, S., Russo, S., Catania, S., De Pellegin, M., Di Luzio, L., Ferrari, M., Tortora, C., Meazzini, M. C., Brusati, R., Milani, D., Zampino, G., Montirosso, R., Riccio, A., Selicorni, A., Cocchi, G., & Ferrero, G. (2016). Genetic forum: Recommendations of the Scientific Committee of the Italian Beckwith-Wiedemann Syndrome Association on the diagnosis, management, and follow-up of the syndrome. *European Journal of Medical Genetics, 59*, 52–64. https://doi.org/10.1016/j.ejmg.2015.11.008

Nahle, A. A., Hamdar, H., Soqia, J., Diab, M., Ataya, J., & Al-Dairy, A. (2024). Factors associated with early postoperative mortality after total anomalous pulmonary venous connection repair: A retrospective cohort study. *Medicine, 103*(21), e38285–e38285. https://doi.org/10.1097/MD.0000000000038285

Nakano, H., Fajardo, V. M., & Nakano, A. (2021). The role of glucose in physiological and pathological heart formation. *Developmental Biology, 475*, 222–233. https://doi.org/10.1016/j.ydbio.2021.01.020

National Institutes of Health. (2011). *Genetic conditions: VACTERL association*. https://medlineplus.gov/genetics/condition/vacterl-association/#frequency

National Institutes of Health. (2020). *Genetic conditions: Down syndrome*. https://medlineplus.gov/genetics/condition/down-syndrome/#frequency

National Institutes of Health. (2021a). *Genetics condition: Beckwith-Wiedemann syndrome*. https://medlineplus.gov/genetics/condition/beckwith-wiedemann-syndrome/#frequency

National Institutes of Health. (2021b). *Genetic conditions: Trisomy 18.* https://medlineplus.gov/genetics/condition/trisomy-18/#frequency

National Institutes of Health. (2022). *Genetic conditions: Williams syndrome.* https://medlineplus.gov/genetics/condition/williams-syndrome/#frequency

National Institutes of Health. (2023a). Genetic conditions: Jacobsen syndrome. https://medlineplus.gov/genetics/condition/jacobsen-syndrome/#frequency

National Institutes of Health. (2023b). *Genetic conditions: Turner syndrome.* https://medlineplus.gov/genetics/condition/turner-syndrome/#frequency

National Organization for Rare Disorders. (2007). *Trisomy 13 syndrome.* https://rarediseases.org/rare-diseases/trisomy-13-syndrome

National Organization for Rare Disorders. (2020). *VACTERL association.* https://rarediseases.org/rare-diseases/vacterl-association/

National Organization for Rare Disorders. (2024). *Trisomy 18.* https://rarediseases.org/rare-diseases/trisomy-18-syndrome.

Nies, M., & Brenner, J. I. (2013). Tetralogy of Fallot: Epidemiology meets real-world management: Lessons from the Baltimore–Washington infant study. *Cardiology in the Young, 23*(6), 867–869. https://doi.org/10.1017/S1047951113001698

Noori, S., Friedlich, P. S., & Seri, I. (2022). Pathophysiology of shock in the fetus and neonate. In R. A. Polin, S. H. Abman., D. H. Rowitch, W. E. Benitz, & W. W. Fox (Eds.), *Fetal and neonatal physiology* (6th ed., pp. 1662–1671). Elsevier.

Novack M. L., Zubair, M. (2025). Natriuretic peptide B type test. [Updated 2025 Aug 2]. *In StatPearls.* https://www.ncbi.nlm.nih.gov/books/NBK556136/

Ornoy, A., Reece, E., Pavlinkova, G., Kappen, C., & Miller, R. (2015). Effect of maternal diabetes on the embryo, fetus, and children: Congenital anomalies, genetic and epigenetic changes and developmental outcomes. *Birth Defects Research. Part C, Embryo Today, 105*(1), 53–72. https://doi.org/10.1002/bdrc.21090

Oster, M. E., Pinto, N. M., Pramanik, A. K., Markowsky, A., Schwartz, B. N., Kemper, A. R., Hom, L. A., Martin, G. R., and the Section on Cardiology and Cardiac Surgery, Section on Hospital Medicine, & Committee on Fetus and Newborn. (2025). Newborn screening for critical congenital heart disease: A new algorithm and other updated recommendations: Clinical report. *Pediatrics, 155*(1), e2024069667. https://doi.org/10.1542/peds.2024-069667

Ottolia, M., Torres, N., Bridge, J. H. B., Philipson, K. D., & Goldhaber, J. I. (2013). Na/Ca exchange and contraction of the heart. *Journal of Molecular and Cellular Cardiology, 61,* 28–33. https://doi.org/10.1016/j.yjmcc.2013.06.001

Patorno, E., Huybrechts, K. F., Bateman, B. T., Cohen, J. M., Desai, R. J., Mogun, H., Cohen, L. S., & Hernandez-Diaz, S. (2017). Lithium use in pregnancy and the risk of cardiac malformations. *New England Journal of Medicine, 376*(23), 2245–2254. https://doi.org/10.1056/NEJMoa1612222Peter, A. K., Cheng, H., Ross, R. S., Knowlton, K. U., & Chen, J. (2011). The costamere bridges sarcomeres to the sarcolemma in striated muscle. *Progress in Pediatric Cardiology, 31*(2), 83–88. https://doi.org/10.1016/j.ppedcard.2011.02.003

Pigula, F. A., & Mettler, B. (2017). Management of tricuspid regurgitation in patients with hypoplastic left heart syndrome. *Seminars in Thoracic and Cardiovascular Surgery, 29*(1), 64–69. https://doi.org/10.1053/j.semtcvs.2017.02.004

Puri, K., Allen, H. D., & Qureshi, A. M. (2017). Congenital heart disease. *Pediatrics in Review, 38*(1), 471–486. https://doi.org/10.1542/pir.2017-0032

Robbins, N., & Arruda, J. (2025). Congenital defects of the cardiovascular system. In R. J. Martin & A. A. Fanaroff (Eds.), *Fanaroff and Martin's neonatal-perinatal medicine: Diseases of the fetus and infant* (12th ed., pp. 1411–1432). Elsevier.

Rolfo, A., Nuzzo, A. M., De Amicis, R., Moretti, L., Bertoli, S., & Leone, A. (2020). Fetal-maternal exposure to endocrine disruptors: Correlation with diet intake and pregnancy outcomes. *Nutrients, 12*(6), 1744. https://doi.org/10.3390/nu12061744

Romeo, J. L. R., Etnel, J. R. G., Takkenberg, J. J. M., Roos-Hesselink, J. W., Helbing, W. A., van de Woestijne, P., Bogers, A. J. J. C., & Mokhles, M. M. (2020). Outcome after surgical repair of tetralogy of Fallot: A systematic review and meta-analysis. *The Journal of Thoracic and Cardiovascular Surgery, 159*(1), 220–236.e8. https://doi.org/10.1016/j.jtcvs.2019.08.127

Ryan, T. D., Kindel, S. J., & O'Connor, M. J. (2018). Heart failure in the neonate. In J. Rossano, J. L. Jeffries, A. C. Chang, J. A. Towbin, & R. E. Shaddy (Eds.), *Heart failure in the child and young adult: From bench to bedside* (1st ed., pp. 383–397). Elsevier Inc. https://doi.org/10.1016/B978-0-12-802393-8.00029-6

Sahni, M., Asrani, P., & Jain, S. K. (2015). Role of the renin-angiotensin-aldosterone system in the management of neonatal heart failure. *Neoreviews, 16*(10), e575–e585. https://doi.org/10.1542/neo.16-10-e575

Sakamoto, T., Nagashima, M., Umezu, K., Houki, R., Ikarashi, J., Katagiri, J., & Yamazaki, K. (2018). Long-term outcomes of total correction for isolated total anomalous pulmonary venous connection: Lessons from 50-years' experience. *Interact Cardiovasc Thorac Surg, 27*(1), 20–26. doi:10.1093/icvts/ivy034

Schumacher, K., Marin Cuartas, M., Meier, S., Aydin, M. I., Borger, M. A., Dähnert, I., Kostelka, M., & Vollroth, M. (2023). Long-term results following atrioventricular septal defect repair. *Journal of Cardiothoracic Surgery, 18*(1), 1–7. https://doi.org/10.1186/s13019-023-02355-6

Senartne, T. N., Zackai, E. H., & Saitta, S. C. (2024). Chromosome disorders. In C. A. Gleason & T. Sawyer (Eds.), Avery's diseases of the newborn (11th ed., pp. 347–361). Elsevier.

Shuman, C., Kalish, J. M., & Weksberg, R. (2000, March 3). Beckwith-Wiedemann syndrome. In M. P. Adam, J. Feldman, G. M. Mirzaa, R. A. Pagon, S. E. Wallace, & A. Amemiya (Eds.), *GeneReviews.* University of Washington. https://www.ncbi.nlm.nih.gov/sites/books/NBK1394/

Shuman, C., Beckwith, J. B., & Weksberg, R. (2016). Beckwith-Wiedemann syndrome. In M. Adams, H. Ardlinger, R. Pagon, M. Adam, H. Ardinger, R. Pagon, & S. Wallace (Eds.), *GeneReviews.* University of Washington. https://www.ncbi.nlm.nih.gov/books/NBK1394

Simeone, R., Tinker, S., Gilboa, S., Agopian, A., Oster, M., Devine, O., Honein, M., & the National Birth Defects Prevention Study. (2016). Proportion of selected congenital heart defects attributable to recognized risk factors. *Annals of Epidemiology, 26,* 838–845. https://doi.org/10.1016/j.annepidem.2016.10.003

Sneeringer, M. R., Vadlaputi, P., Lakshminrusimha, S., & Siefkes, H. (2022). Lower pass threshold (≥93%) for critical congenital heart disease screening at high altitude prevents repeat screening and reduces false positives. *Journal of Perinatology, 42*(9), 1176–1182. https://doi.org/10.1038/s41372-022-01491-6

Society for Maternal-Fetal Medicine, Silver, R., Craigo, S., Porter, F., Osmundson, S. S., Kuller, J. A., Norton, M. E., & Publications Committee. (2023). Society for Maternal-Fetal Medicine Consult series #64 systemic lupus erythematosus in pregnancy. *American Journal of Obstetrics and Gynecology, 228*(3), B41–B60. https://doi.org/10.1016/j.ajog.2022.09.001

Solomon, B. D., Baker, L. A., Bear, K. A., Cunningham, B. K., Giampietro, P. F., Hadigan, C., Hadley, D. W., Harrison, S., Levitt, M. A., Niforatos, N., Paul, S. M., Raggio, C., Reutter, H., & Warren-Mora, N. (2014). An approach to the identification of anomalies and etiologies in neonates with identified or suspected VACTERL (vertebral defects, anal atresia, tracheaesophageal fistula with esophageal atresia, cardiac defects, renal and limb anomalies) association. *Journal of Pediatrics, 163*(3), 451–457. https://doi.org/10.1016/j.jpeds.2013.10.086

Starling, E. H. (1918). The linacre lecture on the law of the heart given at Cambridge, 1915. *Nature, 101*, 43. https://doi.org/10.1038/101043a0

Strainic, J. (2025). Prenatal diagnosis of congenital heart disease. In R. J. Martin & A. A. Fanaroff (Eds.), *Fanaroff and Martin's neonatal-perinatal medicine: Diseases of the fetus and infant* (12th ed., pp.1387–1400). Elsevier.

Strasburger, J. F., Wacker-Gussmann, A., & Schellpfeffer, M. A. (2022). Developmental electrophysiology in the fetus and neonate. In R. A. Polin, S. H. Abman., D. H. Rowitch, W. E. Benitz, & W. W. Fox (Eds.), *Fetal and neonatal physiology* (6th ed., pp. 482–501.e4). Elsevier.

Sun, J., Brizard, C., Winlaw, D., Alphonso, N., d'Udekem, Y., Eastaugh, L., Marathe, S., Bell, D., & Ayer, J. (2019). Biventricular repair versus Fontan completion for patients with d- or l-transposition of the great arteries with ventricular septal defect and left ventricular outflow tract obstruction. *Journal of Thoracic and Cardiovascular Surgery, 158*(4), 1158–1167.e1. https://doi.org/10.1016/j.jtcvs.2019.05.061

Swamy, P., Bharadwaj, A., Varadarajan, P., & Pai, R. G. (2015). Echocardiographic evaluation of tetralogy of Fallot. *Echocardiography, 32*, 40–48. https://doi.org/10.1111/echo.12437

Torchia, M. G., & Persaud, T. V. N. (Ed). (2025). *The developing human: Clinically oriented embryology.* (12th ed.). Elsevier.

van den Hoff, M. J. B., & Wessels, A. (2022). Cardiovascular development. In R. A. Polin, S. H. Abman, D. H. Rowitch, W. E. Benitz, & W. W. Fox (Eds.), *Fetal and neonatal physiology* (6th ed., pp. 472–482.e2). Elsevier.

Villafañe, J., Feinstein, J. A., Jenkins, K. J., Vincent, R. N., Walsh, E. P., Dubin, A. M., Geva, T., Towbin, J. A., Cohen, M. S., Fraser, C., Dearani, J., Rosenthal, D., Kaufman, B., Graham Jr, T. P., & Adult Congenital and Pediatric Cardiology Section, American College of Cardiology. (2013). Hot topics in tetralogy of Fallot. *Journal of the American College of Cardiology, 62*(23), 2155–2166. https://doi.org/10.1016/j.jacc.2013.07.100

Wallis, G., & Fricker, F. J. (2012). Neonatal cardiomyopathy. *NeoReviews, 13*(12), e711–e723. https://doi.org/10.1542/neo.13-12-e711

Wijesekera, V. A. (2024). Tetralogy of fallot in adults. *Australian Journal of General Practice, 53*(7), 449–452. https://doi.org/10.31128/AJGP-06-23-6875

Wilkinson, J. D., Westphal, J. A., Bansal, N., Czachor, J. D., Razoky, H., & Lipshultz, S. E. (2015). Lessons learned from the Pediatric Cardiomyopathy Registry (PCMR) Study Group. *Cardiology in the Young, 25*(Suppl. 2), 140–153. https://doi.org/10.1017/S1047951115000943

Williams, K., Carson, J., & Lo, C. (2019). Genetics of congenital heart disease. *Biomolecules, 9(12)*, 879. https://doi.org/10.3390/biom9120879

Wu, W., He, J., & Shao, X. (2020). Incidence and mortality trend of congenital heart disease at the global, regional, and national level, 1990–2017. *Medicine, 99*(23), e20593. https://doi.org/10.1097/MD.0000000000020593

Yang, J., Qiu, H., Qu, P., Zhang, R., Zeng, L., & Yan, H. (2015). Prenatal alcohol exposure and congenital heart defects: A meta-analysis. *PLOS One, 10*(6), e0130681. https://doi.org/10.1371/journal.pone.0130681

Yazigi, A., De Pecoulas, A., Vauloup-Fellous, C., Grangeot-Keros, L., Ayoubi, J.-M., & Picone, O. (2017). Fetal and neonatal abnormalities due to congenital rubella syndrome: A review of literature. *Journal of Maternal-Fetal & Neonatal Medicine, 30*(3), 274–278. https://doi.org/10.3109/14767058.2016.1169526

Ye, X. T., Buratto, E., Schulz, A., Macalister, S. J., Weintraub, R. G., Brizard, C. P., & Konstantinov, I. E. (2023). Long-term outcomes of staged repair of tetralogy of Fallot. *The Journal of Thoracic and Cardiovascular Surgery, 165*(6), 2169–2180.e3. https://doi.org/10.1016/j.jtcvs.2022.07.026

Yeh, J., & Berger, S. (2015). Cardiac findings in infants of diabetic mothers. *NeoReviews, 16*(11), e624-e630. https://doi.org/10.1542/neo.16-11-e624

Zeliger, H. I. (2023). *Oxidative stress: Its mechanisms and impacts on human health and disease onset* (pp. 71–76). Elsevier. https://doi.org/10.1016/B978-0-323-91890-9.00011-8

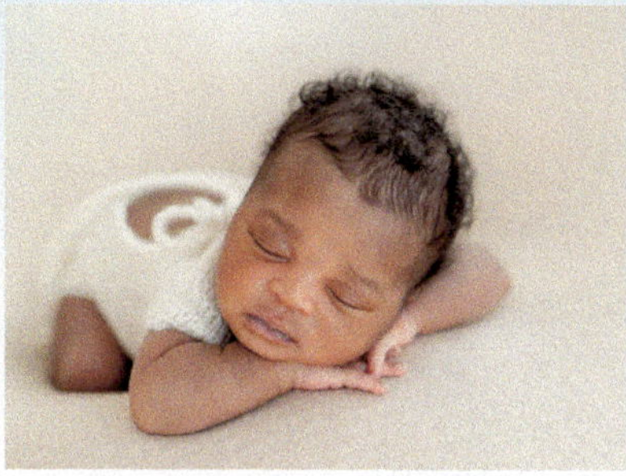

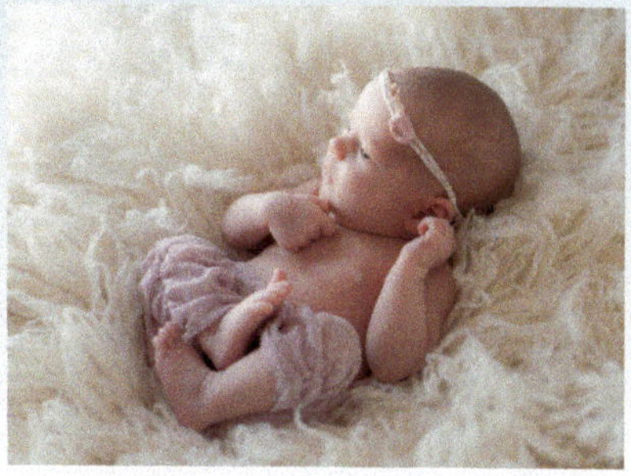

6

THE GASTROINTESTINAL SYSTEM

Jacqui Hoffman, Colleen R. Moss, and Amy J. Jnah

LEARNING OBJECTIVES

After completing this chapter, the reader should be able to:

- Understand normal gastrointestinal (GI) system development.
- Analyze the physiologic function of the fetal and neonatal GI system.
- Discuss common inherited disorders and their effect on fetal and neonatal GI system development and function.
- Identify health issues in XX pregnant patients that have a potential impact on fetal and postnatal GI system development and function.
- Evaluate common disorders that affect the GI system and their implications across the life span.

INTRODUCTION

This chapter is designed to provide knowledge of the embryologic, genetic, and physiologic development of the gastrointestinal (GI) tract. The environmental, maternal, and paternal risk factors that commonly influence GI development are discussed. Included in the chapter are the common abnormalities of GI development and the implications of these abnormalities in the newborn and across the life span. This knowledge provides the foundation for management of feeding and GI disorders in the newborn.

Vital functions of the GI system are the intake, digestion, and absorption of nutrients; the elimination of waste in stool and bile; participation in the maintenance of water balance; and the development of beneficial intestinal microbiota. Normal anatomic development and the functional maturity of the GI tract are crucial in establishing and maintaining these vital functions (Neu & Poindexter, 2024). The alimentary tract is the key component in providing nutrients to the body and plays an essential role in regulating energy homeostasis. It is a primary component of the GI system and consists of the mouth, pharynx, esophagus, stomach, small and large intestine, rectum, and anus (**Figure 6.1**).

TIMELINE FOR ORGAN DEVELOPMENT

Primitive Gut Development

Similar to the heart (see Chapter 5), GI development begins during week 4 of gestation. The three germ layers (endoderm, mesoderm, ectoderm) differentiate to form various GI structures. The endoderm gives rise to the gut, epithelium, and glands. The mesoderm gives rise to the parietal and visceral peritoneum. These mesenteries will cover and suspend the gut within the abdominal cavity. The ectoderm gives rise to the epithelium of the upper and lower GI tract; the distal portion of the anal canal also arises from the ectoderm. In addition, the neural crest gives rise to the nerves and neurons that innervate the walls of the GI tract and comprise the enteric nervous system (ENS; Sadler, 2023; Torchia & Persaud, 2025).

Early cranial and caudal folding, during week 4 of gestation, causes the ends of the primitive GI tube to come

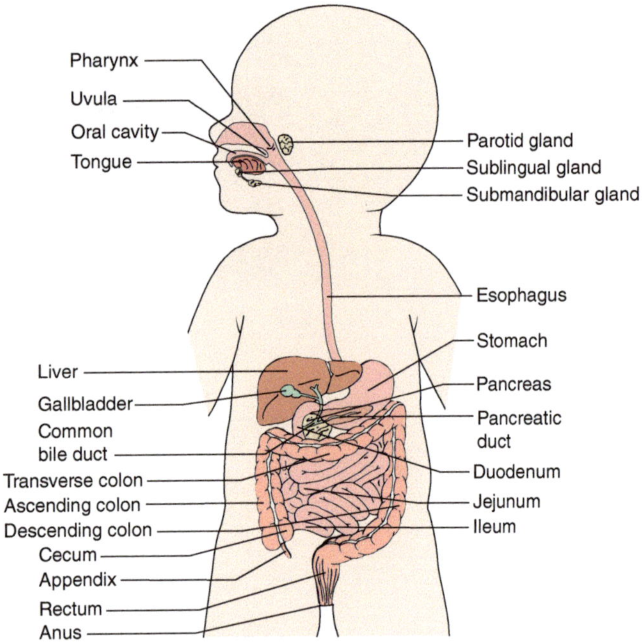

Figure 6.1 The alimentary tract.

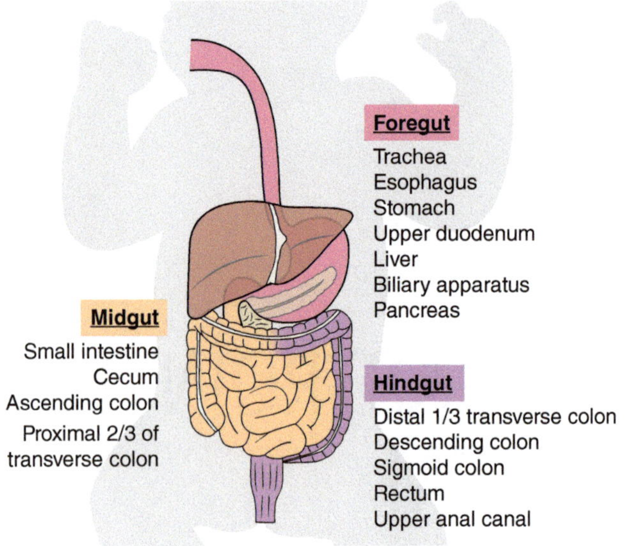

Figure 6.2 Structures that arise from foregut, midgut, and hindgut.

together like purse strings, incorporating the dorsal side of the umbilicus (yolk sac) within the tube. Initially, this creates a physical barrier at both the cranial and caudal ends of the tube (Torchia & Persaud, 2025). An oropharyngeal membrane covers the cranial end, which regresses during later development and gives rise to the anterior intestinal portal, or foregut, as well as the pharyngeal area (Faure & de Santa Barbara, 2011). Subsequent rupture of the oropharyngeal membrane creates an opening between the pharynx and foregut with the amniotic cavity, making way for the oral cavity (Torchia & Persaud, 2025). For the purposes of GI development, the pharyngeal area gives rise to the upper portion of the esophagus.

A cloacal membrane covers the caudal end of the GI tube, which regresses over time to permit formation of the posterior intestinal portal, or hindgut (Faure & de Santa Barbara, 2011). The middle of the primitive gut, or midgut, remains connected to the yolk sac through the vitelline duct (yolk stalk). During lateral-edge fusion, the vitelline duct regresses. Failed regression is associated with the formation of Meckel diverticulum, a remnant of the yolk stalk that presents as an outpouching of the ileum and often with gross bleeding from the bowel (Schoenwolf et al., 2021; Torchia & Persaud, 2025). Of note, Meckel diverticulum presents in infancy, usually around 4 months of age; a male 3:1 to 5:1 prevalence is reported.

The early events just described permit primitive gut development, or the formation of the foregut, midgut, and hindgut (Figure 6.2; Mahe et al., 2022; Torchia & Persaud, 2025). While the structures that comprise each region will be described categorically in the text that follows, it is important to understand that the development of the adult structures that arise from each primitive structure often overlap (Table 6.1). Most GI development occurs during the embryonic phase of development; maturation of the muscular layer and mesenteric attachments, and the formation of meconium occur during the fetal phase of development.

Foregut Development

The foregut is located between the upper part of the duodenum and the tracheobronchial diverticulum. It gives rise to the esophagus and stomach, upper portion of the duodenum, liver and biliary system, gallbladder, pancreas, and spleen (Sadler, 2023; Schoenwolf et al., 2021; Torchia & Persaud, 2025). Embryologic development of the diaphragm was discussed in Chapter 4, development of the spleen is discussed in Chapter 7, and pancreatic development is covered in Chapter 10.

Esophagus. The esophagus arises during week 4 of gestation from bifurcation of the trachea, by way of the tracheoesophageal septum (Figure 6.3). Next, a process of growth and stretching of the esophagus ensues. By week 6 of gestation, ciliated epithelia cluster and transform into esophageal glands. During week 7 of gestation, the esophagus reaches its final length; however, due to rapid cellular proliferation, it becomes temporarily obliterated. By week 8 to 9 of gestation, the esophagus is recanalized and achieves patency. By this time, vascular innervations matriculate to the submucosa. The muscular wall of the upper two thirds of the esophagus becomes striated and innervated by the vagus nerve, while the splanchnic plexus innervates the lower third of the esophagus (Neu & Poindexter, 2024; Schoenwolf et al., 2021; Torchia & Persaud, 2025).

Several esophageal anomalies may arise during this period of complex and overlapping development. Errors in partition of the foregut into respiratory and digestive parts during weeks 4 and 5 of gestation, resulting from

TABLE 6.1 Embryologic-to-Adult Gastrointestinal Differentiation

Primitive Structure	Vascular Innervation	Adult Structures
Foregut	Celiac artery	• Esophagus • Stomach • Upper duodenum (distal to the entry of the bile duct) • Liver and biliary system • Gallbladder • Pancreas
Midgut	Superior mesenteric artery	• Lower duodenum • Small intestine • Cecum • Appendix • Ascending colon • Proximal two-thirds of transverse colon
Hindgut	Inferior mesenteric artery	• Distal one-third of transverse colon • Descending colon • Sigmoid colon • Rectum • Upper anal canal

Note: The foregut also gives rise to the lower respiratory system and the hindgut also gives rise to the urinary bladder, urethra, and male and female reproductive systems.

Sources: Flynn-O'Brien, K. T., & Rice-Townsend, S. E. (2024). Structural anomalies of the gastrointestinal tract. In C. A. Gleason & D. O. Sawyer (Eds.), *Avery's diseases of the newborn* (11th ed.). Elsevier; Torchia, M. G. & Persaud, T. V. N. (2025). *The developing human* (12th ed.). Elsevier.

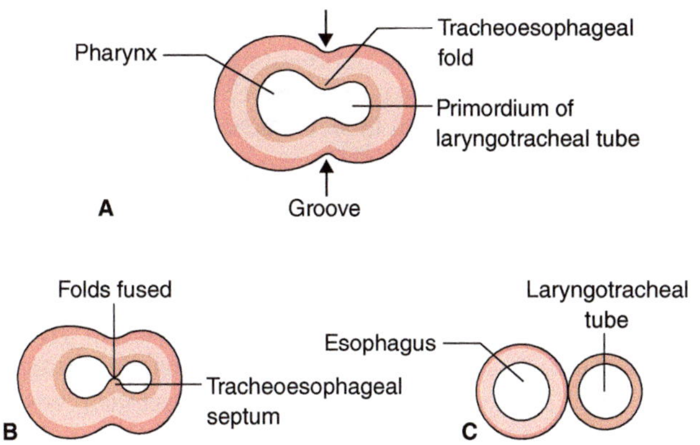

Figure 6.3 The tracheoesophageal septum. The drawing illustrates successful stages in development of the tracheoesophageal septum during the fourth and fifth weeks of gestation in the transverse view. (**A**) Beginning of partitioning of primordial laryngotracheal tube from primordial pharynx. (**B**) Developing the tracheoesophageal septum by fusion of tracheoesophageal folds. (**C**) Formation of the tracheoesophageal septum and complete separation of the foregut into the laryngotracheal tube and esophagus.

either spontaneous posterior deviation of the tracheoesophageal septum or from mechanical forces pushing the dorsal wall of the foregut anteriorly, lead to isolated esophageal atresia (EA) or EA combined with a tracheoesophageal fistula (TEF). Atresia or stenosis of the esophagus results from incomplete recanalization or narrowing of the lumen during week 8 of gestation. Failure of esophageal elongation pulls the stomach through the diaphragm into the esophageal hiatus and leads to a congenital hiatal hernia (Neu & Poindexter, 2024; Sadler, 2023; Schoenwolf et al., 2021; Torchia & Persaud, 2025).

Stomach. The stomach arises during week 4 of gestation. The endoderm of the foregut dilates and migrates 90 degrees on its long axis, and in a clockwise direction around the dorso-ventral axis (Figure 6.4; Sadler, 2023; Torchia & Persaud, 2025). This phenomenon creates the greater and lesser curvatures of the stomach. During this rotation, the cephalic and caudal ends, initially located on the midline, relocate. The caudal (pyloric) end moves upward and to the right, and the cephalic (cardiac) end moves downward and to the left. Once movement is complete, the stomach initially resides at the C3 to C5 level. Over time, the stomach slowly descends to a final location below the diaphragm, between T5 and L3 (Mahe et al., 2022).

Next, the greater and lesser omenta (sheets of fat covered by the peritoneum that connect the stomach to the abdominal viscera) arise from the dorsal and ventral mesenteries, respectively (Sadler, 2023). Finally, the pyloric sphincter forms at the caudal end of the stomach, through the proliferation of mesoderm-derived smooth muscles. The pylorus is a muscle located between the stomach and

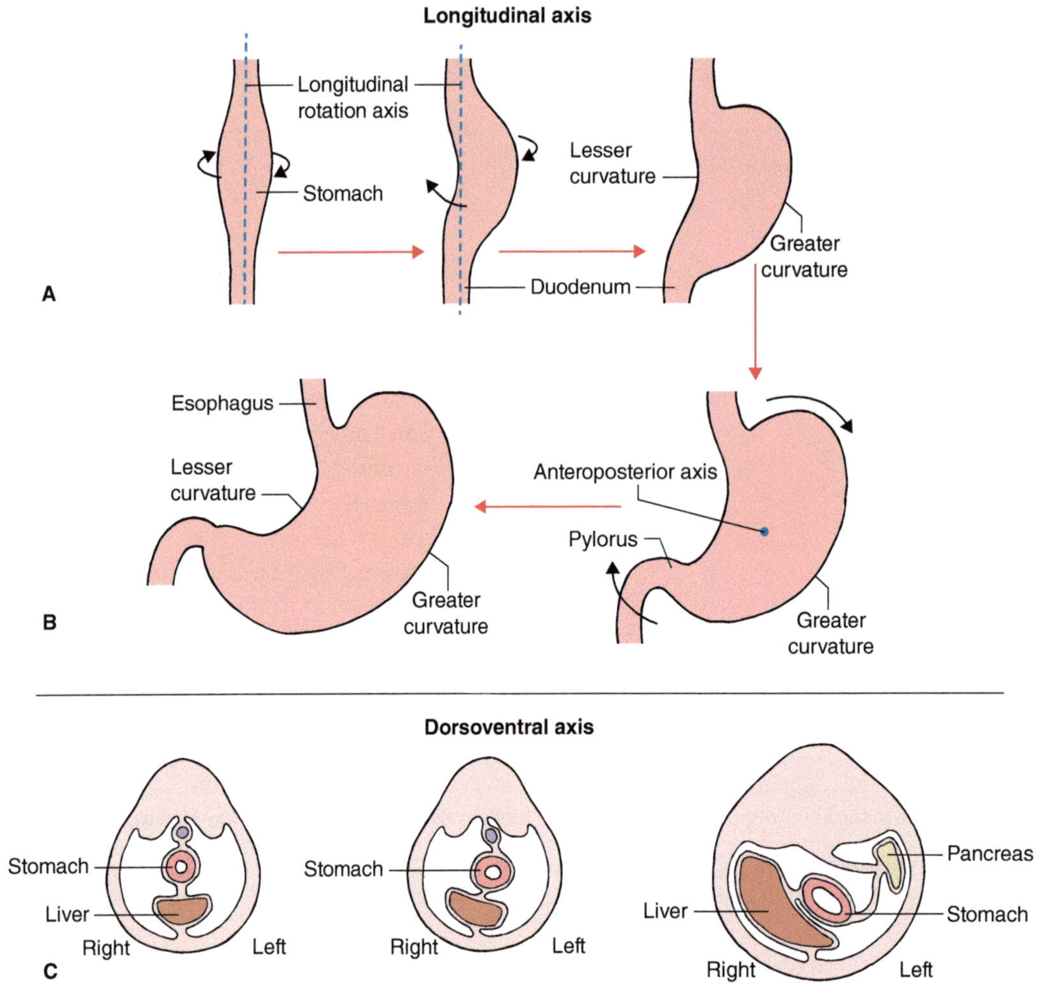

Figure 6.4 Rotation of stomach (longitudinal axis). (**A**) Original position of primitive stomach, before rotation. (**B**) Ventral border begins moving in rightward direction while dorsal border moves leftward. (**C**) Continued migration. Once relocated, the stomach resides on the left side of midline and the liver resides primarily on the right side of midline. Invagination shows early development of the pancreas.

duodenum which modulates the movement of intestinal contents by way of preventing retrograde reentry from the small intestine back into the stomach. Merely 2 weeks after its inception, at 6 weeks of gestation, the stomach is structurally intact (Mahe et al., 2022). Morphologic development of the stomach is rather simple, and as such, congenital anomalies are comparatively rare. Incomplete rotation and a developmental arrest in the caudal region may result in microgastria. Hypertrophy, mainly in circular muscles in the pylorus area, leads to *hypertrophic pyloric stenosis*, the most common stomach abnormality in neonates (Torchia & Persaud, 2025).

Duodenum. Similar to the esophagus and stomach, the duodenum arises during week 4 of gestation. The duodenum arises from the caudal end of the foregut, the cranial aspect of the midgut, and a segment of the splanchnic mesenchyme (Torchia & Persaud, 2025). During its evolution, the duodenum develops into a C-shaped loop (Figure 6.5). Following the normal rotation of the stomach, the duodenal loop rotates to the right and moves to the right upper abdominal quadrant, where it presses against the posterior abdominal wall (along with the pancreas) and assumes a retroperitoneal position (Sadler, 2023).

Similar to the esophagus, rapid proliferation of the endothelial lining of the duodenum temporarily obliterates its lumen. This occlusion typically occurs between weeks 5 and 6 of gestation, with subsequent recanalization between weeks 6 and 7 of gestation (Figure 6.6). Failed or partial recanalization is associated with duodenal stenosis and/or atresia. Although rare, duodenal atresia (DA) is the most common congenital small bowel obstruction diagnosed prenatally and genetic involvement (e.g., trisomy 21) is reported (Torchia & Persaud, 2025).

Clinical Application. DA is thought to be from failure of recanalization of the intestinal lumen. About one third of cases of DA have been associated with trisomy 21; other congenital anomalies including cardiovascular defects and anorectal malformations (ARMs) may be present; therefore, it is prudent for the advanced practice provider to

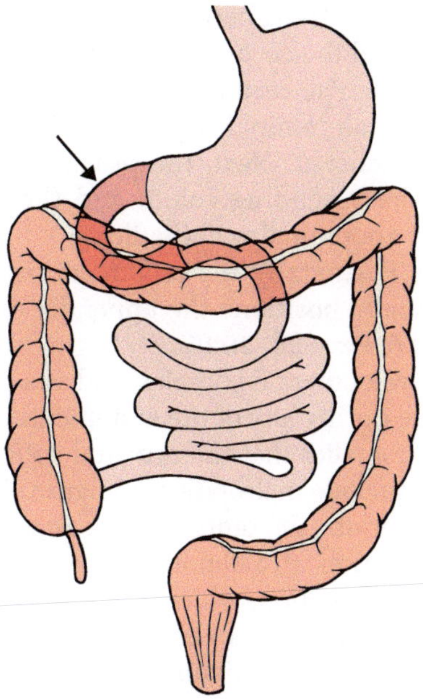

Figure 6.5 The C-shaped duodenum.

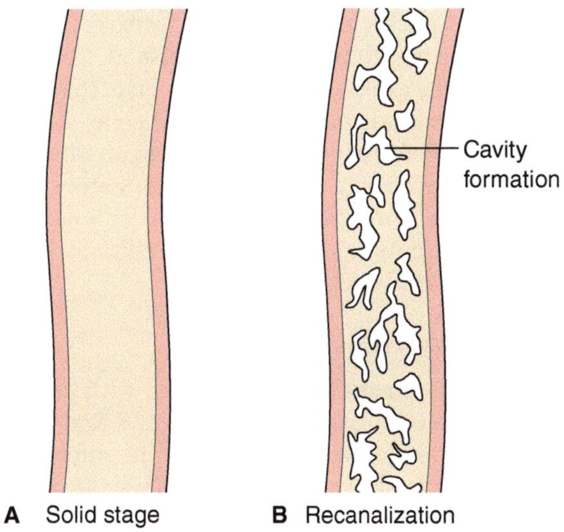

Figure 6.6 Recanalization of the duodenal lumen.

evaluate closely. The occurrence in families suggests an autosomal recessive inheritance pattern. Fetal ultrasound and postnatal x-ray demonstrate the hallmark findings of a large stomach bubble and dilated proximal duodenum; this is referred to as the "double bubble." When no air is noted in the intestine on the imaging, this is consistent with duodena atresia; however, if air is noted in the intestines, this is consistent with a duodenal stenosis. The neonate with DA often presents with distention isolated to the epigastrium and early onset emesis within a few hours of birth. Placement of a replogle to low continuous suction, parenteral support, and an evaluation for other anomalies are important aspects of management prior to surgery.

Liver, Gallbladder, and Biliary System. The liver, gallbladder, and biliary duct appear during week 4 of gestation. The liver arises as a small bud off the hepatic diverticulum, at a position adjacent to the heart (Sadler, 2023; Torchia & Persaud, 2025). From weeks 5 to 10 of gestation, the liver undergoes rapid growth, occupying a significant portion of the upper abdominal cavity. During this time, the cranial portion of the diverticulum differentiates into the liver and biliary system, whereas the caudal segment differentiates into the gallbladder. Next, the stalk of the diverticulum differentiates into the bile duct. Functional segmentation is determined by oxygen intake from the fetal umbilical veins, one of two major blood supplies to the liver (the other being the portal vein). Over time, the right lobe typically exceeds the size of the left. By week 10 of gestation, the liver has descended into the abdominal cavity and accounts for about 10% of total body weight (Torchia & Persaud, 2025).

Similar to the esophagus and duodenum, epithelial cells initially clog the extrahepatic biliary apparatus. Recanalization occurs shortly thereafter, and by week 13 of gestation, bile enters the duodenum through the common bile duct and *meconium production begins*. Failed recanalization leads to extrahepatic biliary atresia (BA), the most serious anomaly of the extrahepatic biliary system and cause for direct hyperbilirubinemia (cholestasis). Alternatively, intrahepatic BA and hypoplasia may arise during embryonic development, affecting duct formation. Benign variations in liver lobulation are common, yet of little clinical relevance (Sadler, 2023; Torchia & Persaud, 2025).

Pancreas. The pancreas begins as dorsal and ventral primorida (buds) within the duodenal endoderm around week 5 of gestation. The dorsal pancreatic bud just opposite the hepatic diverticulum appears first and becomes considerably larger than the two ventral pancreatic buds located caudal to the developing gallbladder. At about the same time, when the duodenum forms a C-shaped loop, the ventral pancreatic buds and common bile ducts are carried behind it into the dorsal mesentery. During week 6 of gestation, the ventral pancreas contacts the dorsal pancreas, and both become fused. When the two buds fuse normally, the main duct of the ventral pancreas (duct of Wirsung) persists, creating an egress pathway between the pancreas into the duodenum at the ampulla of Vater. When normal fusion does not occur, because the two lobes of the ventral pancreas migrate in opposite directions around the duodenum and fuse to the dorsal pancreatic bud, an annular pancreas arises. Of importance, annular pancreas can lead to a partial or complete duodenal obstruction.

The pancreas exhibits both exocrine and endocrine functions. Pancreatic acinar cells are the functional units of the exocrine portion of the pancreas. Acinar cells synthesize, store, and secrete digestive enzymes including amylase and elactase. These digestive enzymes are ushered into the duodenum by way of pancreatic ductal cells and help neutralize stomach acids. Islet of Langerhans cells are the functional units of the endocrine portion of the pancreas. These cells give rise to two types of committed precursor cells which will eventually be responsible for producing insulin, glucagon, pancreatic polypeptide, and somatostatin. Insulin secretion is produced as early as week 10 of gestation and glucagon by week 15 of gestation. Hypertrophy of the insulin secreting beta-cells can occur when exposed to high levels of glucose as seen with diabetes mellitus (DM) in XX pregnant patients (Carlson, 2024; Schoenwolf et al., 2021; Torchia & Persaud, 2025). Recall that maternally synthesized glucose can cross the placenta, whereas insulin cannot.

Midgut Development

The midgut originates from the dorsal abdominal wall during week 5 of gestation, initially as a linear tube, and receives oxygen and nutrients from the superior mesenteric artery (Torchia & Persaud, 2025). Derivatives of the midgut include the lower segment of the duodenum, jejunum, ileum, cecum, appendix, ascending colon, and two thirds of the transverse colon.

Around week 5 of gestation, the primitive ileum elongates and quickly exceeds the capacity of the abdominal cavity of the embryo. As a result, U-shaped looping occurs, creating the primary intestinal loop. The primary intestinal loop connects to the yolk sac, at the apex, by the vitelline duct. The cephalic portion of the loop transforms into the distal part of the duodenum, the jejunum, and the ileum. The caudal portion rises to the ascending colon and proximal two thirds of the transverse colon (Dingeldein, 2025; Torchia & Persaud, 2025). Midgut development then proceeds as four sequential stages: *herniation, rotation, retraction*, and *fixation*.

Because of the rapid growth described previously, the U-shaped midgut loop challenges the strength and capacity of the abdominal cavity. During week 6 of gestation, likely due to excess pressure, *herniation* of the midgut into the umbilicus occurs (Sadler, 2023; Torchia & Persaud, 2025). During this time, the midgut rotates 90 degrees in a counterclockwise direction, around the axis of the superior mesenteric artery (within the umbilical cord). Rotation is complete by week 8 of gestation, yet the abdominal contents remain in the herniated location, continuously elongating and folding. This proliferation gives rise to the cecum and, shortly after, the appendix, which arises as a small pouch off the dorsal end of the cecum and elongates over time. *Retraction* begins during week 10 of gestation. During this time, the midgut undergoes an *additional 180 degrees of counterclockwise rotation, totaling 270 degrees of rotational movement around the superior mesenteric pedicle* (Sadler, 2023; Torchia & Persaud, 2025). By week 11 of gestation, and under normal circumstances, all abdominal contents are situated back within the abdomen (Figure 6.7). *Fixation* thereby occurs during week 12 of gestation. The duodenum merges with the jejunum and becomes suspended by the ligament of Treitz between the left upper abdominal quadrant and the cecum in the right lower quadrant of the abdomen. The cecum and appendix descend into the subhepatic abdominal region and further into the right lower quadrant. Next, the proximal colon transforms into the ascending colon, and the mesenteries fuse with the abdominal wall (Sadler, 2023; Schoenwolf et al., 2021). Postnatally, the cecum continues to grow, which eventually positions the appendix on its medial side (Torchia & Persaud, 2025).

Midgut development is complex, and as a result, anomalies can arise during any of the aforementioned sequential stages. Anomalies that the neonatal APRN should be familiar with include malrotation, midgut volvulus, intestinal stenosis or atresia, omphalocele, and gastroschisis. Incomplete rotation with abnormal fixation can give rise to intestinal malrotation, which is a surgical abdominal catastrophe. Malrotation can be complicated by a midgut volvulus, which involves twisting of the intestines around the superior mesenteric artery. This abnormal twisting of intestine constricts the mesenteric artery and compromises blood supply to the small intestine. If left untreated, necrosis will quickly ensue and can progress to death (Schoenwolf et al., 2021; Torchia & Persaud, 2025). This pathology will be explored in a later section of this chapter.

Intestinal stenosis or atresia may arise as a primary defect, from failed recanalization, or from an interrupted blood supply affecting morphogenesis. Errors during intestinal retraction may create persistently herniated bowel, namely, omphalocele or gastroschisis, which are discussed later in this chapter.

Hindgut Development

Hindgut development is interconnected with genitourinary system development (see Chapters 8 and 11). The hindgut receives its blood supply from the inferior mesenteric artery. The derivatives of the hindgut are noted in Table 6.1, for visual reference (Torchia & Persaud, 2025). This discussion focuses on the development of the anorectal canal, which is an integral part of the GI system.

The cloaca is regarded as the most developmentally complex portion of the hindgut and arises as early as the end of week 1 of gestation. Between weeks 5 and 7 of gestation, a wall of mesenchyme develops between the allantois and hindgut and divides the cloaca into three separate structures: the (a) urogenital sinus (which differentiates into the bladder), (b) rectum, and (c) anal canal (Schoenwolf et al., 2021; Torchia & Persaud, 2025). Around week 8 of gestation, the cloacal membrane ruptures and the lumen of the superior portion of the anorectal canal becomes transiently obliterated with epithelial cells (Figure 6.8; Schoenwolf et al., 2021; Torchia & Persaud, 2025). This process of clogging mimics the normal development of other structures, including the esophagus and GI tract. Over time, proliferation of the mesenchyme raises the surface ectoderm enough that the clogging subsides and recanalization occurs. Subsequently, the primitive anal pit forms, and

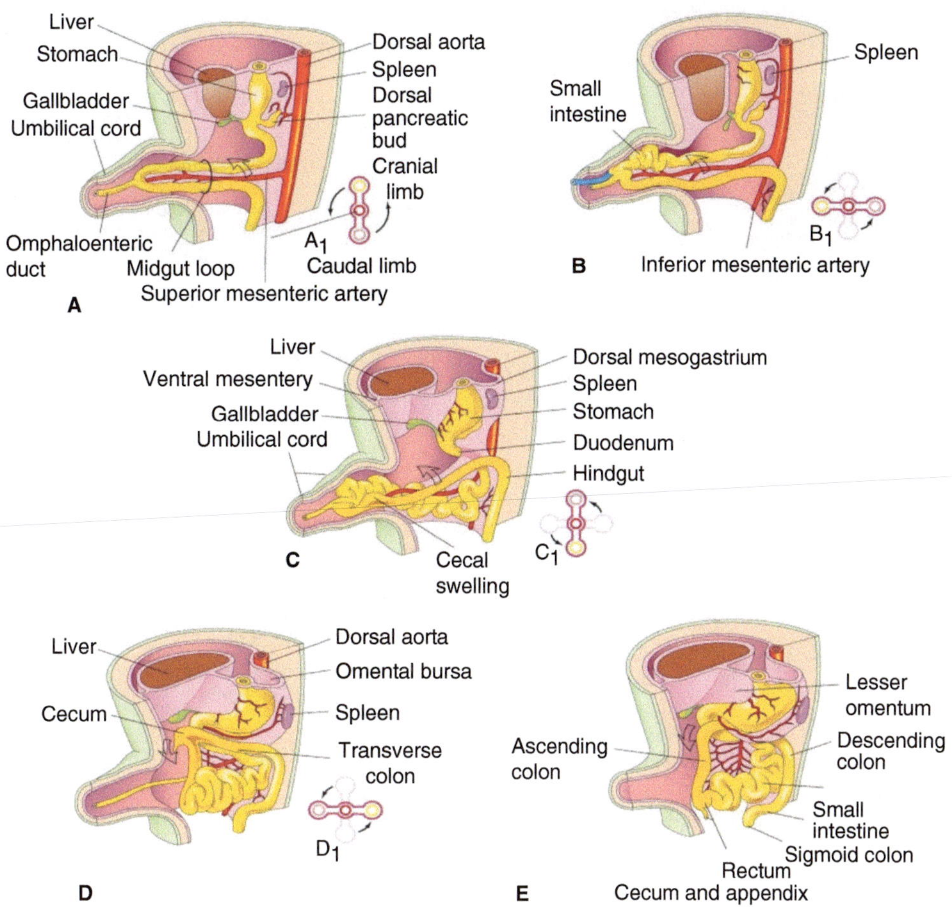

Figure 6.7 Herniation and rotation of the midgut. (**A**) At the beginning of the sixth week. (A1) Transverse section through the midgut loop, illustrating the initial relationship of the limbs of the loop to the superior mesenteric artery. Note that the midgut loop is in the proximal part of the umbilical cord. (**B**) Later stage showing the beginning of midgut rotation. (B1) Illustration of the 90-degree counterclockwise rotation that carries the cranial limb of the midgut to the right. (**C**) At approximately 10 weeks, showing the intestine returning to the abdomen. (C1) Illustration of a further rotation of 90 degrees. (**D**) At approximately 11 weeks, showing the location of the viscera after retraction of the intestine. (D1) Illustration of a further 90-degree rotation of the viscera, for a total of 270 degrees. (**E**) Later in the fetal period, showing the cecum rotating to its normal position in the lower right quadrant of the abdomen.
Source: Torchia, M. G. & Persaud, T. V. N. (2025). *The developing human* (12th ed.). Elsevier.

continues, in partnership with the hindgut, to give rise to the inferior portion of the anal canal (proctodeum) and, later, the anal sphincter (Torchia & Persaud, 2025).

Once anal formation is well underway, the superior rectal artery innervates the superior portion of the anal canal and provides an incoming blood supply, while the superior rectal vein innervates and offers a point of egress. Comparatively, the inferior rectal arteries and inferior rectal vein arise and supply the lower segment of the anal canal. Nervous system innervation differs by location. The superior portion of the anal canal is innervated by the autonomic nervous system (ANS). The inferior portion of the anal canal is innervated by the inferior rectal nerve (Torchia & Persaud, 2025).

Disrupted development of the hindgut may give rise to developmental abnormalities. Most anorectal anomalies result from errors of cloacal septation, the most common being an imperforate anus. Cases of imperforate anus may be associated with a urorectal fistula, and 50% of affected infants present with a VACTERL association. It is imperative that the neonatal APRN evaluate the anal wink in all newborns. If an imperforate anus is identified, it is essential to assess for the presence (or absence) of a fistula (rectovaginal or rectourinary), using ultrasound, to determine if pediatric surgical involvement and the creation of a temporary colostomy is indicated. Other defects involving disrupted hindgut development include anal stenosis and rectal atresia (Schoenwolf et al., 2021; Torchia & Persaud, 2025).

DEVELOPMENTAL PHYSIOLOGY

Molecular Regulation of Gut Tube Development

Signaling from multiple genes is necessary for the correct organ to form in the correct place. Readers are cautioned that molecular signaling patterns are complex, and de-

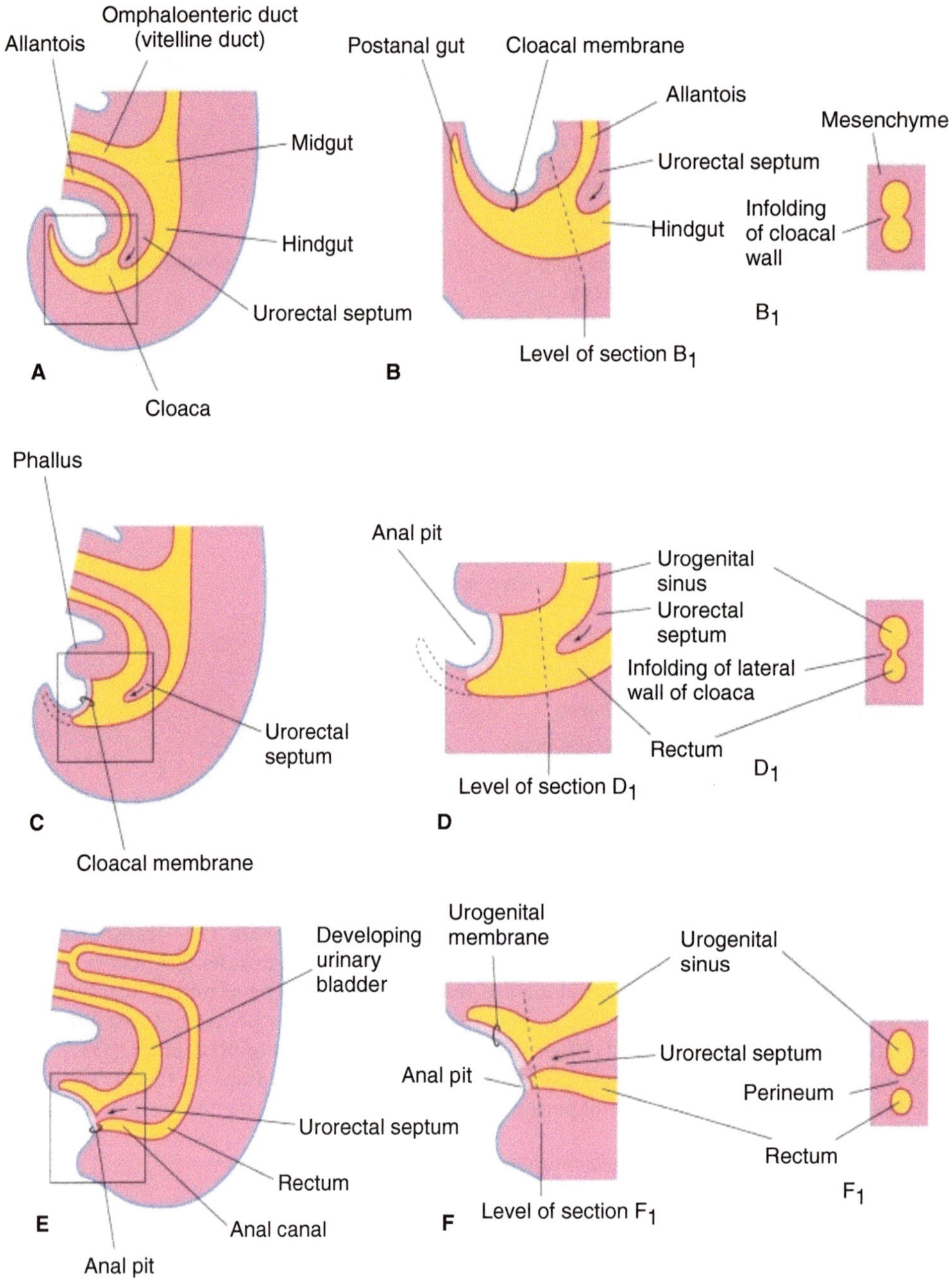

Figure 6.8 Successive stages in the partitioning of the cloaca into the rectum and urogenital sinus by the urorectal septum. (**A**, **C**, and **E**) Views from the left side at 4, 6, and 7 weeks, respectively. (**B**, **D**, and **F**) Enlargements of the cloacal region. (B1 and D1) Transverse sections of the cloaca at the levels shown in **B** and **D**. Note that the postanal portion (shown in **B**) degenerates and disappears as the rectum forms.
Source: Torchia, M. G. & Persaud, T. V. N. (2025). *The developing human* (12th ed.). Elsevier.

tailed explanations exceed the scope of this textbook. We provide a high-level overview of major signaling proteins (sonic hedgehog [SHH], Wingless-type mouse mammary tumor [Wnt] virus, fibroblast growth factor-4 [FGF4], retinoic acid [RA], and bone morphogenic protein 4 [BMP4]) and reference several reports that can be explored for additional context (Batts et al., 2006; Chin et al., 2017; G. M. Kelly & Drysdale, 2015; Logan & Nusse, 2004; Zorn, 2008).

Recall that GI tract development involves three major developmental milestones: (a) initial specification of endoderm, (b) formation of the gut tube, and (c) configuration of organs expanding beyond the gut tube (pancreas and liver). During this developmental process, endodermal tissues are pluripotent, meaning they can develop into any organ that arises from the endoderm. The aforementioned signaling proteins might be upregulated or downregulated in various sections of the GI tract, to control the pattern of organ formation. We discuss them in greater detail next.

SHH is a signaling protein that is expressed throughout the gut tube and stimulates interactions between the endoderm and spatially related mesoderm. Upregulation of SHH stimulates mesodermal growth and differentiation, as well as organogenesis (Walton & Gumucio, 2021). Inhibition of SHH signaling at the foregut endoderm allows for the formation of the dorsal and ventral pancreatic buds (Figure 6.9). Wnt and FGF4 are expressed at the gastric epithelium and regulate cellular proliferation, differentiation, migration, and apoptosis (de Santa Barbara et al., 2003). Together, Wnt and FGF4 promote posterior gut development and must be inhibited for the foregut to form (Chin et al., 2017).

We know that vitamin A is an essential micronutrient, and dietary intake of vitamin A during pregnancy is important to the developing embryo. Vitamin A is oxidized through a series of chemical reactions to RA, a signaling protein. The highest level of RA signaling occurs in the mesoderm, near the developing dorsal pancreatic buds and lungs. RA signaling is also essential for proper development of the anterior foregut, pharynx, liver, and stomach (in addition to the lungs!). BMP4 signaling contributes to hindgut formation, as well as the lengthening of the intestines (G. M. Kelly & Drysdale, 2015; Twaroski et al., 2015). The combinations of these signals determine the secondary genes controlling the development of different parts of the gut tube. *SOX2* specifies esophagus and stomach, *PDX1* the duodenum, *CDXC* the small intestine, and *CDXA* the large intestine and rectum (Sadler, 2023).

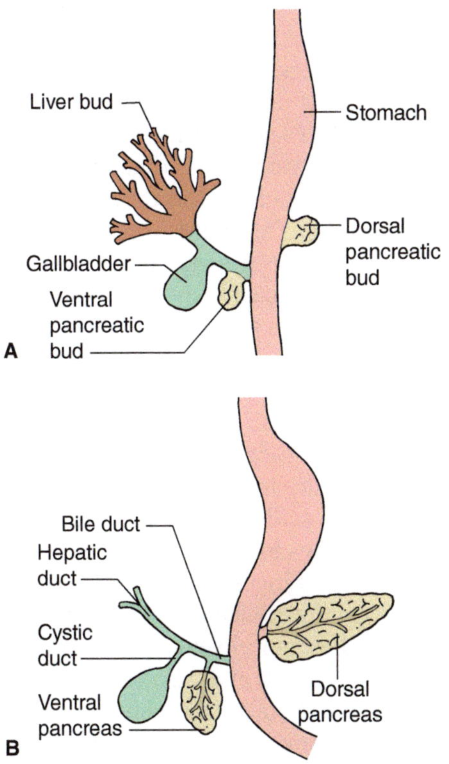

Figure 6.9 Formation of dorsal and ventral pancreatic buds. (**A**) Early development of pancreatic buds. (**B**) Progressive development of dorsal and ventral pancreas.

Clinical Application. RA is a primary regulator of lung development and homeostasis. In fact, RA regulates the development of the trachea, airways, lungs, and the diaphragm. Insufficient RA levels are associated with the development of TEF, tracheomalacia, congenital diaphragmatic hernia, and pulmonary hypoplasia or agenesis. Among preterm infants, retinol deficiency (vitamin A deficiency) is associated with an increased risk for bronchopulmonary dysplasia (BPD). Therefore, some clinicians opt to administer prophylactic vitamin A to preterm infants at-risk for BPD. As it turns out, vitamin A is metabolized into RA, and RA can attenuate the effect of hyperoxia on lung tissues in preterm infants. Vitamin A is administered intramuscularly, three times weekly, for a total of 12 doses.

Innervation of the Digestive Tract: Function of the Enteric Nervous System

The ENS is a complex network of both neurons and glia that are positioned across the GI tract, from the esophagus to the rectum. This system arises during early embryogenesis, by way of the neural crest, and is considered the "brain of the gastrointestinal system" (Avetisyan et al., 2015, p. 899). The neurons become situated and interconnected within both the myenteric plexus (muscle layers) and submucosal plexus (region between muscle and mucosa). These ENS neurons ultimately initiate and disseminate GI reflexes, which modulate GI motility, secretion, and blood flow.

Development of the ENS begins with the process of *migration*. ENS precursors migrate from the vagal neural crest cells to the foregut, and subsequently to the rest of the digestive tract in a rostral-to-caudal progression (Figure 6.10; Uesaka et al., 2016). These cells first enter the myenteric plexus, or outer region, of the gut, and later enter the deeper submucosal plexus, found only in the small and large intestine. The neurons in the myenteric plexus reside between the longitudinal and circular muscle in the bowel wall, and control muscle contraction and relaxation. The neurons in the submucosal plexus reside between the circular muscle and the bowel mucosa, and modulate fluid and electrolyte secretion and absorption, supporting bowel function (Diposarosa et al., 2021; Torchia & Persaud, 2025).

Incomplete development of the ENS has been implicated in several diseases of the bowel, which are referred to as neurocristopathies. These diseases are associated with a deficiency or absence of enteric ganglion cells which leads to dysfunctional peristalsis, blood flow, and often deficient GI secretions (Bondurand & Southard-Smith, 2016). Common diseases include

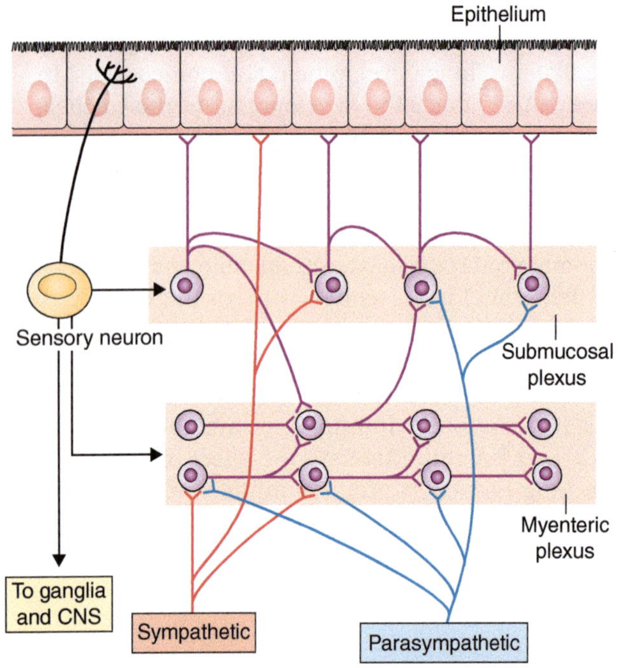

Figure 6.10 Enteric nervous system innervation.

Hirschsprung disease, small left colon syndrome, gastroparesis, cystic fibrosis, and irritable bowel syndrome.

> **Clinical Application.** Under normal circumstances, the ENS develops in a caudal direction and involves migration, proliferation, and differentiation. Failed migration of neural crest cells in the bowel wall can lead to diseases including Hirschsprung disease. This typically affects the distal colon. Lack of these intestinal ganglion cells prevents the inhibitory relaxation normally regulated by parasympathetic nerves. Since the area affected is unable to relax, a functional obstruction ensues (Flynn-O'Brien & Rice-Townsend, 2024). This is one of the hallmark findings, lack of stool within the first 48 hours after birth, in addition to other signs of obstruction such as abdominal distention and nonbilious emesis (usually recurrent emesis of ingested breast milk or formula during or shortly after feeding sessions).

Digestive Function of the Gastrointestinal Tract

The alimentary canal, or GI tract, is the system where food enters the body, nutrients are digested and absorbed, and waste is eliminated. The four primary functions of the GI tract are (a) digestion and absorption, (b) fluid and electrolyte balance, (c) protection against invaders, and (d) elimination of waste; each function is essential to the health of the newborn. From the esophagus to the anus, the GI tract contains the same histologic cell layers. The GI mucosa has four major layers and modifies these layers in various GI segments regarding the functions of digestion, absorption, and secretion. The GI *mucosa* is comprised of three sublayers: the outermost epithelium, lamina propria (comprised of blood vessels), and muscularis mucosa (a double layer of smooth muscle). The *submucosa* is collagenous tissue with nerves and blood vessels. The GI *muscularis propria* is primarily responsible for moving bulk food. GI *adventitia* is collagenous tissue with larger vasculature and nerves that regulate the entire tract (Mahe et al., 2022). The esophagus is a tunnel or "covered bridge" from the mouth to the stomach. Impulses from the swallowing center, where the nuclei of cranial nerves IX and X are located, activate swallowing. Digestion and absorption do not occur in the esophagus, but rather, a bolus of food is propelled through the esophagus and toward the stomach (Dingeldein, 2025).

The GI tract secretes many digestive hormones, including cholecystokinin, gastrin, secretin, and gastrin inhibitory peptide. It is important to note that the cells producing glucagon are present only in fetal and neonatal glands, indicating a role in growth. Gastric secretions are present by 10 weeks of gestation. Gastrin, hydrochloric acid, pepsin, and intrinsic factor (IF) are present early along with mucus and bicarbonate at about 16 weeks of gestation. While in utero, gastric pH is alkaline (approximately pH 7.05) because amniotic fluid is neutral. After birth, the gastric pH in term newborns falls to a pH of 3.5 within hours of birth, and by 48 hours, the pH is approximately 3.0. In contrast, preterm newborns exhibit GI immaturity and it takes upwards of 5 to 7 postnatal days for gastric pH to acidify (Khlevner et al., 2022).

Among orally fed newborns, digestion begins when food (human milk/formula) enters the mouth. Swallowing is divided into sequential phases: oral, pharyngeal, and esophageal. During the oral transit phase, the infant takes milk into the oral cavity and the tongue thrusts the bolus of milk toward the pharynx. It is here that salivary amylase begins to break down carbohydrates and lipases begin to break down fats (see Figure 6.11).

Next, the bolus of milk passes from the mouth, past the pharynx, into the esophagus and then the stomach. Once milk reaches the stomach, parietal cells secrete hydrochloric stomach acid and this activates pepsinogen, which is produced by chief cells. Pepsinogen inactivates bacteria inadvertently ingested with the milk and is then degraded to pepsin, a molecule capable of hydrolyzing proteins into smaller peptide chains and funneling them into the duodenum (Jnah et al., 2024).

The partially digested milk is ushered to the duodenum (and further into the intestinal tract) by way of migrating motor complexes, small waves of peristaltic contractions that encourage the migration of food toward the colon. The duodenum and remainder of the

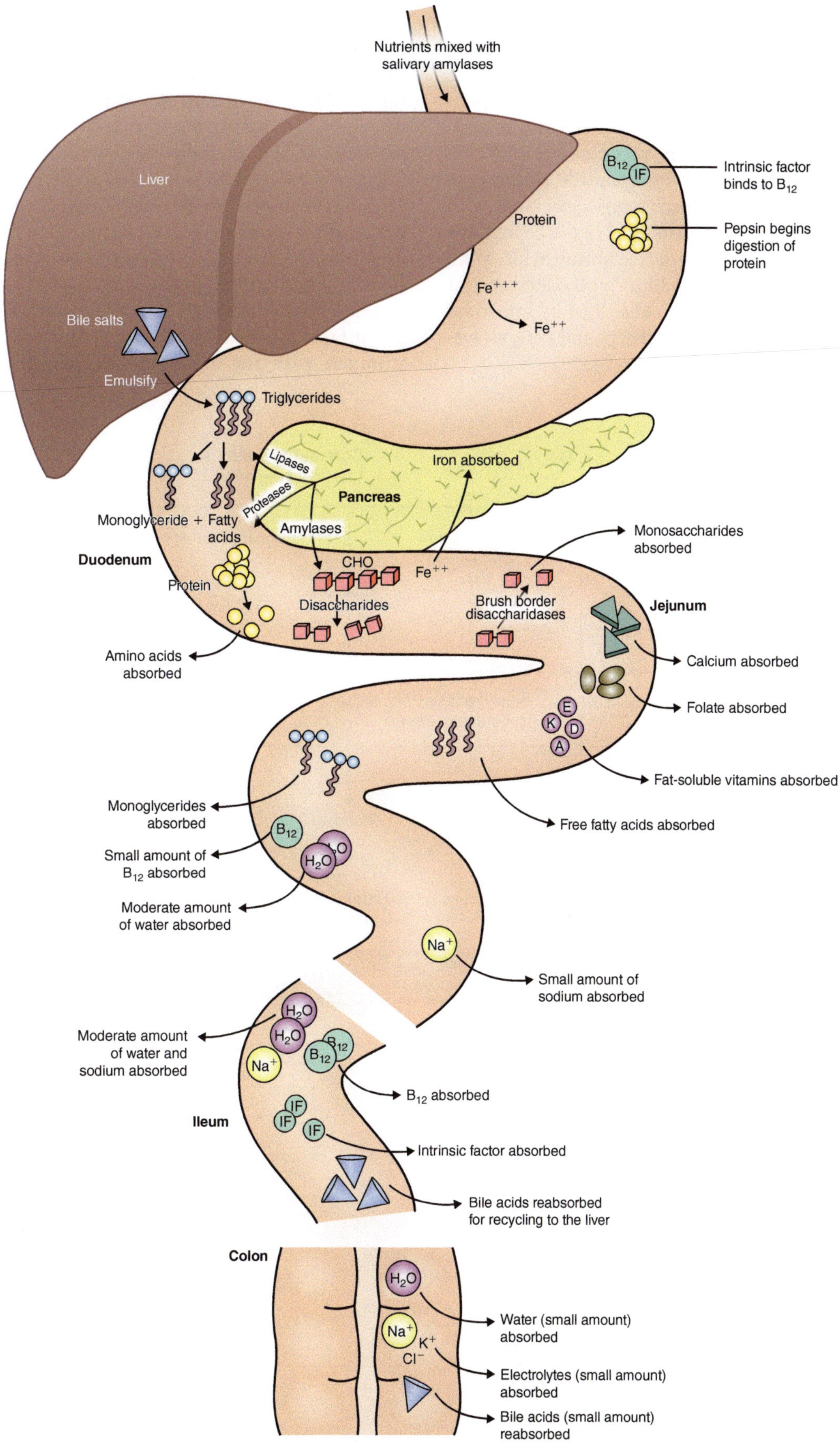

Figure 6.11 Overview of digestion.

small intestine is coated by a single layer of mucus, produced by goblet cells. This mucus lining is comprised of antimicrobial proteins, which help keep any ingested bacteria away from the epithelial lining of the small intestine to maintain its integrity and ability to digest food. Once the bolus of food reaches the small intestine, pancreatic enzymes are synthesized. These enzymes include trypsinogen, chymotrypsinogen, proelastase, and procarboxypeptidase, which hydrolyze peptide chains into oligopeptides; enzyme deficiencies are associated with some inborn errors of metabolism (Table 6.2). Next, the oligopeptides are hydrolyzed into free amino acids. With the help of transporters (e.g., sodium-amino acid carrier system), the free amino acids are absorbed by intestinal epithelial cells and released into the portal venous system (Neu & Singh, 2022; Taylor & Neu, 2021).

Next, carbohydrate digestion and absorption, which began in the mouth (among orally fed infants), continues in the small intestine. Importantly, the complement of pancreatic enzymes required for carbohydrate digestion increases with advancing gestational and postnatal age (Jnah et al., 2024). Starches are broken down by pancreatic amylase and brush border enzymes into disaccharides and then absorbable monosaccharides (Figure 6.12; Neu & Singh, 2022; Taylor & Neu, 2021). Monosaccharides can be transported through the membrane of the small intestine epithelium using specialized membrane porters and both active and passive transport (Neu & Singh, 2022; Taylor & Neu, 2021).

Lipid digestion begins in the mouth (among orally fed infants) with lingual lipase and continues in the stomach with the churning actions of gastric motil-

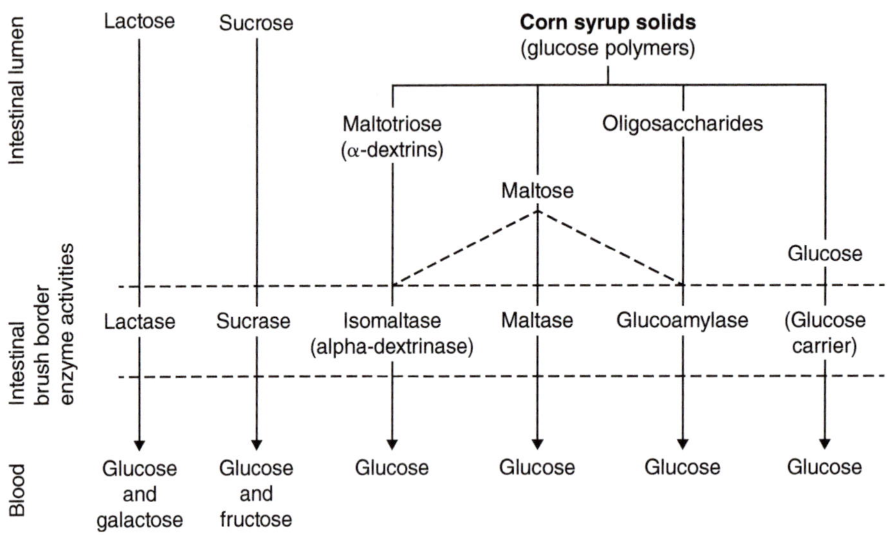

Figure 6.12 Overview of carbohydrate digestion.

TABLE 6.2 Protein Digestion and Inborn Errors of Metabolism

Pancreatic Enzyme	Target Protein(s)	Enzyme Deficiency and IEM(s)
Trypsinogen	• Arginine • Lysine	• Hyperammonemia • Urea cycle defect
Chymotrypsinogen	• Leucine • Phenylalanine • Tryptophane • Tyrosine	• Homocystinuria • Maple syrup urine disease • Phenylketonuria • Tyrosinemia
Proelastase	• Alanine • Glycine • Serine	• Nonketotic hyperglycinemia • 3-phosphoglycerate dehydrogenase deficiency
Procarboxypeptidases	• Arginine • Lysine	• Hyperammonemia • Urea cycle defect

Source: Sperling, M. A., Majzoub, J. A., Menon, R. K., & Stratakis, C. A. (2020). *Sperling pediatric endocrinology* (5th ed.). Elsevier.

ity and gastric lipase; the remainder of lipid digestion occurs in the small intestine. It is important to distinguish that lipid digestion is relatively mature in term infants; however, preterm infants demonstrate reduced lipid absorption due to low levels of pancreatic lipase and bile acids, which assist with emulsifying lipids in the small intestine into monoglycerides and free fatty acids. Under normal circumstances, once lipids are emulsified, the molecules can diffuse across the small intestine brush border and into the circulation. Of note, medium-chain triglycerides (MCTs) do not require bile acids or pancreatic lipase for intestinal absorption; therefore, these fats are found in most preterm infant nutrition products. See **Figure 6.13** for a contrast between MCT and long chain triglyceride absorption (Jnah et al., 2024).

The GI tract also absorbs small-molecule vitamins. Fat-soluble vitamins (A, D, E, K) can be absorbed in the presence of other lipids in the jejunum. Water-soluble vitamins can be absorbed throughout the small intestine without the need for simultaneous fat intake (Neu & Singh, 2022; Taylor & Neu, 2021). Recall that infants with cholestasis or chronic liver disease can develop a fat-soluble vitamin deficiency because they might lack adequate synthesis and secretion of bile acids necessary for fat-soluble vitamin absorption. Therefore, clinicians will supplement the enteral feeding regimen with an aqueous preparation of vitamin A, D, E, and K ("ADEK"), which is a water miscible form of these fat-soluble vitamins, to optimize intestinal absorption despite the deficit of bile acids and prevent the onset of a vitamin deficiency.

Water and electrolyte absorption and secretion occur in the small and large intestines. Sodium absorption occurs primarily in the duodenum and jejunum and, to a lesser extent with the assistance of aldosterone, in the large intestine. Chloride absorption occurs in the small intestine, particularly in the duodenum and jejunum, through passive diffusion. Glucose absorption occurs across the intestine, although it is less efficient in newborns and even more so in premature infants. Water is absorbed through passive osmosis in the GI tract and is enhanced by the absorption of osmotic electrolytes, namely sodium (Taylor & Neu, 2021).

The Postnatal Gut Microbiota. The microbial complex living with an individual is referred to as the *microbiota.* Fetuses and newborns have a relatively sterile gut, but after birth, numerous microbial organisms infiltrate the gut and establish a microbiome in the newborn. The gut microbiota is an important regulator of health, and as such, the establishment of a diverse and *healthy* microbiome is important after birth. The newborn's microbiome is influenced by several factors including gestational age

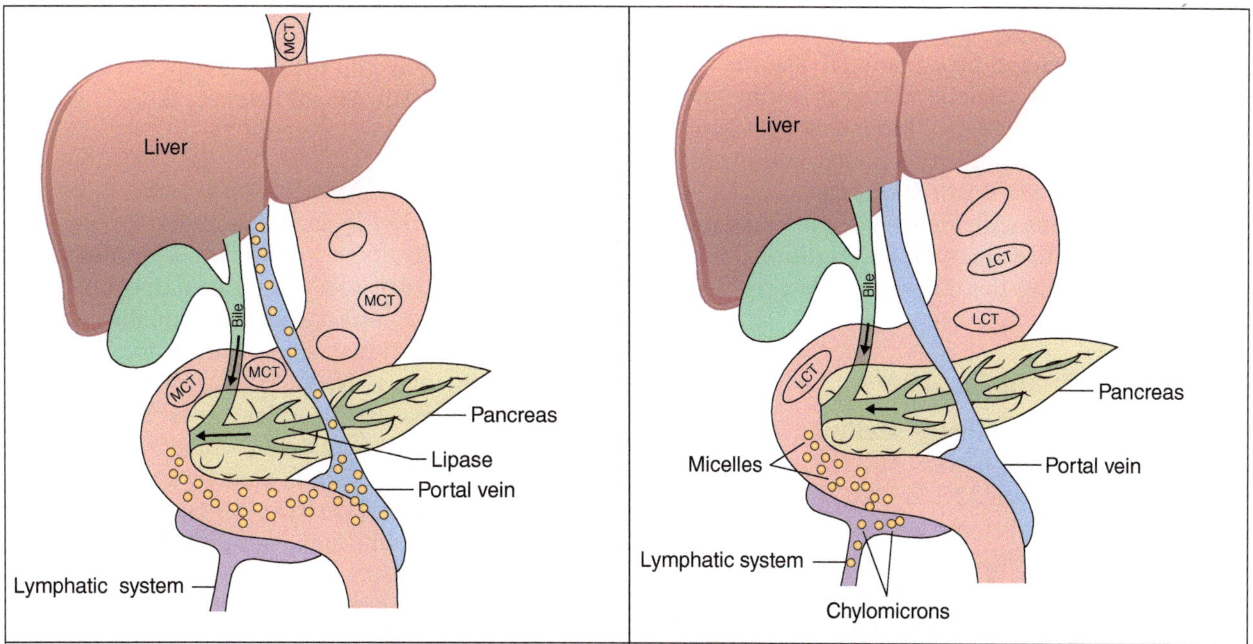

The absorption of medium chain triglycerides (MCT) occurs rapidly and directly through the portal vein. MCTs require much less pancreatic lipase and bile salts for effective digestion compared to long chain triglycerides (LCT). MCTs do not require micellar or chylomicron formation for absorption and digestion.

Long chain triglycerides (LCT) are emulsified by bile salts into micelles and hydrolyzed to fatty acids and glycerol by pancreatic lipase. The emulsified fat enters the epithelial cells, combining with protein to form chylomicrons, which are directly transferred into the lymphatic system (through the thoracic duct), into the blood stream, and finally to the liver.

Figure 6.13 Medium-chain and long-chain triglyceride digestion and absorption.
LCT, long-chain triglyceride; MCT, medium-chain triglyceride.

at birth, mode of delivery, enteral feeding pattern and type, antibiotic exposure, and postnatal environment (Healy et al., 2022). For example, studies have indicated that preterm infants are at increased risk for excess colonization with *Klebsiella* species, a gram-negative bacteria associated with necrotizing enterocolitis (NEC). Preterm infants are also at risk for developing reduced microbial diversity within the gut microbiota as compared to term counterparts (Paveglio et al., 2020). Further, preterm infants exposed to antibiotics can present with resistant strains of *Enterococcus* in stool samples.

Ultimately, it is important to promote the establishment of a healthy microbiota, as this can enhance immune function (e.g., maturation of T-cells and natural killer cells) among the most vulnerable infants and discourage the development of disease (Tamburini et al., 2016). Early enteral feeding is known to stimulate the production of digestive enzymes, which can aid in upregulating the production of gastric acid and lower gastric pH. Gastric acid protects the upper tract and insulates the bacteria in the intestine against contamination (Jnah et al., 2024; Kamada et al., 2013; Neu & Singh, 2022).

GENETIC INFLUENCES

Many diseases of the GI tract have genetic predispositions. Numerous genes responsible for pathologic GI conditions have been discovered; researchers continue to uncover genes associated with GI diseases whose causes had not previously been fully understood. These discoveries have changed how many GI disorders are diagnosed and treated. Genetic testing is commercially available for many of the GI conditions that have genetic involvement; testing facilitates screening and diagnosing predisposed persons (Roath & Di Palma, 2012). Several such GI conditions with known genetic foundations are discussed in the text that follows. Additional inherited disorders affecting the GI system are provided in Box 6.1.

BOX 6.1 Other Inherited Disorders of the Gastrointestinal System

- 22q11.2 deletion syndrome (DiGeorge syndrome)
- Accessory pancreas
- Alpers syndrome
- Alpha-1 antitrypsin deficiency
- Annular pancreas
- Aplasia cutis
- Cholestasis, progressive familial
- Congenital bile duct acid synthesis defects
- Cornelia de Lange syndrome (type 1 and 2)
- Dandy-Walker cyst with renal–hepatic–pancreatic dysplasia
- Hepatoblastoma
- Pentalogy of Cantrell
- Whipple disease
- Zellweger syndrome

Note: A more comprehensive list is provided by the National Institutes of Health, Genetic and Rare Diseases Information Center at https://rarediseases.info.nih.gov/diseases.

Autosomal Dominant Disorders

Permanent Neonatal Diabetes Mellitus. Permanent neonatal DM affects one in every 400,000 infants (National Library of Medicine [NLM], 2024g). Autosomal dominant inheritance is most common. Mutations in the *KCNJ11, INS*, and *ABCC8* genes are reported, which disrupt normal pancreatic function. Essentially, gene dysfunction causes failed closure of K^+–adenosine triphosphate (ATP) channels, which provokes decreased beta cell synthesis of insulin. In about 90% of cases, new gene mutations are identified in the absence of a family history of the disease (NLM, 2024g). Prenatal manifestations include poor fetal growth and intrauterine growth restriction (IUGR). After birth, hyperglycemia with dehydration and failure to thrive result secondary to decreased insulin secretion (NLM, 2024g). Epilepsy and developmental delay, known as *DEND syndrome* (**D**evelopmental delay—**E**pilepsy—**N**eonatal **D**iabetes), is associated with this genetic disorder. Patients with an underdeveloped pancreas may manifest with fatty stools and the inability to absorb fat-soluble vitamins (NLM, 2024g). Lifelong insulin therapy is required for adequate weight gain and nutritional balance; there is no chance for remission (Polak & Cave, 2007).

Biliary Hypoplasia (Alagille Syndrome). Biliary hypoplasia, characterized by incomplete development of the biliary system, results in a reduction in intrahepatic bile ducts. This disorder affects approximately one in every 30,000 live births; boys and girls are equally represented (Figure 6.14; National Organization for Rare Disorders [NORD], 2024; NLM, 2024a). Most cases involve mutations in the *JAG1* gene (chromosome 20p12); less than 1% of cases are caused by mutations in *NOTCH2* (National Institute of Health Genetic and Rare Diseases Information Center [GARD], 2025). Gene mutations lead to insufficient bile flow. This provokes liver dysfunction, which manifests as jaundice, pale stools, malabsorption, pruritus, and xanthelasma (soft yellow plaques on eyelids; Kamoth & Piccoli, 2008; Taylor & Neu, 2021). Lifelong continuing care is required.

Autosomal Recessive

Cystic Fibrosis. Recall from Chapter 4 that cystic fibrosis (CF) is an inherited condition characterized by the accumulation of thick, sticky mucus that damages many organs. It is estimated to occur in one in 2,500 to 3,500

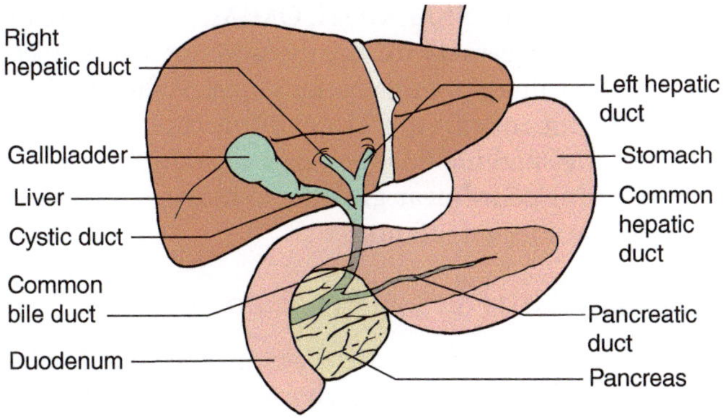

Figure 6.14 Normal anatomy of the biliary system. In cases of abnormal formation of the bile ducts (e.g., Alagille syndrome), failed passage of bile causes buildup of bile within the liver and subsequent hepatic injury.

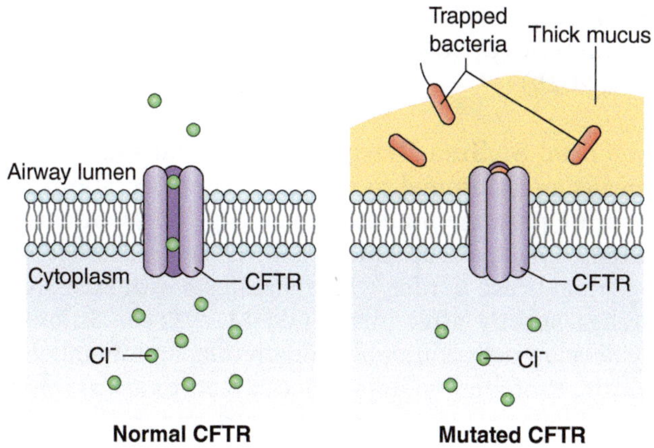

Figure 6.15 Impact of functioning CFTR (left) and nonfunctional CFTR (right). CFTR regulates Chloride (Cl^-) ion flow in and out of the cells. When CFTR is mutated (nonfunctional), ion flow is impaired, which allows for mucus accumulation. Stagnation of the mucous accumulation may occur in the pancreatic and bile ducts, as well as the respiratory system.
CFTR, cystic fibrosis transmembrane conductance regulator.

Caucasian infants and is less common in African American (1/17,000) and Asian (1/31,000) races (NLM, 2024b). CF is caused by mutations in the *CFTR* (CF transmembrane regulator) gene. Normally, CFTR protein works as a channel that allows cells to release chloride and other ions. When the *CFTR* gene is defective, it prevents cells from releasing the chloride (Figure 6.15; NLM, 2024b). The outcome is an improper salt balance in the cells and thick, sticky mucus that clogs and damages body organs, especially the GI and respiratory systems. The disease causes alterations in exocrine gland function and pancreatic enzyme deficiency (NLM, 2024b; Salar-Khalil & Sferra, 2025).

In the newborn, GI symptoms include failure to pass meconium and jaundice, which may be prolonged (Salar-Khalil & Sferra, 2025). The failure to pass meconium is typically the result of the accumulation of multiple meconium plugs within the ileum or distal colon (meconium plug syndrome [MPS]). The presence of a meconium ileus affects approximately 50% of infants with CF and may lead to further complications, including microcolon, abdominal distention, peritonitis, or even volvulus. Radiographically, neonatal APRNs may identify small loops of bowel that take on a honeycomb-like ground-glass appearance and low air-fluid levels. The ground glass appearance is due to an accumulation of air bubbles ("soap bubble appearance") trapped around thick meconium (also known as the Nehauser sign). Complementary low air-fluid levels are a classic manifestation of meconium ileus (due to the presence of tenacious meconium and abnormal mucous-gland secretion) compared to other abdominal obstructions and should raise the index of suspicion for CF. Respiratory symptoms include chronic respiratory failure with wheezing, cough, and recurrent pneumonia (NLM, 2024b, 2024c).

Life expectancy has improved with earlier diagnosis and treatment; a multidisciplinary approach is critical to optimize outcomes and must be customized according to disease severity and comorbidities. Common life-span implications include acquired pancreatic insufficiency, which typically requires lifelong supplementation of pancreatic enzyme and fat-soluble vitamin supplementation, in addition to a high-calorie diet (Salar-Khalil & Sferra, 2025). Males may be affected by infertility, secondary to an absence of the vas deferens (NLM, 2024b).

Shwachman–Diamond Syndrome. Shwachman–Diamond syndrome is an autosomal recessive disorder that affects one in 50,000 North American infants (NLM, 2024h; Online Mendelian Inheritance in Men [OMIM], 2024g). Alterations in the *RPS19* gene and *SBDS* gene located on chromosome 7 alter normal development of the pancreas, bone marrow, and skeletal system. Pancreatic insufficiency and bone marrow failure result. Clinical manifestations include failure to thrive, malabsorption, and steatorrhea. Cyclic neutropenia is the most common hematologic finding; these infants are at risk for frequent bacterial infections. Similar to CF, pancreatic insufficiency requires lifelong pancreatic enzyme and fat-soluble vitamin supplementation and high caloric diet (NLM, 2024h; Salar-Khalil & Sferra, 2025).

Congenital Chloride Diarrhea. Congenital chloride diarrhea is an autosomal recessive form of severe chronic diarrhea characterized by voluminous, watery stools with high chloride concentration (GARD, 2024a). Mutation in the *SLC26A3* gene on chromosome 7 disrupts chloride transport within the distal ileum and colon (OMIM, 2024a). Postnatal clinical manifestations include dehydration, metabolic alkalosis, hyperbilirubinemia, abdominal distention, hyperactive renin–angiotensin system, and hyperaldosteronism. Older infants may present with failure to thrive (GARD, 2024a; OMIM, 2024a). The disease affects infants across the life span and no cure is available; treatment is supportive and targets the normalization of electrolyte absorption in the jejunum (GARD, 2024b; OMIM, 2024a; Salar-Khalil & Sferra, 2025).

Congenital Sodium Diarrhea. Congenital sodium diarrhea is an autosomal recessive disorder. Mutations in the serine protease inhibitor gene (*SPLINT2*) on chromosome 19q13 disrupt sodium–hydrogen exchange at the jejunal brush border, which manifests with excessive diarrhea shortly after birth (OMIM, 2024b). Infants may develop dehydration, hyponatremia, and metabolic acidosis. Profound volume loss can lead to acute renal failure. Lifelong monitoring is required, and treatment is focused on fluid and electrolyte replacement and managing individual symptoms (Salar-Khalil & Sferra, 2025).

Glucose–Galactose Malabsorption. Malabsorption of glucose and galactose is an autosomal recessive disorder (NLM, 2024d). Mutations in the *SLC5A1* gene lead to altered transport of glucose, galactose, and sodium across the intestinal epithelium (NLM, 2024d). As a result, glucose, galactose, and water accumulate within the intestinal tract and are lost in the stool (NLM, 2024d). Hallmark manifestations among infants include severe diarrhea, dehydration, metabolic acidosis, and weight loss (NLM, 2024d). Life-span implications include the risk for development of kidney stones with calcium deposits throughout the kidneys. Lifelong avoidance of glucose and galactose sugars may be required (NLM, 2024d; OMIM, 2024c).

Congenital Lactase Deficiency. Congenital lactase deficiency is an autosomal recessive disorder characterized by an impaired ability to digest lactose. This is considered a rare genetic disorder within the United States; one in 60,000 Finnish-born infants are affected (NLM, 2024f; OMIM, 2024d). Congenital lactase deficiency is linked to mutations in the *LCT* gene, which modulates lactase production (NLM, 2024f; OMIM, 2024d). Recall that lactase is necessary for the digestion of lactose (see Chapter 10). Clinical manifestations present shortly after the establishment of enteral nutrition (breast or formula feeding) and include the onset of watery diarrhea with resultant poor linear growth; vomiting is reported among some affected infants.

Disorders With Familial Predisposition

Large bowel obstructions are diseases associated with a familial predisposition. Newborns will present with symptoms including progressively worsening abdominal distention, feeding intolerance, bilious emesis, and failure to pass meconium within the first 48 hours after birth. Neonatal APRNs must consider the differential diagnosis associated with this type of presentation to quickly and accurately diagnose the pathology. Diseases to consider include Hirschsprung disease, small left colon syndrome, CF, MPS, and ARMs. We present relevant information specific to Hirschsprung disease and small left colon syndrome.

Congenital Megacolon (Hirschsprung Disease). Hirschsprung disease involves a congenital absence of enteric ganglia and, as a result of this deficiency, is the most common cause for intestinal obstruction in newborns (NLM, 2024e). The incidence of this congenital aganglionosis is one in every 5,000 live births; a prevalence among males (4:1) and association with trisomy 21, is reported (NLM, 2024e). The pathogenesis involves gene mutations (*RET*, *EDNRB*, or *EDN3*) which alter the normal development and signaling of enteric nerves (ganglia; Figure 6.16; NLM, 2024e). The result is a deficiency in normal functioning of the enteric nerves as well as segments of bowel that lack enteric nerves (aganglionic segments), which prevents the normal evacuation of stool. The majority of cases involve the rectosigmoid

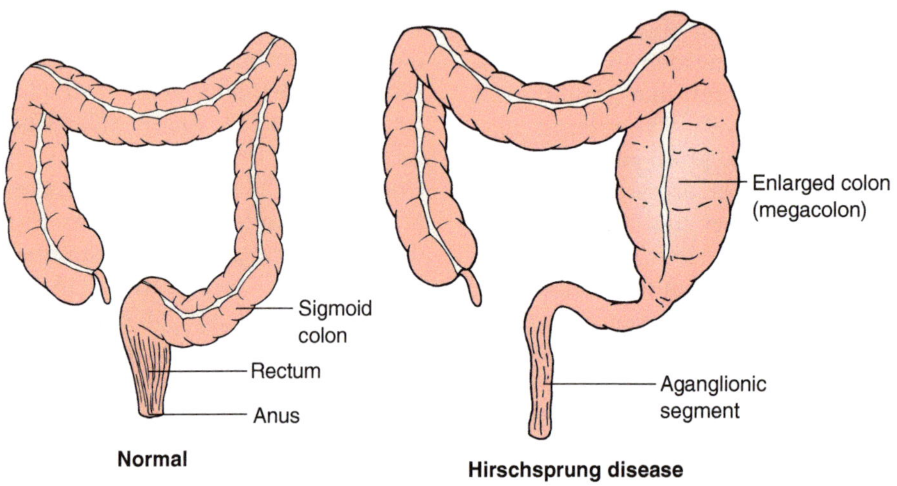

Figure 6.16 Normal intestine and manifestations of Hirschsprung disease. Hirschsprung disease results from failed migration of neural crest cells to the distal colon. As a result, submucosal and myenteric plexuses fail to develop, rendering the distal colon nonfunctional.

colon. Most affected infants (80%–90%) present with abdominal distention, emesis, and failure to pass meconium within the first 48 hours of life. *Meconium plugs* are strongly associated with Hirschsprung disease, whereas *meconium ileus* is strongly associated with CF. In contrast, MPS is a mechanical obstruction of the distal colon and rectum from thick meconium that usually results from colonic dysmotility secondary to fetal exposure to magnesium sulfate therapy, diabetes, hypothyroidism, or hypotonia and sepsis.

Long-term outcomes are reassuring, as 90% of patients achieve normal or near-normal bowel function (Dingeldein, 2025; Huang et al., 2017). Mortality and morbidity risks are associated with the length of bowel involvement and presence or absence of colonic atresia (Sloan & Wagener, 2016). Infants with microcolon or megacolon may incur lifelong bowel dysfunction, including constipation and fecal incontinence, as well as an increased risk for enterocolitis (Sloan & Wagener, 2016).

Small Left Colon Syndrome. Small left colon syndrome (SLCS) is considered a functional disease of the lower colon region. A strong association between diabetes in XX pregnant patients and SLCS is reported, which can help narrow the differential diagnosis. Common manifestations, which mimic the presentation of Hirschsprung disease early after birth, include progressively worsening abdominal distention with bilious emesis and failure to pass meconium within the first 48 hours after birth. Radiographic findings include a rectum of regular width and a normal rectosigmoid ratio with a notably large change in the caliber of the intestinal tract at the splenic flexure, which differentiates this type of bowel obstruction from Hirschsprung disease. It is common for affected infants to pass meconium plugs which resemble "casts" of the intestinal tract, particularly after a contrast enema or rectal irrigations are administered. SLCS typically resolves spontaneously within a few days of birth, and more invasive treatment (e.g., surgery) is typically only indicated if the obstruction precipitates bowel perforation (Qumsieh et al., 2023).

NOTEWORTHY DISEASES IN THE XX PREGNANT PATIENT THAT INFLUENCE FETAL GASTROINTESTINAL DEVELOPMENT AND FUNCTION

Genetic makeup, the uterine environment, chronic diseases of the XX pregnant patient, and the external environment all impact the fetus during gestation and may program the baby for lifelong morbidities. The developing GI system may be impacted directly or indirectly (Baker, 2022; Schierding et al., 2022).

External Environmental Factors

Environmental factors with impact on the GI system include drugs, chemicals, radiation, and infections. Common drugs associated with IUGR and/or prematurity in the fetus are alcohol, aminopterin, cocaine, and phenytoin. Alcohol and tobacco smoke containing nicotine, carbon monoxide, and other substances enter the birthing parent's blood and are transported to the placenta. From the placenta, those toxic substances enter the baby's bloodstream. These substances are associated with growth restriction (Torchia & Persaud, 2025). Individuals of child-bearing age are commonly exposed to reproductive toxins such as polychlorinated biphenyls and possible ionizing radiation. Furthermore, the modifications of sperm secondary to environmental exposures via epigenetic processes is associated with GI defects such as EA and TEF (Day et al., 2016). All of these factors are associated with premature birth, IUGR infants, and birth defects. These exposures increase the risk for prenatal and postnatal GI problems, including poor absorption of nutrients, NEC, faulty glucose regulation, and cholestasis secondary to altered liver metabolism (Baker, 2022; Torchia & Persaud, 2025). The exact mechanism of environmental factors resulting in fetal disruption, prematurity, and IUGR infants is unknown; however, epigenetic processes are increasingly implicated (Day et al., 2016; Torchia & Persaud, 2025).

The Microbiome

Recall the earlier discussion focused on the newborn microbiota. Microbes are present in the amniotic fluid, the placenta, and meconium (Neu & Singh, 2022). Although microbes in the placenta are associated with postnatal infection, exposure does not always lead to morbidity. The pregnant XX pregnant individual, embryo, fetus, and neonate live with several commensal microbes; interactions between microbes and the host are often beneficial to the developing fetus (Neu & Singh, 2022; Tourneur & Chassin, 2013; Wu & Wu, 2012).

The fetal intestine is considered an immunoreactive organ. The interaction of microbes and fetal intestines may be part of early intestinal immune development; however, the mechanism is not understood, and research is needed (Gritz & Bhandari, 2015; Wu & Wu, 2012). The microbes in meconium are representative of organisms contained in the amniotic fluid. However, there is limited data to explain how these microbes impact the developing intestine of the fetus and newborn. It is known, however, that a dysbiotic microbial environment may result in an intestine-initiated inflammatory response, which can precipitate premature labor and delivery or increase the risk for NEC (Gritz & Bhandari, 2015; Neu & Singh, 2022). Early population of the neonatal gut microbiome indicates exposure to the XX pregnant patient. However, the preterm infant has reduced microbial diversity and an increase in pathogenic organisms; thus, the fragile preterm is at risk for dysbiosis (Gritz & Bhandari, 2015).

Long-term implications focus on the fetal intestine's role in priming the intestinal immune responses that result in tolerance or exacerbation of immune responses. These interactions may be important to autoimmunity and allergic responses later in life. In addition, intestinal microbes in the XX pregnant patient may produce metabolic products that are transferred to the fetus via the hematogenous route. Very-low-birthweight infants have increased risk for obesity later in life, perhaps due to metabolic programing toward energy storage or altered nutrient utilization; more research is needed (Gritz & Bhandari, 2015; Neu & Singh, 2022; Wu & Wu, 2012). The oligosaccharides in human milk may enhance the intestinal microbiome of the newborn. Early studies indicate the oligosaccharides promote growth of certain taxa of bacteria and positively impact the infant's GI tract (Neu & Singh, 2022).

Bacterial and Viral Infections in the Pregnant Patient

The gut microbiota is a complex, unique, multifunction system that shapes the immune system of the baby. The development of this system begins during antenatal life and continues throughout the neonatal period. External factors, including breastfeeding, environment, delivery mode, and genetic factors, influence this process. Microbiota and microbes plus intestinal epithelial cells are responsible for the development of homeostasis in the neonate. This foundation may allow homeostasis maintenance during adult life. When the immune tolerance balance is upset, inflammatory disease and susceptibility to infections and sepsis may occur (Tourneur & Chassin, 2013; Wu & Wu, 2012).

Despite a protected environment, intraamniotic infection (IAI), commonly referred to as chorioamnionitis, can occur with or without rupture of membranes. Microorganisms may enter the amniotic space by (a) ascending through the vagina; (b) accidental introduction during invasive procedures such as amniocentesis, chorionic villus sampling, fetal blood sampling, or transfusion; (c) blood infection circulating through the placenta; or (d) peritoneal cavity infection through the fallopian tubes (Jung et al., 2022). The infection may be bacterial or viral, with *Ureaplasma urealyticum* and *Mycoplasma hominis* the most commonly cultured bacteria. Amniotic compartment infection, bacterial or viral, sets up an inflammatory response that may be acute or chronic. This inflammatory process is known as systemic fetal inflammatory response syndrome (FIRS), which can progress to multiple-organ failure and death. Preterm delivery is associated with FIRS with risks to the GI system including NEC, poor nutrient absorption, and late-onset sepsis (Jung et al., 2022).

Gut flora contributes to changes in the immune system and energy balance. Human microbe colonization accelerates at birth and is important in resistance to pathogen invasion, immune stimulation, and other developmental cues. Babies experiencing vaginal birth receive inoculation with vaginal and other urogenital microbes, including *Lactobacillus* and *Prevotella* types. Cesarean-section babies have intestinal colonization with epidermal species, including *Clostridium, Staphylococcus, Propionibacterium*, and *Corynebacterium*. C-section babies also have fewer anaerobes such as *Bacteroides* and *Bifidobacterium*. The exact impact on the newborn GI tract is unknown (Gritz & Bhandari, 2015; Neu & Singh, 2022). Meconium also has bacteria and Ardissone et al. (2014) found the species were the same as bacteria in the amniotic fluid. The influence of gut colonization may be the programming for adult disease, including autoimmune disorders, obesity, diabetes, cardiovascular disease, and hypertension (Aaguard et al., 2014; Jung et al., 2022; Wu & Wu, 2012). Shifts or dysbiosis in microbe composition can occur secondary to diet, antibiotics, or infection. The growth of pathogens may disrupt the inflammatory balance and lead to the development of NEC, a multifactorial condition (Gritz & Bhandari, 2015; Wu & Wu, 2012).

Gestational Diabetes Mellitus. Gestational diabetes mellitus (GDM) presents during pregnancy and usually disappears after birth; however, the birth parent remains at risk for type 2 diabetes. Placental overgrowth increases glucose transfer to the fetus with increased levels of GLUT1 protein. GDM increases the risk of premature delivery, hyperinsulinemia, and hypoglycemia in the newborn. Lifelong implications for the fetus include developing type 2 diabetes and obesity (Simmons et al., 2017; Weiner et al., 2025).

Diabetes Mellitus in the Pregnant Patient. DM is a constellation of metabolic disorders with high blood glucose levels, either due to inadequate insulin sensitivity or insulin resistance. As in GDM, with DM there is increased glucose transfer with an increase in basal plasma membrane GUT1 levels (Simmons et al., 2017). The effect on blood vessels of the pregnant patient may cause fetal growth restriction or macrosomia (Weiner et al., 2025). DM also increases the risk of preterm birth and macrosomia with mild to severe hypoglycemia from elevated glucose levels in utero. GI disturbances include hypoglycemia, altered absorption, poor insulin regulation, and increased risk for NEC (Navathe et al., 2016). DM may also result in IUGR babies with altered cell proliferation in pancreatic beta-islet cells resulting in glucose intolerance. This metabolic change results in dyslipidemia, hepatic cholestasis, and hepatic dysfunction in the fetus and newborn. The consequences of the DM fetal environment include coronary disease, obesity, and diabetes type 2 as adults (Baker, 2022).

Obesity in the Pregnant Patient. The Centers for Disease Control and Prevention (CDC) defines *overweight* as a body mass index (BMI) between 25 to 29.9 and *obese* as a BMI greater than 30 (CDC, 2024a). The impact of obesity begins before conception as a chronic health condition with comorbidities (Correa & Marcinkevage, 2013; Navathe et al., 2016). The impact on the fetus is the increased risk for preeclampsia in the pregnant patient. Owens et al. (2010) found that preeclampsia is nearly five times greater in obese pregnant patients, frequently ending in preterm delivery; delivery at less than 33 weeks' gestation occurs twice as often. Preterm delivery increases the risk of altered immunity, feeding intolerance, and NEC. Gut morbidity increases with decreasing gestational age at birth (Owens et al., 2010; Williams et al., 2014). Initiation and duration of lactation are decreased in obese postpartum patients; therefore, fewer infants benefit from the protections/enhancements of breast milk (Amir & Donath, 2007; Gussler & Arensberg, 2011). Lifelong implications include the risk of obesity, diabetes mellitus, stroke, asthma, and heart disease in the baby. In addition, some evidence implies poorer cognitive function and neurodevelopmental disorders. Preliminary evidence supports a long-term negative impact on the immune and infectious-disease outcomes via epigenetic processes changing the gut microbiome (Baker, 2022; Godfrey et al., 2017; Perdu et al., 2016).

Hypertension in the Pregnant Patient. There are currently four types of hypertension diagnosed in pregnant patients: gestational hypertension, preeclampsia, chronic hypertension, and preeclampsia superimposed on chronic hypertension. Preeclampsia accounts for approximately 12% to 25% of IUGR and small-for-gestational-age (SGA) infants and 15% to 20% of preterm babies. Prematurity, IUGR, and SGA status increase the risk for altered immune status, NEC, impaired absorption, and feeding intolerance. Lifelong implications include insulin resistance, hypertension, and cardiovascular disease (Jeyabalan, 2025).

In conclusion, any chronic disease process which causes preterm birth, IUGR, or macrosomia imposes a negative impact on the newborn's GI system. The impact correlates with gestational age and severity of the disease in the XX pregnant patient, and may program the fetus for adult-onset disease.

COMMON PROBLEMS WITH IMPLICATIONS ACROSS THE LIFE SPAN

Disorders of the Foregut

Esophageal Atresia and Tracheoesophageal Fistula. EA and TEF occur as a consequence of failed septation of the foregut into separate esophageal and tracheal structures (see Chapter 4, Table 4.9). EA affects one in 4,100 births; approximately 90% of all cases are associated with TEF (CDC, 2024b). According to population studies (CDC, 2024b), increased risk of EA/TEF is associated with advanced paternal age (sperm abnormalities) and assisted reproductive technology (CDC, 2024b; Chia & Shi, 2002; Day et al., 2016). A history of polyhydramnios supports the inability of the fetus to swallow amniotic fluid in utero, and should increase the index of suspicion for EA/TEF (Dingeldein, 2025; Guandalini & Dhawan, 2022; Wolfe & Jnah, 2024).

Although a complete understanding of genetic influences remains to be determined, the pathogenesis of some cases of EA and TEF is influenced by gene defects. Research demonstrates that teratogens induce alterations in the expression of genes involved with certain signaling pathways within the dorsal and ventral foregut. This disrupts normal septation of the foregut into the trachea (anteriorly) and the esophagus (posteriorly), between weeks 4 and 7 of gestation (Rayyan et al., 2017).

EA/TEF can be associated with trisomy 13, 18, or 21; Pierre Robin sequence; DiGeorge syndrome; Fanconi syndrome; and polysplenia syndrome; as well as VACTERL spectrum (**V**ertebral defects, anal **A**tresia, **C**ardiac defects, **TEF**, **R**enal anomalies, and **L**imb abnormalities) and CHARGE syndromes (**C**oloboma, **H**eart defects, choanal **A**tresia, **R**etardation of growth/development, **G**enital/urinary defects, and **E**ar anomalies). Associated anatomic defects include DA, annular pancreas, jejunoileal atresia, malrotation, diaphragmatic hernia, and abdominal wall defects (Dingeldein, 2025; Wolfe & Jnah, 2024).

Clinical manifestations of EA/TEF are usually evident soon after birth, with the exception of type E (see Chapter 4). The affected infant may exhibit excessive oral secretions that occlude the airway, causing coughing and mild to severe respiratory distress. Radiographic studies display a feeding tube that stops or coils above the stomach. The gut will be gasless if no connection between the trachea and lower esophagus exists, as with types A and B. On the contrary, the stomach may be distended if a distal fistula connects the stomach to the trachea.

Life-span implications include esophageal strictures and gastroesophageal reflux (GER) with chronic esophageal inflammation. Esophageal dysmotility and dysphagia occur secondary to abnormal neural development, or from the EA repair. Approximately 10% to 20% of patients develop clinically significant tracheomalacia. Recurrent bronchitis, pneumonia, wheezing, and daily coughing are also reported (Wolfe & Jnah, 2024).

Infantile Hypertrophic Pyloric Stenosis. Infantile hypertrophic pyloric stenosis (IHPS) is the most common cause of gastric outlet obstruction in infants (Ross & Johnson, 2016). It occurs in about two to 3.5 births per 1,000 live births. The incidence is lowest in urban versus rural areas. IHPS is more common in males (4–5:1) and premature infants. The incidence is reported as 0.1% to 1% in the general population and varies by region (Ranells et al., 2011).

There is a convincing familial tendency; the risk for the sibling of a child diagnosed with IHPS increases 20-fold, or almost 200-fold for an identical twin (Feenstra et al., 2012). Although this condition does not fall under the category of Mendelian inheritance, genetic heterogeneity and multiple loci have been implicated in IHPS, including IHPS1 on chromosome 12, IHPS2 on chromosome 16, IHPS3 on chromosome 11, IHPS4 on chromosome X, and IHPS5 on chromosome 16 (OMIM, 2024f). Some reports indicate that 30% to 40% of cases occur among first-born children; additional data is needed to generalize these findings (Dingeldein, 2025; Ranells et al., 2011).

The etiology of IHPS is unclear; however, immaturity of the ENS with aberrant innervation and altered levels of neuropeptides at the pylorus is one possibility (Ranells et al., 2011). Recall that the pylorus muscle is located where the stomach innervates with the intestine. The pathogenesis of IHPS involves overgrowth and tightening of the circumferential muscle around the pyloric channel. This leads to narrowing and elongation of the pylorus, a gastric outlet obstruction, and dilation and hyperperistalsis of the stomach (Ranells et al., 2011; Ross & Johnson, 2016; Torchia & Persaud, 2025).

IHPS characteristically manifests in otherwise healthy newborns, usually between 3 and 6 weeks of age (Dingeldein, 2025). Classically, these infants present with persistent nonbilious vomiting, dehydration, weight loss, hypoglycemia, hyperbilirubinemia, and hypokalemic, hypochloremic metabolic alkalosis. IHPS may be diagnosed during palpation of the epigastric region; a small, mobile mass or "palpable olive," is identified and confers 97% selectivity (Dingeldein, 2025; Taylor & Neu, 2021). Ultrasound and/or upper GI contrast radiographs support the diagnosis. Fluid and electrolyte imbalance require urgent attention. Surgical correction is considered curative (Ross & Johnson, 2016).

Jejunoileal Atresia. Jejunoileal atresia is a rare condition that involves the absence of the fold of the stomach membrane that connects the small intestine to the dorsal abdominal wall. Classified as a rare disorder, jejunal atresia occurs equally in males and females (NORD, 2020). Cases are typically sporadic or follow an autosomal recessive inheritance pattern. Polyhydramnios, fetal distress, and drug exposure are known prenatal risk factors for this type of GI obstruction.

Jejunoileal atresia occurs due to a vascular accident in utero, likely between weeks 8 and 12 of gestation. Because the membrane connecting the small intestine to the abdominal wall is absent, the jejunum twists around the marginal artery of the colon, creating the atresia (NORD, 2020). The resultant loss of blood flow to that particular segment of bowel increases the risk for necrosis, volvulus, or strangulation (Torchia & Persaud, 2025). Jejunal and ileal stenosis, on the other hand, are thought to occur from failed recanalization of the intestinal lumen. Failure of recanalization and vascular insults lead to necrosis and reabsorption of the affected segments (Dingeldein, 2025).

Jejunoileal atresia is classified based on primary anatomic derangement (Table 6.3; Dingeldein, 2025). Clinical manifestations include bilious vomiting, varying degrees of dilated bowel proximal to the atretic area, and much smaller bowel loops downstream from the obstruction, as well as failure to pass meconium. On physical exam, the abdomen may be swollen in the epigastric region (NORD, 2020). A contrast enema usually shows microcolon, which occurs due to the lack of intestinal contents passing beyond the obstructed area. On abdominal radiography, jejunoileal atresia presents as a "triple bubble" of distended air-filled bowel loops (Dingeldein, 2025).

Life-span implications include bowel leak at postsurgical anastomosis sites and sepsis in the short-term postoperative period. Extensive bowel involvement may lead to significant bowel resection and short gut syndrome, long-term parenteral nutrition, and anastomotic strictures (Dingeldein, 2025; Nusinovich et al., 2013).

Duodenal Atresia. DA affects one to nine in every 100,000 births; as high as one in 11,000 births within Europe (Orphanet, 2021). DA most often occurs sporadically; however, in some cases, it is inherited as an autosomal recessive trait. Approximately 30% of affected infants are diagnosed with trisomy 21 (GARD, 2024b; Orphanet, 2021; Pritchard & Korf, 2016).

DA may be the result of intrinsic or extrinsic derangements. The pathogenesis of intrinsic DA involves failed duodenal recanalization. Extrinsic DA is associated with malrotation with Ladd's bands, annular pancreas, cysts, and duplications near the duodenum (Dingeldein, 2025; Pritchard & Korf, 2016). Annular pancreas occurs when the pancreatic bud fails to rotate behind the duodenum, creating a ring around a segment of the duodenum.

Similar to other proximal GI obstructions, a history of polyhydramnios is suspicious for DA. Affected infants may present with abdominal distention (or nondistention), bilious emesis (or nonbilious emesis), and dilated proximal bowel. Neonatal APRNs should recognize that classic manifestations include abdominal distention paired with non-bilious vomiting. Radiographic findings include the classic "double bubble" appearance of the gas-filled stomach and the gas-filled proximal duodenum. The distal intestine is usually gasless. DA and malrotation with midgut volvulus may have similar clinical presentations. However, midgut volvulus is an intestinal emergency requiring prompt intervention. The point of obstruction, in relation to the ampulla of Vater (where the common bile duct innervates with the bowel), is important during repair of DA to protect the duct. Surgical correction is highly successful (Orphanet, 2021).

Life-span implications include delayed stomach emptying and GER, which occurs postsurgically. Late complications include peptic ulcer, esophagitis, duodenal–gastric

TABLE 6.3 Five Classifications of Jejunoileal Atresia

Type	Common Clinical Manifestations	Visual Depiction
Type I	Mucosal (membranous) web	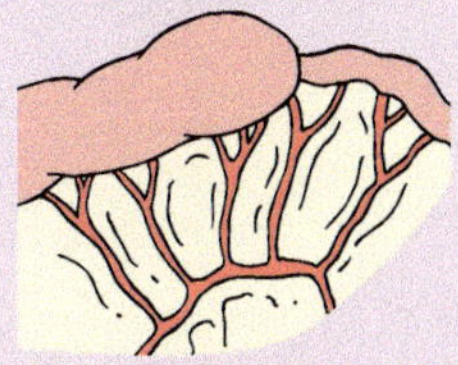
Type II	Blind ends connected by a fibrous cord	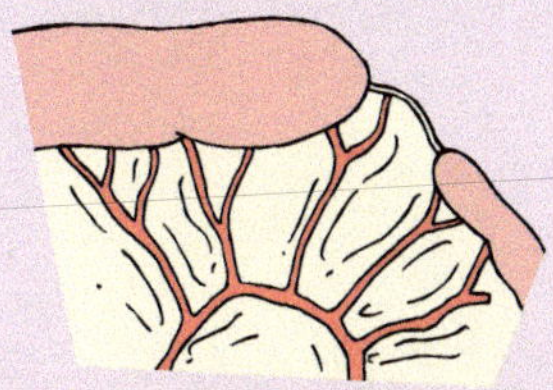
Type IIIa	Blind ends separated by a V-shaped mesenteric defect	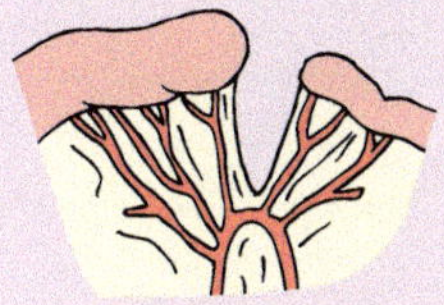
Type IIIb	Apple-peel or Christmas-tree deformity (blind ends; distal small bowel segment forms corkscrew around ileocecal artery terminus)	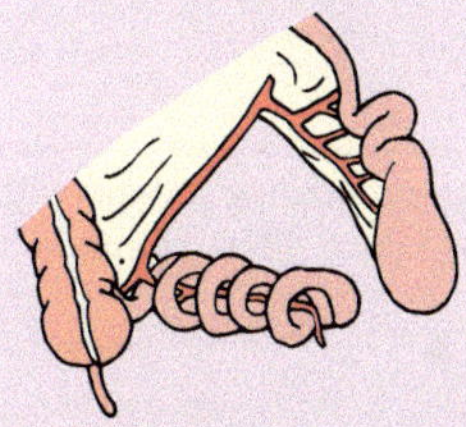
Type IV	Multiple atresias (string of sausages)	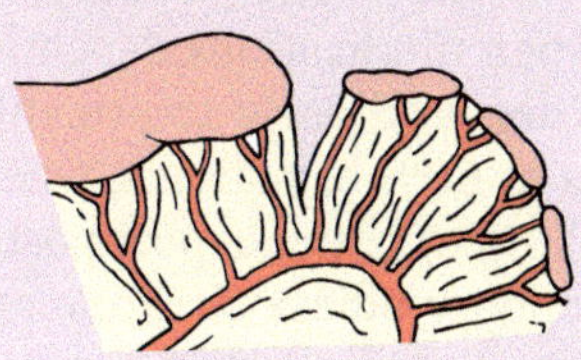

reflux, pancreatitis, and cholecystitis. Blind-loop syndrome, an overgrowth of normal bacterial flora that impairs normal function, and mega-duodenum, an elongation/dilatation of the duodenum impairing the movement of waste, have been reported (Orphanet, 2021).

Biliary Atresia. BA is the most common cause of obstructive jaundice in the newborn and the leading cause for liver transplantation among children (Lupo et al., 2017). The incidence is estimated at 0.5 to 0.8 per 10,000 births. African Americans have a twofold higher risk than Caucasians, and females more often than males.

BA is characterized by inflammation and obliteration of the extrahepatic or intrahepatic biliary system, which results in an obstruction of bile excretion from the gallbladder and bile duct into the small intestine (Lupo et al., 2017; Sanchez-Valle et al., 2017). The defect is typically an isolated finding; approximately 15% to 30% of cases occur in patients with situs inversus, polysplenia, asplenia, or other congenital anomalies.

The classification of extrahepatic BA is based on the site of the atresia (Table 6.4; Lupo et al., 2017). The fetal type presents within the first 2 weeks of life, and the postnatal type presents between the first and second month of life. Common clinical manifestations include hyperbilirubinemia, dark urine, and acholic stools. Jaundice may progress to conjugated or direct hyperbilirubinemia; unconjugated hyperbilirubinemia is rarely present after 2 weeks. Hepatosplenomegaly may develop, and an enlarging spleen may be a sign of cirrhosis and portal

TABLE 6.4 Three Classifications of Biliary Atresia

Type	Incidence	Common Clinical Manifestations	Visual Depiction
Type I	5%	Obliteration of the common duct; the proximal ducts are patent	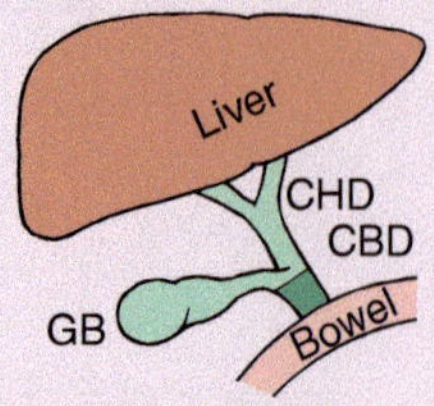
Type II	3%	Atresia of the hepatic duct, with cystic structures found in the porta hepatis	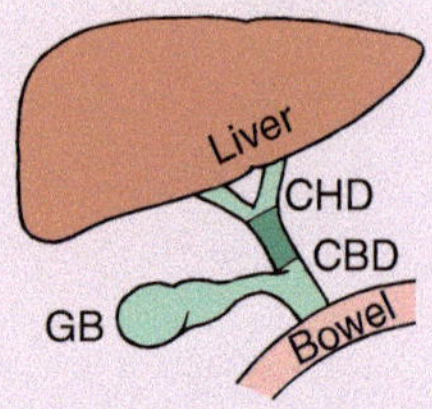
Type III (>90%)	90%	Atresia of the right and left hepatic ducts to the level of the porta hepatis	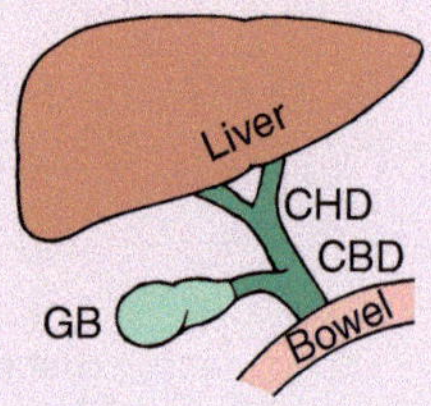

Note: The dark green shading present within each respective drawing corresponds with the locus of the atresia.
CBD, common bile duct; CHD, common hepatic duct; GB, gallbladder.

hypertension. Treatment by 2 months improves the outcome (Sanchez-Valle et al., 2017).

Life-span implications depend on the type of BA, comorbidities, and early treatment. Portal hypertension develops in 60% of patients, whereas cholangitis manifests in 50% of patients post portoenterostomy. Fibrosis and secondary biliary cirrhosis results if the disorder is not surgically corrected (Sanchez-Valle et al., 2017). For patients who develop cirrhosis, hepatocellular cancer is a risk. Liver transplantation is a treatment for long-term survival (Sanchez-Valle et al., 2017).

Disorders of the Midgut

Umbilical Hernia. Umbilical hernia is classified as a central fascial defect that occurs underneath the umbilicus. It affects 4% of Caucasian infants and 30% of African American infants. Umbilical hernia is more common in premature and low-birthweight neonates and newborns with congenital thyroid hormone deficiencies and trisomy 21; there is high familial tendency (Bohara, 2024; Flynn-O'Brien & Rice-Townsend, 2024; K. B. Kelly & Ponsky, 2013).

An umbilical hernia typically forms during week 10 of gestation, as the intestines return to the abdominal cavity. The pathology is well understood. A portion of intestine abnormally herniates through the umbilical ring, giving rise to this defect (Torchia & Persaud, 2025). The herniated tissue includes the greater omentum, a portion of the small intestine, and is covered by subcutaneous tissue and skin. Umbilical hernias average between 1 and 5 cm in diameter, and can increase in size during crying, straining, or coughing. Typically, they can be easily reduced into the abdomen or preperitoneal fat with gentle digital pressure during the physical examination (Bohara, 2024). The risk of incarceration is low, and most umbilical hernias close spontaneously. Surgical correction is only required with large defects, or when a hernia persists in a child over 4 years of age (Boardman et al., 2021; Flynn-O'Brien & Rice-Townsend, 2024). The recurrence risk is low (Bendavid et al., 2001; Boardman et al., 2021).

Omphalocele. Omphalocele is classified as a persistent herniation of bowel (and in some cases, other organs) *into the umbilical cord* and that is covered by a peritoneal sac (Bence & Wagner, 2021; Mowrer et al., 2022; Stallings et al., 2019). This is considered a central herniation of abdominal contents. The peritoneal sac covering the omphalocele is comprised of an amnion membrane, peritoneum, and Wharton's jelly; the umbilical cord connects to the central portion of the membrane (Bohara, 2024). Omphalocele is reported in 1.5 to 1.7 per 10,000 live births within the United States (Bhatt et al., 2022; CDC, 2024d); many pregnancies are associated with spontaneous abortions or stillbirths.

The pathology of omphalocele involves abnormal formation of the umbilical ring, such that between weeks 6 and 10 of gestation, as the abdominal contents herniate outside the abdominal compartment and return, some intestine (and possibly other nearby organs) remain outside the abdominal cavity. An abdominal wall defect greater than 5 cm and that includes liver tissue is considered a giant omphalocele. Genetic and teratogenic influences (e.g., alcohol, tobacco, or selective serotonin-reuptake inhibitor use during pregnancy, obesity) likely play a role in the pathology of this disease (CDC, 2024d). Importantly, *omphalocele is frequently associated with genetic disorders (e.g., Beckwith-Wiedemann syndrome, trisomy 13, 18, 21) as well as other midline defects (e.g., neurologic, cardiac, skeletal, genitourinary).* In fact, 50% to 75% of infants with omphalocele have other structural or genetic anomalies, including trisomy 13, trisomy 18, and trisomy 21; VACTERL association; Beckwith-Wiedemann syndrome; ectrodactyly–ectodermal dysplasia–cleft (EEC) syndrome (ectodermal dysplasia, ectrodactyly, cleft palate); and OEIS (omphalocele, exstrophy, imperforate anus, spinal defects). In rare instances, the defect is more cephalic, causing pentalogy of Cantrell: diaphragmatic hernia, sternal cleft, omphalocele, exstrophy of the heart, and intracardiac defects (Jnah et al., 2015). When the defect occurs below the umbilicus, bladder or cloacal exstrophy results (Dingeldein, 2025). Life-span implications are highly dependent on the presence and severity of comorbidities.

Gastroschisis. This defect is classified as a congenital extravasation of viscera through an opening that is lateral and to the right of an intact umbilical cord (Dingeldein, 2025). Varying amounts of small and large bowel, which may be edematous and thickened, and rarely the liver, are eviscerated through a small (2–4 cm) abdominal wall defect with no protective covering (Bohara, 2024). Gastroschisis is reported in 3.4 per 10,000 live births in the United States (Bhatt et al., 2022; Sadler, 2023; Schoenwolf et al., 2021) and commonly presents as an isolated defect; associated anomalies are reported in only 5% to 10% of all cases (Bhatt et al., 2022; CDC, 2024c). Risk factors include low socioeconomic status, young age at conception, and exposure to vasoconstriction as with some decongestants, nonsteroidal anti-inflammatory medications, cocaine, methamphetamine, and marijuana (Souther et al., 2017).

Several theories attempt to explain the pathology of this defect. One theory focuses upon a failed attachment between the umbilical cord and the umbilical ring. A second theory proposes that an infarction of the abdominal wall leads to gastroschisis. A third theory suggests that failure of mesenchymal migration during early development causes the defect (Mahe et al., 2022). Neonates with gastroschisis may present with signs of dehydration and gastric dilatation at birth, as well as varying degrees of edema, matting, and ischemia of the exposed bowel. Rarely do infants with gastroschisis have other associated birth defects or chromosomal/genetic problems. GI defects, including intestinal atresia or mechanical injury to the eviscerated bowel, may be seen. These complications may affect long-term morbidity. Dysmotility, adhesions, or strictures at points of resection put the neonate at risk for partial or complete obstruction later in life (Dingeldein, 2025).

CLINICAL APPLICATION. Stabilization in the delivery room and the immediate neonatal time period for an infant with a gastroschisis requires several important steps. The infant should be placed directly into a bowel bag to keep a barrier between the external environment and to allow visualization of the intestines. If a bowel bag is not available, the intestines can be wrapped in a sterile dressing soaked in warm saline and covered with a plastic coating. Think about the disadvantages with this method; first, as the wrap cools, hypothermia may occur; second, the dressing has to have saline reapplied, otherwise, as it dries, it can adhere to the intestinal mucosa causing pain and injury; and third, kinking of the bowel can occur as the dressing is applied and since the intestine is covered, visualization of compromise is not possible. Keep the infant lying on the right side to minimize the risk of occlusion of the superior mesenteric artery. Place a Replogle or sump tube to suction; if distention of the bowel occurs, there will be compromised blood flow to the intestinal wall resulting in ischemia. Obtain IV access and start maintenance fluids at increased total milliliters per kilogram per day; these infants are at risk for significant insensible water loss until surgical closure extending into the immediate postoperative period at which time the increased total fluids are related to third spacing. Empiric antibiotics are recommended until surgical closure occurs.

Malrotation. Malrotation is classified as an abnormal position of the small bowel within the abdomen. It affects one in every 500 live births, and most cases are subtle and subclinical. Symptomatic malrotation occurs in one in every 6,000 live births; a male prevalence is reported (Alani, 2023; Appaji et al., 2013; Martin & Shaw-Smith, 2010). Risk factors include imperforate anus; Marfan syndrome; cardiac anomalies; intestinal atresias; and trisomy 13, 18, and 21, as well as Meckel diverticulum and other congenital anomalies. It is estimated that 75% of all cases occur in newborns and young infants; 90% of symptomatic cases are diagnosed within the first year (Martin & Shaw-Smith, 2010).

Recall that between weeks 4 and 6 of gestation, the midgut portion of the intestine undergoes normal rotation. During this time, the intestine rapidly proliferates and quickly exceeds the constraints of the abdominal cavity. As such, a portion of the intestine herniates into the umbilical cord. A 270-degree counterclockwise intestinal rotation thereby occurs around the superior mesenteric artery. When the bowel rotates correctly, it fixes itself in the abdomen, eliminating the risk for twisting and obstruction. However, if the bowel does not rotate and properly fix itself, a malrotation occurs, which increases the risk for vascular compromise, or volvulus (Figure 6.17; Alani, 2023; Bohara, 2024). Genetic mutations in the gene *BCL6* are thought to disrupt the signaling pathway critical for normal intestinal rotation; however, this is poorly understood (Alani, 2023).

Midgut Volvulus. Midgut volvulus is an intestinal emergency. Intestinal twisting causes a blockage of blood flow to a segment of bowel, leading to occlusion and necrosis (Dingeldein, 2025; Taylor & Neu, 2021). A volvulus can occur at any age and may also be identified on prenatal ultrasound; however, the defect is more frequently observed among infants and children (Coste & Anand, 2022).

A wide range of clinical manifestations are reported among infants and include symptoms similar to NEC, including persistent bilious emesis, abdominal distention, and hematochezia. It is important for neonatal APRN students to recognize that *bilious emesis should always be considered malrotation with a midgut volvulus until proven otherwise by an upper GI study*, which will assess the position of the ligament of Treitz and duodenojejunal flexure (normal position is the left side of the abdomen) to evaluate for malrotation and assess for bowel obstruction (to evaluate for volvulus).

Mortality and morbidity are dependent upon the timing of the diagnosis; a higher mortality risk is associated with bowel necrosis. Associated congenital anomalies significantly impact the outcome. If surgery is required, the postoperative course influences the outcome. Intermittent bilious emesis, adhesions, and short gut syndrome are possible lifelong consequences (Coste & Anand, 2022).

Clinical Application. Sudden, bilious emesis in an otherwise well-appearing infant is a volvulus until proven otherwise. An upper GI contrast study is the gold standard to rule out this disorder. Contrast will highlight the abnormal location of the duodenojejunal flexure and malplacement of the ligament of Treitz; the abnormal placement of the proximal jejunal loops will be seen in the right hemiabdomen. Another finding that is typically described is the "whirlpool sign," a corkscrew constriction of the third portion of the duodenum (Choi et al., 2022). These findings support immediate surgery to prevent necrosis and loss of bowel.

Gastrointestinal Duplications. GI duplications are rare congenital anomalies characterized by a coating of smooth muscle and epithelial lining that represents some

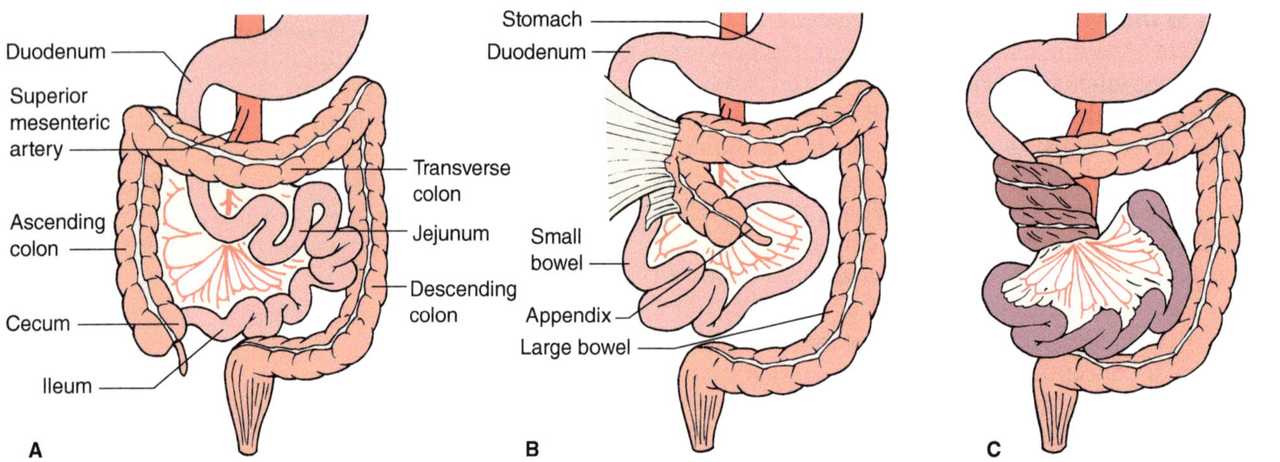

Figure 6.17 Intestinal malrotation and volvulus: (**A**) Normal positioning of the small and large intestine. (**B**) Impaired twisting (malrotation) of the midgut around its mesentery, as it returns into the abdominal cavity. Abnormal fixation of the cecum to the right abdominal wall, with obstruction of the duodenum by Ladd bands (bands of peritoneum), occurs. (**C**) Wrapping of bowel around the superior mesenteric artery causes ischemia (volvulus).

portion of the alimentary tract. The duplication usually requires surgical intervention (Dingeldein, 2020). The etiology is unknown. When present, duplications commonly occur at the ileum, esophagus, or colon, and can be cystic or tubular (R. Liu & Adler, 2014). Clinical manifestations vary, and presenting symptoms depend on the site of the duplication. Four pathologic criteria are necessary to establish the diagnosis: (a) anatomical continuity with the stomach, (b) presence of an outer smooth muscle layer, (c) a shared vascular supply with the stomach, and (d) a lining composed of gastric epithelial (Dingeldein, 2025; Taylor & Neu, 2021).

Surgery is generally curative and likewise carries a good prognosis. However, perforation and peritonitis may occur. Pancreatitis, neoplastic changes, rectal bleeding, and stool incontinence are potential complications of surgery (Rattan et al., 2017).

Disorders of the Hindgut

Anorectal Malformations. ARMs comprise a group of conditions that affect the lower intestinal tract and urogenital systems. The incidence is approximately one in every 5,000 births; a slightly higher male predominance is reported (Sloan & Wagener, 2016). Seventy percent of cases are associated with other defects, including abnormal or missing vertebrae or a tethered cord, as well as cardiac defects and EA, VACTERL, trisomy 21, Currarino syndrome, or cat eye syndrome (Sloan & Wagener, 2016).

The spectrum of ARMs includes a mildly stenotic anus, imperforate anus with genitourinary fistula, and congenital cloaca. Imperforate anus with genitourinary fistula, which is the most common anorectal defect, is known to affect approximately 80% of males (Sloan & Wagener, 2016). Rarely, ARMs are devoid of a fistula and the rectum ends in a blind pouch within the pelvis. Affected females may present with a perineal fistula at the skin level, vestibular or posterior vaginal fistula, or a more complex malformation where the urethra, vagina, and rectum have a common opening onto the perineum, known as a *congenital cloaca* (Pena, 2019).

The pathogenesis of ARMs is poorly understood (Sloan & Wegener, 2016). It is believed that ARMs result from arrested development of the urorectal septum, which normally divides the cloacal cavity into the anterior urogenital sinus and the posterior rectum; this normally occurs between weeks 4 and 8 of gestation. The precise etiology for this developmental arrest is not clear. One theory cites differences in the homeobox and SHH signaling pathways (see the section "Developmental Physiology"; Sloan & Wagener, 2016).

Infants with anorectal defects should be identified during the initial newborn physical examination. Infants who are affected, yet undiagnosed, may present with signs of bowel obstruction if a fistula is absent or too small to allow passage of stool (Sloan & Wagener, 2016). Comorbidities include urosepsis and metabolic acidosis, necessitating monitoring of all involved organs (Pena, 2019). Life-span implications include constipation, incontinence, and poor bowel and bladder control, as well as the psychosocial concerns that accompany these issues (Pena, 2019; Sloan & Wagener, 2016).

Other Disorders of the Gastrointestinal System

Necrotizing Enterocolitis. NEC is the most common acquired GI disease and GI surgical emergency in neonates and carries significant mortality and morbidity risks (Dominguez & Moss, 2012). The foremost risk factor is prematurity. Approximately 7% to 8% of premature infants are diagnosed with NEC during the birth hospitalization and the disease is associated with a 20% to 30% mortality risk (Singh et al., 2023). Prenatal risk factors include smoking, ampicillin exposure during labor, incomplete antenatal steroid exposure (Wong et al., 2014), inflammation (Lee et al., 2017), preeclampsia (Cetinkaya et al., 2012), IUGR (Kamoji et al., 2008), and DM (Grandi et al., 2015). Postnatal risk factors specific to infants born prematurely include SGA status at birth (Ree et al., 2014), intestinal dysbiosis and GI tract ischemia (Frazer & Good, 2022), bovine-based feeding (Shulhan et al., 2017), congenital heart defects (most notable is patent ductus arteriosus), polycythemia, red blood cell transfusion, and repeated nosocomial infections/antibiotic exposure (Markel et al., 2014; Weintraub et al., 2012). Thirty percent of all affected infants manifest a mild form of NEC that does not require aggressive treatment; however, 40% of infants require treatment, which may include surgical drain placement or bowel resection, and 30% of infants develop NEC totalis. Among surviving infants, postoperative risks include intestinal stricture and infection (de la Cruz, D., & Neu, 2025).

The etiology and pathogenesis of NEC is currently focused upon the vertical transfer of immunity from birth parent to newborn, presence of immature innate immune barriers, and lack of adequate GI immune defenses (Singh et al., 2023). Consider that IgG antibodies can cross the placenta and augment the fetus and newborn's immature immune system. However, the majority of IgG transfer occurs between week 28 and 32 of gestation and represents only half of the birth parent antibody levels (Singh et al., 2023). Therefore, infants born before this threshold exhibit a critically immature immune system. In addition, consider that IgA and human milk oligosaccharides (HMO) are only transferrable through human milk. Preterm infants who do not receive IgA-rich human milk cannot effectively bind IgA with bacteria in the GI tract and stave off NEC. The lack of IgA predisposes a preterm infant to dysbiosis, inflammatory disease, and infection (Gopalakrishna et al., 2019). The lack of HMOs contributes to a less diverse microbiome and inability of the preterm GI tract to block the adhesion of pathogens to the gut epithelium (Abbas et al., 2021). Other protective characteristics found only in significant amounts in freshly expressed human milk include the presence of Bacteroides species, casein, lactoferrin, and lysozymes.

Next, consider that immature innate immune responses are associated with a higher risk for NEC. Recall from the discussion of digestion and absorption that the small intestine is coated by a layer of mucus which is in part comprised of antimicrobial proteins. This mucus layer extends from the small to large intestine and colon, offering full-length protection from bacterial adhesion. A deficiency of this protective mucus is associated with NEC as well as the inability to effectively mount a defense to gut inflammation in cases of NEC (Vieten et al., 2005). In addition, complement activity is, in part, diminished in preterm infants, which reduces the body's ability to opsonize bacteria. On the other hand, one particular complement component, C5, appears to be upregulated in NEC and is posited to precipitate the inflammatory response seen with this disease (Tayman et al., 2011). It is possible that real-time trending of C5 levels will be used in the future to help diagnose NEC. Toll-like receptors (TLR) hold another role in the pathogenesis of NEC. Although there are numerous types of TLR, organized numerically, we will focus on the relationship between TLR4 and NEC. During fetal development, increased concentrations of TLR4 encourage the formation and migration of enterocytes, which form the intestinal epithelium. TLR4 also maintains the sterility of the intestinal tract during fetal development; high concentrations resist bacterial aggregation. Among term infants, TLR4 levels drop after birth, which permits the establishment of the gut microflora. Thereafter, TLR4 concentrations fluctuate, as needed, to maintain homeostasis between microbial load (lower TLR4 concentrations) and the immune response (higher TLR4 concentrations). In comparison, TLR4 levels remain elevated among preterm infants, which alters postnatal gut maturation and colonization, as well as exacerbates the immune response. Among premature infants affected by NEC, markedly elevated concentrations of TLR4 lead to apoptosis of existing enterocytes and reduce the synthesis of new enterocytes, which would normally be recruited during the healing process (Egan et al., 2016; Sodhi et al., 2012).

In addition, recent research suggests that alterations in intestinal colonization, by way of microbial imbalance, encouraged inflammation, increased TLR4 concentrations, and led to degradation of the intestinal epithelium (de la Cruz, D., & Neu, 2025; Markel et al., 2014). In fact, preterm infants who require life support (e.g., mechanical ventilatory support, isolette) tend to develop an abundance of pathogenic bacteria within the gut including *Enterobacteriaceae* species, *Klebsiella, Neisseria, Staphylococcus,* and *Streptococcus.* Gammaproteobacteria (*Klebsiella, Escherichia coli*) and even viruses including adenovirus have been identified in the stool of preterm infants with NEC (Sim et al., 2015). When present, intestinal ischemia and inflammation weaken the bowel and increase its propensity for perforation. Perforation, which may be localized or diffuse, leads to leakage of GI contents into the peritoneal cavity and subsequent peritonitis (de la Cruz, D., & Neu, 2025). Radiographic findings include the presence of air in the bowel wall, which may track across the liver (portal venous gas).

Clinical manifestations include abdominal distention and any combination of the following: hematochezia, bilious emesis, increased gastric residuals, lethargy, apnea, bradycardia, tachycardia, neutropenia, low peripheral monocyte count (due to recruitment from the peripheral circulation and to the diseased bowel), thrombocytopenia, metabolic acidosis, abdominal tenderness/erythema, respiratory failure, and shock (Singh et al., 2023). Erythema of the abdominal wall may be caused by necrotic bowel loops abutting up against the thin abdominal wall; a bluish discoloration is due to intraperitoneal stool seen through the thin abdominal wall. The diagnosis is confirmed in the presence of pneumatosis intestinalis with dissection of bacterial toxins into the bowel wall and/or portal venous gas on radiograph (de la Cruz, D., & Neu, 2025; Taylor & Neu, 2021).

Disease severity is graded by modified Bell staging, which is summarized in Table 6.5. Kliegman and Walsh (1987) modified the original Bell staging to aid clinicians in differentiating between mild and more severe disease states. Laboratory findings are included with staging criteria to alert clinicians of correlations among acidosis, hyponatremia, thrombocytopenia, neutropenia, disseminated intravascular coagulation, and disease severity. While it is well beyond the scope of this textbook to comprehensively address emerging treatments for NEC, new data suggest that the use of two cytokines, interleukin 22 (IL-22) and interleukin 37 (IL-37); TLR inhibitors; stem cell therapy; probiotics; and possibly fecal microbiota transplants could reduce the incidence and/or severity of NEC (Cho et al., 2020; Drucker et al., 2018; J. Liu et al., 2020; Lu et al., 2021; Mihi et al., 2021; Nolan et al., 2020; Rager et al., 2016; Tayman et al., 2011; Wu et al., 2022). Experts continue to emphasize that the use of freshly expressed colostrum or breast milk, rich with human milk oligosaccharides and immunoglobulins (e.g., IgA), is protective against NEC because the milk positively shifts the gut microbiota and enhances immune defenses.

Life-span implications for surgically treated infants include short gut syndrome, a condition where surgical bowel resection leads to the removal of the ileocecal valve and minimal residual intact bowel. Affected infants battle with "dumping" of gastric contents and poor nutrient absorption, leading to weight loss and nutrient deficits, long-term parental nutrition use, increased infectious risk, and chronic liver injury. In addition, hearing and visual impairments, as well as recurrent infections, are reported (Arnold et al., 2010).

TABLE 6.5 Modified Bell Staging

Stage	Classification	Common Clinical Findings	Common Radiographic Findings
I	Suspected NEC	• Abdominal distention • Apnea • Bloody stools • Bradycardia • Emesis/gastric residuals • Lethargy • Temperature instability	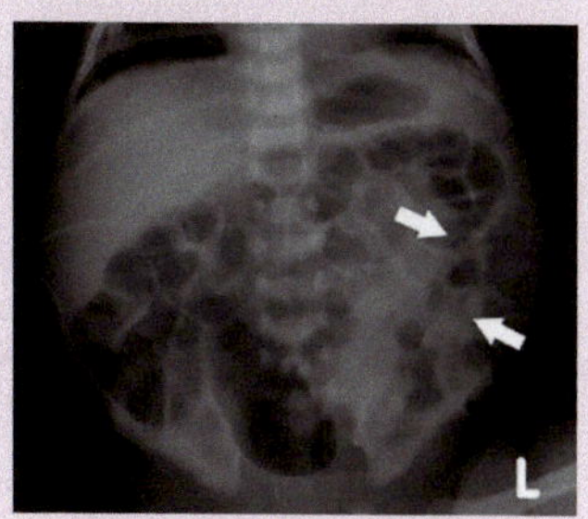 Ileus, gastric dilatation, asymmetric bowel loops
II	Proven NEC	Clinical findings from stage I *plus*: • Abdominal tenderness • Peritonitis • Possible metabolic acidosis • Possible cellulitis • Right lower quadrant mass • Thrombocytopenia	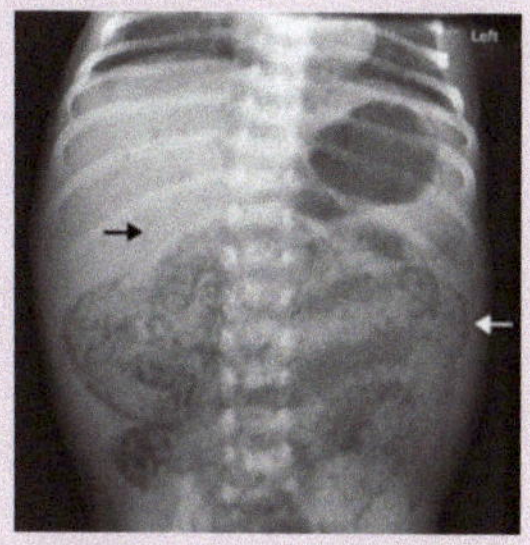 Pneumatosis intestinalis (white arrow) with portal venous gas (black arrow)
III	Advanced NEC	Clinical findings from stages I and II *plus*: • Acidosis (combined respiratory and metabolic) • Abdominal tenderness and distention (severe) • Apnea (severe) • DIC • Hypotension • Neutropenia • Thrombocytopenia	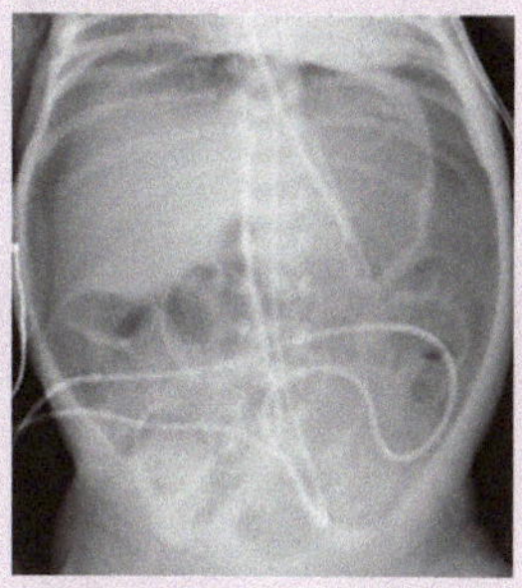 Pneumoperitoneum with free intraperitoneal air, ascites

DIC, disseminated intravascular coagulation; NEC, necrotizing enterocolitis.

Sources: Dominguez, K. M., & Moss, R. L. (2012). Necrotizing enterocolitis. *Clinics in Perinatology, 39*(2), 387–401. https://doi.org/10.1016/j.clp.2012.04.011; Esposito, F., Mamone, R., Di Serafino, M., Mercogliano, C., Vitale, V., Vallone, G., & Oresta, P. (2017). Diagnostic imaging features of necrotizing enterocolitis: A narrative review. *Quantitative Imaging in Medicine and Surgery, 7*(3), 336–344. https://doi.org/10.21037/qims.2017.03.01; Metzler, M., Burns, W., Mitchell, C., Napolitano, S., & Chaudhari, B. P. (2023). A case report of necrotizing enterocolitis in a moderately preterm neonate with LCHADD-A call to focus on the basics while utilizing advanced new therapies. *Frontiers in Pediatrics, 11*, 1081802. https://doi.org/10.3389/fped.2023.1081802

Clinical Application. In the infant that presents with early concerns of NEC such as abdominal distention and emesis, you want to get a basic metabolic panel (evaluating for hyponatremia and acidosis), a blood gas (evaluating for metabolic acidosis), complete blood count and coagulation panel (evaluating for anemia, thrombocytopenia, and/or evidence of disseminated intravascular coagulation), and a two-view abdominal x-ray (anterior-posterior [AP] flat plate and left lateral decubitus) or abdominal ultrasound. The AP-view is used to assess for the presence of pneumatosis, bowel gas pattern, and portal venous gas. Pneumatosis is the collection of hydrogen gas in the bowel wall as a result of breakdown of carbohydrates by the bacteria; the intramural air may look like thin black areas within the bowel wall (subserosal) or may look like a cystic bubbly pattern within the bowel wall (submucosa); see Figure 6.18. Other findings to look for include intraperitoneal air that outlines the falciform ligament, the "football sign," and the presence of air outlining both sides of the bowel lumen, known as the "Rigler sign." When assessing for portal venous gas, it is important to pay close attention to the area over the liver as the lucencies can be subtle and easily overlooked. A pneumoperitoneum can sometimes be subtle on the AP-view, however, with a left lateral decubitus view (placing the infant with the left side down so that if free air is present, it will rise and can be seen above the liver). Keep in mind that a pneumoperitoneum can be from other causes that should be considered if the infant has not had other clinical or radiographical concerns for NEC.

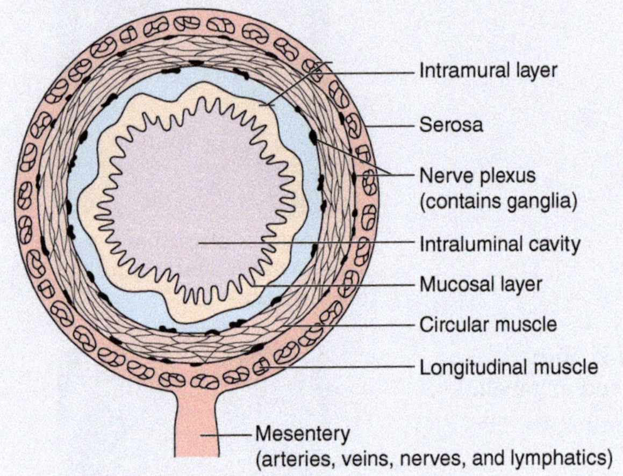

Figure 6.18 Cross section of the gut lumen.

Meckel Diverticulum. Meckel diverticulum, the most common congenital malformation of the GI tract, is characterized by an outpouching of the small intestine (ileum) caused by persistence of the omphalomesenteric (vitelline) duct. Approximately 2% to 4% of individuals are affected by Meckel diverticulum (Sagar et al., 2006). Failed regression of the omphalomesenteric duct, which normally occurs by week 7 of gestation, leads to the formation of a fibrous band that connects the (ileal) diverticulum to the umbilicus, as well as a cyst or a fistula that opens to the anterior abdomen. Although rare, Meckel diverticulum may become clinically significant during the neonatal period or infancy. Manifestations include GI bleeding, intestinal obstruction, intussusception, volvulus, bands, internal hernias, or Littre hernia. Typically, the diverticulum is devoid of clinical significance, and among individuals who require treatment, no long-term complications are reported (Obasi et al., 2015).

Meconium Plug Syndrome. The meconium plug is a thick tubular accumulation of meconium at the level of the colon. The epidemiology is rather illusive; Keckler et al. (2008) identified 77 newborns with meconium plug; 68% were males and 38% were females. Risk factors include prematurity, infants of diabetic XX pregnant patients, hypermagnesemia, and hypoglycemia (Dingeldein, 2025). Meconium plug is not considered a genetic disorder. The pathogenesis involves a functional immaturity of the colon and small intestine (hypomotility). As a result, the large colon may become dilated as meconium accumulates, becomes thick, and forms a plug (Figure 6.19; Dingeldein, 2025).

Clinical manifestations include delayed passage of meconium beyond the first 48 hours of life and abdominal distention. The plug may be difficult to pass and neonates may pass one or more meconium plugs. Life-span implications are related to associated conditions; CF and Hirschsprung disease are both positively associated with meconium plug and warrant further investigation (Dingeldein, 2025).

Meconium Ileus. Meconium ileus is an obstruction of the terminal ileum by tenacious, thick meconium, and accounts for about 33% of all small bowel obstructions in neonates. The obstruction occurs at the terminal ileum and the bowel distal to the obstruction may be empty and small, to the level of microcolon; the reduced size of the colon is secondary to disuse.

The majority of cases of meconium ileus are associated with CF (OMIM, 2024e). Clinical manifestations include abdominal distention, palpable bowel loops, poor feeding, and bilious emesis. If left untreated, meconium ileus may progress to volvulus, necrosis, peritonitis, and perforation. Life-span implications are dependent on the etiology and associated complications. If CF is present, lifelong treatment is required (Dingeldein, 2025; Taylor & Neu, 2021).

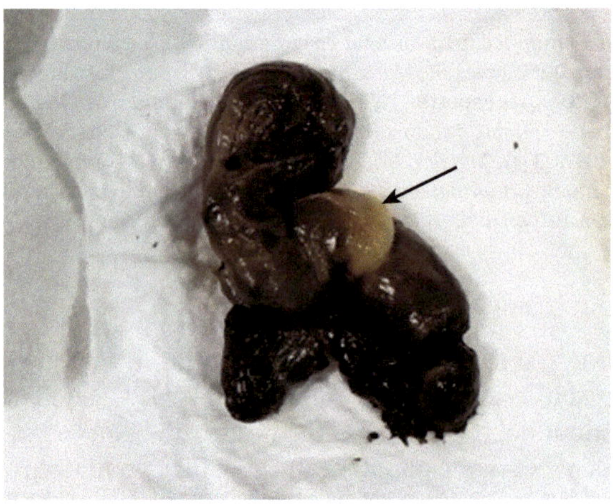

Figure 6.19 Colon of infant with evidence of one meconium plug (arrow).

CONCLUSION

The development, physiology, and functioning of the GI system are complex and the transition from fetus to newborn has lifelong implications. The primary GI functions of absorption of nutrients, fluid and electrolyte maintenance, protection from invaders, and waste elimination are essential to health. Careful attention to GI function is vital to the well-being of the newborn.

LEARNING TOOLS AND RESOURCES

CourseConnect

To access self-assessment questions and interactive, competency-based learning activities for this chapter, visit www.springerpub.com/courseconnect. See inside front cover and tear-out card for CourseConnect details.

Podcast

This podcast is available online by visiting www.springerpub.com/courseconnect. See inside front cover and tear-out card for CourseConnect details.

Intestinal Immunity

Rani Delaney, Lauren Fraser, Maryellen Lane, and Melissa Bauserman

DISCUSSION PROMPTS

1. How/why is the fetal gut considered an immunoreactive agent?
2. Discuss major components of the digestive process (mechanical, secretory, absorption) and how this implicates the premature infant.
3. Discuss the pathogenesis of NEC and the role of emerging treatments in mitigating the effects of the disease process.

MIND MAP

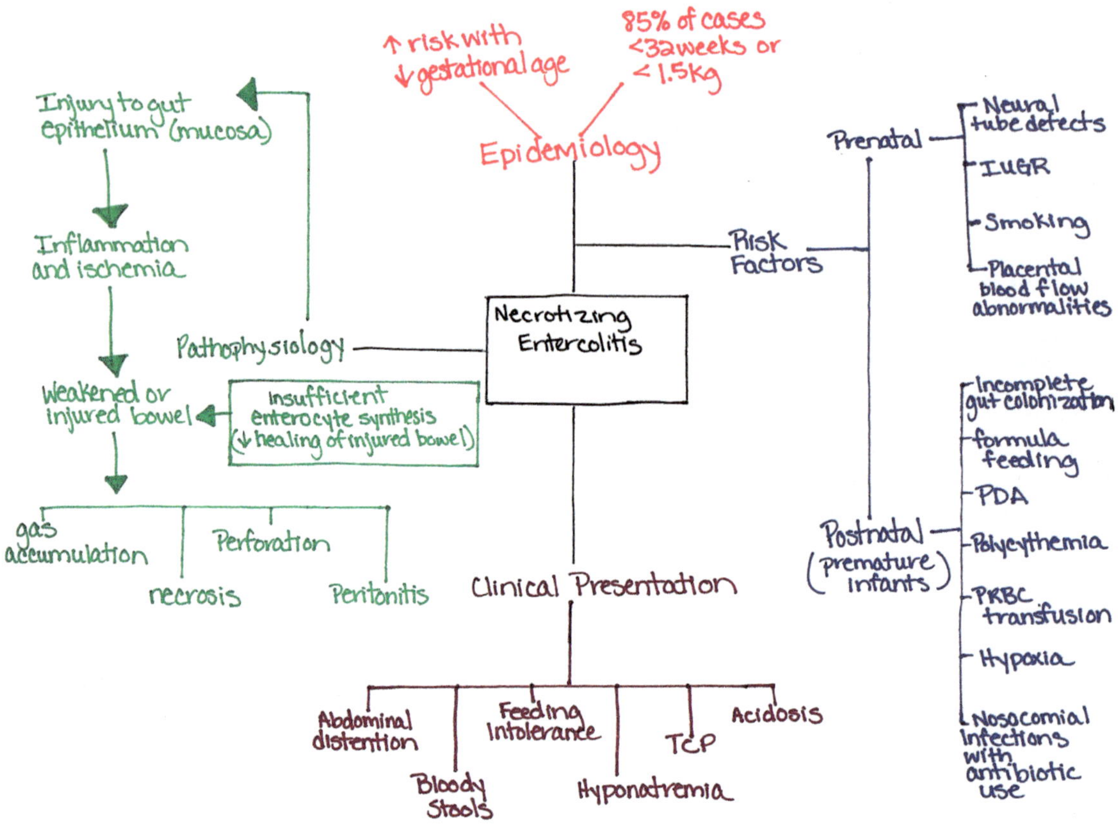

Note: *This mind map reflects one neonatal nurse practitioner student's interpretation of a concept addressed in this chapter. Readers should regard the mind maps woven throughout this textbook as examples of multisensory study tools that can be developed to aid conceptual understanding. Readers are encouraged to develop their own unique mind maps in consultation with academic faculty or clinical preceptors.*

Image Credit: Lisa Clevenger, DNP, APRN, NNP-BC.

TIMELINE OF ORGAN DEVELOPMENT

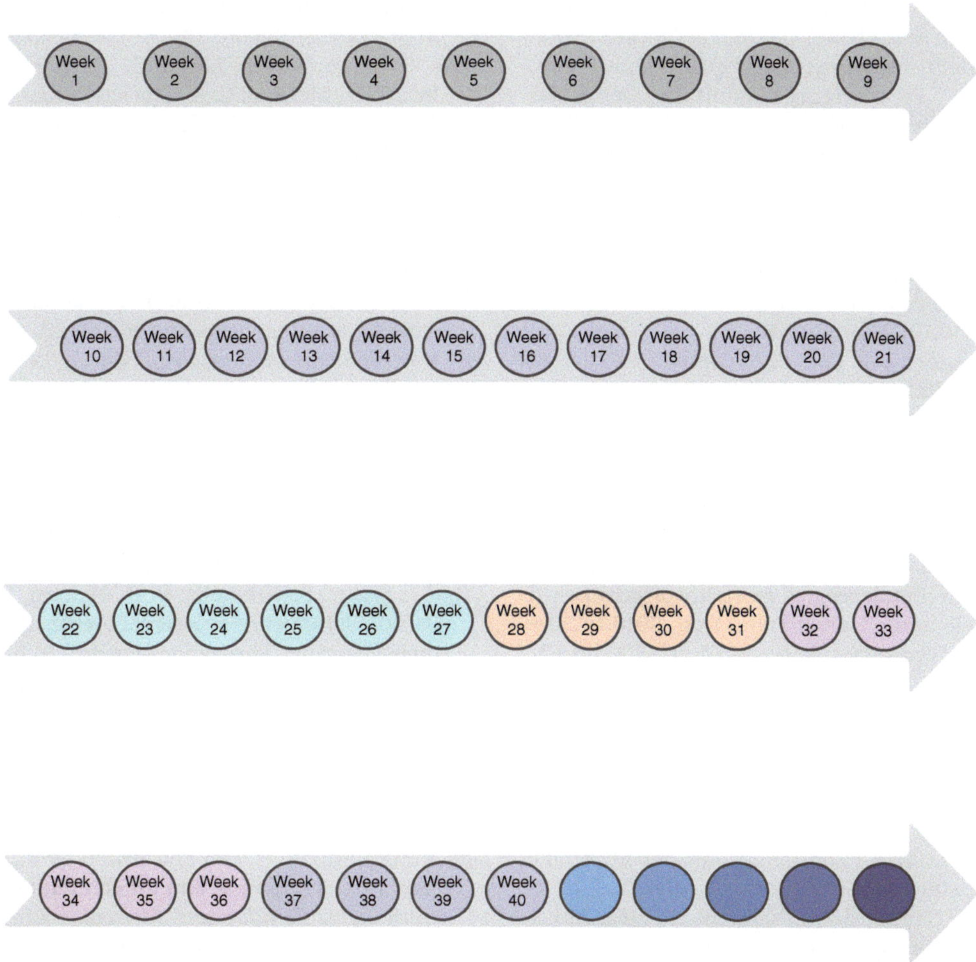

Note: Placement of common problems is meant to offer visual/ conceptual perspective on the timing of onset of these commonly reported malformations. Variation exists across the literature.	***Legend:*** <22 – 27 6/7 weeks = extremely preterm 28 – 31 6/7 weeks = very preterm 32 – 36 6/7 weeks = late/moderate preterm 37 – 40 weeks = term

Note: Readers should annotate the blank timeline during studying, self-directed learning, and creation of feedback loops with mentors. To access the blank and completed timelines visit www.springerpub.com/courseconnect. See inside front cover and tear-out card for CourseConnect details.

REFERENCES

Aaguard, K., Ma, J., Antony, K. M., Ganu, R., Petrosino, J., & Versalvovic, J. (2014). The placenta harbors a unique microbiome. *Science Translational Medicine, 6*, 237ra65. https://doi.org/10.1126/scitranslmed.3008599

Abbas, S., Keir, A. K., Makrides, M., Klein, L. D., Grzeskowiak, L. E., McPhee, A. J., & Rumbold, A. R. (2021). Tailoring human milk oligosaccharides to prevent necrotising enterocolitis among preterm infants. *Frontiers in Nutrition, 8*, 702888. https://doi.org/10.3389/fnut.2021.702888

Alani, M. (2023). *Midgut malrotation.* https://www.statpearls.com/point-of-care/25138

Amir, L. H., & Donath, S. (2007). A systematic review of maternal obesity and breastfeeding intention, initiation, and duration. *BMC Pregnancy and Childbirth, 7*, 9. https://doi.org/10.1186/1471-2393-7-9

Appaji, A. C., Kulkami, R., & Kadaba, J. S. (2013). Nonrotation of intestine: A case report. *Journal of Diagnostic Research, 7*(11), 2575–2576. https://doi.org/10.7860/JCDR/2013/6177.3616

Ardissone, A. N., de la Cruz, D. M., Davis-Richardson, A. G., Rechcigl, K. T., Li, N., Drew, J. C., Murgas-Torrazza, R., Sharma, R., Hudak, M. L., Triplett, E. W., & Neu, J. (2014). Meconium microbiome analysis identifies bacteria correlated with premature birth. *PLoS One, 26*, 141–147. https://doi.org/10.1371/journal.pone.0090784

Arnold, M., Moore, S. W., Sidler, D., & Kirsten, G. F. (2010). Long-term outcome of surgically managed necrotizing enterocolitis in a developing country. *Pediatric Surgery*

International, 26(4), 355–360. https://doi.org/10.1007/s00383-010-2583-8

Avetisyan, M., Schill, E. M., & Heuckeroth, R. O. (2015). Building a second brain in the bowel. *Journal of Clinical Investigation, 125*(3), 899–907. https://doi.org/10.1172/JCI76307

Baker, P. R. (2022). Fetal origins of adult disease: A classic hypothesis with new relevance. In R. A. Polin, S. H. Abman, D. H. Rowitch, W. E. Benitz, & W. W. Fox (Eds.), *Fetal and neonatal physiology* (6th ed., Vols. 1 & 2, pp. 129–137). Elsevier.

Batts, L. E., Polk, D. B., Dubois, R. N., & Kulessa, H. (2006). BMP signaling is required for intestinal growth and morphogenesis. *Developmental Dynamics, 235*(6), 1563–1570. https://doi.org/10.1002/dvdy.20741

Bence, C. M., & Wagner, A. J. (2021). Abdominal wall defects. *Translational Pediatrics, 10*(5), 1461–1469. https://doi.org/10.21037/tp-20-94

Bendavid, R., Abrahamson, J., Arregui, M. E., Flament, J. B., & Phillips, E. H. (Eds.). (2001). *Abdominal wall hernias: Principles and management.* Springer Science.

Bhatt, P., Poku, F. A., Umscheid, J., Ayensu, M., Parmar, N., Vasudeva, R., Donda, K., Doshi, H., & Dapaah-Siakwan, F. (2022). Trends in prevalence and mortality of gastroschisis and omphalocele in the United States from 2010 to 2018. *World Journal of Pediatrics: WJP, 18*(7), 511–514. https://doi.org/10.1007/s12519-022-00544-2

Boardman, J., Groves, A., & Ramasethu, J. (2021). *Avery & McDonald's neonatology: Pathophysiology and management of the newborn* (8th ed.). Wolters Kluwer.

Bohara, B. (2024). Abdominal assessment. In C. L. Witt & C. H. Wallman (Eds.), *Physical assessment of the newborn* (pp. 125–134). Springer Publishing Company. https://doi.org/10.1891/9780826140606 30

Bondurand, N., & Southard-Smith, E. M. (2016). Mouse models of Hirschsprung disease and other developmental disorders of the enteric nervous system: Old and new players. *Developmental Biology, 417*(2), 139–157. https://doi.org/10.1016/j.ydbio.2016.06.042

Carlson, B. M. (2024). Digestive and respiratory systems and body cavities. In B. M. Carlson (Ed.), *Human embryology and developmental biology* (7th ed., pp. 341–383). Elsevier.

Centers for Disease Control and Prevention. (2024a). *Weight gain during pregnancy.* https://www.cdc.gov/maternal-infant-health/pregnancy-weight/index.html

Centers for Disease Control and Prevention. (2024b). *Facts about esophageal atresia.* https://www.cdc.gov/ncbddd/birthdefects/esophagealatresia.html

Centers for Disease Control and Prevention. (2024c). *Facts about gastroschisis.* https://www.cdc.gov/ncbddd/birthdefects/gastroschisis.html

Centers for Disease Control and Prevention. (2024d). *Facts about omphalocele.* https://www.cdc.gov/ncbddd/birthdefects/omphalocele.html

Cetinkaya, M., Ozkan, H., & Koksal, N. (2012). Maternal preeclampsia is associated with increased risk of necrotizing enterocolitis in preterm infants. *Early Human Development, 88*, 893–898. https://doi.org/10.1016/j.earlhumdev.2012.07.004

Chia, S. E., & Shi, L. M. (2002). Review of recent epidemiological studies on paternal occupations and birth defects. *Occupational Environmental Medicine, 59*(3), 149–155. https://doi.org/10.1136/oem.59.3.149

Chin, A. M., Hill, D. R., Aurora, M., & Spence, J. (2017). Morphogenesis and maturation of the embryonic and postnatal intestine. *Seminars in Cell & Developmental Biology, 66*, 81–93. https://doi.org/10.1016/j.semcdb.2017.01.011

Cho, S. X., Rudloff, I., Lao, J. C., Pang, M. A., Goldberg, R., Bui, C. B., McLean, C. A., Stock, M., Klassert, T. E., Slevogt, H. S., Mangan, N. E., Cheng, W., Fischer, D., Gfroerer, S., Sandhu, M. K., Ngo, D., Bujotzek, A., Lariviere, L., Schumacher, F., . . . Nold, M. F. (2020). Characterization of the pathoimmunology of necrotizing enterocolitis reveals novel therapeutic opportunities. *Nature Communications, 11*(1), 5794. https://doi.org/10.1038/s41467-020-19400-w

Choi, G., Je, B-K., & Kim, Y. J. (2022). Gastrointestinal emergency in neonates and infants: A pictorial essay. *Korean Journal of Radiology, 23*(1), 124–138. https://doi.org/10.3348/kjr.2021.0111

Correa, A., & Marcinkevage, J. (2013). Prepregnancy obesity and the risk of birth defects: an update. *Nutrition reviews, 71 Suppl 1*(Suppl 1), S68–S77. https://doi.org/10.1111/nure.12058

Coste, A. H., & Anand, S. (2022). *Midgut volvulus.* StatPearls. www.statpearls.com/point-of-care/25139

Day, J., Savani, S., Krempley, B. D., Nguyen, M., & Kitlinska, J. B. (2016). Influence of paternal preconception exposures on their offspring: Through epigenetics to phenotype. *American Journal of Stem Cells, 5*(1), 11–18. PMID: 27335698; PMCID: PMC4913293.

de la Cruz, D., & Neu, J. (2025). Neonatal necrotizing enterocolitis. In In R. J. Martin & A. A. Fanaroff (Eds.), *Fanaroff & Martin's neonatal-perinatal medicine* (12th ed., pp. 1653–1669). Elsevier.

de Santa Barbara, P., van den Brink, G. R., & Roberts, D. J. (2003). Development and differentiation of the intestinal epithelium. *Cellular and Molecular Life Sciences, 60*(7), 1322–1332. https://doi.org/10.1007/s00018-003-2289-3

Dingeldein, M. (2025). Selected gastrointestinal anomalies in the neonate. In R. J. Martin & A. A. Fanaroff (Eds.), *Fanaroff & Martin's neonatal-perinatal medicine* (12th ed., pp. 1626–1652). Elsevier.

Diposarosa, R., Bustam, N. A., Sahiratmadja, E., Susanto, P. S., & Sribudiani, Y. (2021). Literature review: Enteric nervous system development, genetic and epigenetic regulation in the etiology of Hirschsprung's disease. *Heliyon, 7*(6), e07308. https://doi.org/10.1016/j.heliyon.2021.e07308

Dominguez, K. M., & Moss, R. L. (2012). Necrotizing enterocolitis. *Clinics in Perinatology, 39*(2), 387–401. https://doi.org/10.1016/j.clp.2012.04.011

Drucker, N. A., McCulloh, C. J., Li, B., Pierro, A., Besner, G. E., & Markel, T. A. (2018). Stem cell therapy in necrotizing enterocolitis: Current state and future directions. *Seminars in Pediatric Surgery, 27*, 57–64. https://doi.org/10.1053/j.sempedsurg.2017.11.011

Egan, C. E., Sodhi, C. P., Good, M., Lin, J., Jia, H., Yamaguchi, Y., Lu, P., Ma, C., Branca, M. F., Weyandt, S., Fulton, W. B., Niño, D. F., Prindle, T., Jr, Ozolek, J. A., & Hackam, D. J. (2016). Toll-like receptor 4-mediated lymphocyte influx induces neonatal necrotizing enterocolitis. *Journal of Clinical Investigation, 126*(2), 495. https://doi.org/10.1172/JCI83356

Faure, S., & de Santa Barbara, P. (2011). Molecular embryology of the foregut. *Journal of Pediatric Gastroenterology and Nutrition, 52*(Suppl. 1), S2–S3. https://doi.org/10.1097/MPG.0b013e3182105a1a

Feenstra, B., Geller, F., Krogh, C., Hollegaard, M. V., Gortz, S., Boyd, H. A., Murray, J. C., Hougaard, D. M., & Melbye, M. (2012). Common variants near MBNL1 and NKX2-5 are associated with infantile hypertrophic pyloric stenosis. *Nature Genetics, 44*, 224–337. https://doi.org/10.1038/ng.1067

Flynn-O'Brien, K. T., & Rice-Townsend, S. E. (2024). Structual anomalies of the gastrointestinal tract. In C. A. Gleason & D. O. Sawyer (Eds.), *Avery's diseases of the newborn* (11th ed., pp. 897–912). Elsevier.

Frazer, L. C., & Good, M. (2022). Intestinal epithelium in early life. *Mucosal Immunol, 15*(6), 1181–1187. https://doi.org/10.1038/s41385-022-00579-8

Genetic and Rare Diseases Information Center. (2024a). *Congenital chloride diarrhea.* https://rarediseases.info.nih.gov/diseases/10001/congenital-chloride-diarrhea

Genetic and Rare Diseases Information Center. (2024b). *Duodenal atresia.* https://rarediseases.info.nih.gov/diseases/54/duodenal-atresia

Godfrey, K. M., Reynolds, R. M., Prescott, S. L., Nyirenda, M., Jaddoe, V. W., Eriksson, J. G., & Broekman, B. F. (2017). Influence of maternal obesity of the long-term health of offspring. *Lancet Diabetes Endocrinology, 5*(1), 53–64. https://doi.org/10.1016/s2213-8587(16)30107-3

Gopalakrishna, K. P., Macadangdang, B. R., Rogers, M. B., Tometich, J. T., Firek, B. A., Baker, R., Ji, J., Burr, A. H. P., Ma, C., Good, M., Morowitz, M. J., & Hand, T. W. (2019). Maternal IgA protects against the development of necrotizing enterocolitis in preterm infants. *Natural Medicine, 25*(7), 1110–1115. https://doi.org/10.1038/s41591-019-0480-9

Grandi, C., Tapia, J. L., & Cardoso, V. C. (2015). Impact of maternal diabetes mellitus on mortality and morbidity of very low birth weight infants: A multicenter Latin America study. *Jornal de Pediatria (Rio J), 91*(3), 234–241. https://doi.org/10.1016/j.jped.2014.08.007

Gritz, E. C., & Bhandari, V. (2015). The human neonatal gut microbiome: A brief review. *Frontiers in Pediatrics, 3*, 1–12. https://doi.org/10.3389/fped.2015.00017

Guandalini, S., & Dhawan, A. (2022). *Textbook of pediatric gastroenterology, hepatology and nutrition: A comprehensive guide to practice* (2nd ed.). Springer Publishing Company.

Gussler, J., & Arensberg, M. B. (2011). Impact of maternal obesity on pregnancy and lactation: The health care challenge. *Nutrition Today, 46*(1), 6–11. https://doi.org/10.1097/NT.0b013e3181e988ea

Healy, D. B., Ryan C. A., Ross R. P., Stanton C., & Dempsey, E. M. (2022). Clinical implications of preterm infant gut microbiome development. *Nature Microbiology, 7*, 22–33. https://doi.org/10.1038/s41564-021-01025-4

Huang, W., Li, X., Zhang, J., & Zhang, S. (2017). Prevalence, risk factors, and prognosis of postoperative complications after surgery for Hirschsprung disease. *Journal of Gastrointestinal Surgery, 22*(2), 335–343. https://doi.org/10.1007/s11605-017-3596-6

Jeyabalan, A. (2025). Hypertensive disorders of pregnancy. In R. J. Martin, A. A. Fanaroff, & M. C. Walsh (Eds.), *Fanaroff & Martin's neonatal-perinatal medicine* (12th ed., pp. 290–306). Elsevier.

Jnah, A. J., Newberry, D. M., & England, A. (2015). Pentalogy of Cantrell: Case report with review of the literature. *Advances in Neonatal Care, 15*(4), 261–268. https://doi.org/10.1097/ANC.0000000000000209

Jnah, A. J., Smith, C., & Barr, S. M. (2024). Enteral nutrition and gastrointestinal problems: Formulas, supplements, and pharmacotherapeutics. In A. J. Jnah & C. McPherson (Eds.), *Fetal and neonatal pharmacology for the advanced practice nurse* (pp. 475–476). Springer Publishing Company.

Jung, E., Romero, R., Chaemsaithong, P., & Gomez-Lopez, N. (2022). Intra-amniotic infection/inflammation and the fetal inflammatory response syndrome. In R. A. Polin, S. H. Abman, D. H. Rowitch, W. E. Benitz, & W. W. Fox (Eds.), *Fetal and neonatal physiology* (6th ed., Vols. 1 & 2, pp. 111–129). Elsevier.

Kamada, N., Chen, G., Inohara, N., & Nunez, G. (2013). Control of pathogens and pathobionts by the gut microbiota. *Nature Immunology, 14*(7), 685–690. https://doi.org/10.1038/ni.2608

Kamoji, V. M., Dorling, J. S., Manktelow, B., Draper, E. S., & Field, D. J. (2008). Antenatal umbilical Doppler abnormalities: An independent risk factor for early onset neonatal necrotizing enterocolitis in premature infants. *Acta Paediatr, 97*(3), 327–331. https://doi.org/10.1111/j.1651-2227.2008.00671.x

Kamoth, B. M., & Piccoli, D. A. (2008). Alagille syndrome. In C. A. Liacouras & D. A. Piccoli (Eds.), *Pediatric gastroenterology: Requisites* (pp. 227–232). Mosby Elsevier.

Keckler, S. J., St. Peter, S. D., Spilde, T. L., Tsao, K.-J., Ostlie, D. J., & Snyder, C. L. (2008). Current significance of meconium plug syndrome. *Journal of Pediatric Surgery, 43*(5), 896–898. https://doi.org/10.1016/j.jpedsurg.2007.12.035

Kelly, G. M., & Drysdale, T. A. (2015). Retinoic acid and the development of the endoderm. *Journal of Developmental Biology, 3*(2), 25–56. https://doi.org/10.3390/jdb3020025

Kelly, K. B., & Ponsky, T. A. (2013). Pediatric abdominal wall defects. *Surgical Clinics of North America, 93*(5), 1255–1267. https://doi.org/10.1016/j.suc.2013.06.016

Khlevner, J., Del Collis, A., & Margolis, K. G. (2022). Development of the enteric nervous system and gastrointestinal motility. In R. A. Polin, S. H. Abman, D. H. Rowitch, W. E. Benitz, & W. W. Fox (Eds.), *Fetal and neonatal physiology* (6th ed., Vols. 1 & 2, pp. 859–868). Elsevier.

Kliegman, R. M., & Walsh, M. C. (1987). Neonatal necrotizing enterocolitis: Pathogenesis, classification, and spectrum of illness. *Current Problems in Pediatrics, 17*(4), 213. https://doi.org/10.1016/0045-9380(87)90031-4

Larson-Nath, C., Gurram, B., & Chelimsky, G. (2020). Disorders of digestion in the neonate. In R. J. Martin, A. A. Fanaroff, & M. C. Walsh (Eds.), *Fanaroff & Martin's neonatal-perinatal medicine* (11th ed., pp. 1522–1540). Elsevier.

Liu, J., Miyake, H., Zhu, H., Li, B., Alganabi, M., Lee, C., & Pierro, A. (2020). Fecal microbiota transplantation by enema reduces intestinal injury in experimental necrotizing enterocolitis. *Journal of Pediatric Surgery, 55*(6), 1094–1098. https://doi.org/10.1016/j.jpedsurg.2020.02.035

Liu, R., & Adler, D. G. (2014). Duplication cysts: Diagnosis, management, and the role of endoscopic ultrasound. *Endoscopic Ultrasound, 3*(3), 152–160. https://doi.org/10.4103/2303-9027. 138783

Logan, C. Y., & Nusse, R. (2004). The Wnt signaling pathway in development and disease. *Annual Review Cell Developmental Biology, 20*, 781–810. https://doi.org/10.1146/annurev.cellbio.20.010403.113126

Lu, P., Yamaguchi, Y., Fulton, W. B., Wang, S., Zhou, Q., Jia H, Kovler, M. L., Salazar, A. G., Sampah, M., Prindle, T., Jr,

Wipf, P., Sodhi, C. P., & Hackam, D. J. (2021). Maternal aryl hydrocarbon receptor activation protects newborns against necrotizing enterocolitis. *Nature Communications, 12*(1), 1042. https://doi.org/10.1038/s41467-021-21356-4

Lupo, P. J., Isenburd, J. L., Salemi, J. L., Mai, C. T., Liberman, R. F., Canfield, M. A., Copeland, G., Haight, S., Harpavat, S., Hoyt, A. T., Moore, C. A., Nembhard, W. N., Nguyen, H. N., Rutkowski, R. E., Steele, A., Alverson, C. J., Stallings, E. B., & Kirby, R. S., & The National Birth Defects Prevention Network. (2017). Population-based birth defects data in the United States, 2010–2014: A focus on gastrointestinal defects [Special issue]. *Birth Defects Research, 109*(18), 1504–1515. https://doi.org/10.1002/bdr2.1145

Mahe, M. M., Helmraph, M. A., & Shroyer, N. F. (2022). Organogenesis of the gastrointestinal tract. In R. A. Polin, S. H. Abman, D. H. Rowitch, W. E. Benitz, & W. W. Fox (Eds.), *Fetal and neonatal physiology* (6th ed., Vols. 1 & 2, pp. 845–854). Elsevier.

Markel, T. A., Engelstad, H., & Poindexter, B. B. (2014). Predicting disease severity of necrotizing enterocolitis: How to identify infants for future novel therapies. *Journal of Clinical Neonatology, 3*(1), 1–9. https://doi.org/10.4103/2249-4847.128717

Martin, V., & Shaw-Smith, C. (2010). Review of genetic factors in intestinal malrotation. *Pediatric Surgery International, 26*(8), 769–781. https://doi.org/10.1007/s00383-010-2622-5

Mihi, B., Gong, Q., Nolan, L. S., Gale, S. E., Goree, M., Hu, E., Lanik, W. E., Rimer, J. M., Liu, V., Parks, O. B., Lewis, A. N., Agrawal, P., Laury, M. L., Kumar, P., Huang, E., Bidani, S. S., Luke, C. J., Kolls, J. K., & Good. M. (2021). Interleukin-22 signaling attenuates necrotizing enterocolitis by promoting epithelial cell regeneration. *Cell Report. Medicine, 2*, 100320. https://doi.org/10.1016/j.xcrm.2021.100320

Mowrer, A. R., DeUgarte, D. A., & Wagner, A. J. (2022). Abdominal wall defects: A review of current practice guidelines. *Clinics in Perinatology, 49*(4), 943–953. https://doi.org/10.1016/j.clp.2022.07.004

National Institute of Health Genetic and Rare Diseases Information Center. (2025). *Arteriohepatic dysplasia*. https://rarediseases.info.nih.gov/diseases/804/arteriohepatic-dysplasia

National Library of Medicine. (2024a). *Alagille syndrome*. MedlinePlus, https://medlineplus.gov/genetics/condition/alagille-syndrome

National Library of Medicine. (2024b). *Cystic fibrosis*. MedlinePlus. https://medlineplus.gov/genetics/condition/cystic-fibrosis

National Library of Medicine. (2024c). *Sweat test for cystic fibrosis*. https://medlineplus.gov/lab-tests/sweat-test-for-cystic-fibrosis/

National Library of Medicine. (2024d). *Glucose-galactose malabsorption*. MedlinePlus. https://medlineplus.gov/genetics/condition/glucose-galactose-malabsorption

National Library of Medicine. (2024e). *Hirschsprung disease*. MedlinePlus. https://medlineplus.gov/genetics/condition/hirschsprung-disease

National Library of Medicine. (2024f). *Lactose intolerance*. MedlinePlus. https://medlineplus.gov/genetics/condition/lactose-intolerance

National Library of Medicine. (2024g). *Permanent neonatal diabetes*. MedlinePlus. https://medlineplus.gov/genetics/condition/permanent-neonatal-diabetes-mellitus

National Library of Medicine. (2024h). *Shwachman–Diamond syndrome*. MedlinePlus. https://medlineplus.gov/genetics/condition/shwachman-diamond-syndrome

National Organization for Rare Disorders. (2020). *Jejunal atresia*. https://rarediseases.org/rare-diseases/jejunal-atresia

National Organization for Rare Disorders. (2024). *Alagille syndrome*. https://rarediseases.org/rare-diseases/alagille-syndrome

Navathe, R., Gerli, S., Pacella, E., & Berghella, V. (2016). Diabetes in pregnancy. In A. Malvasi, A. Tinelli, & G. C. Di Renzo (Eds.), *Management and therapy of early pregnancy complications: First and second trimesters* (pp. 315–331). Springer International.

Neu, J., & Singh, N. K. (2022). The developing microbe of the fetus and neonate: A multiomic approach. In R. A. Polin, S. H. Abman, D. H. Rowitch, W. E. Benitz, & W. W. Fox (Eds.), *Fetal and neonatal physiology* (6th ed., Vols. 1 & 2, pp. 888–895). Elsevier.

Nolan, L. S., Rimer, J. M., & Good, M. (2020). The role of human milk oligosaccharides and probiotics on the neonatal microbiome and risk of necrotizing enterocolitis: A narrative review. *Nutrients, 12*(10), 3052. https://doi.org/10.3390/nu12103052

Nusinovich, Y., Revenis, M., & Torres, C. (2013). Long-term outcomes for infants with intestinal atresia followed at Children's National Medical Center, Washington, DC. *Journal of Pediatric Gastroenterology and Nutrition, 57*(3), 324–329. https://doi.org/10.1097/MPG.0b013e318299fd9f

Obasi, A. A., Ekenze, S. O., & Ogbobe, U. (2015). Ileal obstruction from Meckel's diverticulum in a neonate: A case report and review of literature. *Journal of Pediatric Surgery Case Reports, 3*(10), 423–425. https://doi.org/10.1016/j.epsc.2015.08.013

Online Mendelian Inheritance in Men. (2024a). *Diarrhea 1, secretory chloride, congenital, with or without other congenital anomalies, DIAR3*. https://www.omim .org/entry/214700

Online Mendelian Inheritance in Men. (2024b). *Diarrhea 3, secretory sodium, congenital, DIAR1*. https://www.omim.org/entry/270420

Online Mendelian Inheritance in Men. (2024c). *Glucose/galactose malabsorption; GGM*. https://www .omim.org/entry/606824

Online Mendelian Inheritance in Men. (2024d). *Lactase deficiency, congenital*. https://omim.org/entry/223000

Online Mendelian Inheritance in Men. (2024e). *Meconium ileus*. https://www.omim.org/entry/614665

Online Mendelian Inheritance in Men. (2024f). *Pyloric stenosis, infantile hypertrophic*. https://www.omim.org/entry/179010

Online Mendelian Inheritance in Men. (2024g). *Shwachman–Diamond syndrome; SDS*. www/omim.org/entry/260400

Orphanet. (2021). *Duodenal atresia*. https://www.orpha.net/en/disease/detail/1203?name=duodenal%20atresia&mode=name

Owens, L. A., O'Sullivan, E. P., Kirwan, B., Avalos, G., Gaffney, G., & Dunne, F. (2010). For the ATLANTIC DIP collaborators: The impact of obesity on pregnancy outcome in glucose-tolerant women. *Diabetes Care, 33*, 577–579. https://doi.org/10.2337/dc09-0911

Paveglio, S., Ledala, N., Rezaul, K., Lin, Q., Zhou, Y., Provatas, A. A., Bennett, E., Lindberg, T., Caimano, M. J., & Matson, A. (2020). Cytotoxin-producing Klebsiella oxytoca in the preterm gut and its association with necrotizing enterocolitis. *Emerging Microbes and Infections, 9*, 1321–1329. https://doi.org/10.1080/22221751.2020.1773743

Pena, A. (2019). Anorectal atresia and cloacal malformations. In G. W. Holcomb, J. P. Murphy, & S. D. St. Peter (Eds.), *Holcomb & Ashcroft's pediatric surgery* (7th ed., pp. 577–598). Elsevier.

Perdu, S., Castellana, B., Kim, Y., Chan, K., DeLuca, L., & Beristain, A. G. (2016). Maternal obesity drives functional alterations in uterine NK cells. *Journal of Clinical Investigation: Insight, 1*(11), e85560. https://doi.org/10.1172/jci.insight.85560

Polak, M., & Cave, H. (2007). Neonatal diabetes mellitus: A disease linked to multiple mechanisms. *Orphanet Journal of Rare Diseases, 2*, 12. https://doi.org/10.1186/1750-1172-2-12

Pritchard, D. J., & Korf, B. R. (2016). *Medical genetics at a glance* (3rd ed., pp. 229–233). Wiley-Blackwell.

Qumsieh, U., Jaber, M. S., Emran, W., Abdelghani, I., Manasra, F., Ahmad, N., & Shawar, B. (2023). A neonatal small left colon syndrome of nondiabetic mother. *Journal of Pediatric Surgery Case Reports, 89*, 102524. https://doi.org/10.1016/j.epsc.2022.102524

Rager, T. M., Olson, J. K., Zhou, Y., Wang, Y., & Besner, G. E. (2016). Exosomes secreted from bone marrow-derived mesenchymal stem cells protect the intestines from experimental necrotizing enterocolitis. *Journal of Pediatric Surgery, 51*, 942–947. https://doi.org/10.1016/j.jpedsurg.2016.02.061

Ranells, J. D., Carver, J. D., & Kirby, R. S. (2011). Infantile hypertrophic pyloric stenosis: Epidemiology, genetics, and clinical update. *Advances in Pediatrics, 58*(1), 195–206. https://doi.org/10.1016/j.yapd.2011.03.005

Rattan, K. N., Bansal, S., & Dhamija, A. (2017). Gastrointestinal duplication presenting as neonatal intestinal obstruction: An experience of 15 years at a tertiary care center. *Journal of Neonatal Surgery, 6*(1), 5. https://doi.org/10.21699/jns.v5i4432

Rayyan, M., Rommel, N., Tack, J., Deprest, J., & Allegaert, K. (2017). Esophageal atresia: Future directions for research on the digestive tract. *European Journal Pediatric Surgery, 27*(4), 306–312. https://doi.org/10.1055/s-0036-1587330

Ree, I. M. C., Smits-Wintjens, V. E. H. J., Rijntjes-Jacobs, E. G. J., Pelsma, I. C. M., Steggerda, S. J., Walther, F. J., & Lopriore, E. (2014). Necrotizing enterocolitis in small-for-gestational-age neonates: A matched case-control study. *Neonatology, 105*, 74–78. https://doi.org/10.1159/000356033

Roath, M. C., & Di Palma, J. A. (2012). Genetics in gastroenterology: What you need to know. *Consultant, 52*(2), 99–105.

Ross, A., & Johnson, R. V. R. (2016). Infantile hypertrophic pyloric stenosis. *Surgery, 34*(12), 609–611. https://doi.org/10.1016/j.mpsur.2016.09.003

Sadler, T. W. (2023). *Langman's medical embryology* (15th ed.). Wolters Kluwer.

Sagar, J., Kumar, V., & Shah, D. K. (2006). Meckel's diverticulum: A systematic review. *Journal of the Royal Society of Medicine, 99*(10), 501–505. https://doi.org/10.1258/jrsm.99.10.501

Salar-Khalil, A., & Sferra, T. J. (2025). Disorders of digestion in the Neonate. In R. J. Martin & A. A. Fanaroff (Eds.), *Fanaroff & Martin's neonatal-perinatal medicine* (12th ed., pp. 1615–1625). Elsevier.

Sanchez-Valle, A., Kassira, N., Vardla, V. C., Radu, S. C., Paidas, C., & Kirby, R. S. (2017). Biliary atresia: Epidemiology, genetics, clinical update, and public health perspective. *Advances in Pediatrics, 64*(1), 285–305. https://doi.org/10.1016/j.yapd.2017.03.012

Schierding, W., Vickers, M. H., O' Sullivan, J. M., & Cutfield, W. S. (2022). Epigenetics. In R. A. Polin, S. H. Abman, D. H. Rowitch, W. E. Benitz, & W. W. Fox (Eds.), *Fetal and neonatal physiology* (6th ed., Vols. 1 & 2, pp. 11–22). Elsevier.

Schoenwolf, G. C., Bleyl, S. B., Brauer, P. R., & Francis-West, P. H. (2021). Development of the gastrointestinal tract. In G. C. Schoenwolf, S. B. Bleyl, P. R. Brauer, & P. H. Francis-West (Eds.), *Larsen's human embryology* (6th ed., pp. 335–367). Elsevier.

Shulhan, J., Dicken, B., Hartling, L., & Larsen, B. M. (2017). Current knowledge of necrotizing enterocolitis in preterm infants and the impact of different types of enteral nutrition products. *Advances in Nutrition, 8*, 80–91. https://doi.org/10.3945/an.116.013193

Sim, K., Shaw, A. G., Randell, P., Cox, M. J., McClure, Z. E., Li, M.-S., Haddad, M., Langford, P. R., Cookson, W. O. C. M., Moffatt, M. F., & Kroll, J. S. (2015). Dysbiosis anticipating necrotizing enterocolitis in very premature infants. *Clinical Infectious Diseases, 60*, 389–397. https://doi.org/10.1093/cid/ciu822

Simmons, R. K., Griffin, S. J., Witte, D. R., Borch-Johnsen, K., Lauritzen, T., & Sandbæk, A. (2017). Effect of population screening for type 2 diabetes and cardiovasular risk factors on mortality rate and cardiovascular events: A controlled trial among 1,912,392 Danish adults. *Diabetologia, 60*(11), 2183–2191. https://doi.org/10.1007/s00125-017-4323-2

Singh, D. K., Miller, C. M., Orgel, K. A., Dave, M., Mackay, S., & Good, M. (2023). Necrotizing enterocolitis: Bench to bedside approaches and advancing our understanding of disease pathogenesis. *Frontiers in Pediatrics, 10*, 1107404. https://doi.org/10.3389/fped.2022.1107404

Sloan, K., & Wagener, S. (2016). Updates in Hirschsprung's disease and anorectal malformations. *Journal of Pediatric Surgical Specialties, 10*(3), 43–51. https://api.semanticscholar.org/CorpusID:202608379

Sodhi, C. P., Neal, M. D., Siggers, R., Sho, S., Ma, C., Branca, M. F., Prindle, T., Jr, Russo, A. M., Afrazi, A., Good, M., Brower-Sinning, R., Firek, B., Morowitz, M. J., Ozolek, J. A., Gittes, G. K., Billiar, T. R., & Hackam, D. J. (2012). Intestinal epithelial toll-like receptor 4 regulates goblet cell development and is required for necrotizing enterocolitis in mice. *Gastroenterology, 143*(3), 708. https://doi.org/10.1053/j.gastro.2012.05.053

Souther, C., Puapong, D. P., Woo, R., & Johnson, S. M. (2017). Possible etiologies of increased incidence of gastroschisis. *Pediatric Surgery International, 33*(11), 1209–1213. https://doi.org/10.1007/s00383-017-4166-4

Stallings, E. B., Isenburg, J. L., Short, T. D., Heinke, D., Kirby, R. S., Romitti, P. A., Canfield, M. A., O'Leary, L. A., Liberman, R. F., Forestieri, N. E., Nembhard, W. N., Sandidge, T., Nestoridi, E., Salemi, J. L., Nance, A. E., Duckett, K., Ramirez, G. M., Shan, X., Shi, J., & Lupo, P. J. (2019). Population-based birth defects data in the United States, 2012–2016: A focus on abdominal wall defects. *Birth Defects Research, 111*(18), 1436–1447. https://doi.org/10.1002/bdr2.1607

Tamburini, S., Shen, N., Wu, H. C., & Clemente, J. C. (2016). The microbiome in early life: Implications for health outcomes. *Nature Medicine, 22*(7), 713–722. https://doi.org/10.1038/nm.4142

Taylor, J. A., & Neu, J. (2021). Disorders of the gastrointestinal tract. In J. Boardman, A. Groves, & J. Ramasethu (Eds.), *Avery and MacDonald's neonatology: Pathophysiology and management of the newborn* (8th ed., pp. 546–563). Wolters Kluwer.

Tayman, C., Uckan, D., Kilic, E., Ulus, A. T., Tonbul, A., Murat Hirfanoglu, I., Helvacioglu, F., Haltas, H., Koseoglu, B., & Tatli, M. M. (2011). Mesenchymal stem cell therapy in necrotizing enterocolitis: A rat study. *Pediatric Research, 70*, 489–494. https://doi.org/10.1203/PDR.0b013e31822d7ef2

Torchia, M. G., & Persaud, T. V. N. (2025). *The developing human* (12th ed.). Elsevier.

Tourneur, E., & Chassin, C. (2013). Neonatal immune adaptation of the gut and its role during infections. *Clinical and Developmental Immunology, 2013*, 270301. https://doi.org/10.1155/2013/ 270301

Twaroski, K., Mallana, S. K., Jing, R., DiFurio, F., Urick, A., & Duncan, S. A. (2015). FGF2 mediates hepatic progenitor cell formation during human pluripotent stem cell differentiation by inducing the WNT antagonist NKD1. *Genes & Development, 29*(23), 2463–2474. https://doi.org/10.1101/gad.268961.115

Uesaka, T., Young, H. M., Pachnis, V., & Emomoto, H. (2016). Development of the intrinsic and extrinsic innervation of the gut. *Developmental Biology, 417*(2), 158–167. https://doi.org/10.1016/j.ydbio.2016.04.016

Vieten, D., Corfield, A., Carroll, D., Ramani, P., & Spicer, R. (2005). Impaired mucosal regeneration in neonatal necrotising enterocolitis. *Pediatric Surgery International, 21*(3), 153–160. https://doi.org/10.1007/s00383-004-1312-6

Walton, K. D., & Gumucio, D. L. (2021). Hedgehog signaling in intestinal development and homeostasis. *Annual Review of Physiology, 83*, 359–380. https://doi.org/10.1146/annurev-physiol-031620-094324

Weinder, M. R., Gurevich, P., Shinwell, E. S., & Yogev, Y. (2025). *Fanaroff & Martin's neonatal-perinatal medicine* (12th ed., pp. 307–317). Elsevier.

Weintraub, A. S., Ferrara, L., Deluca, L., Moshier, E., Green, R. S., Oakman, E., Lee, M-J., & Rand, L. (2012). Antenatal antibiotic exposure in preterm infants with necrotizing enterocolitis. *Journal of Perinatology, 32*, 705–709. https://doi.org/10.1038/jp.2011.180

Williams, C. B., Mackenzie, K. C., & Gahagan, S. (2014). The effect of maternal obesity on the offspring. *Clinical Obstetric Gynecology, 57*(3), 508–515. https://doi.org/10.1097/GRF.0000000000000043

Wolfe, C., & Jnah, A. J. (2024). Tracheoesophageal fistula with esophageal atresia: A case series. *Neonatal Network, 43*(2), 65–75. http://dx.doi.org/10.1891/NN-2023-0051

Wong, D., Abdel-Latif, M., Kent, A., & NICUS Network. (2014). Antenatal steroid exposure and outcomes of very premature infants: A regional cohort study. *Archives of Disease in Childhood. Fetal and Neonatal Edition, 99*(1), F12–F20. https://doi.org/10.1136/archdischild-2013-304705

Wu, H., Guo, K., Zhuo, Z., Zeng, R., Luo, Y., Yang, Q., Li, J., Jiang, R., Huang, Z., Sha, W., & Chen, H. (2022). Current therapy option for necrotizing enterocolitis: Practicalities and challenge. *Frontiers in Pediatrics, 10*, 954735. https://doi.org/10.3389/fped.2022.954735

Wu, H., & Wu, E. (2012). The role of gut microbiota in immune homeostasis and autoimmunity. *Gut Microbes, 3*(1), 4–14. https://doi.org/10.4161/gmic.19320

Zorn, A. M. (Ed.). (2008). Liver development. In *StemBook*. https://www.ncbi.nlm.nih.gov/books/NBK27068

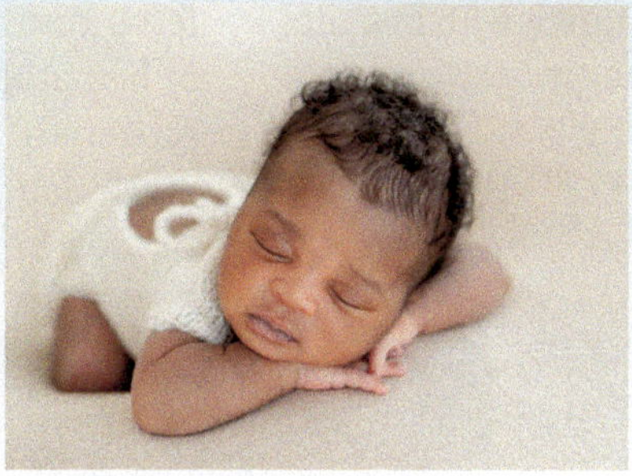

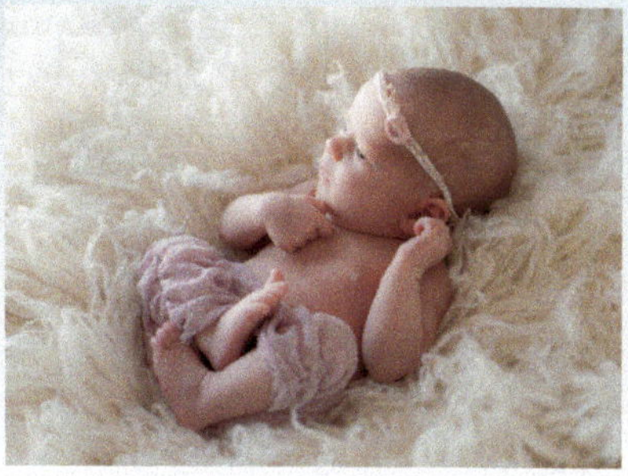

7 THE HEMATOPOIETIC SYSTEM

Jennifer Fitzgerald, Jacqui Hoffman, and Amy J. Jnah

LEARNING OBJECTIVES

After completing this chapter, the reader should be able to:

- Understand normal hematopoietic system development.
- Analyze the physiologic function of the fetal and neonatal hematopoietic system.
- Discuss common inherited disorders and their effect on fetal and neonatal hematopoietic system development and function.
- Identify health issues in XX pregnant patients that have a potential impact on fetal and postnatal hematopoietic system development and function.
- Evaluate common disorders that affect the hematopoietic system and their implications across the life span.

INTRODUCTION

The hematologic system is one of the first to achieve operational activity in utero, available to support life, growth, and well-being. Hematopoiesis, or the formation of blood cells, begins during early embryonic development and continues across the life span. Epigenetic, genetic, or environmental shocks may impact hematologic development or function and impose pathophysiologic dysfunction. A developmentally and functionally competent hematologic system is critical to survival of life in utero and after birth.

TIMELINE OF ORGAN DEVELOPMENT

The study of hematopoiesis allows clinicians to understand normal development across the life span, which aids in understanding the pathogenesis of blood disorders and certain cancers. All cellular components of the hematologic system originate from hematopoietic stem cells (HSCs), also known as pluripotent cells, of the embryonic mesoderm. The initial site for hematopoiesis is the extraembryonic yolk sac, with blood cells noted as early as week 3 of gestation. The progenitor cells seen in the yolk sac migrate to the aorta-gonad-mesonephros (AGM) of the embryo prior to arrival in the placenta and to the liver by the fourth week of pregnancy (Owusu-Ansah et al., 2025). These progenitor cells are subsequently noted in the fetal bone marrow by week 11 of gestation (Owusu-Ansah et al., 2025; Palis & Segel, 2021).

Embryonic HSCs are ultimately capable of self-renewal and differentiation into either myeloid or lymphoid lineages. When these HSCs proliferate, some persist as stem cells for autonomous regeneration. The remaining cells form various blood cell lineages: erythroid (red blood cell [RBC]), lymphoid (T cells and B cells), and myeloid (granulocytes and platelets).

Given the complexity involved with the proliferation and maturation of the hematologic system, we offer an integrated approach to the study of this system. Major embryologic milestones are woven into the following discussion of functional maturation.

DEVELOPMENTAL PHYSIOLOGY

There are three phases of hematopoiesis: primitive, transient, and definitive (**Figure 7.1**). The yolk sac is the first hematopoietic site in the developing human with hematopoietic cell production limited to primitive erythroblasts (or RBCs), macrophages, and megakaryocytes (MKs; Palis & Segel, 2021; Sommer & Perdiguero, 2024). Evidence points to these primitive cells migrating to the liver as the fetus transitions through the transient-definitive phase of hematopoiesis with the production of erythro-myeloid progenitor (EMP) cells (D'Souza et al., 2021; Palis & Segel, 2021; Sommer & Perdiguero, 2024). Finally, hematopoiesis moves into the definitive phase with the arrival of HSCs

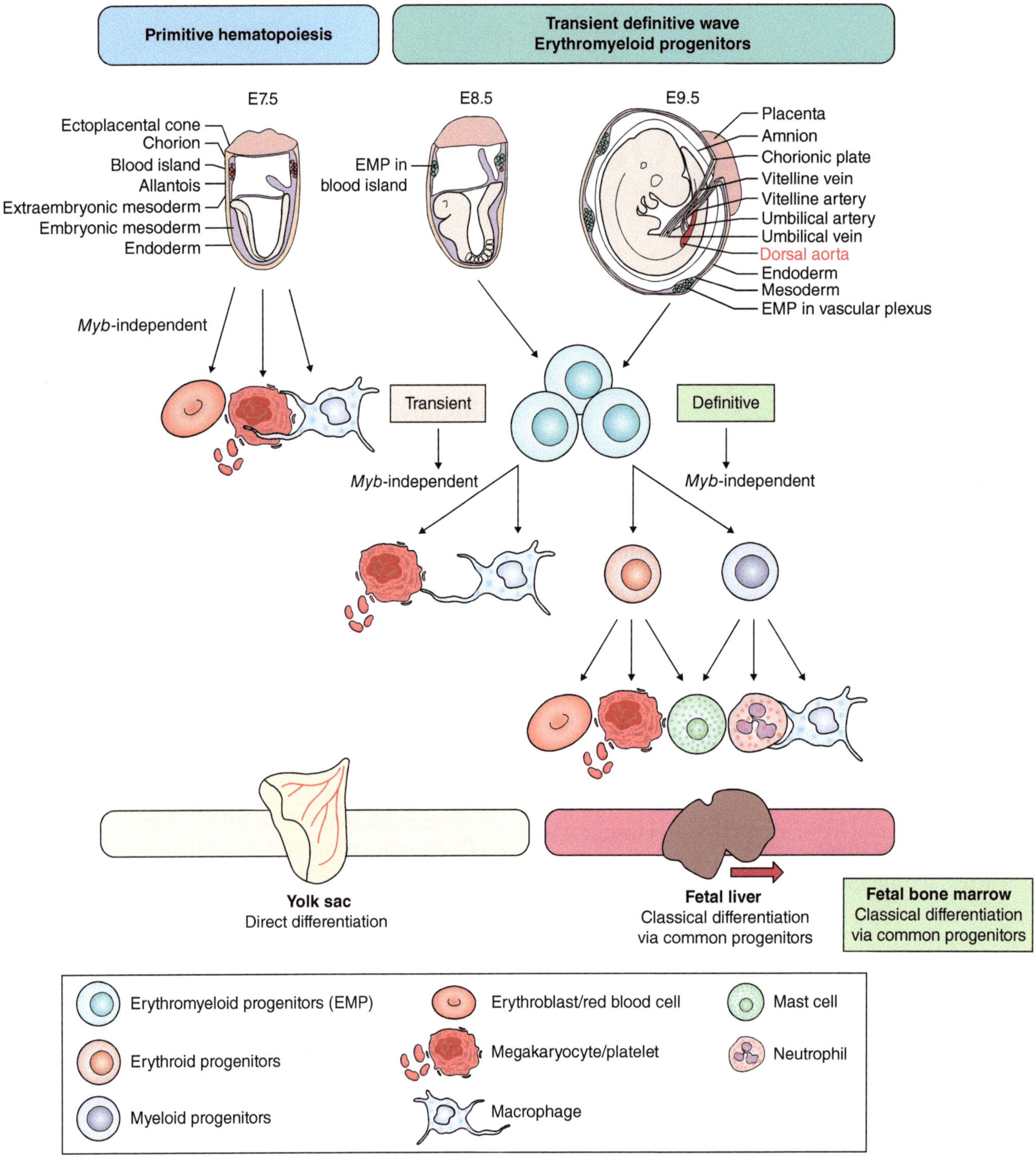

Figure 7.1 Phases of hematopoiesis: Primitive, transient, and definitive. Dorsal aorta is labeled in red font to denote development within the extraembryonic yolk sac. All other labels denote structures that form within the embryo.

HSC, hematopoietic stem cells.

Source: Adapted from Sommer, A., & Perdiguero, E. G. (2024). Extraembryonic hematopoietic lineages-to macrophages and beyond. *Experimental Hematology, 136*, 104285. https://doi.org/10.1016/j.exphem.2024.104285

and multipotent progenitor cells within the liver and ultimately the bone marrow, marking the transition to life-sustaining hematopoiesis (Palis & Segel, 2021; Sommer & Perdiguero, 2024). Through the successful interplay of gene, glycoprotein, growth, and transcription factor expression, the fetus moves through the three phases of hematopoiesis necessary to facilitate functional maturation of the hematologic system (Sommer & Perdiguero, 2024) The major functions of the hematologic system are summarized in Table 7.1.

Physiology of Hematopoiesis

Red Blood Cells. The RBC is an anucleated, biconcave cell that is responsible for oxygen delivery to, and carbon dioxide removal from, organs and tissues. Primitive RBCs, erythroblasts, are detectable during week 2 of gestation and are distinguished by their larger size, hemoglobin configuration, and retention of a nucleus (D'Souza et al., 2021; Owusu-Ansah et al., 2025; Sommer & Perdiguero, 2024). As one of the earliest differentiated cell lines, RBCs play a vital role in embryonic and fetal development. Without the development of early RBCs, life could not be sustained (Owusu-Ansah et al., 2025). In fact, to maintain normal RBC numbers in the adult human, HSCs produce 2.4 million new cells each second (Cosgrove et al., 2021).

Erythropoiesis defines the process of RBC development, which occurs in two distinct waves. In the first trimester, hematopoietic precursors undergo primitive erythropoiesis, primarily within the yolk sac and, to a lesser degree, within the liver and bone marrow. Mesodermal cells migrate to the yolk sac, enter, and interact with cells within the endoderm (cells with vascular endothelial and hematopoietic potential), forming blood islands. It is here, within the blood islands of the yolk sac, that erythroid progenitor cells emerge and give rise to primitive erythrocytes, termed erythroblasts. Erythroblasts are necessary to promote embryonic tissue oxygenation and development yet are subject to a short life span (Owusu-Ansah et al., 2025). Because these cells are transient, this period of hematopoiesis is considered primitive. Generally, primitive erythrocytes are noted within the yolk sac between weeks 2 and 10 of gestation, within the liver between weeks 4 and 5 of gestation, and within the bone marrow between weeks 8 and 9 of gestation (Figure 7.2). A continuous transition toward the production of mature erythroblasts continues within the liver and bone marrow, while production within the yolk sac terminates around week 10 of gestation.

The second wave of erythropoiesis is termed the definitive wave. This wave involves the production of lineage-committed, multipotent, and ultimately pluripotent definitive HSCs and progenitors that can give rise to all cell types in the body (Figure 7.3). Lineage-committed progenitors are EMPs, which first arise within

TABLE 7.1 Major Physiologic Functions of the Hematologic System

Major Function	Examples
Transport	• Antibodies • Carbon dioxide • Electrolytes • Heat • Hormones • Oxygen • Waste products
Modulation	• Acid–base homeostasis • Body temperature • Coagulation • Fluid homeostasis
Protection	• Infectious response (white blood cells)

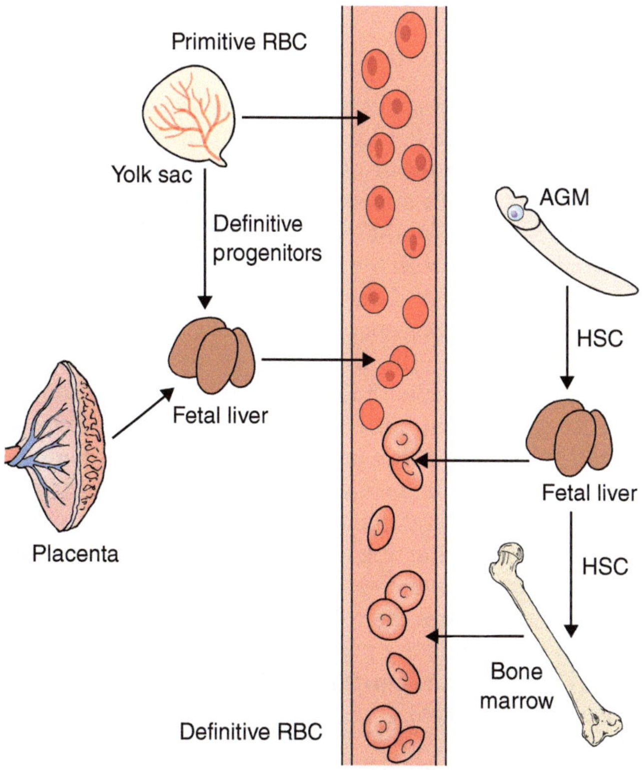

Figure 7.2 Transition of RBC production during development. Initially, larger, nucleated primitive erythrocytes are produced in the yolk sac. The location of HSCs shifts during development from the AGM to the liver and they ultimately reside in the bone marrow throughout adult life.

AGM, aorta-gonad-mesonephros region; HSC, hematopoietic stem cells; RBC, red blood cell.

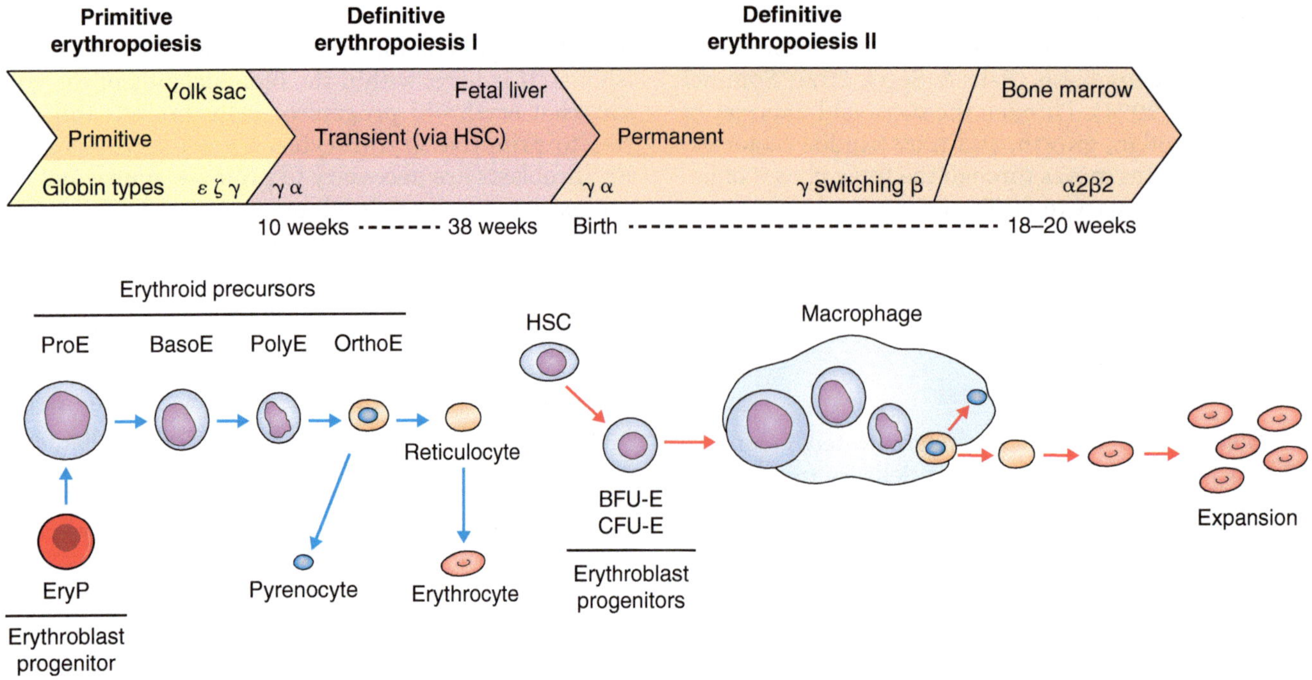

Figure 7.3 Process of erythropoiesis from HSC to fully differentiated anucleated RBC.
BFU-E, burst-forming unit–erythrocyte; CFU-E, colony-forming unit–erythrocyte; CFU-GEMM, colony-forming unit–granulocyte, erythrocyte, monocyte, megakaryocyte; EPO, erythropoietin; HSC, hematopoietic stem cell; NK, natural killer cells; RBC, red blood cell.
Source: Lee, S.-J., Jung, C., Oh, J. E., Kim, S., Lee, S., Lee, J. Y., & Yoon, Y.-s. (2023). Generation of red blood cells from human pluripotent stem cells—An update. *Cells, 12*(11), 1554. https://doi.org/10.3390/cells12111554.

the yolk sac (D'Souza et al., 2021; Owusu-Ansah et al., 2025; Sommer & Perdiguero, 2024). By day 23 (concurrent with the onset of the heartbeat and primitive circulation), EMPs appear within the aorta-gonad-mesonephros region (AGM), vitelline veins, umbilical arteries, and vasculature in the head. It is within the primitive heart (aortic region of the AGM) that multipotent definitive HSCs arise (Sommer & Perdiguero, 2024). By week 6, EMPs colonize the liver, leading to erythropoiesis shifting to the liver, with the liver being the major source of RBC production until 24 weeks of gestation (Palis & Segel, 2021). The RBCs produced in the liver and entering the fetal circulation eject their nucleus and contain a more mature hemoglobin configuration (Sommer & Perdiguero, 2024). Starting around 20 weeks of gestation, the bone marrow increases its RBC production proficiency and assumes the role of primary site for erythropoiesis; it remains the primary locus for hematopoiesis across the life span (Owusu-Ansah et al., 2025; Sommer & Perdiguero, 2024).

Erythropoietin. Erythropoietin (EPO) is a glyco-protein hormone that regulates RBC production through the Janus kinase 2 (JAK2) pathway (Palis & Segel, 2021). During fetal development, EPO does not cross the placenta and is initially produced in neural crest cells prior to initiation of fetal circulation (Carlberg, 2024). As hematopoiesis transitions to the liver, so too does the production of EPO. Ultimately, EPO production transitions to the fetal kidney by 30 weeks' gestation with levels of EPO production increasing with gestational age (Carlberg, 2024).

EPO holds a significant role in definitive erythropoiesis across the life span. An inverse correlation exists with EPO synthesis and secretion, and tissue oxygenation (Figure 7.4; Carlberg, 2024). When oxygen levels are high, EPO activity is low. Conversely, when oxygen levels are low, transcription factors including hypoxia-inducible factor (HIF) and hepatic nuclear factor 4, stimulate an increase in EPO production (Aster & Scadden, 2017; Owusu-Ansah et al., 2025). These principles are discussed later in this chapter, relative to the pathophysiology of anemia.

Hemoglobin

Hemoglobin provides the RBC with the capability to carry and release oxygen to the tissues. Hemoglobin is a protein composed of two pairs of globin chains that are connected to the heme molecule and are required for oxygen binding. Different forms of globin peptides are expressed throughout fetal development and into adult life and determine the type of hemoglobin produced. Adult hemoglobin contains α-like globin peptides and β-like globin peptides which work in conjunction to regulate oxygen delivery. During the embryonic phase, primitive erythrocytes produce the β-like globin known

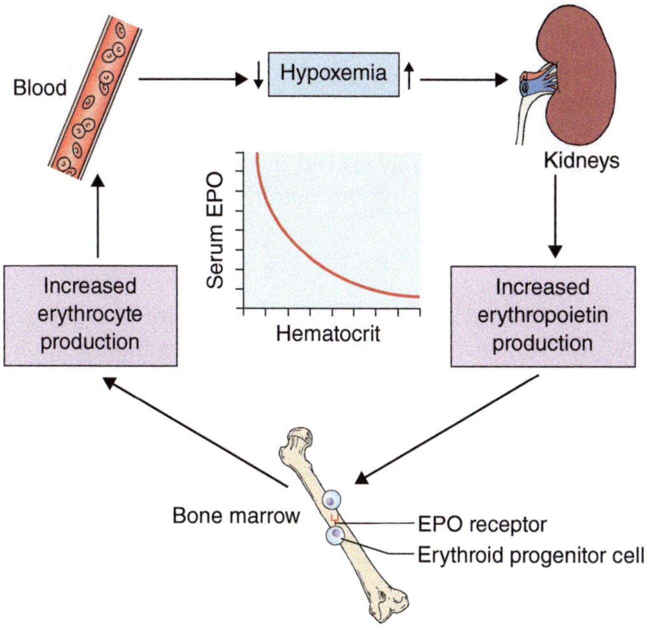

Figure 7.4 Feedback loop between hypoxia and EPO production. Response of EPO production in the presence of low oxygen levels. HIF located in the kidney responds to increased tissue hypoxia and increases EPO production. The EPO then stimulates bone marrow to produce and release more RBCs into circulation to deliver oxygen. The inset graph shows the relationship between hematocrit and EPO production; the left of the graph demonstrates low hematocrit and increased EPO levels while the right of the graph demonstrates normal hematocrit and low EPO levels. More EPO is produced as a result of tissue hypoxia that occurs at lower hemoglobin/hematocrit levels. At higher hemoglobin/hematocrit levels, less EPO is produced due to adequate tissue perfusion.

EPO, erytropoietin; Hb, hemoglobin; HIF, hypoxia-inducible factor; RBC, red blood cell.

Source: Adapted from Spivak, J. L. (2005). The anaemia of cancer: Death by a thousand cuts. *Nature Reviews Cancer, 5*, 543–555. https://doi.org/10.1038/nrc1648

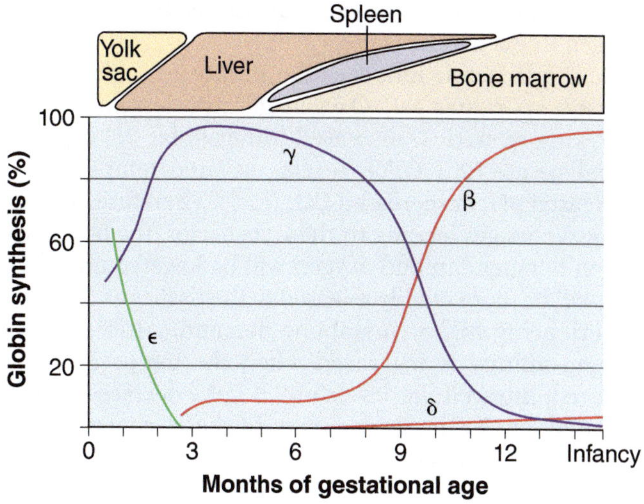

Figure 7.5 Globulin peptide synthesis and hemoglobin. Timing of β-like gene expression from embryonic period to infancy. The β-like subunits, when paired with the α-like subunits, form different types of hemoglobin produced during gestation. Green line: embryonic hemoglobin which disappears with the resolution of the yolk sac. Purple line: fetal hemoglobin which gradually decreases as hemoglobin production moves from the liver to the bone marrow. Red line: adult hemoglobin which increases in production near term and becomes the primary hemoglobin produced throughout the life span.

Source: Data from Sankaran, V. G., & Orkin, S. H. (2013). Genome-wide association studies of hematologic phenotypes: A window into human hematopoiesis. *Current Opinion in Genetics & Development, 23*(3), 339–344. https://doi.org/10.1016/j.gde.2013.02.006

as ε-*globin*. Hemoglobin produced during this embryonic phase are Hb Gower 1, Hb Gower 2, and Hb Portland (Owusu-Ansah et al., 2025). With the transition to definitive erythropoiesis, the major β-like globin produced is Gamma (γ)-globin. The combination of γ-globin and α-globin produces fetal hemoglobin (Hb F; Palis & Segel, 2021). Hb F is the primary hemoglobin produced during the remainder of fetal life and has higher oxygen-binding capabilities than adult hemoglobin. As RBC production transitions from the liver to the bone marrow, γ-globin production decreases and is replaced by production of β-globin heterodimers (Figure 7.5). The resulting tetramer, two pairs of α-globin and two pairs of β-globin, is known as hemoglobin A (*Hb A*). Hb A will remain the primary form of hemoglobin through adult life. By 6 months of postnatal life, Hb F comprises less than 1% of total hemoglobin (Owusu-Ansah et al., 2025).

Clinical Application. The APRN should recall that the life span of the fetal RBC is shorter than the adult RBC. The average life span of the fetal RBC (Hb F) ranges from 60 to 80 days (30–50 days in the extremely low birthweight [ELBW] neonate) compared to the 120-day life span of the adult RBC (Hb A). Delayed cord clamping (DCC), or umbilical cord management following delivery, enables a transfusion of fetal RBCs at the time of delivery. This practice has been demonstrated to improve blood pressure regulation and decrease the need for RBC transfusions in premature neonates, while decreasing the incidence of iron-deficiency anemia in full-term neonates.

As stated previously, hemoglobin allows RBCs to carry oxygen to the tissues. The affinity for oxygen binding determines how well the hemoglobin picks up oxygen and releases it to the tissues and is a finely orchestrated balance. When affinity is high, the hemoglobin can hold onto oxygen more easily. But high oxygen affinity means the hemoglobin will not release oxygen at the tissue level as readily. When oxygen affinity is lowered, the hemoglobin does not bind oxygen as well but will readily release the oxygen to the tissues.

Multiple factors influence the affinity hemoglobin has for oxygen (Figure 7.6). Oxygen affinity is lessened in the following scenarios: increased intracellular 2,3 diphosphoglycerate (2,3 DPG) levels, elevated temperature, decreased pH, or increased CO_2 levels. Therefore, during clinical changes leading to these scenarios, the bond between hemoglobin and oxygen will be lowered and oxygen will be more readily released to the tissues as they are experiencing higher metabolic demand. Alternatively, oxygen affinity is increased when the temperature is lowered, intracellular levels of 2,3 DPG decrease, pH is elevated, or CO_2 levels decrease. In these scenarios, the bond between hemoglobin and oxygen will be stronger; therefore, oxygen delivery to the tissues is decreased.

Clinical Application. The APRN should always remember how the differences between fetal and adult hemoglobin impact the neonate and that excessive oxygen delivery to the tissues can be damaging. Consider the neonate with bronchopulmonary dysplasia who has received multiple packed RBC transfusions during the course of their NICU hospitalization. Attention to oxygen levels is key to reducing oxidative injury. As these neonates live in a state of permissive hypercapnia and are working with increased amounts of Hb A, oxygen is more easily released to the tissues. Due to the lower affinity adult hemoglobin has to hold onto oxygen molecules, delivery of oxygen to the tissues is increased and may exceed the need despite these neonates having a higher metabolic demand.

Recall from Chapter 2 that the structure of Hb F allows for higher oxygen delivery to the developing fetus. In utero, under normal circumstances, blood from the XX pregnant patient and fetal blood do not mix and the placenta acts as the site for oxygen exchange. However, the blood coming to the placenta contains a lower oxygen content. Therefore, the fetal RBCs need to have a stronger ability to capture as much of the available oxygen as possible. The fetus has a higher number of RBCs to assist in oxygen delivery to tissues.

Red Blood Cell Indices. RBC indices include the *mean cell volume* (MCV), *mean cell hemoglobin* (MCH), and *mean corpuscular hemoglobin concentration* (MCHC). The MCV defines the size of the RBC. The MCH and MCHC define the hemoglobin concentration within the RBC. More specifically, MCH quantifies the concentration of hemoglobin per individual RBC, whereas

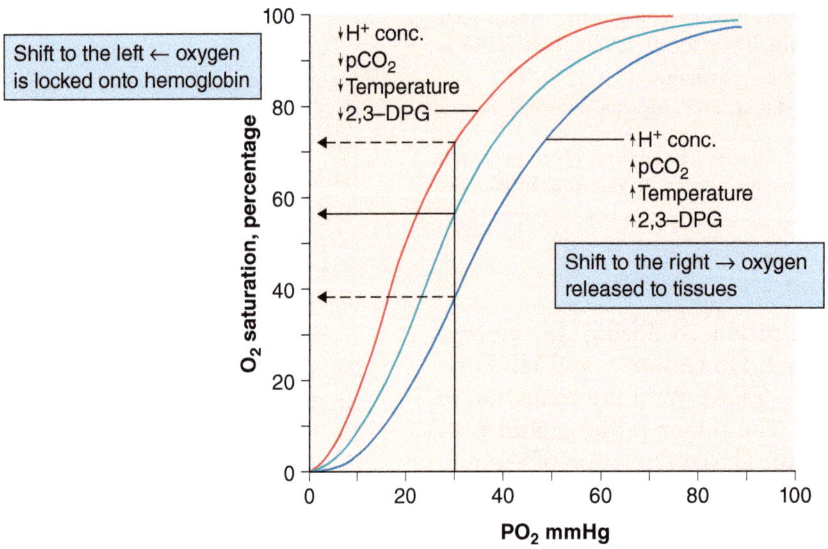

Figure 7.6 Oxyhemoglobin dissociation curve. At the same PO_2, the percentage of oxygen saturation changes by shift of the curve. A shift in the oxygen-hemoglobin dissociation curve to the left (red line) is illustrated here with hemoglobin having a higher affinity for oxygen. This means that hemoglobin holds on to oxygen more tightly, resulting in hemoglobin being more saturated with oxygen (70%) at the PaO_2 of 30 mmHg. A shift in the curve to the right (blue line) signifies that hemoglobin is less eager to hold onto oxygen. This change makes it easier for hemoglobin to release oxygen to the tissues. However, as illustrated here, the same PaO_2 of 30 mmHg results in lower oxygen saturation of hemoglobin (39%). The factors affecting the shifts in the curve are hydrogen ion concentration (pH), carbon dioxide content (CO_2), temperature, and intracellular levels of 2,3 DPG.

DPG, diphosphoglycerate.

Source: Adapted from Humes, H. D., & Kelley, W. N. (2000). *Kelly's textbook of internal medicine* (4th ed.). Lippincott, Williams, & Wilkins.

the MCHC quantifies the concentration of hemoglobin per unit volume. In that regard, the MCHC offers a correlation between the volume of the cell (MCV) and hemoglobin content. The neonate demonstrates both an increased size (MCV) and hemoglobin concentration (MCH; Owusu-Ansah et al., 2025). Each of these indices can be calculated if the RBC count, hemoglobin, and hematocrit are known.

MCV and MCHC values are classified as low, normal, or elevated. Therefore, when referring to size, RBCs are termed microcytic, normocytic, or macrocytic, based upon the calculated MCV. The RBCs' description of hemoglobin concentration (MCHC) are termed either hypochromic (low hemoglobin), normochromic, or hyperchromic (increased hemoglobin).

To calculate the MCV, the following formula is used:

$$\text{MCV} = \frac{\text{hematocrit (\%)} \times 10}{\text{RBC count (millions/mm}^3\text{)}}$$

To calculate the MCH, the following formula is used:

$$\text{MCH} = \frac{\text{hemoglobin (g/100 mL)} \times 10}{\text{RBC count (millions/mm}^3\text{)}}$$

To calculate the MCHC, the following formula is used:

$$\text{MCHC} = \frac{\text{hemoglobin (g/100 mL)} \times 100}{\text{hematocrit (\%)}}$$

APRNs may be asked to analyze RBC indices. Recall from prior discussions that RBC indices of a term newborn immediately after birth often reflect a nonpathologic and transient state of macrocytosis, which may be paired with polycythemia and polychromasia. This slowly transitions to a state of anemia as erythropoiesis is suppressed, secondary to increased extrauterine tissue oxygenation and other factors (see physiologic anemia of infancy, physiology anemia of prematurity). Less common etiologies associated with macrocytosis include congenital hypothyroidism (macrocytic, normochromic RBCs) and megaloblastic anemia (Bunn & Heeney, 2017). Conditions associated with microcytosis include hereditary spherocytosis (HS), iron deficiency, and the thalassemias.

Physiology of Clotting

Clotting factors are vital to the formation of clots when hemostasis (*heme* = blood; *stasi* = stopping) is required. As part of its normal development, the human fetus begins expressing most clotting factors by week 10 of gestation as coagulation proteins cannot cross from mother to fetus through the placenta. Concentration differences exist between neonatal and adult levels of clotting factors. For example, vitamin K-dependent factors (II, VII, IX, and X) and contact factors (XI and XII) are all about 50% of normal adult values at birth (Ostilla et al., 2024). Factors V, VIII, and XIII are equivalent to adult normal values, while von Willebrand factor levels are increased (Ostilla et al., 2024). Fibrinogen (factor I) is present by 3 to 5 weeks of gestation and is present in concentrations equivalent to adult normal values (Albisetti et al., 2021). However, the fetal fibrinogen is distinct in its makeup and has decreased capability of clot formation due to decreased fibrin polymerization (Moiseiwitsch & Brown, 2021; Nellenbach et al., 2020).

Two pathways lead to clot formation, *intrinsic* and *extrinsic* coagulation, before converging into the common pathway (Figure 7.7). The intrinsic coagulation pathway is a series of steps that are activated by trauma to the cells. This slower pathway begins with the activation of factor XII to its active form, XIIa. Activated factor XIIa, in the presence of high-molecular-weight kininogen (HMWK), converts factor XI to its active form, XIa. Next, factor XIa, in the presence of calcium, elicits the activation of factor IX. Active factor IXa, in the presence of activated factor VIIIa and calcium, prompts the conversion of factor X into its active form, Xa. Finally, activated factor Xa, in the presence of calcium and factor V, forms the prothrombin activator (Bunn & Furie, 2017; Grover & Mackman, 2019; Moiseiwitsch & Brown, 2021).

The extrinsic pathway is activated by way of trauma to the vascular endothelium or tissue. This faster pathway begins with the activation of tissue factor (TF), a membrane-bound protein located in the endothelium. TF modulates the conversion of factor VII to activated factor VIIa. Next, TF and activated factor VIIa combine with calcium and convert factor X to activated factor Xa. Activated factor Xa, in the presence of calcium and factor V, forms the prothrombin activator (Bunn & Furie, 2017; Grover & Mackman, 2019; Moiseiwitsch & Brown, 2021).

Both intrinsic and extrinsic pathways converge, forming the common pathway, when prothrombin activator is formed. Prothrombin activator, in the presence of calcium, converts prothrombin into thrombin, the active enzyme. When sufficient thrombin concentrations are present in the plasma, it leads to the conversion of fibrinogen into fibrin monomers. Through an interaction with calcium and fibrinogen stabilizing factor (factor XIII), fibrin polymers are created. These fibrin polymers aggregate with platelets and phospholipids, which forms a clot and achieves hemostasis. The maturation process of the coagulation system continues throughout childhood (Table 7.2; Bunn & Furie, 2017; Grover & Mackman, 2019; Moiseiwitsch & Brown, 2021).

Platelet Production

MK progenitor cells are first noted in the embryonic yolk sac with platelets noted in fetal circulation as early as 8 weeks postconception (Davenport et al., 2022). MKs are the precursors of platelets and they are large cells, though smaller in the fetus and newborn than the

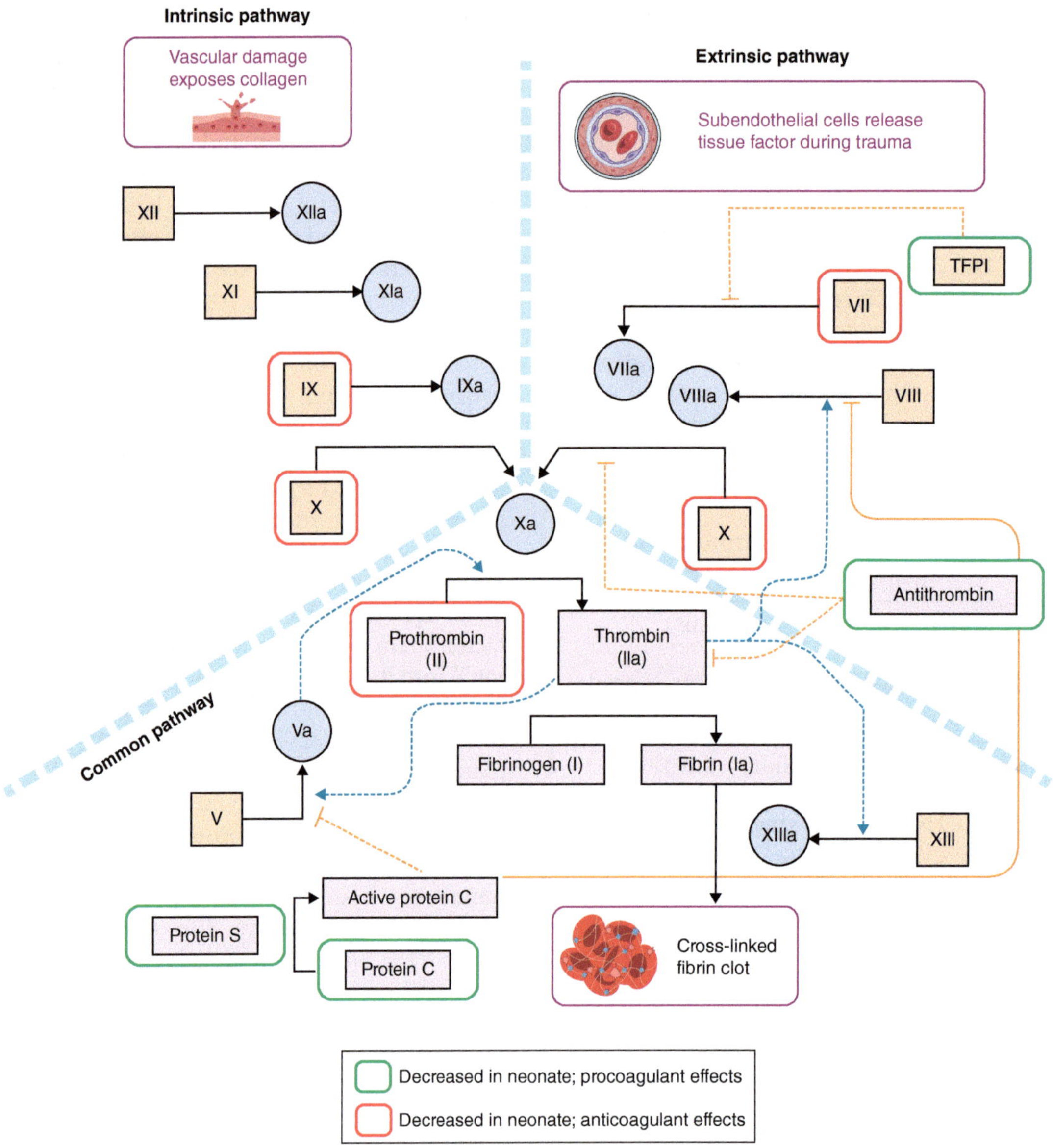

Figure 7.7 Coagulation pathway.

Source: Moiseiwitsch, N., & Brown, A. C. (2021). Neonatal coagulopathies: A review of established and emerging treatments. *Experimental Biology and Medicine, 246*, 1447–1457. https://doi.org/10.1177/15353702211006046

TFPI, tissue factor pathway inhibitor.

adult, and exist in small numbers in the bone marrow at the time of birth (Davenport et al., 2022). Megakaryocytopoiesis is the process by which bone marrow progenitor cells develop into mature MKs. Fragmentation of the cytoplasm of mature MKs leads to the release of platelets, which are small anucleated cells that are the first cells to respond to injury to the vascular endothelium. Following an event, there is platelet activation and migration to the site of injury. The process of platelet production is as follows: production of thrombopoietic factors (thrombopoietin [TPO]) → increase of MK progenitors → differentiation and development of MKs → production and release of platelets into the circulation (Figure 7.8; Davenport & Sola-Visner, 2021; Deschmann & Sola-Visner, 2024). The platelet count is dependent on the size and number of MKs. In contrast to the adult MK, neonatal MKs are smaller and have lower ploidy levels and thus make fewer platelets per MK (Davenport & Sola-Visner, 2021). The healthy fetus and neonate compensates for this limitation by having higher TPO levels and creates more MKs per MK progenitor (Davenport & Sola-Visner, 2021). The period between maturation of MK to release of platelets is about 5 days in humans.

In the classic model of differentiation, it is believed that MKs are developed from a committed, common myeloid progenitor cell (CMP), the CFU-GEMM cell. This committed CMP gives rise to a common MK–erythroid progenitor (Davenport et al., 2022). The MK–erythroid progenitor subsequently separates into different cell

TABLE 7.2 Functional Maturation of Major Hemostatic Factors

Major Hemostatic Factors	Maturation (Postnatal Age)
Tissue plasminogen activator	5 days
Platelet	2–4 weeks
Coagulation factor VIII	1 month
Protein S	1 month
Coagulation factor VIII	1 month
Antithrombin	3 months
Von Willebrand factor	3 months
Plasminogen	6 months
Coagulation factor XI	1 year
Fibrinogen	5 years
Coagulation factor II, VII, IX, X	16 years
Coagulation factor V	16 years
Coagulation factor XII	16 years
Protein C	16 years

Source: Adapted from Diaz-Miron, J., Miller, J., & Vogel, A. M. (2013). Neonatal hematology. *Seminars in Pediatric Surgery, 22*(4), 199–204. https://doi.org/10.1053/j.sempedsurg.2013.10.009

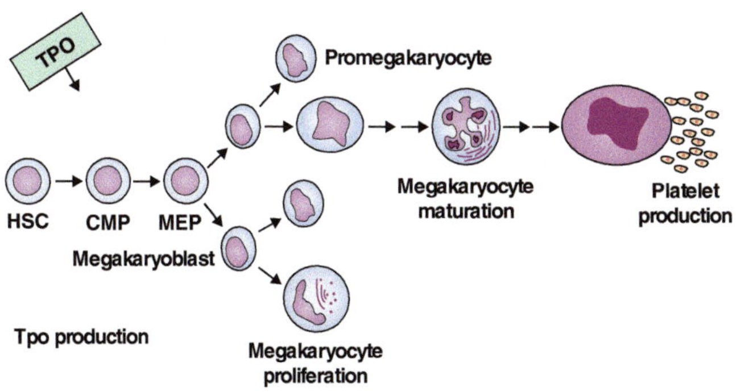

Figure 7.8 Representation of platelet production.

CMP, common myeloid progenitor; HSC, hematopoietic stem cell; MEP, megakaryocyte-erythrocyte progenitor; TPO, thrombopoietin.

Source: Davenport, P. E., & Sola-Visner, M. C. (2021). Acquired thrombocytopenias. In P. A. de Alarcon, E. J. Werner, R. D. Christensen, & M. C. Sola-Visner (Eds.), *Neonatal hematology: Pathogenesis, diagnosis, and management of hematologic problems* (3rd ed., pp. 210–222). Cambridge University Press.

lineages that result in the production of RBCs and platelets. Recently, there is evidence that other pathways may exist that end in the formation of MKs directly from the HSC (Davenport et al., 2022). There are two types of MK progenitors: the burst-forming unit-megakaryocyte (BFU-MK), which is the most primitive cell committed to the MK line, and the more differentiated colony-forming-unit megakaryocyte (CFU-MK; Juul & Christensen, 2024; Palis & Segel, 2021). MK progenitor concentrations are inversely proportional to gestational age and this persists in neonatal life in babies born prematurely, with the concentration decreasing with increasing postnatal age (Davenport et al., 2022). These progenitor cells exist in a high proliferative state. Proliferation occurs at the expense of further differentiation; as such, fetal MKs are more immature and produce significantly fewer platelets than adult MKs (Davenport & Sola-Visner, 2021).

Unlike MK progenitors, MK precursors (megakaryoblasts) have lost their ability to proliferate and instead undergo a process known as endomitosis or endoreduplication, by which they evolve from small mononuclear cells to large polyploidal cells (Mazzi et al., 2018). This process involves cycles of DNA replication (doubling of chromosomes within cells) without cell division and is called polyploidization. MK differentiation occurs in four stages. These stages are as follows: megakaryoblast (Stage I) → promegakaryocyte (Stage II) → granular MK (Stage III) → mature MK (Stage IV). Functional maturation of MKs occurs across fetal development, with low ploidy MK cells common in the embryo, and increased ploidy observed in cells in the fetus and highest among adults (Mazzi et al., 2018). This unique pattern of MK maturation in the fetus enables rapid proliferation to meet the demands of an expanding blood volume and maintenance of normal platelet counts (Deschmann & Sola-Visner, 2024). As the MK progresses through the stages of maturation, the cell grows in size with a nucleus that is multilobed as the platelet field is developed (Juul & Christensen, 2024). Platelet counts reach normal values by the second trimester (Ostilla et al., 2024).

Several cytokines affect the development of MKs. Those that stimulate the development of MKs include TPO, interleukin-3 (IL-3), interleukin-6 (IL-6), and interleukin-11 (IL-11), which stimulate differentiation and maturation of the MK (Huang et al., 2024; Jeon, 2022). Others appear to inhibit MK development and include platelet factor 4 and transforming growth factor-β (TGF-β). TPO is primarily produced in the liver throughout the life span (Ostilla et al., 2024). TPO levels peak on day 2 of postnatal life, remain elevated for about a month, and then gradually decline to adult levels (Jeon, 2022). Preterm neonates, both healthy and thrombocytopenic, show increased sensitivity to TPO compared to term neonates; however, this does not translate to increased platelet production given the limitations of MK size and ploidy (Jeon, 2022; Ostilla et al., 2024). The major differences noted between neonatal and adult megakaryopoiesis are presented in Table 7.3.

Neonatal thrombocytopenia is common, especially in preterm infants. Fetal MKs are ultimately smaller than those in infants, which are in turn smaller than those seen in children and adults. The point at which MKs attain normal adult sizes is unknown, as there is insufficient data in children from birth to 1 year of age. However, adult-size MKs have been identified in the bone marrow of children around 2 years of age (Fuchs et al., 2012).

Physiology of Phagocytes

As we have previously discussed, hematopoiesis begins in the yolk sac with the first macrophages noted between 2 to 5 weeks of gestation before they are recognized in the fetal liver as Kupffer cells by week 6 (O'Connell et al., 2021). The arrival of macrophages in the fetal bone marrow facilitates the hollowing out of the bone marrow space facilitating the initiation of hematopoiesis within the fetal bone marrow. Neutrophils first appear in the fetal bone marrow between weeks 11 and 12 of gestation with mature neutrophils, the most common leukocyte making up 40% of the hematopoietic cells in the fetal bone marrow, being seen after week 14 (Juul & Christensen, 2024; O'Connell et al., 2021), HSCs are situated within the bone marrow near osteoblasts, which secrete chemokines and growth factors needed in the process of generating, regulating, and maintaining the HSC (Lawrence et al., 2017, 2018). By the end of the first trimester, neutrophil precursors can be detected in the peripheral blood (Lawrence et al. 2017, 2018). The neutrophil count doubles by 18 weeks with a further doubling by 32 weeks (Figure 7.9; Thomas & Yoffey, 1962)

Mature blood cells (leukocytes) are of two separate lineages—lymphoid and myeloid. The lymphoid lineage consists of T cells, B cells, and natural killer (NK) cells and is covered in Chapter 9. The myeloid line includes the white blood cells (WBCs)—granulocytes (neutrophils, eosinophils, basophils), monocytes, and macrophages, as well as erythrocytes, MKs, and mast cells. The function of the granular and agranular leukocytes is summarized in Table 7.4. In the classic model of stem cell differentiation, multipotent progenitor cells differentiate into either the lymphoid progenitor cell (CLP) or the CMP. This is the earliest process exhibited by a developing multipotent progenitor cell.

The process for differentiation between the myeloid and lymphoid lineage remains a topic for debate with rapid advancements occurring over the past 20 years. Myeloid differentiation appears to be predominant and, if lymphoid gene expression is not achieved, the multipotent cell differentiates into a CMP with further differentiation into a granulocyte, monocyte, MK, or erythrocyte (Lawrence et al., 2017, 2018). Cells committed to the lymphoid line have been noted prior to the development of the fetal thymus and are noted within the thymus by 9 weeks postconception (O'Connell et al., 2021). T-cell production migrates to occur within the bone marrow and thymus from hematopoietic precursors in the fetal liver. Once in the thymus, T cells undergo a process of differentiation

TABLE 7.3 Major Differences in Megakaryopoiesis Between Neonates and Adults

	Neonates	Adults
TPO concentrations	Slightly higher in healthy neonates than in healthy adults	Lower in healthy adults than in healthy neonates
Megakaryocyte progenitors	Abundant in the blood	Sparse in the blood
	Give rise to large colonies	Give rise to small colonies
	More sensitive to TPO	Less sensitive to TPO
Megakaryocytes	Small	Large
	Low ploidy levels	High ploidy levels
Effects of rTPO	Inhibits MK polyploidization	Stimulates MK polyploidization
	Stimulates cytoplasmic maturation	Stimulates cytoplasmic maturation

MK, megakaryocyte; rTPO, recombinant thrombopoietin; TPO, thrombopoietin.

Source: Liu, Z., & Sola-Visner, M. (2011). Neonatal and adult megakaryopoiesis. *Current Opinion in Hematology, 18*(5), 330–337. https://doi.org/10.1097/MOH.0b013e3283497ed5

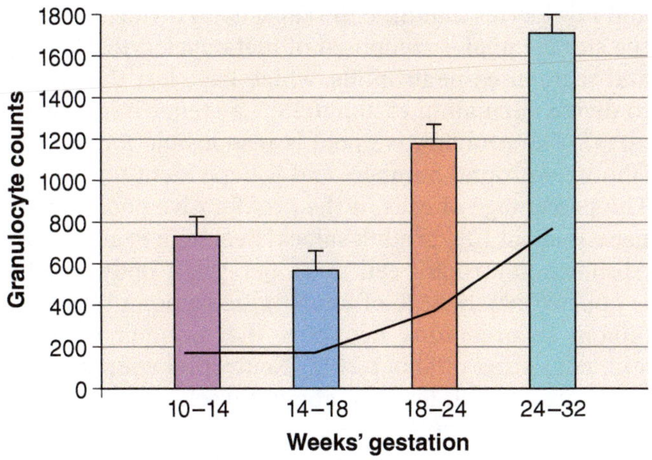

Figure 7.9 Neutrophil counts across gestation. Mean and range of neutrophil counts at 10 to 14, 14 to 18, 18 to 24, and 24 to 32 weeks' gestational age.

Source: Data from Thomas, D. B., & Yoffey, J. M. (1962). Human foetal haemo-poiesis. I. The cellular composition of foetal blood. *British Journal of Haematology*, *8*(3), 290–295. https://doi.org/10.1111/j.1365-2141.1962.tb06523.x

into macrophages, NK cells, or dendritic cells prior to being released into the bloodstream where they migrate to the secondary lymphoid organs: spleen, lymph nodes, and mucosal tissue (O'Connell et al., 2021).

The fetal liver and omentum are the first sites of B-cell development. The first recognizable cell in the B-cell lineage is the pre-B cell. This is first identified in the fetal liver around week 8 of gestation. From week 12, the bone marrow gradually takes over the function of B cell production and this is sustained until adulthood (Nielsen & Boyd, 2022). B cells are released from the bone marrow into the circulation once they have begun to express immunoglobulin on their cell surface (Benjamin et al., 2024). The APRN should understand that cord blood has higher concentrations of lymphocytes (B cells and T cells) than what is circulating in the adult peripheral system (Benjamin et al., 2024).

As discussed previously, progenitor cells, also known as pluripotent CFU-GEMM (colony-forming unit granulocyte–erythrocyte–megakaryocyte–monocyte) and the myeloid committed CFU-GM (CFU granulocyte–macrophage) are present in the fetal liver between weeks 12 and 14; they appear later in the fetal marrow, around weeks 15 to 16 with few immature neutrophils noted in fetal circulation at this time (Juul & Christensen, 2024; O'Connell et al., 2021). The concentration of both progenitors is also greatly increased in the blood of neonates, preterm more than term; however, this does not translate into increases in neutrophil counts.

Highly specific protein factors called colony-stimulating factors (CSFs) regulate and control the white cell lineage by stimulating the proliferation and differentiation of the CMP. Research has increased the types of CSFs identified in the past 20 years. Granulocyte-macrophage colony-stimulating factor (GM-CSF) stimulates the proliferation of pluripotent and immature progenitor cells with the capability of producing cells of different lineages, while granulocyte colony-stimulating factor (G-CSF) and macrophage colony-stimulating factor (M-CSF) act late in the developmental cycle, leading to proliferation and differentiation of late progenitor cells. The growth factors G-CSF and GM-CSF are the most frequent and are noted in higher concentrations in neonatal cord blood than adult peripheral blood (Laver et al., 1990; Michniacki & Walkovich, 2021).

Granulocytopoiesis is the process of production and maturation of granulocytes (neutrophils, eosinophils, and basophils). G-CSF is the major cytokine involved in the regulation of granulocytopoiesis. G-CSF is produced in many cells, mainly mature macrophages and monocytes, and production is stimulated by other cytokines such as tumor necrosis factor α (TNFα), interferon γ (IFN-γ), and lipopolysaccharides (present on the cell membrane of Gram-negative bacteria). In emergency situations, the concentration of G-CSF increases to

TABLE 7.4 Function of Granular and Agranular Leukocytes

Category of Leukocyte	Site of Production	Type of Cell	Mature Life Span	Function
Granulocyte	Bone marrow	Basophil	24–48 hours	Allergic histamine inflammatory response
		Eosinophil	12–72 hours	Allergic detoxifying response
		Neutrophil	10 hours	Phagocytosis
Agranulocyte	Bone marrow/ thymus	Lymphocyte	4–12 months	Immune response
	Bone marrow	Monocyte	4–12 months	Phagocytosis

Note: Basophils contain histamine, which is released during a hypersensitivity reaction. Eosinophils are released during an allergic (hypersensitivity) reaction to detoxify the body. Neutrophils are referred to as polymorphonuclear (PMN) cells or segmented neutrophils. Because neutrophils phagocytize bacteria, yet are the shortest-living leukocyte, increased bone marrow production of immature neutrophils (myelocytes, metamyelocytes, and bands) may be observed. Monocytes are converted into macrophages, the phagocytic form of that cell line; elevated counts suggest an acute viral, fungal, or chronic disease state.

allow production of an increased number of neutrophils. G-CSF concentrations in term infants are higher than for preterm infants, though these increases do not translate into increased numbers of mature neutrophils. Instead, the result is an increased release, from the proliferative pool, of immature neutrophil forms which have a diminished capacity for an immune response, and which are quickly depleted. The effects of G-CSF are mediated via the G-CSF receptor (G-CSFR), which regulates the production of committed myeloid progenitors, and enhances bactericidal and phagocytic activity (Mehta & Corey, 2021). In healthy neonates, both preterm and term, serial G-CSF concentrations show a peak between the first 4 to 7 hours of life, with subsequent decrease to normal adult range by days 4 to 7 (Benjamin et al., 2025). Once committed to the CFU-GM lineage, granulocytes move through proliferation, differentiation, and maturational phases with the increased production of granules noted during maturation. The types of granules expressed within each granulocyte (neutrophil, eosinophil, and basophil) differ, but for the purpose of this text, neutrophils will be discussed.

Neutrophils retain the ability to proliferate through the first few divisions from myeloblast to early myelocyte (Lawrence et al., 2017, 2018). Granule production begins during the proliferative period with myeloblasts, promylelocytes, and early myelocytes producing *azurophilic* granules, such as myeloperoxidase (MPO; Benjamin et al., 2025; Lawrence et al., 2017, 2018). As the neutrophil matures, additional granules begin to appear, such as *specific* granules during the period of myelocyte and metamyelocyte stage and *gelatinase* granules as the cell matures from a metamyelocyte to a band neutrophil (Lawrence et al., 2017, 2018). Once the neutrophil has matured into a segmented cell, additional granules (*ficolin-1*) are noted (Lawrence et al., 2017, 2018). The APRN should recall that during this maturational period the nucleus of the maturing neutrophil moves from a large, round nucleus to its characteristic segmented shape in the mature neutrophil. The maturation of the neutrophil, and associated increase in granule expression, enhances the immune properties of the neutrophil. Neutrophilic granules have essential microbicidal, proteolytic, and antimicrobial properties necessary for defense from bacteria, viruses, fungi, and other organisms (Lawrence et al., 2017, 2018).

PMNs are the most prominent of the circulating leukocytes in the human body and exist in three states, the proliferative pool, the maturing pool, and the storage pool within the bone marrow. Once the neutrophil has left the bone marrow, the cells exist in the circulating pool, vascular pool, and the tissue pool (Pateva et al., 2025). PMNs are the first immune cells to respond to pathogens; however, once released into the circulating pool, they have a short half-life of about 7 hours, requiring constant replenishment from the storage pool. The proliferative pool consists of myeloblasts, promyelocytes, and myelocytes that have the capacity to divide, whereas the storage pool is composed of metamyelocytes, bands, and segmented neutrophils, which have lost the ability to divide (Benjamin et al., 2025; Lawrence et al., 2017, 2018). The proliferative pool is responsible for replenishing neutrophil numbers and is dependent on G-CSF. The percentage of cells in the proliferative pool in neonates is about 10% of adult values (Benjamin et al., 2025). Absolute neutrophil cell mass per gram body weight is approximately 25% of adult values among term neonates. In premature neonates, that number is lower still, consisting of about 20%. Neutrophil counts eventually attain adult levels at about 4 weeks postnatal age (Lawrence et al., 2017, 2018).

It is important that learners understand that unlike adults, granulocytic progenitors do not increase during an infection in neonates. In addition, the storage pool is significantly smaller in premature infants compared to term neonates and adults. Similar to G-CSF concentrations, there is a surge in circulating neutrophils during the peripartum period that will never happen again in the life span of an individual (Lawrence et al., 2017, 2018). This surge occurs at 6 to 12 hours of life in neonates born at greater than 28 weeks of gestation and by 24 hours in those born at younger gestational ages. From the storage pool, available mature neutrophils are released into the circulation. Therefore, the combination of the small percentage of cells in the proliferative pool, inability to increase proliferation rates due to the already high rates, and low numbers of granulocytes in the storage pool leads to an increased risk for neutropenia in the face of infections. The neonate responds to infection by releasing into circulation more immature neutrophils which have a diminished ability to respond to invading pathogens. This contributes to the increased sepsis-associated morbidity and mortality seen in neonates.

Clinical Application. The APRN should understand that the surge of neutrophils following delivery will be reflected in lab values obtained during this time. Secondary to the stress associated with labor and delivery, circulating catecholamines and cortisol are believed to stimulate this neutrophilic surge. The WBC from a complete blood count (CBC) may reflect this surge if drawn within the first 6 to 12 hours. Elevated WBC values should be interpreted within the context of clinical presentation of the neonate and should not be used in isolation to determine clinical management strategies.

The high rate of proliferation of cells negatively affects their normal protective function, namely, their bacterial killing effect. MPO is produced in the promyelocyte, which then divides. Human neonatal neutrophils undergo several divisions to increase the number of cells in the storage pool. However, each division leads to a halving of the MPO content. When immature cells are released into the circulation without developing the necessary granules needed for bacterial killing, the neonate remains at risk for adverse sequelae. A summary of blood cell types and their differentiation is offered in Figure 7.10.

GENETIC INFLUENCES

Numerous genetic conditions impact the neonate's hematologic system; therefore, clinicians should always consider the hematologic system at risk until proven otherwise. Three common genetic defects that affect normal hematopoietic cell development, synthesis, and function are presented in the text that follows. Additional inherited disorders affecting the hematopoietic system are provided in Table 7.5.

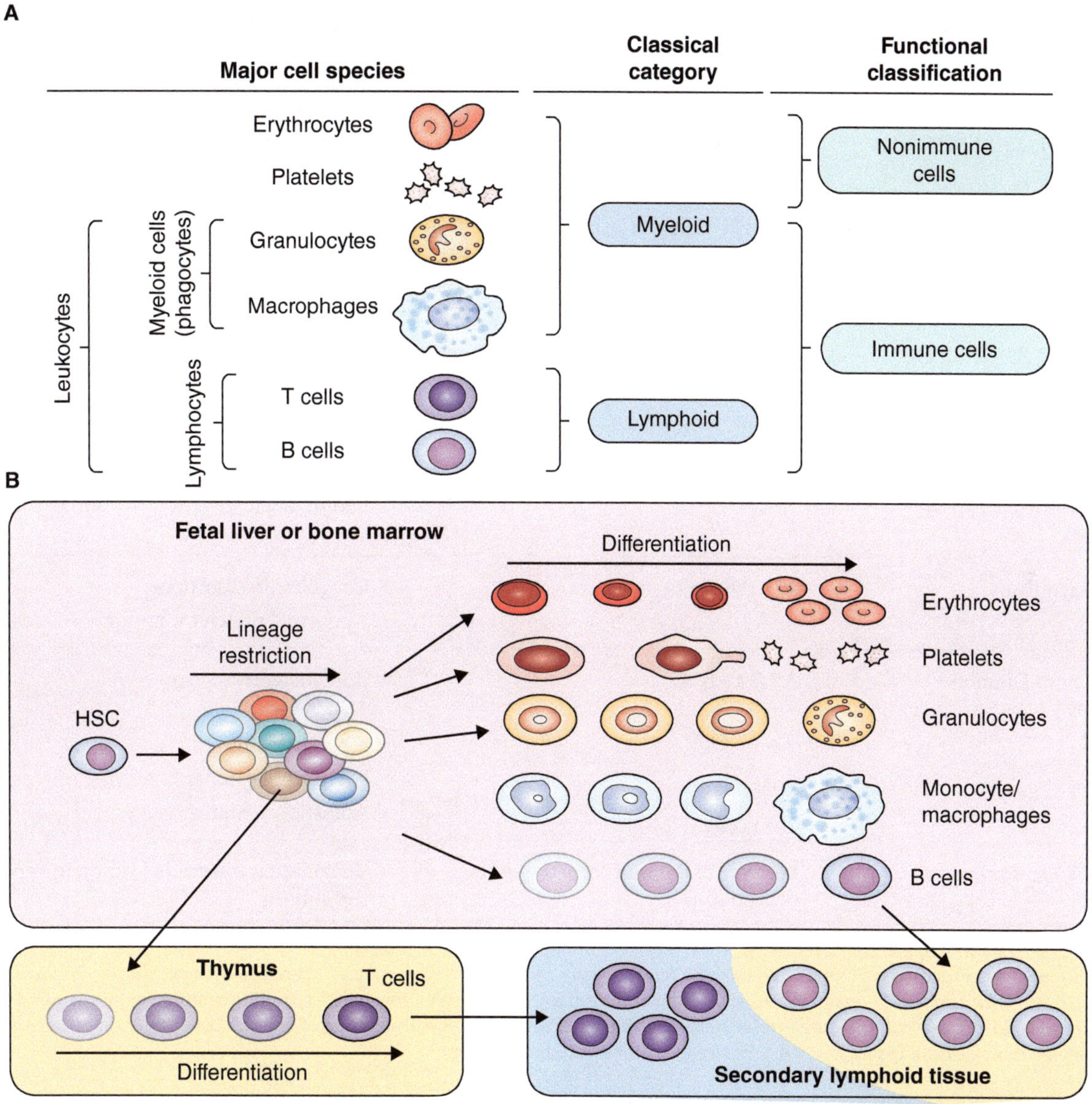

Figure 7.10 Blood cell types and their differentiation. (**A**) Major types of hematopoietic cells. Historically, erythroid and myeloid cells have been grouped into the "myeloid" lineage, and T and B lymphocytes into the "lymphoid"' lineage. Functionally, blood cells can be classified into "nonimmune" cells and "immune" cells. For the sake of simplicity, we group hematopoietic cells here into four major classes: (a) erythroid, including erythrocytes and platelets; (b) myeloid, including granulocytes and macrophages; (c) T lymphoid; and (d) B lymphoid. (**B**) Sites of hematopoiesis. Extensive proliferation occurs during both lineage restriction and differentiation phases. T cells and B cells undergo further maturation in secondary lymphoid organs such as the spleen or lymph nodes upon encountering specific antigens.

HSC, hematopoietic stem cell.

Source: Adapted from Kawamoto, H., & Yoshimoto K. (2009). A new paradigm for hematopoietic cell lineages: Revision of the classical concept of the myeloid–lymphoid dichotomy. *Trends in Immunology, 30*(5), 193–200. https://doi.org/10.1016/j.it.2009.03.001

TABLE 7.5 Other Inherited Disorders of the Hematologic System

Disorder	Inheritance Pattern	Hematologic Impact
Aplasia cutis congenita	AD, AR, or spontaneous mutation	• Prolonged bleeding
Diamond–Blackfan anemia	Isolated mutation; autosomal dominant; occasionally X-linked	• Decreased RBC production in the bone marrow/aplasia • Increased MCV (macrocytosis) • Leukopenia • Persistence of hemoglobin F (Hgb F)
Ehlers–Danlos syndrome-Vascular type	Varies by type: Vascular type is autosomal dominant	• Increased bleeding due to vascular, platelet, or coagulation defects • Increased bruising from vascular rupture
Factor V, VII, X, XI, XII, XIII deficiencies		• Coagulation disorders

Fanconi anemia	AR or X-linked	• Pancytopenia
		  ◦ Anemia
		  ◦ Leukopenia
		  ◦ Thrombocytopenia
		• Bone marrow failure

Neonatal hemochromatosis	AR	• Prolonged neonatal jaundice
Klippel–Trenaunay (angioosteohypertrophic) syndrome	AD	• Coagulation disorders leading to increased hemorrhagic or venous thrombosis risk
Noonan syndrome	AD; AR	• Coagulation disorders • Abnormal platelet function

Shwachman–Diamond syndrome	AR; rarely AD	• Bone marrow failure
		  ◦ Anemia
		  ◦ Neutropenia
		  ◦ Thrombocytopenia
		• Aplastic anemia

Sturge–Weber syndrome	Somatic mutation (occurring after conception)	• Coagulation disorders leading to venous thrombosis

AD, autosomal dominant; AR, autosomal recessive; MCV, mean cell volume; RBC, red blood cell.

Sources: National Institutes of Health. (n.d.). *Genetic and Rare Diseases Information Center.* https://rarediseases.info.nih.gov; National Library of Medicine. (n.d.-a). *Schwachman-Diamond syndrome.* MedlinePlus. https://medlineplus.gov/genetics/condition/shwachman-diamond-syndrome; National Library of Medicine. (n.d.-b). *Sturge-Weber syndrome.* MedlinePlus. https://medlineplus.gov/genetics/condition/sturge-weber-syndrome; National Organization for Rare Disorders. (n.d.). *Homepage.* https://rarediseases.org

Thalassemias

The thalassemias are a heterogeneous grouping of inherited hemolytic anemias that occur secondary to defective synthesis of globin chains and are regarded as the single most common inherited (single-gene) disorder in the world. The two most common types of thalassemia are classified according to which globin chain is impacted; alpha (α) or beta (β) thalassemia. Alpha thalassemia most often presents in the neonatal period owing to the fact that there are defects in the α globin chains which are present in both fetal and adult hemoglobin configurations (Blankenhorn & Strumph, 2024). Beta thalassemia more often presents after 3 months of age due to an impaired synthesis of the β globin chains which becomes more prominent as the neonate works to replace fetal hemoglobin (Blankenhorn & Strumph, 2024). Both alpha (α) and beta (β) thalassemia are classified according to severity and will be presented separately.

The pathogenesis of the thalassemias involves deficient, defective, or completely deleted (absent) globin genes. This destabilizes the normal 1:1 (ratio of α:β) globin chain and causes a variable degree of dysfunction with globin formation resulting in RBC membrane damage, insufficient erythropoiesis in the face of increased hemolysis, and hypochromic, microcytic anemia (Figure 7.11; Owusu-Ansah et al., 2025). We present an overview of the two most common thalassemias: alpha (α) and beta (β) thalassemia.

Alpha Thalassemia. Alpha (α) thalassemia is defined as a deficiency or absence of alpha globin chains, which is usually the result of one or more α gene deletions. Alpha globin deficits are a result of defects on chromosome 16 and lead to the production of unstable hemoglobin chains. The result is the formation of alternate β globin chains as there is an excess of β and gamma globin chains (Blankenhorn & Strumph, 2024; Rai et al., 2021). Recall that alpha chains are synthesized during fetal development and shared by fetal and adult hemoglobin (Hb); therefore, α thalassemia can manifest during fetal development and present as early as the immediate postnatal period.

In some cases, affected infants possess no defective α globin genes, and display a normal phenotype, normal hematologic findings, and require no medical intervention. However, most infants inherit one to four alpha gene deletions, which leads to an inability to cleave an appropriate number of alpha globin chains. α thalassemia can be classified genetically or clinically. The three clinical classifications are: (a) minor disease (silent carrier status), (b) α thalassemia trait (HbH disease), or (c) major disease (Hb Bart syndrome; Table 7.6; Owusu-Ansah et al. 2025; Rai et al., 2021). These hemoglobin pairs manifest clinically with tissue hypoxia as a result of the increased affinity for oxygen and resultant tissue hypoxemia (Rai et al., 2021). Hemoglobin H (HbH) disease typically manifests with hemolytic anemia, microcytosis, and splenomegaly. Hb Bart syndrome typically leads to fetal demise secondary to fatal hydrops fetalis.

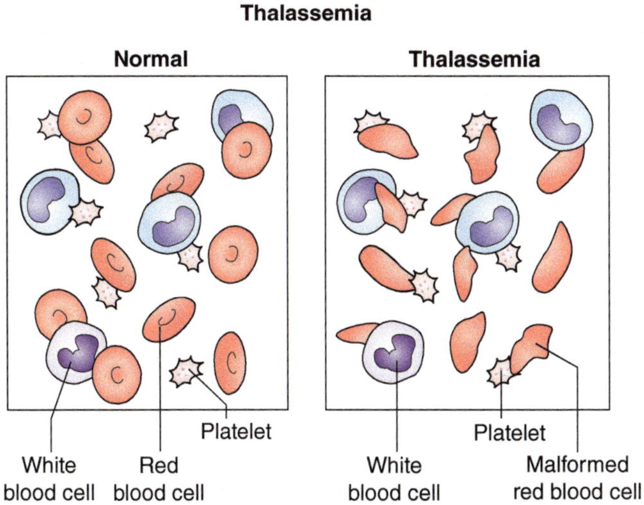

Figure 7.11 Cell morphology: Normal versus thalassemias. The malformed RBC depicted in the thalassemia image is unable to deliver oxygen to the tissues due to either an increased affinity for oxygen, decreased erythropoiesis, or increased RBC destruction (Rai et al., 2021). The malformed RBC is subsequently removed from circulation earlier leading to increased rates of hemolysis and anemia.

Beta Thalassemia. Beta thalassemia results from deficient or, in rare circumstances, absent synthesis of beta globin chains, which is usually the result of β gene deletions on chromosome 11. This leads to the formation of excess alpha and, in some circumstances, excess gamma globin chains. Similar to α thalassemia, β thalassemia can be classified genetically or clinically. The three classic clinical classifications are: (a) minor disease, (b) β thalassemia intermedia, or (c) major disease; however, more recent classifications are based on the need for transfusions and are referred to as transfusion-dependent β thalassemia (TDT) or non-transfusion dependent β thalassemia (NTDT; Blankenhorn & Strumph, 2024). Table 7.7 provides further information on clinical manifestations of β thalassemia.

TABLE 7.6 Effect of Gene Dysfunction With Alpha Thalassemia

Type of Alpha Thalassemia	Number of Defective α Genes	Common Clinical Manifestations
Minor	1	• Asymptomatic
α trait	2	• Mild hemolytic anemia • Childhood iron deficiency anemia • Low MCV and MCHC
Hb H disease	3	• Bone marrow expansion • Moderate hemolytic anemia • Hyperbilirubinemia • Iron hyperabsorption • Splenomegaly
Major disease (Hb Bart syndrome)	4	• Congestive heart failure • Genitourinary abnormalities • Hepatomegaly • Hydrops fetalis • Severe hemolytic anemia • Splenomegaly • Intrauterine demise

α, alpha; Hb, hemoglobin; MCHC, mean corpuscular hemoglobin concentration; MCV, mean corpuscular volume.

Neonatal APRNs should recognize that unlike α thalassemia, most cases of β thalassemia do not manifest during the birth hospitalization or the neonatal period due to the predominance of HbF at the time of delivery. The exception to this principle involves situations where infants require extensive postnatal blood transfusions. In these circumstances, HbF is rapidly replaced with HbA. This provokes early stimulation and expression of this inherited genetic disorder that would otherwise manifest during late infancy, childhood, or adulthood.

For older children, beta thalassemia minor (one gene defect) is associated with asymptomatic microcytic, hypochromic anemia, and erythrocytosis. The manifestations of beta thalassemia intermedia (two gene defects) and beta thalassemia major (two gene defects) are similar, albeit less severe among children with the intermediate disease state. Manifestations include microcytic and hypochromic anemia, hepatosplenomegaly, extramedullary erythropoiesis, lifelong blood transfusions, jaundice, and growth restriction (Blankenhorn & Strumph, 2024; Owusu-Ansah et al., 2025). Chelation therapy is indicated to prevent iron overload.

Hereditary Spherocytosis

HS is the third most common inherited defect in RBC membrane structure, superseded only by glucose-6-phosphate dehydrogenase deficiency (G6PD) and ABO isoimmunization (Glader & Kamdar, 2021; Will et al., 2017). In the United States, the overall incidence of spherocytosis is one in every 5,000 infants; however, the incidence increases to as high as one in every 1,000 to 2,000 births to families of Northern European descent (Glader & Kamdar, 2021; Will et al., 2017). The majority of cases are inherited in an autosomal dominant (AD) manner (75%), though spontaneous mutations and autosomal recessive (AR) inheritance have been described in about 25% of cases (Christensen, Yaish, & Gallagher, 2015; Owusu-Ansah et al., 2025). This defect may occur in one of several membrane proteins, including Ankryn-1 (ANK1; most common AD protein defect), alpha and beta Spectrin (SPTA1, SPTB), Band 3 (SCL4A1), and protein 4.2 (EBP42). Defective Ankryn-1 protein is reported in 40% to 50% of all HS cases (Christensen, Yaish, & Gallagher, 2015; Glader & Kamdar, 2021; Will et al., 2017). These proteins provide the RBC with its biconcave shape and membrane integrity, and, when deficient, they lead to RBC membrane instability, decreased deformability, and the characteristic spherical shape identified with this disorder (Figure 7.12).

The abnormally formed RBCs are sequestered in the spleen, where they are prematurely broken down by macrophages, resulting in hemolytic anemia, neonatal jaundice, and splenomegaly (Glader & Kamdar, 2021; Will et al., 2017). Jaundice is reported in more than 80% of affected infants, whereas 28% to 43% of infants are anemic at birth (Will et al., 2017). Commonly, MCH concentrations (MCHC greater than 36.5) are elevated among affected infants with a low MCV, reflecting membrane loss and RBC dehydration. The MCHC/MCV ratio has been demonstrated to be a positive predictor of HS with values greater than 0.36 demonstrating strong sensitivity, specificity, and a negative predictive value (Glader & Kamdar, 2021). An elevated reticulocyte count (3%–7%) is common within the first 72 hours of life, indicating early hemolysis

TABLE 7.7 Effect of Gene Dysfunction With Beta Thalassemia

Type of Beta Thalassemia	Number of Defective β Genes	Common Clinical Manifestations
Minor	1	• Asymptomatic to mild hemolytic anemia • Increased HbF
Intermediate	2	• Increased HbF • Iron hyperabsorption • Hepatosplenomegaly • Moderate to severe hemolytic anemia that may require lifelong blood transfusions
Major	2	• Iron hyperabsorption • Hepatosplenomegaly • Severe decrease in β globulin synthesis • Severe hemolytic anemia that will require lifelong blood transfusions

β, beta; HbF, fetal hemoglobin.

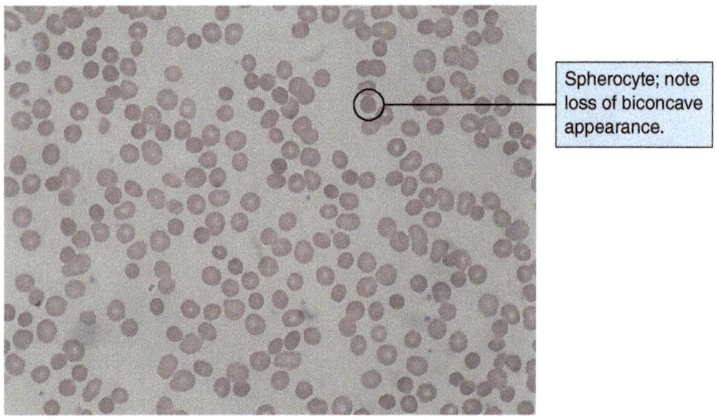

Figure 7.12 Peripheral blood smear of patient with hereditary spherocytosis.

Source: Mourao, P. H. O. (2010). *Hereditary spherocytosis smear.* https://commons.wikimedia.org/wiki/File:Hereditary_Spherocytosis_smear_2010-03-17.JPG

with compensatory cleavage of immature cells. These RBC indices make powerful screening tools (Christensen, Juul, & Del Vecchio, 2015; Will et al., 2017). Table 7.8 describes other common clinical laboratory findings indicative of HS.

There are several life-span implications for children with moderate to severe spherocytosis. Affected individuals have ongoing anemia, sometimes requiring blood transfusions. Up to 50% of patients develop gallstones (Will et al., 2017). Aplastic crises may occur as a result of viral infections such as parvovirus B19 (Christensen, Juul, & Del Vecchio, 2015). Splenic sequestration of abnormal RBCs results in splenomegaly and hypersplenism and may eventually require splenectomy once the child reaches school age or adolescence. Asplenic or functionally asplenic individuals are at an increased lifelong risk of sepsis with encapsulated organisms, such as *Streptococcus pneumoniae* and *Haemophilus influenza*, necessitating vaccination and anticipatory guidance for children and families (Glader & Kamdar, 2021). Growth failure, folate deficiency, and bony abnormalities may occur in children with severe disease due to increased hematopoiesis in the bone marrow in the setting of severe, chronic anemia (Christensen, Juul, & Del Vecchio, 2015). Life expectancy is typically unaffected.

Sickle Cell Disease

Sickle cell disease (SCD) is one of the most common AR, single-gene blood disorders reported within in the United States and across the globe. Within the United States, approximately 100,000 people are living with SCD, with SCD particularly impacting African American (one out of 365) and Hispanic American (one out of 16,000) infants each year (Centers for Disease Control and Prevention [CDC], 2024; National Library of Medicine, 2024). On a global scale, SCD affects approximately 300,000 infants each year; experts posit that the incidence may continue to rise, to upward of 400,000 infants by the year 2050 (Figure 7.13; Kavanagh et al., 2022). Global risk factors include African, Mediterranean, Arabian, Indian, South and Central American, and Caribbean descent (Kavanagh et al., 2022; National Library of Medicine, 2024). Hemoglobin S inheritance is due to a mutation on chromosome 11 and is either expressed as sickle cell trait (inheritance of one hemoglobin S [*HgB S*] gene) or SCD. For individuals to demonstrate SCD, the individual either inherits two abnormal genes for hemoglobin S or inherits one faulty *HgB S* gene with another abnormal β-globin mutation (such as β Thalassemia; Blankenhorn & Strumph, 2024).

Hemoglobin S (HbS) was first discovered by Linus Pauling in 1949, and its presence is the root cause for sickling of RBCs. The pathogenesis involves the deoxygenation and polymerization of HbS, which deforms the RBC, turning it from a normal biconcave cell into an oblong, stiff, and fragile, "sickle" shaped cell (Figure 7.14; Kavanagh et al., 2022). The sickle cell has difficulty traversing the vasculature, which leads to clogging of the vascular lumen. The occlusion provokes a vascular occlusive event, the hallmark manifestation of SCD. Although a discussion of the complex cellular responses that are elicited with a vascular occlusive event are beyond the scope of this textbook, it is important to understand that sickle cells readily adhere to the vascular endothelium and this propensity, along with several cellular processes,

TABLE 7.8 RBC Indices and HS

Lab Value	Definition	Associated Laboratory Finding	Rationale
MCHC	Represents the average gram per deciliter (g/dL) of hemoglobin within the RBC	MCHC >36 g/dL	Mild cellular dehydration causes increased cellular hyperdensity.
MCV	Represents the average volume or size in fL of the RBC	MCV<100 fL in case of HS	Caused by decreased spectrin content on the RBC membrane
MCHC/MCV ratio	MCHC ÷ MCV = MCHC/MCV ratio which is represented as a percentage	MCHC/MCV ratio >36% (0.36)	
RDW percentile	Reflects the average width of the RBC based on fL	RDW >14 fL	Caused by a greater variation in the size of RBC, known as anistocytes

fL, femtoliter; HS, hereditary spherocytosis; MCHC, mean corpuscular hemoglobin concentration; MCV, mean corpuscular volume; RBC, red blood cell; RDW, red blood cell distribution width.

Source: Will, A., Henderson, C. A., Jnah, A. J., & Newberry, D. (2017). Hereditary spherocytosis in the neonatal period: A case report. *Neonatal Network, 36*(5), 280–288. https://doi.org/10.1891/0730-0832.36.5.280

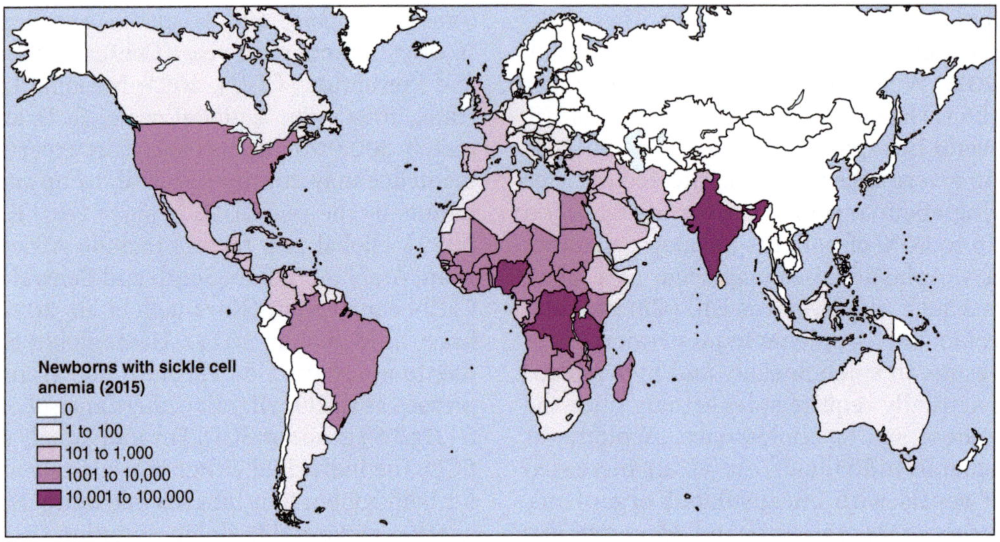

Figure 7.13 Number of newborns with sickle cell anemia in each country in 2015.

Source: Adapted from Kato, G. J., Piel, F. B., Reid, C. D., Gaston, M. H., Ohene-Frempong, K., Krishnamurti, L., Smith, W. R., Panepinto, J. A., Weatherall, D. J., Costa, F. F., & Vichinsky, E. P. (2018). Sickle cell disease. *Nature Reviews: Disease Primers, 4*, 18010. https://doi.org/10.1038/nrdp.2018.10

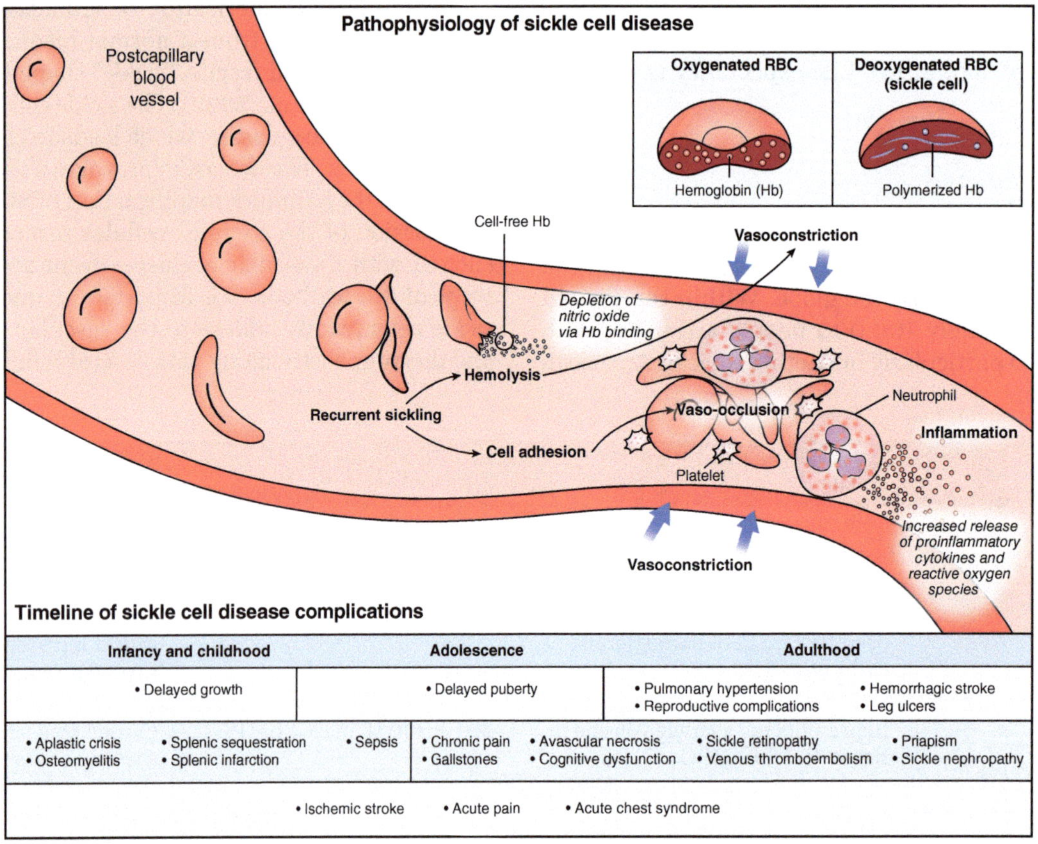

Figure 7.14 Note normal, biconcave RBC versus abnormal oblong and stiff, sickled RBC.

Note: HbS polymerizes when deoxygenated, inducing recurrent RBC sickling and hemolysis (top portion of figure). The sickled RBCs interact with white blood cells and platelets on vascular endothelium via adhesion molecules which leads to vaso-occlusion. The free Hb and heme released from RBC hemolysis trigger endothelial dysfunction due to depletion of nitric oxide and resultant vasoconstriction. The dual processes of vaso-occlusion and endothelial dysfunction activate inflammatory responses, via increased cytokines and reactive oxygen species, which perpetuates further vaso-occlusion. The morbidity of sickle cell disease is progressive throughout the life span (bottom portion of figure). Early on, most complications occur in acute recurrent episodes. Additionally, growth and puberty are delayed due to the increased metabolic demands secondary to ongoing hemolytic anemia. In adulthood, organ damage is prominent in addition to acute complications. Acute pain episodes, acute chest syndrome, and ischemic stroke can occur at any life stage. HbS, hemoglobin S; RBC, red blood cell.

Source: Adapted from Kavanagh, P. L., Fasipe, T. A., & Wun, T. (2022). Sickle cell disease: A review. *Journal of the American Medical Association, 328*(1), 57–68. https://doi.org/10.1001/jama.2022.10233

encourages a painful, proinflammatory state within the blood vessels (Kavanagh et al., 2022).

Associated clinical manifestations are summarized in Figure 7.15. Symptoms usually do not manifest until late infancy when fetal hemoglobin levels have reached their lowest level and hemoglobin S production has increased. Symptoms may vary from mild to severe. Factors that affect disease severity include climate, outside air quality, smoking, and viral infections; most notable are pneumococcus, *Haemophilus influenzae*, and malaria. Life-span implications include increased risk for priapism, stroke, acute anemia, delayed growth and development in children, and increased risk for activity-induced fatigue. Affected individuals typically fare better in temperate climates, as extreme heat or extreme cold temperatures seem to provoke acute complications of SCD (Rees et al., 2022). New evidence related to gene therapy is showing improvements in sequelae and long-term morbidity data in a small sample of patients (Kavanagh et al., 2022; Owusu-Ansah et al., 2025).

Thrombocytopenia-Absent Radii Syndrome

Thrombocytopenia-absent radius (TAR) syndrome is characterized by limb anomalies, including bilateral absence of radii (with normally developed thumbs) and thrombocytopenia. The platelet count is typically less than 50×10^9/L (normal 150–400 $\times 10^9$/L; Petit & Boussion, 2023). The incidence of TAR is less than one per 100,000 infants (National Institutes of Health [NIH], 2025). Inheritance is AR, although de novo cases have been described (NIH, 2025).

Affected infants may have other limb anomalies affecting upper and/or lower extremities as well as involvement of other organ systems, including cardiac and renal anomalies. Thrombocytopenia may be congenital or may develop in the months after birth and is usually transient and self-limited (Petit & Boussion, 2023). However, severe thrombocytopenia may result in life-threatening bleeding such as intracranial hemorrhage (ICH). The pathogenesis of thrombocytopenia in TAR is not well

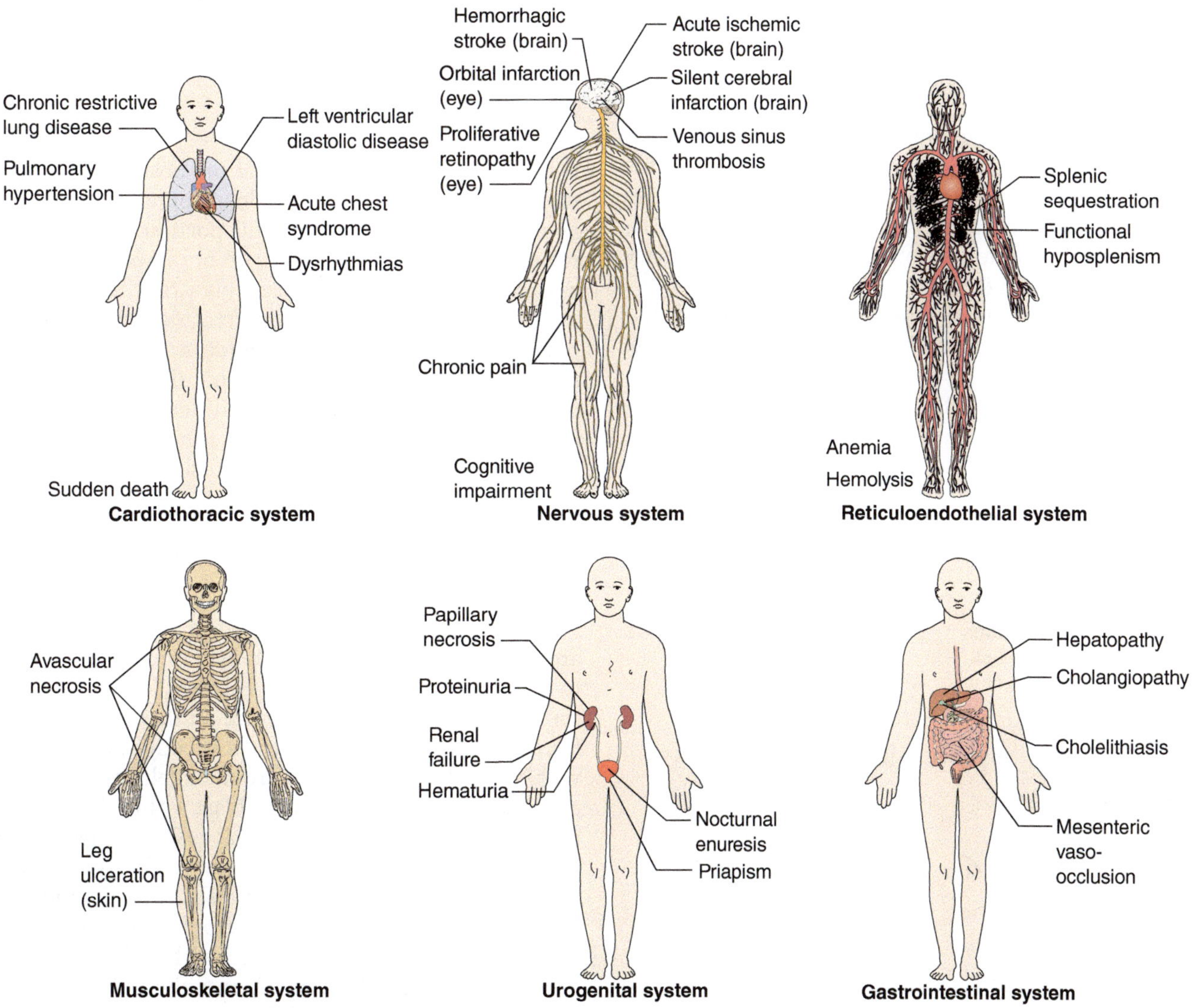

Figure 7.15 Common complications of sickle cell disease.

understood, but it is thought to be related to a poor response to TPO leading to abnormal maturation of the MK (Petit & Boussion, 2023).

There are several life-span implications related to TAR. First, it is possible for thrombocytopenia to recur intermittently during childhood. In addition, 67% of individuals with TAR syndrome exhibit an allergy to cow's milk; exposure is associated with thrombocytic episodes (Petit & Boussion, 2023). Individuals with TAR may also develop transient leukemoid reactions, with WBC counts greater than 35×10^9/L. There have also been case reports of individuals with TAR developing acute lymphocytic or myeloid leukemia, but it remains unclear if this is directly related to the underlying TAR syndrome (Petit & Boussion, 2023).

Von Willebrand Disease

Von Willebrand disease is the most common inherited bleeding disorder with a prevalence of one in every 100 individuals, although only 1% of those individuals experience symptomatic disease (1/1000; Weyand & Flood, 2021). Males and females are equally affected. The mutation results in a decrease in quantity or function of von Willebrand factor (vWF).

vWF facilitates adherence of platelets to areas of endothelial injury within blood vessels, formation of a platelet plug at the site of injury, and initiation of platelet aggregation (Figure 7.16; Weyand & Flood, 2021). This process is known as *primary hemostasis.* vWF is also involved in the stabilization and binding of factor VIII, which is essential in formation of fibrin clots (secondary hemostasis; Weyand & Flood, 2021).

There are three major types of von Willebrand disease. Type I involves decreased concentrations of vWF, and is responsible for 75% of cases; type II results from abnormal function of vWF, and may present with thrombocytopenia. Type III, the most severe form, is characterized by the absence or near-complete deficiency of vWB, and may present similarly to hemophilia A due to its effects on factor VIII. Types I and II are inherited in an AD manner and type III is typically AR (Ding et al., 2025; Weyand & Flood, 2021).

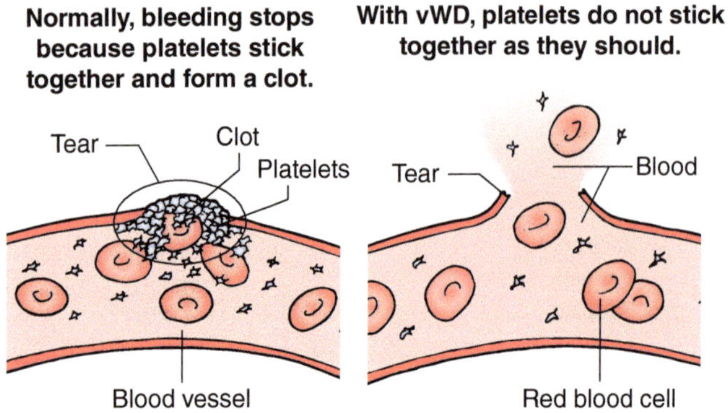

Figure 7.16 Von Willebrand disease.
vWD, von Willebrand disease.

Symptoms include mucosal bleeding and easy bruising, which can range from mild to severe and life-threatening (Weyand & Flood, 2021). Less common, hematomas and hemarthrosis (bleeding into the joints) may occur (Weyand & Flood, 2021). Von Willebrand disease commonly presents after the neonatal period, although types II and III may present soon after birth due to their severity (Ding et al., 2025). Unexplained or excessive bleeding after procedures, such as circumcision, should prompt concern. Usually, the disease will become clinically apparent later in childhood or early in adulthood with chronic mucosal bleeding such as recurrent epistaxis, gastrointestinal bleeding, or increased bleeding after trauma or procedures, including dental surgery, or may present as menorrhagia in younger patients of childbearing age (Weyand & Flood, 2021). Von Willebrand disease is a lifelong disease that requires ongoing medical management and prophylactic treatment prior to invasive procedures (Weyand & Flood, 2021).

NOTEWORTHY DISEASES IN THE XX PREGNANT PATIENT THAT INFLUENCE FETAL HEMATOPOIETIC DEVELOPMENT AND FUNCTION

It has been well established that the health of XX pregnant patients influences the development of fetal and neonatal disease. Therefore, this portion of the chapter reviews infectious etiologies, immune-mediated processes, and the effect of drug ingestion and diseases in XX pregnant patients on fetal/neonatal hematopoiesis. Future directions include understanding the mechanisms for neutropenia and thrombocytopenia in non–antibody-mediated conditions in XX pregnant patients, including pregnancy-induced hypertension (PIH), systemic lupus erythematosus (SLE), diabetes mellitus, and hyperthyroidism.

Maternal Antibodies and the Fetus and Neonate

Antibodies, commonly referred to as *immunoglobulins*, are glycoproteins that are naturally produced in response to a foreign antigen. Through a process known as receptor-mediated endocytosis, intact antibodies are transferred to the fetus. Initially, the antibody is internalized within vesicles. The vesicles are then delivered from the cytoplasm of the syncytiotrophoblast within the placenta through the capillary endothelial cell and given entry into the fetal circulation (Figure 7.17). Importantly, *IgG (immunoglobulin G) is the only antibody that can be transported across the placenta to the developing fetus.*

Several diseases are described within the "Common Problems With Implications Across the Life Span" section of this chapter that highlight the hematologic effects

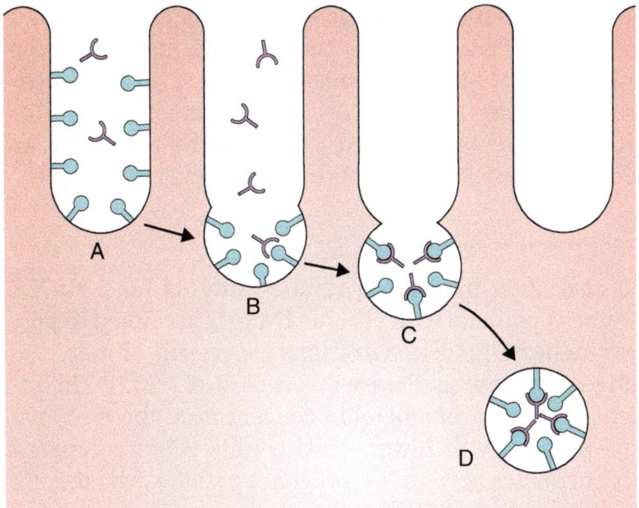

Figure 7.17 Receptor-mediated endocytosis.

of maternal antibodies targeting RBCs, neutrophils, lymphocytes, and platelets. These diseases include hemolytic disease of the fetus and newborn, ABO incompatibility, Rh (D) hemolytic disease, neonatal neutropenia, and thrombocytopenia.

Viral Infections

STORCH and Other Related Infections. As a group, neonatal STORCH infections traditionally include **S**yphilis (*Treponema pallidum*), ***T**oxoplasma gondii*, "**O**ther" (HIV, enterovirus [coxsackie B and echovirus], parvovirus, and hepatitis), **R**ubella virus, **C**ytomegalovirus (CMV–human herpes virus 5), and **H**erpes simplex virus (HSV) because of their similar presentations. CMV is the most common of the congenital viral infections. These infections can alter the hematologic profile of infected neonates resulting in anemia, neutropenia, thrombocytopenia, and disseminated intravascular coagulation (DIC). In some cases, particularly among neonates with congenital HSV, coxsackie B virus, and echovirus infections, DIC can be profound. An overview of the major clinical manifestations of STORCH infections is provided in the text that follows.

Anemia is a well-recognized manifestation among neonates and infants with parvovirus B19 and congenital syphilis, and sometimes occurs in congenital CMV infection. The anemia is due to hemolysis of the RBCs as evidenced by increased reticulocytes and hyperbilirubinemia with elevations in both the direct and indirect components (Desai et al., 2025; Glader & Kamdar, 2021). With parvovirus B19 and congenital syphilis, severe fetal and neonatal anemia may result in fetal nonimmune hydrops. Although hemolytic anemia is commonly reported in those infants with symptomatic congenital CMV, the presence of anemia is variable. In CMV, infection of hematopoietic precursor cells may result in a more pronounced anemia secondary to diminished RBC production (Werner et al., 2021). In neonates with HIV infection, a transient anemia may occur from intrauterine exposure to antiretroviral therapy in the XX pregnant patient, altering neonatal hematopoiesis (Werner et al., 2021). In addition, postnatal treatment with antiretrovirals is well recognized for its effect on the development of anemia and neutropenia in the infant (Werner et al., 2021).

Elevated leukocyte counts, lower CD4 and CD8 lymphocytes, and thromobocytopenia have been described in neonates and infants with congenital toxoplasmosis and congenital rubella (Werner et al., 2021). Eosinophilia has been reported in as many as 18% to 25% of neonates with congenital toxoplasmosis (Werner et al., 2021). In congenital toxoplasmosis, cerebral spinal fluid evaluation reveals an elevated WBC count (pleocytosis) with specific elevation of lymphocyte counts (Kaufman et al., 2025). Similarly, extreme variability in WBC count has been described in newborn infants with congenital syphilis. Several leukocyte abnormalities have been associated with congenital CMV, including lymphocytosis and neutrophilia (Werner et al., 2021). Neutropenia has also been reported in infants with congenital CMV infection (Werner et al., 2021). Enteroviral infections have been associated with leukocytosis, neutrophilia, and an increase in immature WBC forms (Werner et al., 2021). Although the literature is limited on the impact of the SARS-CoV-2 virus in neonates, intrapartum transmission is low, and most infections are postnatally acquired and result in leukocytosis and thrombocytopenia.

Thrombocytopenia is the most common manifestation of many of the viral infections described previously. Of those neonates with congenital CMV, thrombocytopenia may manifest in up to 80% of symptomatic CMV infections and is multifactorial. Thrombocytopenia is likely the result of more than one pathology such as increased platelet consumption or impairment to platelet production from MKs (Moiseiwitsch & Brown, 2021; Werner et al., 2021). In neonates infected with the protozoan parasite *T. gondii*, thrombocytopenia affects approximately 10%. Thrombocytopenia should be interpreted within the clinical picture. Symptomatic congenital infections present with features of clinical illness such as petechiae, prolonged bleeding from puncture sites, and hemorrhagic lesions or events.

Multiorgan involvement is a common feature of severe congenital infections and is often seen with both neonatal enterovirus and neonatal HSV infections. In neonatal HSV, up to 25% of infections are disseminated and involve multiple organs and account for the highest mortality of the three types of neonatal HSV infection (Desai et al., 2025). DIC, neutropenia, and thrombocytopenia are frequently reported in conjunction with congenital HSV infection. The presence of DIC increases the infant's risk of death, which may be as high as 80% in untreated patients with neonatal HSV (Desai et al., 2025; Werner et al., 2021). DIC, neutrophilia, and thrombocytopenia are commonly observed with enteroviral infection (Werner et al., 2021).

Autoimmune Disorders

Autoimmune Hemolytic Anemia. Autoimmune hemolytic anemia may occur during pregnancy and is recognized by Coombs's positivity in the XX pregnant patient and the infant in the absence of a setup for Rh or ABO incompatibility. The anemia in the fetus results from the passive transfer of IgG antibodies. In this manner, autoimmune hemolytic disease is similar to immune diseases including SLE and rheumatoid arthritis, which may also transfer IgG antibodies to the fetus. In addition to causing anemia, the IgG antibodies may not be specific to antigens on the fetal RBC and may affect neutrophils and platelets.

Systemic Lupus Erythematosus. SLE is commonly defined as a multisystem autoimmune disorder. The neonate can passively acquire the disorder by way of antibody acquisition from the XX pregnant patient and genetic/environmental factors which lead to neonatal lupus (Biron-Shental & Hershkovich-Shporen, 2025). The antibodies which impose pathogenic function upon the developing fetus are usually anti-Ro (SS-A) or anti-La (SS-B), which begin crossing the placenta around week 12 of gestation and matriculate into fetal tissues (Ballas & Kelly, 2024). This gives rise to a spectrum of disorders which may include hemolytic anemia, thrombocytopenia, and neutropenia; each have been reported in 10% to 20% of all affected neonates (Biron-Shental & Hershkovich-Shporen, 2025). In addition, congestive heart failure may develop secondary to anemia and immune-mediated myocarditis. Fetal heart block may develop secondary to antibody complement deposition within the myocardium, which leads to fibrosis and a blockage of the cardiac conduction system (Biron-Shental & Hershkovich-Shporen, 2025). For those infants with thrombocytopenia, the degree of the condition may be severe with platelet counts as low as 30,000/mm^3. The specific cause of the thrombocytopenia is not known in all cases, but in at least some, anti-SS-A/Ro antibodies are involved. The occurrence of DIC has been reported as well as hepatosplenomegaly and pericarditis. Hematologic manifestations of neonatal lupus are self-limited; the timing of resolution mirrors the disappearance of circulating antibodies in the neonate from the XX pregnant patient.

Leukemia and Malignancies

Cancer during pregnancy is more frequent than the occurrence of appendicitis, thyrotoxicosis, nephrolithiasis, and deep vein thrombosis, complicating one in every 1,000 to 1,500 pregnancies (Ballas & Kelly, 2024; Werner et al., 2021). Cases of leukemia, lymphoma, breast, cervical, and ovarian cancers have all been reported during pregnancy. Chemotherapeutic medications used to treat cancers can cross the placenta and have been linked to fetal malformations if used during the first trimester (Ballas & Kelly, 2024; Werner et al., 2021). Additional evidence is needed to understand the impact of cancer therapies on the unborn fetus.

Cardiac Disease

Compared to unaffected infants, infants born to XX pregnant patients with chronic hypoxia are noted to possess higher HgF concentrations as a result of maternal congenital cardiac disease (Werner et al., 2021). In addition to higher hemoglobin concentrates, these infants also present with lower WBC counts when compared with neonates born to XX pregnant patients who did not have heart disease. When the bone marrow of these infants was examined, increased erythropoiesis was noted (Werner et al., 2021).

Metabolic Disorders

Hyperthyroidism. Thyroid disease in the XX pregnant patient can result in neonatal hyperviscosity syndrome and thrombocytopenia (van der Kaay et al., 2016). The precise mechanisms are not clearly understood.

Diabetes Mellitus. Infants born to pregnant patients with diabetes mellitus can present with a variety of hematologic abnormalities, including increased RBC mass (resulting in hyperviscosity syndrome), hyperaggregable platelets (resulting in thrombosis), and neutropenia (Werner et al., 2021). The etiology of the increased incidence of thrombosis is felt to be multifactorial.

Infants with increased RBC mass and those with hyperviscosity syndrome had increased plasma concentrations of EPO associated with fetal hypoxia (Werner et al., 2021). Insulin may also contribute to the increased RBC mass as it may further promote erythropoiesis (Werner et al., 2021).

The etiology for increased thrombosis is multifactorial. Unlike the relationship between EPO concentrations and hyperviscosity, evaluation of IDM with thrombosis did not demonstrate any abnormalities in plasma coagulation factors. To be specific, no difference in the prothrombin time, activated partial thromboplastin time, or fibrinogen; von Willebrand antigen; or factors V, X, or XII were found (Werner et al., 2021).

Increased insulin concentrations found in pregnant patients with gestational diabetes and hyperglycemia may contribute to impaired platelet function, as has been demonstrated in animal studies. The proposed mechanisms may include inhibition of platelet-activating factor biosynthesis, reduction of the levels of platelet-activating factor, and impairment of thromboxane synthesis.

Neonatal thrombocytopenia that is self-limiting (resolving within 10 days) has been described in infants born to pregnant patients with diabetes during pregnancy. The mechanism is thought to involve fetal hypoxia, similar to that occurring in PIH, preeclampsia, and intrauterine growth restriction. Although common in these infants, the platelet count is usually greater than 50,000/mcL.

For infants with neutropenia related to diabetes in the XX pregnant patient, the duration is generally brief (2–3 days) and self-resolving. The precise cause of the neutropenia remains unknown but is believed to relate to fetal-tissue hypoxia.

Pregnancy-Related Conditions and Common Hematologic Problems

Gestational Hypertension. Gestational hypertension (GH) can affect fetal and neonatal hematologic function and is defined as blood pressure elevations in previously normotensive pregnant patients, without proteinuria, after 20 weeks of pregnancy (Werner et al., 2021). Neutropenia, thrombocytopenia, and DIC are commonly reported, and are the focus of this discussion.

Neutropenia is reported in approximately 40% to 50% of offspring born to XX pregnant patients with GH (Werner et al., 2021). The severity of neutropenia increases with the severity of hypertension in the XX pregnant patient and is most evident in those neonates delivered of XX pregnant patients with severe or prolonged hypertension associated with fetal intrauterine growth restriction. The kinetic mechanism for the neutropenia is decreased neutrophil production, but the specific etiology of the decreased production remains under debate. Possible etiologies include a placentally derived inhibitor of neutrophil production, a decreased responsiveness of precursor cells to G-CSF, the erythrocyte steal phenomena seen with intrauterine hypoxia, and/or downregulation of white cell production due to placental dysfunction and FAS–FAS ligand interaction abnormalities (Werner et al., 2021). Although some have reported that these infants have an increased incidence of nosocomial infection that may be as high as 6% compared to nonneutropenic infants, the published literature is conflicting (Werner et al., 2021). Stoll and colleagues noted that the presence of hypertension/preeclampsia actually decreased the risk of neonatal infection (Stoll & Hansen, 2003; Werner et al., 2021).

Thrombocytopenia, or impaired platelet function, is also reported among offspring of pregnant patients with GH. Thrombocytopenia is felt to be the direct result of chronic fetal hypoxia, similar to that reported in infants of diabetic mothers and those with preeclampsia (Werner et al., 2021). Thrombocytopenia may occur in 15% to 36% of infants born to pregnant patients with GH (Werner et al., 2021). Although the precise mechanism for reduced platelet function is not known, proposed mechanisms include altered metabolism of calcium, alteration of platelet membrane glycoproteins, increased release of plasma β-thromboglobulin, and altered nitric oxide bioavailability (Christensen, Juul, & Del Vecchio, 2015). The platelet surface expression of P-selectin and CD63, GPIIb/IIIa, and CD9 are diminished in neonates born to pregnant patients with GH (Christensen, Juul, & Del Vecchio, 2015). TPO levels did not differ between those infants born to mothers with and without GH (Tsao et al., 2002).

In addition, DIC has been identified among offspring of pregnant patients with GH, preeclampsia, and platelet counts less than 50,000/mcL (Werner et al., 2021). The pathogenesis of DIC in the neonate is not fully understood, is complex, and is secondary to a variety of underlying diseases and conditions including congenital viral infections and adverse events that affect the feto-placental unit. The diagnosis is confirmed by prolongation of the prothrombin time, activated partial thromboplastin time, thrombocytopenia, and decreased fibrinogen with increased concentrations of fibrinogen degradation products (Werner et al., 2021).

Placental Insufficiency. Placental insufficiency is felt to be an underlying cause for fetal and neonatal thrombocytopenia. Megakaryocytopoiesis is severely impaired as shown by a marked reduction in circulating MKs and their precursor/progenitor cells. The reduced megakaryocytopoiesis results in reduced fetal platelet production and the resultant thrombocytopenia (Davenport & Sola-Visner, 2021).

Intra-Amniotic Infection. In addition to the viral infections previously discussed, intra-amniotic infection affects fetal and neonatal hematopoietic function. Numerous cytokine concentrations, including interleukins (IL)-1, IL-6, IL-8, TNF, and G-CSF, are significantly increased with intra-amniotic infection. Recall that G-CSF is recognized as a lineage-specific growth factor and the primary regulator of neutrophil production, differentiation, and function. Concentrations of G-CSF may be 10- to 100-fold higher in the amniotic fluid obtained from preterm pregnancies with culture-proven infection (Werner et al., 2021).

Therapeutics for Common Conditions Affecting Pregnant Patients

Betamethasone Administration. Antenatal betamethasone exposure has been reported to have a variable effect on neutrophil counts in neonates. Historically, both neutrophilia and neutropenia have been reported in infants whose mothers had received antenatal betamethasone (Werner et al., 2021). In those infants experiencing a leukemoid reaction (absolute neutrophil count [ANC] greater than 50,000/mcL), some of the XX pregnant patients were noted to have received betamethasone. Larger studies are necessary in order to determine whether the effect of antenatal betamethasone consistently results in an increase in WBC counts in infants who are exposed prior to delivery. At this time, monitoring of the WBC count and neutrophil count after birth should be considered.

Indomethacin Administration. Limited information exists related to indomethacin exposure during pregnancy and the effect on the fetal hematologic system; however, some experts contend that exposure can increase the risk for fetal and neonatal neutropenia. Indomethacin has also been implicated in platelet dysfunction (Ostilla et al., 2024).

Intravenous Immunoglobulin (IVIG) Administration. Neonatal thrombocytopenia may occur as the direct result of the placental transfer of IgG antibodies to the fetus. Immune thrombocytopenia purpura (ITP) in XX pregnant patients results in autoimmune IgG antibodies crossing the placenta and destroying fetal platelets. Alternatively, alloimmune thrombocytopenia is caused by IgG antibodies that have been produced secondary to exposure to platelet-specific fetal antigens of paternal origin, most commonly human platelet antigen 1a (HPA-1a). These alloimmune (antiplatelet) IgG antibodies cross the placenta resulting in the destruction of fetal platelets. The use of IVIG remains the primary antenatal treatment of both ITP and fetal/neonatal alloimmune thrombocytopenia (FNAIT). Weekly infusions of IVIG (with or without concomitant steroid therapy) continue to be the most commonly used therapeutic regimen (Christensen, Juul, & Del Vecchio, 2015). IVIG may act by several proposed mechanisms, which include suppressing platelet antibody synthesis, blocking antiplatelet antibody transfer across the placenta, and interfering with phagocyte-mediated immune clearance by the reticulo-endothelial system. Recommendations for using IVIG and steroid administration together are supported when platelet counts are less than 10,000 to 30,000 in XX pregnant patients or for those fetuses where fetal blood sampling demonstrates a platelet count less than 20K (Biron-Shental & Hershkovich-Shporen, 2025). The American College of Obstetricians and Gynecologists (ACOG) recommends treatment approaches individualized based on patient presentation. Prednisone therapy with dosing ranging between 0.5 and 2 mg/kg is the standard first line of therapy for XX pregnant patients with ITP, with the addition of IVIG (1 gm/kg) when platelet counts are refractory to steroids alone or a faster increase in platelet count is desired (ACOG, 2019). However, IVIG therapy is the preferred first-line therapy in cases of FNAIT (ACOG, 2019).

Clinical Application. In the well-appearing neonate presenting with thrombocytopenia, the APRN should look to the history and laboratory evaluation of the XX pregnant patient for potential explanation. When considering platelet transfusion in the neonate, evaluating the platelet count in the XX pregnant patient is critical as HPA negative platelets should be ordered for fetal/neonatal transfusion in cases of FNAIT. In neonates born to XX pregnant patients with ITP, the platelet count will be low because of autoimmune antibodies responsible for the destruction of platelets in both the XX pregnant patient and the fetus/neonate. However, in the fetus/neonate with FNAIT the platelet count in the XX pregnant patient is normal. The physiology of these two diagnoses will be presented later in this chapter.

Folic Acid and Vitamin B_{12} Deficiency. Both folate and vitamin B_{12} are effectively transported across the placenta (Werner et al., 2021). Folate deficiency results in a megaloblastic anemia and is associated with impaired nuclear maturation of the hematopoietic cells in the marrow. The characteristic marrow finding is a delay of nuclear maturation compared with cytoplasmic maturation, resulting in a macrocytic anemia, thrombocytopenia, and hypersegmentation of neutrophils and a reduction in the number of granulocytes (Werner et al., 2021).

Prolonged breastfeeding by mothers with vitamin B_{12} deficiency (pernicious anemia) or dietary restrictions (e.g., strict vegetarians and vegans) limiting B_{12} intake may also cause megaloblastic anemia, which is observed later during infancy (Werner et al., 2021).

Zidovudine Administration. Zidovudine treatment for HIV infection in XX pregnant patients has been associated with fetal and neonatal anemia. However, treatment of pregnant patients with zidovudine is the standard of care in those who are HIV positive in order to prevent vertical transmission of the virus to the fetus. Zidovudine crosses the placenta to the fetus by active transport that is energy-dependent (Werner et al., 2021). The reduction in transmission of infection to the fetus was found in seropositive pregnant patients who were treated with oral zidovudine during the pregnancy and then intravenous zidovudine during labor. Zidovudine provokes anemia by inhibiting fetal erythropoiesis; neonates whose birthing parent received treatment have lower hemoglobin concentrations and hematocrits, though it is uncommon to see clinically significant anemia (Werner et al., 2021).

COMMON PROBLEMS WITH IMPLICATIONS ACROSS THE LIFE SPAN

Hematologic diseases have the potential to involve RBCs, granulocytes, lymphocytes, and monocytes, as well as platelets and clotting proteins. Here we present common disorders of the hematologic system with implications across the life span.

Disorders of Red Blood Cells

Polycythemia. *Polycythemia* is defined as hematocrit and hemoglobin levels more than 2 *SDs* above the norm, or more simply, a hemoglobin greater than 20 g/dL and a hematocrit greater than 65% (Fay et al., 2024; Owusu-Ansah et al., 2025). Polycythemia is thought to occur in about 2% to 5% of all term infants, and is associated with hyperviscosity syndrome, which leads to impairment of the circulatory system.

Infants at highest risk for developing polycythemia include postterm infants; infants who are small for gestational age (SGA) and large for gestational age (LGA); those born at high altitude; IDM; and infants with genetic syndromes, including trisomy 21 and Beckwith-Weidemann syndrome. Placental transfusion, such as maternal–fetal transfusion or twin-to-twin transfusion, contributes, as does prolonged intrauterine tobacco exposure (Owusu-Ansah et al., 2025; Rosenkrantz & Oh, 2021). Neonatal thyrotoxicosis, perinatal asphyxia, DCC, and postnatal dehydration may increase the risk for polycythemia (Owusu-Ansah et al., 2025; Rosenkrantz & Oh, 2021).

The pathogenesis of polycythemia involves one of two pathways: (a) increased fetal erythropoiesis or (b) erythrocyte transfusion. Conditions that increase fetal erythropoiesis include preeclampsia, chronic placental abruption, heart disease, smoking or alcohol abuse, and diabetes. Inherited conditions that lead to increased fetal erythropoiesis include trisomy 13, 18, 21, and Beckwith-Wiedemann syndrome, yet the pathogenesis is poorly understood. Many of the aforementioned conditions give rise to placental insufficiency, fetal hypoxia, decreased fetal tissue oxygenation, and a resultant increase in fetal erythropoiesis. Polycythemia caused by erythrocyte transfusion is associated with oxytocin administration, DCC (greater than 3 minute delay), placenta-to-fetus transfusion (lowering infant more than 15 cm below level of placenta after birth), and among fetuses affected by twin anemia polycythemia syndrome (TAPS).

After birth, an infant's hematocrit level will increase. Levels peak at about 2 hours of age, and then demonstrate a steady decrease to normal levels by 24 hours of age (Rosenkrantz & Oh, 2021). Symptomatic infants may display plethora, respiratory distress, lethargy, poor feeding, hypoglycemia, thrombocytopenia, hyperbilirubinemia, and, rarely, thrombosis. Possible complications include acute kidney injury and cerebral infarction as a result of venous thrombosis, sludging, or thromboembolic events (Rosenkrantz & Oh, 2021).

The long-term outcomes for infants with polycythemia are controversial. Some studies suggest that infants with polycythemia have worse neurodevelopmental outcomes compared to infants without polycythemia. This may be reflective of the underlying cause (hypoxemic environment or asphyxia) rather than the presence of polycythemia given the currently available evidence (Rosenkrantz & Oh, 2021).

Anemia. *Anemia* is defined as decreased RBC mass with hemoglobin or hematocrit measurement 2 *SD*s below the mean for age (Carlberg, 2024; Owusu-Ansah et al., 2025). Risk factors range from health risks in the XX pregnant patient (e.g., PIH, preeclampsia, and nutritional deficiencies), to blood loss or sequestration, underproduction, or increased destruction of RBCs (**Table 7.9**). The mean corpuscular volume (MCV) of RBCs and degree of reticulocytosis are important in differentiating among the various etiologies of anemia. The following sections will review the most common causes of anemia resulting from diminished production, accelerated destruction, or blood loss.

Anemia Due to Diminished Production. Typical causes for decreased RBC production include aplastic or hypoplastic anemia, bone marrow suppression, and iron deficiency. Aplastic or hypoplastic anemias may be the result of a wide array of rare congenital and acquired conditions. Examples include Diamond–Blackfan and Fanconi anemias. Diamond–Blackfan is a rare AD condition that causes bone marrow failure and a pure RBC aplasia. This leads to anemia and deficient erythropoiesis; laboratory findings include a low hematocrit and low reticulocyte count. Diamond-Blackfan is known to present in the neonatal period or during infancy. Fanconi anemia results from a defect in any of the genes that are responsible for the repair of DNA. Of the 22 genes identified, the majority of the defects are inherited in an AR pattern (Owusu-Ansah et al., 2025). Individuals with FA often experience severe anemia that typically presents around school age rather than in the neonatal period, although birth defects may also be present. Both of these conditions may be associated with other physical findings, such as growth failure; microcephaly; and skeletal, cardiac, ophthalmologic, and genitourinary anomalies (Gallagher, 2022).

In addition to genetic conditions, a transient deficiency of EPO synthesis observed during the early postnatal period may occur. Among term infants, this is named physiologic anemia of infancy. Among premature infants, this is named physiologic anemia of prematurity.

Anemia of infancy is a normocytic, normochromic anemia that afflicts term infants. Recall that hypoxia and anemia stimulate erythropoiesis, and the fetus resides in a relatively hypoxic intrauterine environment. Birth exposes the newborn to a new environment, rich in oxygen. Tissue oxygenation quickly increases, which transiently suppresses EPO production and the synthesis of new RBCs. In addition, the birth process typically causes an increased rate of turnover among existing RBCs. Remaining RBCs are subject to a shortened life span (60–80 days among term infants and 30–50 days for extremely low gestational age neonates [ELGAN]), as compared to adults (100–120 days). Therefore, the reduced ability to establish normal hematopoiesis after birth, and compensate for any RBC losses imposed during the birth process, gives rise to a transient state of physiologic anemia while the body adjusts to life outside the womb. Physiologic anemia of infancy typically presents

TABLE 7.9 Causes of Neonatal Anemia

Blood Loss	Diminished Production of RBCs	Increased Destruction of RBCs

• Coagulation defect
• Fetal-maternal hemorrhage
• Twin-to-twin transfusion
• Abnormal placentation
• Placental abruption
• Cord accidents
• Traumatic birth
• Iatrogenic blood draws
• Sequestration
  ◦ Subdural hematoma
  ◦ Cephalohematoma
  ◦ Hemangioma
  ◦ Vascular malformations
  ◦ Extensive ecchymosis
  ◦ Subgaleal hemorrhage
	• Anemia of prematurity
	• Congenital underproduction related to chronic disease
	  ◦ Hypothyroidism
	  ◦ Adrenal insufficiency
	  ◦ Hypopituitarism
	• Congenital bone marrow failure syndromes
	  ◦ Diamond–Blackfan
	  ◦ Fanconi anemia
	  ◦ Aplastic anemia
	• Infection-related
	  ◦ Parvovirus B19
	  ◦ Hepatitis
	  ◦ HIV
	  ◦ Syphilis
	• Nutritional deficiency
	  ◦ Iron
	  ◦ Folate
	  ◦ Vitamin B_{12}
		• Immune mediated
		  ◦ ABO/Rh incompatibility
		• Nonimmune mediated structural erythrocyte defects
		  ◦ Hereditary spherocytosis
		  ◦ Hereditary eliptocytosis
		• Erythrocyte enzyme defects
		  ◦ G6PD deficiency
		  ◦ Pyruvate kinase deficiency
		• Hemoglobinopathies
		  ◦ Microangiopathic hemolytic anemia
		• Infection (bacterial, viral, fungal)

RBC, red blood cell.
Sources: Gleason, C. A., & Sawyer, T. (Eds.). (2024). *Avery's diseases of the newborn* (11th ed.). Elsevier; Martin, R. J., & Fanaroff, A. A. (Eds.). (2025). *Fanaroff & Martin's neonatal-perinatal medicine: Diseases of the fetus and infant* (12th ed.). Elsevier Saunders.

during the first 2 to 3 months of postnatal life (8–12 weeks); a hemoglobin nadir of 10 to 12 mg/dL, paired with low reticulocyte counts, is observed (Owusu-Ansah et al., 2025). Postnatal iron ingestion aids in establishing normal iron stores, as EPO production shifts from the liver to the kidneys and normalizes.

Physiologic anemia of prematurity is a normocytic, normochromic anemia that afflicts premature infants (younger than 32 weeks' gestation). Birth exposes the premature newborn to a new environment, rich in oxygen. Tissue oxygenation quickly increases, which transiently suppresses EPO production and the synthesis of new RBCs. In addition, the birth process typically causes an increased rate of turnover among existing RBCs. Remaining RBCs are subject to a shortened life span (fewer than 60 days among premature infants; likely shorter in proportion to gestational age), as compared to 60 to 80 days among term infants (Owusu-Ansah et al., 2025). Therefore, the reduced ability to establish normal hematopoiesis after birth, and compensate for any RBC losses imposed during the birth process or as a result of iatrogenic losses, gives rise to a transient state of physiologic anemia of prematurity, while the body adjusts to life outside the womb.

Additional factors often exacerbate the pathogenesis of anemia of prematurity. First, consider the short life span of the RBC among premature infants (when compared to term counterparts). Second, consider that premature infants are, in part or in full, deprived of third trimester iron transfer; 80% of iron is transferred to the fetus during this third trimester (Owusu-Ansah et al., 2025). Next, recall that erythropoiesis is modulated by transcription factors, which may be poorly developed among premature infants. These factors, in combination with other comorbid states (e.g., illness), place premature infants at-risk for a more severe and prolonged physiologic anemia of prematurity. A hemoglobin nadir of 7 to 10 g/dL, with a low reticulocyte count, is often observed at 6 weeks postnatal age (Owusu-Ansah et al., 2025). Factors such as ongoing blood loss and repeated blood transfusions may further prolong the recovery of intrinsic erythropoiesis and necessitate intervention.

Anemia Due to Blood Loss. Anemia from blood loss may occur in utero, intrapartum, or postnatally. Several etiologies are known and described here. Prenatally, blood loss may occur due to transfusion from the fetus to the XX pregnant patient; this occurs in approximately 8% of all pregnancies. Significant blood loss (greater than 50 mL) is noted in approximately 1% of pregnancies. (Carlberg, 2024). Alternatively, anemia may occur due to monochorionic–diamniotic placentation (twin–twin transfusion syndrome [TTTS] or twin anemia polycythemia sequence [TAPS]). In TTTS there is blood volume loss between the donor (hypovolemic) and recipient (volume overloaded), although the hemoglobin and hematocrit are concordant; however, in TAPS there are significant differences in hemoglobin and hematocrit between the donor (anemic) and recipient (polycythemic) twin (Shlomai et al., 2025). Traumatic births may result in intracranial bleeding or bleeding within solid organs, such as the liver or spleen. Iatrogenic losses secondary to frequent blood draws may predispose the infant to anemia; this is particularly problematic among premature infants with reduced circulating blood volume (Kling, 2021). Blood loss in these cases may be profound. There is also the potential for significant blood loss within sequestrations, such as cephalohematomas or subgaleal hemorrhages. Acute blood loss typically results in normocytic anemia without reticulocytosis, whereas chronic blood loss leads to reticulocytosis to compensate for ongoing losses (Owusu-Ansah et al., 2025).

Clinical Application. When acute blood loss is suspected without a clear source (such as loss that occurs with placental abruption, placenta previa, or uterine rupture), the APRN should be suspicious of a fetal-maternal hemorrhage (FMH). Hemorrhage of fetal blood into the circulation of the XX pregnant patient occurs secondary to abnormal placental vessels, trauma, or following invasive procedures. Feto-maternal hemorrhages vary in blood volume but may lead to life-threatening blood loss in the fetus. Prenatal identification is challenging due to subtle clinical signs including decreased fetal movement and abnormal fetal heart tracings. The APRN should include a request for a Kleihauer-Betke (KB) test when concerned for this type of acute blood loss. A sample of the blood of the XX pregnant patient is evaluated to identify the presence of fetal blood (Hb F) in the maternal circulation.

Anemia Due to Accelerated Destruction. The pathogenesis of hemolytic anemia involves the destruction of RBCs by a variety of mechanisms. Most hemolytic anemias will present within the first week of life. Generally, hemolytic anemias are normocytic with increased reticulocyte counts. Nonimmune hemolytic anemias include structural defects, such as HS, enzyme defects such as G6PD deficiency and pyruvate kinase deficiency, and hemoglobinopathies such as SCD and the thalassemias. Some hemoglobinopathies, particularly those affecting the beta globin chains, do not present until after the neonatal period.

Hemolysis in nonimmune cases may be intravascular, with RBC rupture within small blood vessels due to decreased deformability, or extravascular, with breakdown in the RES occurring earlier than normal due to the inherent RBC abnormalities. In contrast, immune-mediated hemolysis is caused by antibodies transferred from the XX pregnant patient (IgG) recognizing fetal blood cells as foreign due to antigens expressed on their surface. Examples include hemolytic disease of the newborn (HDFN) such as ABO or Rh incompatibility, with Rh disease being more severe. Hemolysis is extravascular, with phagocytosis of immunoglobulin-bound RBCs in the spleen and liver. These immune-mediated hemolytic anemias typically improve over time as antibodies fro the XX pregnant patient are gradually cleared from the neonate's bloodstream, typically within 3 to 4 months.

Hemolytic Disease of the Fetus and Newborn. HDFN relates to pathology associated with the destruction of fetal or neonatal RBCs, by maternal IgG antibodies, that subsequently results in anemia. HDFN involves the major blood groups of Rhesus (Rh), A, B, AB, and O. However, minor blood group incompatibilities, including Kell, Duffy, MNS, P, and Diego systems, can also result in significant disease. For this review, because of the low frequency of HDFN related to the minor blood groups, they will not be discussed.

ABO Incompatibility. Four major blood groups make up the ABO system in humans—A, B, AB, and O. Individuals with an O blood type innately develop antibodies to A and/or B antigens beginning at approximately 3 to 6 months. Antibody production can occur in the first pregnancy as there is no requirement for prior exposure. If there has been prior exposure through previous pregnancies or iatrogenic exposure to A, B, or AB blood types (during a previous pregnancy or fetal-maternal hemorrhage) there may be IgG antibodies present that are able to cross into the fetal circulation (Owusu-Ansah et al., 2025). Subsequent pregnancies, with the same partner, can be expected to be affected to a similar or more severe degree.

Although ABO incompatibility may occur in up to 15% of all pregnancies, it results in neonatal hemolytic anemia in only 3% of affected pregnancies (Owusu-Ansah et al., 2025). ABO incompatibility likely results in less severe anemia than Rh incompatibility, as A and B antigens are present on other tissues in addition to fewer sites on the RBC (Owusu-Ansah et al., 2025). Additionally, anti-A and anti-B immunoglobulin is mostly represented by IgM antibodies which are unable to cross into the fetal circulation. Infants with ABO incompatibility are generally asymptomatic at birth, but may develop hyperbilirubinemia in the first 24 hours due to cell deformation and destruction. Hydrops fetalis is rare, and most infants will have either no anemia or mild anemia. Use of phototherapy, intravenous immune globulin (IVIg), or exchange transfusion may be necessary for those neonates with the most severe hemolysis who develop hyperbilirubinemia. Recommendations for management of affected infants is based on the guidelines from the American Academy of Pediatrics (AAP; Kemper et al., 2022).

Clinical Application. A simple method to use to remember the relationship that sets up a mother and baby for ABO incompatibility involves spelling Mom ("O" in m**O**m) and baby (**B-A**-by or b-**AB**y). The APRN should be alert to the at-risk neonate and routinely follow all infants born to mothers with an O blood type with specific attention paid to maternal history, previous pregnancy history and outcomes, neonatal blood type with antibody screening, and for signs and symptoms of hyperbilirubinemia

Rh (D) Hemolytic Disease. The best recognized cause of HDFN is secondary to Rh (D) incompatibility as it results in the most severe (and rare) form of the disease, hydrops fetalis. Individuals are classified as Rhesus (Rh) negative or positive based on the expression of the major D antigen on their RBCs. Rh negative results from either the absence of the Rh (D) gene or alterations in the gene that result in its inactivation (Ross et al., 2021).

Mothers who are Rh negative become sensitized due to a prior exposure to the Rh antigen. This can occur through blood transfusion or a previous pregnancy with a Rh-positive fetus. As such, the occurrence of HDFN does not usually occur during the first pregnancy (Figure 7.18). The obstetrical practice of providing Rh (D) immune globulin prophylaxis to pregnant patients who are Rh negative during pregnancy has significantly reduced the rate of alloimmune sensitization.

Although Rh (D) incompatibility remains the most frequent cause of HDFN, there are more than 44 Rh antigens. Careful review of the blood type of the XX pregnant patient and antibody panel is essential to identify at-risk pregnancies and those neonates who may be at risk for hyperbilirubinemia in the neonatal period.

Affected neonates may exhibit the full spectrum from mild self-limited hemolytic disease to severe life-threatening anemia as is seen in hydrops fetalis. Fetal elevations in bilirubin levels are infrequent secondary to placental clearing of bilirubin; cord blood bilirubin levels greater than 4 mg/dL are highly suspicious for severe isoimmunization. Extramedullary hematopoiesis, or the recruitment of other tissues into the production of RBCs outside of the bone marrow, namely occurs within the liver, spleen, lymph nodes, and integumentary system in response to severe anemia. Hepatosplenomegaly may be present in cases of severe isoimmunization due to increased need for RBC production by the liver and spleen as well as increased removal, from the circulation, of damaged RBCs by the spleen. Therefore, affected fetuses incur a higher risk for rupture of the spleen as well as hypoxia due to decreased circulating RBCs. The severity of the HDFN from Rh isoimmunization increases with subsequent pregnancies. Common postnatal clinical manifestations are summarized in Table 7.10.

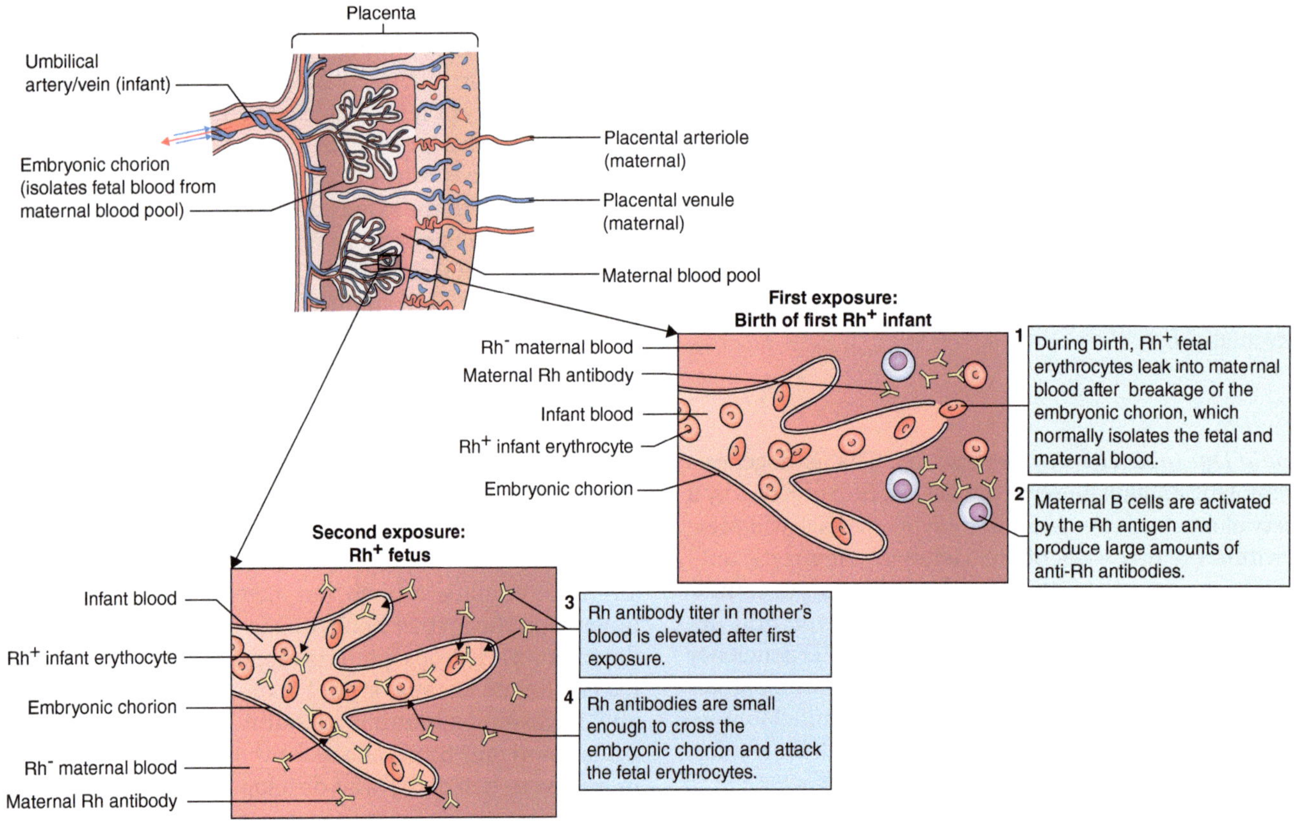

Figure 7.18 Hemolytic disease of the newborn secondary to Rh isoimmunization.
Rh, Rhesus.

TABLE 7.10 Common Postnatal Manifestations of Rh (D) Hemolytic Disease

Clinical Manifestation	Etiology
Coagulopathies	• Thrombocytopenia • Decreased clotting factors
Edema	• Hydrops fetalis • Thrombocytopenia
Hyperbilirubinemia	• Increased RBC destruction
Hypoglycemia	• Hyperinsulinemia
Kernicterus	• Severe hyperbilirubinemia

RBC, red blood cell.

Neonates affected by HDFN should be monitored closely for the development of hyperbilirubinemia and late anemia (anemia at 4–6 weeks of age) due to the persistence of antibodies from the XX pregnant patient within the neonatal circulation. Attention to adequate hydration, use of phototherapy, and administration of supplemental iron may be important interventions for neonates affected by hemolysis as a result of maternal Rh alloimmunization.

Clinical Application. The APRN should be diligent in reviewing the blood type and antibody test results for both the XX pregnant patient and fetus/neonate. Recognition and early intervention for neonates exhibiting signs of HDFN improves morbidity and mortality of this disease. Additional clinical management of the neonate with HDFN may also include IVIg administration and exchange transfusion (ET), with the goal of either decreasing the impact or removal of maternal IgG antibodies from neonatal circulation, respectively. IVIg administration works by binding to the antibody receptor on the fetal RBC, preventing the circulating IgG antibodies from binding to these sites and causing hemolysis. While ET removes fetal whole blood, thereby subsequently removing fetal RBCs that have been coated with antibodies from the XX pregnant patient leading to hemolysis, and replaces them with Oneg RBCs. Replacing with O- RBCs negates the impact of the circulating antibodies until the antibody quantity gradually diminishes, a process that can take up to 3 to 4 months to completely resolve.

Hyperbilirubinemia

We begin with a review of bilirubin metabolism. Bilirubin is derived from heme-containing proteins (hemoglobin) during RBC turnover, which occurs within the reticuloendothelial system (RES). Bilirubin production begins when the enzyme heme oxygenase converts heme into biliverdin. The enzyme biliverdin reductase then converts the biliverdin into bilirubin. In this fat-soluble and unconjugated state, bilirubin readily binds with albumin and is transported to the liver. Once within the hepatic microcirculation, albumin dissociates from the bilirubin. This permits bilirubin uptake into the hepatocyte, a process facilitated by ligandin (a receptor protein). Ligandin transports the bilirubin to the smooth endoplasmic reticulum (SER). It is here that bilirubin undergoes glucuronidation (or conjugation), a process modulated by the enzyme *uridine diphosphoglucuronate (UDP) glucuronyltransferase (UGT1A1)*. Conjugation changes bilirubin from a fat-soluble to a water-soluble molecule. The bilirubin is thereby excreted into the bile and travels down the common bile duct and into the intestine, where it is converted (by bacterial action) into urobilinogen. The majority continues to the colon, is oxidized into stercobilinogen (brown pigment), and is eliminated from the body via the stool. A small portion of urobilinogen is excreted from the urine (Kaplan et al., 2025). Bilirubin is a known antioxidant and may provide protection from oxidative injuries, at physiologic levels, which is especially important in the premature neonate (Kaplan et al., 2025).

During fetal development, bilirubin that reaches the intestinal tract is reversed to its unconjugated state by the enzyme beta-glucuronidase. This is necessary for the bilirubin to travel to the placenta for excretion and is known as enterohepatic circulation. Postnatally, conjugated bilirubin is primarily excreted by the stool (98%), with a small amount of bilirubin eliminated in the urine (2%). Several factors contribute to elevations of bilirubin levels in term and preterm neonates. High concentrations of beta-glucuronidase combined with low enzymatic activity (specifically *UGT1A1)*, limited bacterial flora in the intestines, slow enteric motility, and increased concentrations of beta-glucuronidase in freshly expressed colostrum or breast milk all contribute to bilirubin elevations through the same enterohepatic circulation pathway. Risk factors for severe hyperbilirubinemia are summarized in Table 7.11, whereas Table 7.12 summarizes the major causes for unconjugated hyperbilirubinemia.

Neonatal APRNs employed within primary care facilities, community hospitals, and larger centers must recognize hyperbilirubinemia as one of the most common, yet preventable, causes for hospital readmission within the first week of life. Noteworthy risk factors for readmission secondary to hyperbilirubinemia include exclusive breastfeeding, discharge to home within the first 2 days of life, primigravida status, and pregnancy occurring at an age younger than 20 years (Kaplan et al., 2025; Kemper et al., 2022).

Physiologic Hyperbilirubinemia. Approximately 80% of premature and term infants develop clinically

TABLE 7.11 Risk Factors for Developing Significant Hyperbilirubinemia

Clinical jaundice and discharge timing	• **Clinical jaundice apparent in first 24 hours** • Phototherapy prior to discharge • Predischarge bilirubin level close to phototherapy threshold
Infant medical conditions	• **Hemolysis from any cause (rate of rise greater than 0.3 mg/dL per hour in first 24 hours or greater than 0.2 mg/dL per hour thereafter)** • Macrosomic infant of diabetic mother • **Cephalohematoma, significant bruising, or other blood sequestration** • Trisomy 21 (Down syndrome)
Gestational age	• Lower gestational age (risk increases for each week less than 40 weeks' gestation)
Family history	• **History of parent or sibling requiring phototherapy or exchange transfusion** • Family history or genetic concern for inherited RBC enzyme disorders (G6PD deficiency)
Feeding	• **Exclusive breastfeeding with suboptimal oral intake (poor feeding, excessive weight loss)**

Note: Major risk factors identified in bold font.
G6PD, glucose-6-phosphate dehydrogenase.
Source: Adapted from Kemper, A. R., Newman, T. B., Slaughter, J. L., Maisels, M. J., Watchko, J. F., Downs, S. M., Grout, R. W., Bundy, D. G., Stark, A. R., Bogen, D. L., Holmes, A. V., Feldman-Winter, L. B., Bhutani, V. K., Brown, S. R., Maradiaga Panayotti, G. M., Okechukwu, K., Rappo, P. D., & Russel, T. L. (2022). Clinical practice guideline revision: Management of hyperbilirubinemia in the newborn infant 35 or more weeks of gestation. *Pediatrics, 150*(3), e2022058859. https://doi.org/10.1542/peds.2022-058859

TABLE 7.12 Causes for Neonatal Hyperbilirubinemia

Increased Production or Destruction of Bilirubin	Decreased Excretion of Bilirubin
• ABO/Rh incompatibility (isoimmunization)	• Dehydration-induced jaundice
• Structural abnormalities of erythrocytes (e.g., spherocytosis, elliptocytosis)	• Disorders of hepatic uptake (e.g., Gilbert syndrome)
• Erythrocyte enzyme defects (e.g., G6PD deficiency, pyruvate kinase deficiency)	• Disorders of conjugation (e.g., Crigler–Najjar)
• Sequestered blood (e.g., cephalohematoma, ecchymoses, hemangiomas)	• GI obstructive processes (e.g., pyloric stenosis, duodenal, or jejunal obstruction)
• Polycythemia	• Hypothyroidism
• Sepsis/infection	• Breast-milk jaundice

GI, gastrointestinal; G6PD, glucose-6-phosphate dehydrogenase.

apparent unconjugated (indirect) hyperbilirubinemia within the first week of life (Kaplan et al., 2025). The pathogenesis involves increased bilirubin production, impaired conjugation, or delayed clearance during the peripartum period. Of these etiologies, the majority of cases are attributed to increased bilirubin production (twofold higher than adults) and physiologic immaturity of hepatic bilirubin metabolic pathways. Low hepatic UDP-glucuronyl transferase (or glucuronyltransferase) levels limit the liver's ability to conjugate bilirubin into a water-soluble entity, which limits movement through the common bile duct and into the intestinal tract for excretion. Delayed passage of meconium stalls its excretion.

For term infants, serum bilirubin levels peak between days 3 and 5 of postnatal life, with an average concentration of 8 mg/dL to 10 mg/dL. For most infants, subsequent regression occurs; this regression can be delayed among infants who develop breast-milk jaundice. Premature infants tend to garner higher peak bilirubin levels, between days 4 and 7 of postnatal life. A slower return to normalcy among premature neonates, when compared to term neonates, is common (Kaplan et al., 2025).

Pathologic Hyperbilirubinemia. Pathologic hyperbilirubinemia may result from hemolytic diseases of the newborn, altered bilirubin conjugation and recirculation, or structural or other problems that impede normal excretion of conjugated bilirubin (cholestatic jaundice). *Hemolytic* causes for increased bilirubin levels include the previously described Rh and ABO incompatibility as well as enzyme defects, such as glucose-6-phosphate dehydrogenase (G6PD) deficiency. Recall that with Rh incompatibility, the anti-Rh IgG antibodies from the XX pregnant patient cross the placenta and destroy fetal RBCs. The increased destruction of cells causes an increase in circulating bilirubin, which extends into the peripartum period. The most common enzyme defect is G6PD deficiency. Cases of G6PD deficiency can be linked to spontaneous mutations or as X-linked inherited genetic defects and impacts predominantly male individuals, although in rare instances (inheritance from both parents) female individuals are also affected. A deficient amount of this enzyme weakens the RBC membrane, resulting in an increased risk for oxidative injury and (premature) rate of destruction when exposed to certain triggers. Although G6PD impacts individuals from all ethnic and racial groups, the highest prevalence of G6PD is noted in individuals descended from the Middle East, Africa, Asia, and parts of the Mediterranean. In the United States, the incidence is higher in the African American population with 10% to 14% of African American males and approximately 4% of African American females being impacted (Kaplan et al., 2025; Kemper et al., 2022; NORD, 2017).

Clinical Application. Although individuals with a deficiency of the G6PD enzyme may not experience a hemolytic event and lead normal lives, exposure to certain triggers are known to incite episodes of hemolysis leading to anemia, and in the neonate profound hyperbilirubinemia. Triggers known to impact individuals with G6PD deficiency include diagnoses (sepsis), medications (sulfa drugs and herbal medicines), chemicals (naphthalene—ingredient in "moth balls), and foods (fava beans). G6PD deficiency is a leading cause of kernicterus; therefore, the APRN should be suspicious of the diagnosis in at-risk neonates (family history or ethnicity) or in neonates with a rapid rise in bilirubin levels with evidence of anemia.

Nonhemolytic causes for indirect hyperbilirubinemia include bruising secondary to the birth process; blood sequestrations, including cephalohematoma and subgaleal bleeding; and polycythemia. Infections, including sepsis and urinary tract infections, inherited disorders, congenital hypothyroidism, poor nutritional intake, and breast-milk jaundice, are also causative factors (Kaplan et al., 2025; Kemper et al., 2022). Inherited disorders, such as Gilbert syndrome and Crigler–Najiir syndrome, involve a reduction in available UDP-glucoruronyl transferase and resultant hyperbilirubinemia. Congenital hypothyroidism typically manifests with reduced tone, including gastrointestinal tone. This provokes reduced enteral intake among some affected infants as well as decreased gastrointestinal motility.

Exclusively breastfed infants are considered at higher risk for pathologic hyperbilirubinemia secondary to dehydration from delayed onset of lactogenesis II (dehydration-induced jaundice). Delayed lactogenesis II stalls the establishment of adequate enteral intake and stooling and voiding patterns and encourages enterohepatic recirculation of bilirubin. Some breastfed infants may develop a more prolonged unconjugated hyperbilirubinemia, even after the onset of lactogenesis II (breast-milk jaundice). Particular substances found in the breast milk, glucouronidases and nonesterified fatty acids, are understood to modulate the deconjugation of bilirubin and perpetuate enterohepatic recirculation of bilirubin. Breast-milk jaundice may persist for several weeks before resolution is observed. Other pathologic causes for increased enterohepatic circulation include gastrointestinal obstructions, intestinal atresia, meconium ileus, and Hirschsprung disease.

Clinical Manifestations. Jaundice typically progresses in a cranial to caudal direction, yet visual severity and progression cannot be relied on for diagnostic or management purposes. Most infants with mild to moderate jaundice are well appearing during the physical examination. However, severe hyperbilirubinemia has the potential to manifest with signs of bilirubin-induced neurologic dysfunction (BIND), a spectrum of findings that includes lethargy, poor feeding, high-pitched crying, and hypotonia followed by the development of hypertonicity and opisthotonos (back arching) as the condition progresses (Kaplan et al., 2025). Although a discussion of management is beyond the scope of this book, it is essential that clinicians recognize bilirubin-induced encephalopathy as abnormal and time-sensitive in order to prevent the development of kernicterus. Criteria for exchange transfusion have been established by the AAP (Kemper et al., 2022).

Fortunately, the AAP offers a phototherapy and hour-specific nomogram for hyperbilirubinemia. This promotes the early identification, treatment, and timely postdischarge follow-up for at-risk or affected infants (Kemper et al., 2022). APRNs must align postdischarge follow-up plans for interval repeat serum bilirubin testing among infants at 35 weeks or more gestation with the guidance provided by the AAP (Kemper et al., 2022). The hour-specific risk zone and other clinical risk factors (previously highlighted in Table 7.13) must be jointly considered when formulating a plan for treatment and discharge. The APRN should also consider clinical decision-making tools which have been developed to assist neonatal providers in determining treatment thresholds, escalation of therapy, and recommendations for outpatient follow-up. The BiliTool (https://bilitool.org) was developed based on the updated 2022 AAP Hyperbilirubinemia guidelines for management of neonates older than 35 weeks' gestation. Additionally, Premie BiliRecs (pbr.stanfordchildrens.org) has been developed to aide

TABLE 7.13 Common Manifestations of Cholestasis

Clinical Manifestation	Etiology
Acholic stools	• Decreased stercobilin
Jaundice	• Aggregation of conjugated bilirubin
Hepatomegaly	• Hepatic obstruction

clinicians in the management of premature neonates younger than 35 weeks' gestation. 35 weeks of gestation and who are greater than 48 hours old. Clinicians can refer to Maisels and colleagues (2012) phototherapy and exchange transfusion guidelines for preterm infants who are less than 48 hours old.

Life-Span Implications. The aim of treatment is to prevent BIND and kernicterus, or irreversible damage to the basal ganglia, brainstem, and cerebellum, by neurotoxic bilirubin that crossed the blood–brain barrier (Kaplan et al., 2025; Kemper et al., 2022). Most cases of mild to moderate unconjugated hyperbilirubinemia are benign and associated with no long-term effects. Severe neurotoxicity may result in kernicterus, which is fatal in about 10% of infants; the majority of surviving infants develop cerebral palsy, sensorineural hearing loss, and other neurodevelopmental disabilities (Kaplan et al., 2025; Kemper et al., 2022). There is evidence to suggest that those infants with acute bilirubin encephalopathy in the setting of hemolysis have worse neurologic outcomes than those without hemolysis (Kaplan et al., 2025).

Cholestasis. Cholestasis, or impaired bile flow, affects one in every 2,500 infants (Kaplan et al., 2025; NORD, 2024). Premature infants are particularly susceptible to cholestasis due to immaturity of the hepatobiliary system and the need for prolonged parenteral nutrition.

The presence of conjugated hyperbilirubinemia is always pathologic and should raise suspicion for underlying hepatobiliary disease. Etiologies include structural anomalies such as biliary atresia, neonatal hepatitis, viral or bacterial infections, endocrinopathies, and metabolic diseases (Kaplan et al., 2025). Clinical manifestations of conjugated hyperbilirubinemia are summarized in Table 7.13. Laboratory findings point to the elevation of the conjugated form of bilirubin greater than 1 mg/dL, or greater than 20% of the total bilirubin level (Kemper et al., 2022).

Lifelong medical surveillance and management is indicated, as symptoms may recur. Certain cholestatic processes resulting in conjugated hyperbilirubinemia resolve spontaneously or with treatment of the underlying cause without further sequelae. Other etiologies are chronic with some cases requiring prompt operative management, as in the case of biliary atresia.

Disorders Associated With Hemostatic Elements

Neonatal Thrombocytopenia. Neonatal thrombocytopenia is traditionally defined as a platelet count less than 150,000/mcL. Mild thrombocytopenia is a platelet count between 100,000 to 150,000/mcL, moderate thrombocytopenia is 50,000 to 100,000/mcL, and severe neonatal thrombocytopenia presents with a platelet count less than 50,000/mcL (Deschmann & Sola-Visner, 2021; Ding et al., 2025). However, despite the definitions, the evaluation of neonates and the specific platelet concentration for treatment varies on whether the patient is actively bleeding, their gestational age (term versus preterm), whether they are sick/ill, or whether they are being prepared for an invasive procedure.

Alloimmune Thrombocytopenia. Similar to the presentation of Rh and ABO hemolytic disease of the newborn, sensitization to paternally derived fetal platelet antigens by the XX pregnant patient results in IgG antibodies that cross the placenta and subsequently destroy the fetal platelets. However, unlike the maternal antibody-related hemolytic anemia, cases of alloimmune thrombocytopenia occur in the first pregnancy in nearly 50% of cases (ACOG, 2019). The incidence of NAIT has been estimated to be one in 1,000 to 2,000 live births (Ding et al., 2025; Mitchell & Bussel, 2021; Norton et al., 2020). The most serious complication of NAIT is ICH, which occurs in 10% to 20% of affected newborns, with one quarter of these occurring in utero (ACOG, 2019; Ding et al., 2025; Mitchell & Bussel, 2021).

The pathophysiology of alloimmune thrombocytopenia involves the expression of a paternally inherited antigen on the fetus's platelets, against which the XX pregnant patient produces antibodies. During the pregnancy, there is placental transfer of these IgG antibodies to the fetus's bloodstream. The antibodies recognize the paternal antigen on fetal platelets as foreign, resulting in platelet destruction within the fetus's RES (Ding et al., 2025; Mitchell & Bussel, 2021; Norton et al., 2020). HPA-1a is the most common antigen to result in this process, accounting for 85% of cases among Caucasians (Ding et al., 2025; Mitchell & Bussel, 2021). Of note, maternal platelets are unaffected, and the maternal platelet count is normal, helping to distinguish alloimmune thrombocytopenia from immune thrombocytopenia (ITP; Ding et al., 2025; Mitchell & Bussel, 2021; Norton et al., 2020).

The diagnosis should be considered in any well-appearing term infant who presents with severe unexplained thrombocytopenia during the first 48 hours of life. However, a high index of suspicion should also be considered in ill-appearing infants (Mitchell & Bussel, 2021). Clinical manifestations of alloimmune thrombocytopenia range from asymptomatic to catastrophic. Thrombocytopenia is often severe (less than $50 \times 10^9/L$; normal $150–400 \times 10^9/L$) and signs may include petechiae, bruising, hematomas, melena, or ICH (Ding et al., 2025;

Mitchell & Bussel, 2021; Norton et al., 2020). Many infants will not display overt signs at birth, and the diagnosis may go unrecognized even though the infant is at risk for significant bleeding. In severe cases, the effects occur in utero and the fetus may experience ICH or even intrauterine demise. The estimated incidence of ICH related to NAIT is 10 to 20 per every 100,000 newborns, with nearly half of ICH's occurring in utero (Mitchell & Bussel, 2021). The mortality rate for NAIT-related ICH is estimated at 33% (Ding et al., 2025).

Without treatments aimed at platelet recovery, platelet counts continue to fall for several days after birth, followed by recovery over days to weeks. During this time the neonate remains at-risk for adverse sequelae, especially if platelet counts fall to less than 20,000. Circulating antiplatelet antibodies from the XX pregnant patient remain in the neonate's circulation up to 3 months following birth; once removed from the neonate's circulation, the infant should not experience further thrombocytopenia or complications related to NAIT (Norton et al., 2020). If ICH has occurred, the infant's long-term neurodevelopmental outcome can be negatively impacted depending on the degree of neurologic injury sustained (Ding et al., 2025; Mitchell & Bussel, 2021). Parents should be counseled about the high risk of recurrence in subsequent pregnancies. A 50% (heterozygous father) to 100% (homozygous father) recurrence risk is understood to implicate future family planning (Deschmann & Sola-Visner, 2024).

Autoimmune Thrombocytopenia. When the XX pregnant patient has thrombocytopenia that is the direct result of antibodies directed against her own platelets, those antibodies may also cross the placenta and bind to fetal platelets, resulting in their destruction. This condition occurs in autoimmune disorders (e.g., ITP and SLE). Affected infants are otherwise well appearing. Those with moderate to severe thrombocytopenia may present with petechiae, bruising, and bleeding. While most infants will have platelet counts greater than 50,000/mcL, in a series of cases of XX pregnant patient with ITP, there is a risk of 4% to 10% that the infant will have a platelet count that is less than this (Davenport & Sola-Visner, 2021). Table 7.14 contrasts NAIT and autoimmune thrombocytopenia.

TABLE 7.14 Contrast of Findings Between Neonatal Alloimmune Thrombocytopenia and Autoimmune Thrombocytopenia

Clinical Feature	Neonatal Alloimmune Thrombocytopenia	Autoimmune Thrombocytopenia
Birthing parent platelet count	Normal	Decreased
Neonatal platelet count	Severely decreased	Moderately decreased
Physical manifestations	• Bruising • Petechiae • Bleeding from wounds • Intracranial hemorrhage	• Well appearing • Bruising • Petechiae • Bleeding
Time to resolution	1–3 months of life	2–3 years of life
Management	• IVIg (prenatally or postnatally) • Transfusion of HPA negative platelets postnatally	• IVIg • Platelet transfusion for severe thrombocytopenia

HPA, human platelet antigen; IVIg, intravenous immune globulin.

Disseminated Intravascular Coagulopathy. The pathophysiology of DIC is not fully understood, and the actual incidence of DIC is unknown as it is thought to be widely underdiagnosed. No one laboratory test can be used to diagnose DIC early. However, it is known that the neonatal population is at higher risk of developing DIC when compared to older patients (Davenport & Sola-Visner, 2021). DIC occurs secondary to other diagnoses or risk factors including sepsis, perinatal hypoxic ischemia, respiratory disorders, NEC, metabolic disorders, and vascular anomalies (Davenport & Sola-Visner, 2021; Saxonhouse & Hinson, 2024). The process seems to be triggered by damaged TF and cytokines that are released, causing widespread activation of the coagulation cascade and fibrinolysis (Ding et al., 2025). Clinical manifestations include petechiae, bruising, generalized bleeding, persistent oozing from puncture sites, and pulmonary hemorrhage (Ding et al., 2025). DIC represents a continuum of severity of symptoms. Although there is no single definitive test to diagnose DIC, common laboratory findings include thrombocytopenia, prolonged prothrombin time (PT) and activated partial thromboplastin time (aPTT), and low fibrinogen (Ding et al., 2025).

Clinical Application. Consider the neonate with NEC. This diagnosis leads to the activation of the inflammatory response, referred to as systemic inflammatory response syndrome (SIRS); triggers the release of cytokines; and activates the coagulation cascade. As premature neonates have limited abilities to downregulate this inflammatory process, consumption of platelets and clotting factors occurs, increasing the risk for development of DIC. Neonates with extensive NEC are at the highest risk for DIC due to the strength of the inflammatory response and rapid exhaustion of stores.

DIC is a common feature of neonatal sepsis and is especially noted with congenital viral infections such as enterovirus and HSV due to multiorgan involvement. In neonatal HSV, approximately one fourth of infections are the disseminated form involving multiple organs. DIC along with neutropenia and thrombocytopenia are frequently reported with congenital HSV infection, whereas DIC, neutrophilia, and thrombocytopenia are noted with enteroviral infection (Werner et al., 2021). The presence of DIC increases the infant's risk of death in both viral infections and may be as high as 80% in untreated patients with neonatal HSV (Werner et al., 2021).

Vitamin K Deficiency Bleeding (Formerly Hemorrhagic Disease of the Newborn). Vitamin K deficiency in the neonate leads to an unexpected bleeding diathesis known as vitamin K deficiency bleeding (VKDB). Risk factors include lack of placental transfer, poor neonatal hepatic reserves, and parental refusal of intramuscular (IM) vitamin K prophylaxis immediately after birth (Guzzardo & Regling, 2022). The incidence of late VKDB among infants receiving prophylaxis is estimated to be 0.25 to 2.8 per 100,000 infants, in contrast to 5.8 to 80 per 100,000 infants among those who do not receive prophylaxis (Sankar et al., 2016).

Vitamin K is a fat-soluble vitamin that has two forms: (a) K1, which is available in green vegetables, and (b) K2, which is synthesized by gut bacteria and contributes to the daily requirement in humans (Albisetti & Monagle, 2021). Vitamin K is an essential cofactor for several coagulation factors, including procoagulant factors II, VII, IX, and X as well as anticoagulant proteins C and S, and its absence, therefore, leads to defective coagulation (Ding et al., 2025).

Early-onset disease typically presents within the first 24 hours of age and is seen in neonates who do not receive exogenous vitamin K or those who have intrauterine exposure to medications that affect vitamin K utilization or production, such as anticonvulsants, warfarin, and antibiotics. Classic hemorrhagic disease presents between 2 to 7 days postnatal age and is commonly a result of inadequate postnatal prophylaxis or inadequate exogenous intake of vitamin K. Breastfed infants are at risk due to poor passage of vitamin K into breast milk. Late-onset disease presents between 2 and 12 weeks of age, as a result of inadequate postnatal prophylaxis or exogenous vitamin K intake, malabsorption, or hepatobiliary disease affecting coagulation factor synthesis and absorption of fat-soluble vitamins (Albisetti & Monagle, 2021; Ding et al., 2025; Guzzardo & Regling, 2022). Symptoms may include gastrointestinal bleeding, umbilical cord bleeding, intracranial hemorrhage, or prolonged bleeding after blood draws or procedures, such as circumcision (Albisetti & Monagle, 2021; Ding et al., 2025; Guzzardo & Regling, 2022).

Given the decreased endogenous levels of vitamin K at birth, the risk for VKDB is increased. This underpins the need for IM postnatal vitamin K prophylaxis. Oral vitamin K is available off label and is considered effective for preventing the classic form of VKDB, but less efficacious for preventing late-onset disease based on observational studies; thus, the IM formulation remains the standard of care (Gwartney & Ierardi, 2024). Life-span implications depend on the severity of bleeding. Irreversible cerebral injury or death is associated with the development of ICH.

Hemophilia. Hemophilia is an X-linked inherited bleeding disorder that results from a deficiency of factor VIII (hemophilia A) or factor IX (hemophilia B). Hemophilia type A is reported in one in every 5,000 males, whereas hemophilia B is reported in one out of every 30,000 males (Ding et al., 2025; Ostilla et al., 2024). The deficiency of factor VIII or IX causes reduced thrombin formation, which leads to excessive bleeding.

Clinical manifestations primarily present in the neonatal period and may be the result of injections, punctures, or birth trauma; most affected infants are diagnosed within the first month of life (Figure 7.19). Intracranial and extracranial hemorrhage occur in up to one third of severe cases of hemophilia (Ding et al., 2025; Ostilla et al., 2024). Bleeding can be minimized by tailoring care to avoid exposure to any type of trauma, for example, injections, punctures, and unnecessary procedures (circumcision). Hemophilia is a lifelong condition and care should be coordinated through a hemophilia center.

Thrombotic Disorders

Due to a decreased concentration of the inhibitory factors of coagulation, ill neonates, particularly those born

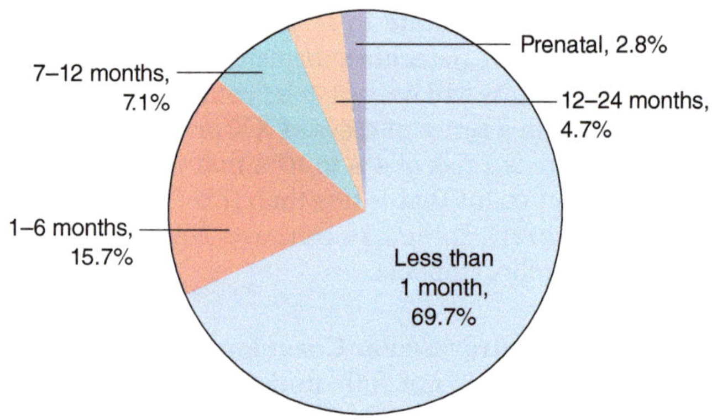

Figure 7.19 Age of diagnosis of hemophilia among children less than 2 years of age. The median age at diagnosis is 36 months (mild hemophilia), 8 months (moderate hemophilia), and 1 month (severe hemophilia). Approximately one third of affected infants have no family history of hemophilia; unusual bleeding patterns lead to the diagnostic evaluation.

Source: Centers for Disease Control and Prevention. (2024). *Hemophilia: Data & statistics.* https://www.cdc.gov/hemophilia/data-research/index.html

preterm, are at an increased risk of thrombotic events. Coupled with a significant need for vascular access devices, it is estimated that 7.5/1,000 infants admitted to the NICU will have a thrombotic complication (Knopoff et al., 2024). Predisposing factors to thrombosis include mechanical devices, such as intravascular catheters, hypotension, hyperviscosity, severe genetic and acquired deficiencies and/or mutations of specific anticoagulation factors, sepsis, and diabetes mellitus in the XX pregnant patient. In critically ill neonates, approximately 90% of thrombotic events in the NICU are catheter related, with umbilical venous and arterial catheters conferring anywhere from 12% to 35% risk of thrombosis (Knopoff et al., 2024). Both venous and arterial catheters may lead to thromboses. Infants may be asymptomatic; however, erythema, pain, swelling, decreased pulses, and discoloration may be present.

Renal Vein Thrombosis. The most common non–catheter-related thrombotic event is renal vein thrombosis (RVT), which accounts for up to 20% of all thrombosis in the NICU (Ding et al., 2025). Males are most likely to be affected. Risk factors include perinatal asphyxia, prematurity, dehydration, sepsis, congenital heart disease, and gestational diabetes (Ding et al., 2025). Depending on the severity of the occlusion, the infant may present with the following key clinical features: hematuria, thrombocytopenia, and palpable flank mass (Ding et al., 2025). Long-term complications of RVT include chronic renal impairment and hypertension; nephrology follow-up is imperative.

Disorders of White Blood Cells

Neutropenia. Neutropenia is common among infants and children. It is generally defined as an ANC less than the fifth percentile for postnatal age (1,500/mcL; Pateva et al., 2025). Calculation of the ANC is determined by the following formula: ANC = total WBC (cells/mcL) × percentage (neutrophils + bands) ÷ 100. Mild neutropenia is considered to be 1,000 to 1,500/mcL, moderate is 500 to 1,000/mcL, and severe is less than 500/mcL. Neutrophil count norms are dynamic in early life. After birth, infants' neutrophil counts rise for the first 48 to 72 hours, followed by a gradual decrease until reaching adult norms by about 2 months of age (Pateva et al., 2025).

There is a wide array of etiologies of neutropenia, ranging from congenital to acquired and transient to chronic. Neutropenia is a more common finding among premature infants compared to term infants, particularly those of low birthweight, although otherwise healthy term infants may also be affected. Around 22 weeks of gestation, the fetal bone marrow assumes hematopoiesis; however, neutrophil production does not become well established until the third trimester, thereby putting premature infants at higher risk for neutropenia. As described earlier in this chapter, these early neutrophils may not function as effectively as neutrophils of term infants or older children and may increase the risk of sepsis.

Risk factors for other acquired neutropenias include intrauterine factors, such as growth restriction and preeclampsia, each of which relates to decreased placental blood flow and hypoxia leading to decreased neutrophil production in favor of increased erythrocyte precursor production in the bone marrow (Lawrence et al., 2017). Sepsis may cause neutropenia due to consumption of the neutrophil supply and the neonate's inability to appropriately upregulate neutrophil production in the bone marrow in times of stress. Drug-induced neutropenia may be caused by a wide variety of medications that lead to bone marrow suppression or direct neutrophil destruction (Pateva et al., 2025). Neutropenia in neonates may also be immune mediated, including alloimmune and autoimmune neutropenias. Each of the immune-mediated neutropenias is the result of accelerated neutrophil destruction that begins before birth or shortly after birth of the infant.

Although the common immune-mediated neutropenias will be described individually, infection is a common manifestation of forms of neutropenia. In fact, neutropenia confers an increased risk for infection, particularly bacterial and fungal infections, which may be severe or life-threatening. Common organisms include staphylococci, streptococci, pneumococci, enterococci, Gram-negative organisms, and Candida species (Pateva et al., 2025). Infants with neutropenia most commonly acquire infections in cutaneous, mucosal, and pulmonary sites (Pateva et al., 2025). Immune-mediated neutropenias may present with fever in the first few days of life and may develop pneumonia, cutaneous infections, omphalitis, or sepsis. Congenital neutropenia tends to have more of a chronic course with signs that include recurrent oral ulcers, gingivostomatitis, cellulitis, pharyngitis, respiratory infections, and perianal disease (Pateva et al., 2025).

Neonatal Alloimmune Neutropenia. Neonatal alloimmune neutropenia (NAIN) has an incidence of 0.5 to two cases per 1,000 births (Schibler & Christensen, 2021). This form of neutropenia is also known as *neonatal isoimmune neutropenia*. The disorder is the result of maternally produced antibodies of the IVIG type directed against antigens on fetal neutrophils (Pateva et al., 2025; Schibler & Christensen, 2021). The antigens are paternally derived. Like Rh hemolytic disease of the newborn, sensitization to fetal neutrophil antigens by the XX pregnant patient results in antibodies that cross the placenta and subsequently destroy the fetal neutrophils. However, unlike antibody-related hemolytic anemia, cases of alloimmune neutropenia can occur in the first pregnancy. Human neutrophil antigens (HNAs) of the groups HNA1, HNA2, HNB1, and HNC1 are most frequently involved (Pateva et al., 2025; Schibler & Christensen, 2021).

This form of neutropenia should be suspected in neonates with unexplained neutropenia that persists for several days. Often the infants are well appearing. Although the condition is self-limited, and the duration of the neutropenia can range from a few weeks to months, the neutropenia may not be benign. Infants with severe neutropenia are at risk for serious bacterial infections such as cellulitis, omphalitis, pneumonia, and meningitis from organisms including *Staphylococcus aureus, Beta-hemolytic Streptococcus, and Escherichia coli* (Pateva et al., 2025; Schibler & Christensen, 2021).

Autoimmune Neutropenia of Infancy. Autoimmune neutropenia of infancy (AINI) occurs when infants produce antibodies that attack their own neutrophils; no maternal antibodies are to blame for this form of neutropenia (Pateva et al., 2025). The development of autoimmune antibodies can occur as an isolated phenomenon resulting in AINI. Some cases have been associated with parvovirus B19 infection, whereas others have been linked to the use of beta-lactam antibiotics, molecular mimicry, changes in endogenous antigens, enhanced human leucocyte antigen (HLA) expression, or loss of suppression of clones of self-reacting lymphocytes (Schibler & Christensen, 2021). This condition is self-limiting, with a median duration of 30 months. Common clinical manifestations include isolated neutropenia, lack of dysmorphic features, no hepatosplenomegaly, absence of bone pain, no diarrhea, no severe or unusual infections, and no other signs suggestive of a significant underlying disorder (Black & Maheshwari, 2009). At least 95% of affected infants recover by 4 years of age. Like infants with alloimmune neutropenia, infections, including cellulitis, gastroenteritis, otitis media, and respiratory infections, may be present at the time of diagnosis (Schibler & Christensen, 2021).

Neonatal Neutropenia Resulting From Autoimmune Neutropenia. This form of immune neutropenia is found in neonates who are born to pregnant patients with autoimmune neutropenia, such as in cases of SLE. The condition in the neonate tends to be transient and generally is mild. However, in some cases infection may occur.

CONCLUSION

The hematologic system performs some of the most critical functions of the body—oxygen transport, protection against infections, and hemostatic regulation. Development of this system begins very early in fetal life. In the fetus, hematopoiesis takes place in several locations. The process begins in the yolk sac, eventually ending in the bone marrow, which then carries out hematopoiesis through adulthood. Fetal and neonatal hematologic cells are less mature compared to adult cells, leading to decreased function of these cells. This knowledge is important in understanding the difference in response to certain conditions, such as infections, anemia, or clotting problems in the neonate, as compared to the adult human. Maternal influences—genetic, metabolic, and autoimmune, among others—could lead to dysfunction of the hematologic system and thus illness. Therefore, complete evaluation of any hematologic disorder in the neonate involves careful history and possibly laboratory testing of the xx pregnant patient. Although some diseases of the hematologic system are transient or curable, they may have long-term sequelae; for example, RVT leads to chronic renal disease or intraventricular hemorrhage results in neurodevelopmental impairment. Some other diseases, such as hemophilia, are chronic and persist for the lifetime of the individual. Understanding the development, physiology, and function of the hematologic system is instrumental in the long-term management of these disorders.

LEARNING TOOLS AND RESOURCES

CourseConnect

To access self-assessment questions and interactive, competency-based learning activities for this chapter, visit www.springerpub.com/courseconnect. See inside front cover and tear-out card for CourseConnect details.

Podcast

This podcast is available online by visiting www.springerpub.com/courseconnect. See inside front cover and tear-out card for CourseConnect details.

Physiologic Hyperbilirubinemia
Christie del Castillo-Hegyi

Discussion Prompts

1. Discuss the role of genetics in the pathogenesis of neonatal hemophilia.
2. Review the pathogenesis of neonatal thrombocytopenia.
3. Compare and contrast the various methods by which maternal antibodies may lead to immune-mediated hemolysis of fetal blood cells.

MIND MAP

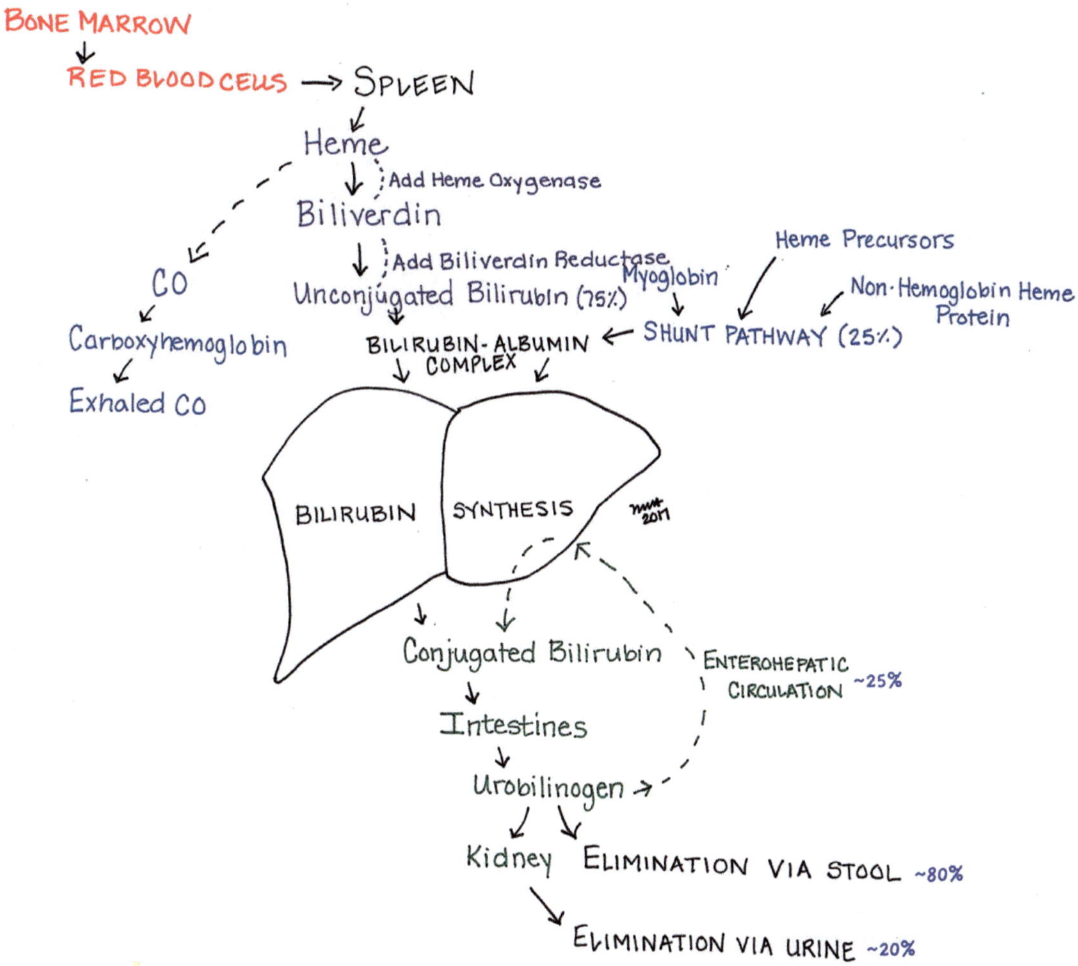

Note: This mind map reflects a former neonatal nurse practitioner student's interpretation of a concept addressed in this chapter. Readers should regard the mind maps woven throughout this textbook as examples of multisensory study tools that can be developed to aid conceptual understanding. Readers are encouraged to develop their own unique mind maps in consultation with academic faculty or clinical preceptors.

Image Credit: Nicole Harvey, MSN, APRN, NNP-BC.

REFERENCES

Albisetti, M., & Monagle, P. (2021). Bleeding disorders. In P. A. de Alarcon, E. J. Werner, R. D. Christensen, & M. C. Sola-Visner (Eds.), *Neonatal hematology: Pathogenesis, diagnosis, and management of hematologic problems* (3rd ed., pp. 293–310). Cambridge University Press.

American College of Obstetricians and Gynecologists. (2019). ACOG practice bulletin No. 207: Thrombocytopenia in pregnancy. *Obstetrics & Gynecology, 133*(3), 1–13. https://doi.org/10.1097/AOG.0000000000003100

Aster, J. C., & Scadden, D. T. (2017). Hematopoiesis. In J. C. Aster & H. Bunn (Eds.), *Pathophysiology of blood disorders* (2nd ed., pp. 1–11). McGraw-Hill Education. https://accessmedicine.mhmedical.com/content.aspx?bookid=1900&sectionid=137394642

Ballas, J., & Kelly, T. F. (2024). Maternal medical disorders of fetal significance. In C. A. Gleason & T. Sawyer (Eds.), *Avery's diseases of the newborn* (11th ed., pp. 82–98). Elsevier.

Benjamin, J. T., Molloy, E. J., & Maheshwari, A. (2025). Developmental immunology. In R. J. Martin & A. A. Fanaroff (Eds.), *Fanaroff and Martin's neonatal-perinatal medicine: Diseases of the fetus and infant* (pp. 2838–2954). Elsevier.

Benjamin, J. T., Torres, B. A., & Maheshwari, A. (2024). Neonatal leukocyte physiology and disorders. In C. A. Gleason, & T. Sawyer (Eds.), *Avery's diseases of the newborn* (11th ed., pp. 1033–1044). Elsevier.

Biron-Shental, T., & Hershkovich-Shporen, C. (2025). Fetal effects of autoimmune disease. In R. J. Martin & A. A. Fanaroff (Eds.), *Fanaroff and Martin's neonatal-perinatal medicine: Diseases of the fetus and infant* (12th ed., pp. 1275–1304). Elsevier.

Black, L. V., & Maheshwari, A. (2009). Immune-mediated neutropenia in the neonate. *NeoReviews, 10*(9), e446–e453. https://doi.org/10.1542/neo.10-9-e446

Blankenhorn, K., & Strumph, K. (2024). Hemoglobinopathies in the neonate. *NeoReviews, 25* (11), e720–e728. https://doi.org/10.1542/neo.25-11-e720

Bunn, H. F., & Furie, B. (2017). Overview of homeostasis. In J. C. Aster & H. Bunn (Eds.), *Pathophysiology of blood disorders* (2nd ed, pp. 1–14). McGraw-Hill Education. https://accessmedicine.mhmedical.com/content.aspx?bookid=1900&sectionid=137395249

Bunn, H. F., & Heeney, M. M. (2017). Iron homeostasis: Deficiency and overload. In J. C. Aster & H. Bunn (Eds.), *Pathophysiology of blood disorders* (2nd ed, pp. 1–11). McGraw-Hill Education. https://accessmedicine.mhmedical.com/content.aspx?bookid=1900&sectionid=137394788

Carlberg, K. (2024). *Neonatal erythrocyte disorders.* In C. A. Gleason & T. Sawyer (Eds.), *Avery's diseases of the newborn* (11th ed., pp. 996–1024). Elsevier.

Centers for Disease Control and Prevention. (2024). *Sickle cell disease.* Data and Statistics on Sickle Cell Disease. https://www.cdc.gov/sickle-cell/data/index.html

Christensen, R. D., Juul, S. E., & Del Vecchio, A. (2015). Neonatal hematology and transfusion medicine. *Clinics in Perinatology, 42*(3), i. https://doi.org/10.1016/S0095-5108(15)00068-8

Christensen, R. D., Yaish, H. M., & Gallagher, P. G. (2015). A pediatrician's practical guide to diagnosing and treating hereditary spherocytosis in neonates. *Pediatrics, 135*(6), 1107–1114. https://doi.org/10.1542/peds.2014-3516

Cosgrove, J., Hustin, L. S. P., de Boer, R. J., & Perié, L. (2021). Hematopoiesis in numbers. *Trends in Immunology, 42*(12), 1100–1112. https://doi.org/10.1016/j.it.2021.10.006

Davenport, P., Liu, Z., & Sola-Visner, M. (2022). Fetal vs adult megakaryopoiesis. *Blood, 139*(22), 3233–3244. https://doi.org/10.1182/blood.2020009301

Davenport, P. E., & Sola-Visner, M. C. (2021). Acquired thrombocytopenias. In P. A. de Alarcon, E. J. Werner, R. D. Christensen, & M. C. Sola-Visner (Eds.), *Neonatal hematology: Pathogenesis, diagnosis, and management of hematologic problems* (3rd ed., pp. 210–222). Cambridge University Press.

Desai, A. P., Lim, P. P. C., Ogundare, M. O., & Gonzalez, B. E. (2025). Viral infections in the neonate. In R. J. Martin & A. A. Fanaroff (Eds.), *Fanaroff and Martin's neonatal-perinatal medicine: Diseases of the fetus and infant* (pp. 3155–3366). Elsevier.

Deschmann, E., & Sola-Visner, M. (2021). Approach to the thrombocytopenic neonate. In P. A. de Alarcon, E. J. Werner, R. D. Christensen, & M. C. Sola-Visner (Eds.), *Neonatal hematology: Pathogenesis, diagnosis, and management of hematologic problems* (3rd ed., pp. 201–208). Cambridge University Press.

Deschmann, E., & Sola-Visner, M. (2024). Neonatal platelet disorders. In C. A. Gleason & T. Sawyer (Eds.), *Avery's diseases of the newborn* (11th ed., pp. 982–995). Elsevier.

Ding, H., Citla-Sridhar, D., & Ahuja, S. P. (2025). The hematopoietic system. In R. J. Martin & A. A. Fanaroff (Eds.), *Fanaroff and Martin's neonatal-perinatal medicine: Diseases of the fetus and infant* (pp. 5098–5160). Elsevier.

D'Souza, A. M., de Alarcon, P. A., & Yoder, M. C. (2021). Hematopoiesis. In P. A. de Alarcon, E. J. Werner, R. D. Christensen, & M. C. Sola-Visner (Eds.), *Neonatal hematology: Pathogenesis, diagnosis, and management of hematologic problems* (3rd ed., pp. 10–24). Cambridge University Press.

Fay, E., Simmons, L., & Brown, C. (2024). Maternal diabetes. In C. A. Gleason & T. Sawyer (Eds.), *Avery's diseases of the newborn* (11th ed., pp. 67–81). Elsevier.

Fuchs, D. A., McGinn, S. G., Cantu, C. L., Klein, R. R., Sola-Visner, M. C., & Rimsza, L. M. (2012). Developmental differences in megakaryocyte size in infants and children. *American Journal of Clinical Pathology, 138*(1), 140–145. https://doi.org/10.1309/AJCP4EMTJYA0VGYE

Gallagher, P. G. (2022). Anemia in the pediatric patient. *Blood, 140*(6), 571–593. https://doi.org/10.1182/blood.2020006479

Glader, B., & Kamdar, A. (2021). Neonatal hemolysis. In P. A. de Alarcon, E. J. Werner, R. D. Christensen, & M. C. Sola-Visner, *Neonatal hematology: Pathogenesis, diagnosis, and management of hematologic problems* (3rd ed., pp. 154–183). Cambridge University Press.

Grover, S. P., & Mackman, N. (2019). Intrinsic pathway of coagulation and thrombosis: Insights from animal models. *Arteriosclerosis, Thrombosis, and Vascular Biology, 39*, 331–338. https://doi.org/10.1161/ATVBAHA.118.312130

Guzzardo, G. M., & Regling, K. (2022). Developmental hemostasis: The evolution of our coagulation system. *NeoReviews, 32*(2), e82–e95. https://doi.org/10.1542/neo.23-2-e82

Gwartney, T., & Ierardi, J. (2024). Common medications prescribed in the newborn nursery. In A. J. Jnah & C. McPherson (Eds.), *Fetal and neonatal pharmacology for the advanced practice nurse* (pp. 128–150). Springer Publishing Company.

Huang, M., Wang, L., Zhang, Q., Zhou, L., Liao, R., Wu, A., Wang, X., Luo, J., Huang, F., Zou, W., & Wu, J. (2024). Interleukins in platelet biology: Unraveling the complex regulatory network. *Pharmaceuticals, 17*(1), 109. https://doi.org/10.3390/ph17010109

Jeon, G. W. (2022). Pathophysiology, classification, and complications of common asymptomatic thrombocytosis in newborn infants. *Clinical and Experimental Pediatrics, 65*(4), 182–187. https://doi.org/10.3345/cep.2021.00864

Juul, S. E., & Christensen, R. D. (2024). Developmental hematology. In C. A. Gleason & T. Sawyer (Eds.), *Avery's diseases of the newborn* (11th ed., pp. 957–964). Elsevier.

Kaplan, M., Wong, R. J., Bensen, R., Sibley, E., & Stevenson, D. K. (2025). Neonatal jaundice and liver disease. In R. J. Martin & A. A. Fanaroff (Eds.), *Fanaroff and Martin's neonatal-perinatal medicine: Diseases of the fetus and infant* (12th ed., pp. 6302–6549). Elsevier.

Kaufman, D. A., Nadipuram, S. M., & Manzoni, P. (2025). Fungal and protozoal infections of the neonate. In R. J. Martin & A. A. Fanaroff (Eds.), *Fanaroff and Martin's neonatal-perinatal medicine: Diseases of the fetus and infant* (12th ed., pp. 3039–3154). Elsevier.

Kavanagh, P. L., Fasipe, T. A., & Wun, T. (2022). Sickle cell disease: A review. *Journal of the American Medical Association, 328*(1), 57–68. https://doi.org/10.1001/jama.2022.10233

Kemper, A. R., Newman, T. B., Slaughter, J. L., Maisels, M. J., Watchko, J. F., Downs, S. M., Grout, R. W., Bundy, D. G., Stark, A. R., Bogen, D. L., Holmes, A. V., Feldman-Winter, L. B., Bhutani, V. K., Brown, S. R., Maradiaga Panayotti, G. M., Okechukwu, K., Rappo, P. D., & Russel, T. L. (2022). Clinical practice guideline revision: Management of hyperbilirubinemia in the newborn infant 35 or more weeks of gestation. *Pediatrics, 150*(3), e2022058859. https://doi.org/10.1542/peds.2022-058859

Kling, P. J. (2021). Anemia of prematurity and indications for erythropoietin therapy. In P. A. de Alarcon, E. J. Werner, R. D. Christensen, & M. C. Sola-Visner (Eds.), *Neonatal hematology: Pathogenesis, diagnosis, and management of hematologic problems* (3rd ed., pp. 120–131). Cambridge University Press.

Knopoff, K., Ostilla, L., Morocco, P., & Myers, P. (2024). Thrombotic disorders in the newborn. *NeoReviews, 25*(11), e710–e719. https://doi.org/10.1542/neo.25-11-e710

Laver, J., Duncan, E., Abboud, M., Gasparetto, C., Sahdev, I., Warren, D., Bussel, J., Auld, P., O'Reilly, R. J., & Moore, M. A. (1990). High levels of granulocyte and granulocyte-macrophage colony-stimulating factors in cord blood of normal full-term neonates. *Journal of Pediatrics, 116*(4), 627–632. https://doi.org/10.1016/S0022-3476(05)81617-8

Lawrence, S. M., Corriden, R., & Nizet, V. (2017). Age-appropriate functions and dysfunctions of the neonatal neutrophil. *Frontiers in Pediatrics, 5,* 2296–2360. https://doi.org/10.3389/fped.2017.00023

Lawrence, S. M., Corriden, R., & Nizet, V. (2018). The ontogeny of a neutrophil: Mechanisms of granulopoiesis and homeostasis. *Microbiology & Molecular Biology Reviews, 82*(1), e00057-17. https://doi.org/10.1128/MMBR.00057-17

Maisels, M. J., Watchko, J. F., Bhutani, V. K., & Stevenson, D. K. (2012). An approach to the management of hyperbilirubinemia in the preterm infant less than 35 weeks of gestation. *Journal of Perinatology: Official Journal of the California Perinatal Association, 32*(9), 660–664. https://doi.org/10.1038/jp.2012.71

Mazzi, S., Lordier, L., Debili, N., Raslova, H., & Vainchenker, W. (2018). Megakaryocyte and polyploidization. *Experimental Hematology, 57,* 1–13. https://doi.org/10.1016/j.exphem.2017.10.001

Mehta, H. M., & Corey, S. J. (2021). G-CSF, the guardian of granulopoiesis. *Seminars in Immunology, 54,* 101515. https://doi.org/10.1016/j.smim.2021.101515

Michniacki, T. F., & Walkovich, K. (2021). Functional phagocyte disorders in the neonate. In P. A. de Alarcon, E. J. Werner, R. D. Christensen, & M. C. Sola-Visner (Eds.), *Neonatal hematology: Pathogenesis, diagnosis, and management of hematologic problems* (3rd ed., pp. 279–291). Cambridge University Press.

Mitchell, W. B., & Bussel, J. B. (2021). Fetal and neonatal alloimmune thrombocytopenias. In P. A. de Alarcon, E. J. Werner, R. D. Christensen, & M. C. Sola-Visner (Eds.), *Neonatal hematology: Pathogenesis, diagnosis, and management of hematologic problems* (3rd ed., pp. 222–241). Cambridge University Press.

Moiseiwitsch, N., & Brown, A. C. (2021). Neonatal coagulopathies: A review of established and emerging treatments. *Experimental Biology and Medicine, 246,* 1447–1457. https://doi.org/10.1177/15353702211006046

National Institutes of Health. (2025). *Thrombocytopenia-absent radius syndrome.* Genetic and Rare Diseases (GARD) Information Center. https://rarediseases.info.nih.gov/diseases/5116/thrombocytopenia-absent-radius-syndrome

National Library of Medicine. (2024). *Medline Plus: Sickle cell disease.* https://medlineplus.gov/genetics/condition/sickle-cell-disease

National Organization for Rare Disorders. (2017). *Glucose-6-dehydrogenase deficiency.* https://rarediseases.org/rare-diseases/glucose-6-phosphate-dehydrogenase-deficiency/#disease-overview-main

National Organization for Rare Disorders. (2024). *Neonatal cholestasis.*https://rarediseases.org/rare-diseases/idiopathic-neonatal-hepatitis/#complete-report

Nellenbach, K. A., Nandi, S., Kyu, A., Sivadanam, S., Guzzetta, N. A., & Brown, A. C. (2020). Comparison of neonatal and adult fibrin clot properties between porcine and human plasma. *Anesthesiology, 132*(5), 1091–1101. https://doi.org/10.1097/ALN.0000000000003165

Nielsen, S. C. A., & Boyd, S. D. (2022). B cell development. In R. A. Polin, S. H. Abman, D. H. Rowitch, W. E. Benitz, & W. W. Fox (Eds.), *Fetal and neonatal physiology* (6th ed., pp. 1200–1206). Saunders.

Norton, T., Newberry, D., & Jnah, A. (2020). Neonatal alloimmune thrombocytopenia: A concise review. *Advances in Neonatal Care, 21*(2), 115–121. https://doi.org/10.1097/ANC.0000000000000775

O'Connell, A. E., Rivers, A. E., & Slayton, W. B. (2021). The development of the human immune system. In P. A. de Alarcon, E. J. Werner, R. D. Christensen, & M. C. Sola-Visner (Eds.), *Neonatal hematology: Pathogenesis, diagnosis, and management of hematologic problems* (3rd ed., pp. 24–41). Cambridge University Press.

Ostilla, L., Knopoff, K., Myers, P., & Morocco, P. (2024). Disorders of coagulation in the newborn. *NeoReviews, 25*(11), e694–e709. https://doi.org/10.1542/neo.25-11-e694

Owusu-Ansah, A., Letterio, J., & Ahuja, S. P. (2025). Red blood cell disorders in the fetus and neonate. In R. J. Martin & A. A. Fanaroff (Eds.), *Fanaroff and Martin's neonatal-perinatal medicine: Diseases of the fetus and infant* (pp. 5162–5262). Elsevier.

Palis, J., & Segel, G. B. (2021). Hematology of the fetus and newborn. In K. Kaushansky, M. A. Lichtman, J. T. Prchal, M. Levi, L. J. Burns, & D. Lynch (Eds.), *Williams hematology* (10th ed., pp. 93–110). McGraw Hill Education.

Pateva, I., Huerta Urrutia, V. Y., Letterio, J., & Ajuja, S. P. (2025). White blood cells and immune disorders. In R. J. Martin & A. A. Fanaroff (Eds.), *Fanaroff and Martin's neonatal-perinatal medicine: Diseases of the fetus and infant* (pp. 5262–5302). Elsevier.

Petit, F., & Boussion, S. (2023). Thrombocytopenia absent radius syndrome. In M. P. Adam, J. Feldman, G. M. Mirzaa, R. A. Pagon, S. A. Wallace, & A. Amemiya (Eds.), *GeneReviews*. University of Washington, Seattle. https://www.ncbi.nlm.nih.gov/books/NBK23758/

Rai, P., Mamcarz, E. K., & Hankins, J. S. (2021). Newborn genetic screening for blood disorders. In P. A. de Alarcon, E. J. Werner, R. D. Christensen, & M. C. Sola-Visner, *Neonatal hematology: Pathogenesis, diagnosis, and management of hematologic problems* (3rd ed., pp. 93–112). Cambridge University Press.

Rees, D. C., Brousse, V. A. M., & Brewin, J. N. (2022). Determinants of severity in sickle cell disease. *Blood Reviews, 56*, 100983. https://doi.org/10.1016/j.blre.2022.100983

Rosenkrantz, T. S., & Oh, W. (2021). Polycythemia and hyperviscosity in the newborn. In P. A. de Alarcon, E. J. Werner, R. D. Christensen, & M. C. Sola-Visner (Eds.), *Neonatal hematology: Pathogenesis, diagnosis, and management of hematologic problems* (3rd ed., pp. 184–200). Cambridge University Press.

Ross, M. E., Emery, A. P., de Alarcón, P. A., & Watchko, J. F. (2021). Hemolytic disease of the fetus and newborn. In P. A. de Alarcon, E. J. Werner, R. D. Christensen, & M. C. Sola-Visner (Eds.), *Neonatal hematology: Pathogenesis, diagnosis, and management of hematologic problems* (3rd ed., pp. 132–153). Cambridge University Press.

Sankar, M. J., Chandrasekaran, A., Kumar, P., Thukral, A., Agarwal, R., & Paul, V. K. (2016). Vitamin K prophylaxis for prevention of vitamin K deficiency bleeding: A systematic review. *Journal of Perinatology: Official Journal of the California Perinatal Association, 36*(Suppl. 1), S29–S35. https://doi.org/10.1038/jp.2016.30

Saxonhouse, M. A., & Hinson, A. P. (2024). Neonatal bleeding and thrombotic disorders. In C. A. Gleason & T. Sawyer (Eds.), *Avery's diseases of the newborn* (11th ed., pp. 965–981). Elsevier.

Schibler, K. R., & Christensen, R. D. (2021). Eosinophils and neutrophils. In P. A. de Alarcon, E. J. Werner, R. D. Christensen, & M. C. Sola-Visner (Eds.), *Neonatal hematology: Pathogenesis, diagnosis, and management of hematologic problems* (3rd ed., pp. 261–277). Cambridge University Press.

Shlomai, N. O., Friedman, S. E., & Gielchinsky, Y. (2025). Multiple gestation: Fetal and maternal conditions. In R. J. Martin & A. A. Fanaroff (Eds.), *Fanaroff and Martin's neonatal-perinatal medicine: Diseases of the fetus and infant* (12th ed., pp. 1305–1344). Elsevier.

Sommer, A., & Perdiguero, E. G. (2024). Extraembryonic hematopoietic lineages—to macrophages and beyond. *Experimental Hematology, 136*, 104285. https://doi.org/10.1016/j.exphem.2024.104285

Stoll, B. J., & Hansen, N. (2003). Infections in VLBW infants: Studies from the NICHD neonatal research network. *Seminars in Perinatology, 27*(4), 293–301. https://doi.org/10.1016/S0146-0005(03)00046-6

Thomas, D. B., & Yoffey, J. M. (1962). Human foetal haemopoiesis. I. The cellular composition of foetal blood. *British Journal of Haematology, 8*(3), 290–295. https://doi.org/10.1111/j.1365-2141.1962.tb06523.x

Tsao, P., Teng, R., Chou, H., & Tsou, K. (2002). The thrombopoietin level in the cord blood in premature infants born to mothers with pregnancy-induced hypertension. *Biology of the Neonate, 82*(4), 217–221. https://doi.org/10.1159/000065888

van der Kaay, D. C. M., Wasserman, J. D., & Palmert, M. R. (2016). Management of neonates born to mothers with Graves' disease. *Pediatrics,* 137(4), 1–10. https://doi.org/10.1542/peds.2015-1878

Werner, E. J., Chescheir, N. C., & Fisher, R. G. (2021). Disorders of the fetomaternal unit. In P. A. de Alarcon, E. J. Werner, R. D. Christensen, & M. C. Sola-Visner, *Neonatal hematology: Pathogenesis, diagnosis, and management of hematologic problems* (3rd ed., pp. 401–438). Cambridge University Press.

Weyand, A. C., & Flood, V. H. (2021). Von Willebrand disease: Current status of diagnosis and management. *Hematology/Oncology Clinics of North America, 35*(6), 1085–1101. https://doi.org/10.1016/j.hoc.2021.07.004

Will, A., Henderson, C. A., Jnah, A. J., & Newberry, D. (2017). Hereditary spherocytosis in the neonatal period: A case report. *Neonatal Network, 36*(5), 280–288. https://doi.org/10.1891/0730-0832.36.5.280

8

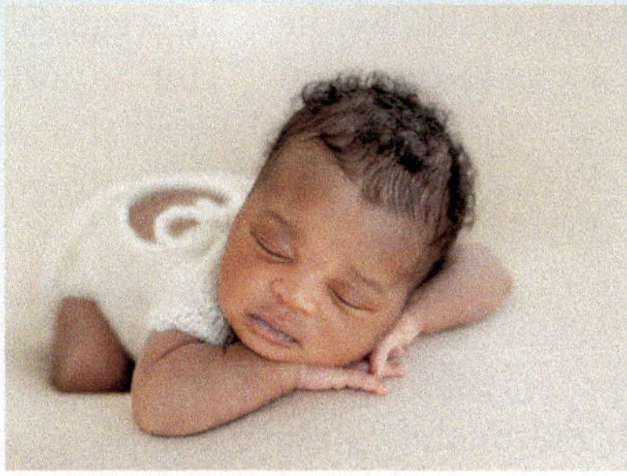

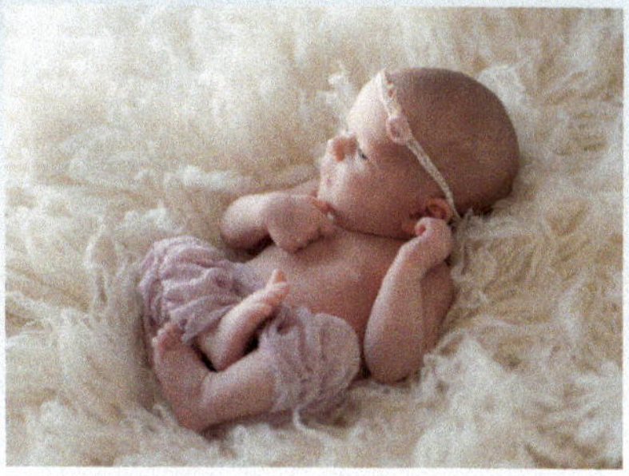

THE RENAL SYSTEM

Colleen R. Moss, Amy Williford, and Amy J. Jnah

LEARNING OBJECTIVES

After completing this chapter, the reader should be able to:

- Understand normal renal organ development.
- Analyze the physiologic function of the fetal and neonatal kidney and bladder.
- Discuss common inherited disorders and their effect on fetal and neonatal renal system development and function.
- Identify health conditions in XX pregnant patients that have a potential impact on fetal and postnatal renal system development and function.
- Evaluate common disorders that affect the renal system and their implications across the life span.

INTRODUCTION

Morphologic and physiologic development of the renal system involves complex, genetically influenced adaptations that span from early gestation to postnatal life. Once functional, the kidneys modulate ion concentrations, hormone levels, and the excretion of metabolic waste products as well as blood pressure, the composition of blood, and blood volume. Therefore, appropriate renal function is critical to maintaining physiologic homeostasis. A lack of architectural precision during fetal development, or that which occurs secondary to premature birth, as well as epigenetic errors, may give rise to renal dysfunction. Problems, including acute kidney injury (AKI) and electrolyte imbalances, are commonly observed among premature and critically ill newborns and require astute identification, diagnosis, and timely treatment by advanced practice clinicians. This is essential to prevent long-term renal damage. Understanding normal morphologic development and physiologic function of the fetal and neonatal kidney helps clinicians associate normal function with renal maladaptation.

TIMELINE OF ORGAN DEVELOPMENT

The renal system consists of the kidneys, bladder, ureters, and urethra. Each structure arises from either the pronephros, mesonephros, or metanephros and is explained in linear progression from early embryonic development through maturation. Normal development of the renal system is contingent upon the activity of numerous genes, transcription factors, and other molecules and proteins. Any disruption to this normal process can impede development and cause anomalies to form at the kidneys or urinary tract.

Embryonic Period

Kidneys. The renal system arises from the intermediate mesenchyme, which is located at the dorsal wall of the embryo (Torchia & Persaud, 2025). Renal development is commonly organized into three phases known as the *pronephros, mesonephros*, and *metanephros*.

The pronephros phase begins and ends during week 4 of gestation (Torchia & Persaud, 2025). It gives rise to balls of epithelial tubular cells, or nephrotomes, which drain into the primary nephric duct ("Wolffian duct").

The nephrotomes make contact with the cloaca by the end of week 4 of gestation and, in a caudo-cephalad direction, form primitive canals and then regress (Figure 8.1; Torchia & Persaud, 2025).

The mesonephros appears next, during week 5 of gestation, and will ultimately become the mature kidney (Torchia & Persaud, 2025). The mesonephric ducts stretch (elongate), and during this process undergo a process of S-looping (Figure 8.2). This ultimately gives rise to four critical structures: the (a) glomeruli, (b) mesonephric tubules, (c) mesonephric ducts, and (d) cloaca (Torchia & Persaud, 2025). The primitive glomeruli and Bowman's capsule sit at the proximal end of the S-loop, whereas the Wolffian duct resides at its distal end (Vogt, 2025). This early and programmed shaping of the nephron permits primitive renal function, which typically commences after day 23 of gestation, just after early cardiac contractions (heart beats) begin.

Next, hypertrophy of the caudal end of the mesonephric duct permits the genesis of the ureteric bud (Figure 8.3). The ureteric bud grows laterally, toward the mesenchyme, and ultimately invades and embeds itself within the mesenchyme (the primitive renal parenchyma, or kidney). Once embedded, the ureteric bud undergoes a process of branching, which forms the collecting system and major and minor calyces (Figure 8.4). Proximal ends of the metanephric tubules approximate with the existing glomeruli and the tube differentiates into its adult structures: the (a) proximal tubule, (b) loop of Henle (LOH), (c) distal convoluted tubule (DCT), and (d) collecting duct (Torchia & Persaud, 2025). In addition, some metanephric mesenchyme cells undergo mesenchymal-to-epithelial conversion and form the epithelial lining of the nephron (Torchia & Persaud, 2025; Scott et al., 2020). It is within week 8 of gestation that nephrons form, and a process of structural elongation and functional maturation begins.

Ureters and Bladder. The ureters and bladder develop between weeks 8 and 12 of gestation (Vogt, 2025). First, the cloaca is partitioned by the urorectal septum. The anterior portion of the cloaca becomes the urogenital sinus, and the posterior portion becomes the anorectal canal. The urogenital sinus then goes on to differentiate into the primitive bladder and membranous urethra (males) or vestibule for the vagina (females). Finally, urine formation and excretion begin between weeks 6 and 10 of gestation (Torchia & Persaud, 2025; Schoenwolf et al., 2021).

Fetal Period

Kidneys. The fetal period of development marks a period of vertical ascent and shift in blood supply for each kidney; failed ascent leads to pelvic (ectopic) kidney formation. These two structures, once nestled within the pelvis and receiving nourishment from the common iliac arteries, migrate upward and outward from one another as a result of normal embryonic growth toward the thoracolumbar region. Once the migration is finished, each kidney resides on either side of the spine and receives its blood supply from a dedicated renal artery. Each renal artery is a branch off the abdominal aorta (Torchia & Persaud, 2025).

Concurrent with migration, glomerular proliferation occurs. The nephrons' glomerular filtration barrier (GFB), glomeruli, and glomerular vasculature develop centrifugally, beginning with the juxtamedullary glomeruli and with progressive maturation of the cortical glomeruli. In other words, the superficial cortical nephrons are the newest nephrons, and the deeper juxtamedullary nephrons are more mature. Glomerular filtration commences during week 9 of gestation, and between weeks 10 through 18 of gestation, significant and steady proliferation occurs. Weeks 19 through 36 of gestation involve an exponential increase in the number of glomeruli, as the fetus begins to prepare for the demands of extrauterine life (Torchia & Persaud, 2025). Nephrogenesis is considered complete at week 34 of gestation (Vogt, 2025).

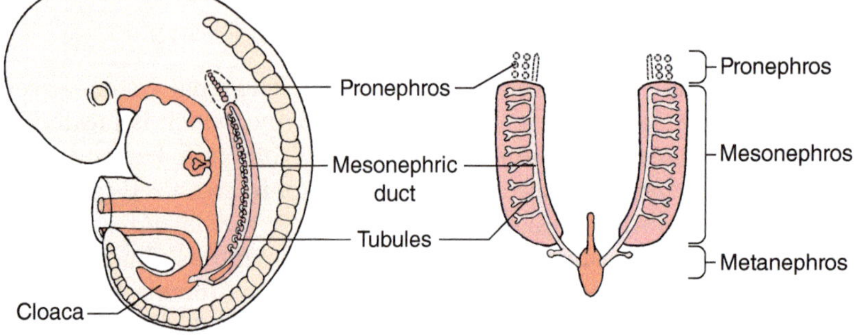

Figure 8.1 Regression of the pronephros during week 4 of gestation.

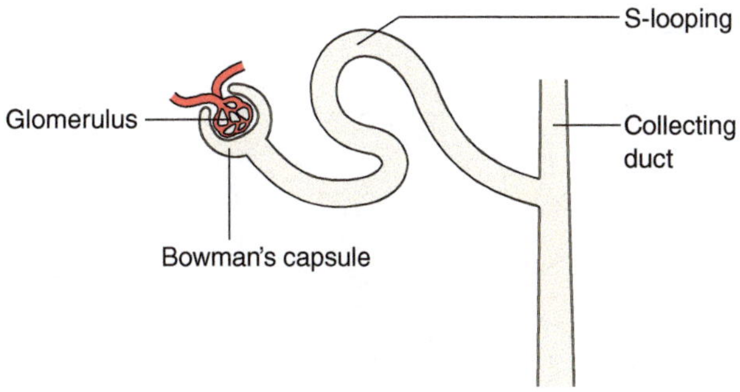

Figure 8.2 S-looping of primitive kidney.

Ureters and Bladder. The end of the fetal period of development (week 8 of gestation) through week 12 of gestation involves continued development and differentiation of the cloaca. In addition, the anatomic development of other portions of the urogenital system occurs. The caudal end of the mesonephric duct melds into the nearby wall of the bladder and becomes a portion of connective tissue within the trigone, or triangular region, of the bladder (Torchia & Persaud, 2025). The caudal portions of the left and right ureters begin to migrate down and into the developing urinary bladder, giving rise to two of three trigone regions. Shortly thereafter, an opening appears, one at each vertex of the inverted triangle. The right and left upper vertices (openings) permit the innervation of the corresponding ureter, while the third opening communicates with the urethra. Once the ureter innervates with the trigone, a muscular band, or internal urethral sphincter, encircles this opening.

During weeks 13 to 17 of gestation, the urinary bladder epithelium undergoes thickening and transforms from two layers of cuboidal epithelial cells into a trilayered urothelium. The urothelium expresses the growth factor sonic hedgehog (SHH), which is likely the signal that stimulates mesenchymal proliferation and smooth muscle differentiation in the urinary bladder (Tasian et al., 2010). Throughout the rest of fetal development, the bladder differentiates into a structure comprising three linings. The innermost mucosal layer of the bladder is affixed with the identical epithelium as each ureter. When empty, this mucosa folds in a rugated, or accordionlike, fashion, which allows for later expansion secondary to the accumulation of urine. The middle layer of the bladder is affixed with connective and elastic tissue. The outermost layer becomes the muscular layer of the bladder, responsible for expelling urine from the bladder.

Neonatal Period

Nephrogenesis is considered complete by week 34 of gestation, as greater than 80% of nephrons have formed (Vogt, 2025). Once mature, each healthy kidney contains between 800,000 and 2 million nephrons, although variability is reported and may occur as a result of altered epigenetic programming, the number of nephron progenitors present during nephrogenesis, and prematurity (Torchia & Persaud, 2025; Vogt, 2025). In fact,

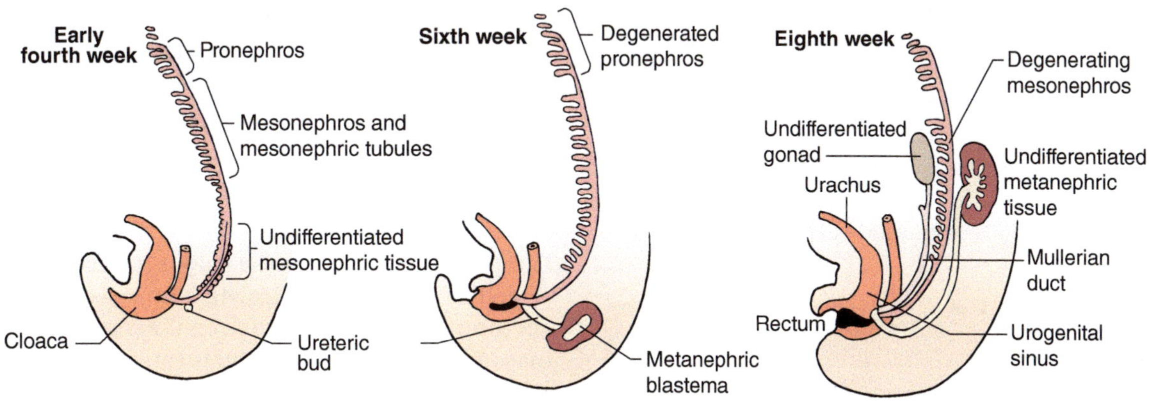

Figure 8.3 Early kidney development. The pronephros and mesonephros regress by the time the metanephros is well-developed. ***Source:*** Adapted from Scott, R. P., Maezawa, Y., Kreidberg, J., & Quaggin, S. E. (2020). Embryology of the kidney. In A.S.L. Yu, G. M. Chertow, V. A. Luyckx, P. A. Marsden, K. Shorecki, & M. W. Taal (Eds.), *Brenner and Rector's the kidney* (11th ed., pp. 2–37). Elsevier.

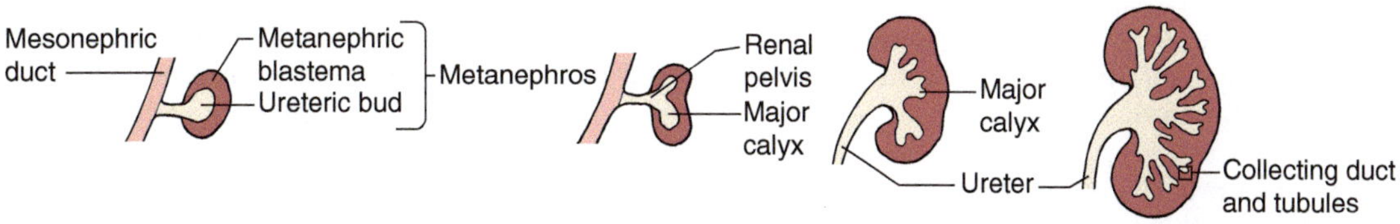

Figure 8.4 Ureteric bud branching. The ureteric bud gives rise to the ureter, major calyx, minor calyx, and collecting system.

premature infants born prior to week 36 of gestation undergo active extrauterine nephrogenesis. This continued development, which occurs due to glomerular hypertrophy and renal tubular elongation (not by postnatal nephrogenesis), is influenced by the fetal and/or maternal factors that initiated the premature birth, maintenance of adequate renal blood flow and oxygenation, and toxic exposure to medications (Kliegman et al., 2025).

DEVELOPMENTAL PHYSIOLOGY

The kidneys are one of the most astute organ systems, intricately equipped to modulate fluid, electrolyte, and acid–base homeostasis in the face of minimal to severe pathological threats. In addition, the renal vascular system participates in the modulation of arterial blood pressure through the secretion of various vasoregulators. In order to understand the core concepts related to fetal and neonatal renal physiology discussed in this section of the chapter, several core terms are presented in Table 8.1.

Renal Blood Flow

Blood flow to the kidneys occurs by way of the afferent arteriole (Figure 8.5). Fetal blood flow to the kidney is low (3%–5% of cardiac output) because of high renal vascular resistance caused by high renin–angiotensin–aldosterone activity, low perfusion pressure, and the diversion of 65% of fetal cardiac output to the placenta (Solhaug & Jose, 2022). This preferential blood-flow pattern explains why most developing organ systems acclimate to a persistent state of increased vascular resistance in utero. With maturation during gestation and after birth, renal vascular resistance decreases, most likely due to an increase in the number of glomeruli and increased renin–angiotensin–aldosterone system (RAAS) activity, as well as increases in renal blood flow. By day 7 of life, renal blood flow accounts for 10% of cardiac output. By age 2, renal blood flow is commensurate with adult levels, accounting for 25% of cardiac output (Vogt, 2025).

TABLE 8.1 Core Terminology

Term	Definition
Glomerular filtration	Filtration of plasma from the glomerulus into the Bowman's capsule.
Tubular reabsorption	Reabsorption of solute from the tubular lumen back into the peritubular capillaries. This occurs by simple, facilitated, or active transport.
Tubular secretion	Movement of solute from the peritubular capillaries into the tubular lumen.

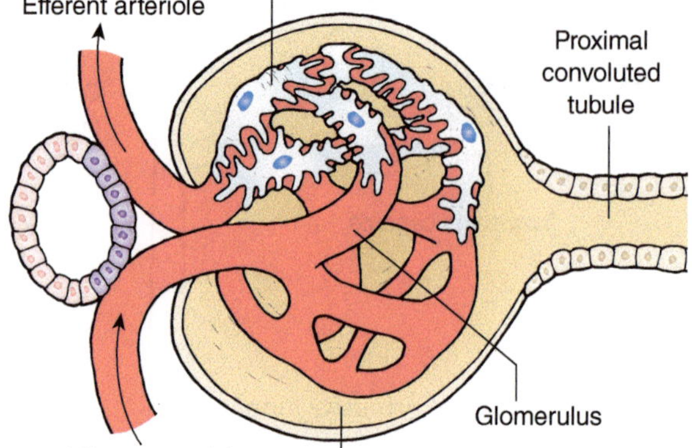

Figure 8.5 Renal blood flow (afferent and efferent arterioles). Note direction of blood flow: Afferent arterioles carry blood into the glomerulus, and blood flows out of the glomerulus through the efferent arterioles.

Postnatally, renal blood flow steadily increases through the second year of life (Vogt, 2025). Renal blood flow is approximately 4% to 6% of total cardiac output within the first 12 hours and increases to 8% to 10% of cardiac output by the first week of life (Nada et al., 2017; Vogt, 2025). This phenomenon is the result of decreased perfusion pressure due to increased renal vascular resistance, which is initially low in the newborn period and increases steadily over the first 2 years of life. In fact, high renal vascular resistance accounts for the decreased GFR after birth and may affect the newborn's ability to respond to any untoward events, such as hypoxic–ischemic insults, that may precede AKI and/or renal failure. By 2 years of age, renal blood flow reaches the adult status of about 20% to 25% of cardiac output (Nada et al., 2017).

Glomerular Filtration

The placenta serves as the major source of filtration, as well as fluid and electrolyte homeostasis, for the developing fetus, offering the renal system a margin for anatomic and functional maturation throughout the first 16 weeks of gestation. Early glomerular filtration commences at approximately 8 weeks of gestation and continues to advance throughout fetal and postnatal development (Matsell & Hiatt, 2017; Rosenblum et al., 2017). Several factors influence the maturation of the glomerular filtration rate (GFR), including ongoing anatomic kidney maturation and expansion of the glomerular bed, increasing fetal body mass index, increasing hydrostatic pressure at the glomerulus, increasing renal blood flow, and functional integration of vasoregulators (Kliegman et al., 2025). Risk factors for alterations in normal maturation of GFR include placental insufficiency; fetal intrauterine exposure to environmental toxins;

dietary protein restriction in XX pregnant patients; and structural anomalies, including urinary tract obstruction (Guignard & Iacobelli, 2022).

Expansion of glomerular surface area offers a wider capillary bed for glomerular filtration and urine formation. Mean arterial pressure increases as the fetus matures, which increases glomerular capillary hydrostatic pressure. This process, in synergy with increasing renal blood flow, increases the pressure gradient at the glomerulus and facilitates increasing filtration. In the newborn, adequate glomerular filtration is essential for body fluid homeostasis, electrolyte homeostasis, and elimination of drugs (Guignard & Iacobelli, 2022). Postnatal GFR is estimated at 15 mL/min/1.73 m^2 to 25 mL/min/1.73 m^2 among term infants (Abitbol et al., 2016; Vogt, 2025). Adult renal function of GFR of 110 to 120 mL/min/1.73 m^2 to 120 mL/min/1.73 m^2 is achieved by approximately 2 years of age in the healthy infant and directly determined by the maturation and growth of the kidney based on the increasing surface area of the glomeruli present at birth (Abitbol et al., 2016; Alpern et al., 2013; Matsell & Hiatt, 2017; Vogt, 2025).

Factors that may impair or delay postnatal functional maturation of glomerular filtration include fetal exposure to hypertensive drugs and prostaglandin inhibitors, perinatal hypoxemia and asphyxia, and mechanical ventilation. Mothers with hypertensive disorders may require treatment with angiontensin-converting enzyme (ACE) inhibitors, and mothers in preterm labor may receive prostaglandin synthesis inhibitors; these drugs inhibit vasodilation at the afferent arteriole (Guignard & Iacobelli, 2022). Perinatal hypoxemia is associated with upregulated RAAS activity, which can decrease GFR (Alpern et al., 2013). Mechanical ventilation can decrease venous return and bring about low cardiac output, thus decreasing renal blood flow and GFR (Guignard & Iacobelli, 2022).

CLINICAL APPLICATION. It is important to recognize that GFR is currently measured by creatinine clearance, *the most consistent marker of GFR in the fetus and neonate* (Kastl, 2017). Around 20 weeks of gestation, creatinine clearance is estimated to be less than 1 mL/min, but with rapid nephrogenesis it increases to 4 to 5 mL/min at term and doubles to 8 to 10 mL/min by 2 weeks of postnatal age (Guignard & Iacobelli, 2022). The best way to assess renal function/creatinine clearance is by ordering a basic metabolic panel or comprehensive metabolic panel. These tests will provide both a blood urea nitrogen level and creatinine level, which can be considered along with the infant's renal output and other morbidities that may affect renal function. In some circumstances (e.g., pharmacologic treatment of a patent ductus arteriosus, treatment of sepsis with an aminoglycoside), an elevated creatinine level may prompt cessation of treatment or the use of alternative (e.g., cephalosporin) pharmacologic agents that are less renal toxic.

Renal Vasoregulators

Vaso-regulatory factors play an important role in *regulating* GFR both during fetal development and postnatally. Major vasoactive factors include nitric oxide (NO), prostaglandins, atrial natriuretic peptide (ANP), the sympathetic nervous system, catecholamines, and the RAAS (Solhaug & Jose, 2022). These factors either increase or decrease GFR, and often work to modulate the effects of one another to preserve homeostatic renal function.

Nitric Oxide. NO is a potent vasodilator and is derived from endothelium in the early embryonic kidney, especially in the glomeruli and intrarenal capillaries (Vogt, 2025). NO inhibits the strong vasoconstrictive effects of angiotensin II in the fetal kidney and promotes blood flow through smooth muscle relaxation (Solhaug & Jose, 2022).

Prostaglandins. Prostaglandins affect both renal development and function. Recent studies indicate that prostaglandins are important in the normal development of the kidneys by maintaining cyclooxygenase activity to prevent severe renal anomalies. Similar to NO, prostaglandins are potent vasodilators. They serve to inhibit the strong vasoconstrictive effects of angiotensin II and decrease afferent (incoming) arteriolar tone through vasodilation, thus improving blood flow into the glomerulus (Matsell & Hiatt, 2017).

Atrial Natriuretic Peptide. ANP is a vasoactive hormone produced in the atria and ventricles of the heart in response to stretching associated with fluid overload. ANP may help regulate GFR by dilating the afferent arterioles and constricting the efferent arterioles simultaneously (Partin et al., 2021). ANP levels are highest during fetal development and decrease to adult levels within the first few weeks after birth. Although ANP has important vascular and renal effects in mature kidneys, it does not increase renal blood flow in the newborn period (Solhaug & Jose, 2022).

Endothelin. Endothelin is a peptide produced by the vascular epithelium. Peptide levels increase throughout fetal development. Endothelin functions to increase efferent (outgoing) arteriolar tone through vasoconstriction, thus improving blood flow to the glomerulus (Solhaug & Jose, 2022).

Renin-Angiotensin-Aldosterone System. The RAAS is a negative feedback hormonal system in the human body that regulates many biologic processes, including cell growth and remodeling, blood pressure, and fluid and electrolyte homeostasis. The vasculature, kidneys, liver, heart, lungs, brain, and adrenal glands orchestrate the actions of the RAAS. Decreased glomerular flow, in combination with decreased blood pressure, activates the RAAS (Goyal & Banerjee, 2020). The RAAS serves a key role in maintaining systemic blood pressure during fetal and postnatal development by regulating systemic and renal vascular tone (resistance within the vessels); mechanisms that regulate on-and-off switching of this system are poorly understood (Figure 8.6; Sparks et al., 2014).

Juxtaglomerular (JG) cells, located within the afferent arteriole in the glomerulus, are the main source for the storage and release of renin. Any decrease in pressure to the afferent arteriole may decrease glomerular filtration and sodium chloride concentrations in the distal tubules, triggering the release of renin by the JG cells. Renin is the highly sensitive baroreceptor secreted by the JG cells in response to alterations in blood pressure or sodium chloride levels. It is considered the rate-limiting step of the RAAS and is secreted as early as week 2 of gestation (Sparks et al., 2014). Initially, renin is found scattered along the intralobular artery and afferent arterioles. Throughout gestational development and into the postnatal period, renin release is narrowed to only the terminal lip of the afferent arteriole.

Events that comprise the RAAS response to hypotension include the following: Renin is secreted at the afferent arteriole and acts on circulating angiotensinogen to cleave angiotensin I (Figure 8.6; Klabunde, 2012). Next, angiotensin I traverses the portal and cardiovascular systems in order to reach the pulmonary circuit. Here, ACE, found mainly within the pulmonary vascular epithelium, cleaves two amino acids from angiotensin I, converting it into angiotensin II (Klabunde, 2012). Angiotensin II is the biologically active hormone produced by the RAAS and initiates three key processes: (a) an increase in vascular resistance; (b) water and solute reabsorption in the nephron; and (c) the release of vasopressin, which promotes vascular retention of fluid (Sands et al., 2020).

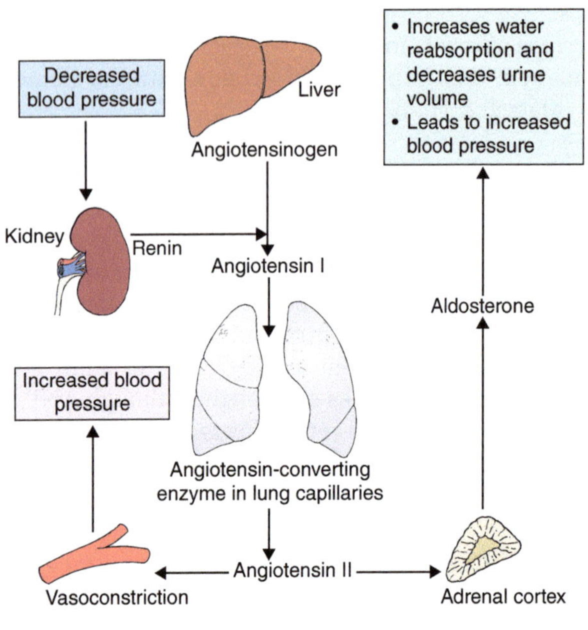

Figure 8.6 Renin-angiotensin-aldosterone system. The outcome of the activation of RAAS is water and sodium retention, leading to increased blood pressure.

Increased vascular resistance (vasopressive effects) occurs by way of specialized receptors (AGTR1 and AGTR2) that transmit a vaso-stimulating effect at the efferent arteriole. As a result, renal blood flow increases. Water and solute reabsorption occur through two pathways: (a) aldosterone release and (b) vasopressin release. Aldosterone release occurs secondary to stimulation of the adrenal cortex. Aldosterone facilitates reabsorption of sodium and water at the distal convoluting tubules and the cortical collecting ducts, thereby increasing circulating blood volume and blood pressure (Klabunde, 2012). Vasopressin (antidiuretic hormone [ADH]) release occurs secondary to stimulation of the posterior pituitary gland. Circulating ADH increases solute-free water reabsorption through the DCTs and collecting ducts and increases systemic blood pressure (Klabunde, 2012; Sands et al., 2020). Additional effects of ADH include increased sodium reabsorption and potassium excretion, increased prostaglandin synthesis, and increased adrenocorticotropic hormone secretion; this serves to increase fluid volume and renal blood flow (Partin et al., 2021).

Prenatal factors that affect RAAS function include malnutrition in XX pregnant patients and placental insufficiency; both conditions are regarded as perinatal shocks (see Chapter 1) and may negatively impact fetal programming and thereby contribute to the development of latent chronic disease (Alexander et al., 2015). Postnatally, any issue that decreases blood flow to the glomeruli, such as a decrease in systemic blood pressure, renal artery stenosis, or a decrease in filtrate sodium chloride concentration, may implicate orderly RAAS function (Klabunde, 2012).

Acid–Base Homeostasis

The fetal kidney is capable of reabsorbing filtered bicarbonate, delivered by way of the placenta. However, the fetal kidney is less capable of generating bicarbonate. As such, acid–base regulation is immature during early fetal development (and handled by way of the placenta) and increases throughout gestation. The synthesis of bicarbonate requires the reciprocal excretion of acid and ammonia and a mature, elongated proximal tubule (Azhibekov et al., 2022).

Postnatally, bicarbonate is a critical component of acid-based homeostasis. Acute changes to the pH call on the carbonic–anhydrase buffering system to exchange hydrogen ions (H^+) and potassium (K^+). Acidemia provokes H^+ influx into the cell, buffered primarily by bone apatite. Alkalemia prompts an efflux of H^+ from the cell in exchange for K^+. Long-term acid–base compensation relies on balanced intake and excretion of acid, or a balance of carbon dioxide (CO_2) and bicarbonate. Acid intake occurs through the production of CO_2 (volatile acid) and metabolic acids, as well as the ingestion of acids through enteral feedings (nonvolatile acids; Curtis, 2025). Acid–base homeostasis (long-term) occurs through chemical buffering, which facilitates the "blowing off" of CO_2 through respiration and renal reabsorption, excretion, and supplemental generation of bicarbonate.

Buffer System Modulation. Buffers are substances that can minimize changes in pH when acid or base is added to the system. Intracellular buffers facilitate entry of H^+ into the cell and include hemoglobin, organic phosphates, and bone apatite. Bone apatite is responsible for nearly 50% of all intracellular buffering among premature infants, and in some cases may explain poor linear growth among infants with frequent acid–base imbalance. Extracellular buffers include phosphates, plasma proteins, and the bicarbonate–carbonic acid system, the most important extracellular buffer system (Azhibekov et al., 2022; Curtis, 2025).

Carbonic acid buffering primarily implicates the respiratory system. An increase in H^+ levels prompt its binding with bicarbonate, facilitated by the enzyme carbonic anhydrase and the formation of carbonic acid. The molecules thereby cross the blood–brain barrier, where the hydrogen ions disassociate and stimulate chemoreceptors. Because the majority of the daily acid load consists of volatile acids, this buffering system is critically important to acid–base homeostasis and is utilized to normalize acute acid–base imbalances.

Bicarbonate buffering in the kidneys facilitates modulation of bicarbonate reabsorption, excretion, and new production. The two primary regions that acidify the urine are the proximal tubule and thick ascending LOH. This buffering system is slower compared to the bicarbonate–carbonic acid system and participates in long-term acid–base compensation (Curtis, 2025).

Respiratory Modulation. Respiratory modulation of acid–base balance involves the elimination of CO_2 (volatile acid). This is modulated by alveolar ventilation, which adjusts to ensure appropriate elimination of CO_2. This process is regulated by the effect of H^+ and CO_2 on central and peripheral chemoreceptors, located within the medulla oblongata of the brain. Central chemoreceptors regulate respiration at the level of the brainstem. Increased partial pressure of carbon dioxide, or hypercarbia, causes an increase in CO_2 influx into the cerebrospinal fluid (CSF). Once immersed within the CSF, CO_2 combines with water and forms carbonic acid (Figure 8.7). The H^+ at the ends of the carbonic acid molecule disassociate. This increase in H^+ upregulates the central chemoreceptors. Simultaneously, the hypercarbic state lowers the pH, which alerts peripheral chemoreceptors, located within the aortic arch. The net result is an increase in the respiratory rate, which redirects the pH toward homeostasis (Figure 8.8).

Renal Modulation. Renal modulation of acid–base balance involves permissive excretion of normal daily acid load, with the prevention of excessive bicarbonate losses into the urine. The majority of bicarbonate (80%) is reabsorbed within the proximal tubule and the remainder is primarily reabsorbed within the thick ascending LOH (10%) and more distal segments (10%; Azhibekov et al., 2022). Bicarbonate reabsorption increases during acidic states and under the influence of adrenergic agonists and angiotensin II as well as parathyroid hormone. Reabsorption decreases during alkaline states (Curtis, 2025).

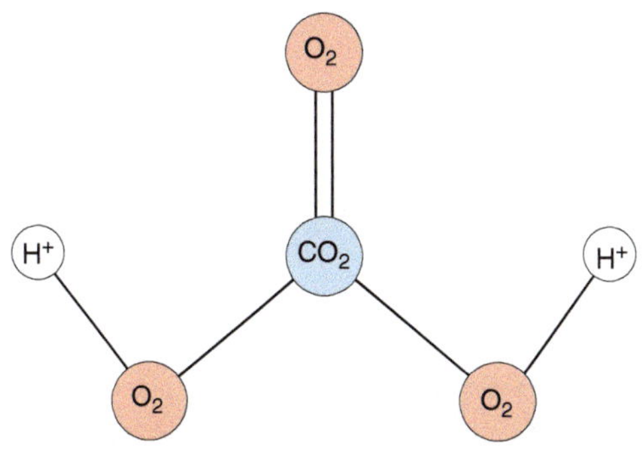

Figure 8.7 Carbonic acid molecule.

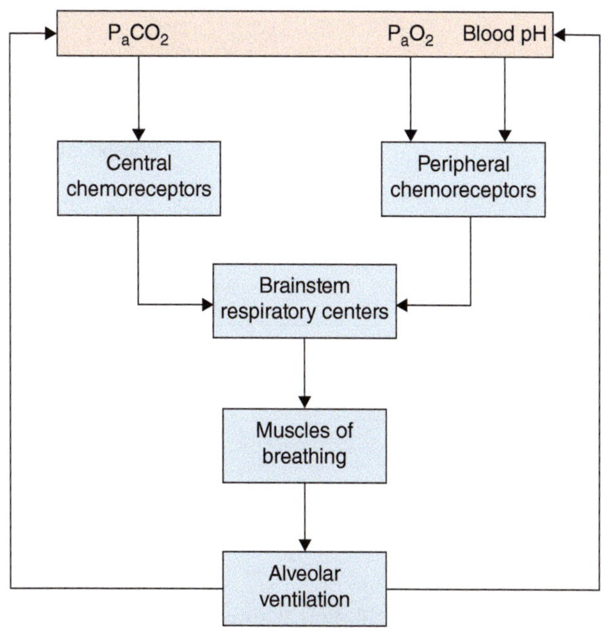

Figure 8.8 The role of central and peripheral chemoreceptors on acid–base balance.

In addition, the kidneys are responsible for the production of new bicarbonate. The production of new bicarbonate occurs through the exchange of acid (H^+ ions) for bicarbonate; the amount of acid excreted into the urine typically equals the amount of new bicarbonate generated by the kidneys. However, during illness or other pathological states, the kidneys may be tasked with generating additional bicarbonate to compensate for acid load. In these circumstances, net acid and ammonium excretion increases to permit more rapid cleavage of bicarbonate.

Tubular Regulation of Solutes Within the Nephron

The basic functions of the tubular system include reabsorption (transport of substances from the lumen to the blood), secretion (transport of substances from blood to the lumen), and transport of solute through the nephron and into the ureters for excretion as urine (Figure 8.9). Substances can follow one of two pathways: (a) transcellular (across the lumen and cell membrane) or (b) paracellular (between cells). The proximal duct, LOH, distal tubules, and collecting ducts primarily serve to reabsorb solutes from glomerular filtration, secrete other ions, concentrate and dilute urine, and maintain fluid and electrolyte homeostasis. Multiple pathways, genes, pumps, and transcriptors facilitate this process; a discussion of each is beyond the scope of this textbook. Factors that influence the movement of water and major substrates are described in the following section of this chapter.

Tubular Transport of Solutes Within the Nephron

Proximal Convoluting Tubule. The proximal convoluting tubule (PCT) consists of two parts, the pars convoluta and the pars recta, spread over three segments (Baum, 2017). The PCT consists of a brush border with tight cell junctions, a network of mitochondria, and low

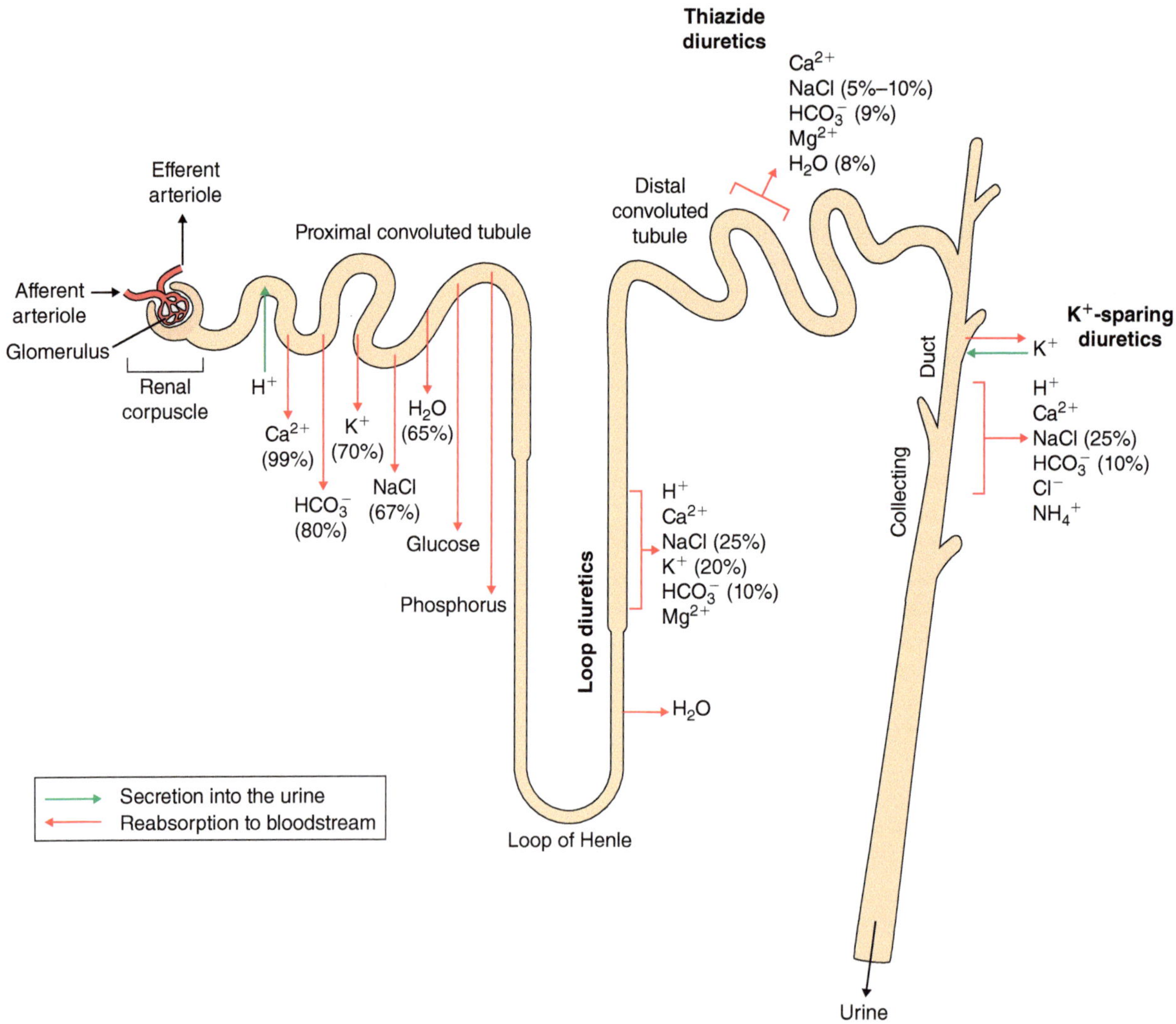

Figure 8.9 Movement of solute within the nephron.

Note: This diagram should be used to establish a conceptual understanding of the movement of solute in the nephron. Percentage of reabsorption of solute may vary across the literature. The site of action of common diuretics is included to enhance the learning process.

Ca^2, calcium ion; Cl^-, chloride ion; H^+, hydrogen ion; HCO_3, bicarbonate ion; K^+, potassium ion; Mg^{2+}, magnesium ion; NH_4^+, ammonium ion.

Image Credit: Mya Jnah.

transepithelial cell resistance that allows ample paracellular transport. For that reason, the PCT is often referred to as a *leaky epithelium* (Baum, 2022). Approximately 60% of water, sodium (67%), potassium (70%), bicarbonate (80%), chloride (65%), calcium (>90%), phosphate (85%), and 100% of filtered glucose and amino acids are reabsorbed as the filtrate passes through the proximal tubule (Gattineni & Baum, 2015; Johnson et al., 2017; Wright et al., 2024). That makes this portion of the nephron particularly influential in maintaining acid–base balance.

The active transport of sodium occurs through the sodium–potassium–adenosine triphosphatase (Na^+-K^+-ATPase) pump at the PCT and NKCC2 (Na^+, K^+, $2Cl^-$) pathways at the thick ascending LOH. Passive reabsorption of sodium in the proximal tubule occurs by way of Cl^-Na^+ transport within the distal and collecting tubules and occurs by way of the epithelial sodium channels (ENaC).

Bicarbonate reabsorption also predominantly occurs at the proximal tubule by way of sodium–hydrogen (Na^+-H^+) exchangers and sodium–bicarbonate (Na^+-HCO_3^-) cotransporters. The process that must take place for bicarbonate reabsorption involves numerous sequential steps. Na^+-H^+ exchangers secrete hydrogen into the proximal tubule. From within the tubule, H+ combines with filtered HCO_3^- to form carbonic acid ($H^+ + HCO_3^- = H_2CO_3$), and then (with the help of carbonic anhydrase) splits into water and carbon dioxide ($H_2CO_3 \rightarrow H_2O + CO_2$). The H_2O molecule stays within the tubule while CO_2 diffuses across the apical membrane of the proximal tubule and combines with intracellular H_2O to again form H_2CO_3. The newly reformed H_2CO_3 found inside the cells now splits into H^+ and HCO_3^-. This intracellular HCO_3^- ion interacts with the Na^+-HCO_3 cotransporter, and as a result, both sodium and bicarbonate are transported into the interstitial space and then reabsorbed into the circulation.

The proximal tubule is also the primary site for the *synthesis* and secretion of ammonia into the tubule, which occurs within the mitochondria (**Figure 8.10**). The newly formed ammonia ions begin to travel through

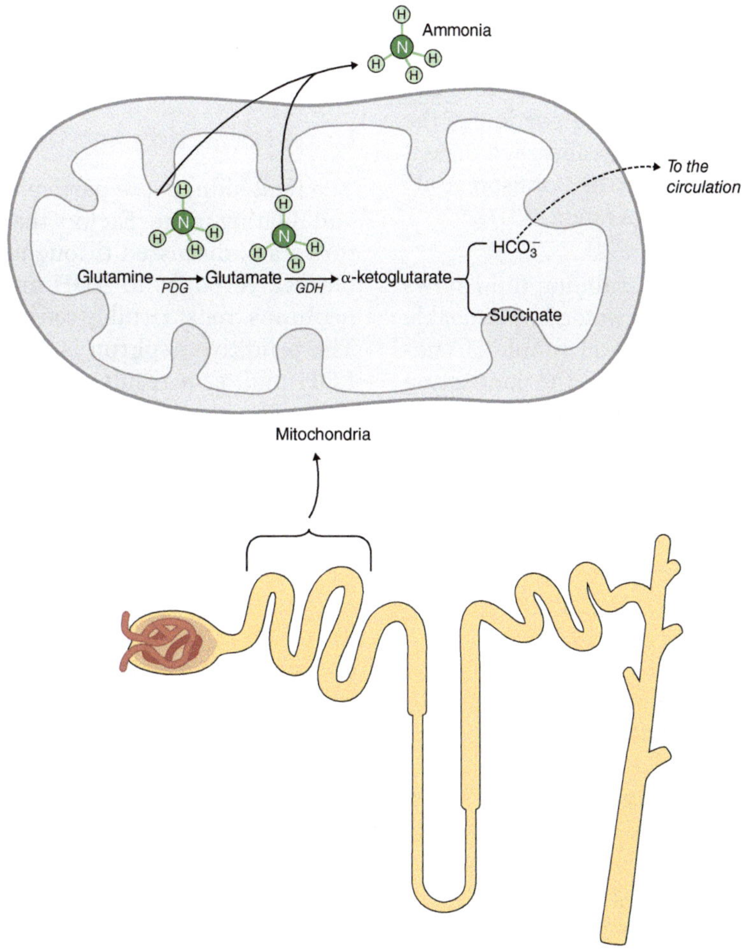

Figure 8.10 Renal ammonia production at the proximal tubule.

Note: Glutamine interacts with the PDG enzyme and is converted into glutamate. Then, glutamate interacts with GDH enzyme and is converted into alpha ketoglutarate. This process cleaves ammonia, which can be used to buffer hydrogen ions. The reduction of glutamate into alpha ketoglutarate leads to the formation of a new bicarbonate ion and succinate. The bicarbonate ion is then reabsorbed into the circulation. GDH, glutamate dehydrogenase; HCO_3^-, bicarbonate ion; PDG, phosphate-dependent glutaminase.

Image Credit: Amy J. Jnah.

the tubule in search of hydrogen ions because ammonia serves as a buffer to hydrogen ions and facilitates hydrogen elimination in the urine. This will be discussed further in the "distal tubule" section.

Loop of Henle. The proximal tubule leads directly to the LOH, which consists of four segments: the (a) thin descending limb (TDL), (b) thin ascending limb (TAL), (c) medullary thick ascending limb (mTAL), and (d) cortical thick ascending limb (cTAL; Partin et al., 2021). The TDL descends and forms a boundary between the inner and outer strips of the medulla. This descending limb is known for its high water permeability; no active transport of solutes occurs in this portion of the nephron (Baum, 2022). As filtered solute curves toward the TAL, the water permeability of the nephron disappears. Here, at the TAL, a high permeability to sodium is observed. As fluid moves from the TAL into the mTAL, significant solute reabsorption occurs. Cellular transport mechanisms aid in the reabsorption of water (15%), sodium (25%), potassium (20%), and bicarbonate (10%), as well as in the reabsorption of chloride and calcium (Gattineni & Baum, 2015; Johnson et al., 2017; Partin et al., 2021; Wright et al., 2024). Loop diuretics act on this portion of the nephron, inhibiting the reabsorption of sodium, potassium, and chloride through off-switching of the Na^+-K^+-$2Cl^-$-cotransporter; in these circumstances, a portion of the filtered sodium may be captured and reabsorbed once it reaches the distal tubule (Holmes, 2016: Johnson et al., 2017; Taketomo et al., 2017; Yaffe & Aranda, 2011).

Distal Tubule. From the mTAL, tubular fluid flows through the distal DCT, a relatively water-impermeable environment (Baum, 2017). The distal tubule is anatomically subdivided into the DCT and the connecting tubule (CNT); the DCT is of primary significance as this is the major location for solute reabsorption (Partin et al, 2021). Sodium (5%–10%), calcium (10%–15%), bicarbonate (8%–9%), magnesium (5%–10%), and water reabsorption occurs within the DCT. Thiazide diuretics act on this portion of the nephron, inhibiting the reabsorption of sodium and chloride through off-switching of the Na^+Cl^- cotransporter (Holmes, 2016; Taketomo et al., 2017; Yaffe & Aranda, 2011).

Recall from the earlier review of bicarbonate reabsorption at the proximal tubule that 80% of bicarbonate is absorbed at that location. Under normal physiologic conditions, a much smaller percentage (~10%) of bicarbonate is also reabsorbed at the distal tubule. A similar physiologic process occurs here as at the proximal tubule, again driven primarily by hydrogen ions interacting with bicarbonate ions within the tubule and in the presence of carbonic anhydrase, which prompts the sequence of events necessary for bicarbonate reabsorption into the circulation.

Also recall from the earlier review that ammonia is formed within mitochondria located at the proximal tubule. From there, ammonia travels through the tubule, in search of hydrogen ions to buffer. The distal tubule is a location where hydrogen ions are secreted. It is here that ammonia combines with hydrogen ions and facilitates the loss of hydrogen ions (acid) in the urine.

Collecting Ducts. From the CNT, filtrate approaches the collecting ducts. This segment of the nephron is subdivided into three regions: (a) the cortex connecting duct (CCD), (b) the outer medulla collecting duct (OMCD), and (c) the inner medulla collecting duct (IMCD; Baum, 2017). Sodium reabsorption (1%–3%), acid secretion, and K^+ regulation occurs in the CCD. Acidification of the urine occurs between the OMCD and IMCD by way of H^+ secretion and reciprocal reabsorption of bicarbonate (Baum, 2022).

Aldosterone and vasopressin exert effects on water and solute traversing the collecting ducts. Increased aldosterone secretion increases the excretion of K^+. Increased levels of circulating vasopressin open water channels, thereby facilitating water reabsorption. Potassium-sparing diuretics act on this portion of the nephron, inhibiting the reabsorption of Na^+ and therefore decreasing the secretion of K^+ into the filtrate (Holmes, 2016; Partin et al., 2021; Taketomo et al., 2017; Yaffe & Aranda, 2011).

Urine Formation and Composition

The fetal kidneys are particularly inept at concentrating and dilating urine. Factors that contribute to this immature state, discussed throughout this chapter, include a blunted response to ADH and anatomically immature nephrons, most notably during early fetal development. The primitive nephron is devoid of a deeply extending LOH and, as a result, is devoid of its thick ascending limb. Their superficial location renders the nephrons functionally immature at water and solute reabsorption. For example, fetal urinary excretion of sodium, expressed as fractional excretion of sodium (FE_{Na}), is much higher in the fetus than in the newborn (Segar, 2016). Around 30 weeks of gestation, FE_{Na} is about 14% to 15%, near term it is approximately 5%, and a term newborn has a FE_{Na} of 1% or less. Maturational changes, including an increase in tubular transporters, increased functional (intracellular and extracellular) transport of sodium, and increased sensitivity to angiotensin II, glucocorticoids, and catecholamines, explain the progressive maturational process.

Fortunately, the placenta is the principal source of fluid and electrolyte homeostasis during early fetal development (Segar, 2016). Urine formation occurs early in fetal development, between 9 and 12 weeks of gestation, and is essentially composed of free water with small amounts of solutes (Scott et al., 2020). Filtration, reabsorption, and secretion of solutes begin at week 14 of gestation (Chestnut et al., 2014). After 16 to 20 weeks of gestation, GFR contributes to adequate fetal urine production (up to 300 mL/kg fetal weight/day; Rosenblum et al., 2017). By 20 weeks of gestation, renal function is demonstrably improved, as the volume of amniotic fluid measures approximately 320 mL (90% of total amniotic fluid at term) and thereby increases to around 800 mL from 28 weeks until term (Lindower, 2017). Urine formation guarantees appropriate circulating amniotic fluid levels, which are essential for normal development of many body systems, including the pulmonary and gastrointestinal systems (Curtis, 2025). Urinalysis reference ranges are provided in Table 8.2.

Clinical Application. There are several problems that are associated with abnormal urinalysis results. Consider a situation involving hematuria (or blood in the urine). This can occur from nonrenal etiologies including a severe diaper dermatitis and bleeding that spills into the urine, or renal pathologies including urinary tract infection, renal vein thrombosis, or acute tubular necrosis (often associated with perinatal asphyxia). Proteinuria is defined as at least 1+ protein with urine pH 1.015 or 2+ protein with urine pH greater than 1.015. Possible etiologies include acute tubular necrosis, dehydration, and Fanconi syndrome (when there is concurrent glucosuria, phosphaturia, and metabolic acidosis). Glycosuria should raise suspicion for hyperglycemia and sepsis, among other pathologies (e.g., renal dysplasia). The presence of urine ketones should alert the NNP to consider a variety of inborn errors of metabolism. For example, laboratory findings in infants affected with methylmalonic acidemia include metabolic acidosis, hyperammonemia, and plasma and urine ketones with or without hypoglycemia.

TABLE 8.2 Urinalysis Components and Reference Ranges in Preterm and Term Newborns

Indices	Preterm	Term
Specific gravity	1.002–1.015	1.001–1.020
pH	5–8	4.5–8
Maximal concentration ability (mOsmol/L)	500	800
Maximal diluting ability (mOsmol/L)	25–30	25–30
Glucose	(-) or 2+	(-)
Protein (100 mg/dL)	(-) or 2+	(-) or 1+
Blood	(-)	(-)
Leukocytes	(-)	(-)

Note: The dipstick urine test provides levels of glucose, blood, protein, and leukocytes in the urine; (-) represents "none" or "negative" for these values.
Sources: Adapted from Curtis, S. N. (2025). Fluid, electrolytes, and acid-base homeostasis. In R. Martin & A. A. Fanaroff (Eds.), *Fanaroff and Martin's neonatal-perinatal medicine: Diseases of the fetus and infant* (12th ed., pp. 1948–1965). Elsevier; Whiteseal, E. (2023). Fluid and electrolyte management. In E. C. Eichenwald, A. R. Hansen, C. R. Martin, & A. R. Stark (Eds.), *Cloherty & Stark's manual of neonatal care* (9th ed., pp. 301–317). Wolters Kluwer; Wright, C. J., Posencheg, M. A., & Seri, I. (2024). Fluid, electrolyte, and acid–base balance. In C. A. Gleason & S. E. Juul (Eds.), *Avery's diseases of the newborn* (11th ed., pp. 231–252). Elsevier Saunders.

GENETIC INFLUENCES

Congenital abnormalities of the kidneys and urinary tract (CAKUT) comprise 20% to 50% of all cases of pediatric end-stage renal disease and account for 20% of all birth defects (Capone et al., 2017; dos Santos et al., 2014). There are more than 500 CAKUT; a positive family history of renal or urinary anomalies occurs in about 10% of all renal anomalies (dos Santos et al., 2014). Common CAKUT disorders will be presented in this section of the chapter. Additional inherited disorders affecting the renal system are provided in Box 8.1.

Autosomal Dominant Polycystic Kidney Disease

Autosomal dominant polycystic kidney disease (ADPKD) is a severe malformation of one or both kidneys involving the formation of multiple, nonfunctioning cysts that dominate normal functioning renal tissue (Figure 8.11). It is a multisystem disorder. Cysts may present in other locations, including the liver, seminal vesicles, pancreas, and arachnoid membrane. Vascular abnormalities, in-

BOX 8.1 Other Inherited Disorders of the Renal System

- Alagille syndrome
- Fanconi syndrome
- Meckel syndrome
- Systemic lupus erythematosus
- Nephrotic syndrome
- Renal agenesis
- Trisomy 13, 18, 21
- Zellweger syndrome

Note: A more comprehensive list is provided by the National Institute of Health, Genetic and Rare Diseases Information Center (GARD); https://globalgenes.org/rare-list/

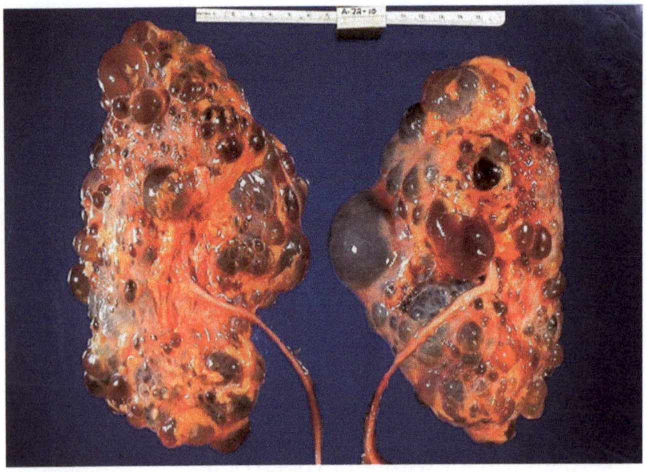

Figure 8.11 Polycystic kidneys.

Source: Ewing, E. P. (1972). *Gross pathologic changes in a case of polycystic kidney disease.* Centers for Disease Control and Prevention. https://phil.cdc.gov/details.aspx?pid=861

cluding intracranial aneurysms, dilatation of the aortic root, and dissection of the thoracic aorta, have been reported (Harris & Torres, 2022).

ADPKD is the most common Mendelian kidney disease; offspring of parental carriers incur a 50% inheritance risk (dos Santos et al., 2014). ADPKD is reported in one of every 500 to 1,000 live births; males and females are equally affected (Chebib & Torres, 2016; National Institutes of Health [NIH], 2018; Rogers, 2023). In 95% of patients with ADPKD, there is an affected parent; 10% of cases involve de novo mutations. Two genes, *PKD1* and *PKD2*, are associated with ADPKD. Approximately 85% of cases are associated with *PKD1*, and the remaining 15% of cases involve *PKD2* (Baker & Jnah, 2024; Chebib & Torres, 2016). *PKD2* gene mutations are associated with milder disease, whereas *PKD1* mutations correlate with more severe disease states.

The etiology for ADPKD involves mutations in the aforementioned genes, which disrupt normal coding for proteins (in this case, polycystins) that reside on the primary cilia within the collecting duct and modulate intracellular calcium levels. Disrupted coding decreases intracellular calcium levels, increases cyclic adenosine monophosphate levels, and increases vasopressin sensitivity at the collecting duct (Chebib & Torres, 2016). These factors alter tubular formation and differentiation of the primary cilia as well as increase fluid secretion within the distal tubule of the nephron (Chebib & Torres, 2016; Harris & Torres, 2022; NIH, 2024b). As the cysts matriculate, they increase in size with some detaching into the tubules. This causes a secondary release of cytokines and chemokines and subsequent inflammation. Persistent inflammation can alter the renal vascular network and increase the risk for fibrosis.

ADPKD rarely presents in the neonatal period; manifestations during this period include vesicoureteral reflux (VUR) and renal failure. More commonly, fluid accumulation within the distal tubule and collecting ducts progresses throughout infancy and even into childhood, leading to the formation of more and more cysts, localized to the epithelia. Latent manifestations include hypertension, hematuria, and renal pain (Harris & Torres, 2022). Approximately 50% of affected individuals with ADPKD will develop end-stage renal disease before 60 years of age (Harris & Torres, 2022; Reule et al., 2014).

Multicystic Dysplastic Kidney Disease

Multicystic dysplastic kidney (MCDK) disease is one of the most common causes of CAKUT and the most common cause of cystic disease in children. The incidence of unilateral disease is estimated at one in every 1,000 to 4,300 live births; bilateral disease is rare (Baker & Jnah, 2024; Cooper et al., 2013; Engen & Hingorani, 2024).

The pathogenesis of MCDK is poorly understood. Recall that under normal circumstances the ureteric bud grows laterally during early development and invades the nearby renal parenchyma. One widely published explanation for MCDK suggests that failed invasion of the metanephric blastema (parenchyma) predisposes the kidney to MCDK (Holcomb et al., 2020). An alternative explanation suggests an atresia or obstruction of the ureters causes MCDK. Environmental shocks, including viral infections, have been reported as other potential triggers for MCDK (Cardona-Grau & Kogan, 2015).

MCDK manifests as severe hydronephrosis secondary to ureteropelvic junction (UPJ) obstruction. Hydronephrosis, secondary to UPJ obstruction, may implicate the contralateral, otherwise structurally normal, kidney. Radiographic scans may yield a renal parenchyma notably "saturated" with fluid (echogenic). Cysts may be irregularly placed on one or both kidneys. It is also not uncommon for MCDK to occur in association with other renal anomalies, including fetal aplastic kidney (cystic remnants on a ureter), horseshoe, or ectopic kidney disease. Life-span implications vary depending on the degree of cystic matriculation as well as the degree of involution. Most cysts involute during fetal development or over the first 2 years of life (Holcomb et al., 2020). Malignancy risk, or the risk for acquired Wilms tumor or renal cell carcinoma, is very low among children affected by MCDK (Eickmeyer et al., 2014).

Wilms Tumor (Nephroblastoma)

Nephroblastoma, also known as Wilms tumor, is a solid and malignant tumor of the kidney (Figure 8.12). Nephroblastoma is caused by a mutation of the *WT1* gene, located on chromosome 11p15. The incidence of Wilms tumor in neonates is rare, at 0.2%, due to its subclinical presentation during early infancy (Kenner & Lott, 2014). However, Wilms tumor accounts for 92% of all pediatric renal tumors diagnosed among children less than 5 years of age; an increased prevalence among females is reported (Ward et al., 2014). Clinical manifes-

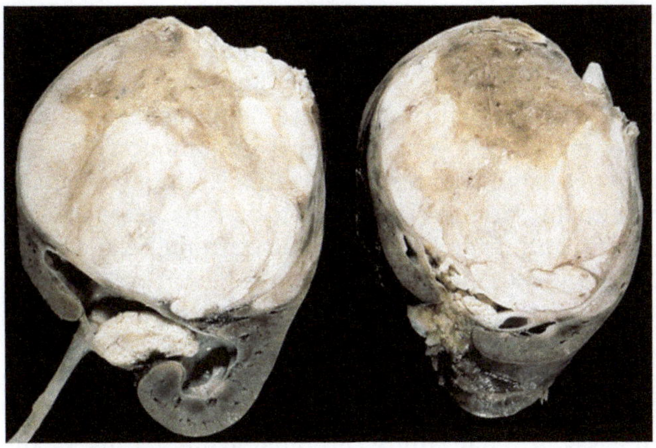

Figure 8.12 Wilms tumor.
Source: The Armed Forces Institute of Pathology.

tations include a large abdominal mass, vomiting, and hematuria. Life-span implications include intellectual disability, genitourinary abnormalities, kyphosis and scoliosis, end-stage renal failure, and recurrence risk; survival is estimated at 90%.

Bartter Syndrome

Bartter syndrome is a rare constellation of renal disorders that derange ion channels and renal tubular cotransporters within the distal segments of the nephron. The incidence is estimated at one per every 1 million individuals worldwide (NIH, 2024a). This leads to failed Na^+ and Cl^- reabsorption within the thick ascending LOH and DCT and resultant wasting into the urine. This salt-wasting is also associated with hypokalemia and metabolic alkalosis. Bartter syndrome, specifically types 1, 2, 4a, and 4b, manifests during fetal development or infancy, whereas the other subtypes commonly manifest during adulthood (Phadke et al., 2014).

During fetal development, this syndrome manifests as polyhydramnios; affected fetuses are often subject to premature birth. Postnatally, Bartter syndrome may manifest with physical abnormalities, including a triangular face, prominent occiput, proptosis, and pointed ears. Affected infants often fail to thrive and develop nephrocalcinosis and renal calcifications and are at risk for osteopenia. Life-span implications associated with chronic electrolyte imbalance include sensorineural hearing loss and deafness as well as cognitive deficits. There is currently no cure for Bartter syndrome (Phadke et al., 2014).

NOTEWORTHY DISEASES IN THE XX PREGNANT PATIENT THAT INFLUENCE FETAL RENAL DEVELOPMENT AND FUNCTION

Research indicates that the intrauterine environment has a significant impact on determining the number of nephrons a baby has at birth. A low nephron count or endowment is associated with chronic renal disease (CRD) in childhood and adult life (McAleer & Chiang, 2024; Rosenblum et al., 2017). Several health factors observed in XX pregnant patients implicate the developing renal system and will be discussed here.

Recall from Chapter 2 that fetal exposure to various toxins can provoke intrauterine growth restriction, premature delivery, and low birth weight (LBW; Calkins & Devaskar, 2011). Specific to the renal system, prematurity and LBW have been positively correlated with reduced nephrogenesis, childhood hypertension, and reduced insulin reactivity. In fact, a direct linear association exists between birth weight and nephron number; infants are affixed with approximately 250,000 additional nephrons for each 1 kg increase in birth weight (Smyth et al., 2022). *Infants born prior to 34 weeks of gestation or those weighing less than 2.5 kg are deficient in nephrons and incur a 70% higher risk for latent kidney disease* (Brophy, 2017). Given the integral role that the renal system holds in cardiovascular and endocrine homeostasis, and 31 to 36 weeks of gestation as the critical renal programming period, the reduction in total number of nephrons either due to altered perinatal programming or prematurity offers a reasonable explanation for later pancreatic insufficiency and latent chronic disease (McAleer & Chiang, 2024). Essentially, fewer nephrons offer a reduced landscape for glomerular filtration and sodium excretion, despite any compensatory glomerular hypertrophy, which favors hypertension (Luyckx et al., 2013).

Other health factors that may influence perinatal programming and low fetal nephron endowment include prior LBW status as an infant, hypertensive disorders during pregnancy, gestational diabetes, smoking, vitamin A deficiency, low socioeconomic status, and minority status (Brophy, 2017; Collins et al., 2011; McAleer & Chiang, 2024). Mothers born weighing less than 2.5 kg are more likely to deliver offspring of similar LBW (odds ratio [OR] 1.8, 95% CI, 1.3–2.5; Collins et al., 2011). Transgenerational passage of genetic determinants of chronic kidney disease, defined as low nephron number, has been reported among Cuban pregnant patients (Collins et al., 2011). Gestational diabetes incurs a threefold increase in risk for altered fetal renal development (renal agenesis or renal dysgenesis) and increased fetal growth with resultant increased birth weight greater than 4 kg (large for gestational age [LGA]). Increased birth weight is associated with an increased risk for latent cardiovascular disease and diabetes. Smoking and alcohol consumption have also been positively correlated with reduced nephrogenesis (Davis et al., 2010).

Malnutrition, specific to caloric, protein, and vitamin A deficiency in XX pregnant patients, has been linked to reduced nephrogenesis. This is particularly significant in resource-poor countries where micronutrient and protein deficiencies are common or during periods of widespread famine. Specific to the developing renal system, a dose-dependent relationship between micronutrients, such as vitamin A, and nephrogenesis has been reported. Retinoic acid, the active metabolite of vitamin A, is responsible for modulating nephrogenesis. Therefore, insufficient vitamin A intake during pregnancy has been linked to LBW and a reduction in fetal nephrogenesis, thereby increasing the risk for latent chronic cardiovascular and renal disease. Recent studies using animal models also suggest a dose-dependent relationship between vitamin D intake and nephrogenesis (Nascimento et al., 2012).

Several medications, as well as ingestion of licit and illicit drugs, have been associated with renal anomalies. ACE inhibitors or angiotensin receptor blockers have been associated with renal agenesis or anomalies, and cocaine, tobacco, and alcohol use are risk factors for diminished nephron endowment and renal anomalies (Good et al., 2022). Ingestion of nonsteroidal anti-inflammatory drugs, such as indomethacin for preterm labor, interferes with the production of prostaglandins necessary for vasodilation in renal blood flow, thereby reducing nephrogenesis and predisposing the fetus to kidney dysfunction (Good et al., 2022).

Clinicians must consider the increase in survivability among extremely premature infants during modern times, as well as those born to mothers with risk factors, as noted previously. A thorough investigation into the past medical and prenatal medical history is essential for neonatal clinicians to appraise the relative risk for altered kidney function among newborns. As noted, premature, LBW, and LGA infants are at increased risk for low nephron counts, childhood hypertension, and progressive chronic kidney disease in addition to diabetes and coronary artery disease. Therefore, risks must be communicated to pediatric primary care providers, and kidney function must be followed closely throughout childhood.

COMMON PROBLEMS WITH IMPLICATIONS ACROSS THE LIFE SPAN

The kidney is vulnerable to a host of insults during fetal development, which may give rise to a number of defects that affect renal development and function. Common problems that may affect the renal system are discussed here.

Acute Kidney Injury

AKI, also known as *acute renal failure*, is characterized as the abrupt deterioration in renal function resulting in the inability to maintain fluid and electrolyte homeostasis. Approximately 26% of extremely LBW infants (fewer than 1,500 grams) and 56% of infants with perinatal asphyxia develop AKI (Nada et al., 2017). A 25% to 50% mortality risk is conferred (Kenner & Lott, 2014). Risk factors for the development of AKI are multifactorial and include very LBW status and prematurity; both are associated with incomplete nephrogenesis. Other risks include exposures to anti-inflammatory agents and nephrotoxic antibiotics (e.g., aminoglycosides), patent ductus arteriosus, phototherapy, neonatal diuretics, and respiratory distress syndrome (Nada et al., 2017; Vogt, 2025).

AKI is classified as prerenal (hemodynamic), renal (intrinsic), or postrenal (obstructive), and the pathogenesis of each subtype is unique (Table 8.3). Prerenal failure (prerenal azotemia) is reported in up to 70% of all cases of renal failure; prerenal azotemia marks the earliest phase of kidney failure. Decreased blood flow to the kidney causes a reduction in glomerular filtration and an induced state of oliguria. Given that the renal tubules are intact at this stage, enhanced reabsorption of sodium and water is observed with increased urine osmolarity. FE_{Na} is often less than 2.5% among premature infants and less than 1% among term infants with prerenal azotemia (Holcomb et al., 2020). If recognized in a timely manner, prerenal failure is considered curable.

Intrinsic renal failure affects 6% to 8% of all hospitalized neonates requiring inpatient intensive care. Intrinsic failure occurs secondary to cellular damage to the glomerulus or renal parenchyma. Sloughing of epithelial cells precedes the loss of renal function, as sodium and water reabsorption are impaired and decreased urine osmolarity is observed. Intrinsic failure manifests as one of four possible subtypes, which are summarized in Table 8.4.

Postrenal failure involves an obstruction to the flow of urine. This prevents the evacuation of urine from the body and may affect one or both kidneys. Three common causes for obstructive failure are (a) UPJ obstruction, (b) posterior urethral valves (PUVs), and (c) ureterovesical obstruction (Holcomb et al., 2020). Although typically reversible, long-standing obstructions may progress to intrinsic renal failure and permanent kidney damage (Nada et al., 2017; Vogt, 2025).

Clinical manifestations of AKI include elevated serum BUN and creatinine (greater than 1.5 mg/dL), hyperkalemia (peaked T waves or ventricular fibrillation on electrocardiogram), and metabolic acidosis. In particular, metabolic acidosis accumulates due to insufficient renal H^+ production and resultant reduction of serum bicarbonate. These children may hyperventilate to attempt respiratory compensation; however, this is not sustainable in most situations (Holcomb et al., 2020; Vogt, 2025).

Life-span implications include cystic kidney disease, altered glomerular filtration, hyperfiltration, proteinuria, and hypertension (Nada et al., 2017). In the aging post-AKI patient, latent chronic hypertension and other cardiovascular problems may arise.

TABLE 8.3 Categories of Acute Kidney Injury

Category of AKI	Etiology	Incidence	Common Predisposing Factors
Prerenal	Decreased renal blood flow to kidney	85%	• Asphyxia • Cardiac tamponade • Central nephrogenic diabetes insipidus • Congestive heart failure • Dehydration • Hemorrhagic conditions • Pericarditis • Respiratory distress • Salt-wasting diseases • Septic shock (third space losses)
Intrinsic	Structural damage and loss of renal function	11%	• Acute tubular necrosis[a] • Congenital renal anomalies • Direct nephrotoxic injury • Hypoxemia • Infection • Inflammatory conditions • Perinatal asphyxia • Prolonged renal hypoperfusion • Vascular conditions
Postrenal	Obstruction altering normal renal outflow	3%	• Meningomyelocele • Neurogenic bladder • Posterior urethral valves • Prolonged administration of paralytic agents or sedatives • Spina bifida • Ureteropelvic juncture obstruction

[a]Acute tubular necrosis, which commonly manifests secondary to perinatal asphyxia, is the most common cause for intrinsic acute renal failure. Incidences cited in this table are estimations and may not reflect the most current data.
AKI, acute kidney injury.
Source: Vogt, B. A. (2025). The kidney and urinary tract of the neonate. In R. Martin & A. A. Fanaroff (Eds.), *Fanaroff and Martin's neonatal–perinatal medicine: Diseases of the fetus and infant* (12th ed., pp. 1966–1989). Elsevier.

TABLE 8.4 Intrinsic Renal Failure

Subtype	Common Predisposing Factors
Ischemic	• Acute tubular necrosis
Nephrotoxic	• Aminoglycoside administration • Indomethacin administration
Congenital	• Autosomal recessive polycystic disease
Vascular	• Renal artery thrombosis • Renal vein thrombosis

Source: Steflik, H. J., Askenazi, D., & Selewski, D. (2024). Acute kidney injury. In C. A. Gleason & S. E. Juul (Eds.), *Avery's diseases of the newborn* (11th ed., pp. 1125–1138). Elsevier.

Clinical Application. Newborns who require the insertion of an umbilical arterial catheter are considered at-risk for the development of renal artery thrombosis. Likewise, newborns who require the insertion of an umbilical venous catheter are considered at-risk for the development of renal vein thrombosis. In both cases, the thrombus often develops at the tip of the catheter and can partially or completely obstruct blood flow and lead to the onset of systolic hypertension. The diagnostic evaluation will include a renal ultrasound with Doppler flow and four-extremity blood pressures, along with interval assessments of blood pressure. In some circumstances, when hypertension is sustained at greater than the 95th to 99th percentile, pharmacologic agents (e.g., amlodipine) may be required to normalize blood pressure.

Renal Tubular Acidosis

When the renal system cannot maintain a stable acid–base balance, the term *renal tubular acidosis* (RTA) is used to define the disorder. RTA occurs from impaired bicarbonate reabsorption at the proximal tubule, impaired buffering and excretion of hydrogen (H^+) ions at the distal tubule, or both problems concurrently (Curtis, 2025; Eichenwald et al., 2023; Gil-Peña et al., 2014). Normal glomerular function is present, meaning there is no evidence of overt renal failure. Risk factors for RTA include fetal exposure to toxins (e.g., toluene, found in glue and paint), inheritance risks, aberrant fetal development, premature birth, and birth-related injuries (Maguire, 2021).

The three most common types of RTA are type I (distal), type II (proximal), and type IV (hyperkalemic; Table 8.5 and Figure 8.13). Type I RTA is caused by impaired secretion of acid (hydrogen ions) into the DCT. This can be attributed to autosomal recessive disorders (primary RTA type I) or distal tubular injury (secondary RTA type I). Typically, faulty genes alter solute cotransport mechanisms in the distal tubule and disrupt bicarbonate reabsorption or H^+ secretion. The end result is impaired distal tubular acidification and acidosis yielding alkalotic urine with a pH greater than 5.5. Neonates may present with hypotonia and irritability, and demonstrate poor feeding ability.

Type II RTA disrupts bicarbonate reabsorption within the proximal tubule. Failed bicarbonate reabsorption yields increased losses into the urine and will manifest biochemically as a downtrending serum bicarbonate level. In preterm infants with immature renal function, serum bicarbonate levels often drop to 15 mEq/L before physiologic reabsorption is triggered. The threshold for bicarbonate reabsorption in term infants with type II RTA is usually 20 mEq/L. Reduced bicarbonate reabsorption encourages a persistent acidotic state. This can

TABLE 8.5 Renal Tubular Acidosis

Category of RTA	Primary Problem	Lab Indices
Type I (primary distal)	Deficient H^+ (acid) secretion in distal renal tubule	Biochemical indices • Non-anion gap metabolic acidosis • High serum Cl^- • Low serum HCO_3^- • Low or normal serum K^+ Urinary indices • Hypercalciuria • Low urine ammonium • Positive urine anion gap • Urine pH >5.5
Type II (proximal)	Deficient HCO_3^- (base) reabsorption at the proximal tubule	Biochemical indices • Non-anion gap metabolic acidosis • High serum Cl^- • Low serum HCO_3^- • Low or normal serum K^+ Urinary indices • Negative urine anion gap • Urine pH variable, but usually is <5.5
Type IV (hyperkalemic)	Deficient mineralocorticoid level or renal aldosterone resistance	Biochemical indices • Non-anion gap metabolic acidosis • Low serum Na^+ • High serum Cl^- • High serum K^+ Urinary indices • Negative urine anion gap • Low urine K^+ • High urine Na^+

Cl^-, chloride ion; H^+, hydrogen ion; HCO_3^-, bicarbonate ion; K^+, potassium ion; Na^+, sodium ion; RTA, renal tubular acidosis.

Source: Yu, E., & Yonekawa, K. (2024). Glomerulonephropathies and disorders of tubular function. In C. A. Gleason & S. E. Juul (Eds.), *Avery's diseases of the newborn* (11th ed., pp. 1148–1154). Elsevier.

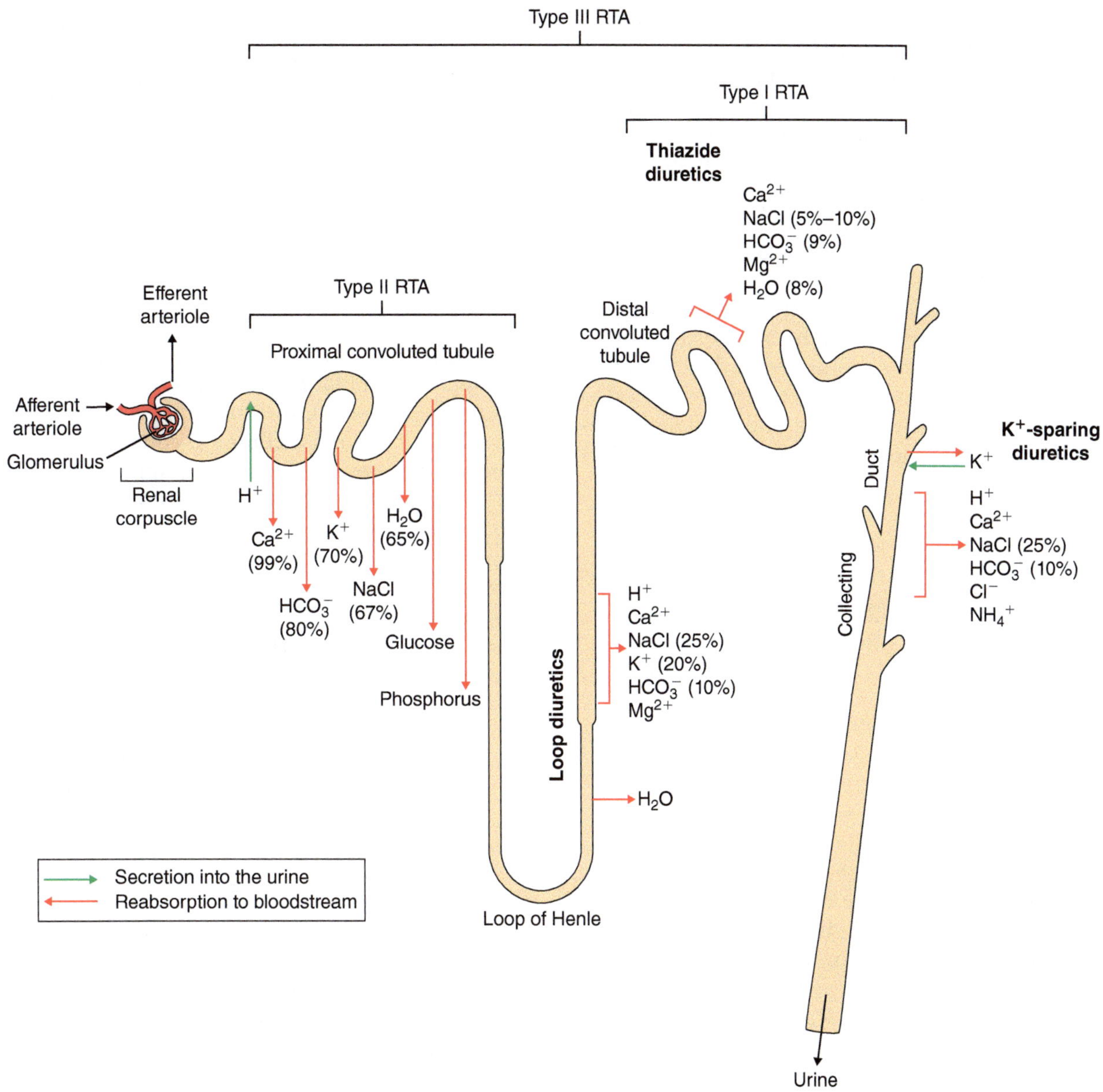

Figure 8.13 Locus for type I to III RTA.

Ca^{2}, calcium ion; Cl^-, chloride ion; H^+, hydrogen ion; HCO_3^-, bicarbonate ion; K^+, potassium ion; Mg^{2+}, magnesium ion; NH_4^+, ammonium ion; RTA, renal tubular acidosis.

Image Credit: Mya Jnah.

be attributed to gene mutations or X-linked inheritance as well as inborn errors of metabolism (e.g., galactosemia, hereditary fructose intolerance, tyrosinemia) that cause a pathological accumulation of metabolites, which impair proximal tubular function. Similar to type I RTA, affected neonates may present with hypotonia and irritability, and demonstrate poor feeding ability.

Type IV RTA is caused by a genetically inherited or transient form of aldosterone resistance or mineralocorticoid deficiency. Recall that aldosterone regulation involves the actions of a cascade of hormones (in the adrenal glands and kidneys, liver, and lungs). Angiotensinogen, a participant in the cascade, is produced in the liver and interacts with renin in order to be converted to angiotensin 1. Next, angiotensin 1 travels through the circulation and enters the pulmonary vasculature, where it interacts with ACE and is converted into biologically active angiotensin 2. Angiotensin 2 enters the circulation and travels to the adrenal gland and interacts at the zona glomerulosa (see Chapter 10) to stimulate the production of aldosterone. Both angiotensin 2 and aldosterone affect acid–base regulation in the kidneys. Both increase sodium reabsorption, whereas aldosterone also encourages potassium secretion in the renal tubule by interacting with mineralocorticoid receptors in the proximal tubule and sodium channels in the distal tubule. Angiotensin 2 specifically increases bicarbonate reabsorption (in addition to the aforementioned effect of increasing sodium reabsorption). The net result is a change in acid–base balance toward metabolic alkalosis. Therefore, any disease state (transient or permanent) that inhibits renin or aldosterone production can cause the opposite effect—metabolic acidosis. Common causes for RTA type IV include aldosterone deficiency (hypoaldosteronism), renal parenchymal damage secondary to obstructive kidney disease, nephrotoxic medication administration, and congenital adrenal hyperplasia (Curtis, 2025; Gil-Peña et al., 2014; Holcomb et al., 2020; Maguire, 2021). In addition, preterm infants commonly present with a transient, physiologic aldosterone resistance at birth, which tends to resolve by the third day of life. Affected neonates may present with hyponatremia-induced dehydration, lethargy, emesis, and poor feeding ability. When differentiating between the etiologies for type IV RTA, a mineralocorticoid deficiency will be associated with low serum aldosterone and elevated ACTH. In contrast, cases of aldosterone resistance present with high serum aldosterone and decreased ACTH (Lee, 2024).

Clinical Application. When RTA is suspected in a newborn, it is important to obtain both a blood gas and an electrolyte panel. Obtaining both of these lab panels allows the opportunity to confirm the true presence of metabolic acidosis. Remember that all newborns with any form of RTA will demonstrate a hyperchloremic non-anion gap metabolic acidosis. Determining the anion gap requires some simple arithmetic. The serum anion gap is calculated as the mathematical difference between the sum of positively and negatively charged anions found in the blood. The cations commonly found in the blood are sodium and potassium. The anions commonly found in the blood are chloride and bicarbonate. Therefore, the anion gap calculation for the serum is: $(Na^+) - (Cl^- + HCO_3^-)$. While potassium, calcium and magnesium (cations), and phosphates and sulfates (anions) are also found in the serum, they are considered "unmeasured" ions.

For example, consider the following results on a serum chemistry panel: Na^+ 142, K^+ 4.6, Cl^- 108, HCO_3^- 20. The serum anion gap would be calculated in this manner: (142) - (112 + 20) = 10. This value reflects a "normal" (non-anion gap) acidosis, because the normal range for anion gap is 8 to 16 mEq/L.

Note that the urine anion gap calculation is slightly different: $(Na^+ + K^+) - Cl^-$. This calculation gives us the difference between positively and negatively charged anions found in the urine. While ammonium (cation), phosphates, and sulfates (anions) are also found in the urine, they are considered "unmeasured" ions. In the case of RTA, which brings about a metabolic acidosis, as the kidneys attempt to secrete as much acid as possible into the urine, the amount of ammonium increases (since it buffers hydrogen ions). This excess of ammonium in the urine will increase the amount of unmeasured cations and yield a normal or negative urine anion gap.

Urinary Tract Dilation

Urinary tract dilation (UTD), the *most common cause of nephron loss among neonates*, is characterized by abnormal accumulation of urine within the collecting system (renal pelvis), resulting in renal cavity distention. UTD is the most common congenital condition identified on prenatal ultrasonography and affects 1% to 4.5% of all pregnancies (Vincent et al., 2022). Approximately 30% to 40% of all cases persist into the postnatal period; of that statistic, 40% spontaneously resolve (Ferri, 2025; Good et al., 2022; Vogt, 2025). Risk factors for UTD in the fetal and neonatal period include the aforementioned obstructive disorders, renal calculi, renal thrombosis, and renal tumors; however, UTD may also be the result of obstructive or nonobstructive abnormalities and affect one or both kidneys (Vogt, 2025). It is essential that clinicians recognize that UTD is not a primary disorder; the underlying pathogenesis is attributed to the primary disease process.

The Society of Fetal Urology offers a severity scale for UTD (Table 8.6). In most cases, UTD is detected on prenatal ultrasound as a consequence of oligohydramnios (Vogt, 2025). Although most radiologists use terminology commensurate with the severity scale (mild, moderate, and severe) when rendering radiographic reports, poor interrater reliability and subjectivity confound a standardized approach to interpretation and reporting; this can make classification challenging (Hagen-Ansert, 2023; Rickard et al., 2017).

Postnatal manifestations include a large, firm, palpable abdominal mass in the kidney region. Renal function is dependent on disease severity and unilateral or bilateral presentation. Infants with unilateral involvement, or mild to moderate hydronephrosis, may demonstrate normal renal function.

Most cases of hydronephrosis self-resolve and are considered a benign finding. Life-span implications of clinically significant moderate to severe hydronephrosis include recurrent urinary tract infection, hypertension, and urinary reflux. VUR, if severe, may cause glomerulosclerosis and progressive renal insufficiency (Good et al., 2022; Kenner & Lott, 2014). Severe bilateral hydronephrosis may manifest with renal failure, pulmonary hyperplasia, or recurrent urinary tract infections and progress to end-stage renal disease (Kenner & Lott, 2014).

TABLE 8.6 Grading and Severity of UTD

Grade	Severity	Clinical Finding	Visual Depiction
I	Mild	Slight splitting of the central renal echo complex with normal calyces	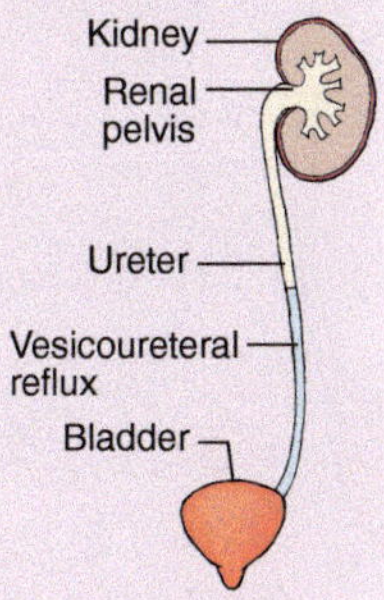
II	Mild	Dilated renal pelvis with marginal fluid in calyces	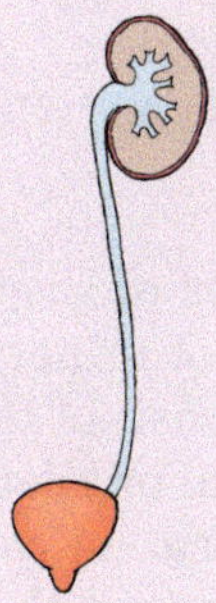
III	Moderate	Dilated renal pelvis beyond sinus with equally dilated calyces	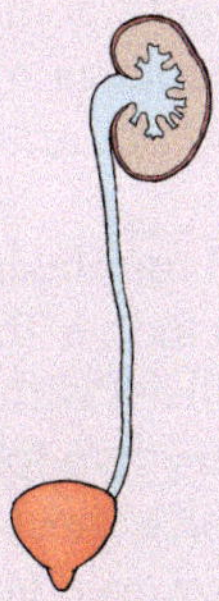
IV	Severe	Thinning of renal parenchyma with dilated pelvis and calyces	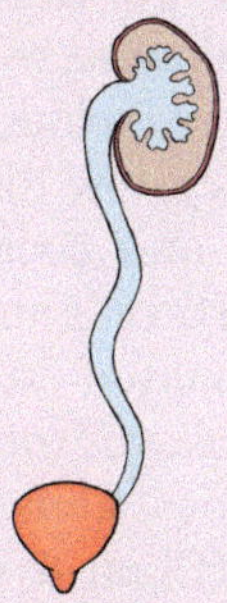
V	Severe	Severe dilation with atrophic cortex	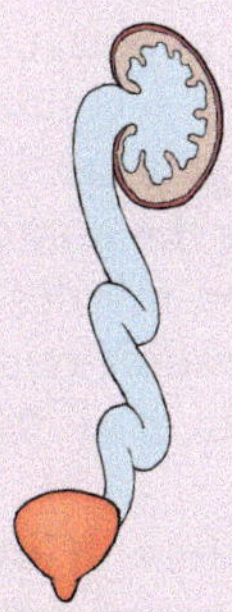

UTD, urinary tract dilation.

Developmental and Positional Anomalies

Developmental and positional disorders of the renal system may include complete absence of renal tissue, alterations in the functional number of nephrons, or renal parenchymal malformations. Associated diagnoses include renal agenesis, supernumerary kidneys, renal ectopia, fusion defects, renal tumors, and cystic renal diseases. We will focus our attention on renal agenesis, renal dysplasia and hypoplasia, and horseshoe kidney, the more common developmental and positional anomalies that affect the renal system.

Renal Agenesis. Renal agenesis is the congenital absence of one or both kidneys (**Figure 8.14**). Unilateral renal agenesis occurs in one in 2,000 live births with bilateral renal agenesis occurring in one in 8,500 births; a higher incidence of left-sided agenesis is reported (Fong & De Beritto, 2024; Torchia & Persaud, 2025). A male prevalence is reported, with a ratio of 1.7 to every one affected female (Rogers, 2023; Torchia & Persaud, 2025).

Risk factors include genetic and environmental agents. Mutations in many genes, such as *RET, BMP4, FRAS1, FREM1*, or *UPK3A*, correlate with unilateral renal agenesis, whereas mutations in *RET, FGF20*, or *ITGA8* genes are reported with bilateral renal agenesis (NIH, 2024b). Renal agenesis may be associated with other structural defects, such as vertebral and anal abnormalities, tracheoesophageal atresia, renal agenesis or dysplasia, and limb defects (VACTERL), CAKUT, and extrarenal anomalies (Fong & De Beritto, 2024; Vogt, 2025). Alcohol, cocaine, thalidomide, and warfarin use during pregnancy has been associated with fetal renal agenesis.

Renal agenesis results when the ureteric bud fails to differentiate into the ureters, renal pelvis, and collecting ducts, and the mesenchyme fails to differentiate into the nephrons (Torchia & Persaud, 2025). This results in failed renal differentiation and nephrogenesis. As such, reduced or absent urine formation causes a significantly decreased (oligohydramnios) or absent (anhydramnios) amniotic fluid level. Oligohydramnios is a common finding in prenatal ultrasound.

Renal agenesis may be associated with other CAKUT disorders or extrarenal complications. Common associated CAKUT disorders include VUR (24%), 22q11 syndrome, and extrarenal malformations (Fong & De Beritto, 2024; Westland et al., 2013). Associated extrarenal anomalies may include malformations of the skeletal, auditory, respiratory, and cardiovascular systems, as well as the genitalia.

Unilateral renal agenesis is often asymptomatic during the infancy period; the unaffected kidney hypertrophies as a compensatory mechanism (Torchia & Persaud, 2025). Manifestations of bilateral agenesis are more severe and include visible yet grossly dysmorphic (cystic) kidneys with or without a bladder outlet obstruction and absence of urine formation.

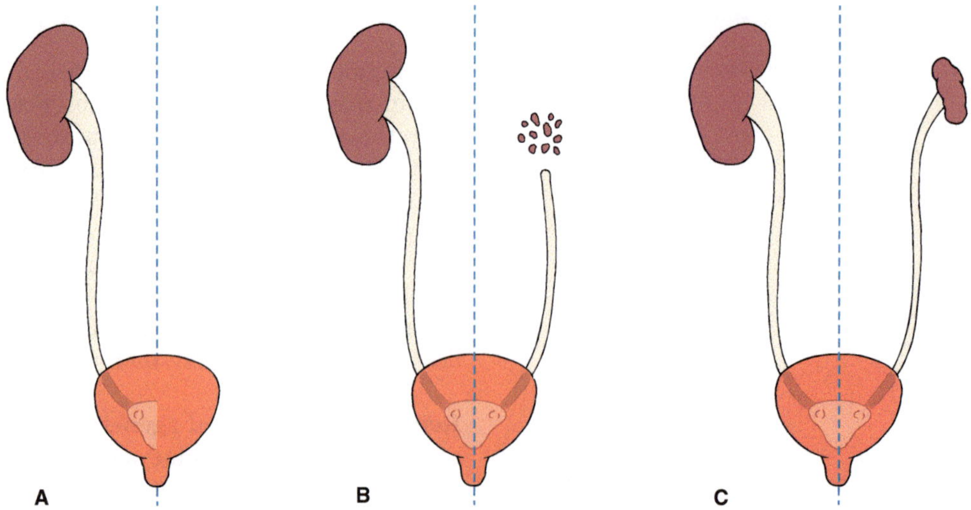

Figure 8.14 (**A**) Renal agenesis, (**B**) dysplasia, and (**C**) hypoplasia.

Life-span implications include hypertension, persistent hypertrophy of the unaffected kidney (considered normal compensation), hydronephrosis, altered GFR, and evidence of CRD (Torchia & Persaud, 2025; Vogt, 2025).

Renal Dysplasia. Renal dysplasia is characterized by errors in renal induction. Approximately 4% of fetuses and infants are affected by renal dysplasia, with unilateral disease reported in one of every 2,000 live births and bilateral dysplasia in one of every 4,000 live births (Vogt, 2025). Renal dysplasia may be confounded by other associated congenital diseases, including VATER sequence, Meckel syndrome, renal–coloboma syndrome, and prune belly syndrome. Furthermore, renal dysplasia is regarded as the most common cause for chronic kidney disease and end-stage renal failure among children, with a prevalence of 34% and 2:1 male to female preference (Chen & Chang, 2015; Fong & De Beritto, 2024; Phua & Ho, 2016). Epigenetic, genetic, and environmental factors are postulated to implicate this disease process.

Renal dysplasia involves aberrant metanephric development (Chen & Chang, 2015). The pathogenesis of renal dysplasia involves defective differentiation of the renal parenchyma. Less common, renal dysplasia occurs secondary to other obstructive pathologies, including PUV or UPJ obstruction. Regardless of the pathogenesis, the end result is the persistence of immature, primitive tubules and parenchymal damage secondary to cyst formation or interstitial fibrosis (Phua & Ho, 2016).

Fetal manifestations of renal dysplasia include oligohydramnios and hydronephrosis. Neonatal manifestations may include a palpable mass associated with the affected kidney and reflux to the affected (and possibly the normal) kidney. Later manifestations include persistent urinary incontinence and dysfunction, urinary infections, and renal failure. Adult females are more likely to report urinary incontinence, which should increase the index of suspicion for a congenital anomaly of the kidneys or urinary tract (Chen & Chang, 2015).

Prognosis of infants with renal dysplasia is related to unilateral or bilateral disease presentation (Vogt, 2025). Long-term outcomes for unilateral dysplasia are positive. Infants with bilateral dysplasia disease exhibit more complicated comorbidities and symptoms. Infants with renal dysplasia may present with oligohydramnios prenatally, UTD, and impaired renal function.

Renal Hypoplasia. Primary renal hypoplasia is characterized by a kidney that is normally developed, yet abnormally small, affixed with a decreased number of intact nephrons. Secondary hypoplasia manifests as a consequence of infection or a mechanical obstruction. Most cases are sporadic; however, genetic and environmental influences are reported. For example, mutations in the *PAX2* gene have been linked to reductions in kidney size. Environmental influences include uteroplacental insufficiency, vitamin A deficiency, low dietary protein intake during pregnancy, alcohol and cocaine ingestion, and fetal exposure to glucocorticoids and thalidomide (Cain et al., 2010).

Associated inherited disorders include branchio-oto-renal syndrome, renal–coloboma syndrome, trisomy syndromes, Cenani–Lenz syndrome, and CHARGE syndrome (Chen & Chang, 2015; Gribouval et al., 2012). Histological studies offer insight into the pathogenesis of renal hypoplasia. A reduction in ureteral bud branches is observed, secondary to an increased apoptosis. Although nephrogenesis is possible, fewer nephrons develop, yielding the anatomically small kidney. The clinical presentation mimics renal dysplasia. Life-span implications include adult-onset hypertension and chronic renal failure (Cain et al., 2010).

Horseshoe Kidney. A horseshoe-shaped kidney is characterized by fusion of the lower poles, causing the formation of a U-shaped kidney (Figure 8.15; Torchia

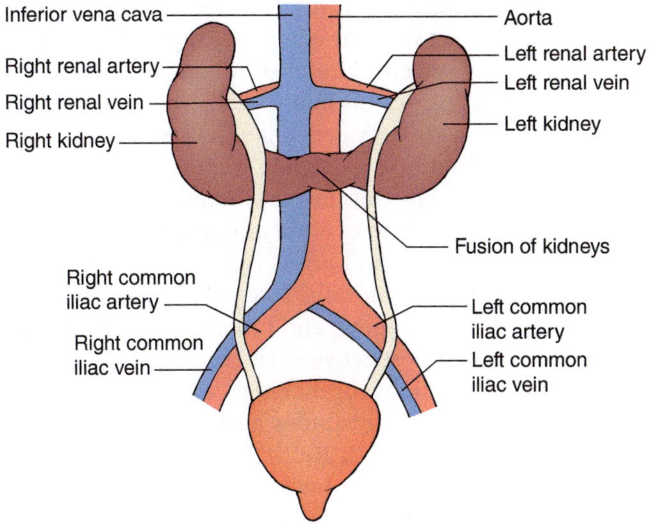

Figure 8.15 Horseshoe kidney. Note the abnormal fusion of the kidneys at the inferior lobes.

& Persaud, 2025). The incidence of horseshoe kidney is approximately one in 500 live births, with a 2:1 male to female preference reported in the literature (Fong & De Beritto, 2024; Holcomb et al., 2020). Associated renal defects include VUR, UPJ obstruction, and renal duplication. The most common genetic association is Turner syndrome (Zitelli et al., 2023).

Recall that the early fetal period of development involves the vertical ascent of each kidney. Both kidneys migrate upward and outward from one another toward the thoracolumbar region, ultimately situating on either side of the spine. Horseshoe shaping of the kidney occurs as a result of fusion of the metanephric blastemal prior to vertical ascent (Rumack & Levine, 2024). The process of fusion creates a structural barrier to normal ascent as the inferior mesenteric artery lies within the pathway of the abnormally merged kidneys (Torchia & Persaud, 2025). This causes abnormal rotation and axial position changes with anterior positioning of each kidney. Each kidney typically remains affixed with a normal collection system and ureter; however, the abnormal rotation of the renal pelves increases the risk for UPJ obstruction. As a result, affected individuals incur a higher risk for kidney stones and infection.

Hydronephrosis should increase the index of suspicion for horseshoe kidney (Rumack & Levine, 2024). Up to 33% of affected infants who are not diagnosed during fetal development are clinically asymptomatic (Torchia & Persaud, 2025). Children or adults may present with idiopathic back or abdominal pain. Kidney stones and hypocitraturia are commonly reported among affected individuals and may recur across the life span.

Ureteropelvic Junction Obstruction. UPJ obstruction is the most common cause of lower urinary tract obstruction and hydronephrosis in infants. The incidence of UPJ obstruction is approximately one in every 1,500 live births; a male prevalence is reported (Vogt, 2025). UPJ may be associated with genetic syndromes, congenital anomalies, or genitourinary malformations.

Congenital UPJ obstruction is caused by anatomic or functional disturbances restricting urinary flow through the UPJ (Figure 8.16; Kenner & Lott, 2014). This obstruction is typically a result of intrinsic proximal ureter stenosis or extrinsic compression (less common; Greenbaum, 2025). Intrinsic stenosis occurs if the upper segment is narrow or kinked as the ureter enters the pelvis (Rogers, 2023). Extrinsic compression occurs from the compression of the UPJ by an aberrant or accessory artery crossing the lower pole of the kidney. Glomerular function may be reduced due to the effects of mechanical compression; however, normal glomerular function is reported in up to 50% of all cases (Greenbaum, 2025; Vogt, 2025).

Fetal hydronephrosis with or without a dilated ureter should raise the index of suspicion for UPJ obstruction. Manifestations during the newborn period or infancy include a palpable mass, hematuria, or, in older children, flank pain (60% of cases affect the left kidney; Greenbaum, 2025). As pyeloplasty is associated with a 91% to 98% success rate, long-term sequelae are uncommon.

Posterior Urethral Valve Disease. PUV disorder is the most common obstructive anomaly of the urethra and urinary system (Greenbaum, 2025; Vogt, 2025). PUV occurs in one in 5,000 to 8,000 live births and typically affects male infants (Fong & De Beritto, 2024; Greenbaum, 2025; Vincent et al., 2022).

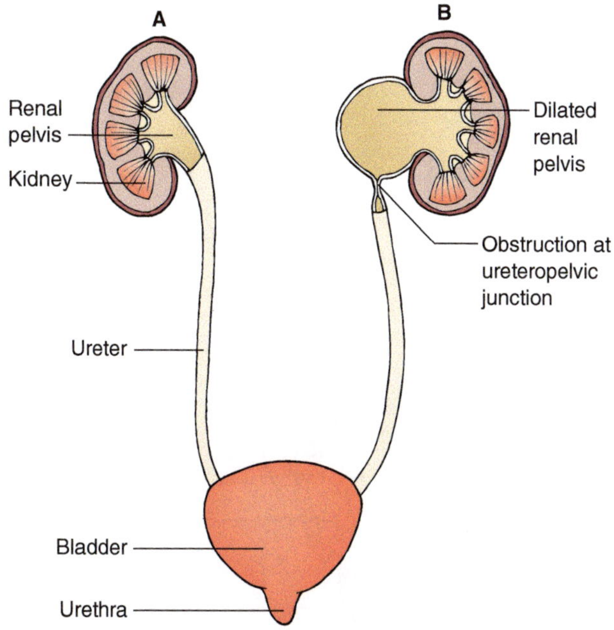

Figure 8.16 Ureteropelvic junction (UPJ) obstruction. (**A**) Normal kidney; (**B**) kidney affected by UPJ obstruction.

Recall that the male urethra develops during the early fetal period of development. A portion of that process includes the generation of urethral valves. Normally, during the downward evacuation of urine from bladder to the penis, pressure from the solute pushes the valves open and allows outflow of urine. With PUV, the anterior fusion of the valves obstructs outflow of urine from the bladder. As a result, persistent urinary pressure induces thickening, trabeculations, sacculations, diverticula, and hypertrophy of the bladder wall with urethral dilatation (**Figure 8.17**; Dogra et al., 2014). Antenatal ultrasound findings include bilateral hydronephrosis, dilated urethra, and distended bladder with thickened wall (Fong & De Beritto, 2024).

Fetal manifestations of PUV include hydronephrosis and oligohydramnios; more severe manifestations include urinoma, urine ascites, and dilated ureters (Vogt, 2025). Male newborns frequently present with a visible or palpable distended bladder and weak urinary stream; as the onset of urinary output may extend into the second postnatal day, diagnosis may be delayed accordingly (Maguire, 2021). Life-span implications include urinary incontinence, urosepsis, and VUR (Talabi et al., 2015). Between 25% to 40% of affected males exhibit renal insufficiency, which progresses to end-stage renal disease within 10 years of diagnosis (Bhadoo et al., 2014; Fong & De Beritto, 2024; Kenner & Lott, 2014).

Ureteral Anomalies

Errors in ureteral bud development and differentiation may give rise to several ureteral anomalies. These include ureteral duplication, ureteral triplication, megaureter, and ectopic ureters. The focus for this section will be on ureteral duplication, the most common ureteral anomaly.

Renal Duplication. Renal duplication (also known as *renal duplex*) is a partial or complete duplication of the renal collecting system. Ureteral anomaly is the most common urinary tract anomaly, with an incidence of 1% to 10%; a female prevalence is reported (Fong & De Beritto, 2024; Partin et al., 2021). Females are twice as likely to be affected by this defect in renal development.

Recall from our review of embryologic kidney development that the ureteric bud arises from the mesonephric duct. The bud grows laterally, toward the metanephric blastema (or future kidney), and innervates it. Once embedded within the mesenchyme, the ureteric bud undergoes a series of divisions (branching), which gives rise to the collecting ducts and tubules and major and minor calyces (Torchia & Persaud, 2025). If the ureteric bud begins its process of division before innervating with the mesenchyme, a ureteral duplication occurs.

Ureteral duplications may be complete or partial. A complete duplication involves the genesis of two separate and independent ureters, both of which drain urine from the kidney and innervate the bladder (**Figure 8.18**). A partial duplication, or "bifid collecting system," may present in two forms. A bifid pelvis involves the genesis of two separate ureters that fuse together at the UPJ and then innervate the bladder as one conjoined unit (**Figure 8.19**). A bifid ureter involves the genesis of two separate ureters that fuse together below the UPJ, yet above the bladder, and thereby innervate the bladder as one conjoined unit (**Figure 8.20**; Doery et al., 2015; Rodriguez, 2014).

Infants with uncomplicated or partial renal duplication may be asymptomatic. More complex or complete duplication may result in obstructive disorders or VUR.

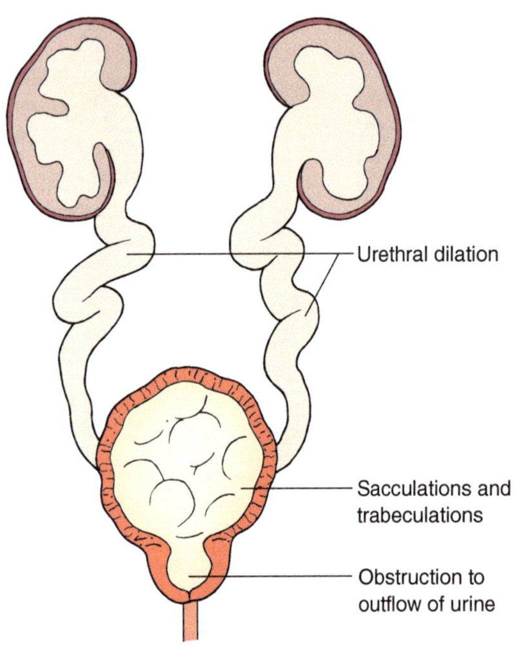

Figure 8.17 Posterior urethral valves.

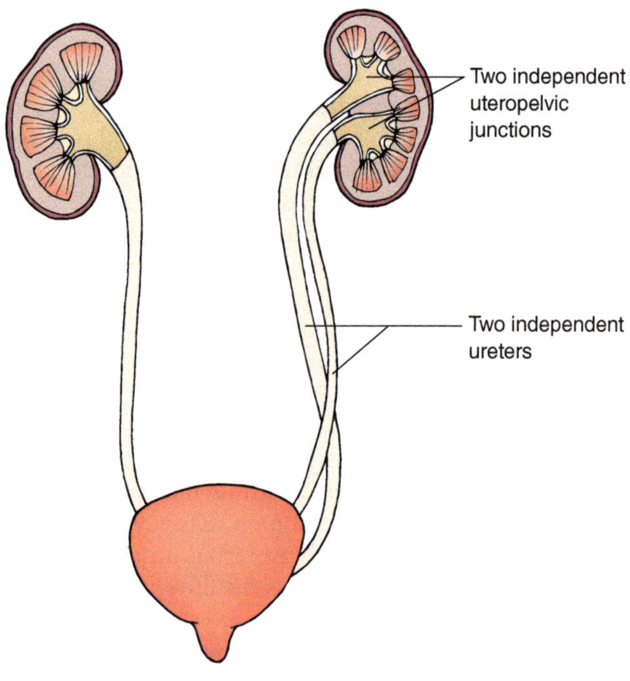

Figure 8.18 Complete ureteral duplication.

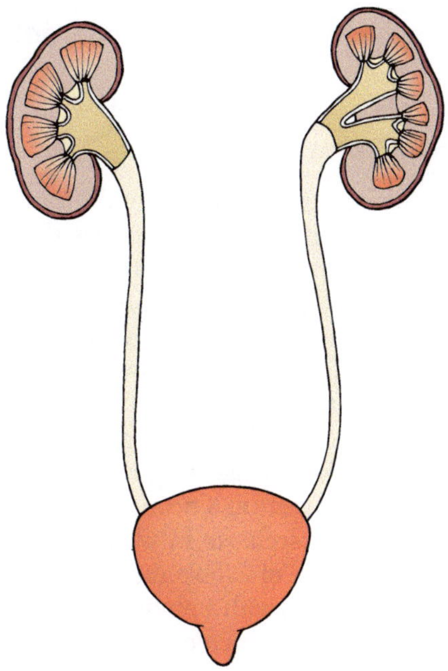

Figure 8.19 Partial ureteral duplication (bifid pelvis). A bifid pelvis involves the fusion of two separate ureters at the ureteropelvic junction. The fused ureter innervates the bladder as one conjoined unit.

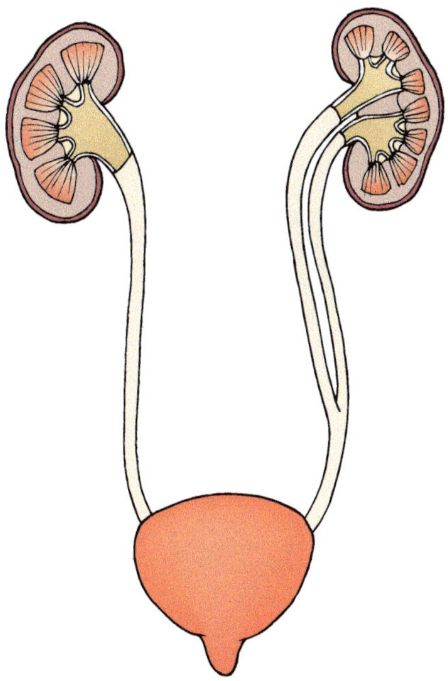

Figure 8.20 Partial ureteral duplication (bifid ureter). A bifid ureter involves the creation of two separate ureters that fuse together below the ureteropelvic junction, yet above the bladder, and thereby innervate the bladder as one conjoined unit.

Based on ectopic insertion location in complete duplication, sexual dysfunction and urinary incontinence may occur. Additional evaluation is warranted for patients with a history of urinary tract infection, renal system dilation, or alterations in urine flow.

Urachal Anomalies

Recall that the allantois, a fingerlike projection of the yolk sac, develops during early embryologic development and connects the umbilicus to the ventral cloaca (bladder). Between weeks 5 and 7 of gestation, the allantois canalizes into the urachus, a primitive conduit for the evacuation of liquid waste and exchange of gases in the time frame preceding the genesis of the umbilical cord and bladder. Once these structures develop and renal function begins, the urachus shifts from a functionally significant duct to a remnant of early embryologic development. As the bladder descends toward the pelvic region, between weeks 16 and 20 of gestation, the urachus is stretched between both poles and into a closed, fibrous ligament. This ligament typically ranges between 8 and 10 cm in length and 8 to 10 mm in diameter, and after birth rests on top of the obliterated umbilical arteries (de Queiroz Garcia et al., 2015; Partin et al., 2021).

Four types of congenital urachal anomalies are known: patent urachus (50%), urachal cysts (30%), umbilical–urachal sinus (15%), and vesicourethral diverticula (3%–5%; Partin et al., 2021).

Patent Urachus. A host of urachal anomalies may present during embryologic development or in later adulthood. Patent urachus, first identified by Bartholomaeus Cabrolius in 1550, involves persistent canalization of the urachus and backflow of urine from the bladder out the umbilicus. Associated defects include Meckel diverticulum, umbilical hernia, PUV, and urethral atresia (Partin et al., 2021). Manifestations of patent urachus include drainage or edema from the umbilicus and delayed detachment of the umbilical stump during the first weeks of life. Fever should raise the index of suspicion for infection; common pathogens include *Staphylococcus aureus*, *Escherichia coli*, and *Enterococcus* (Partin et al., 2021). Surgical correction is considered curative.

CONCLUSION

The renal system is a complex, yet exquisitely organized system designed to regulate fluid and electrolytes, assist in acid–base regulation, filter waste products, and respond to hemodynamic instability. Glomerular precursors arise during the early embryonic period, and glomerulogenesis is complete by 34 to 36 weeks. As the urinary system develops, the ureters, bladder, and urethra develop, providing a route of excretion for water and waste products. Renal blood flow, hormonal development, and increasing gestational age contribute to renal and urinary maturation. Genetic disorders, environmental and developmental disorders, low nephron endowment, infection, and prematurity may contribute to prenatal or postnatal renal or urinary injury. Unlike other body systems, birth halts renal (glomerular) proliferation, placing premature infants at a particularly high risk for renal dysfunction and later injury. Most newborns, especially premature newborns who require neonatal intensive care, will require regular outpatient monitoring. Clinicians must be vigilant, yet mindful of therapies that risk nephrotoxicity or intrinsic injury, when managing critically ill infants.

LEARNING TOOLS AND RESOURCES

CourseConnect

To access self-assessment questions and interactive, competency-based learning activities for this chapter, visit www.springerpub.com/courseconnect. See inside front cover and tear-out card for CourseConnect details.

Podcast

This podcast is available online by visiting www.springerpub.com/courseconnect. See inside front cover and tear-out card for CourseConnect details.

The Renin-Angiotensin-Aldosterone
Amy J. Jnah

Discussion Prompts

1. Interruption of nephrogenesis by preterm birth may interfere with renal function. Discuss the short- and long-term effects of preterm birth on renal function. Choose a common problem that premature infants face during the postnatal period; how might renal hypertrophy affect the infant's ability to maintain homeostasis?
2. Acute renal failure may manifest as a consequence of premature birth, or as a result of a pathological condition. Apply your knowledge of acute renal failure by reflecting upon your years as a neonatal nurse or clinician. Describe a clinical scenario in which an infant manifested with each type of failure and associate the clinical or laboratory findings with a physiologic explanation.
3. Discuss scenarios that increase the index of suspicion for PUVs in a term neonate.

MIND MAP

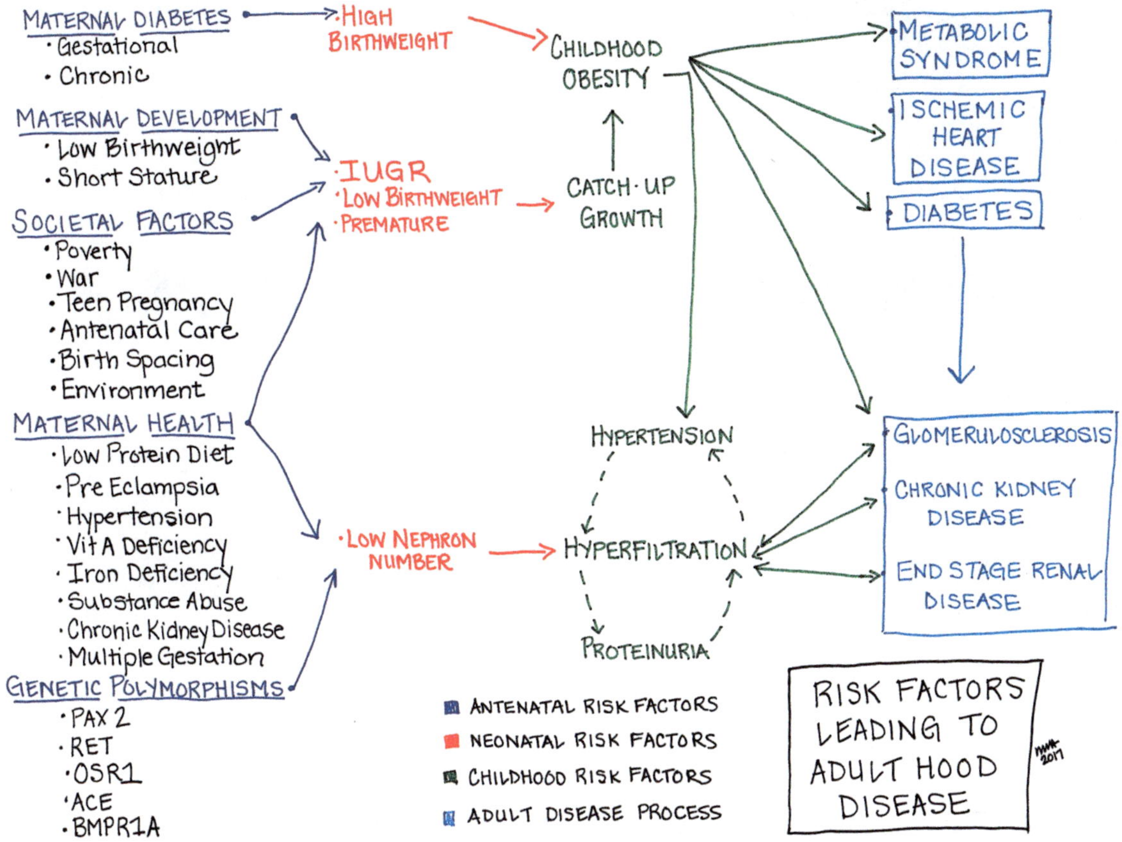

Note: This mind map reflects a former neonatal nurse practitioner student's interpretation of a concept addressed in this chapter. Readers should regard the mind maps woven throughout this textbook as examples of multisensory study tools that can be developed to aid conceptual understanding. Readers are encouraged to develop their own unique mind maps in consultation with academic faculty or clinical preceptors.

Image Credit: Nicole Harvey, MSN, APRN, NNP-BC.

TIMELINE OF ORGAN DEVELOPMENT

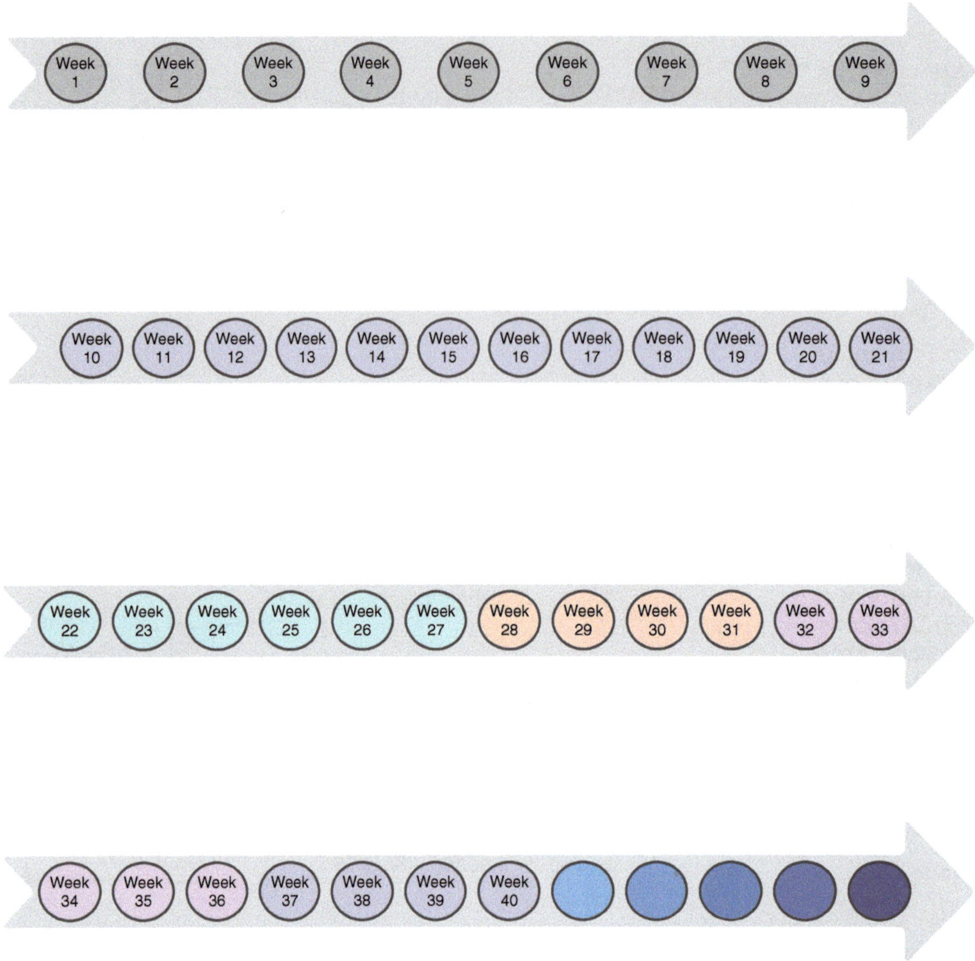

Note: Placement of common problems is meant to offer visual/conceptual perspective on the timing of onset of these commonly reported malformations. Variation exists across the literature.	***Legend:*** <22–27 6/7 weeks = extremely preterm 28–31 6/7 weeks = very preterm 32–36 6/7 weeks = late/moderate preterm 37–40 weeks = term

Note: Readers should annotate the blank timeline during studying, self-directed learning, and creation of feedback loops with mentors.
To access the blank and completed timelines visit www.springerpub.com/courseconnect. See inside front cover and tear-out card for CourseConnect details.

REFERENCES

Abitbol, C. L., DeFreitas, M. J., & Strauss, J. (2016). Assessment of kidney function in preterm infants: Lifelong implications. *Journal of Pediatric Nephrology, 31*(12), 2213–2222. https://doi.org/10.1007/s00467-016-3320-x

Alexander, B. T., Dasinger, J. H., & Intapad, S. (2015). Fetal programming and cardiovascular pathology. *Comprehensive Physiology, 5*(2), 997–1025. https://doi.org/10.1002/cphy.c140036

Alpern, R. J., Caplan, M. J., & Moe, O. W. (Eds.). (2013). *Seldin and Giebisch's the kidney: Physiology & pathophysiology* (5th ed.). Elsevier Science.

Azhibekov, A., Philippe, S., & Seri, I. (2022). Regulation of acid-base balance in the fetus and neonate. In R. A. Polin, S.H. Abman, D. H. Rowitch, & W. Benitz (Eds.), *Fetal and neonatal physiology* (6th ed., pp. 1076–1081). Elsevier.

Baker, H. M., & Jnah, A. J. (2024). Supporting infants with multicystic dysplastic kidney disease: A comprehensive approach. *Neonatal Network, 43*(5), 286–294. https://doi.org/10.1891/NN-2024-0007

Baum, M. (2022). Renal transport of sodium during development. In R. A. Polin, S. H. Abman, D. H. Rowitch, & W. E. Benitz (Eds.), *Fetal and neonatal physiology* (6th ed., pp. 984–992). Elsevier.

Baum, M. (2017). Renal transport of sodium during development. In R. A. Polin, S. H. Abman, D. H. Rowitch, W. E. Benitz, & W. W. Fox (Eds.), *Fetal and neonatal physiology* (5th ed., pp. 1002–1010). Elsevier.

Bhadoo, D., Bajpai, M., & Panda, S. S. (2014). Posterior urethral valve: Prognostic factors and renal outcome. *Journal of Indian Association of Pediatric Surgeons, 19*(3), 133–137. https://doi.org/10.4103/0971-9261.136459

Brophy, P. (2017). Maternal determinants of renal mass and function in the fetus and neonate. *Seminars in Fetal & Neonatal Medicine, 22*(2), 67–70. https://doi.org/10.1016/j.siny.2017.01.004

Cain, J. E., Di Giovanni, V., Smeeton, J., & Rosenblum, N. D. (2010). Genetics of renal hypoplasia: Insights into the mechanisms controlling nephron endowment. *Pediatric Research, 68*(2), 91–98. https://doi.org/10.1203/PDR.0b013e3181e35a88

Calkins, K., & Devaskar, S. U. (2011). Fetal origins of adult disease. *Current Problems in Pediatric and Adolescent Health Care, 41*(6), 158–176. https://doi.org/10.1016/j.cppeds.2011.01.001

Capone, V. P., Morello, W., Taroni, F., & Montini, G. (2017). Genetics of congenital anomalies of the kidney and urinary tract: The current state of play. *International Journal of Molecular Science, 18*(4), 796. https://doi.org/10.3390/ijms18040796

Cardona-Grau, D., & Kogan, B. A. (2015). Update on multicystic dysplastic kidney. *Current Urology Reports, 16*(10), 1–5. https://doi.org/10.1007/s11934-015-0541-7

Chebib, F. T., & Torres, V. E. (2016). Autosomal dominant polycystic kidney disease: Core curriculum 2016. *American Journal of Kidney Diseases, 67*(5), 792–810. https://doi.org/10.1053/j.ajkd.2015.07.037

Chen, R., & Chang, C. (2015). Renal dysplasia. *Archives of Pathology & Laboratory Medicine, 139*(4), 547–551. https://doi.org/10.5858/arpa.2013-0660-RS

Chestnut, D. H., Wong, C. A., Tsen, L. C., Kee, W. D., Beilin, Y., & Mhyre, J. (Eds.). (2014). *Chestnut's obstetric anesthesia: Principles and practice e-book* (5th ed.). Saunders.

Collins, J. W., Rankin, K. M., & David, R. J. (2011). Low birth weight across generations: The effect of economic environment. *Maternal and Child Health Journal, 15*(4), 438–445. https://doi.org/10.1007/s10995-010-0603-x

Cooper, C. J., Said, S., Khalillullah, S., Salameh, H. J., & Hernandez, G. T. (2013). Multicystic dysplastic kidney complicated by pyelonephritis. *American Journal of Case Reports, 14*, 412–415. https://doi.org/10.12659/AJCR.889557

Curtis, S. N. (2025). Fluid, electrolytes, and acid-base homeostasis. In R. Martin & A. A. Fanaroff (Eds.), *Fanaroff and Martin's neonatal-perinatal medicine: Diseases of the fetus and infant* (12th ed., pp. 1948–1965). Elsevier.

Davis, E. M., Peck, J. D., Thompson, D., Wild, R. A., & Langlois, P. (2010). Maternal diabetes and renal agenesis/dysgenesis. *Birth Defects Research: Part A. Clinical and Molecular Teratology, 88*(9), 722–727. https://doi.org/10.1002/bdra.20702

de Queiroz Garcia, M., de Queiroz Garcia, M., & Barral, C. M. (2015). Patent urachus presenting as acute abdomen. *Journal of Medical Ultrasound, 23*(4), 189–192. https://doi.org/10.1016/j.jmu.2015.08.003

Doery, A. J., Ang, E., & Ditchfield, M. R. (2015). Duplex kidney: Not just a drooping lily. *Journal of Medical Imaging and Radiation Oncology, 59*(2), 149–153. https://doi.org/10.1111/1754-9485.12285

Dogra, V., MacLennan, G. T., Turgut, A. T., Canacci, A., & Onur, M. R. (2014). *Genitourinary radiology: Kidney, bladder and urethra: The pathologic basis*. Springer.

dos Santos, J. A. C. S., de Miranda, D. M., & Simoes e Silva, A. C. (2014). Congenital anomalies of the kidney and urinary tract: An embryogenetic review. *Birth Defects Research: Part C, 102*, 374–381. https://doi.org/10.1002/bdrc.21084

Eichenwald, E. C., Hansen, A. R., Martin, C. R., & Stark, A. R. (Eds.). (2023). *Cloherty and Stark's manual of neonatal care* (9th ed.). Lippincott Williams & Wilkins.

Eickmeyer, A. B., Casanova, N. F., He, C., Smith, E. A., Wan, J., Bloom, D. A., & Dillman, J. R. (2014). The natural history of the multicystic dysplastic kidney–Is limited follow-up warranted? *Journal of Pediatric Urology, 10*(4), 655–661. https://doi.org/10.1016/j.jpurol.2014.06.001

Engen, R., & Hingorani, S. (2024). Developmental abnormalities of the kidneys. In C. A. Gleason & S. E. Juul (Eds.), *Avery's diseases of the newborn* (11th ed., pp. 1100–1110). Elsevier Saunders.

Ferri, F. F. (2025). *Ferri's clinical advisor 2025: 5 books in 1*. Elsevier.

Fong, J., & De Beritto, T. (2024). Congenital anomalies of the kidneys and urinary tract. *Neoreviews, 25*(2), e78–e85. https://doi.org/10.1542/neo.25-2-e78

Gattineni, J., & Baum, M. (2015). Developmental changes in renal tubular transport—An overview. *Pediatric Nephrology, 30*, 2085–2098. https://doi.org/10.1007/s00467-013-2666-6

Gil-Peña, H., Mejía, N., & Santos, F. (2014). Renal tubular acidosis. *Journal of Pediatrics, 164*(4), 691–698.e1. https://doi.org/10.1016/j.jpeds.2013.10.085

Good, P. I., Lin, F., & Charlton, J. R. (2022). Response to nephron loss in early development. In R. A. Polin, S. H. Abman, D. H. Rowitch, W. E. Benitz, & W. W. Fox (Eds.), *Fetal and neonatal physiology* (6th ed., pp. 1056–1063). Elsevier.

Goyal, S., & Banerjee, S. (2020). Fluid, electrolyte and early nutritional management in the preterm neonate with very low birth weight. *Paediatrics and Child Health, 31*(1), 7–17. https://doi.org/10.1016/j.paed.2020.10.002

Greenbaum, L. A. (2025). Electrolyte and acid-base disorders. In R. M. Kliegman, B. F. Stanton, J. W. St Geme, & N. F. Schor (Eds.), *Nelson textbook of pediatrics* (22nd ed., pp. 485–525). Elsevier.

Gribouval, O., Morinière, V., Pawtowski, A., Arrondel, C., Sallinen, S.-L., Saloranta, C., Clericuzio, C., Viot, G., Tantau, J., Blesson, S., Cloarec, S., Christine Machet, M., Chitayat, D., Thauvin, C., Laurent, N., Sampson, J. R., Bernstein, J. A., Clemenson, A., Prieur, F., ... Gubler, M. C. (2012). Spectrum of mutations in the renin–angiotensin system genes in autosomal recessive renal tubular dysgenesis. *Human Mutation: Variation, Informatics, and Disease, 33*, 316–326. https://doi.org/10.1002/humu.21661

Guignard, J-P. & Iacobelli, S. (2022). Postnatal development of glomerular filtration rate in neonates. In R. A. Polin, S.H. Abman, D. H. Rowitch, & W. Benitz (Eds.), *Fetal and neonatal physiology* (6th edition., pp. 975–984). Elsevier.

Hagen-Ansert, S. L. (2023). *Textbook of diagnostic sonography* (9th ed.). Elsevier.

Harris, P. C., & Torres, P. C. (2022). Polycystic kidney disease, autosomal dominant. In M. P. Adam, J. Feldman, & G. M.

Mirzaa (Eds.), *GeneReviews*. University of Washington. https://www.ncbi.nlm.nih.gov/books/NBK1246

Holcomb, G. W., Murphy, J. P., & Ostlie, D. J. (Eds.). (2020). *Ashcraft's pediatric surgery* (7th ed.). Saunders/Elsevier.

Holmes, A. P. (Ed.). (2016). *NICU primer for pharmacists*. American Society of Health-System Pharmacists.

Johnson, A. K., Lynch, N., Newberry, D., & Jnah, A. J. (2017). Impact of diuretic therapy in the treatment of bronchopulmonary dysplasia and acute kidney injury in the neonatal population. *Advances in Neonatal Care, 17*(5), 337–346. https://doi.org/10.1097/ANC.0000000000000427

Kastl, J. T. (2017). Renal function in the fetus and neonate–The creatinine enigma. *Seminars in Fetal & Neonatal Medicine, 22*(2), 82–89. https://doi.org/10.1016/j.siny.2016.12.002

Kenner, C., & Lott, J. W. (Eds.). (2014). *Comprehensive neonatal nursing care* (5th ed.). Springer Publishing Company.

Klabunde, R. E. (2012). *Cardiovascular physiology concepts* (2nd ed., pp. 137–140). Lippincott, Williams & Wilkins.

Kliegman, R. M., St. Geme, J. W., Blum, N. J., Tasker, R. C., Wilson, K. M., Schuh, A. M., & Mack, C. L. (2025). Introduction to glomerular diseases. In R. M. Kliegman, B. F. Stanton, J. W. St Geme, & N. F. Schor (Eds.), *Nelson textbook of pediatrics* (22nd ed., pp. 3180–3183). Elsevier.

Lee, B. R. (2024). Renal tubular acidosis in the neonate. *Neoreviews, 25*(2), e99–e106. https://doi.org/10.1542/neo.25-2-e99

Lindower, J. B. (2017). Water balance in the fetus and neonate. *Seminars in Fetal & Neonatal Medicine, 22*(2), 71–75. https://doi.org/10.1016/j.siny.2017.01.002

Luyckx, V. A., Bertram, J. F., Brenner, B. M., Fall, C., Hoy, W. E., Ozanne, S. E., & Vikse, B. E. (2013). Effect of fetal and child health on kidney development and long-term risk of hypertension and kidney disease. *Lancet, 382*(9888), 273. https://doi.org/10.1016/S0140-6736(13)60311-6

Maguire, D. (2021). Renal and genitourinary disorders. In T. W. Verklan & M. Walden (Eds.), *Core curriculum for neonatal intensive care nursing* (6th ed., pp. 617–628). Elsevier.

Matsell, D. G., & Hiatt, M. J. (2017). Functional development of the kidney in utero. In R. A. Polin, S. H. Abman, D. H. Rowitch, W. E. Benitz, & W. W. Fox (Eds.), *Fetal and neonatal physiology* (5th ed., pp. 965–976). Elsevier.

McAleer, I., & Chiang, K-W. (2024). Renal development. In C. A. Gleason & S. E. Juul (Eds.), *Avery's diseases of the newborn* (11th ed., pp. 1087–1099). Elsevier Saunders.

Nada, A., Bonachea, E. M., & Askenazi, D. J. (2017). Acute kidney injury in the fetus and neonate. *Seminars in Fetal & Neonatal Medicine, 22*(2), 90–97. https://doi.org/10.1016/j.siny.2016.12.001

Nascimento, F. A. M., Ceciliano, T. C., Aguila, M. B., & Mandarim-de-Lacerda, C. A. (2012). Maternal vitamin D deficiency delays glomerular maturity in F1 and F2 offspring. *PLoS One, 7*(8), e41740. https://doi.org/10.1371/journal.pone.0041740

National Institutes of Health. (2018). *Genetics home reference: Polycystic kidney disease*. https://ghr.nlm.nih.gov/condition/polycystic-kidney-disease#statistics

National Institutes of Health. (2024a). *Genetic and rare diseases information center: Bartter syndrome*. https://rarediseases.info.nih.gov/diseases/5893/bartter-syndrome

National Institutes of Health. (2024b). *Genetic and rare diseases information center: Renal agenesis*. https://rarediseases.info.nih.gov/diseases/9228/renal-agenesis

Partin, A. W., Dmochowski, R. R., Kavoussi, L. R., & Peters, C. A. (Eds.). (2021). *Campbell-Walsh urology* (12th ed.). Elsevier.

Phadke, K., Goodyer, P., & Bitzan, M. (Eds.). (2014). *Manual of pediatric nephrology* (1st ed.). Springer Verlag. https://doi.org/10.1007/978-3-642-12483-9

Phua, Y. L., & Ho, J. (2016). Renal dysplasia in the neonate. *Current Opinion in Pediatrics, 28*(2), 209–215. https://doi.org/10.1097/MOP.0000000000000324

Reule, S., Sexton, D. J., Solid, C. A., Chen, S., Collins, A. J., & Foley, R. N. (2014). ESRD from autosomal dominant polycystic kidney disease in the United States, 2001–2010. *American Journal of Kidney Diseases, 64*(4), 592–599. https://doi.org/10.1053/j.ajkd.2014.05.020

Rickard, M., Easterbrook, B., Kim, S., Farrokhyar, F., Stein, N., Arora, S., Belostotsky, V., DeMaria, J., Lorenzo, A. J., & Braga, L. H. (2017). Six of one, half a dozen of the other: A measure of multidisciplinary inter/intra-rater reliability of the society for fetal urology and urinary tract dilation grading systems for hydronephrosis. *Journal of Pediatric Urology, 13*(1), 80–80.e5. https://doi.org/10.1016/j.jpurol.2016.09.005

Rogers, J. (2023). Alterations of renal and urinary tract function in children. In K. L. McCance & S. E. Huether (Eds.), *Pathophysiology: The biologic basis for disease in adults and children* (9th ed., pp. 1270–1284). Elsevier.

Rodriguez, M. M. (2014). Congenital anomalies of the kidney and the urinary tract (CAKUT). *Fetal & Pediatric Pathology, 33*(5–6), 293–320. https://doi.org/10.3109/15513815.2014.959678

Rosenblum, S., Pal, A., & Reidy, K. (2017). Renal development in the fetus and premature infant. *Seminars in Fetal & Neonatal Medicine, 22*(2), 58–66. https://doi.org/10.1016/j.siny.2017.01.001

Rumack, C. M., & Levine, D. (Eds.). (2024). *Diagnostic ultrasound* (6th ed.). Elsevier.

Sands, J. M., Layton, H. E., & Fenton, R. A. (2020). Urine concentration and dilution. In A. S. L. Yu, G. M. Chertow, V. A. Luychx, P. A. Marsden, K. Shorecki, & M. W. Taal (Eds.), *Brenner and Rector's the kidney* (11th ed., pp. 274–302). Elsevier.

Schoenwolf, G. C., Bleyl, S. B., Brauer, P. R., & Francis-West, P. H. (2021). *Larsen's human embryology* (6th ed.). Churchill Livingstone.

Scott, R. P., Maezawa, Y., Kreidberg, J., & Quaggin, S. E. (2020). Embryology of the kidney. In A. S. L. Yu, G. M. Chertow, V. A. Luychx, P. A. Marsden, K. Shorecki, & M. W. Taal (Eds.), *Brenner and Rector's the kidney* (11th ed., pp. 2–37). Elsevier.

Segar, J. L. (2016). Renal adaptive changes and sodium handling in the fetal-to-newborn transition. *Seminars in Fetal and Neonatal Medicine, 22*(2), 76–82. https://doi.org/10.1016/j.siny.2016.11.002

Smyth, I. M., Cullen-McEwen, L. A., Combes, A. N., O'Brien, L. L., Black, M. J., & Bertram, J. F. (2022). Development of the kidney: Morphology and mechanisms. In R. A. Polin, S. H. Abman, D. H. Rowitch, W. E. Benitz, & W. W. Fox (Eds.), *Fetal and neonatal physiology* (6th ed., 941–954). Elsevier.

Solhaug, M. & Jose, P. A. (2022). Development and refgulation of renal blood flow in the neonate. In R. A. Polin, S. H. Abman, D. H. Rowitch, & W. Benitz (Eds.), *Fetal and neonatal physiology* (6th ed., pp. 965–974). Elsevier.

Sparks, M., Crowley, S. D., Gurley, S. B., Mirotsou, M., & Coffman, T. M. (2014). Classical renin-angiotensin system in kidney physiology. *Comprehensive Physiology, 4*(3), 1201–1228. https://doi.org/10.1002/cphy.c130040

Taketomo, C. K., Hodding, J. H., & Kraus, D. M. (2017). *Lexicomp pediatric & neonatal dosage handbook with international trade names index: A global resource for clinicians treating pediatric and neonatal patients* (24th ed.). Wolters Kluwer.

Talabi, A. O., Sowande, O. A., Etonyeaku, A. C., Salako, A. A., & Adejuyigbe, O. (2015). Posterior urethral valves in children: Pattern of presentation and outcome of initial treatment in Ile-Ife, Nigeria. *Nigerian Journal of Surgery, 21*(2), 151–156. https://doi.org/10.4103/1117-6806.162591

Tasian, G., Cunha, G., & Baskin, L. (2010). Smooth muscle differentiation and patterning in the urinary bladder. *Differentiation, 80*(2–3), 106–117. https://doi.org/10.1016/j.diff.2010.05.004

Torchia, M. G., & Persaud, T. V. N. (2025). *The developing human: Clinically oriented embryology* (12th ed.). Elsevier.

Torchia, M. G., & Persaud, T. V. N. (Ed.). (2025). *The developing human: Clinically oriented embryology* (12th ed.). Elsevier.

Vincent, K., Murphy, H. J, & Twombley, K. E. (2022). Urinary tract dilation in the fetus and neonate. *Neoreviews, 23*(3), e159–172. https://doi.org/10.1542/neo.23-3-e159

Vogt, B. A. (2025). The kidney and urinary tract of the neonate. In R. Martin & A. A. Fanaroff (Eds.), *Fanaroff and Martin's neonatal–perinatal medicine: Diseases of the fetus and infant* (12th ed., pp. 1966–1989). Elsevier.

Ward, E., DeSantis, C., Robbins, A., Kohler, B., & Jemal, A. (2014). Childhood and adolescent cancer statistics, 2014. *CA: A Cancer Journal for Clinicians, 64*(2), 83–103. https://doi.org/10.3322/caac.21219

Westland, R., Schreuder, M. F., Ket, J. C., & van Wijk, J. A. (2013). Unilateral renal agenesis: A systematic review on associated anomalies and renal injury. *Nephrology, Dialysis, and Transplantation, 28*(7), 1844–1855. https://doi.org/10.1093/ndt/gft012

Wright, C. J., Posencheg, M. A., & Seri, I. (2024). Fluid, electrolyte, and acid–base balance. In C. A. Gleason & S. E. Juul (Eds.), *Avery's diseases of the newborn* (11th ed., pp. 231–252). Elsevier Saunders.

Yaffe, S. J., & Aranda, J. V. (Eds.). (2011). *Neonatal and pediatric pharmacology: Therapeutic principles in practice* (4th ed.). Lippincott Williams & Wilkins.

Zitelli, B. J., McIntire, S. C., & Nowalk, A. J. (Eds.). (2023). *Zitelli and Davis' atlas of pediatric physical diagnosis* (8th ed.). Elsevier.

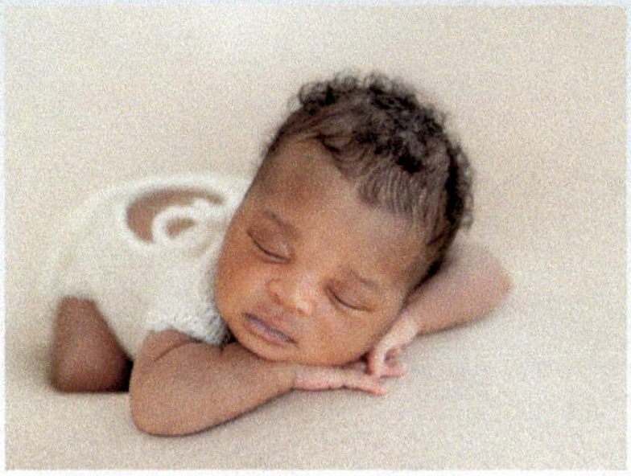 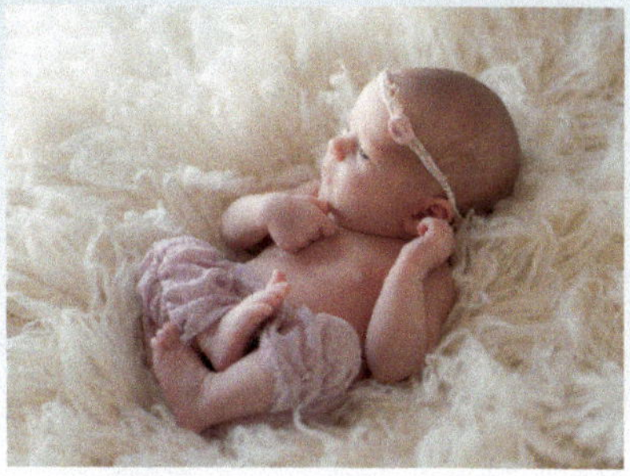

9

THE IMMUNE SYSTEM

Jacqui Hoffman, Colleen R. Moss, and Amy J. Jnah

LEARNING OBJECTIVES

After completing this chapter, the reader should be able to:

- Understand normal immune system development.
- Analyze the physiologic function of the fetal and neonatal immune system.
- Discuss common inherited disorders and their effect on fetal and neonatal immune system development and function.
- Identify health issues in XX pregnant patients that have a potential impact on fetal and postnatal immune system development and function.
- Evaluate common disorders that affect the immune system and their implications across the life span.

INTRODUCTION

The human immune system is composed of a heterogenous network of cells, tissues, and organs that work together to defend the body against a wide variety of foreign pathogens—from bacteria to parasites—that have the potential to cause disease or even death. During pregnancy, the fetus develops within the sterile intrauterine environment; however, after birth (and in some cases even before) the neonate is immediately exposed to several potentially pathogenic organisms and possesses limited innate defenses. Although maternal antibodies acquired through the placenta and through breast milk provide some (time-limited) protection to the newborn, many of the components of the innate and adaptive immune system are functionally immature, rendering the neonate vulnerable to infectious diseases. All newborns encounter antigens after birth, and these exposures prompt maturation of the neonatal immune system over the first 3 to 6 months of life; however, full maturation does not occur until early childhood. Consequently, sepsis (e.g., bacteremia, bacteruria, fungemia, viremia) in the newborn represents a major cause of mortality and morbidity worldwide. In this chapter, we review the developmental physiology of the innate and adaptive arms of the immune system; maternal and genetic influences on neonatal immune function; and common bacterial, viral, fungal, and protozoal pathogens implicated in neonatal infections, including their potential implications across the life span.

TIMELINE OF IMMUNE SYSTEM DEVELOPMENT

Recall from Chapter 7 that white blood cells (WBCs) develop from pluripotent stem cells that serve as a renewable source for the production of mature erythrocytes, platelets, and WBCs throughout life (**Figure 9.1**). The site of fetal hematopoiesis (blood cell production) changes several times during gestation as stem cells migrate from one site to another. From weeks 3 through 6 of gestation, stem cell progenitors appear in the blood islands of the yolk sac. From weeks 4 to 24 of gestation,

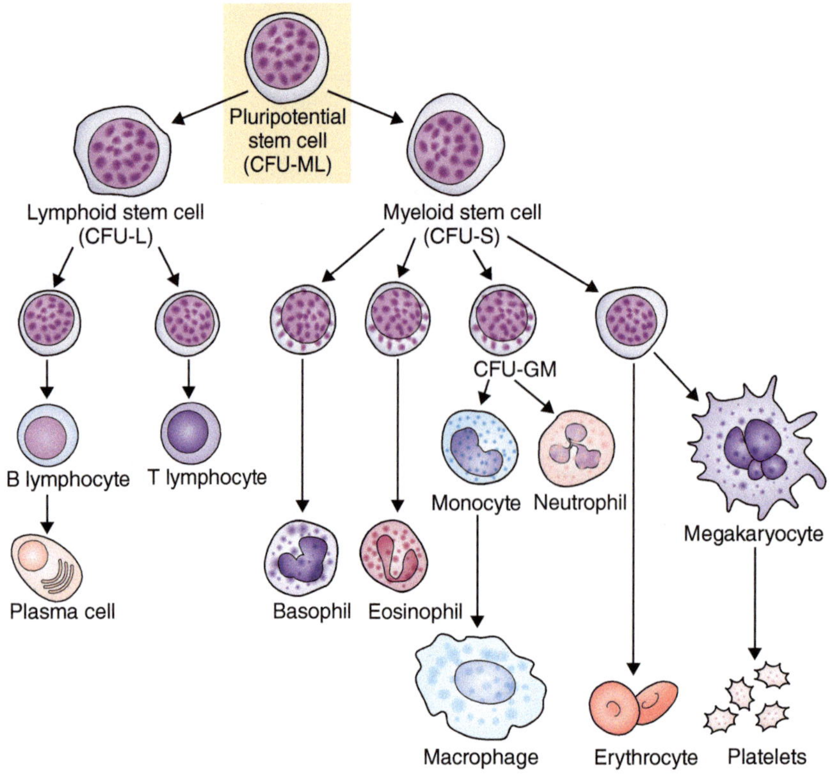

Figure 9.1 The first progenitor stem cells appear in the fetal yolk sac as early as 3 weeks' gestation. All blood cell lines originate from pluripotent stem cells. Lymphoid stem cells go on to differentiate into B lymphocytes and T lymphocytes. Myeloid stem cells are the precursors to neutrophils, macrophages, and dendritic cells.

CFU, colony-forming unit; GM, granulocyte and monocyte; L, lymphocyte; ML, myeloid and lymphoid; S, spleen.

Source: Adapted from Carlson, B. M. (2024). *Human embryology and developmental biology* (7th ed.). Elsevier/Saunders.

hematopoiesis occurs within the liver, with increasing contributions from the bone marrow. The bone marrow ultimately becomes a primary site for hematopoiesis near 24 weeks of gestation (Fernandez & de Alarcon, 2013; Lewis et al., 2025). The cell lines that comprise the immune system are the lymphoid and myeloid lines. Lymphoid stem cells give rise to two types of lymphocytes: B lymphocytes or B cells, which produce antibodies; and T lymphocytes or T cells, which are responsible for cell-mediated immune responses. Myeloid stem cells are precursors to other cell lines, including neutrophils, macrophages, and dendritic cells (Carlson, 2024). Growth factors and cellular interactions that occur in the bone marrow influence the differentiation of immune progenitors into their final cell lineage.

While many immune cells arise from bone marrow, T cells (named for the thymus gland) are produced in the thymus, which begins to develop from the third pharyngeal pouch during week 4 of gestation (Figure 9.2) and descends to its final position in the mediastinum near week 7 (Haddad et al., 2006; Schoenwolf et al., 2021). Around week 8 of gestation, progenitor cells that arise from the bone marrow migrate to the thymus and initiate a process of cell colonization (Erdos & Maródi, 2022; Haddad et al., 2006). Naïve T cells subsequently arise from the thymus and differentiate into specific subtypes based on interactions with antigens presented by myeloid cells and the cytokine milieu. By week 14 of gestation, the thymus is capable of modulating the complex processes necessary for the formation of diverse T-cell receptors (TCRs) necessary for self-tolerance (recognition of endogenously produced antigens as nonthreats and foreign antigens as threats), the prevention of infection, and the prevention of autoimmune disease (Haddad et al., 2006).

B cells are produced in the fetal liver by 8 weeks of gestation and the bone marrow by week 13 (S. C. A. Nielsen & Boyd, 2022). B-cell numbers continue to increase in the bone marrow, circulation, and peripheral lymphoid tissues with levels similar to adults reached by 22 weeks of gestation (S. C. A. Nielsen & Boyd, 2022). B-cell receptors (BCRs) undergo a complex process of gene rearrangement similar to that of T cells with the goal of promoting the formation of a diverse array of BCRs with strong affinity for foreign antigens. Naïve B cells subsequently differentiate into plasma cells, which serve as the source of antibody production throughout life.

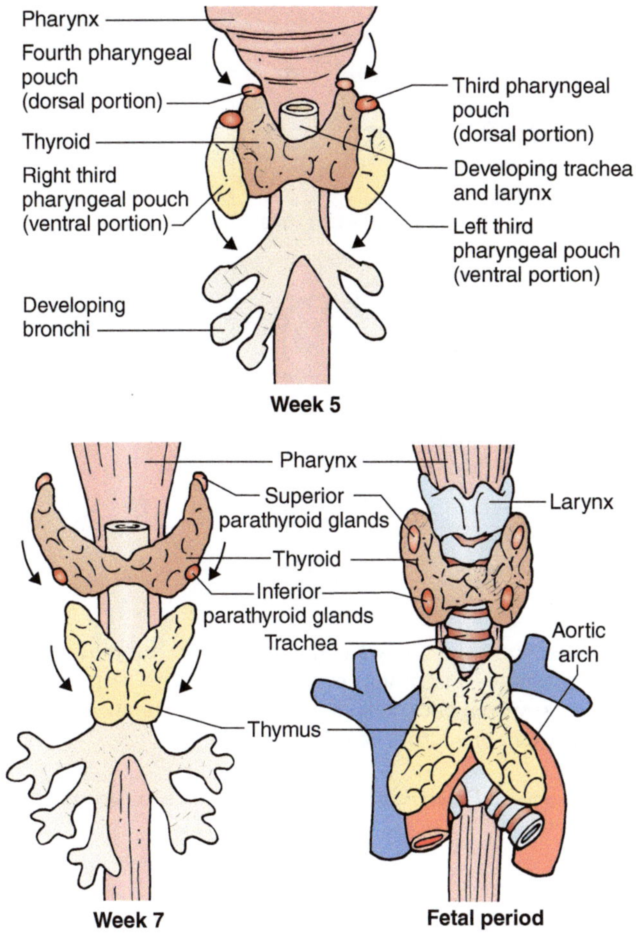

Figure 9.2 Beginning in week 4 of gestation, the fetal thymus begins to form from the third pharyngeal pouch. By week 5, the ventral portions of the left and right pharyngeal pouches begin to migrate inferiorly. By week 7 of gestation, the left and right third pharyngeal pouches fuse to form the bilobed thymus, which descends into its final position in the mediastinum.

DEVELOPMENTAL PHYSIOLOGY OF THE IMMUNE SYSTEM

The neonatal immune system has two major lines of protection: innate and adaptive immunity. The innate immune system is the first line of defense against potentially infectious organisms. The adaptive immune system confers specificity and immunologic memory but can take days to mount an appropriate antigenic response (Figure 9.3). Together, innate and adaptive immune responses function interdependently to provide host protection against invasive infection.

Innate Immunity

The body's first line of defense from infection is referred to as *innate immunity*, which can operate without any prior exposure to a pathogen. The defense mechanisms that comprise the innate immune response include anatomical barriers (e.g., skin and mucous membranes) and chemical barriers (e.g., gastrointestinal [GI] enzymes and gastric acid). These barriers help to prevent the invasion of microbes (Table 9.1).

The innate cells that recognize foreign antigens are termed *pattern recognition receptors (PRRs)*, and they are highly effective at initiating inflammatory responses (Medzhitov, 2013). Most foreign antigens take on a similar molecular structure, which often includes a cell wall and inner single- and double-stranded nucleic acids and unmethylated DNA (deoxyribonucleic acid). This structure is labeled a *pathogen-associated molecular pattern* (PAMPs). PRRs can recognize PAMPs (found on any foreign material that may be comprised of proteins, protein fragments, polysaccharides, or lipids) and initiate an inflammatory cascade consisting of cellular and soluble defenses, which will be discussed in the text that follows.

Clinical Application. The biggest organ in the body is the skin. Mature and intact skin offers outstanding innate defenses. For example, the outer surface of the skin is dry, which offers limited nutrients for pathogen proliferation. Skin layers normally shed or slough off, which removes pathogens. The skin also secretes toxic lipids and acids, which neutralize pathogens. In addition, intact skin is colonized with nonpathogenic, commensal flora with whom incoming microbes must compete, and it is replete with infection-fighting cells (e.g., Langerhans cells) as well as antimicrobial peptides that kill bacteria, viruses, and fungi. While it would be ideal for all neonates to have mature skin defenses, we must recognize that very preterm and extremely preterm neonates are born with fragile skin that is vulnerable to injury and less capable of limiting and neutralizing pathogen activity. In fact, the outermost layer of their skin (stratum corneum) is often highly porous/gelatinous and frail. The use of antimicrobial agents (e.g., betadine, chlorhexidine), while an essential part of the performance of invasive procedures, can irritate the skin and/or induce burns if not completely wiped away. Routine handling can also induce trauma to the skin and increase the risk for the penetration of pathogens through the skin layers.

Cellular Components of Innate Immunity. Celluluar components, or soluble mediators, of the immune system include *phagocytic* cells that are capable of engulfing and absorbing foreign antigens. There are multiple types of phagocytes present in the human body, in various body compartments (Table 9.2). Neutrophils, mononuclear phagocytes, dendritic cells, natural killer (NK) cells, and

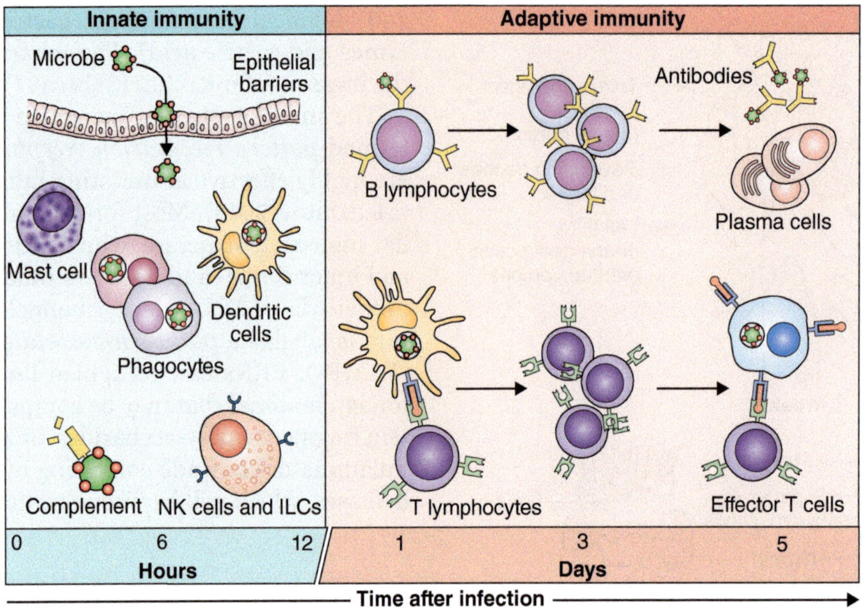

Figure 9.3 The innate immune response and the adaptive immune response comprise the two major arms of the immune system. The innate immune system responds to infection within hours and requires no previous exposure to mount a response. The adaptive immune system can take days to mount an immune response; however, once activated it confers specificity and immunologic memory to ensure a more robust and efficient response in the event of a future exposure.
ILC, innate lymphoid cells; NK, natural killer.
Source: Adapted from Abbas, A. K., Lichtman, A. H., & Pillai, S. (2024). *Basic immunology: Functions and disorders of the immune system* (7th ed.). Elsevier.

TABLE 9.1 Innate Defenses to Invading Pathogens

Defense Mechanism		Description
Anatomic barriers	Intact skin	Fatty acids and sweat glands offer antimicrobial protection.
		Skin flora (resident microbes) compete with pathogens.
	Mucous membranes and cilia	Mucous membranes trap particles and pathogens. Cilia facilitate pathogen removal.
	Nasal passages	Hair and mucus filter airborne particles and microbes.
Chemical barriers	Gastric acidity/pH	Normal acidity (hydrochloric acid, pepsin) kills pathogens (greater than 99% of gram-negative pathogens are killed within 30 minutes).
	Mucus	Limits pathogen binding and neutralizes pathogens.
	Microbiota/Flora	Inhibits pathogen colonization.
	Saliva	Lactoferrins bind to iron and limit bacterial proliferation.
		Lysozymes break down the bacterial cell wall.
		Peroxidases neutralize harmful microorganisms.

TABLE 9.2 Cells of the Innate Immune System

Cell Type	Characteristics	Location
Neutrophil 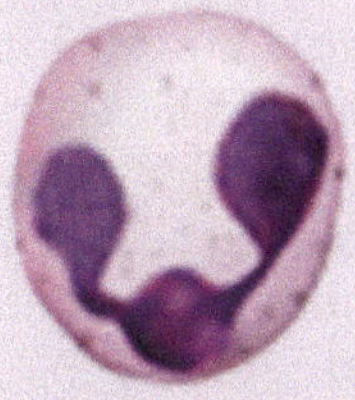	First responder to the site of infection or trauma. Neutrophils are the most abundant WBC in humans. They participate in the innate immune response through phagocytosis as well as the expression and release of cytokines that amplify the immune reaction in other cells.	Migrates from the bone marrow and the blood vessels to the site of infection.
Macrophage 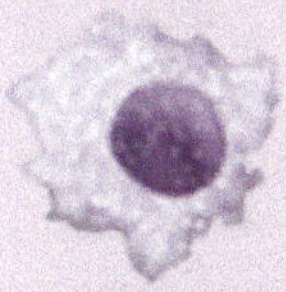	Phagocytic cell that also produces cytokines, participates in tissue repair, and serves as an APC.	Migrates from blood vessels into the tissues.
Dendritic cell 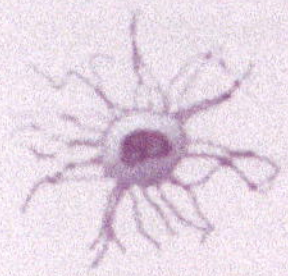	Phagocytic cell that also interacts with the adaptive immune system by serving as an APC.	Present on epithelial tissue including the skin, lungs, and tissues of the digestive tract. Migrates to lymph nodes upon activation.
Natural killer cell 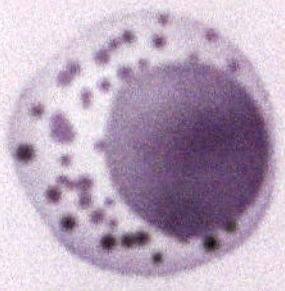	Recognizes and kills viral-infected cells. Releases cytokines that increase the microbicidal activity of macrophages.	Circulates in the blood and migrates into the tissues.
Mast cell 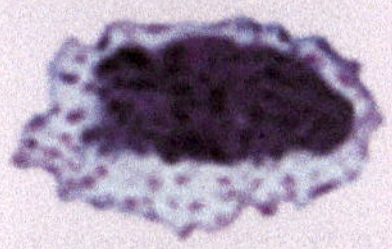	Dilates blood vessels and induces inflammation through the release of histamine. Recruits macrophages and neutrophils. Can participate in phagocytosis and plays a role in allergic reactions.	Present on the skin, GI tract, and respiratory tract.
Basophil 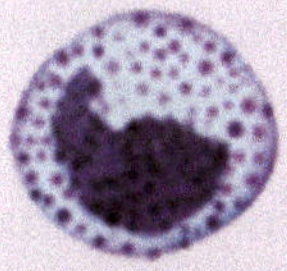	Responsible for defense against parasites. Releases histamine that induces inflammation.	Circulates in the blood and migrates to the tissues.
Eosinophil 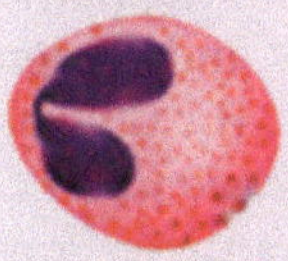	Releases toxins that kill bacteria and parasites but can also cause tissue damage.	Circulates in the blood and migrates to the tissues.

APC, antigen-presenting cell; GI, gastrointestinal; WBC, white blood cell.

mast cells are the most common cells that participate in the innate immune response and will be discussed in this chapter.

Neutrophils. Beginning at approximately week 14 of gestation, bone marrow production of neutrophils begins. Neutrophils are the first cells to respond to infection and likewise play a key role in the acute response. During the acute phase, cytokines, also known as *colony-stimulating factors (CSF)*, stimulate the bone marrow to increase neutrophil production. Upon release into the bloodstream, nearly half of the newly produced neutrophils "roll" through the circulation, with 50% adhering to the endothelium of the respiratory tract and the remainder continuing to circulate throughout the body. After approximately 6 to 8 hours, neutrophils undergo chemotaxis (migration) into target tissues and participate in phagocytosis. Importantly, chemotaxis is immature in term and preterm newborns, with more preterm infants exhibiting the weakest response. Preterm infants exhibit appropriate chemotaxis between 40 to 42 weeks post conceptual age, and term infants demonstrate competence within 2 weeks of birth (J. T. Benjamin et al., 2025). Within 24 hours of arrival at target tissues, neutrophils are cleared by the reticuloendothelial system (Abbas et al., 2024; Rich et al., 2023).

The lineage of neutrophils is important to investigate (and memorize!) because the proportion of immature to mature neutrophils can offer insight into the likelihood of neonatal sepsis. There are several types of immature neutrophils shown in the image tha follows. The mature neutrophil is titled the *segmented neutrophil (segs) or polymorphonuclear leukocyte (PMN)* on lab reports. During the acute phase, the bone marrow will rapidly and nonselectively attempt to increase the complement of circulating neutrophils to optimize phagocytosis. As such, a disproportionate number of immature cells may be released into the circulation.

Promyelocyte → myelocyte → metamyelocyte → band → segmented neutrophil

Immature (promyelocyte through band) ↓ Mature (segmented neutrophil)

Monocytes and Macrophages. Mononuclear phagocytes include monocytes and macrophages. Like neutrophils, monocytes originate from the bone marrow and then migrate into the circulation and remain there for approximately 72 hours. Next, monocytes migrate toward target tissues (the site of an infection). This process of chemotaxis (migration) is much slower compared to neutrophils, as it takes monocytes between 6 to 12 hours to reach the site of an infection. Next, monocytes expand by 300% (3x the original diameter) and differentiate into macrophages (Abbas et al., 2024; Rich et al., 2023). Macrophages are also produced from the bone marrow and hold several important roles in innate immune function. They are particularly adept at phagocytizing Group B *Streptococcus (GBS)*, *Escherichia coli*, *Staphylococcus epididymis*, and *Candida albicans* pathogens. In addition, they stimulate the production of cytokines and the destruction of microbes, which helps to regulate the inflammatory response. Next, macrophages can process antigens and present fragments of them on their exterior surface. As such, macrophages are also considered *professional antigen-presenting cells* (APC). These antigen fragments are recognized by naïve T cells and this kickstarts adaptive immune responses. Lastly, macrophages exhibit a longer life span than neutrophils and can participate in tissue debridement and repair after pathogens have been neutralized (Abbas et al., 2024; Rich et al., 2023).

> **Clinical Application.** There is a natural "rise and fall" of WBC, absolute neutrophil count (ANC), and immature to total neutrophil counts over the first 72 hours after birth. We must consider this postnatal surge and normalization of values in situations that may involve concerns for early onset sepsis (EOS). The WBC and ANC counts reliably predict EOS when values are abnormally low (WBC <5,000 and ANC <1,000). A disproportionate ratio of immature-to-total (I:T) neutrophils also can increase the index of suspicion for sepsis. Remember that these cell counts are recorded as percentages on a lab report. You will need to convert the percentage to the appropriate decimal form to accurately calculate the I:T ratio. The equation is: [% immature neutrophils ÷ % mature] + immature neutrophils. An I/T ratio >0.3 is positively associated with EOS. Even more telling is an elevated I/T (>0.3) and an abnormally low ANC (<1), findings that are predictive of EOS in newborns.

Dendritic Cells. Dendritic cells originate from progenitor cells found in the bone marrow. Dendritic cells appear in fetal tissues (e.g., yolk sac) by 4 to 6 weeks of gestation and on the fetal skin by week 7 of gestation (J. T. Benjamin et al., 2025). Once released into the circulation, they are widely distributed throughout the body and typically found in higher concentrations within tissues that interface with the environment, like the skin (Heath & Carbone, 2009). Like macrophages, dendritic cells participate in phagocytosis by engulfing and killing pathogens. Dendritic cells also process antigens and present fragments of them on their exterior surface. For this reason, dendritic cells are also considered *professional APCs* (Table 9.3). As previously described, the antigen fragments are recognized by naïve T cells and this kickstarts adaptive immune responses.

Natural Killer Cells. NK cells are derived from lymphoid progenitor cells found in the bone marrow and are released into the circulation by week 6 of gestation. The

TABLE 9.3 Professional Antigen-Presenting Cells

	Dendritic Cell	Macrophage	B Cell
Cell type	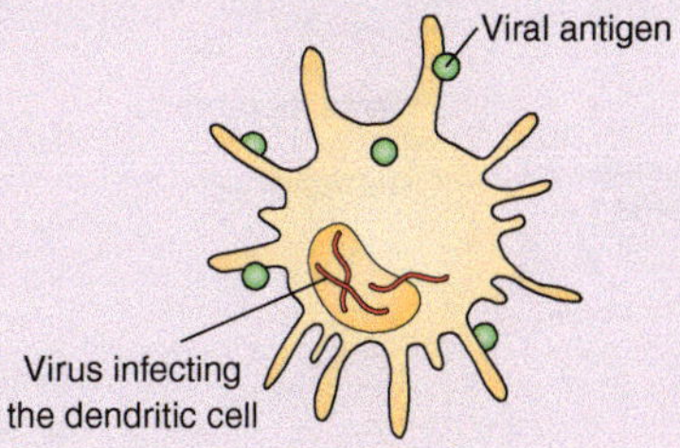	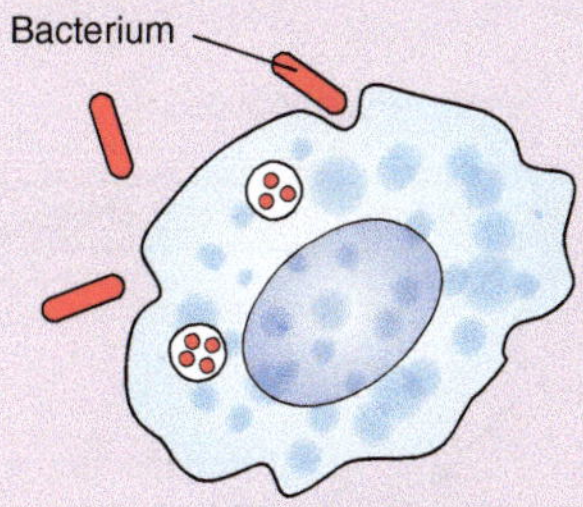	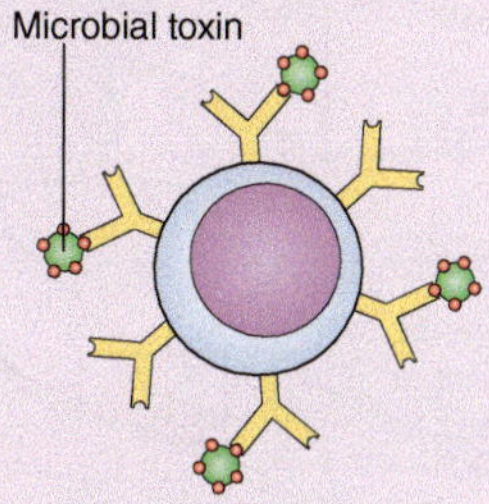
Location in lymph node	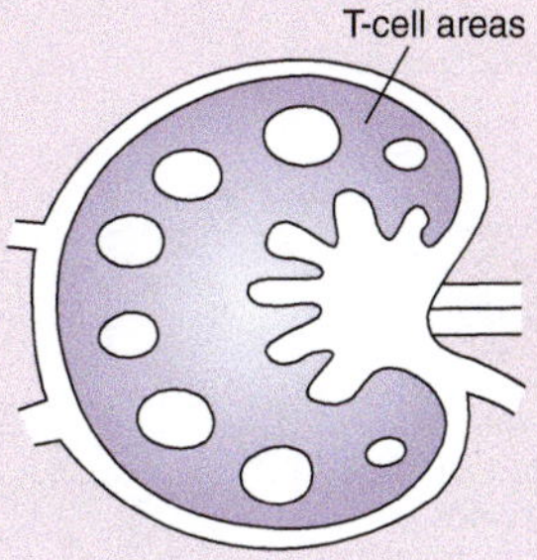	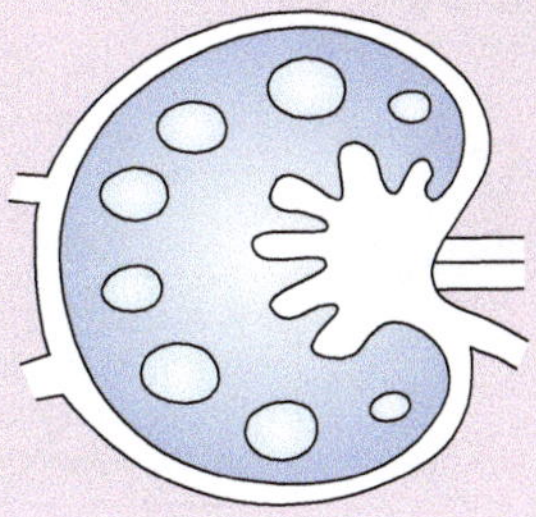	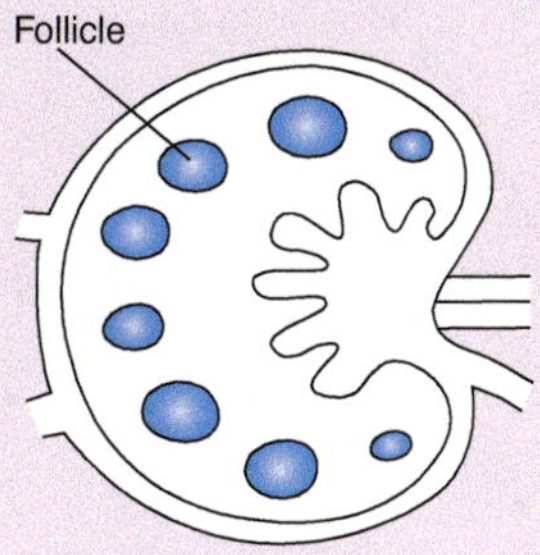
Antigen presented	• Peptides • Viral antigens • Allergens	• Particulate antigens • Intracellular and extracellular pathogens	• Soluble antigens • Toxins • Viruses

Note: Dendritic cells, macrophages, and B cells are all professional APCs found in secondary lymphoid tissues, but are distributed in different locations, reflecting the variation in their functions. In lymph nodes, dendritic cells are confined to the cortical T cell areas and play an important role in viral antigen presentation. Macrophages are found throughout the cortex of lymph nodes and respond to particulate antigens, while B cells only reside in the lymphoid follicles of lymph nodes and acquire soluble antigens. The three cells also vary in their relative effectiveness in presenting antigens to naïve T cells. Dendritic cells are most effective, followed by macrophages and then B cells.
Source: Adapted from Parham, P. (2021). *The immune system* (5th ed.). W. W. Norton & Company.

name NK is used because these cells are highly adept at recognizing infected cells and killing pathogens. Once an infected cell is identified, NK cells release cytoplasmic granules that enter the infected cell and induce apoptosis. Activated NK cells also synthesize the cytokine interferon-g (IFN-g), which enhances the complementary microbicidal activity of macrophages (Abbas et al., 2024). These cells should not be confused with NK T cells, a different subgroup, which participate in allergy-mediated inflammatory responses.

Mast Cells. Mast cells, which are produced in the bone marrow and present in the skin, GI tract, and respiratory tract, are another type of phagocytic cell known for involvement in allergic reactions as well as physiologic angiogenesis, vasodilation, and wound healing. Mast cells are activated when microbial products, such as PAMP, bind to cellular receptors. This induces the synthesis and secretion of proinflammatory cytokines and chemokines.

Clinical Application. Infantile hemangioma is the most common benign vascular tumor diagnosed during infancy. The etiology remains unclear. Newborns with a hemangioma require monitoring particularly if the hemangioma is located near a fontanelle, in the oral cavity, or neck. This is because the tumor will proliferate for approximately the first 5 months of life. As it turns out, one of the cells that contributes to the proliferation phase, when the tumor rapidly grows in size, is the mast cell. Next, the tumor will plateau in size for several months, and then nearly 90% undergo spontaneous involution beginning around 12 months of life. Some tumors will leave residual scarring or hyperpigmented tissue behind, after regressing.

Phagocytosis. Phagocytosis, the manner by which phagocytic cells of the innate immune system ingest and kill microbes, is a well-orchestrated, multistep process that leads to the destruction of pathogens (**Figure 9.4**). The first step of phagocytosis is activation of immune responses. This involves the release of inflammatory mediators, such as bacterial products, cytokines, and complement proteins. The second step, *chemotaxis*, involves movement of phagocytic cells toward target

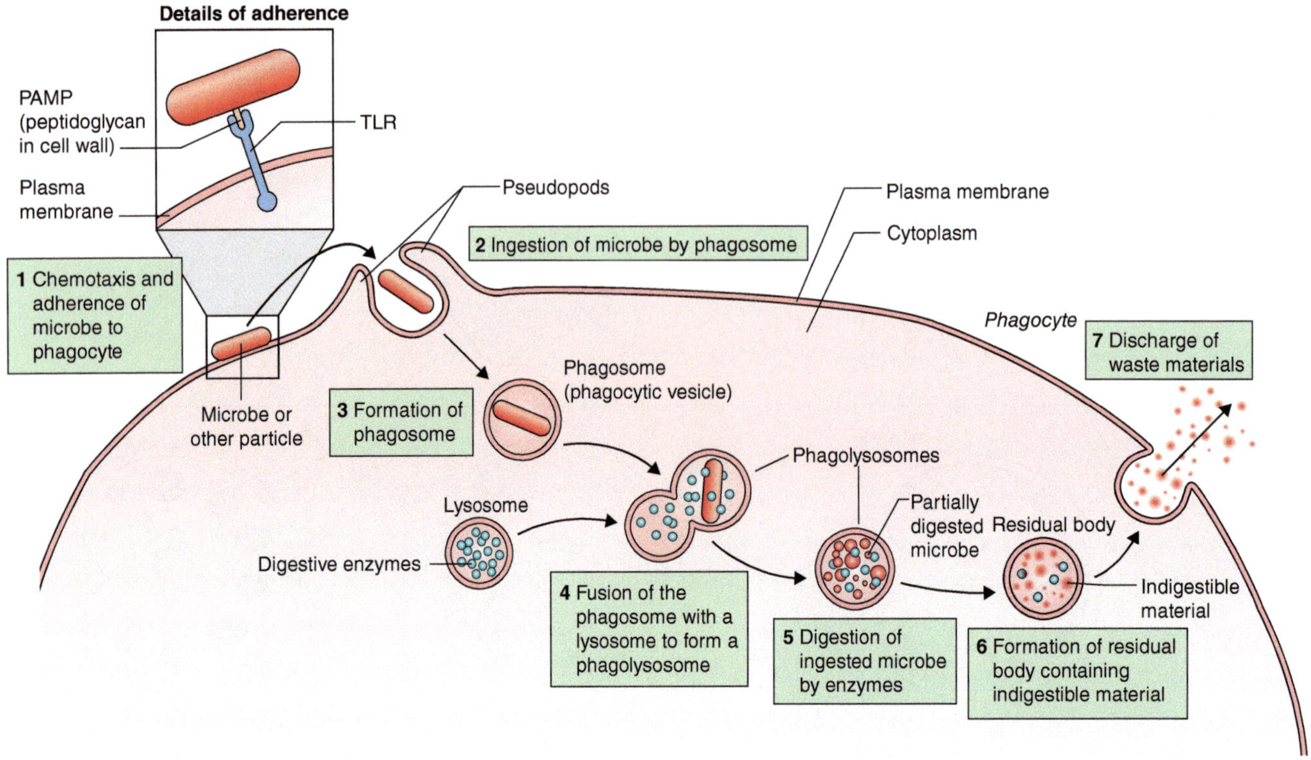

Figure 9.4 Phagocytosis is the process by which phagocytes ingest and kill pathogens. Once activated, the phagocyte moves toward the microbe and attaches itself to it. Once attached, the phagocyte forms pseudopods that envelop the organism to create a phagosome. The phagosome then fuses with a lysosome to form a phagolysosome. The microbe is subsequently destroyed by the release of lytic enzymes. A residual body is formed, and the waste materials are discharged from the cell.
PAMP, pathogen-associated molecular pattern; TLR, toll-like receptor.

bacteria or circulating cytokines. Next, phagocytes attach to microbes using the PRR. Each phagocyte thereby forms armlike structures, called *pseudopodia*, which engulf each microbe and bring it into a vesicle called a *phagosome*. The phagosome then fuses with a lysosome, becoming a *phagolysosome*. Once contained inside of the phagolysosome, the microbe is exposed to noxious substances that degrade and ultimately destroy it. The phagolysosome then forms a residual body that contains cellular waste products that are eventually expelled from the cell (Swanson, 2013).

Soluble Components of Innate Immunity.

Cytokines. Cytokines are small glycoproteins synthesized by mononuclear phagocytes (e.g., macrophages, mast cells) and nonimmune cells (e.g., endothelial cells). Types of cytokine cells include interleukins, interferons, chemokines, tumor necrosis factor, CSFs, and transforming growth factor-beta (Table 9.4). Each of these families of cytokines participates in the systemic inflammatory cascade and overall immune response to an invading pathogen.

Once synthesized by mononuclear phagocytes, cytokines elicit the activation, proliferation, and differentiation of other immune cells. For example, cytokines trigger neutrophils and T cells to produce secondary inflammatory mediators. Neutrophils will participate in phagocytosis and release preformed mediators named elastase and myeloperoxidase. These enzymes participate in the formation of extracellular networks that trap and kill bacteria (Papayannopoulos et al., 2010). The net result is a robust inflammatory response that occurs during the onset of sepsis. While this inflammatory response can be protective, excessive inflammation is detrimental and can lead to tissue and organ damage (Sugitharini et al., 2013).

Cytokines also stimulate increased hepatic production of chemokines and innate immune proteins known as acute phase reactants (APR; Sugitharini et al., 2013). APR production is induced by the activity of IL-1, IL-6, and TNF-a. Two common APRs are C-reactive protein (CRP) and procalcitonin (PCT), which function to reduce host bacterial load through improved cellular recruitment, opsonin function, and direct antimicrobial activity (Fattah et al., 2017; Wynn & Levy, 2010). CRP levels typically begin to rise within 6 to 8 hours of exposure to an infection and peak at 24 to 48 hours before gradually returning to normal as the initial inflammatory response resolves. A recently published retrospective cohort study by Dhudasia and colleagues (2023) reported that CRP levels offer poor sensitivity and specificity with the diagnosis of EOS. In addition, the authors noted that use of CRP levels in the formal evaluation and treatment

TABLE 9.4 Cytokine Types and Major Activities

Cytokine	Cellular Source(s)	Major Activities
Chemokines	Hepatocytes	Regulate the migration (chemotaxis) of granulocytes, monocytes, and lymphocytes
CSF	Helper T cells and macrophages	Stimulates the proliferation and maturation of myeloid precursor cells
IL-1	Macrophages	Activation of T cells and macrophages; promotion of inflammation
IL-2	Helper T cells	Activation of lymphocytes, NK cells, and macrophages
IL-4	Helper T cells, mast cells, basophils, and eosinophils	Activation of lymphocytes, monocytes, and IgE class switching
IL-5	Helper T cells, mast cells, and eosinophils	Differentiation of eosinophils
IL-6	Helper T cells and macrophages	Activation of lymphocytes; differentiation of B cells; stimulation of the production of acute-phase proteins
IL-8	T cells and macrophages	Chemotaxis of neutrophils, basophils, and T cells
IL-11	Bone marrow and stromal cells	Stimulation of the production of acute-phase proteins
IL-12	Macrophages, B cells, and dendritic cells	Stimulation of the production of IFN-g by helper T cells and by NK cells; induction of helper T cells
TNF-α	Macrophages, NK cells, T cells, B cells, and mast cells	Promotion of inflammation
IFN- α	Virally infected cells	Induction of resistance of cells to viral infection
IFN- β	Virally infected cells	Induction of resistance of cells to viral infection
IFN-γ	Helper T cells and NK cells	Activation of macrophages

CSF; colony-stimulating factor; IFN; interferon; IgE, immunoglobulin E; NK, natural killer; TNF, tumor necrosis factor.
Source: Adapted from Dhama, K., Saminathan, M., Jacob, S. S., Singh, M., Karthik, K., Amarpal, R. T., Sunkara, L. T., Malik, Y. S., & Singh, R. S. (2015). Effect of immunomodulation and immunomodulatory agents on health with some bioactive principles, modes of action and potent biomedical applications. *International Journal of Pharmacology, 11*, 253–290. https://doi.org/10.3923/ijp.2015.253.290

for suspected EOS was associated with increased antibiotic use and a longer duration of antibiotic therapy (Dhudasia et al., 2023). While decreasing CRP levels may suggest a positive response to treatment, use may lead to prolonged exposure to nephrotoxic and ototoxic medications and a prolonged hospital stay.

PCT is currently regarded as the best biomarker for determining length of antibiotic treatment for EOS to date. Similar to CRP, PCT levels begin to rise within 6 to 8 hours of exposure to an infection and peak within 24 to 48 hours of birth before gradually returning to normal as the initial inflammatory response resolves (J. T. Benjamin et al., 2025; Naramura et al., 2020; Stocker et al., 2017). An exception to this trend involves neonates with respiratory disease, which may lead to persistently elevated PCT levels for the first 36 hours after birth (Naramura et al., 2020). The negative predictive value for PCT is 87% to 100%, making PCT trending superior to CRP in determining length of antibiotic therapy in the treatment of suspected EOS. PCT use is associated with a reduced duration of antibiotic exposure (55 hours vs. 65 hours; *p less than* 0.0001) and reduced length of stay (123 hours vs. 126 hours; $p = 0.0039$) in the treatment of suspected EOS in term and late-preterm neonates (Stocker et al., 2017).

Complement. The complement system is an essential component of the innate immune system that works in conjunction with the antibody response of the acquired immune system (Walport, 2001a, 2001b). The goal of the complement system is to identify foreign particles for elimination and identify damaged parts of the host, or to identify debris that can promote inflammatory or immune responses. This system must be tightly regulated to avoid deficient or overproduction of complement proteins, as these situations can precipitate autoimmune diseases (Abbas et al., 2024).

The proteins that make up the complement system are named with a capital C and a number indicating the order in which they were discovered (e.g., C1, C2, C3, C4; Kemper et al., 2014). The formation of complement proteins occurs through three major pathways that involve sequential chemical reactions: the (a) classical pathway, (b) alternative pathway, or (c) lectin pathway. The *classical pathway* is triggered by antibodies and/or plasma proteins (e.g., CRP) and becomes engaged when immunoglobulin M (IgM) or immunoglobulin G (IgG) antibodies bind antigens. In other words, the binding of antibody to antigen triggers this pathway. This initiates a sequential process whereby C1 produces the next complement (C4), which produces C2, and then C2 initiates the production of C3 (as depicted in Figure 9.5). The *alternative pathway* is the most primitive portion of the immune system and represents a set of proteins (C3) that continuously survey the blood and tissue looking for pathogens and injured tissues. The *lectin pathway* uniquely recognizes arrangements of carbohydrates found only on microbial pathogens. Examples of lectins that perform this function include mannose-binding lectin (MBL), ficolin 1, ficolin 2, and ficolin 3. MBL, for example, recognizes fructose, mannose, and N-acetylglucosamine that are exposed on the cell wall of a pathogen. MBL will form a complex with one of those sugars, which initiates the cleavage of complement proteins. The lectin pathway merges with the classic and alternative pathways with the cleavage of C3b, and in that way assists with the formation of MACs. While each of these pathways is independently activated, they merge (perform the same actions) once C3b is formed. Next steps result in the formation of factors that intensify the function of phagocytic cells by promoting local inflammation and opsonization as well as activation of a set of proteins (C5, C6, C7, C8, C9) called the *membrane attack complex (MAC)* occurs. The MAC disrupts cell walls of bacteria leading to lysis while also creating an inflammatory response.

Clinical Application. Consider a case of GBS sepsis in a neonate. Under normal circumstances, the alternative complement pathway recognizes gram-positive bacteria, such as GBS. Fragments of C3 are deposited on the surface of this gram-positive bacteria, and this primes them for subsequent phagocytosis through opsonization. Through chemotaxis, small peptides (C3a and C5a) attract neutrophils to the site of inflammation, stimulating them to release active mediators such as reactive oxygen species and enzymes. Meanwhile, the C5b-9 complex provides the lytic activity of complement. Together, these actions facilitate the destruction and clearance of the pathogen and demonstrate an important and efficient means of host defense. However, we know that immune defenses are immature in newborns (and particularly preterm newborns), and this limits the ability of the complement pathways to opsonize

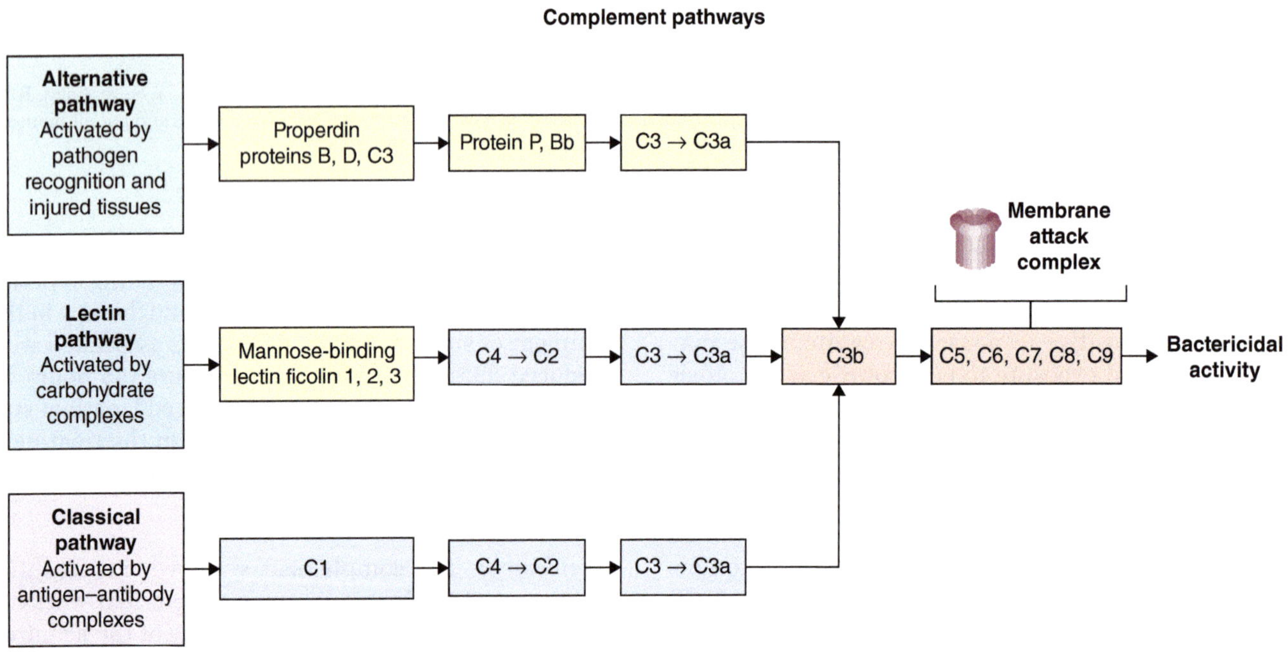

Figure 9.5 Complement activation. The image depicts a simplified overview of complement activation and the formation of the membrane attack complex.

and lyse pathogens. This underpins the importance of early recognition of the newborn at-risk for sepsis, close clinical monitoring, a surveillance blood culture, and potentially additional laboratory testing and empiric antimicrobial prophylaxis to prevent multiplication of pathogens and evolving overwhelming sepsis. While it is essential that we uphold the tenets of antibiotic stewardship, we must maintain diligence, as signs of sepsis are often nonspecific/elusive.

Acquired or Adaptive Immunity

The acquired immune system has important features that distinguish it from the innate immune system. It must be *induced*, or activated, to mount an immune response. Once activated, it produces a *specific* response to antigens, and *immunologic memory* develops. Simply stated, once a pathogen has been encountered and a response mounted, the adaptive immune system will be ready to act again in the event of a future exposure. The first time a pathogen is encountered, a *primary response* occurs. After the pathogen is cleared, the acquired immune system "remembers" it, allowing subsequent encounters with the same pathogen to occur faster, stronger, and with greater specificity. The subsequent responses are termed *memory responses*. To help learn this concept, consider an XX pregnant patient with a primary viral infection, such as herpes simplex virus (HSV). With primary HSV, there is increased excretion of viral particles, prolonged shedding of the viral particles, and very little or no IgG transfer from the pregnant patient to the fetus. This explains why infants of XX pregnant patients with a primary HSV infection are more likely to acquire the viral infection. In contrast, with recurrent viral infections, there are fewer viral particles excreted and plenty of IgG resulting in less risk of fetal/neonatal infection.

The primary cells involved in the acquired immune system are lymphocytes (B cells and T cells). B cells also participate in the acquired *humoral immune* response, because antibodies are found in the blood and body fluids, the body's so-called *humors*. T cells interact directly with other cells to mediate an adaptive immune response and are therefore considered part of the cell-mediated acquired immune response (Helbert, 2017).

Humoral Immunity. The primary functions of B cells are to make antibodies against antigens, act as APCs, and eventually develop into memory B cells. B lymphocyte production occurs in bone marrow secondary to stimulation from IL-2. IL-4 stimulates maturation within secondary lymphoid tissues, and subsequently goes through an "education process" (stimulated by IL-6) prior to becoming mature antibody-secreting lymphocytes. Once they are mature, they patrol the secondary lymphoid organs for target cells presenting with foreign antigens and the "memory function" is modulated by IL-14 stimulation (J. T. Benjamin et al., 2025; LeBien & Tedder, 2008).

B cell education occurs in two stages in the bone marrow and assures that B cells produce antibodies that can recognize foreign antigens but not self-antigen. The first stage is called *positive selection*. In this stage, BCRs must recognize the protein that will present foreign antigens in the future. It is known as a *major histocompatibility molecule complex* (MHC). MHC can bind to the body's own peptides (self-antigens) as well as pathogenic peptides from invading microorganisms. The second stage in the B cell education process is *negative selection*. If B cells recognize self-antigens presented by the MHC too strongly, they will be deleted or their BCRs will be restructured. This process ensures that dangerous autoreactive B cells are deleted (Helbert, 2017). Once B cells are educated, they are said to be *mature*.

Mature B cells migrate out of the bone marrow to secondary lymphoid organs, such as the lymph nodes and spleen, to be activated. Each B cell must be activated by a series of two signals that induces the B cell to multiply. The first signal involves antigen binding to the BCR (Gauld et al., 2002). The second signal relies on communication from the cell-mediated immune system and is provided by activated T cells (Figure 9.6). Once fully activated, the B cell undergoes clonal expansion, creating antibody-producing plasma cells or memory cells. During the primary/initial immune response, short-term IgM antibodies are produced yet catabolized relatively quickly. During the secondary response, which follows the primary response, long-term IgG antibodies are produced (or with allergies or parasitic infections, IgE is produced).

B cells produce five classes of immunoglobulins or antibodies (IgG, IgM, IgA, IgE, and IgD) that have varying immune functions (Table 9.5; Gleason & Sawyer, 2024). Some antibodies (e.g., IgM, IgG, IgD) bind bacteria directly, which promotes their recognition and phagocytosis by macrophages. This process is called *opsonization* (binding to bacteria). Antibodies can also function by binding to and neutralizing microbes, or by activating other aspects of the immune system to destroy pathogens, through NK cells, complement activation, or cellular activation of eosinophils or mast cells.

Naïve B cells display IgM and IgD on their surface that function as BCRs to recognize antigens. Once a B cell is activated by antigen, a *primary humoral response* leads to IgM production (Peakman & Vergani, 2009). B cells produce IgM as the default antibody until cytokines from the T cells instruct them to produce a different antibody for the specific immune response, a process called *class switching*. For example, IgG will be produced after viral and bacterial infections, whereas IgE will be produced after parasitic or with allergic outbreaks. As activated B cells begin multiplying into plasma B cells and memory B cells, the portion of their DNA that encodes for antibody production is rearranged and only retains the gene that produces the antibody specific to the antigen (Stavnezer et al., 2008). After this transition occurs, the plasma cell,

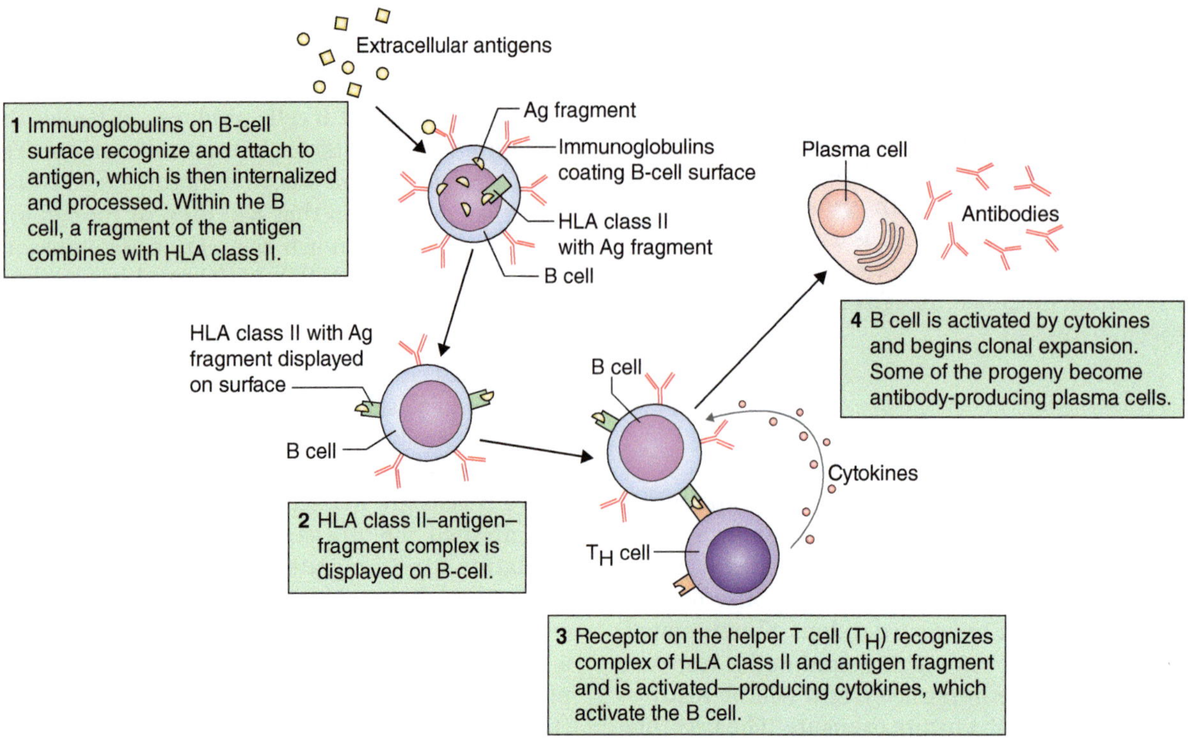

Figure 9.6 It takes two signals for a B cell to be activated and become a plasma cell. The first signal involves the binding of the BCR to an antigen. The second signal comes from cytokines released by a helper T cell that has been activated by the same antigen. Once activated, the B cell undergoes clonal expansion, producing plasma cells and memory cells.
Ag, antigen; HLA, human leucocyte antigen.

or memory cell, will only produce the specific antibody (e.g., IgG) that is required to fight that specific antigen invader. The plasma B cells will continue to fight until they are turned off or destroyed after elimination of the pathogen. Memory B cells will remain in circulation, primed for a repeat exposure to the same infectious organism.

The *secondary immune response* is a rapid response to a previously recognized pathogen. Because class switching of antibodies does not need to occur, this process is much faster than the primary response, taking only 3 to 5 days. In the secondary response, a memory cell does not require a second signal for activation; the BCR binding an antigen and cross-linking alone (first signal) are sufficient to induce the B cell to start producing a specific antibody. The activated memory cell will clonally expand to make plasma cells with specific antibodies and more memory cells (J. T. Benjamin et al., 2025; Peakman & Vergani, 2009; Tangye et al., 2003).

Cell-Mediated Immunity. T cells develop and mature in the thymus, differentiate into CD4+ and CD8+ cells, and then go on to inhabit peripheral tissues including the spleen and lymph nodes. These cells are educated through positive and negative selection in a manner similar to B cells. During negative selection, if a T cell binds too strongly to an antigen it is deleted or changed into a cell capable of shutting down autoreactive immune responses (Haks et al., 1999). Once educated, T cells can inhabit secondary lymphoid organs, such as the spleen and lymph nodes.

Like B cells, mature T cells are naïve until they are activated by a series of two signals. The first signal involves the TCR recognizing and binding to the MHC that is displaying an antigen. The second costimulatory signal is provided when the CD28 receptor on T cells binds to the B7 ligand on APC (Figure 9.7). The expression of B7 proteins on APC is induced by pathogens during the innate immune response to an infection (J. T. Benjamin et al., 2025). Both signals must come from an APC to prompt the naïve T cell to differentiate into an effector T cell. If a T cell is only activated by one signal, it will lead to *anergy*, or become unresponsive until a second signal is received. If, on the other hand, the T cell receives both signals, it will proliferate and differentiate into an effector T cell that migrates to the site of the infection. Effector T cells can either be T helper cells (also known as *CD4+ cells*) or cytotoxic T cells (also known as *CD8+ cells*; Abbas et al., 2024). CD4+ T cells recognize antigens displayed by MHC class II molecules, which are found on APCs. CD8+ T cells recognize antigens presented by MHC class I molecules, which are present on all nucleated cells in the body.

T helper cells are effector T cells whose primary role is to regulate both cellular and humoral immunity. Among other things, T helper cells secrete cytokines that propagate and enhance the response of the innate immune system to the invading organism. They are also essential in the activation

TABLE 9.5 Antibody Isotypes

Name	Properties	Structure
IgA	Found in mucus, saliva, tears, and breast milk. IgA, especially in human milk, protects against pathogens until the infant's own adaptive immune defenses can develop.	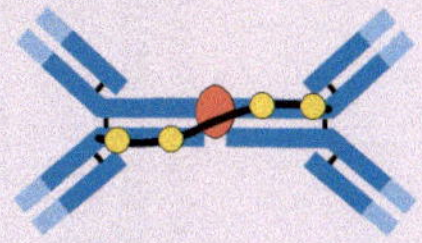
IgD	Part of the BCR. Activates basophils and mast cells.	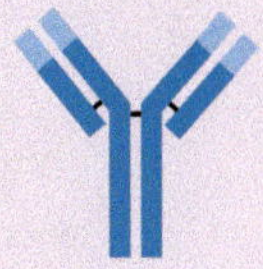
IgE	Protects against parasitic worms. Responsible for allergic reactions.	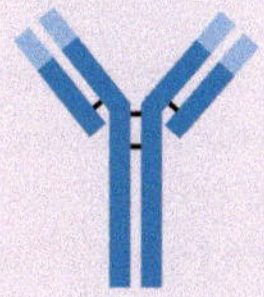
IgG	Secreted by plasma cells in the blood. Able to cross the placenta. Commensurate with long-standing immunity.	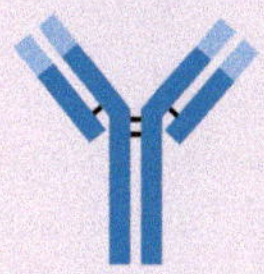
IgM	May be attached to the surface of a B cell or secreted into the blood. Associated with immune responses. Confers short-term immunity.	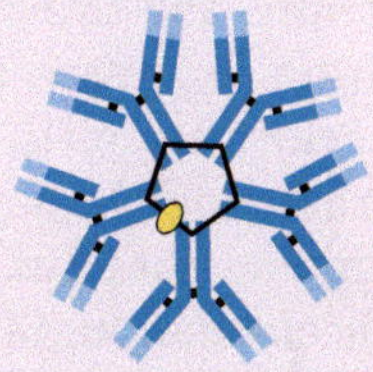

BCR, B-cell receptor; Ig, immunoglobulin.

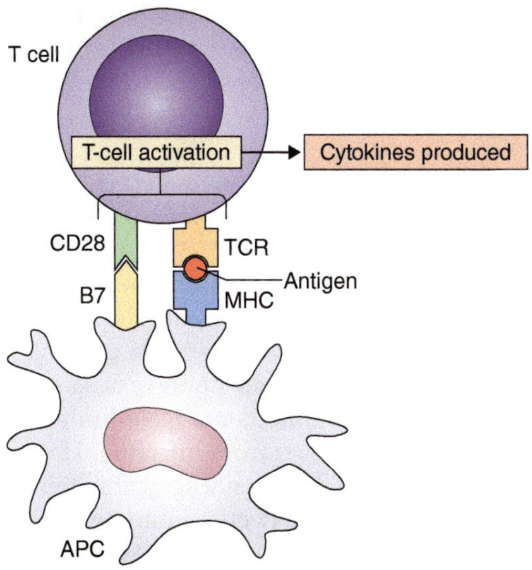

Figure 9.7 Like B cells, T cells require two signals to become activated. The first signal comes from the TCR binding to the MHC on the APC. The second, costimulatory signal is produced when the CD28 receptor on the T cell binds with B7 ligand on the APC.

APC, antigen-presenting cell; MHC, major histocompatibility complex; TCR, T-cell receptor.

of cytotoxic T cells and B cell antibody class switching. The primary role of cytotoxic T cells is to find infected cells and kill them. Upon antigen recognition on the surface of a target cell, cytotoxic T cells release lytic enzymes, or *granzymes*, that induce apoptosis of the infected cell.

A subset of antigen-activated T lymphocytes differentiates into memory cells that survive even after the infection has been eradicated and the antigen cleared. Following activation, both memory CD4+ cells and CD8+ cells only require the first signal to become activated. Therefore, subsequent encounters with the same antigen lead to a secondary response that is quicker and more robust than the primary response (Abbas et al., 2024).

Passive Immunity. *Passive immunity* refers to the process by which a person with no previous antigenic exposure acquires humoral immunity, including specific antibodies or sensitized lymphocytes from another individual. The primary means by which passive immunity is conferred to the fetus is through transplacental acquisition of IgG from the XX pregnant patient. Transfer of IgG begins around week 20 of gestation, with the majority of transfer occurring between weeks 36 and 40 of gestation (J. T. Benjamin et al., 2025). Over time, passively

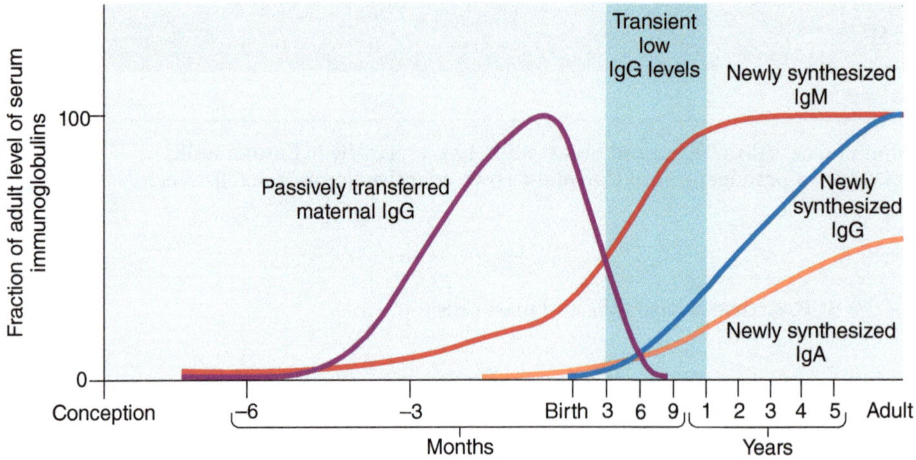

Figure 9.8 Placental transfer of IgG begins early in the second trimester and peaks during the final 4 weeks of pregnancy. After birth, passively acquired IgG degrades over the first few months of life as the infant gains antigenic exposure and begins to produce their own IgG.
IgG, immunoglobulin G; IgM, immunoglobulin M.

acquired IgG degrades and the infant will begin making their own antibodies (Figure 9.8). All antibody classes can be detected in colostrum; however, secretory IgA is the most prominent of the isotypes present in breast milk. Therefore, the transfer of secretory IgA transfer through freshly expressed colostrum and mature breast milk can occur after birth and offer additional passive immune protection. Importantly, there is no evidence that the immunoglobulins present in breast milk enter the systemic circulation; rather, they direct their activity against enteric bacterial and viral pathogens.

Clinical Application. IgG is the only immunoglobulin transported across the placenta. Reduced IgG transfer to the fetus is associated with intrauterine growth restriction ([IUGR]; postnatal small for gestational age [SGA] status), placental insufficiency, and preterm birth less than 36 weeks. Knowing which immunoglobulin crosses the placenta is important when evaluating an infant for a suspected congenital viral infection. The presence of IgG antibodies in the newborn does not confirm congenital infection, since this is transferred from mother to fetus. Rather, elevated levels of IgM or IgA detected by way of cord blood sampling or a postnatal peripheral blood, cerebrospinal fluid, or urine testing, are suspicious for congenital infection. Consider a situation involving concern for congenital cytomegalovirus (CMV) infection. The preferred testing method involves nucleic acid amplification testing, which can detect CMV-positive viral DNA. Urine or peripheral blood testing for CMV should be directed at detecting IgM CMV-specific antibodies.

Communication Within the Adaptive Immune System

The humoral and cell-mediated arms of the immune system interact to coordinate the immune response after an exposure to antigens. APCs from the innate immune system activate both B and T cells during the recognition phase and induce clonal expansion and differentiation. During this activation phase, the cells become antibody-producing plasma cells and effector T cells. These cells eliminate pathogens using antibodies or through cell-mediated immune responses. After the antigen is eliminated, the body returns to homeostasis as the numbers of effector cells decline. Memory B and T cells survive for subsequent interaction with the same pathogen and a quicker secondary response (Figure 9.9).

NEONATAL HOST FACTORS THAT INFLUENCE THE IMMUNE RESPONSE

Both the innate and adaptive immune responses are functionally immature at birth, placing the neonate at increased risk for infection (Table 9.6). In general, neonatal immune function improves with increasing gestational age. Therefore, preterm infants are most limited in their ability to protect themselves from infection. However, all newborns, regardless of gestational age, exhibit limitations in their ability to mount an effective immune response.

As stated earlier in this chapter, the skin and mucous membranes are important elements of the innate immune system and provide a first line of defense against invading organisms. However, the skin of preterm infants exhibits inadequate barrier function and increased permeability to potential pathogens (see Chapter 12). In addition, vernix caseosa, which has been

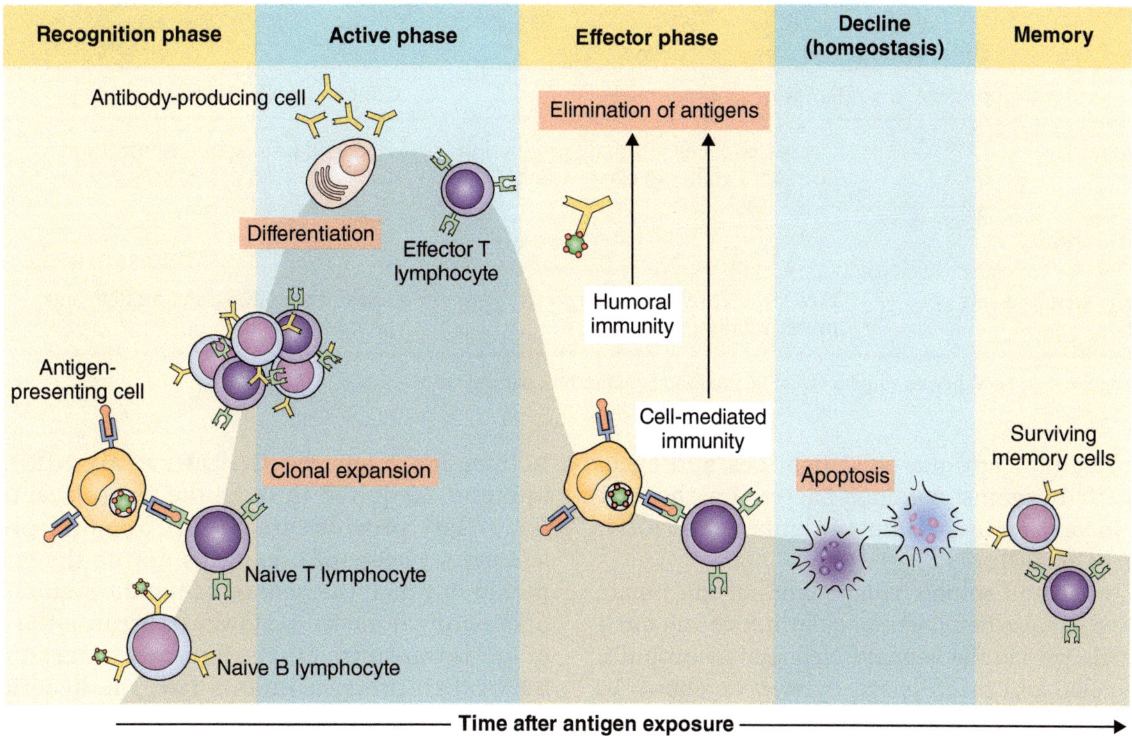

Figure 9.9 Elements of the innate and adaptive immune system interact to successfully mount an immune response. Antigen-presenting cells from the innate immune system activate B cells and T cells to undergo clonal expansion and eliminate the antigen. Once the antigen has been eliminated, the body returns to homeostasis as the effector cells decline in number. A few B and T cells remain as memory cells to mount a stronger and more efficient immune response in the event of a subsequent exposure.
Source: Adapted from Abbas, A. K., Lichtman, A. H., & Pillai, S. (2021). *Cellular and molecular immunology* (10th ed.). Elsevier.

TABLE 9.6 Impairments in Neonatal Immune Function

Immune System Component	Functional Impairment	Clinical Implications
Innate Immunity		
Skin and mucous membranes	Impaired barrier function	Decreased ability to prevent invasion from pathogenic organisms
Neutrophils	Limited pool of neutrophils; impaired chemotaxis and phagocytosis	Decreased ability to respond to and kill pathogens
Macrophages	Decreased antigen presentation and cytokine production	Limited ability to activate T cells
Dendritic cells	Decreased production of inflammatory cytokines	Reduced induction of T cells; decreased activation of NK cells
Complement	Deficient complement proteins	Reduced phagocytosis and impaired pathogen clearance by phagocytes; increased risk of invasive bacterial infection
Adaptive Immunity		
T lymphocytes	Relatively low circulating levels of T cells; greater proportion of naïve T cells to memory T cells	Reduced cell-mediated immunity which increases the risk of infection from intracellular pathogens such as *listeria*, HSV, and CMV

(continued)

TABLE 9.6 Impairments in Neonatal Immune Function *(continued)*

Immune System Component	Functional Impairment	Clinical Implications
B lymphocytes	Decreased B cell antibody production; decreased ability to class-switch	Reduced pathogen opsonization
Passive Immunity		
Maternally acquired IgG	Low circulating levels of IgG in preterm infants	Lack of opsonization and deficient phagocytosis

CMV, cytomegalovirus; HSV, herpes simplex virus; Ig, immunoglobulin; NK, natural killer.

shown to contain antimicrobial peptides and spectrum of activity against common bacterial pathogens, is sparse in very preterm infants (Akinbi et al., 2004; Simonsen et al., 2014).

The cellular and soluble components of the innate immune system also demonstrate quantitative and qualitative deficiencies in the neonate. Neonatal neutrophils, dendritic cells, and macrophages have been shown to be deficient in number and function when compared to older children or adults. For example, in neonates, neutrophils demonstrate diminished response to chemotactic factors and impairment in phagocytosis (Basha et al., 2014; Camacho-Gonzalez et al., 2013). Although the capacity for neonatal dendritic cells to process and present antigens is similar to that of adults, neonatal cells have impaired cytokine production, which may result in blunted activation of T cells and NK cells (Gold et al., 2007). NK cells can be detected in fetal circulation as early as 6 weeks of gestation and are essentially equivalent in number to adults during the neonatal period. However, NK cell cytolytic activity against target cells is diminished during the neonatal period, potentially contributing to an increased vulnerability to viral infections (J. T. Benjamin et al., 2025). Although complement levels increase with increasing gestational age, both preterm and term newborns possess significantly low levels compared to adults. In particular, neonates have extremely low levels of C9, which is critical for the formation of the MAC and is associated with increased susceptibility to *E. coli* (Wynn & Levy, 2010; Zilow et al., 1993). These deficiencies in the cellular and noncellular components of the innate immune system lead to reduced phagocytosis and impaired pathogen clearance (Camacho-Gonzalez et al., 2013; Melville & Moss, 2013).

Maturation of the adaptive immune system is dependent on antigenic exposure; therefore, all newborns have deficiencies in T cell activation and B cell antibody production (Melville & Moss, 2013). The combination of low levels of circulating lymphocytes, increased proportion of naïve T and B cells to memory cells, and impairment in antibody isotype switching limit the neonate's ability to respond effectively to infection (Camacho-Gonzalez et al., 2013). Passive immunity acquired through the transplacental transfer of IgG provides important humoral protection against a variety of organisms during the vulnerable period in which the neonatal immune system is developmentally immature. However, because the majority of IgG is transferred to the fetus late in gestation (after 32 weeks), preterm infants lack the benefit of this protective mechanism conferred to their term counterparts, further increasing their susceptibility to infection (Camacho-Gonzalez et al., 2013; Melville & Moss, 2013).

GENETIC INFLUENCES

Genetic mutations cause an array of immunodeficiencies that range in severity from clinically irrelevant to fatal. One in 2,000 children is diagnosed with an immunodeficiency by the age of 18 (Bousfiha et al., 2018; Boyle & Buckley, 2007). The timing of presentation, between birth and adulthood, depends on which immune cells are involved and the severity of the defect (Cooper et al., 2003). For example, antibody deficiencies generally do not present until after 6 months of age, when the passive immunity wanes. In contrast, deficits in T cells can be detected in infancy when patients present with infection or poor growth. DiGeorge syndrome, Wiskott–Aldrich syndrome (WAS), and X-linked severe combined immunodeficiency (XSCID) are examples of genetic syndromes that can present in the neonatal period.

DiGeorge Syndrome (22q11.2 Deletion Syndrome)

Deletions in 22q11.2 are the most common genetic cause of cleft palate and the second most common genetic cause of developmental delays and congenital heart disease (McDonald-McGinn et al., 2015). Deletions in this region can be found in one in 100 fetuses with serious anomalies on prenatal ultrasound (Grati et al., 2015; Wapner et al., 2012). More than 90% of cases of DiGeorge syndrome occur as the result of a *de novo* mutation on the long arm of chromosome 22, meaning that it is not inherited from either parent (McDonald-McGinn et al., 2001). Embryologically, it is characterized by abnormal development of the third and fourth pharyngeal arches, which are the origin of the palate, thymus, parathyroid glands, and heart (Ford & Wantanabe, 2025; McDonald-McGinn et al., 2015). DiGeorge syndrome should be suspected in any infant presenting with a combination of cleft palate, immunodeficiency, hypocalcemia, and congenital heart disease. Hypocalcemia develops as a consequence of abnormal development of the third-fifth branchial arches and resultant hypoparathyroidism, or more severely as a result of a complete absence of parathyroid development (Abrams & Tiosano, 2025).

DiGeorge syndrome causes a wide spectrum of immunologic compromise. Lymphopenia (low numbers of T cells) is present in 75% of affected infants, but the severity of the lymphopenia ranges from a complete absence of T cells to a T cell count that is near normal (Gennery, 2012). A small fraction (1/1,000) of infants display a complete absence of T cells due to thymic agenesis and may come to attention after a positive newborn screen, which detects decreased T cell production of any etiology (Kwan et al., 2014; Ryan et al., 1997). Infants with less severe lymphopenia may develop recurrent or severe infections despite seemingly normal adaptive immune function in vitro (Morsheimer et al., 2017). Recurrent infections represent a major cause of morbidity in children with DiGeorge syndrome. Cardiac disease and hypocalcemia are responsible for the majority of cases of premature death (McDonald-McGinn et al., 2015; Repetto et al., 2014).

X-Linked Severe Combined Immunodeficiency

Severe combined immunodeficiency (SCID) is a rare and combined group of genetic disorders characterized by impaired development and function of T cells and B cells, which is caused by a variety of gene mutations. XSCID has an X-linked recessive mode of inheritance, meaning that it is either inherited from an asymptomatic maternal carrier or the result of a de novo gene mutation (Puck et al., 1997). It is the result of a mutation of a gene located on the X chromosome called *IL-2 receptor gamma*, which is necessary for cytokine signaling (Pateva et al., 2025). Infants with XSCID develop severe, recurrent, and life-threatening infections within the first few months of life (Buckley, 2002). All newborns with XSCID are lymphopenic and have absent or dramatically reduced T cell function (Buckley, 2002). They may also have absent immunoglobulins and no significant immunologic response to vaccination (Buckley, 2002). As of 2018, all 50 states now have newborn screens that can detect SCID (Immune Deficiency Foundation, 2024). If the newborn state screen is positive, definitive diagnosis is done by whole exome gene sequencing looking for mutations in the genes known to cause SCID. Early diagnosis of these infants is crucial because the infants who receive a bone marrow transplant in the first 3.5 months of life have significantly better outcomes than those transplanted later (Buckley, 2011). Without bone marrow transplantation, XSCID is fatal.

NOTEWORTHY DISEASES IN THE XX PREGNANT PATIENT THAT INFLUENCE FETAL IMMUNE SYSTEM DEVELOPMENT AND FUNCTION

The prenatal period is a delicate time during which maternal health conditions can influence the growth and development of fetal organ systems, including the immune system. HIV infection, autoimmune disease, and immunosuppressive therapy in birthing parents have been shown to impose short- and long-term impacts on neonatal immune function.

HIV Infection

HIV infection in the XX pregnant patient can be passed to the fetus or infant vertically (transplacentally, intrapartum) or horizontally (through breast milk). The availability of antiretroviral agents, access to comprehensive HIV and pregnancy services, and avoidance of breastfeeding when a high viral load is detected have been shown to decrease the risk of mother-to-child HIV transmission. The risk for vertical transmission in the United States is 1% to 2% (HIV.gov, 2023; Nesheim et al., 2012). As of 2021, countries that eliminated vertical transmission included Cuba, Thailand, Belarus, Armenia, Anguilla, Montserrat, Cayman Islands, Bermuda, Antigua and Barbuda, St. Kitts and Nevis, Malaysia, Maldives, Sri Lanka, Dominica, and Oman (Lancet HIV, 2022). In resource poor countries, particularly those in east and southern Africa with high HIV burden, the risk of vertical HIV transmission is 11.94% (Cardenas et al., 2023; UNICEF, 2024).

Infants born with HIV may present with poor growth, recurrent and/or persistent infections, multiorgan dysfunction, or death (Shetty & Maldonado, 2025). These children experience immune defects due to depletion of CD4+ T cells in the periphery and thymus as well as abnormal B cell responses due to the absence of CD4+ T cell help (Shetty & Maldonado, 2025). Although early treatment with antiretroviral therapy (ART) dramatically improves survival, children with HIV face a long-term battle to maintain viral control and immune system function. Even children born to HIV-infected mothers who are not themselves infected are at risk for immunologic deficits, increased mortality, and increased susceptibility to infection (Tobin & Aldrovandi, 2013). For example, these infants have been shown to have a reduced CD4+ T cell count relative to infants born to HIV-uninfected mothers, which is thought to be related to decreased generation of T cells in the thymus during fetal development (S. D. Nielsen et al., 2001).

Autoimmune Disease

Autoimmune diseases are characterized by an immune attack on the body's own tissues in the absence of an infection. Autoimmune disorders are the result of autoantibodies produced by the immune system that are directed at one's own proteins. Maternal autoantibodies that are present in patients with lupus, Sjogren disease, and unspecified connective tissue diseases can cross the placenta and affect the fetus (Zuppa et al., 2017). The most serious complication of these maternal antibodies is third-degree heart block in the fetus or neonate, which can result in bradycardia, pacemaker implantation, or death.

Newborns/infants born to mothers with autoimmune diseases can also develop hematologic abnormalities, including thrombocytopenia, anemia, and neutropenia. In a small study of 50 infants born to mothers with anti-SSA/Ro antibodies, it was determined that the percentage of infants with neutropenia (less than 1,000 neutrophils/mm^3) peaked at 3 months of age, and only a small percentage of children were still neutropenic by 9 months. Despite the presence of neutropenia, and in utero exposure to maternal immunosuppressive therapy, these children did not exhibit an increased susceptibility to infection or require further treatment, suggesting a normal ability to combat infection (Zuppa et al., 2017).

Clinical Application. Antinuclear antibodies are produced when a pregnant patient is diagnosed with an immune disorder. The type of antibodies associated with systemic lupus erythematosus are titled "anti-double-stranded DNA antibodies." These antinuclear antibodies, specifically anti-Ro and anti-La, can cross the placenta and confer passive autoimmunity in the developing fetus. Anti-Ro and anti-La autoantibodies have an affinity for fetal cardiac receptors, and this affinity is the primary reason fetuses can develop heart block as well as inflammation at cardiac conduction tissues that can cause permanent scarring at the atrioventricular (AV) node. Interestingly, the heart block can begin as first-degree and worsen to the potentially fatal third-degree block. The initial evaluation should include an EKG and echocardiogram. Most babies who present with heart block at birth will go on to require a pacemaker.

Biologic Therapy

Treatment of autoimmune diseases in XX pregnant patients with antibodies directed against cytokines or inflammatory mediators continues to increase as research identifies more immunologic targets for treatment. Many of these antibodies are of the IgG subclass and can cross the placenta. Thus, the influence of these antibodies on the developing fetus and newborn is a growing area of study. The use of anti-TNF-a antibodies has been correlated with an increased incidence of infection and neutropenia in infants in a small number of case reports; however, other studies have demonstrated normal immune development and no major complications in these children (Ling & Koren, 2016). The Pregnancy in Inflammatory Bowel Disease and Neonatal Outcomes (PIANO) study, a large and historic registry of 1,000 patients with Crohn disease and ulcerative colitis being treated with anti-TNF-a agents, has shown no difference in infant development or susceptibility to infection in the first year of life (Mahadevan et al., 2012).

Another type of antibody commonly used to treat autoimmune disease and malignancies is anti-CD20, which targets B cells. Infants exposed to these antibodies in the second or third trimester may have reduced circulating B cell numbers and decreased levels of immunoglobulins in the peripheral blood. Despite these reductions, studies have generally shown no increase in rates of infections in exposed infants (Ling & Koren, 2016). As new biologic agents are developed, and an increasing number of patients are being treated with these therapies, the influence on the fetus and infant will need to be monitored for both short- and long-term effects. The potentially adverse effects of immunosuppression will have to be weighed against the risks of uncontrolled autoimmune disease, which in and of itself can have adverse effects.

COMMON PROBLEMS AND IMPLICATIONS ACROSS THE LIFE SPAN

Sepsis is a major cause of neonatal mortality and morbidity. Despite the lack of a universally agreed upon definition, neonatal sepsis typically refers to the isolation of a bacterial, viral, or fungal pathogen from normally sterile body fluids, such as blood or cerebrospinal fluid, on or before 30 days of life (Mukherjee & Ryan, 2025). Neonatal sepsis can be further classified as either early-onset (EOS) or late-onset sepsis (LOS), based on the postnatal days when it is discovered. EOS is defined as an infection which develops within the first 72 hours of life. LOS is defined as an infection that occurs between 72 hours and 30 days of life, and can be attributed to horizontal transmission of pathogens (Mukherjee & Ryan, 2025). We explore EOS and LOS in the following sections of this chapter.

Common Bacterial Pathogens

The overall incidence of EOS in the United States is estimated at 0.77 to 1.08 per 1,000 live births (Stoll et al., 2020) with a higher incidence among preterm and low birthweight infants. In contrast, the incidence of LOS in the United States is estimated at 0.28 to 0.31 per 1,000 live births (Miselli et al., 2022). Several maternal and infant factors have been identified that increase the risk of EOS and LOS (Table 9.7).

Early-Onset Sepsis. *EOS* usually refers to an infection that occurs at less than or equal to 72 hours of life (Mukherjee & Ryan, 2025). Risk factors for EOS include maternal GBS colonization, maternal history of GBS bacteriuria (with or without a positive screen), prolonged rupture of membranes (greater than 18 hours), maternal fever, and preterm birth (American College of Obstetricians and Gynecologists [ACOG], 2020). EOS is most often the result of vertical intraamniotic transmission of an infectious organism, after premature prelabor rupture of membranes, or direct contact with a maternal genitourinary pathogen while descending the vaginal canal. *E. coli* and GBS are the two most common pathogens responsible for cases of EOS of neonates.

Escherichia Coli. Importantly, *E. coli* is now the most commonly identified cause for EOS in both preterm and term infants. *E. coli* are facultative, anaerobic, gram-negative rods that are ubiquitous in the human GI tract (Mukhopadhyay & Puopolo, 2015). Multiple serotypes of *E. coli* exist and are categorized based on their antigenic structure. Strains with the K1 capsular antigen, in particular, have been identified as being important in neonatal sepsis and meningitis (Simonsen et al., 2014; Stenutz et al., 2006). Virulence factors associated with the K1 antigenic strain include the synthesis of polysialic acid, which impairs opsonization and phagocytosis and facilitates complement resistance, as well as surface proteins that facilitate invasion and binding of the brain endothelium (Simonsen et al., 2014).

Group B Streptococcus. GBS is now the second most common pathogen attributed to EOS infection. GBS is a gram-positive, facultative diplococcus known to colonize the genitourinary tract and pharyngeal mucosa of pregnant patients. It was first discovered as a distinct organism in the 1930s; however, it was not until the early 1960s that GBS was recognized as a pathogen commonly responsible for neonatal sepsis (Koenig & Keenan, 2009; Randis et al., 2017). In 1996, the Centers for Disease Control and Prevention (CDC) released a consensus statement that called for identification of pregnant GBS carriers based on prenatal and intrapartum risk factors by obtaining vaginal cultures. They further recommended treatment with intrapartum antibiotic prophylaxis (IAP) for pregnant patients found to be at high risk for GBS carriage or with culture-proven GBS colonization (CDC, 1996). In 2002, the CDC revised and re-released their policy statement, specifically to promote the use of universal screening over the risk-based approach, which had been shown to be less efficacious (Schrag et al., 2002). The most recent treatment guidelines for the prevention of perinatal GBS disease were reaffirmed by ACOG in 2022 and call for the universal GBS screening between 36 0/7 and 37 6/7 weeks of gestation. All pregnant patients whose vaginal-rectal culture is positive should receive IAP (unless cesarean delivery with intact membranes is indicated). Furthermore, the ACOG recommends 4 or more hours of antibiotic prophylaxis prior to delivery of the infant, when possible. The full ACOG recommendations are summarized in Table 9.8 (ACOG, 2020). Since the widespread adoption of universal screening and IAP, rates of EOS due to GBS have declined (allowing for *E. coli* to surpass GBS as the primary pathogen associated with EOS in neonates), but GBS

TABLE 9.7 Risk Factors for Bacterial Sepsis in the Newborn

Early-Onset Sepsis	Late-Onset Sepsis
Chorioamnionitis ("Triple I")	Delayed enteral feedings
Low birthweight	Invasive procedures
Birthing parent GBS colonization	Low birthweight
Birthing parent history of GBS bacteriuria	Poor hand hygiene
Birthing parent intrapartum fever	Prematurity
Prematurity	Prolonged exposure to antibiotics
Premature rupture of membranes	Prolonged indwelling catheter use
Prolonged rupture of membranes (greater than 18 hours)	

GBS, group B *Streptococcus*.

TABLE 9.8 ACOG Recommendations for Intrapartum Antibiotic Prophylaxis to Prevent Early-Onset GBS Sepsis

	Intrapartum GBS Prophylaxis Is Indicated	Intrapartum GBS Prophylaxis Is Not Indicated
Past medical history	Previous infant with invasive GBS disease	Colonization with GBS during a previous pregnancy (unless colonization status in current pregnancy is unknown at onset of labor at term)
Current pregnancy	• Positive GBS culture obtained at 36 0/7 weeks of gestation or more during current pregnancy (unless cesarean birth is performed before onset of labor for a woman with intact amniotic membranes) • GBS bacteruria during any trimester of the current pregnancy	• Negative vaginal-rectal GBS culture obtained on/after 36 0/7 weeks of gestation during the current pregnancy • Cesarean birth performed before onset of labor on a woman with intact amniotic membranes, regardless of GBS colonization status or gestational age
Intrapartum period	• Unknown GBS status at the onset of labor (culture not done or results unknown) AND any of the following intrapartum risk factors: ○ Birth less than 37 0/7 weeks of gestation ○ Amniotic membrane rupture 18+ hours ○ Intrapartum temperature 100.4°F (38.0°C) or higher[a] ○ Intrapartum NAAT positive for GBS ○ Intrapartum NAAT negative for GBS but any of the previously mentioned risk factors develop ○ Known GBS positive status in a prior pregnancy	• Negative vaginal-rectal GBS culture obtained on/after 36 0/7 weeks of gestation during the current pregnancy, regardless of intrapartum risk factors • Unknown GBS status at the onset of labor, NAAT result negative, and no intrapartum risk factors present

[a]If intraamniotic infection is suspected, broad-spectrum antibiotic therapy that includes an agent known to be active against GBS should replace GBS prophylaxis.

ACOG, American College of Obstetricians and Gynecologists; GBS, group B *Streptococcus*; NAAT, nucleic acid amplification test.

Source: Adapted from American College of Obstetricians and Gynecologists. (2020). Committee Opinion, No 797. Prevention of early-onset Group B Streptococcal disease in newborns. *Obstetrics & Gynecology, 135*(2), e51–e72. https://doi.org/10.1097/AOG.0000000000003668

continues to be a common pathogen implicated in EOS (Simonsen et al., 2014).

Fetal and neonatal exposure to GBS typically occurs during the antepartum or intrapartum period during which time the organism can ascend from the vaginal mucosa into the uterus. This most commonly occurs after rupture of the amniotic membranes; however, there is some evidence to suggest that GBS is capable of breaching the intact amnion. Once in the amniotic fluid, the organism replicates and can be aspirated into the fetal lungs (Randis et al., 2017). Vertical transmission can also occur during labor, through direct contact as the infant passes through the vaginal canal (Simonsen et al., 2014). Although the exact mechanisms by which GBS progresses from asymptomatic colonization to invasive disease are not completely understood, the organism is known to possess several characteristics that contribute to its virulence. GBS possesses the ability to adhere to vascular endothelium and epithelium, including rectovaginal tissue, chorionic membranes, and neonatal lungs—a characteristic that is essential in establishing colonization and ultimately invasive disease (Koenig & Keenan, 2009; Rajagopal, 2009). In addition, GBS works to evade and blunt the host's immune response through a variety of processes. It produces a polysaccharide capsule that inhibits the innate immune functions of opsonization and phagocytosis. It also plays a role in the inactivation of complement components and upregulation of inhibitory immune receptors (Rajagopal, 2009; Randis et al., 2017).

Clinical Application. There has been a noteworthy shift in the prevalence of pathogens associated with EOS. Currently *E. coli* is quickly surpassing GBS as the most common organism to blame for EOS. We know that *E. coli* has been the most common pathogen associated with EOS in preterm babies, but now it is the most common pathogen causing EOS in both term and preterm babies. Among very preterm infants, the third and fourth most common pathogens are *Haemophilus* species and *Staphylococcus aureus*. Beyond these top four pathogens, others that commonly affect term and preterm infants include gram-negative species (*Klebsiella*, *Enterobacter*, *Citrobacter*, *Acinetobacter*, and *Pseudomonas*). Interestingly, *Listeria* is no longer ranked as a leading cause for EOS.

Late-Onset Sepsis. *LOS* usually refers to an infection that occurs between 72 hours and 30 days of life (Mukherjee & Ryan, 2025). Risk factors for LOS include prematurity, prolonged use of indwelling catheters, delayed enteral feedings with freshly expressed colostrum or breast milk, and prolonged exposure to empiric antibiotics (Dong & Speer, 2014; Kuppala et al., 2011). LOS is most often acquired through contact with environmental pathogens that commonly colonize NICUs (e.g., methicillin-resistant *Staphylococcus aureus*) or the caregiver's gut microbiome (flora). Gram-positive organisms, most notably coagulase-negative staphylococci, or CoNS (which include the species *S. epidermis, S. haemolyticus, S. capitis,* and *S. hominis*) and *S. aureus* are the predominant pathogens responsible for LOS, particularly in premature and low birthweight infants. GBS is also associated with cases of LOS. Although the implementation of universal screening and routine IAP significantly decreased the incidence of EOS secondary to GBS, it has had no meaningful impact on rates of LOS from GBS (Mukherjee & Ryan, 2025). The incidence of late-onset GBS sepsis is estimated to be 0.28 to 0.31 per 1,000 live born infants (Miselli et al., 2022). Some reports suggest that contaminated human milk from mothers with either clinical or subclinical mastitis may also represent a source of late-onset or recurrent neonatal GBS infections, suggesting bacterial translocation from intestinal sources to the bloodstream as a potential mechanism by which GBS can access sterile sites (Berardi et al., 2013; Randis et al., 2017). A variety of gram-negative bacilli (GNB) also contribute to the burden of LOS, with *E. coli* a common cause for urinary tract infection (Glaser et al., 2021). Importantly, like with EOS, the mortality risk associated with LOS is inversely proportional to gestational age.

Coagulase-Negative Staphyococci and Staphylococcus Aureus. In most humans, CoNS represent commensal organisms that are part of the normal skin flora with relatively low capacity to cause invasive disease. However, neonates requiring intensive care, such as preterm or low-birthweight infants, are vulnerable to CoNS infections secondary to impaired defense barriers, immature immune response, the presence of indwelling devices, and repeated invasive procedures (Becker et al., 2014).

Although CoNS tend to be less virulent and have a more indolent clinical course than other pathogens, *S. epidermis* species have been shown to have the unique capability to form biofilms that permit invasive disease (Becker et al., 2014; Dong & Speer, 2014). Biofilm formation is the process by which bacteria adhere to a foreign body, such as a central venous catheter or indwelling urinary catheter, and form an extracellular matrix (**Figure 9.10**). Once formed, the biofilm allows the organism to evade host defense mechanisms and may even contribute to antimicrobial resistance. As the biofilm matures, intact sections can slough off and seed to other organ systems, leading to systemic infection (Becker et al., 2014; Dong & Speer, 2014; Fey & Olson, 2010).

S. aureus represents both a commensal and infectious pathogen. Approximately 30% of the population are asymptomatic carriers of *S. aureus,* yet it is a common cause of invasive neonatal disease and is associated with myriad complications, including skin and soft tissue infection, brain abscesses, meningitis, osteomyelitis, septic arthritis, infective endocarditis, pneumatoceles, lung abscesses, and death (Dolapo et al., 2014; Tong et al., 2015). *S. aureus* is typically classified as either methicillin susceptible (MSSA) or methicillin resistant (MRSA) based on its sensitivity to beta-lactam antibiotics. Over

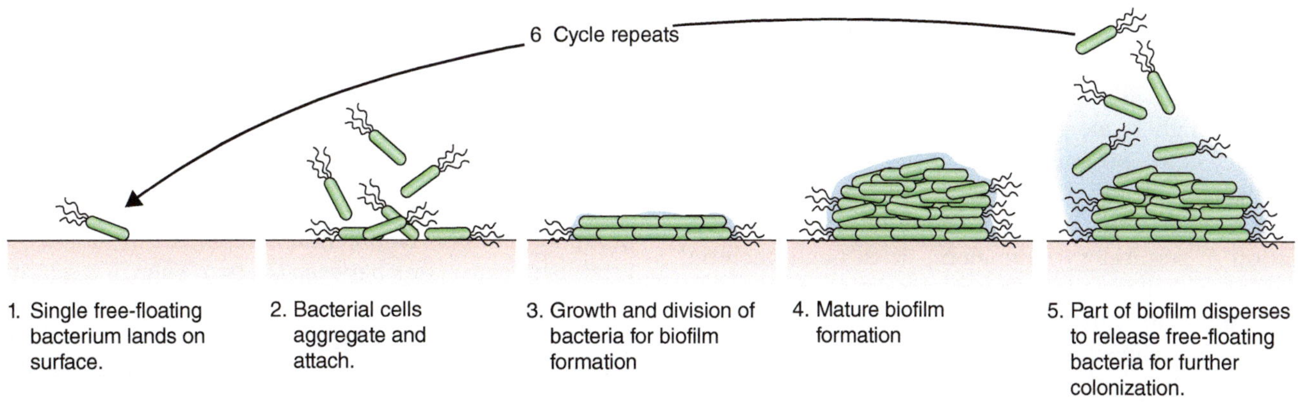

Figure 9.10 The six stages of biofilm formation. *Stage 1:* Single free-floating bacteria adhere to an endothelial or prosthetic surface. *Stage 2:* The bacterial cells aggregate, form microcolonies, and excrete extracellular polymers, creating an irreversible attachment. *Stage 3:* The bacterial cells grow and divide, creating a biofilm. *Stage 4:* The biofilm matures, providing protection to the bacterial colonies against host defense mechanisms and antimicrobials. *Stage 5:* As the biofilm reaches a critical mass, intact portions break off. *Stage 6:* Free-floating bacteria that have detached from the biofilm seed to other parts of the body and repeat the cycle.

the past two decades there have been increasing reports of both hospital-acquired MRSA (HA-MRSA) and community-acquired MRSA (CA-MRSA) outbreaks in NICUs across the country (Dolapo et al., 2014). This underscores the importance of practicing good hand hygiene and strict compliance with infection-control practices in this population.

S. aureus has several characteristics that contribute to its virulence and potential to lead to invasive disease. As with CoNS, *S. aureus* can produce biofilms that adhere to host tissues or foreign materials, enabling it to evade host defense responses and antimicrobials. In addition, *S. aureus* produces a microcapsule that prevents phagocytosis and opsonization from occurring. It also produces proteins that interfere with chemotaxis and limit the extravasation of neutrophils to the site of infection, as well as cytotoxins that cause leukocyte destruction (Gordon & Lowy, 2008; Tong et al., 2015).

There remains some debate as to whether MRSA is more virulent than MSSA. Evidence suggests that there is no significant difference in morbidity and mortality among VLBW infants with MRSA bacteremia when compared to those with MSSA bacteremia (Shane et al., 2012). However, the increase in CA-MRSA outbreaks in NICUs that have been recently observed have been associated with more severe clinical presentation and worse outcomes (Dolapo et al., 2014). Regardless of the strain isolated, MRSA is universally associated with increased healthcare costs and limited treatment options (Gordon & Lowy, 2008).

Gram-Negative Bacilli. As a group, GNB represent the third most common cause of LOS (Camacho-Gonzalez et al., 2013; Downey et al., 2010). Although less prevalent, gram-negative LOS carries a significantly higher risk of mortality, with 19% to 36% of those affected ultimately dying (Downey et al., 2010). Gram-negative pathogens responsible for LOS primarily include *E. coli*, *Klebsiella*, *Enterobacter*, *Serratia*, and *Pseudomonas* (Camacho-Gonzalez et al., 2013; Dong & Speer, 2014). Considered alone, *Pseudomonas aeruginosa*, a gram-negative organism that tends to thrive in moist environments, has been found to have the highest mortality rate among preterm infants (Downey et al., 2010). Horizontal transmission of these pathogens typically occurs via the hands of healthcare workers, contamination of parenteral nutrition, contamination of respiratory equipment, or through bacterial translocation of intestinal flora (Camacho-Gonzalez et al., 2013; Sherman, 2010).

Once introduced, GNB exhibit several virulence factors that enhance their ability to cause systemic disease and evade a host's defenses. One of the most important virulence factors of GNB is endotoxins. Endotoxins are large molecules consisting of a lipid and polysaccharide found on the outer membrane of GNB. Endotoxin expression plays a significant role in the exaggerated release of proinflammatory cytokines (IL-8, IL-6, IL-1b, and TNF-a) that can lead to tissue damage, septic shock, and death (Ramachandran, 2014).

Clinical Application. A fun way to remember β-lactamase resistant gram-negative bacteria responsible for LOS involves the use of this acronym: "SPACE-EK." Sometimes catchy acronyms help in times of stress, when recalling information can be particularly challenging. SPACE-EK stands for **S**erratia, **P**seudomonas, **A**cinetobacter, **C**itrobacter, **E**nterobacter—***E**. coli*, **K**lebsiella.

Clinical Manifestations. The clinical manifestation of EOS and LOS on the neonate is broad and nonspecific. The most common nonspecific symptoms are tachycardia and respiratory distress. Other signs and symptoms include apnea, temperature instability, feeding difficulty, poor perfusion, lethargy, bleeding problems, and metabolic derangements (e.g., hyperglycemia, acidosis). Left untreated, the symptoms of sepsis in preterm and term infants can quickly progress from subtle, vital-sign abnormalities to profound septic shock (Mukherjee & Ryan, 2025).

Implications Across the Life Span. Regardless of the organism isolated or the timing of onset, bacterial sepsis is associated with several serious short- and long-term complications, and the risk for death. For example, the current mortality rate associated with GBS sepsis is 20% in preterm infants and less than 2% in term infants (Flannery et al., 2022). The all-cause mortality risk associated with meningitis is currently 10% to 15% (Ku et al., 2015). Infants who survive are more likely to develop bronchopulmonary dysplasia, visual impairment, and auditory impairment. A history of meningitis is associated with an increased risk for neurologic disease (e.g., cerebral palsy and cognitive impairment). It is important to point out that many of the risk factors for developing sepsis, such as prematurity and low birthweight, are also associated with subsequent poor outcomes. Therefore, although the evidence suggests a strong correlation between sepsis and poor neurodevelopmental outcomes, it is difficult to establish a causal link between the two. There is a relative paucity of data on the outcomes of patients with a history of bacterial sepsis beyond early childhood, and the impact of bacterial sepsis on long-term quality of life and future burden of disease is largely unknown.

Other Bacterial Pathogens

Treponema Pallidum. *T. pallidum* is a thin, tightly coiled, motile spirochete that causes syphilis (Mukherjee & Ryan, 2025). In adult pregnant patients, syphilis is usually acquired through sexual contact and progresses through several well-described stages if left untreated: a primary stage, which presents with a chancre at the site of inoculation; a secondary stage characterized by fever, malaise, and a mucocutaneous rash; an asymptomatic, latent stage; and a late tertiary stage involving damage to multiple organ systems (Janier et al., 2014). The incidence of congenital syphilis generally mirrors that of primary and secondary disease in pregnant patients.

The rate of congenital syphilis has been steadily increasing and has tripled in recent years to more than 3,700 cases (102.5 per 100,000 live births) in 2022 alone (CDC, 2024c). Limited or no prenatal care are risk factors for congenital syphilis. Transmission of *T. pallidum* most often occurs transplacentally but can also occur through direct contact with an infectious lesion during delivery. Although transplacental transfer of *T. pallidum* can occur at any point during gestation, risk of transmission increases with advancing gestational age. Infants born to pregnant patients with primary or secondary disease are more likely to acquire congenital syphilis than infants born to those with latent disease (Mukherjee & Ryan, 2025). Once introduced in the fetal bloodstream, *T. pallidum* multiplies, resulting in spirochetemia and widespread dissemination of the organism to nearly every organ system in the body. Intrauterine syphilis infection can result in spontaneous abortion, stillbirth, or preterm delivery (Mukherjee & Ryan, 2025).

Clinical Manifestations. Congenital syphilis is classified as either early or late disease based on the age at the onset of symptoms. Symptoms of early congenital syphilis are present before 2 years of age; however, 60% to 90% of infants with congenital syphilis are asymptomatic at birth (Bowen et al., 2015; Ortiz-Lopez et al., 2012). When present, clinical manifestations in infected infants include hepatosplenomegaly, maculopapular eruptions, anemia, bone abnormalities, persistent rhinitis (snuffles), chorioretinitis, nonimmune hydrops, and generalized lymphadenopathy (Mukherjee & Ryan, 2025; Ortiz-Lopez et al., 2012).

Implications Across the Life Span. Left untreated, congenital syphilis leads to late-stage disease findings, which typically occur after 2 years of age. APRNs should recognize that "Hutchinson's triad" is a common aggregate of three key clinical manifestations associated with congenital syphilis. This triad manifests during childhood (not at birth) with (a) interstitial keratitis, (b) nerve deafness, and (c) peg-shaped upper incisor teeth ("Hutchinson's teeth"). Eighth-cranial-nerve deafness is common and typically occurs suddenly at 8 to 10 years of age. In addition, abnormalities in permanent dentition characterized by centrally notched Hutchinson's teeth may develop (Mukherjee & Ryan, 2025).

Common Fungal and Protozoal Pathogens

Fungal infections are primarily diagnosed in extremely low birthweight (ELBW) infants and infants with a birthweight lower than 1,000 grams, as well as infants with a history of significant GI disease (e.g., necrotizing enterocolitis; Kaufman et al., 2025). The most common species is *Candida sp.*, followed by *Aspergillus, mucormycosis, Malassezia,* and *Trichosporon.* We will focus our discussion to *Candida sp.*, which is associated primarily with bloodstream (60%) and urinary tract (40%) infection. *Candida* meningitis is rare in ELBW infants (Kimberlin et al., 2024).

Candida organisms are ubiquitous, saprophytic (feeds on dead or decaying matter) yeasts that comprise the normal commensal flora of humans yet can cause disease in immunocompromised patients (Kimberlin et al., 2024). *Candida albicans* is the most common albicans species associated with fungal infections in neonates, accounting for 80% to 90% of invasive Candida infections in neonates admitted to hospital units who do not prescribe antifungal prophylaxis (Kaufman et al., 2025). In contrast, *Candida parapsilosis* has emerged as the most common *nonalbicans* species of Candida that causes infection in neonates (Kimberlin et al., 2024; Kaufman et al., 2025). Other less common species that have been isolated include *C. glabrata, C. tropicalis,* and *C. lusitaniae.*

Like infections caused by bacterial pathogens, *Candida* infections can be the result of vertical transmission from mother to infant during the intrapartum period resulting in early onset of disease. However, the vast majority of invasive *Candida* infections are late onset and the result of horizontal transmission. Risk factors for *Candida* infection include presence of a central catheter, exposure to broad-spectrum antibiotics (particularly third-generation cephalosporins), fungal colonization, exposure to corticosteroids, prematurity, and low birthweight (D. K. Benjamin et al., 2010; Kimberlin et al., 2024). *Candida* infections in neonates and infants can range in severity from superficial cutaneous infection to disseminated disease, and because this pathogen is very slow growing, it can easily and covertly disseminate throughout the body before manifestations become apparent (Kaufman et al., 2025).

Candida species possess several other attributes that support its virulence and ability to cause invasive disease. They have a specialized set of proteins, called *adhesins* and *invasins*, that mediate adherence to and invasion of host cells (Mayer et al., 2013). Adhesion involves the process of "sticking" to invasive catheters, as well as epithelial or endothelial cells. *Candida* organisms then form biofilms that protect the fungus from host defenses and facilitate systemic seeding. Then, sections of the biofilm detach and disseminate to other organ systems, including the heart, kidneys, central nervous system (CNS), eyes, lungs, liver, spleen, bones, and joints, where abscesses can form (Kaufman et al., 2025; Manzoni et al., 2015). Given the attributes just described, it is of no surprise that *Candida sp.* infection is commonly described as a sequence of four predictable steps: (a) adhesion, (b) colonization, (c) dissemination, and (d) abscess formation (Kaufman et al., 2025).

Clinical Manifestations. The clinical manifestations of neonatal fungal infections are similar in nature to the signs and symptoms of bacterial infections and include apnea, respiratory distress, temperature instability, and lethargy. The combination of persistent hyperglycemia and thrombocytopenia are strongly associated with systemic candidiasis in the ELBW infant (Dyke & Ott, 1993).

Implications Across the Life Span. Implications of invasive candidiasis in the neonate are similar to those for bacterial infections. The mortality risk for ELBW infants with candidemia is 28%, and 26% with cases of candiduria. The percentages are even higher at 50% in rare cases of meningitis or peritonitis (Kimberlin et al., 2024). Among survivors, morbidity risks include visual impairment, deafness, and cerebral palsy (Barton et al., 2014; D. K. Benjamin et al., 2006).

> **Clinical Application.** We emphasized in the chapter that ELBW infants are at highest risk for *Candida* infection, which progresses slowly and in a clandestine manner in the body before symptoms appear. The most common symptom in an ELBW infant is persistent hyperglycemia, which should always raise the index of suspicion for *Candida* infection. Recall that this could involve candidemia, candiduria, meningitis, or peritonitis. Therefore, the APRN should be prepared to order a comprehensive evaluation including a blood culture, lumbar puncture, echocardiogram, and ophthalmologic exam, as tolerated. The only appropriate therapy is amphotericin B deoxycholate. (It is important to remember the full name of this medication.)

Toxoplasma Gondii. *Toxoplasma gondii* (*T. gondii*) is an obligate intracellular protozoan parasite that causes the human disease toxoplasmosis. *T. gondii* exist in three forms: oocysts, which are excreted in cat feces; tachyzoites or trophozoites, which proliferate and destroy infected cells during acute infection; and bradyzoites, which multiply in tissue cysts (Kaufman et al., 2025; McAuley, 2014). Therefore, cats are the only known definitive hosts, yet other farm animals (e.g., cattle) can acquire the infection from eating food or water contaminated with cat feces, and spread the disease to humans. Humans can also acquire the infection through ingestion of contaminated meat containing *T. gondii* cysts, ingestion of oocysts through water contaminated by cat feces, organ transplantation, blood transfusion, or via the maternal-fetal transplacental route (McAuley, 2014).

Congenital toxoplasma infections most commonly occur after a primary infection in the XX pregnant patient, although transmission in immunocompromised pregnant patients experiencing reactivation of infection has been described (Lindsay & Dubey, 2011). The incidence of primary infection during pregnancy is estimated to be about 1.1 per 1,000 pregnant patients (Kaufman et al., 2025) and fetal infection in the first trimester is considered most severe (Kimberlin et al., 2024).

In humans, ingesting tissue cysts or oocytes results in the release of sporozoites that disseminate in the body and multiply intracellularly. As the host cell dies, it releases tachyzoites that invade adjacent cells and continue the process. Pressure from the host's immune response ultimately causes the tachyzoites to transform into bradyzoites that form tissue cysts in the skeletal muscle, myocardium, and brain (**Figure 9.11**; McAuley, 2014).

Clinical Manifestations. Most infants with congenital toxoplasmosis are asymptomatic at birth; however, symptoms of disease can manifest within the first few months to years of life. A subset of newborns with congenital toxoplasmosis will have signs of generalized disease at birth that can include chorioretinitis, intracranial calcifications, hydrocephalus, microcephaly, jaundice, thrombocytopenia, anemia, and hepatosplenomegaly (Kaufman et al., 2025; Maldonado & Read, 2017).

Implications Across the Life Span. The long-term implications of congenital toxoplasmosis depend heavily on whether the infant receives prompt treatment for the infection. Without treatment, nearly all infants with symptomatic congenital toxoplasmosis develop long-term sequelae, including cognitive impairment, severe visual impairment, deafness, and seizures (Wilson et al., 1980). Likewise, most infants with subclinical toxoplasmosis who do not receive treatment go on to develop chorioretinitis during childhood that can lead to blindness. They are also at high risk for sensorineural hearing loss (SNHL) and cognitive impairment (Wilson et al., 1980). If, on the other hand, congenital toxoplasmosis is treated immediately, the risks of chorioretinitis and neurologic impairment are substantially decreased, and the prognosis is generally favorable (Berrebi et al., 2010). Most adults with a history of congenital toxoplasmosis who received early treatment report normal to near normal quality of life and minimal visual impairment (Peyron et al., 2011).

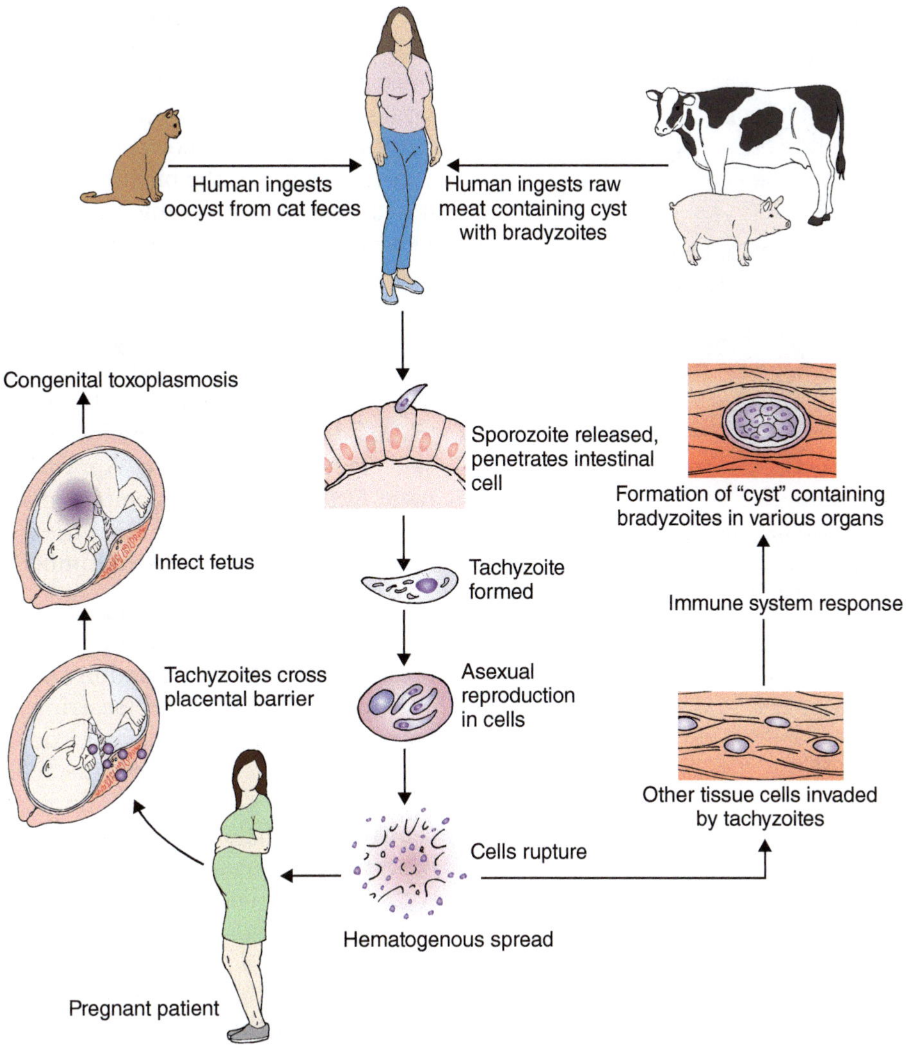

Figure 9.11 The life cycle of *T. gondii.* Humans either ingest tissue cysts from contaminated meat or oocysts from hands, food, or water contaminated by cat feces. Once ingested, the tissue cyst or oocyst ruptures, releasing sporozoites that penetrate the intestinal epithelium, disseminate through the body, and multiply intracellularly. As the host's cells die, they release tachyzoites that invade adjacent cells and continue the process. Pressure from the host's immune response prompts the tachyzoites to transform into bradyzoites that form tissues and cysts in various organs. In pregnant patients with primary infections, tachyzoites cross the placenta, infecting the fetus.

Clinical Application. The classic triad of symptoms of chorioretinitis is important to know. These symptoms include: (a) chorioretinitis (occurs in 70% of cases), (b) intracranial calcifications, and (c) hydrocephalus. Given this triad, it is expected that the diagnostic workup includes a cranial ultrasound and ophthalmologic exam. In addition, a complete blood count, liver function testing, lumbar puncture, and *T. gondii* polymerase chain reaction should be ordered. A positive IgG result is not necessarily confirmation of congenital disease, since IgG crosses the placenta. However, a positive IgM result is predictive of congenital *T. gondii* infection. Closer to discharge, audiology testing should be performed as well as coordination of care for an outpatient audiologic evaluation at approximately 3 months of age.

Common Viral Pathogens

Herpes Simplex Virus. Herpes simplex virus types 1 (HSV-1) and 2 (HSV-2) are members of the herpesvirus family that consist of several closely related viruses. Structurally, the herpesviruses are characterized by a double-stranded DNA core that is enveloped by an icosahedral (20-sided) nucleocapsid consisting of 162 capsomeres (Figure 9.12; Kaufman et al., 2025;

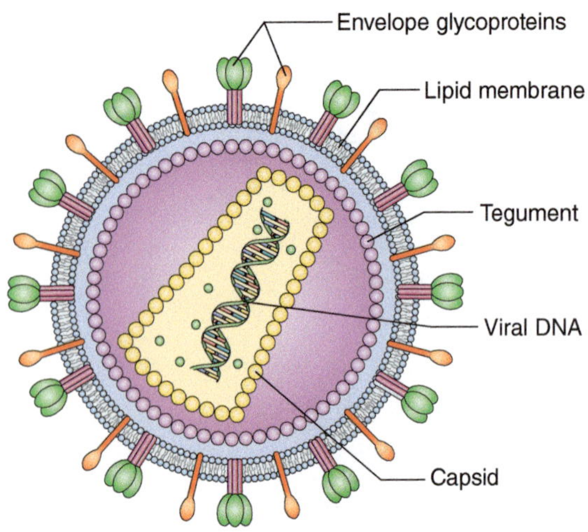

Figure 9.12 All herpes viruses have the same basic structure: an inner core containing large double-stranded viral DNA enclosed within an icosahedral capsid. The capsid is surrounded by a protein coat called the *tegument,* which is encased in a glycoprotein bearing lipid membrane.

Source**:** Adapted from Maldonado, Y. A., Nizet, V., Barnett, E. D., Edwards, K. M., Mally, R., Remington, J. S., & Klein, J. O. (Eds.). (2025). *Remington and Klein's infectious diseases of the fetus and newborn infant* (9th ed.). Elsevier.

Kimberlin et al., 2024). Transmission of HSV most commonly occurs through contact with mucosal surfaces or open areas of skin. Congenital infection can be the cause of a primary infection in the birthing parent or disease recurrence ("flare up"), when the virus is reactivated and migrates from the sensory nerve to the skin or mucous membranes (e.g., vaginal canal). Among individuals in the United States, predominantly those of childbearing age, 48% are positive for HSV-1. Approximately one in 2,000 to 3,200 neonates test positive for HSV, with HSV-1 implicating 50% of all cases (CDC, 2018, 2021a; Kaufman et al., 2025; Kimberlin et al., 2024). Although HSV-1 is most often associated with oral herpes virus, *both HSV-1 and HSV-2 can cause genital herpes.* This means that a birthing parent can pass HSV-1 or HSV-2 to offspring.

Symptomatic or asymptomatic viral shedding of HSV from birthing parent to fetus must occur for the virus to be transmitted to the neonate. When the birth parent is shedding the virus, HSV can be transmitted in utero (transplacental), during the intrapartum period, or postnatally. Transplacental transfer of HSV is rare, accounting for approximately 5% of all cases of neonatal disease. Postnatal transfer is attributed to 10% of cases and is almost always attributed to oral HSV-1 transmission from a host to the newborn (Shetty & Maldonado, 2025).

More concerning is intrapartum transfer of HSV involving direct fetal contact with the genital tract during birth, which accounts for 85% of cases. The worst scenario involves intrapartum transfer of virus after a primary HSV infection in the birthing parent which occurred within 21 days of the onset of labor (25%–60% risk of transmission to the fetus). This is considered most severe because a significantly high level of cervical viral shedding occurs over the first 21 days of the maternal infection (Kaufman et al., 2025). Recurrent/reactivated infection in the birthing parent is associated with a significantly lower amount of viral shedding which persists for 2 to 5 days and is associated with a 2% risk of transmission to the fetus (Kaufman et al., 2025).

Intrapartum transfer of HSV is classified as *disseminated* (affecting multiple organ systems including the lungs, liver, adrenal glands, skin, eyes, and CNS), *CNS disease* with or without skin lesions, or skin-eye-mouth (SEM) disease because the lesions are localized to the skin, eyes, and/or mouth. Approximately 25% of neonatal HSV cases are disseminated and CNS disease accounts for 30% of cases. *SEM disease is most common,* comprising 45% of all cases (Kimberlin et al., 2024).

Clinical Manifestations. Infants who acquire HSV in utero are not typically asymptomatic. Infants usually present a triad of clinical findings at birth that include (a) cutaneous manifestations (scarring, active lesions, cutis aplasia, erythematous macular exanthem); (b) ophthalmologic findings (chorioretinitis, microphthalmia, optic atrophy); and (c) neurologic findings (seizures, microcephaly, encephalomalacia, hydranencephaly). The onset of symptoms usually begins within the first month of life, with SEM and disseminated disease presenting between day 7 and 14 of life and CNS disease between day 14 and 21 of life (Table 9.9; Kimberlin et al., 2024). HSV should be included in the differential diagnosis for all neonates who present within the first 21 days of life with fever, hypothermia, and abnormal cerebrospinal fluid test results with/without seizures, particularly during nonendemic times of the year (Kimberlin et al., 2024). Importantly, *disseminated disease should be suspected when a neonate presents with sepsis syndrome (bacteremia ruled out), hepatic dysfunction, consumptive coagulopathy, and pneumonia (pneumonitis).*

Implications Across the Life Span. Despite the availability of effective antiviral therapy, neonatal HSV infection is a lifelong condition that may be characterized by viral reactivation and recurrence. The short- and long-term sequelae associated with neonatal HSV infection depend on the degree of organ system involvement. Seizures that present before the initiation of antiviral therapy are a poor prognostic indicator and increase the likelihood of neurodevelopmental impairment in patients with CNS disease as well as disseminated disease (Kimberlin, 2007). A history of HSV encephalitis (with either CNS, disseminated, or SEM disease) and confirmed pathologic changes to the temporal lobe, cerebellum, brainstem, and deep grey matter can lead to cystic changes and morbidities including microcephaly, cataracts, or blindless (Kaufman et al., 2025). A history of localized SEM is associated with abnormal ophthalmologic

TABLE 9.9 Hallmark Manifestations of Neonatal Herpes Disease

Body System	Disseminated HSV	Central Nervous System HSV	Skin, Eye, Mucous Membranes HSV
Central nervous system	Apnea, bulging fontanelle, encephalitis, coma, fever, irritability, opisthotonos, seizures	Apnea, bulging fontanelle, fever, irritability, lethargy, seizures, hyperreflexia, spasticity, weakness	
Ophthalmologic			Chorioretinitis, conjunctivitis, keratitis, microphthalmos, retinal dysplasia
Respiratory	Interstitial pneumonitis, pleural effusion, respiratory distress		
Hepatic/Heme	Consumptive coagulopathy with petechiae and purpura, elevated liver enzymes, hepatomegaly, sepsis syndrome with or without shock		
Gastrointestinal	Pneumatosis intestinalis		
Integumentary	Clusters of papulovesicular lesions with an erythematous base usually localized to the presenting part at birth (60%–67% of all cases)	Clusters of papulovesicular lesions with an erythematous base usually localized to the presenting part at birth (67% of all cases)	Clusters of papulovesicular lesions with an erythematous base usually localized to the presenting part at birth (80% of all cases)

Note: This list is not inclusive of all manifestations.
HSV, herpes simplex virus.
Sources: Kaufman, D. A., Nadipuram, S. M., & Manzoni, P. (2025). Fungal and protozoal infections in the neonate. In R. J. Martin & A. A. Fanaroff (Eds.), *Fanaroff and Martin's neonatal-perinatal medicine: Diseases of the fetus and neonate* (12th ed., pp. 881–916). Elsevier; Kimberlin, D. W., Banerjee, R., Barnett, E., Lynfield, R., Sawyer, M. H., & American Academy of Pediatrics Committee on Infectious Diseases. (2024). *Red book: 2024–2027 report of the Committee on Infectious Diseases* (33rd ed.). American Academy of Pediatrics.

findings that can progress to cataracts, as well as neurologic deficits that are likely the result of undiagnosed neurologic damage incurred during the disease process (Kaufman et al., 2025).

Cytomegalovirus. CMV is a ubiquitous herpesvirus spread by close personal contact through blood, saliva, genital secretions, urine, and breast milk. Up to 90% of individuals contract CMV infection at some point during their lifetime, and once introduced, the virus establishes lifelong latency in monocytes and granulocytes (Swanson & Schleiss, 2013). In the immunocompetent host, CMV infection is usually clinically silent, but individuals with impaired cell-mediated immunity may have difficulty controlling CMV infection (Pass & Anderson, 2014). The transmission of a new or reactivated infection to the fetus can occur at any point during gestation, leading to congenital CMV infection.

Congenital CMV is the most common intrauterine infection transmitted from mother to fetus, affecting one in every 200 live births in the United States (Kaufman et al., 2025; Salemi et al., 2024). Vertical transmission can occur in times of viremia and transplacental transfer of infected WBCs, or with placental infection and fetal swallowing of infected amniotic fluid (Salemi et al., 2024). In contrast, postnatal CMV infection has been associated with the ingestion of infected breast milk (20.7% to 87% incidence) and exposure to the saliva of CMV-positive caregivers, including daycare staff (Kimberlin et al., 2024; Salemi et al., 2024).

Clinical Manifestations. Fetal manifestations include growth restriction, intracranial (cerebral) calcifications, and hydrops. Symptoms of congenitally acquired CMV are often ubiquitous, as only 5% to 10% of congenital CMV infections are symptomatic, and they are more likely to be associated with a primary maternal infection (Salemi et al., 2024; van Zuylen et al., 2014). Hallmark manifestations, which include IUGR and SGA, are summarized in Table 9.10 (Salemi et al., 2024). Term infants who acquire CMV during the intrapartum period or through freshly expressed colostrum or breast milk often remain asymptomatic, whereas preterm

TABLE 9.10 Hallmark Clinical Manifestations of CMV Infection

Body System	Congenital CMV	Postnatal CMV
Central nervous system	Intracranial calcifications or cysts, microcephaly	
Ophthalmologic	Chorioretinitis	
Auditory	Sensorineural hearing loss	
Respiratory		Interstitial pneumonitis
Hepatic/Heme	Conjugated hyperbilirubinemia, elevated liver transaminase, hepatitis, petechiae	Sepsislike symptoms, elevated liver transaminase
Gastrointestinal		Colitis, hepatitis
Integumentary	Dermal erythropoiesis ("blueberry muffin rash")	

Note: This list is not inclusive of all manifestations.
CMV, cytomegalovirus.
Source: Salemi, T. F., McLean, V. R., & Jnah, A. J. (2024). Congenital and postnatal cytomegalovirus: Case series and state of the science for neonatal providers. *Neonatal Network, 43*(2), 92–104. https://doi.org/10.1891/NN-2023-0069

VLBW infants who do not have congenital CMV but contract the virus during birth or through breast milk have been reported to have signs of acute illness characterized by respiratory distress, hematologic changes, and abnormal liver function (Kaufman et al., 2025; Pass & Anderson, 2014).

Implications Across the Life Span. Congenital CMV infection is referred to as the "silent virus" because the most common sequelae associated with congenital CMV infection is SNHL (Dreher et al., 2014; Salemi et al., 2024). Upwards of 40% to 60% of newborns with symptomatic infection and 10% to 14% of infants with asymptomatic infection will develop SNHL, which is often progressive (Salemi et al., 2024). Other life-span implications include motor defects, cognitive impairment, and seizures. Many children with chorioretinitis go on to develop strabismus or visual impairment (Kaufman et al., 2025).

Rubella Virus. Rubella virus is an RNA virus in the *Togaviridae* family that, in adults, produces a relatively mild but extremely contagious disease, characterized by a maculopapular rash, lymphadenopathy, conjunctivitis, and malaise (Kimberlin et al., 2024). While the incidence in the United States is extremely low (median = 5 cases per year), it is usually relatively asymptomatic in adults while being extremely contagious (CDC, 2024b). Similar to other viral infections, birthing parent-to-fetal transmission most often occurs with primary infection, and the likelihood of fetal anomalies or death is greatest during the first 20 weeks of pregnancy, with no fetal anomalies or death reported after this time frame (Kaufman et al., 2025). The exact mechanism by which rubella infection leads to teratogenesis is not completely understood, but it is believed to be the result of necrosis or apoptosis, and inhibition of cell division of precursor cells is involved in organogenesis (Lee & Bowden, 2000).

Clinical Manifestations. Most newborns with congenital rubella infection are asymptomatic at birth. However, among infants with *congenital rubella syndrome (CRS)*, early findings may include a history of fetal growth restriction and evolving failure to thrive postnatally. Hallmark clinical manifestations are summarized in **Table 9.11** with dermal extramedullary hematopoiesis reported in over 50% of all cases of CRS (Kaufman et al., 2025). Most symptoms resolve quickly; however, experts caution that fulminant hepatitis or pneumonia, myocarditis, congestive heart failure, and long bone radiolucency are ominous findings (Kaufman et al., 2025).

Implications Across the Life Span. The long-term sequelae associated with CRS include hearing impairment (deafness), ophthalmologic problems (cataracts, blindness), and autoimmune and neurologic disease. Hearing impairment is the single most common defect seen in patients with CRS, which, if left undetected, can go on to affect speech and language development as well as school performance (Reef et al., 2000). Ophthalmologic problems associated with CRS include cataracts, chorioretinopathy, and glaucoma. Adults with a history of congenital rubella have been reported to have a high prevalence of visual problems, including blindness (Forrest et al., 2002). Children and adults with a history of CRS are also at higher risk for developing chronic conditions such as diabetes, thyroid disorders, early menopause, and osteoporosis (Forrest et al., 2002; McIntosh & Menser, 1992). Neurologic sequalae

TABLE 9.11 Hallmark Clinical Manifestations of Congenital Rubella Syndrome

Body System	Manifestations
Central nervous system	Meningoencephalitis, microcephaly
Ophthalmologic	Cataracts, cloudy corneas, congenital glaucoma, microphthalmos, pigmentary retinopathy
Auditory	Sensorineural hearing loss
Cardiovascular	Patent ductus arteriosus; peripheral pulmonary artery stenosis, myocarditis
Respiratory	Interstitial pneumonitis
Hepatic/Heme	Hepatosplenomegaly, thrombocytopenia
Musculoskeletal	Radiolucent bone disease to the long bones
Integumentary	Dermal erythropoiesis ("blueberry muffin rash") to head, neck trunk

Note: This list is not inclusive of all manifestations. Congenital heart diseases only manifest if the disease is acquired within the first 8 weeks of fetal development.
Source: Data from Kimberlin, D. W., Banerjee, R., Barnett, E., Lynfield, R., Sawyer, M. H., & American Academy of Pediatrics Committee on Infectious Diseases. (2024). *Red book: 2024–2027 report of the committee on infectious diseases* (33rd ed.). American Academy of Pediatrics.

include intellectual disability, neurobehavioral problems and autism (Kaufman et al., 2025).

Respiratory Syncytial Virus. Respiratory syncytial virus (RSV) is a single-stranded RNA virus of the *Paramyxoviridae* family. RSV is the most common respiratory virus diagnosed in infants and young children, with an estimated 58,000 to 80,000 children less than age 5 hospitalized from RSV every year in the United States (CDC, 2024a). Results of a cross-sectional surveillance study of 600 infants born in 27 U.S. states offer insight into the clinical characteristics, disease severity, and outcomes of RSV infection (Halasa et al., 2023). The median age at the time of RSV diagnosis is 2.6 months (interquartile range [IQR] 1.4–6 months); the majority (71.1%) of infants diagnosed with RSV were term gestation at birth and 81.2% of infants had no other preexisting conditions (Halasa et al, 2023).

Broadly speaking, RSV is considered endemic between the months of October and April; however, regional trends must be monitored in order to properly guide the timing for initiation of immunoprophylaxis (Hamid et al., 2023). According to the CDC (2024a), sustained positivity of RSV tests occurs between mid-September and mid-November, disease peak occurs between late December and mid-February, and a sustained decrease in positive RSV test results occurs between mid-April to mid-May in the United States. Prior shifts in seasonality were observed during and shortly after the COVID-19 pandemic due to social distancing, lockdowns, and face mask mandates (Hamid et al., 2023). Infants born preterm are considered at 10-fold higher risk for requiring hospitalization for RSV infection. Mortality risk is higher among infants with congenital heart disease, trisomy 21, cystic fibrosis, and those who are immunocompromised.

Recall that IgG antibodies can cross the placenta, and most antibody transfer occurs during the third trimester. While antibody transfer from the birthing parent to fetus and newborn is protective, birthing parent-acquired antibody titers in the newborn are known to wane quickly over the first few months of life. In the case of RSV, this could place the newborn at heightened vulnerability to RSV. Therefore, Abrysvo RSV neutralizing vaccine is recommended in pregnant patients between 32 and 36 weeks of pregnancy to boost RSV neutralizing antibody titers in pregnant patients who will give birth just prior to or during RSV season. This allows for a more robust neutralizing antibody transfer to the fetus and confers 5 months of protection to the newborn when the Abrysvo vaccine is administered at least 14 days prior to birth of the infant (Pfizer, 2024). Administration to pregnant patients at less than 32 weeks' gestation is currently contraindicated due to the possible risk for premature onset of labor; additional studies are indicated to evaluate this relationship (Pfizer, 2024).

Postnatal transmission of RSV occurs through direct inoculation of the nasopharyngeal or conjunctival mucosa with infected secretions or through contact with aerosolized droplets. The structure of the RSV virion helps it evade immune defenses (**Figure 9.13**). Attachment glycoprotein (G) and small hydrophobic protein help RSV evade host defenses, making it more difficult for the body to detect the infection. Fusion glycoprotein F enables *irreversible* attachment of the virion to host

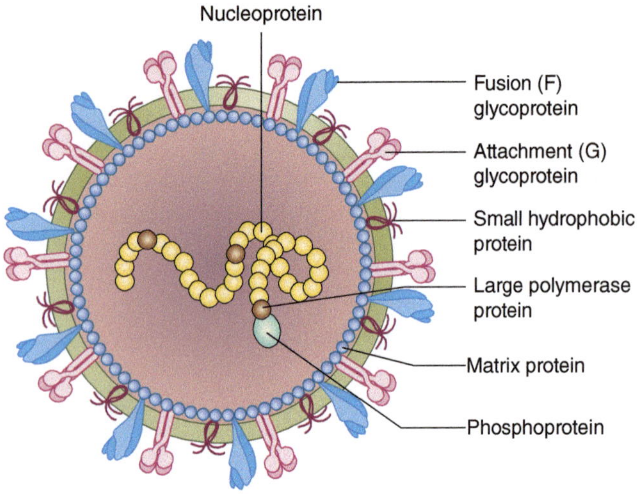

Figure 9.13 Major components of the RSV virion. RSV, respiratory syncytial virus.

cell membranes. Matrix protein assists the formation of the viral particle by offering structural support. The inner nucleoprotein encapsulates the viral RNA and facilitates replication. Phosphoprotein also assists with viral replication as well as offering additional assistance with evading host defenses. The typical incubation period is between 2 and 8 days (Kaufman et al., 2025).

Clinical Application. Prior to the release of nirsevimab, the only immunization available for RSV prevention in newborns was palivizumab. There were few and very strict qualifiers for use (e.g., fewer than 35 weeks at birth and younger than 6 months of age, with bronchopulmonary dysplasia that required treatment, and/or with hemodynamically significant congenital heart disease) and the seasonal cost for 5 monthly injections was approximately $20,000 per infant. Given that we know that most infants diagnosed with RSV are otherwise healthy infants born at term, this population was consistently left unprotected during RSV season until now. As of 2023, a new and cost-effective ($519.75 one-time injection) neutralizing monoclonal antibody achieved U.S. Food and Drug Administration (FDA) approval and is available to infants born preterm and term, who are younger than 8 months of age and entering their first RSV season. Children up to 19 months of age who remain at-risk for severe RSV may receive a second dose during their second RSV season. This vaccine, termed nirsevimab, targets glycoprotein F found on RSV cells. Nirsevimab blocks the virus from irreversibly binding to host cells by doing that very thing before the virus can act—it irreversibly binds to the viral glycoprotein F, thereby neutralizing the virus. Families who qualify for the Vaccines for Children program (VFC) can obtain this immunization completely free of charge, and most insurers eagerly cover the cost of the immunization given that it is known to reduce the risk for hospitalization for an RSV-associated lower respiratory infection by 90%. The most common side effects, which should be reviewed with parents, include pain, edema, and hardness and/or erythema at the injection site. These side effects are self-limiting, and edema/hardness/erythema is known to spontaneously resolve within 10 to 14 days of administration of the immunization.

Clinical Manifestations. Manifestations of RSV are typically nonspecific. Radiographic findings are typically consistent with a lower respiratory tract infection (LRTI)—pulmonary infiltrates, bronchiolitis (67% of all infants), and pneumonia (33% of all infants). Early symptoms of an LRTI include rhinitis and cough, which can worsen to include tachypnea, wheezing, rales, and classic grunting/flaring/retracting associated with respiratory distress (Kimberlin et al., 2024). Approximately 50% of all infants with RSV develop otitis media. Preterm infants often begin by presenting with a nonspecific feeding difficulty, irritability, or lethargy with or without apnea. Preterm infants with bronchiolitis and fever are at high risk for concomitant bacteremia (Kaufman et al., 2025).

Implications Across the Life Span. Nearly all newborns are diagnosed with RSV by the time they reach 2 years of age, and the goal of vaccination/immunization is to prevent severe RSV bronchiolitis that requires hospital admission. Among infants born at term and who are subsequently diagnosed with severe RSV bronchiolitis requiring hospitalization, the most common long-term complications are recurrent wheezing and asthma. Pulmonary function may improve as the child ages (Kaufman et al., 2025).

Human Immunodeficiency Virus. HIV is an RNA-containing retrovirus that causes AIDS. As of 2023, 39.9 million individuals across the globe were living with HIV (HIV.gov, 2024). In the United States, approximately 1.2 million people are living with HIV/AIDS, 280,000 of whom are XX pregnant patients, of which nearly 5,000 give birth annually (Abuogi et al., 2024; Fauci & Folkers, 2012; HIV.gov, 2024). Most newly diagnosed cases are contracted through heterosexual contact (Shetty & Maldonado, 2025). According to the CDC estimates in 2019, over 65% of individuals diagnosed with AIDS are of reproductive age (CDC, 2021b). In the United States, nearly 11,000 children are infected with

HIV and 88% contract the disease through birthing parent-to-child transmission (BPCT; Shetty & Maldonado, 2025).

BPCT of HIV virus can occur in utero (transplacental), during the intrapartum period, or postnatally. In utero transmission is associated with a high degree of viremia, premature prelabor rupture of membranes (PPROM), chorioamnionitis (or "Triple I" infection), and fetal swallowing of infected amniotic fluid (Shetty & Maldonado, 2025). Approximately 20% to 25% of BPCT occurs near the time of delivery or during the intrapartum period, when the vascular integrity of the placenta is disturbed and/or the infant's mucous membranes come in direct contact with cervical and vaginal tissues (Kaufman et al., 2025; Kimberlin et al., 2024; Shetty & Maldonado, 2025). Postnatal BPCT can occur through the ingestion of freshly expressed breast milk or direct breastfeeding. Globally, the risk is highest in lactating parents who are HIV positive and not treated with ART or who have not achieved viral suppression with ART (Abuogi et al., 2024). In high-income countries like the United States, ART compliance by the lactating parent or infant prophylaxis while breastfeeding reduces the risk for HIV horizontal transmission to less than 5%. Even more reassuring is that transmission risk is less than 1% in birthing parent–infant dyads with viral suppression in the birthing parent who is breastfeeding (Abuogi et al., 2024). Therefore, in 2024, the American Academy of Pediatrics (AAP) released a clinical report with revised breastfeeding guidelines in HIV-positive parents living in the United States. The AAP currently supports breastfeeding in HIV-positive birthing parents who initiated ART therapy before or early into the pregnancy; have sustained viral suppression below 50 copies per mL; are committed to compliance (and have no medication access issues) with their own ART; are committed to giving their infant prescribed antiretroviral prophylaxis; and understand the risk for transmission despite all of these measures is less than 1% (Abuogi et al., 2024).

The HIV virus works by using the enzyme *reverse transcriptase* to produce viral DNA that is then integrated into the DNA of host cells containing the surface molecule CD4+ (mostly T helper cells and macrophages; **Figure 9.14**; Weber, 2001). The early, latent phase of HIV infection is characterized by a relative absence of clinical symptoms as CD4+ T cells targeted by the infection are replenished in near equal numbers. Although the latent phase of the disease is clinically quiet, the virus is highly dynamic during this time, actively replicating in the lymph nodes and circulating CD4+ cells. As the concentration of virus in the plasma increases, the pool of CD4+ cells is depleted to a critical threshold at which point cell-mediated immunity becomes impaired (Kaufman et al., 2025; Weber, 2001). The host subsequently becomes vulnerable to pathogens that normally have a low capacity for causing disease.

Left untreated, infants with HIV experience a more rapid progression of disease than adults. HIV infection in the fetus—when T cells and NK are functionally immature—likely facilitates rapid disease progression. Fetal and neonatal immune cells may also provide a better substrate for HIV infection and replication than mature cells. As a result, HIV-infected infants often demonstrate high plasma viral loads, which is a strong predictor of disease manifestation (Kaufman et al., 2025).

Clinical Manifestations. Newborns with congenital HIV infection (perinatal transmission) are rarely symptomatic at birth and do not present with symptoms between 12 and 18 months of age as CD4+ cell counts become depleted; the exception to this involves cases of vertical transmission early in the first trimester when NK and T cells are deficient in the fetus. One of the earliest indications of HIV infection in the infant is *Pneumocystis jirovecii* pneumonia (formerly *Pneumocystis carinii*). Other hallmark signs and symptoms of HIV infection are summarized in **Table 9.12**.

Implications Across the Life Span. Without ART, the infant mortality risk in the United States is 10% to 20% (Shetty & Maldonado, 2025). With the advancements in the efficacy of antiretroviral therapy over the past two decades, HIV has become a chronic yet manageable disease. Overall, survival rates of patients with perinatal HIV infection are good (7%–11% mortality risk) if highly active antiretroviral therapy (HAART) is initiated early. Disease progression typically is faster in cases of vertical (intrauterine, intrapartum) transmission, particularly in infants of birthing parents with a high viral load. In rare circumstances, infants can acquire HIV with a blood transfusion; affected infants are typically asymptomatic for a prolonged period of time, delaying recognition of symptoms, diagnosis, and ART. Among children who do not receive HAART, viremia (greater than 100,000 copies/mL), severe immunosuppression, hepatosplenomegaly, lymphadenopathy (onset less than 3 months of age), and *P. jirovecii* pneumonia are associated with worse outcomes. In contrast, consider the life-span implications of infants exposed to HIV in utero but who remain uninfected. Despite never testing positive for HIV and receiving prophylaxis, experts report an increased risk for poor postnatal growth that slowly resolves into childhood, as well as cognitive, language, and motor deficits in childhood (Shetty & Maldonado, 2025). A single report was published associating fetal exposure to zidovudine and hypertension in infancy.

Common Sites of Infection in the Newborn

Pathogens that cause infection in the newborn may be isolated from the blood (bloodstream infection) or they may be localized in specific tissues or organ systems. **Table 9.13** lists the common sites of infection in the newborn and the organisms typically responsible.

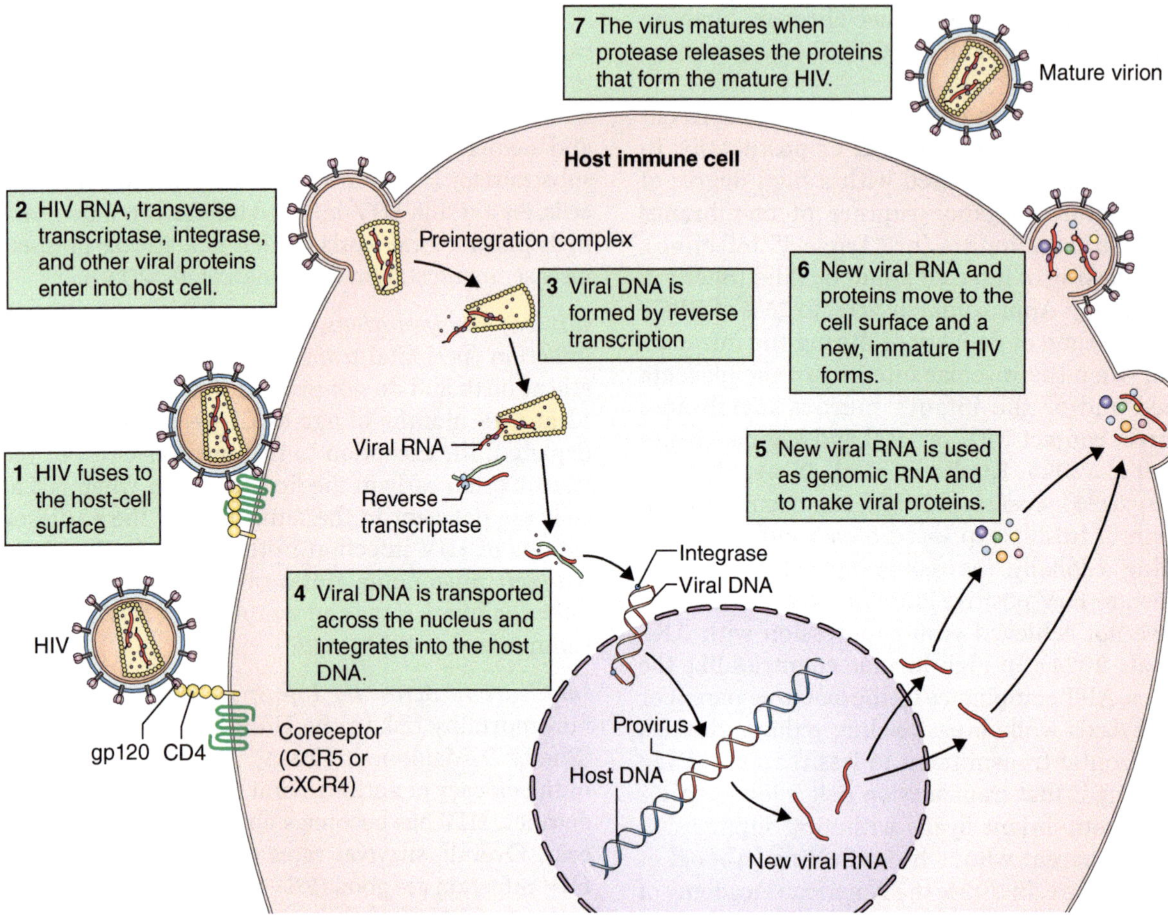

Figure 9.14 The life cycle of HIV. HIV binds to the CD4 receptor of the T cell and fuses to the cell membrane. Inside the cell, HIV uses reverse transcriptase to convert HIV RNA into HIV DNA. HIV DNA is transported into the nucleus of the CD4 cell where it uses the enzyme integrase to integrate the viral DNA into the host DNA. Once integrated into the CD4 DNA, HIV uses the machinery of the CD4 to produce viral proteins. New HIV proteins and viral proteins move to the cell surface and assemble into immature (noninfectious) HIV. The newly formed immature HIV pushes itself out of the CD4 cell and releases the enzyme protease, which breaks up the long protein chains that form the immature (noninfectious) HIV virion. The smaller HIV proteins combine to form the mature (infectious) HIV virion.

CCR5, chemokine receptor type 5; CD4, cluster of differentiation 4; CXCR4, C-X-C chemokine receptor type 4; RNA, ribonucleic acid.

TABLE 9.12 Hallmark Clinical Manifestations of HIV in Infants

Body System	Manifestations
Central nervous system	Encephalopathy, hyperreflexia, hypertonia, floppiness, unexplained fever, failure to thrive
Respiratory	Lymphoid interstitial pneumonia (*Pneumocystis jirovecii*)
Gastrointestinal	Recurrent diarrhea
Hepatic/Heme	Hepatomegaly, lymphadenopathy, splenomegaly, parotitis, recurrent bacterial infections, viral/parasitic/fungal opportunistic infections
Integumentary	Recurrent candidiasis (oral and perianal)

Note: This list is not inclusive of all manifestations.

Source: Data from Kimberlin, D. W., Banerjee, R., Barnett, E., Lynfield, R., Sawyer, M. H., & American Academy of Pediatrics Committee on Infectious Diseases. (2024). *Red book: 2024–2027 report of the Committee on Infectious Diseases* (33rd ed.). American Academy of Pediatrics.

TABLE 9.13 Common Sites of Infection in the Newborn

Site of Infection	Common Pathogens	Potential Sources	Common Clinical Manifestations	Complications
Bloodstream infection	• Early-onset: GBS, *E. coli,* Enterococci *H. influenzae, L. monocytogenes, S. aureus* • Late-onset: *Candida spp.,* CoNS, *E. coli, Enterobacter,* Enterococci, GBS, *Klebsiella,* Pseudomonas *Serratia, S. aureus*	• Early-onset: Vertical transmission from exposure to maternal genital tract • Late-onset: Horizontal transmission through exposure to contaminated objects or hands of healthcare workers/ family members	• Apnea • Hypotension • Lethargy • Respiratory distress • Temperature instability	• Death • Meningitis • Osteomyelitis • Pneumonia
Meningitis	• GBS, *E. coli, L. monocytogenes, Klebsiella,* HSV, *Candida spp.*	• Contamination during lumbar puncture • Hematogenous spread from bloodstream infection • Open neural tube defect	• Apnea • Lethargy • Respiratory distress • Seizures • Temperature instability	• Death • Hearing impairment • Neurologic impairment • Persistent seizures
Pneumonia	• C. trachomatis, *E. coli, GBS, Klebsiella, Pseudomonas, Serratia, S. aureus* • Adenovirus, enterovirus, *Candida spp.,* HSV, CMV, rhinovirus, RSV	• Aspiration of infected amniotic fluid • Aspiration of vaginal organisms • Hematogenous spread from bloodstream infection • Inhalation of aerosolized infectious particles • Prolonged endotracheal intubation	• Apnea • Respiratory distress	• Death • Respiratory failure
Urinary tract	• *Candida spp., E. coli, Enterobacter, Enterococcus, Klebsiella, S. aureus*	• Ascension of skin or intestinal flora into the urinary tract • Hematogenous spread of bloodstream infection • Indwelling urinary catheter	• Hyperbilirubinemia • Poor feeding/weight gain • Temperature instability	• Pyelonephritis • Renal scarring
Cellulitis	• *CoNS, E. coli,* Group A *Streptococcus, S. aureus*	• Invasion of skin flora to the soft tissues through a break in the skin	• Erythema • Tenderness	• Sepsis • Tissue necrosis

(continued)

TABLE 9.13 Common Sites of Infection in the Newborn (*continued*)

Site of Infection	Common Pathogens	Potential Sources	Common Clinical Manifestations	Complications
Omphalitis	• *E. coli* • Group A *Streptococcus, Klebsiella, S. aureus*	• Invasion of umbilical stump by skin or vaginal flora	• Periumbilical erythema and tenderness • Purulent drainage	• Myonecrosis • Necrotizing fasciitis • Sepsis
Osteomyelitis	• *E. coli*, GBS, Klebsiella, *S. aureus*	• Hematogenous spread from bloodstream infection • Invasive procedures • Surgical wounds • Vascular access devices	• Irritability with handling • Localized edema and tenderness	• Bony deformities • Growth plate damage
Endocarditis	• *CoNS*, GBS • *S. aureus, Streptococcus viridans*	• Bacteremia • Central venous catheters	• New murmur • Congestive heart failure	• Death • Persistent bacteremia • Septic emboli • Structural heart damage
Conjunctivitis (ophthalmia neonatorum)	• *C. trachomatis, E. coli, Klebsiella, HSV, N. gonorrhea, S. aureus*	• Exposure to infectious organisms in the maternal genital tract	• Erythema of the palpebral conjunctiva • Eyelid edema • Purulent eye drainage	• Blindness • Visual impairment

CMV, cytomegalovirus; CoNS, coagulase-negative staphylococci; GBS, Group B *Streptococcus;* HSV, herpes simplex virus; RSV, respiratory syncytial virus.

CONCLUSION

The immune system has two major arms: the innate immune system and the adaptive immune system. When confronted with a potentially infectious organism, the innate immune system—which is mediated by various phagocytic cells, cytokines, and the complement system—works quickly to neutralize and remove the threat. The adaptive immune system, on the other hand, can take days to weeks to mount an immune response, but has the added benefit of immunologic memory. Together, the innate and adaptive arms of the immune system protect the host from a range of infectious organisms, including bacteria, viruses, fungi, protozoa, and parasites.

In the fetus, immune system development begins as early as 3 weeks' gestation; however, it is not fully mature until early childhood. The neonate, therefore, is relatively immunocompromised and vulnerable to infection. Consequently, bacterial, fungal, viral, and protozoal infections are a major cause of neonatal mortality and morbidity that have significant implications across the life span. It is important that clinicians who care for neonatal patients are familiar with those organisms commonly implicated in infectious diseases of the newborn and recognize the signs and symptoms associated with infection.

LEARNING TOOLS AND RESOURCES

CourseConnect

To access self-assessment questions and interactive, competency-based learning activities for this chapter, visit www.springerpub.com/courseconnect. See inside front cover and tear-out card for CourseConnect details.

Podcast

This podcast is available online by visiting www.springerpub.com/courseconnect. See inside front cover and tear-out card for CourseConnect details.

Antibiotic Use in the NICU and the Role of the Neonatal Early-Onset Sepsis Calculator in Decreasing Antibiotic Consumption

Rani Delaney, Lauren Fraser, Maryellen Lane, and Melissa Bauserman

Discussion Prompts

1. Discuss the differences between the function and response of the innate immune system and the adaptive immune system.
2. Discuss the host factors specific to the neonatal population that make them more vulnerable to infection.
3. List some of the risk factors for EOS and LOS and the organisms commonly responsible.

MIND MAP

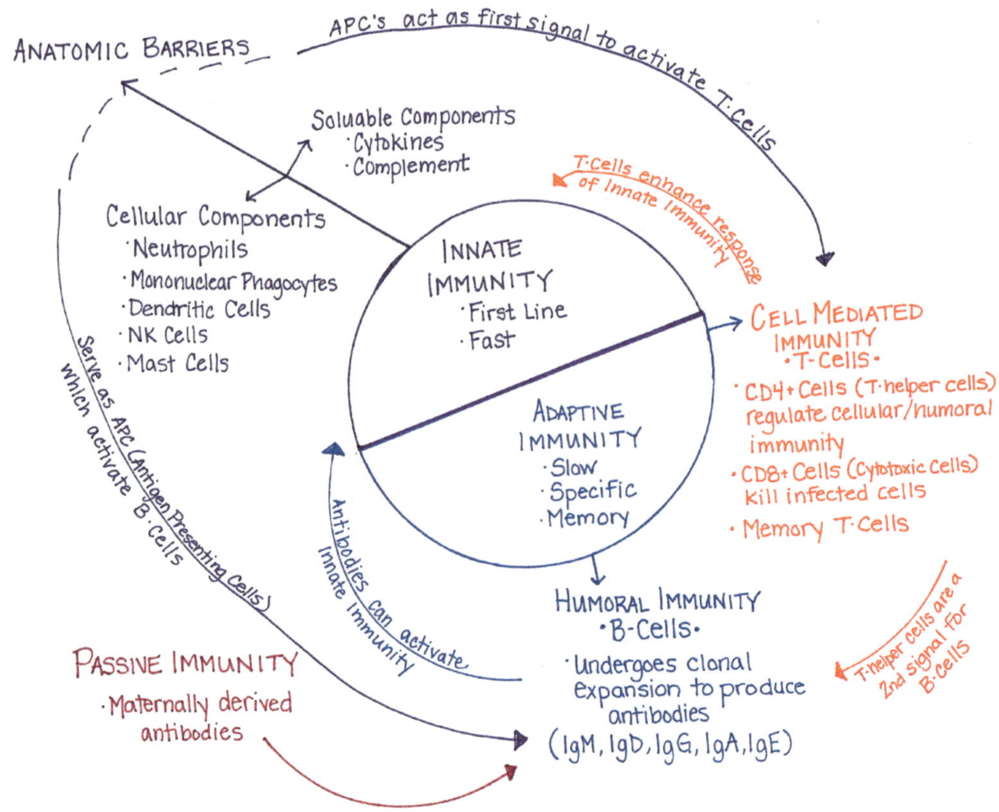

Note: This mind map reflects one physician's interpretation of a portion of one or more concepts addressed in this chapter. Readers should regard the mind maps woven throughout this textbook as examples of multisensory study tools that can be developed to encourage conceptual understanding. Readers are encouraged to develop their own unique mind maps in consultation with academic faculty or clinical preceptors.

Image Credit: *Melissa Bauserman, MD, MPH.*

TIMELINE OF ORGAN DEVELOPMENT

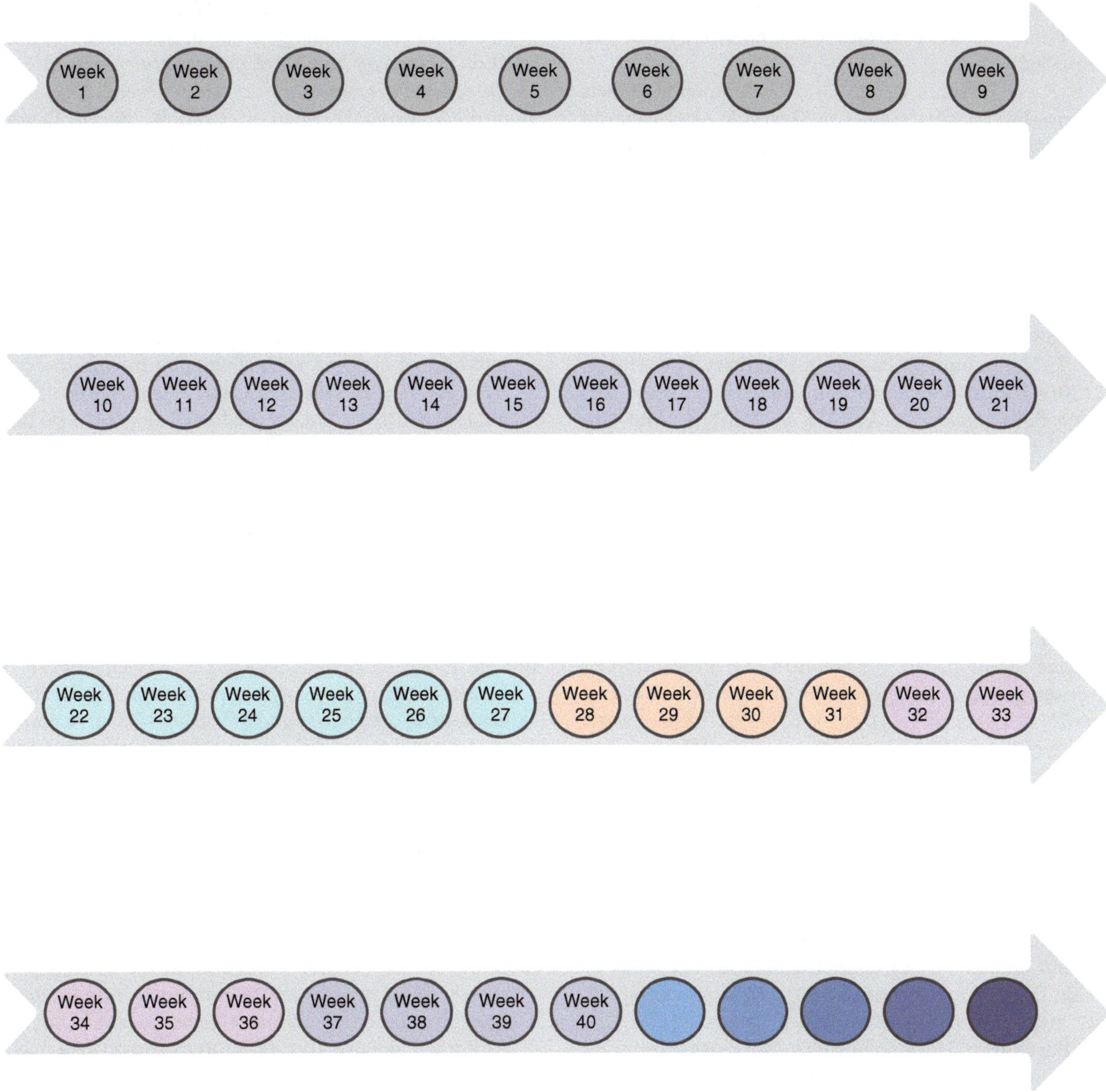

Note: Placement of common problems is meant to offer visual/conceptual perspective on the timing of onset of these commonly reported malformations. Variation exists across the literature.	***Legend:*** <22 – 27 6/7 weeks = extremely preterm 28 – 31 6/7 weeks = very preterm 32 – 36 6/7 weeks = late/moderate preterm 37 – 40 weeks = term

Note: Readers should annotate the blank timeline during studying, self-directed learning, and creation of feedback loops with mentors. To access the blank and completed timelines visit www.springerpub.com/courseconnect. See inside front cover and tear-out card for CourseConnect details.

REFERENCES

Abbas, A. K., Lichtman, A. H., & Pillai, S. (2024). *Basic immunology: Functions and disorders of the immune system* (7th ed.). Elsevier.

Abrams, S. A., & Tiosano, D. (2025). Developmental defects in the parathyroid glands. In R. J. Martin & A. A. Fanaroff (Eds.), *Fanaroff and Martin's neonatal-perinatal medicine: Diseases of the fetus and neonate* (12th ed., pp. 1691–1727). Elsevier.

Abuogi, L., Noble, L., Smith, C., and Committee on Pediatric and Adolescent HIV, Section on Breast Feeding. (2024). Infant feeding for persons living with and at risk for HIV in the United States: Clinical report. *Pediatrics, 153*(6), e2024066843. https://doi.org/10.1542/peds.2024-066843

Akinbi, H. T., Narendran, V., Pass, A. K., Markart, P., & Hoath, S. B. (2004). Host defense proteins in vernix caseosa and amniotic fluid. *American Journal of Obstetrics and Gynecology, 191*(6), 2090–2096. https://doi.org/10.1016/j.ajog.2004.05.002

American College of Obstetricians and Gynecologists. (2020). Committee Opinion, No 797. Prevention of early-onset group B Streptococcal disease in newborns. *Obstetrics & Gynecology, 135*(2), e51–e72. https://doi.org/10.1097/AOG.0000000000003668

American College of Obstetricians and Gynecologists. (2022). Committee Opinion, No 797 (reaffirmed): Prevention of early-onset group B Streptococcal disease in newborns. *Obstetrics & Gynecology, 135*(2), e51–e72. https://www.acog.org/clinical/clinical-guidance/committee-opinion/articles/2020/02/prevention-of-group-b-streptococcal-early-onset-disease-in-newborns

Barton, M., O' Brien, K., Robinson, J. L., Davies, D. H., Simpson, K., Asztalos, E., Langley, J. M., Le Saux, N., Sauve, R., Synnes, A., Tan, B., de Repentigny, L., Rubin, E., Hui, C., Kovacs, L., & Richardson, S. E. (2014). Invasive candidiasis in low birth weight preterm infants: Risk factors, clinical course and outcome in a prospective multicenter study of cases and their matched controls. *BMC Infectious Diseases, 14*, 327. https://doi.org/10.1186/1471-2334-14-327

Basha, S., Surendran, N., & Pichichero, M. (2014). Immune responses in neonates. *Expert Review of Clinical Immunology, 10*(9), 1171–1184. https://doi.org/10.1586/1744666X.2014.942288

Becker, K., Heilmann, C., & Peters, G. (2014). Coagulase-negative staphylococci. *Clinical Microbiology Reviews, 27*(4), 870–926. https://doi.org/10.1128/CMR.00109-13

Benjamin, D. K., Stoll, B. J., Fanaroff, A. A., McDonald, S. A., Oh, W., Higgins, R. D., Duara, S., Poole, K., Laptook, A., Goldberg, R., & National Institute of Child Health and Human Development Neonatal Research Network. (2006). Neonatal candidiasis among extremely low birth weight infants: Risk factors, mortality rates, and neurodevelopmental outcomes at 18 to 22 months. *Pediatrics, 117*(1), 84–92. https://doi.org/10.1542/peds.2004-2292

Benjamin, D. K., Stoll, B. J., Gantz, M. G., Walsh, M. C., Sánchez, P. J., Das, A., Shankaran, S., Higgins, R. D., Auten, K. J., Miller, N. A., Walsh, T. J., Laptook, A. R., Carlo, W. A., Kennedy, K. A., Finer, N. N., Duara, S., Schibler, K., Chapman, R. L., Van Meurs, K. P., ... Goldberg, R. N. (2010). Neonatal candidiasis: Epidemiology, risk factors, and clinical judgment. *Pediatrics, 126*(4), e865–e873. https://doi.org/10.1542/peds.2009-3412

Benjamin, J. T., Molloy, E. J., & Maheshwari, A. (2025). Development immunology. In R. J. Martin & A. A. Fanaroff (Eds.), *Fanaroff and Martin's neonatal-perinatal medicine: Diseases of the fetus and neonate* (12th ed.). Elsevier.

Berardi, A., Rossi, C., Lugli, L., Creti, R., Bacchi Reggiani, M. L., Lanari, M., Memo, L., Pedna, M. F., Venturelli, C., Perrone, E., Ciccia, M., Tridapalli, E., Piepoli, M., Contiero, R., Ferrari, F., & GBS Prevention Working Group, Emilia-Romagna. (2013). Group B *Streptococcus* late-onset disease: 2003–2010. *Pediatrics, 131*(2), e361–e368. https://doi.org/10.1542/peds.2012-1231

Berrebi, A., Assouline, C., Bessieres, M. H., Lathiere, M., Cassaing, S., Minville, V., & Ayoubi, J. M. (2010). Long-term outcome of children with congenital toxoplasmosis. *American Journal of Obstetrics and Gynecology, 203*(6), 552 e551–556. https://doi.org/10.1016/j.ajog.2010.06.002

Bousfiha, A., Jeddane, L., Picard, C., Ailal, F., Bobby Gaspar, H., Al-Herz, W., Chatila, T., Crow, Y. J., Cunningham-Rundles, C., Etzioni, A., Franco, J. L., Holland, S. M., Klein, C., Morio, T., Ochs, H. D., Oksenhendler, E., Puck, J., Tang, M. L. K., Tangye, S. G., ... Sullivan, K. E. (2018). The 2017 IUIS Phenotypic Classification for Primary Immunodeficiencies. *Journal of Clinical Immunology, 38*(1), 129–143. https://doi.org/10.1007/s10875-017-0465-8

Bowen, V., Su, J., Torrone, E., Kidd, S., & Weinstock, H. (2015). Increase in incidence of congenital syphilis—United States, 2012–2014. *Morbidity and Mortality Weekly Report, 64*(44), 1241–1245. https://doi.org/10.15585/mmwr.mm6444a3

Boyle, J. M., & Buckley, R. H. (2007). Population prevalence of diagnosed primary immunodeficiency diseases in the United States. *Journal of Clinical Immunology, 27*(5), 497–502. https://doi.org/10.1007/s10875-007-9103-1

Buckley, R. H. (2002). Primary cellular immunodeficiencies. *Journal of Allergy and Clinical Immunology, 109*(5), 747–757. https://doi.org/10.1067/mai.2002.123617

Buckley, R. H. (2011). Transplantation of hematopoietic stem cells in human severe combined immunodeficiency: Longterm outcomes. *Immunologic Research, 49*(1–3), 25–43. https://doi.org/10.1007/s12026-010-8191-9

Camacho-Gonzalez, A., Spearman, P. W., & Stoll, B. J. (2013). Neonatal infectious diseases: Evaluation of neonatal sepsis. *Pediatric Clinics of North America, 60*(2), 367–389. https://doi.org/10.1016/j.pcl.2012.12.003

Cardenas, M. C., Farnan, S., Hamel, B. L., Mejia Plazas, M. C., Sintim-Aboagye, E., Littlefield, D. R., Behl, S., Punia, S., Enninga, E. A. L., Johnson, E., Temesgen, Z., Theiler, R., Gray, C. M., & Chakraborty, R. (2023). Prevention of the vertical transmission of HIV; A recap of the journey so far. *Viruses, 15*(4), 849. https://doi.org/10.3390/v15040849

Carlson, B. M. (2024). *Human embryology and developmental biology* (7th ed.). Elsevier.

Centers for Disease Control and Prevention. (1996). Prevention of perinatal GBS disease: A public health perspective. *Morbidity and Mortality Weekly Report, 45*(RR-7), 1–24. https://www.cdc.gov/mmwr/preview/mmwrhtml/00043277.htm

Centers for Disease Control and Prevention. (2018). Prevalence of herpes simplex virus type 1 and type 2 in persons aged 14–49: United States, 2015–2016. https://www.cdc.gov/nchs/products/databriefs/db304.htm#:~:

text=The%20prevalence%20of%20HSV%2D1,and%20 40%E2%80%9349%2C%20respectively

Centers for Disease Control and Prevention. (2021a). *Genital herpes.* https://www.cdc.gov/std/treatment-guidelines /herpes.htm

Centers for Disease Control and Prevention. (2021b). *HIV surveillance report: Diagnosis of HIV infections in the United States and dependent areas, 2019.* Vol 32. https://stacks .cdc.gov/view/cdc/149036

Centers for Disease Control and Prevention. (2024a). *RSV in infants and young children.* https://www.cdc.gov/rsv/infants-young-children/?CDC_AAref_Val=https://www.cdc .gov/rsv/high-risk/infants-young-children.html

Centers for Disease Control and Prevention. (2024b). *Rubella (German measles, Three-day measles).* https://www.cdc .gov/rubella/hcp/clinical-overview/index.html

Centers for Disease Control and Prevention. (2024c). *Sexually transmitted infections (STIs).* https://www.cdc.gov/std /statistics/2022/tables/31.htm

Cooper, M. A., Pommering, T. L., & Koranyi, K. (2003). Primary immunodeficiencies. *American Family Physician, 68*(10), 2001–2008. https://www.aafp.org/afp/2003/1115 /p2001.html

Dhudasia, M. B., Benitz, W. E., Flannery, D. D., Christ, L., Rub, D., Remaschi, G., Puopolo, K. M., & Mukhopadhyay, S. (2023). Diagnostic performance and patient outcomes with C-reactive protein use in early-onset sepsis evaluations. *The Journal of Pediatrics, 256*, 98–104.e6. https://doi.org/10.1016/j .jpeds.2022.12.007

Dolapo, O., Dhanireddy, R., & Talati, A. J. (2014). Trends of *Staphylococcus aureus* bloodstream infections in a neonatal intensive care unit from 2000–2009. *BMC Pediatrics, 14*, 121. https://doi.org/10.1186/1471-2431-14-121

Dong, Y., & Speer, C. P. (2014). Late-onset neonatal sepsis: Recent developments. *Archives of Disease in Childhood—Fetal and Neonatal Edition, 100*, F257–F263. https://doi .org/10.1136/archdischild-2014-306213

Downey, L. C., Smith, P. B., & Benjamin, D. K., Jr. (2010). Risk factors and prevention of late-onset sepsis in premature infants. *Early Human Development, 86* (Suppl. 1), 7–12. https://doi .org/10.1016/j.earlhumdev.2010.01.012

Dreher, A. M., Arora, N., Fowler, K. B., Novak, Z., Britt, W. J., Boppana, S. B., & Ross, S. A. (2014). Spectrum of disease and outcome in children with symptomatic congenital cytomegalovirus infection. *Journal of Pediatrics, 164*(4), 855–859. https://doi.org/10.1016/j.jpeds.2013.12.007

Dyke, M. P., & Ott, K. (1993). Severe thrombocytopenia in extremely low birthweight infants with systemic candidiasis. *Journal of Paediatrics and Child Health, 29*(4), 298–301. https://doi.org/10.1111/j.1440-1754.1993.tb00516.x

Erdos, M., & Maródi, L. (2022). T-cell development. In R. A. Polin, S. H. Abman, D. H. Rowitch, W. E. Benitz, & W. W. Fox (Eds.), *Fetal and neonatal physiology* (6th ed., pp. 1195–1199). Elsevier.

Fattah, M. A., Omer, A. F. A., Asaif, S., Manlulu, R., Karar, T., Ahmed, A., Aljada, A., Saleh, A. M., Qureshi, S., & Nasr, A. (2017). Utility of cytokine, adhesion molecule and acute phase proteins in early diagnosis of neonatal sepsis. *Journal of Natural Science, Biology, and Medicine, 8*(1), 32–39. https://doi.org/10.4103/0976-9668.198362

Fauci, A. S., & Folkers, G. K. (2012). Toward an AIDS-free generation. *Journal of the American Medical Association, 308*(4), 343–344. https://doi.org/10.1001/jama.2012.8142

Fernandez, K. S., & de Alarcon, P. A. (2013). Development of the hematopoietic system and disorders of hematopoiesis that present during infancy and early childhood. *Pediatric Clinics of North America, 60*(6), 1273–1289. https://doi .org/10.1016/j.pcl.2013.08.002

Fey, P. D., & Olson, M. E. (2010). Current concepts in biofilm formation of *Staphylococcus epidermidis. Future Microbiology, 5*(6), 917–933. https://doi.org/10.2217/fmb.10.56

Flannery, D. D., Edwards E. M., Coggins S. A., Horbar, J. D., & Puopolo, K. M. (2022). Late-onset sepsis among very preterm infants. *Pediatrics*, 150(6), e2022058813. https:// doi.org/10.1542/peds.2022-058813

Ford, S., & Wantanabe, M. (2025). Cardiac embryology. In R. J. Martin & A. A. Fanaroff (Eds.), *Fanaroff and Martin's neonatal-perinatal medicine: Diseases of the fetus and neonate* (12th ed., pp. 1358–1371). Elsevier.

Forrest, J. M., Turnbull, F. M., Sholler, G. F., Hawker, R. E., Martin, F. J., Doran, T. T., & Burgess, M. A. (2002). Gregg's congenital rubella patients 60 years later. *Medical Journal of Australia, 177*(11–12), 664–667. https://www.mja.com. au/journal/2002/177/11/greggs-congenital-rubella-patients -60-years-later

Gauld, S. B., Dal Porto, J. M., & Cambier, J. C. (2002). B cell antigen receptor signaling: Roles in cell development and disease. *Science, 296*(5573), 1641–1642. https://doi .org/10.1126/science.1071546

Gennery, A. R. (2012). Immunological aspects of 22q11.2 deletion syndrome. *Cellular and Molecular Life Sciences, 69*(1), 17–27. https://doi.org/10.1007/s00018-011-0842-z

Glaser, M. A., Hughes, L. M., Jnah, A., & Newberry, D. (2021). Neonatal sepsis: A review of pathophysiology and current management strategies. *Advances in Neonatal Care: Official Journal of the National Association of Neonatal Nurses, 21*(1), 49–60. https://doi.org/10.1097/ANC.0000 000000000769

Gleason, C. A., & Sawyer, T. (Eds.). (2024). *Avery's diseases of the newborn* (11th ed.). Elsevier.

Gold, M. C., Robinson, T. L., Cook, M. S., Byrd, L. K., Ehlinger, H. D., Lewinsohn, D. M., & Lewinsohn, D. A. (2007). Human neonatal dendritic cells are competent in MHC Class I antigen processing and presentation. *PloS One, 2*(9), e957. https://doi .org/10.1371/journal.pone.0000957

Gordon, R. J., & Lowy, F. D. (2008). Pathogenesis of methicillin-resistant *Staphylococcus aureus* infection. *Clinical Infectious Diseases, 46*(Suppl. 5), S350–S359. https://doi .org/10.1086/533591

Grati, F. R., Molina Gomes, D., Ferreira, J. C., Dupont, C., Alesi, V., Gouas, L., Horelli-Kuitunen, N., Choy, K. W., García-Herrero, S., Gonzalez de la Vega, A., Piotrowski, K., Genesio, R., Queipo, G., Malvestiti, B., Hervé, B., Benzacken, B., Novelli, A., Vago, P., Piippo, K., ... Vialard, F. (2015). Prevalence of recurrent pathogenic microdeletions and microduplications in over 9500 pregnancies. *Prenatal Diagnosis, 35*(8), 801–809. https://doi.org/10.1002/pd.4613

Haddad, R., Guimiot, F., Six, E., Jourquin, F., Setterblad, N., Kahn, E., Yagello, M., Schiffer, C., Andre-Schmutz, I., Cavazzana-Calvo, M., Gluckman, J. C., Delezoide, A.-L., Pflumio, F., & Canque, B. (2006). Dynamics of thymus-colonizing cells during human development. *Immunity, 24*(2), 217–230. https://doi.org/10.1016/j.immuni.2006.01.008

Halasa, N., Zambrano, L. D., Amarin, J. Z., Stewart, L. S., Newhams, M. M., Levy, E. R., Shein, S. L., Carroll, C. L., Fitzgerald, J. C., Michaels, M. G., Bline, K., Cullimore, M. L., Loftis, L., Montgomery, V. L., Jeyapalan, A. S., Pannaraj, P. S., Schwarz, A. J., Cvijanovich, N. Z., Zinter, M. S., ... RSV-PIC Investigators. (2023). Infants admitted to US intensive care units for RSV infection during the 2022 seasonal peak. *JAMA Network Open, 6*(8), e2328950. https://doi.org/10.1001/jamanetworkopen.2023.28950

Haks, M. C., Oosterwegel, M. A., Blom, B., Spits, H. M., & Kruisbeek, A. M. (1999). Cell-fate decisions in early T cell development: Regulation by cytokine receptors and the pre-TCR. *Seminars in Immunology, 11*(1), 23–37. https://doi.org/10.1006/smim.1998.0153

Hamid, S., Winn, A., Parikh, R., Jones, J. M., McMorrow, M., Prill, M. M., Silk, B. J., Scobie, H. M., & Hall, A. J. (2023). Seasonality of respiratory syncytial virus—United States, 2017–2023. *MMWR. Morbidity and Mortality Weekly Report, 72*(14), 355–361. https://doi.org/10.15585/mmwr.mm7214a1

Heath, W. R., & Carbone, F. R. (2009). Dendritic cell subsets in primary and secondary T cell responses at body surfaces. *Nature Immunology, 10*(12), 1237–1244. https://doi.org/10.1038/ni.1822

Helbert, M. (2017). *Immunology for medical students* (3rd ed.). Elsevier.

HIV.gov. (2023). *Preventing perinatal transmission of HIV.* https://www.hiv.gov/hiv-basics/hiv-prevention/reducing-mother-to-child-risk/preventing-mother-to-child-transmission-of-hiv#:~:text=Taking%20HIV%20medicine%20and%20keeping,the%20risk%20is%20not%20zero.

HIV.gov. (2024). *Global statistics.* https://www.hiv.gov/hiv-basics/overview/data-and-trends/global-statistics

Immune Deficiency Foundation. (2024). *IDF SCID newborn screening campaign.* https://primaryimmune.org/resources/news-articles/scid-compass-recognized-supporting-families-through-newborn-screening

Janier, M., Hegyi, V., Dupin, N., Unemo, M., Tiplica, G. S., Potocnik, M., French, P., & Patel, R. (2014). 2014 European guideline on the management of syphilis. *Journal of the European Academy of Dermatology and Venereology, 28*(12), 1581–1593. https://doi.org/10.1111/jdv.12734

Kaufman, D. A., Nadipuram, S. M., & Manzoni, P. (2025). Fungal and protozoal infections in the neonate. In R. J. Martin & A. A. Fanaroff (Eds.), *Fanaroff and Martin's neonatal-perinatal medicine: Diseases of the fetus and neonate* (12th ed., pp. 881–916). Elsevier.

Kemper, C., Pangburn, M. K., & Fishelson, Z. (2014). Complement nomenclature 2014. *Molecular Immunology, 61*(2), 56–58. https://doi.org/10.1016/j.molimm.2014.07.004

Kimberlin, D. W., Banerjee, R., Barnett, E., Lynfield, R., Sawyer, M. H., & American Academy of Pediatrics. Committee on Infectious Diseases. (2024). *Red book: 2024–2027 report of the Committee on Infectious Diseases* (33rd ed.). American Academy of Pediatrics.

Kimberlin, D. W. (2007). Herpes simplex virus infections of the newborn. *Seminars in Perinatology, 31*(1), 19–25. https://doi.org/10.1053/j.semperi.2007.01.003

Koenig, J. M., & Keenan, W. J. (2009). Group B *Streptococcus* and early-onset sepsis in the era of maternal prophylaxis. *Pediatric Clinics of North America, 56*(3), 689–708. https://doi.org/10.1016/j.pcl.2009.04.003

Ku, L.C., Boggess K. A., & Cohen-Wolkowiez, M. (2015). Bacterial meningitis in infants. *Clinics in Perinatology, 42*, 29–45. https://doi.org/10.1016/j.clp.2014.10.004

Kuppala, V. S., Meinzen-Derr, J., Morrow, A. L., & Schibler, K. R. (2011). Prolonged initial empirical antibiotic treatment is associated with adverse outcomes in premature infants. *Journal of Pediatrics, 159*(5), 720–725. https://doi.org/10.1016/j.jpeds.2011.05.033

Kwan, A., Abraham, R. S., Currier, R., Brower, A., Andruszewski, K., Abbott, J. K., Baker, M., Ballow, M., Bartoshesky, L. E., Bonilla, F. A., Brokopp, C., Brooks, E., Caggana, M., Celestin, J., Church, J. A., Comeau, A. M., Connelly, J. A., Cowan, M. J., Cunningham-Rundles, C., ... Bonagura, V. R. (2014). Newborn screening for severe combined immunodeficiency in 11 screening programs in the United States. *Journal of the American Medical Association, 312*(7), 729–738. https://doi.org/10.1001/jama.2014.9132

Lancet HIV. (2022). The path to elimination of vertical transmission of HIV. *The Lancet HIV, 9*(2), e67. https://doi.org/10.1016/S2352-3018(22)00012-1

LeBien, T. W., & Tedder, T. F. (2008). B lymphocytes: How they develop and function. *Blood, 112*(5), 1570–1580. https://doi.org/10.1182/blood-2008-02-078071

Lee, J. Y., & Bowden, D. S. (2000). Rubella virus replication and links to teratogenicity. *Clinical Microbiology Reviews, 13*(4), 571–587. https://doi.org/10.1128/CMR.13.4.571

Lewis, D. B., Weltkamp, J.-H., & Levy, O. (2025). Developmental immunology and role of host defenses in fetal and neonatal susceptibility to infection. In Y. A. Maldonado, V. Nizet, E. D. Barnett, K. M. Edwards, R. Malley, J. S. Remington, & J. O. Klein (Eds.), *Remington and Klein's infectious diseases of the fetus and newborn infant* (9th ed., pp. 73–159). Elsevier.

Lindsay, D. S., & Dubey, J. P. (2011). *Toxoplasma gondii*: The changing paradigm of congenital toxoplasmosis. *Parasitology, 138*(14), 1829–1831. https://doi.org/10.1017/s0031182011001478

Ling, J., & Koren, G. (2016). Challenges in vaccinating infants born to mothers taking immunoglobulin biologicals during pregnancy. *Expert Review of Vaccines, 15*(2), 239–256. https://doi.org/10.1586/14760584.2016.1115351

Mahadevan, U., Martin, C. F., Sandler, R. S., Kane, S. V., Dubinsky, M., Lewis, J. D., Sandborn, W. J., & Sands, B. E. (2012). 865 PIANO: A 1000 patient prospective registry of pregnancy outcomes in women with IBD exposed to immunomodulators and biologic therapy. *Gastroenterology, 142*(5 Suppl. 1), S-149. https://doi.org/10.1016/S0016-5085(12)60561-7

Maldonado, Y. A., & Read, J. S. (2017). Diagnosis, treatment, and prevention of congenital toxoplasmosis in the United States. *Pediatrics, 139*(2). https://doi.org/10.1542/peds.2016-3860

Manzoni, P., Mostert, M., & Castagnola, E. (2015). Update on the management of *Candida* infections in preterm neonates. *Archives of Disease in Childhood: Fetal and Neonatal Edition, 100*(5), F454–F459. https://doi.org/10.1136/archdischild-2012-303350

Mayer, F. L., Wilson, D., & Hube, B. (2013). *Candida albicans* pathogenicity mechanisms. *Virulence, 4*(2), 119–128. https://doi.org/10.4161/viru.22913

McAuley, J. B. (2014). Congenital toxoplasmosis. *Journal of the Pediatric Infectious Disease Society, 3*(Suppl. 1), S30–S35. https://doi.org/10.1093/jpids/piu077

McDonald-McGinn, D. M., Sullivan, K. E., Marino, B., Philip, N., Swillen, A., Vorstman, J. A., Zackai, E. H., Emanuel, B. S., Vermeesch, J. R., Morrow, B. E., Scambler, P. J., & Bassett, A. S. (2015). 22q11.2 deletion syndrome. *Nature Review Disease Primers, 1*, 15071. https://doi.org/10.1038/nrdp.2015.71

McDonald-McGinn, D. M., Tonnesen, M. K., Laufer-Cahana, A., Finucane, B., Driscoll, D. A., Emanuel, B. S., & Zackai, E. H. (2001). Phenotype of the 22q11.2 deletion in individuals identified through an affected relative: Cast a wide FISHing net! *Genetics in Medicine, 3*(1), 23–29. https://doi.org/10.109700125817-200101000-00006

McIntosh, E. D., & Menser, M. A. (1992). A fifty-year follow-up of congenital rubella. *Lancet, 340*(8816), 414–415. https://doi.org/10.1016/ 0140-6736(92)91483-O

Medzhitov, R. (2013). Pattern recognition theory and the launch of modern innate immunity. *Journal of Immunology, 191*(9), 4473–4474. https://doi.org/10.4049/jimmunol.1302427

Melville, J. M., & Moss, T. J. (2013). The immune consequences of preterm birth. *Frontiers in Neuroscience, 7*, 79. https://doi.org/10.3389/fnins.2013.00079

Miselli, F., Creti, R., Lugli, L., & Berardi, A. (2022). Group B *Streptococcus* late-onset neonatal disease: An update in management and prevention. *Pediatric Infectious Disease Journal, 41*, e263–e266. https://doi.org/10.1097/INF.0000000000003517

Morsheimer, M., Brown Whitehorn, T. F., Heimall, J., & Sullivan, K. E. (2017). The immune deficiency of chromosome 22q11.2 deletion syndrome. *American Journal of Medical Genetics Part A, 173*(9), 2366–2372. https://doi.org/10.1002/ajmg.a.38319

Mukherjee, D., & Ryan, R. M. (2025). Postnatal bacterial infections. In R. J. Martin & A. A. Fanaroff (Eds.), *Fanaroff and Martin's neonatal-perinatal medicine: Diseases of the fetus and neonate* (12th ed., pp. 857–880). Elsevier.

Mukhopadhyay, S., & Puopolo, K. M. (2015). Neonatal early-onset sepsis: Epidemiology and risk assessment. *NeoReviews, 16*(4), e221–e230. https://doi.org/10.1542/neo.16-4-e221

Naramura, T., Tanaka, K., Inoue, T., Imamura, H., Yoshimatsu, H., Mitsubuchi, H., Nakamura, K., & Iwai, M. (2020). New reference ranges of procalcitonin excluding respiratory failure in neonates. *Pediatrics International, 62*(10), 1151–1157. https://doi.org/10.1111/ped.14282

Nesheim, S., Taylor, A., Lampe, M. A., Kilmarx, P. H., Fitz Harris, L., Whitmore, S., Griffith, J., Thomas-Proctor, M., Fenton, K., & Mermin, J. (2012). A framework for elimination of perinatal transmission of HIV in the United States. *Pediatrics, 130*(4), 738–744. https://doi.org/10.1542/peds.2012-0194

Nielsen, S. C. A., & Boyd, S. D. (2022). B cell development. In R. A. Polin, S. H. Abman, D. H. Rowitch, W. E. Benitz, & W. W. Fox (Eds.), *Fetal and neonatal physiology* (6th ed., pp. 1200–1206). Saunders.

Nielsen, S. D., Jeppesen, D. L., Kolte, L., Clark, D. R., Sørensen, T. U., Dreves, A. M., Ersbøll, A. K., Ryder, L. P., Valerius, N. H., & Nielsen, J. O. (2001). Impaired progenitor cell function in HIV-negative infants of HIV-positive mothers results in decreased thymic output and low CD4 counts. *Blood, 98*(2), 398–404. https://doi.org/10.1182/blood.V98.2.398

Ortiz-Lopez, N., Diez, M., Diaz, O., Simon, F., & Diaz, A. (2012). Epidemiological surveillance of congenital syphilis in Spain, 2000–2010. *Pediatric Infectious Disease Journal, 31*(9), 988–990. https://doi.org/10.1097/INF.0b013e31825d3152

Papayannopoulos, V., Metzler, K. D., Hakkim, A., & Zychlinsky, A. (2010). Neutrophil elastase and myeloperoxidase regulate the formation of neutrophil extracellular traps. *Journal of Cell Biology, 191*(3), 677–691. https://doi.org/10.1083/jcb.201006052

Pass, R. F., & Anderson, B. (2014). Mother-to-child transmission of cytomegalovirus and prevention of congenital infection. *Journal of the Pediatric Infectious Disease Society, 3*(Suppl. 1), S2–S6. https://doi.org/10.1093/jpids/piu069

Pateva, I., Urrutia, V. Y. H., Letterio, J., & Aguja, S. P. (2025). White blood cells and immune disorders. In R. J. Martin & A. A. Fanaroff (Eds.), *Fanaroff and Martin's neonatal-perinatal medicine: Diseases of the fetus and neonate* (12th ed., pp. 1553–1565). Elsevier.

Peakman, M., & Vergani, D. (2009). *Basic and clinical immunology* (2nd ed.). Churchill Livingstone.

Peyron, F., Garweg, J. G., Wallon, M., Descloux, E., Rolland, M., & Barth, J. (2011). Long-term impact of treated congenital toxoplasmosis on quality of life and visual performance. *Pediatric Infectious Disease Journal, 30*(7), 597–600. https://doi.org/10.1097/INF.0b013e31820bb5f3

Pfizer. (2024). *Abrysvo*. https://www.abrysvo.com

Puck, J. M., Pepper, A. E., Henthorn, P. S., Candotti, F., Isakov, J., Whitwam, T., Conley, M. E., Fischer, R. E., Rosenblatt, H. M., Small, T. N., & Buckley, R. H. (1997). Mutation analysis of IL2RG in human X-linked severe combined immunodeficiency. *Blood, 89*(6), 1968–1977. http://www .bloodjournal.org/content/bloodjournal/89/6/1968.full.pdf

Rajagopal, L. (2009). Understanding the regulation of Group B Streptococcal virulence factors. *Future Microbiology, 4*(2), 201–221. https://doi.org/10.2217/17460913.4.2.201

Ramachandran, G. (2014). Gram-positive and gram-negative bacterial toxins in sepsis: A brief review. *Virulence, 5*(1), 213–218. https://doi.org/10.4161/viru.27024

Randis, T. M., Baker, J. A., & Ratner, A. J. (2017). Group B Streptococcal infections. *Pediatrics in Review, 38*(6), 254–262. https://doi.org/10.1542/pir.2016-0127

Reef, S. E., Plotkin, S., Cordero, J. F., Katz, M., Cooper, L., Schwartz, B., Zimmerman-Swain, L., Danovaro-Holliday, M. C., & Wharton, M. (2000). Preparing for elimination of congenital rubella syndrome (CRS): Summary of a workshop on CRS elimination in the United States. *Clinical Infectious Diseases, 31*(1), 85–95. https://doi.org/10.1086/313928

Repetto, G. M., Guzman, M. L., Delgado, I., Loyola, H., Palomares, M., Lay-Son, G., Vial, C., Benavides, F., Espinoza, K., & Alvarez, P. (2014). Case fatality rate and associated factors in patients with 22q11 microdeletion syndrome: A retrospective cohort study. *BMJ Open, 4*(11), e005041. https://doi.org/10.1136/bmjopen-2014-005041

Rich, R., Fleisher, T. A., Schroeder, H. W., Jr., Weyand, C. M., Corry, D. B., & Puck, J. M. (2023). *Clinical immunology: Principles and practice* (6th ed.). Elsevier.

Ryan, A. K., Goodship, J. A., Wilson, D. I., Philip, N., Levy, A., Seidel, H., Schuffenhauer, S., Oechsler, H., Belohradsky, B., Prieur, M., Aurias, A., Raymond, F. L., Clayton-Smith, J., Hatchwell, E., McKeown, C., Beemer, F. A., Dallapiccola,

B., Novelli, G., Hurst, J. A., ... Scambler, P. J. (1997). Spectrum of clinical features associated with interstitial chromosome 22q11 deletions: A European collaborative study. *Journal of Medical Genetics*, *34*(10), 798–804. https://doi.org/10.1136/jmg.34.10.798

Salemi, T. F., McLean, V. R., & Jnah, A. J. (2024). Congenital and postnatal cytomegalovirus: Case series and state of the science for neonatal providers. *Neonatal Network*, *43*(2), 92–104. https://doi.org/10.1891/NN-2023-0069

Schoenwolf, G. C., Bleyl, S. B., Brauer, P. R., & Francis-West, P. H. (2021). Development of the pharyngeal apparatus and face. In G. C. Schoenwolf, S. B. Bleyl, P. R. Brauer, & P. H. Francis-West (Eds.), *Larsen's human embryology* (6th ed., pp. 419–462). Elsevier.

Schrag, S. J., Gorwitz, R., Fultz-Butts, K., & Schuchat, A. (2002). Prevention of perinatal Group B Streptococcal disease. *Morbidity and Mortality Weekly Report*, *51*(RR-11), 1–22. https://www.cdc.gov/mmwr/preview/mmwrhtml/rr5111a1.htm

Shane, A. L., Hansen, N. I., Stoll, B. J., Bell, E. F., Sanchez, P. J., Shankaran, S., Laptook, A. R., Das, A., Walsh, M. C., Hale, E. C., Newman, N. S., Schrag, S. J., Higgins, R. D., & Eunice Kennedy Shriver National Institute of Child Health and Human Development Neonatal Research Network. (2012). Methicillin-resistant and susceptible *Staphylococcus aureus* bacteremia and meningitis in preterm infants. *Pediatrics*, *129*(4), e914–e922. https://doi.org/10.1542/peds.2011-0966

Sherman, M. P. (2010). New concepts of microbial translocation in the neonatal intestine: Mechanisms and prevention. *Clinics in Perinatology*, *37*(3), 565–579. https://doi.org/10.1016/j .clp.2010.05.006

Shetty, A. K., & Maldonado, Y. A. (2025). Human immunodeficiency virus/acquired immunodeficiency syndrome in the infant. In Y. A. Maldonado, V. Nizet, E. D. Barnett, K. M. Edwards, R. Mally, J. S. Remington, & J. O. Klein (Eds.), *Remington and Klein's infectious diseases of the fetus and newborn infant* (9th ed.). Saunders/Elsevier.

Simonsen, K. A., Anderson-Berry, A. L., Delair, S. F., & Davies, H. D. (2014). Early-onset neonatal sepsis. *Clinical Microbiology Reviews*, *27*(1), 21–47. https://doi.org/10.1128/cmr.00031-13

Stavnezer, J., Guikema, J. E. J., & Schrader, C. E. (2008). Mechanism and regulation of class switch recombination. *Annual Review of Immunology*, *26*, 261–292. https://doi.org/10.1146/annurev.immunol.26.021607.090248

Stenutz, R., Weintraub, A., & Widmalm, G. (2006). The structures of *Escherichia coli* O-polysaccharide antigens. *FEMS Microbiology Reviews*, *30*(3), 382–403. https://doi.org/10.1111/j.1574-6976.2006.00016.x

Stocker, M., van Herk, W., el Helou, S., Dutta, S., Fontana, M. S., Schuerman, F. A. B. A., van den Tooren-de Groot, R. K., Wieringa, J. W., Janota, J., van der Meer-Kappelle, L. H., Moonen, R., Sie, S. D., de Vries, E., Donker, A. E., Zimmerman, U., Schlapbach, L. J., de Mol, A. C., Hoffman-Haringsma, A., Roy, M., . . . NeoPInS Study Group. (2017). Procalcitonin-guided decision making for duration of antibiotic therapy in neonates with suspected early-onset sepsis: A multicentre, randomised controlled trial (NeoPIns). *The Lancet (British Edition)*, *390*(10097), 871–881. https://doi.org/10.1016/S0140-6736(17)31444-7

Stoll, B. J., Puopolo, K. M., Hansen, N. I., Sánchez, P. J., Bell, E. F., Carlo, W. A., Cotten, C. M., D'Angio, C. T., Kazzi, S. N. J., Poindexter, B. B., Van Meurs, K. P., Hale, E. C., Collins, M. V., Das, A., Baker, C. J., Wyckoff, M. H., Yoder, B. A., Watterberg, K. L., Walsh, M. C., ... Eunice Kennedy Shriver National Institute of Child Health and Human Development Neonatal Research Network. (2020). Early-onset sepsis 2015 to 2017, the rise of *Escherichia coli*, and the need for novel prevention strategies. *JAMA Pediatrics*, *174*(7), e200593. https://doi.org/ 10.1001/jamapediatrics.2020.0593

Sugitharini, V., Prema, A., & Berla Thangam, E. (2013). Inflammatory mediators of systemic inflammation in neonatal sepsis. *Inflammation Research*, *62*(12), 1025–1034. https://doi.org/10.1007/s00011-013-0661-9

Swanson, E. C., & Schleiss, M. R. (2013). Congenital cytomegalovirus infection: New prospects for prevention and therapy. *Pediatric Clinics of North America*, *60*(2), 335–349. https://doi.org/10.1016/j.pcl.2012.12.008

Swanson, J. A. (2013). *Macrophage phagocytosis* [electronic resource]. Henry Stewart Talks.

Tangye, S. G., Avery, D. T., Deenick, E. K., & Hodgkin, P. D. (2003). Intrinsic differences in the proliferation of naive and memory human B cells as a mechanism for enhanced secondary immune responses. *Journal of Immunology*, *170*(2), 686–694. https://doi.org/10.4049/jimmunol.170.2.686

Tobin, N. H., & Aldrovandi, G. M. (2013). Immunology of pediatric HIV infection. *Immunology Reviews*, *254*(1), 143–169. https://doi.org/10.1111/imr.12074

Tong, S. Y., Davis, J. S., Eichenberger, E., Holland, T. L., & Fowler, V. G., Jr. (2015). *Staphylococcus aureus* infections: Epidemiology, pathophysiology, clinical manifestations, and management. *Clinical Microbiology Reviews*, *28*(3), 603–661. https://doi.org/10.1128/CMR.00134-14

UNICEF. (2024). *Progress in reducing new HIV infections among children has stagnated in recent years*. https://data.unicef.org/topic/hivaids/emtct/#status

van Zuylen, W. J., Hamilton, S. T., Naing, Z., Hall, B., Shand, A., & Rawlinson, W. D. (2014). Congenital cytomegalovirus infection: Clinical presentation, epidemiology, diagnosis and prevention. *Obstetric Medicine*, *7*(4), 140–146. https://doi.org/10.1177/ 1753495X14552719

Walport, M. J. (2001a). Complement. First of two parts. *New England Journal of Medicine*, *344*(14), 1058–1066. https://doi.org/10.1056/NEJM200104053441406

Walport, M. J. (2001b). Complement. Second of two parts. *New England Journal of Medicine*, *344*(15), 1140–1144. https://doi.org/10.1056/NEJM200104123441506

Wapner, R. J., Martin, C. L., Levy, B., Ballif, B. C., Eng, C. M., Zachary, J. M., Savage, M., Platt, L. D., Saltzman, D., Grobman, W. A., Klugman, S., Scholl, T., Simpson, J. L., McCall, K., Aggarwal, V. S., Bunke, B., Nahum, O., Patel, A., Lamb, A. N., , ... Jackson, L. (2012). Chromosomal microarray versus karyotyping for prenatal diagnosis. *New England Journal of Medicine*, *367*(23), 2175–2184. https://doi.org/10.1056/NEJMoa1203382

Weber, J. (2001). The pathogenesis of HIV-1 infection. *British Medical Bulletin*, *58*(1), 61–72. https://doi.org/10.1093/bmb/58.1.61

Wilson, C. B., Remington, J. S., Stagno, S., & Reynolds, D. W. (1980). Development of adverse sequelae in children born with subclinical congenital toxoplasma infection. *Pediatrics*, *66*(5), 767–774. https://journals.lww.com

/obgynsurvey/Fulltext/1981/08000/Development_of_Adverse_Sequelae_in_Children_Born.13.aspx

Wynn, J. L., & Levy, O. (2010). Role of innate host defenses in susceptibility to early onset neonatal sepsis. *Clinics in Perinatology, 37*(2), 307–337. https://doi.org/10.1016/j.clp.2010.04.001

Zilow, G., Zilow, E. P., Burger, R., & Linderkamp, O. (1993). Complement activation in newborn infants with early onset infection. *Pediatric Research, 34*(2), 199–203. https://doi.org/10 .1203/00006450-199308000-00020

Zuppa, A. A., Riccardi, R., Frezza, S., Gallini, F., Luciano, R. M., Alighieri, G., Romagnoli, C., & De Carolis, S. (2017). Neonatal lupus: Follow-up in infants with anti-SSA/Ro antibodies and review of the literature. *Autoimmunity Reviews, 16*(4), 427–432. https://doi.org/10.1016/j.autrev.2017.02.010

10

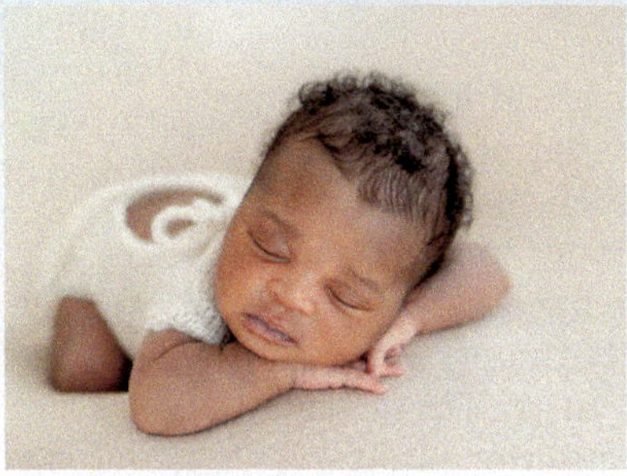

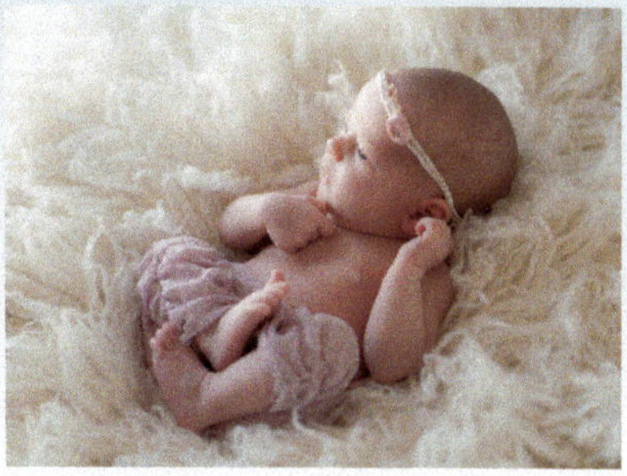

THE METABOLIC AND ENDOCRINE SYSTEM

Jacqui Hoffman, Jennifer Fitzgerald, and Amy J. Jnah

LEARNING OBJECTIVES

After completing this chapter, the reader should be able to:

- Understand normal metabolic and endocrine organ development.
- Describe the effects of hormones produced by metabolic and endocrine organs.
- Discuss common inherited disorders and their effect on fetal and neonatal metabolic and endocrine system development and function.
- Identify health issues in XX pregnant patients that have a potential impact on fetal and postnatal metabolic and endocrine system development and function.
- Evaluate common disorders that affect the metabolic and endocrine system and their implications across the life span.

INTRODUCTION

The human endocrine system is an intricately connected aggregate of glands located throughout the human body. Endocrine glands produce various hormones which regulate human physiology. In fact, the word *hormone* originates from the Greek term *impetus*, or to arouse activity. These hormones, when synthesized and secreted into the bloodstream, bind with target receptors and elicit cellular responses within a target organ. Normal endocrine function is critical for proper physical growth and development, metabolism, fluid and electrolyte homeostasis, stress responses, and reproductive and immune development.

This chapter addresses the hypothalamus as well as the pituitary, adrenal, thyroid, pancreas, pineal, and parathyroid glands. The embryologic development of each gland is summarized and followed by a discussion of the function of each gland. Critical processes, including calcium-magnesium homeostasis and carbohydrate metabolism, are explored. In addition, we present a discussion of glucose metabolism focused to the special populations which align with neonatal intensive care nursing. A discussion of genetic and other maternal health influences, including inherited inborn errors of metabolism, will be identified and discussed. Finally, we present a discussion of common metabolic disorders, their pathogenesis, key clinical manifestations, and lifespan implications. Our intent is to take this perceivably dense content and present it in a clear, concise and multisensory manner for the benefit of neonatal APRN (advanced practice registered nurse) students.

TIMELINE OF ORGAN DEVELOPMENT

The metabolic and endocrine system is a complex network of endocrine glands. The "master glands" include the hypothalamus and pituitary glands. These glands communicate with classical glands, which include the anterior pituitary, thyroid, parathyroids, adrenals, gonads, and pancreas. We begin the chapter with an overview of normal embryologic development of the master and classical endocrine glands.

Hypothalamus

The mature hypothalamus, a master gland located directly above the brainstem, is comprised of a complex collection of nuclei and neurons which modulate homeostasis and hormone synthesis. Under the influence of clusters of neurons which regulate hypothalamic activity, the hypothalamus can secrete hormones into the hypophyseal portal system (**Figure 10.1**). These hormones travel to target glands (e.g., anterior pituitary) and elicit stimulating or inhibiting effects. Stimulating hormones (e.g., growth hormone [GH]-releasing hormone [GHRH]) prompt the anterior pituitary gland to synthesize and secrete hormones in order to correct an imbalance and establish homeostasis. Inhibitory hormones (e.g., dopamine) inhibit further synthesis and secretion of target hormones (e.g., thyroid-stimulating hormone [TSH], prolactin) from the anterior pituitary, to maintain homeostasis.

Embryonic Period. The hypothalamus begins to develop during week 5 of gestation, as the ventral portion of the diencephalon (brain) forms. This gives rise to both the hypothalamus and thalamus. By week 6 of gestation, hypothalamic-releasing hormones, many of which travel through the hypophyseal portal system and to the anterior pituitary, are detected in the systemic circulation (Melmed et al., 2025).

Fetal Period. Maturation of the differentiating structures of the hypothalamus continues from weeks 9 through 14 of gestation. Next, by approximately week 18 of gestation, the hypophyseal portal system, a network of vessels that deliver hypothalamic-releasing neuropeptides to the anterior pituitary, is fully developed. This development gives rise to the future hypothalamic–pituitary–end organ axis (Koutcherov et al., 2002; Melmed et al., 2025).

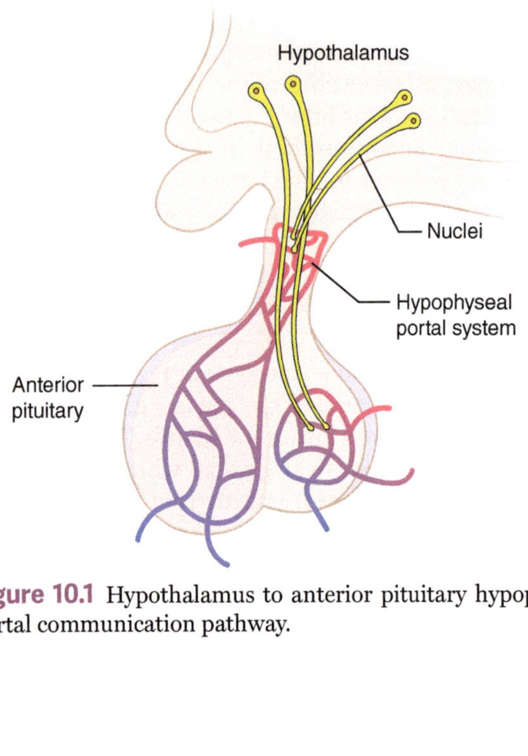

Figure 10.1 Hypothalamus to anterior pituitary hypophyseal portal communication pathway.

Pituitary Gland

The pituitary gland, once mature, is situated just below the hypothalamus at the base of the skull. This gland is comprised of two lobes: an anterior and posterior lobe. The anterior lobe is capable of synthesizing hormones including adrenocorticotropic hormone (ACTH), GH, prolactin, TSH, and luteinizing hormone (LH). These hormones are synthesized when the corresponding hypothalamus-produced stimulating hormone travels through the hypophyseal portal venous system (humoral system) and stimulates specific activity in the anterior pituitary gland. For example, GH-releasing hormone can be released from the hypothalamus, travel through the hypophyseal portal system to the anterior pituitary, and specifically trigger the synthesis of GH. In contrast, the posterior lobe of the pituitary gland is a repository for hormones (e.g., antidiuretic hormone [ADH], oxytocin) that are synthesized by neurons in the hypothalamus. Once produced in the hypothalamus, these hormones travel down nerve fibers (axons) to the posterior pituitary for storage and later secretion into the circulation when stimulated to do so.

Embryonic Period. The pituitary gland begins to develop during week 4 of gestation. First, a fingerlike protrusion ("Rathke's pouch") extends dorsally from the ectoderm and grows in an outward direction, heading toward the diencephalon (brain; S. A. Kaiser & Ho, 2025). This is the early adenohypophysis and future anterior pituitary gland. During week 7 of gestation, a similarly shaped fingerlike protrusion extends ventrally from the ectoderm and grows in an outward direction, heading toward the roof of the mouth. The ventral extension proliferates into the posterior pituitary gland. Evolution of the pituitary gland continues through week 8 of gestation. Shortly thereafter, the anterior walls of both glands merge in tight apposition to one another. Despite this anatomic connection, both glands remain separate, unique structures with differentiated responsibilities.

Fetal Period. Between weeks 9 and 10 of gestation, the anterior pituitary is synthesizing GH, ACTH, TSH, follicle-stimulating hormone (FSH), prolactin, and LH. Oxytocin and vasopressin (ADH) secretion, via the posterior pituitary, can occur by week 10 of gestation (Christ-Crain et al., 2025; Divall & Merjaneh, 2024). By week 16, the pituitary is considered fully formed. As mentioned earlier, by week 18 of gestation, the hypophyseal portal vascular system links the hypothalamus to the pituitary gland. This connection is essential for the hypothalamic–pituitary–adrenal (HPA) interface and is relatively mature by week 20 of gestation (S. A. Kaiser & Ho, 2025). GH levels peak between weeks 20 to 24 of gestation, with a steady decline thereafter (Katugampola et al., 2025).

Adrenal Glands

The adrenal glands are located atop the kidneys and are typically regarded as "fight or flight" glands. Under the direction of the anterior pituitary, the adrenals secrete hormones (e.g., cortisol, aldosterone, androgens) which, during periods of stress (e.g., hypotension, shock, sepsis), seek to assist with maintaining or reestablishing physiologic homeostasis.

Embryonic Period. The adrenal glands (suprarenal glands) arise from a region of intermediate mesoderm adjacent to the kidneys. The adrenal cortex and medulla arise between weeks 5 and 6 of gestation. Beginning with week 5, the outer portion of the adrenal gland epithelium forms the adrenal cortex. The adrenal medulla then forms from a chain of interconnected ganglia that lie both laterally and parallel to the spinal vertebrae extending from the base of the skull to the sacrum. Cortisol synthesis from placental progesterone is evident by the end of week 8 of gestation. The fetal adrenal glands begin producing cortisol at week 10 of gestation and cortisol levels begin to increase around weeks 30 to 32 of gestation (Watterberg, 2006).

Clinical Application. Cortisol levels at birth vary based upon fetal exposure to antepartum or intrapartum corticosteroids and chorioamnionitis, postnatal respiratory distress syndrome, the need for mechanical ventilatory support, postnatal corticosteroid exposure, and time of day. Hospitalized infants (most commonly preterm infants) exposed to several days (usually more than 7 days) of hydrocortisone for profound hypotension or dexamethasone for chronic lung disease management may develop secondary adrenal insufficiency (AI) and require cosyntropin (ACTH) stimulation testing later into the hospitalization. This is most accurate if completed 4 to 6 weeks after the last dose of steroids is administered. In the interim, if an infant requires a surgical procedure before this testing is completed or becomes profoundly ill, prophylactic stress dose hydrocortisone may be required.

Fetal Period. Prior to the third month of gestation, the adrenal gland develops into three distinct zones: the (a) permanent or definitive zone (outer mass of cells) that secretes mineralocorticoids, (b) transient fetal zone (inner mass of cells) that regresses, and the (c) transitional zone that secretes cortisol and androgens (Divall & Merjaneh, 2024; Holmstrom & Jnah, 2021). By midgestation, the adrenal cortex accounts for 80% to 90% of the mass of the gland (Divall & Merjaneh, 2024). The HPA axis is considered formed by week 20 of gestation (Divall & Merjaneh, 2024). Mineralocorticoids are synthesized after 22 weeks of gestation, with glucocorticoid synthesis evident between 25 to 30 weeks of gestation. Migration of neural cells into the adrenal medulla continues until birth (Quintos & Boney, 2010).

Clinical Application. Cortisol is a steroid endogenously synthesized at the adrenal cortex; when production is normal, cortisol can help modulate inflammatory responses and optimize vascular responsiveness. Cortisol deficiency is associated with bronchopulmonary dysplasia and sepsis, as well as a higher risk for death. Preterm infants born before weeks 30 to 32 of gestation are often cortisol deficient, and this is due to AI (immaturity of the adrenal glands at birth). Recent studies have indicated that early use of prophylactic hydrocortisone can mitigate inflammatory responses in preterm infants and reduce the risk for bronchopulmonary dysplasia. Risks associated with hydrocortisone use include spontaneous intestinal perforation, hyperglycemia, necrotizing enterocolitis (NEC), and death.

For more information: Shah, S. D., Shukla, S., Nandula, P. S., Vice, S., Elgendy, M., Gautam, S., Hudak, M. L., & Cortez, J. (2024). Prophylactic early low-dose hydrocortisone and survival without bronchopulmonary dysplasia among extremely preterm infants born at 22–27 weeks' gestation. *Journal of Perinatology, 44*(7), 947–952. https://doi.org/10.1038/s41372-024-01923-5

Thyroid Gland

The thyroid gland is the first endocrine organ to develop and is regarded as one of the larger (if not the largest) endocrine glands. Under the influence of the anterior pituitary gland, this gland releases thyroid hormones, which increase the basal metabolic rate (Kim et al., 2024; Salvatore et al., 2025).

Embryonic Period. Thyroid development begins during week 3 of gestation (Kim et al., 2024). The embryonic thyroid develops from the third and fourth branchial pouch, appearing as an outgrowth at the floor of the primitive buccal cavity (the future site of the mouth and pharynx). Early synthesis of thyroglobulin (thyroid hormone precursor) is evident by the end of week 4 of gestation. Shortly thereafter, the gland descends to a position anterior to the hyoid bone and larynx cartilage (voice box). An isthmus develops and connects the two lateral lobes, measuring approximately 2 inches in length. Evolution of the thyroid gland continues through week 8. At this time, the thyroid exhibits its definitive external form and begins secreting thyroid hormone. Beginning with week 9, iodine absorption is noted.

Fetal Period. By week 13 of gestation, follicular cells secrete thyroid hormones (TSH, T_3, and T_4). Parafollicular cells (C cells) secrete calcitonin by the 16th week. Beginning with week 34 of gestation, total thyroid receptors mature and autoregulation of iodine begins (Katugampola et al., 2025).

Clinical Application. Preterm infants are unable to generate a shivering response at birth (and usually not until 6 months of life), so they must utilize other methods to generate heat. This requires metabolic heat production, and the thyroid gland assists with this process. Consider that the extrauterine environment is colder than the intrauterine environment. This is "shocking" to a newborn, and in response to the cold temperature, the hypothalamus releases thyrotropin-releasing hormone (TRH) into the hypophyseal portal system. Once TRH reaches the anterior pituitary, it stimulates the synthesis of TSH, which causes an overall surge in TSH production in the hours after birth. The extra synthesis of TSH stimulates the thyroid gland to produce thyroxine (T_4) and triiodothyronine (T_3). The T_3 hormones act directly on uncoupling proteins (thermogenin) in brown fat and induce heat production through oxidative mechanisms!

Pancreas

The pancreas resides within the upper left quadrant of the abdomen, behind the stomach. Its function, as an exocrine gland, is to secrete digestive enzymes. The pancreatic islets (islets of Langerhans) secrete glucagon, insulin, somatostatin, and pancreatic polypeptide (Divall & Merjaneh, 2024). As such, the pancreas holds an important role in glucose metabolism.

Embryonic Period. Outgrowths of the duodenum form the ventral and dorsal pancreatic buds, which, in turn, eventually join together to form the adult pancreas. Weeks 4 through 6 of development involve the rotation of the ventral pancreas to the right and invagination of the common bile duct. By week 7, pancreatic hormone secretion is evident and increasing (Cowett, 2012; Divall & Merjaneh, 2024).

Fetal Period. Week 10 of gestation involves rotation of the dorsal and ventral pancreatic buds. The buds thereby fuse and form the pancreas (mostly derived from the larger dorsal pancreatic bud), a flat gland measuring 6 inches long, located between the stomach and spine and connected to the duodenum. Islets of Langerhans bud from the pancreatic duct system, forming clusters of endocrine cells: alpha, then beta, then delta. Insulin secretion thereby begins at approximately 10 weeks, and glucagon is detectable in the fetal plasma by week 15 of gestation. Pancreatic abnormalities, although rare, include failed regression of the left ventral bud and fusion of the bifid ventral bud with the dorsal pancreatic bud. This forms a pancreatic ring, also known as an annular pancreas, which leads to strangulation of the descending portion of the duodenum (Persaud & Torchia, 2025).

Pineal Gland

Posterior to the thalamus is the pineal gland. This gland is responsible for the synthesis and secretion of melatonin, which is understood to occur on a circadian cycle, with darkness the most important signal at which time levels are highest (Lechan, 2025).

Embryonic Period. During weeks 5 and 6 of development, the pineal body forms at the roof of the posterior part of the forebrain. Cellular migration, invagination, and midline epithelial thickening occur during week 7, which gives rise to the gland's distinct anterior lobe. The most caudal part of the roof plate develops into the pineal body or epiphysis (Macchi & Bruce, 2004). Once fully formed, the pineal gland nestles between the two hemispheres of the brain, where the thalami join.

Fetal Period. The pineal gland matures throughout fetal development and into early childhood (age 2). Melatonin synthesis and secretion begins after birth. Among infants born at term, rhythmicity (circadian rhythm) is observed approximately 8 to 12 weeks after birth. Synthesis, secretion, and rhythmicity are often delayed among infants born prematurely (Ferber et al., 2011; Melmed et al., 2025).

Parathyroid Gland

The parathyroid gland is a compilation of four smaller glands which reside posterior to the thyroid gland. Most notably, the parathyroid gland secretes parathyroid hormone (PTH), which facilitates the synthesis and secretion of active vitamin D (1, 25-dihydroxyvitamin D). In addition, the parathyroid gland regulates calcium and phosphorus homeostasis (Katugampola et al., 2025).

Embryonic Period. The parathyroid glands originate from the endoderm of the third and fourth pharyngeal pouches, typically during week 3 of development. The inferior parathyroid glands arise from the third pharyngeal pouch and migrate with the thymus. Separation of the inferior glands occurs just prior to reaching their final anatomic position, at the level of the inferior pole of each thyroid lobe. The superior parathyroid glands arise from the fourth pharyngeal pouch and take their final position along the posterior part of the middle third of each thyroid lobe. Glandular development continues through week 8 of gestation. During this time the inferior parathyroid glands begin producing PTH (Katugampola et al., 2025).

Fetal Period. The parathyroids are mature and physiologically active by week 14 of gestation. Parathyroid abnormalities, such as congenital hypoparathyroidism, are commonly associated with inherited diseases or syndromes, such as DiGeorge syndrome (22q11.2 deletion; Katugampola et al., 2025).

ENDOCRINE SIGNALING

The endocrine system communicates by way of chemical signaling. Signaling cells synthesize and secrete ligands (hormones) into the bloodstream. The circulation carries these hormones to target hormone receptors. Hormones bind with select receptors and a cellular response is observed. Endocrine signaling is primarily modulated by negative feedback loops, which are essential to maintain homeostasis. After all, endocrine function modulates fetal and postnatal growth and development, metabolism, and reproductive development and function, as well as responses to stress and/or injury. In order to better understand how hormones effect body function, and apply that knowledge in clinical practice, a brief discussion of the key components of endocrine signaling, namely hormone receptors, regulation, and negative feedback, is provided.

Hormone Receptors

The process by which hormones are released into the circulation, travel long distances, reach target cells within the body, and elicit cellular responses is known as endocrine signaling. For this to occur, hormones and hormone receptors must be present. Hormones are either water-soluble or fat-soluble. Water-soluble hormones (peptide hormones) cannot permeate the cell membrane and are therefore limited to binding with receptors at the surface of the target cell. Alternatively, fat-soluble hormones (steroid hormones) can penetrate the cell membrane and bind with receptors inside the cell. Likewise, hormone receptors are proteins that either reside within or on the surface of human cells and exhibit an affinity to one or more circulating hormones. Intracellular hormone receptors have an affinity for the fat-soluble hormones (e.g. testosterone), lie within the cell, and regulate gene transcription. Surface hormone receptors have an affinity for water-soluble peptide hormones (e.g. insulin), lie on the surface of the cell, and regulate enzymatic activity. The binding of a hormone to a receptor yields a hormone-receptor complex. These complexes elicit immediate or delayed biological responses; APRNs must recognize that small changes in circulating hormone concentrations can yield a significant (and potentially untoward) effect on the fetus and newborn.

Endocrine signaling can be studied as a stepwise sequence of events. First, a hormone is synthesized and released into the circulation. The circulation "carries" the hormone to a target cell. As the hormone approaches the cell it binds with a target surface or intracellular hormone receptor. This elicits a biological response. Therefore, the relationship between hormones and hormone receptors can be compared to a "lock and key" mechanism. In other words, the affinity of a hormone receptor to a particular hormone draws it near. Once the hormone contacts the receptor, it "locks" with the receptor. When this occurs, the hormone undergoes a conformational change and a cellular response (e.g., metabolic activity) is observed.

Hormone Regulation

Several factors contribute to hormone regulation by increasing, decreasing, or normalizing hormone levels. These factors include (a) blood flow patterns/velocity, (b) rate of metabolism and excretion (of circulating hormones), and (c) feedback loops. Blood flow patterns implicate the rate (or speed) of transport of a hormone to its target organ. The rate at which a hormone is metabolized and excreted from the body affects further synthesis and secretion of additional hormones. Collectively, these factors implicate the negative feedback system.

Negative Feedback

Collectively, the aforementioned components of endocrine signaling implicate the negative feedback system, the primary mechanism by which hormone levels are regulated (**Figure 10.2**). Negative feedback describes a process in which the output of a pathway inhibits the input of a pathway. In other words, as the serum-circulating concentration of a target hormone or output of a feedback loop approaches the upper acceptable limit, a negative message is transmitted to inhibit further release of precursors that encourage the synthesis and secretion of that hormone.

For example, consider the synthesis and secretion of GH. Low-circulating GH alerts the hypothalamus to release GHRH. GHRH travels to the anterior pituitary gland and stimulates the synthesis and secretion of GH. GH, the desirable "end hormone" in this pathway, is released into the circulation. It stimulates

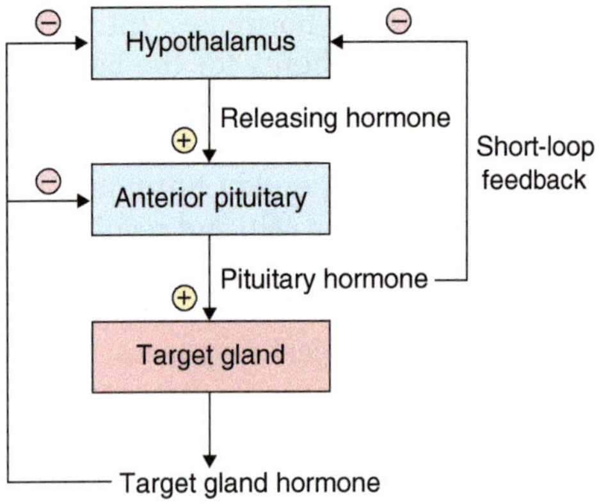

Figure 10.2 The negative feedback loop.

adipose cells to break down stored fat and release free fatty acids to fuel growth. GH also stimulates an increase in amino acid uptake from the circulation, glycogenolysis, and hepatic release of insulinlike growth factor (IGF-1) into the circulation. In aggregate, this encourages the proliferation of bone cells, muscle cells, nervous system cells, and immune cells. However, once IGF-1 levels reach the upper acceptable limit, GHRH secretion stops. In exchange, the hypothalamus secretes GH inhibiting hormone (GHIH). GHIH (also known as somatostatin) inhibits the release of GH and stops the feedback loop. Thyroid hormone and cortisol are also regulated by negative feedback and are discussed later in this chapter.

Clinical Application. The hypothalamus is critical to establishing and maintaining homeostasis with metabolic and endocrine processes, appetite, emotions, and behavior. Among newborns with Prader-Willi syndrome, neurons located within the hypothalamus cannot synthesize adequate prohormones, including pro-GHRH. This leads to deficient production of GH by the pituitary gland and contributes to the characteristic features of Prader-Willi syndrome (e.g., hypotonia, altered body composition, short stature). During fetal development, intrauterine growth restriction (IUGR) is commonly identified. After birth, newborns typically present with hypotonia and feeding difficulties which can progress to failure to thrive if not recognized and treated. With appropriate interventions and nutritional support, infants tend to grow appropriately until age 2, when excessive weight gain sets in despite relatively normal eating habits. Increased fat mass and decreased lean body mass is observed. Between ages 4 and 6, children begin to manifest with hyperphagia, food seeking behaviors, and a lack of satiety after eating meals, which can extend into adulthood. GH replacement initiated within the first year of life (between 3–12 months of age) has been shown to optimize body composition and basal metabolic index, cognition, motor function, height, and head circumference, as well as social-cognitive function.

ENDOCRINE HORMONE CLASSES

Several classes of hormones are produced within the human body and include peptides, polypeptides, proteins, amines, and steroids. These hormone classes differ based on their cell-specific distribution, the type of receptors they bind to, their cellular permeability, and the resultant cellular response.

Peptide, Polypeptide, and Protein Hormones

Most hormones found within the human body are made from peptides and proteins—linked chains of amino acids. These chains range from short (e.g., vasopressin) to long, 200-link chains (Holt et al., 2021). More specific, the short chain amino acids are the peptide hormones, whereas the polypeptide or protein hormones exemplify the longer chains. Both are synthesized like other body proteins: DNA is transcribed into messenger RNA (mRNA), which is translated into an amino acid chain of a certain length and thereby labeled as either a peptide or protein hormone (Holt et al., 2021).

It is worth mentioning one additional type of peptide hormone. Unlike the traditional peptide and polypeptides, the glycoproteins are a blend of peptide and carbohydrate. There are only four known glycoprotein hormones: LH, TSH, human chorionic gonadotropin hormone (HCG), and FSH. Clearly, those hormones affect the developing fetus and neonate and therefore are included in this chapter.

Amine Hormones

Amine hormones are derived from amino acids (tryptophan, tyrosine) or lipids. Amine hormones are secreted from both the adrenal medulla and thyroid gland.

Steroid Hormones

Some steroids originate from the adrenal cortex (e.g., cortisol, aldosterone) and others (e.g., testosterone, progesterone, estrogen) originate in the gonads (testes and ovaries) and are derived primarily from cholesterol. Steroid hormones are not soluble in water (hydrophobic). Rather, because they are composed of lipids, they easily permeate the cell membrane. The receptors for steroid hormones are found within the cell, either in the cytoplasm or the nucleus. Steroid hormones travel to their target cell bound to a transport protein. Once inside the cell, they effect changes that result in the transcription and translation of new proteins inside the cell. Because of this complex structure, the half-life of steroid hormones is much longer than that of those hormones derived from amino acids (Holt et al., 2021).

MAJOR ENDOCRINE GLANDS

Endocrine glands play a major role in maintaining physiologic homeostasis. These glands produce, store, and secrete hormones that evoke specific responses in other cells, tissues, and organs found throughout the body. An investigation into the structure and function of the major glands of the endocrine system is presented next.

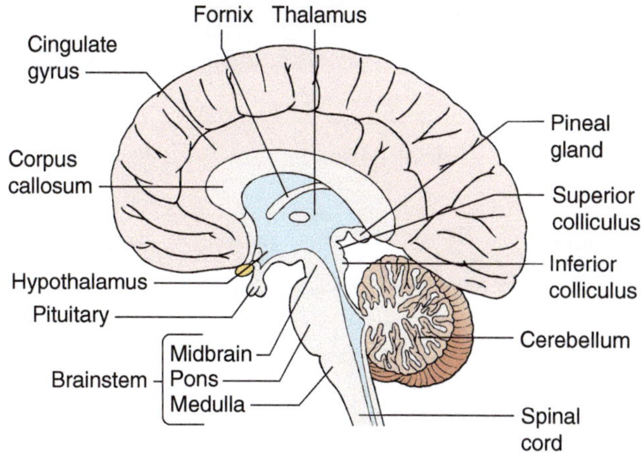

Figure 10.3 Hypothalamus, pituitary, and pineal glands.

Hypothalamus

The hypothalamus is an almond-shaped gland composed of four major substructures: the tuber cinereum, median eminence, infundibulum, and mammillary bodies. It is located below the thalamus and above the pituitary gland and brainstem, in the midbrain region. Albeit one of the smallest (in adults, smaller than 4 cm^3) tissues in the body, the hypothalamus is regarded as one of the most powerful control centers within the human body (**Figure 10.3**). It regulates systemwide physiologic equilibrium (homeostasis) by functioning as a link between the body's endocrine and nervous system, and plays a key role in the regulation of the pituitary and peripheral endocrine organ functions (**Box 10.1**).

The hypothalamus contains neurosecretory neurons that, based on feedback signals from the general circulation and pituitary, synthesize peptides and catecholamines to act as hormones (**Table 10.1**). When indicated, hypothalamic hormones either enter the systemic circulation for systemwide delivery to target cells or enter the hypophyseal portal circulation for focused delivery to the pituitary gland. In these situations, the pituitary responds to the hypothalamic-mediated hormonal communication by stimulating or inhibiting further hormone synthesis and secretion.

BOX 10.1 Major Functions of the Hypothalamus

- ↑ Appetite, body weight, insulin regulation
- ↑ Autonomic control
- ↑ Biological rhythms
- ↑ Emotion and behavior
- ↑ Hormonal control
- ↑ Parturition and human milk let-down
- ↑ Short-term memory
- ↑ Thermoregulation

Pituitary Gland

The pituitary gland is a pea-sized structure, measuring approximately 0.3 inches in adults, located below the hypothalamus at the base of the skull (**Figure 10.4**). Anatomically, the pituitary gland consists of two parts—the *anterior pituitary* lobe (adenohypophysis), which synthesizes and secretes hormones, and the *posterior pituitary* lobe (neurohypophysis), which stores hormones that are synthesized and secreted by the hypothalamus and releases them upon command (**Table 10.2**; Divall & Merjaneh, 2024; Melmed, 2022).

Hypothalamic–Pituitary Interface. The hypothalamic–pituitary (HP) axis is regarded as the "master command center" of the endocrine system. Anatomically connected by the infundibulum, the HP axis is a neuroendocrine communication pathway that mediates signals between the brain and the peripheral hormone-secreting target glands. Stimuli (circadian, pulsatile, or acute brain stimuli) prompt hypothalamic neurons to secrete hypothalamic-releasing or hypothalamic-inhibiting hormones. This regulates hormone synthesis and release by way of positive and negative feedback signals. Hypothalamic-secreted hormones travel to the pituitary by way of the humoral system, or hypophyseal portal system. Hormones secreted by the pituitary in response to the

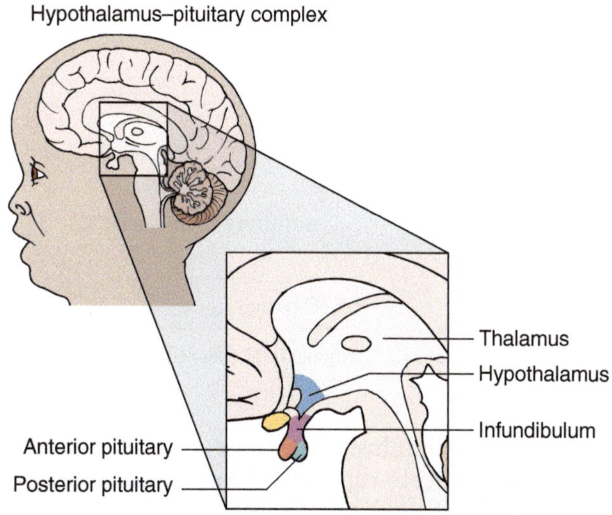

Figure 10.4 The hypothalamic-pituitary interface.

TABLE 10.1 The Hypothalamus

Hormone(s) Synthesized	Hormone Class	Specific Hormone Function(s)
Corticotropin-releasing hormone	Protein	Stimulates the release of ACTH from the anterior pituitary gland (stress response)
Dopamine	Peptide	Inhibits prolactin release; fast-acting transmission of impulses between neurons, which typically produces a short-term response
Gonadotropin-releasing hormone	Amine	Stimulates the release of LH and FSH (sexual and reproductive functions; pregnancy and lactation)
Growth hormone-releasing hormone	Peptide	Most abundant pituitary hormone; controls the body's growth and development; stimulates GH secretion
Somatostatin	Peptide	Inhibits GH and TSH release
Thyrotropin-releasing hormone	Peptide	Assists with hormonal control of lactation (stimulates prolactin release; stimulates TSH secretion

ACTH, adrenocorticotropic hormone; FSH, follicle-stimulating hormone; GH, growth hormone; LH, luteinizing hormone; TSH, thyroid-stimulating hormone.

TABLE 10.2 The Pituitary Gland

Locus	Hormone(s) Synthesized or Stored	Hormone Class	Specific Hormone Function(s)
Anterior pituitary	ACTH	Peptide	Stimulates hormone release from adrenal cortex (stress response)
	FSH	Protein	Is crucial in the promotion of normal gonad function (follicle development or sperm production)
	GH	Protein	Stress hormone; produces somatostatin for body growth and development; promotes glucose release with hypoglycemia and inhibits glucose release with hyperglycemia
	LH	Protein	Excites the gonads to stimulate androgen production (ovulation or testosterone production)
	Prolactin	Peptide	Controls lactation (human milk production)
	TSH	Protein	Stimulates the synthesis and release of thyroid hormone
Posterior pituitary	Antidiuretic hormone	Peptide	Stimulates the reabsorption of water by the kidneys
	Oxytocin	Peptide	Stimulates uterine contractions

ACTH, adrenocorticotropic hormone; FSH, follicle-stimulating hormone; GH, growth hormone; LH, luteinizing hormone; TSH, thyroid-stimulating hormone.

hypothalamic stimulus reach the systemic circulation through an intricate capillary plexus situated between both glands (Holt et al., 2021).

Adrenal Glands

The adrenal glands, or suprarenal glands, are two wedge-shaped glands that measure approximately 1.5 inches by 3 inches in adults. Also known as the *fight-or-flight glands*, these glands sit within the retroperitoneal cavity atop the kidneys.

Structurally, the glands are comprised of a larger outer adrenal cortex and smaller inner adrenal medulla. The adrenal cortex is composed of three layers, each with its own functional responsibilities (**Figure 10.5**). Their importance to establishing and maintaining physiologic homeostasis among neonates, older infants, children, and adults cannot be understated. The outer cortical layer (zona glomerulosa) synthesizes sodium-retaining hormone (aldosterone), the middle cortical layer (zona fasciculata) synthesizes glucocorticoids (cortisol), and the inner cortical layer (zona reticularis) synthesizes androgen hormones (androstenedione, testosterone, estrogen). The adrenal medulla is responsible for the synthesis and secretion of catecholamines, namely, epinephrine and norepinephrine (**Table 10.3**). These hormones enter the systemic circulation by way of the left and right suprarenal veins.

Hypothalamic–Pituitary–Adrenal Axis. Collectively, the paraventricular nucleus of the hypothalamus, anterior pituitary, and adrenal cortex comprise the HPA axis. The HPA axis is activated in response to a stressor and a systematic, complex cascade of hormonal communications follows. This cascade regulates the synthesis and secretion of adrenal hormones in an attempt to restore physiologic equilibrium.

The stress response can be described as a series of carefully executed stimuli. First, neurons within the paraventricular nucleus of the hypothalamus are alerted to an environmental, physical, or physiologic stressor.

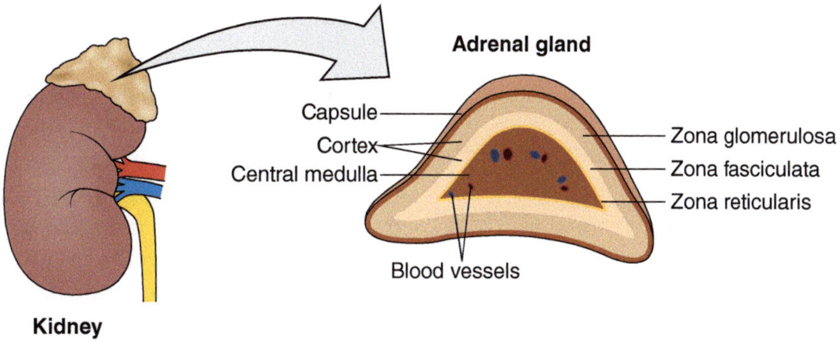

Figure 10.5 The adrenal gland.

TABLE 10.3 The Adrenal Glands

Locus		Hormone(s) Synthesized	Hormone Class	Specific Hormone Function(s)
Adrenal cortex	Zona glomerulosa	Aldosterone	Steroid	Helps regulate salt, water balance, and blood pressure in the body
	Zona fasciculata	Cortisol	Steroid	Released in response to stress
	Zona reticularis	Androstenedione	Steroid	Released to stimulate testosterone or estrogen and maturational changes
Adrenal medulla		Epinephrine, norepinephrine	Amine	Released in response to stress
		Histamine	Amine	Participates in local immune response (allergic reaction) by causing vasodilation and fluid secretion at the site of infection; stimulates gastric acid secretion

The hypothalamus releases corticotropin-releasing hormone (CRH) and arginine vasopressin (AVP). These hormones traverse the median eminence and portal capillary network and reach the anterior pituitary gland. The anterior portion of the pituitary releases ACTH into the circulation. ACTH travels to the adrenal cortex, where it binds to its receptors in the adrenals and triggers the release of glucocorticoids (cortisol and corticosterone). The glucocorticoids travel to and act on target cardiovascular tissues (muscle, adipose tissue, and vasculature). Thereafter, the kidney signals the release of mineralocorticoids, primarily aldosterone, from the adrenal cortex to preserve blood volume. Finally, once homeostasis is restored, feedback is sent to the hypothalamus to inhibit the axis (Figure 10.6; Lechan, 2025). This normal feedback loop may be impaired among premature infants with transient AI, commonly caused by developmental immaturity or critical illness, especially septic shock. These infants may require treatment with corticosteroids to stimulate the HPA axis, in particular during periods of illness or prior to invasive surgical procedures (Fechner, 2024).

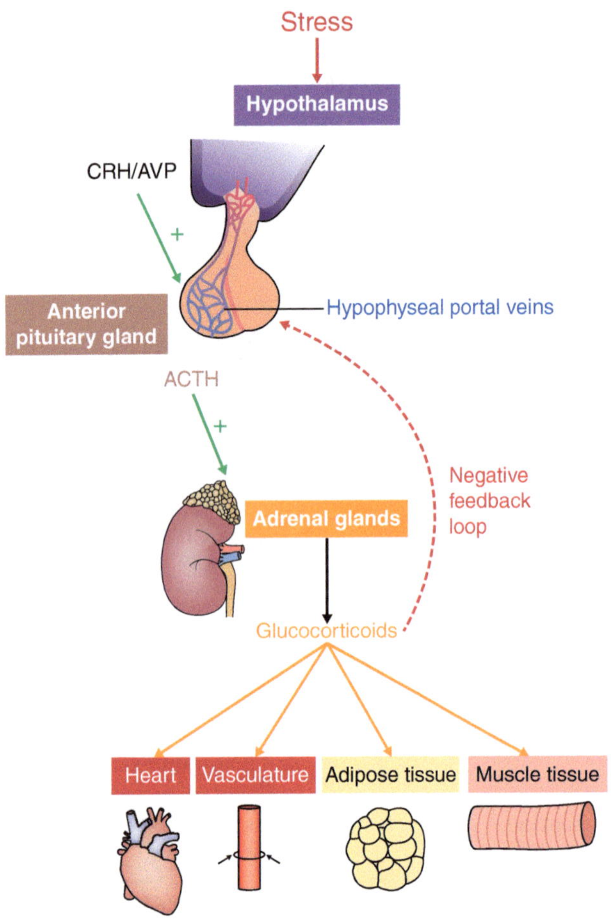

Figure 10.6 Hypothalamic-pituitary-adrenal axis.

ACTH, adrenocorticotropic hormone; AVP, arginine vasopressin; CRH, corticotropin-releasing hormone.

Image Credit: Kerri Rassa, MSN, NNP, RNC-NIC, C-ELBW.

Thyroid Gland

The thyroid gland, one of the largest endocrine glands, is a butterfly-shaped gland that measures approximately 2 inches in length in adults with normal function (thyroid disease causes the gland to swell; Salvatore et al., 2025). The gland is situated inferior to the larynx and just below the thyroid and cricoid cartilage, and is attached to the ventral floor of the pharynx by way of the thyroglossal duct. It is divided into two lobes, which reside on either side of the trachea. This gives them the appearance of two distinct (yet interconnected) wings (American Association of Endocrine Surgeons, 2024b). The thyroid gland is composed primarily of small globular sacs called follicles that house colloid. Colloid is integral to thyroid function, as it influences the processing of iodine and thyroid hormone synthesis. Thyroid tissue may be found anywhere in the body between the tongue and anterior mediastinum. The thyroid begins processing iodine and secreting thyroid hormones (T_3, T_4) and calcitonin by week 10 of gestation (Table 10.4; Kim et al., 2024; Salvatore et al., 2025).

Hypothalamic–Pituitary–Thyroid Axis. The thyroid gland contains the only in vivo cells that absorb iodine, which is then processed in the presence of the amino acid tyrosine to produce the hormones T_4 and T_3. Approximately 80% of thyroid hormone production is in the form of T_4, but it is T_3 that is the more active agent. T_4 consists of four iodine molecules and one tyrosine molecule. These hormones are an integral part of the hypothalamic–pituitary–thyroid (HPT) axis, which controls somatic growth, thermogenesis, and brain development in the fetus and infant.

The HPT axis is activated when the feedback loop notifies the hypothalamus and pituitary of low-circulating T_4 and T_3 levels; this can occur in times of low-circulating thyroid hormone, hypothermia, or increased cortisol or catecholamine synthesis (Figure 10.7). Hypothalamic TRH is then transported through the hypothalamic-hypophyseal portal system to the anterior pituitary gland. This process stimulates the pituitary gland to synthesize and release TSH. TSH secretion stimulates an increase in the organification (biochemical process) of iodine, which triggers organification within the thyroid colloid and synthesis of T_3 and T_4 from the follicle (Figure 10.8). Through a process of proteolysis, regulated by TSH, T_4 is synthesized and secreted into the blood and peripheral tissues. In addition, one of the four iodine molecules bound to T_4 disengages, reducing T_4 to T_3. The unbound iodine atom is returned to the follicle and oxidized by thyroid peroxidase (TPO). Adequate circulating thyroid hormone levels activate the negative feedback loop and inhibit TRH and TSH release (Holt et al., 2021; Khetan, 2014).

As mentioned earlier in the chapter, the hypothalamus responds to hypothermia with secretion of TRH and

TABLE 10.4 The Two Thyroid Glands

Hormone(s) Synthesized	Hormone Class	Specific Hormone Function(s)
Calcitonin	Peptide	Reduces calcium blood levels (calcium metabolism)
Thyroxine and triiodothyronine	Amine	Influences metabolism, body temperature, cell growth, and cellular differentiation (all cells)

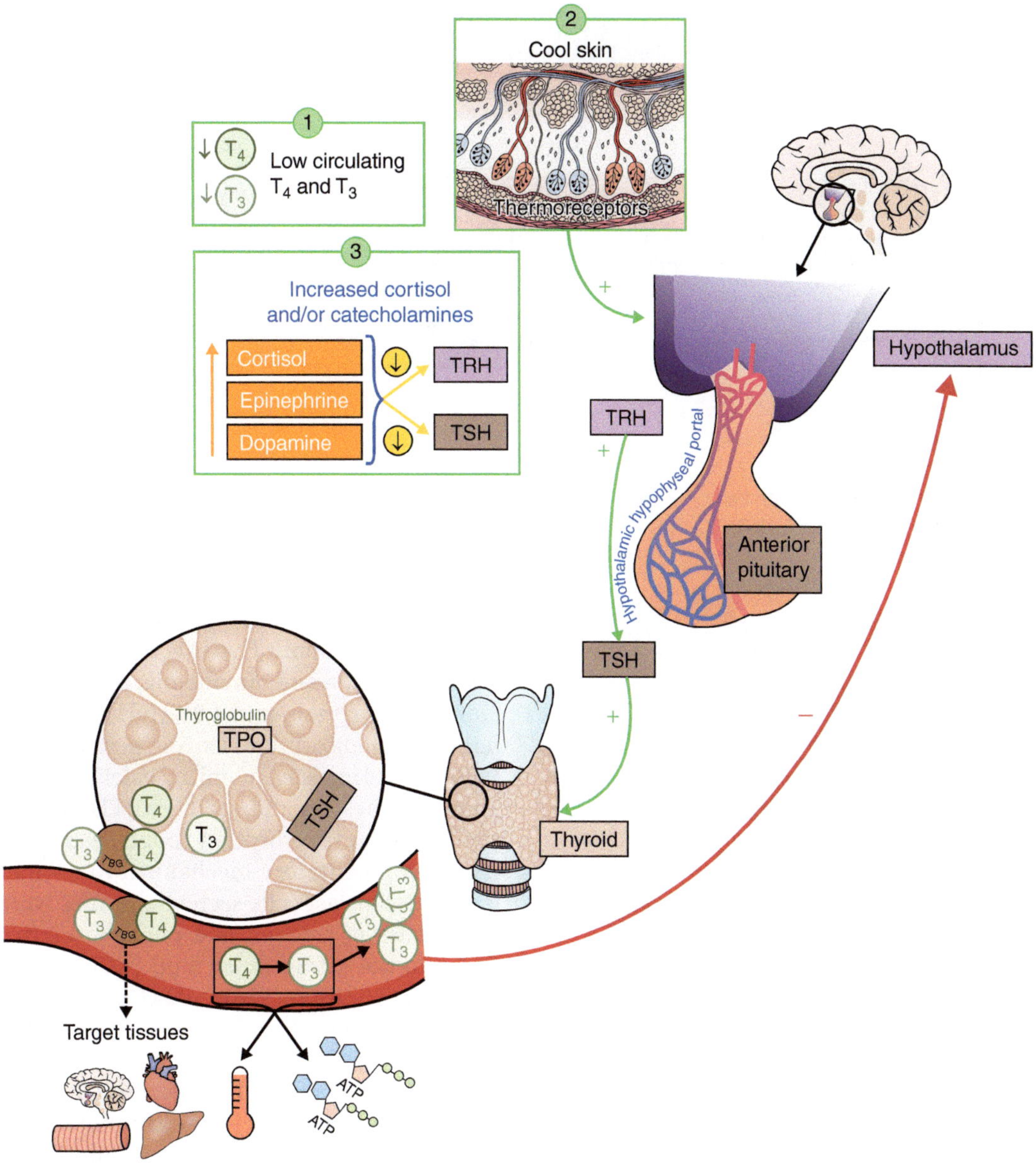

Figure 10.7 Hypothalmic-pituitary-thyroid axis.
ATP, adenosine triphosphate; TBG, thyroid-binding globulin; TRH, thyrotropin-releasing hormone; TSH, thyroid-stimulating hormone.
Image Credit: Kerri Rassa, MSN, NNP, RNC-NIC, C-ELBW.

activation of TSH and T_4 and T_3 synthesis, the upregulation of thermogenin, and production of heat through oxidative mechanisms. In addition, the hypothalamus is sensitive to circulating dopamine, epinephrine, and cortisol levels. Elevated levels of these hormones (as often occurs in neonates with hypotension requiring pharmacologic intervention) lead to decreased secretion of TRH and TSH and downregulation of the feedback loop.

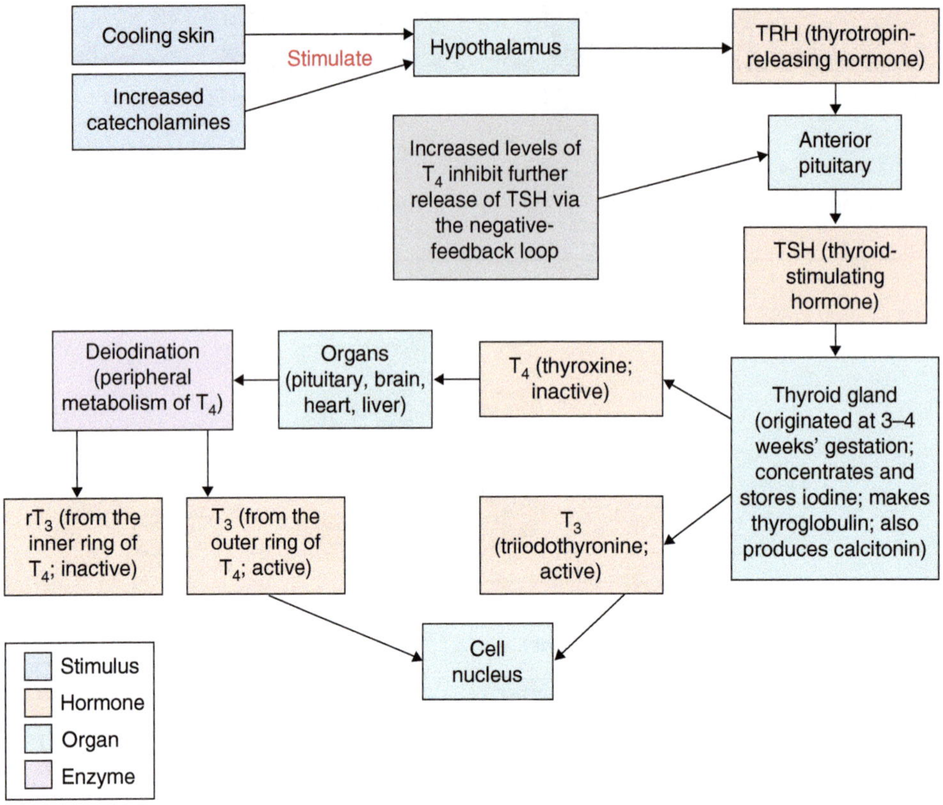

Figure 10.8 Normal thyroid metabolism.
Image Credit: Oksana Kasko, MSN, APRN, NNP-BC.

Clinical Application. Consider the concept of dopamine-induced thyroid feedback loop downregulation. It is true that high circulating dopamine levels can suppress the thyroid feedback loop. This is particularly important for APRNs to be aware of when critically ill newborns require vasoactive drugs during the first 24 hours of life. The administration of IV dopamine in the first 24 hours of life, particularly at high doses, at the same time the postnatal TSH surge is occurring can suppress thyroid gland activity. If a newborn metabolic screening test is obtained at this same time, the high TSH level and low T_4 level might lead to a false positive (exogenous dopamine-induced) result for congenital hypothyroidism (CH).

Parathyroid Glands

The four parathyroid glands are small, yellow-brown–colored glands measuring approximately 2 to 7 mm in length by 2 to 4 mm wide and 0.5 to 2 mm thick in adults (Bilezikian et al., 2015; Polin et al., 2022). These glands modulate calcium homeostasis by stimulating the release of PTH or stimulating the thyroid gland to produce CT (Table 10.5).

Calcium–Parathyroid–Vitamin D Axis. The calcium–parathyroid–vitamin D axis is responsible for regulating bone resorption and remodeling, distal renal tubular calcium reabsorption, and 1,25-$(OH)_2$D-mediated intestinal calcium absorption. During periods of hypocalcemia (low circulating serum ionized calcium), the parathyroid gland synthesizes and secretes PTH. This activates the process of bone resorption (bone destruction) as an intrinsic compensatory mechanism to normalize calcium levels. Osteoclast cells secrete enzymes which stimulate the release of calcium and phosphorus from the bone and into the extracellular fluid (ECF) and systemic circulation. Simultaneously, PTH stimulates the kidney to increase phosphorus excretion through the urine in exchange for the reabsorption of calcium at the distal tubule. In addition, PTH facilitates GI absorption of calcium (among enterally fed newborns) through its effects on synthesis of 1,25-dihydroxyvitamin D (1,25-$[OH]_2$D; American Association of Endocrine Surgeons, 2024a; Polin et al., 2022).

Calcitonin (CT) is a hormone primarily secreted by the thyroid gland; CT is also found in lung and gastrointestinal (GI) tissues. It is primarily metabolized in the kidneys and can rapidly decrease serum calcium levels in infants and children by inactivating osteoclast activity. During periods of hypercalcemia, the calcium-sensing receptor (CaSR) protein is activated. This protein, synthesized within the parathyroid glands, stimulates CT secretion

TABLE 10.5 The Four Parathyroid Glands

Hormone(s) Synthesized	Hormone Class	Specific Hormone Function(s)
Parathyroid hormone	Peptide	Stimulates vitamin D (calcitrol) synthesis, which is an important regulator of blood calcium levels; it helps maintain the proper functioning of cells and builds muscles and bones.

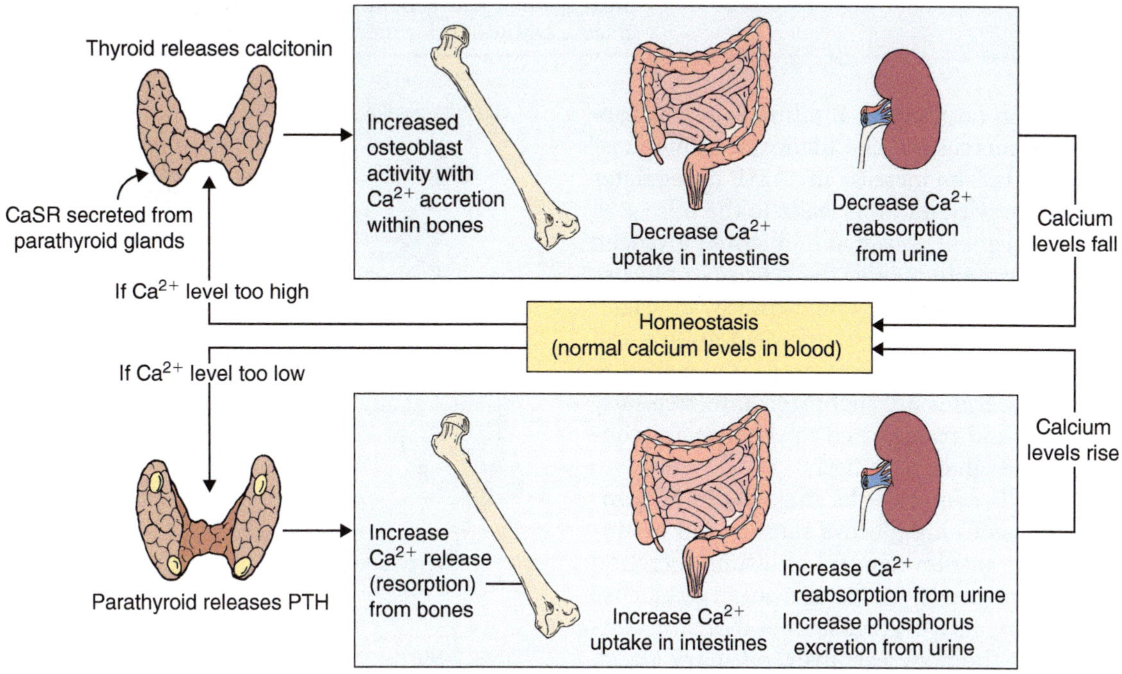

Figure 10.9 Hypocalcemia and hypercalcemia feedback loops.
***Note*:** Parathyroid activity is optimal when serum magnesium levels are within normal range. Hypermagnesemia will suppress parathyroid function. Mild hypomagnesemia will upregulate parathyroid activity, whereas severe hypomagnesemia induces a paradoxical block on parathyroid activity. CaSR, calcium-sensing receptor; PTH, parathyroid hormone.

from the thyroid gland. The net effect of CT secretion is increased calcium deposition in the bones (permitting bone remodeling), decreased intestinal calcium uptake, and decreased renal calcium reabsorption at the distal convoluted tubule (Figure 10.9).

Clinical Application. Think of osteoblasts as the construction crew, working constantly to build and maintain the bones. These cells play a role in bone formation and remodeling by depositing a mixture of collagen, calcium, phosphorus, and other minerals to solidify the broken bone. On the other hand, think of osteoclasts as the demolition crew, responsible for bone resorption. Under normal circumstances, osteoclasts and osteoblasts work in harmony. In situations where serum calcium levels decrease, osteoclast activity increases in order to release more calcium into the bloodstream and normalize serum levels. If this compensation becomes persistent, it can be devastating to bone health in preterm infants.

Pancreas

The pancreas, a flat gland measuring approximately 6 inches in adults, is housed deep in the abdomen between the stomach and spine, near the duodenum. It is composed of clusters of exocrine cells. The green-colored product of these pancreatic exocrine cells is bile, an alkaline fluid comprised of beneficial digestive enzymes. Bile drains into the duodenum by way of the common bile duct and ampulla of Vater. The splenic artery supplies the pancreas, whereas venous blood drains from the pancreas into the hepatic portal vein. Therefore, the liver is the primary recipient of pancreatic hormones and responsible for facilitating first-pass metabolism of those hormones as they approach the heart and systemic circulation (Felsenfeld & Levine, 2015; Holt et al., 2021).

Pancreatic endocrine cells can be subdivided into two major types, each with its own primary function. Pancreatic α-cells account for approximately 20% of pancreatic cells. Their primary function is to secrete glucagon in cases of hypoglycemia to reestablish a state of euglycemia (normal serum glucose level; Table 10.6). This is accomplished when glucagon binds to the G-protein coupled

TABLE 10.6 The Pancreas

Hormone(s) Synthesized	Hormone Class	Specific Hormone Function(s)
Insulin	Protein	Facilitates cellular glucose uptake; regulates carbohydrate, lipid, and protein metabolism
Glucagon	Protein	Responds to hypoglycemia by mobilizing glucose into the circulation by inhibiting glycogen synthesis (glycogenesis), promoting the breakdown of glycogen into glucose (glycogenolysis), and promoting glucose synthesis (gluconeogenesis)

receptor (GPCR) on target cells. Binding activates adenylate cyclase and increases cyclic adenosine monophosphate (cAMP) levels. The increase in cAMP upregulates protein kinase A activity, and this leads to the release of glucagon and subsequent conversion of stored glycogen into glucose (glycogenolysis) and the release of glucose molecules into the circulation. Concurrently, glucagon stimulates the liver to increase amino acid uptake and converts it into glucose (gluconeogenesis). On a smaller scale, stored triglycerides are mobilized into free fatty acids and glycerol and transported to the liver for conversion into glucose (gluconeogenesis).

Pancreatic β-cells comprise the majority of all pancreatic cells; these cells are glucose sensors and modulate the secretion of insulin. Control of insulin secretion during hyperglycemia involves the activation of glucose (glycolysis) and oxidative glucose metabolism. Glucokinase, found in the pancreas, liver, pituitary gland, and brain, is the rate-limiting enzyme in the glycolytic pathway; it has a low affinity for glucose and therefore controls the rate and affinity for glucose entry into the glycolytic pathway and insulin release. Once glucokinase senses increased extracellular glucose load, it activates tyrosine kinase receptors, triggering uptake of glucose by GLUT2 transporters and the phosphorylation and conversion of glucose to glucose-6-phosphate. This process facilitates the rise in the adenosine triphosphate (ATP) to adenosine diphosphate (ADP) ratio, inactivates potassium channels, and depolarizes the beta cell membrane. Calcium channels open, allowing their influx into the cell with subsequent release of insulin (Figure 10.10).

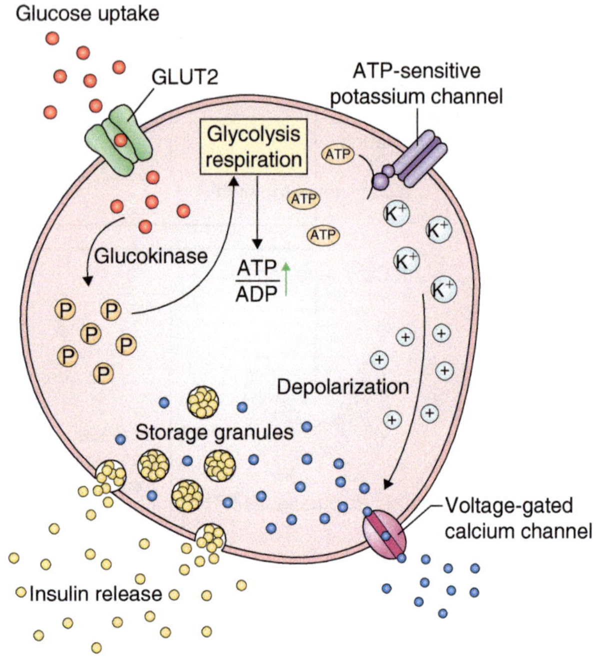

Figure 10.10 Glycolytic pathway.

Note: Two additional subtypes of pancreatic cells are delta and pancreatic polypeptide cells. These cells are responsible for secreting somatostatin and pancreatic polypeptides, respectively (Dingeldien, 2025; Felsenfeld & Levine, 2015; Molina, 2023).

ADP, adenosine monophosphate; ATP, adenosine triphosphate; GLUT2, glucose transporter, type 2.

Pineal Gland

The pineal gland is a small, red-gray–colored and pine-cone-shaped organ that is approximately one third inch in length in adults. It is located distal to the third cerebral ventricle and is composed of pineal and neuroglial cells (Figure 10.3; Lechan, 2025; Molina, 2023). Blood flow to the pineal gland is supplied by the posterior cerebral artery. Despite its seemingly modest role in endocrine function, the pineal gland receives the second-largest blood supply, second only to the kidney. The purpose for this generous circulatory supply is poorly understood, but is likely related to the pineal gland's role in synthesizing and secreting melatonin. Melatonin, derived from the amino acid tryptophan, is responsible for the regulation of circadian rhythm and reproductive hormones as well as skin and eye coloration (Table 10.7; Pfaff & Joëls, 2016).

DEVELOPMENTAL PHYSIOLOGY

Calcium–Phosphorus–Magnesium Homeostasis

Calcium, phosphorus, and magnesium dysregulation can place the neonate at risk for a host of complications, including neurologic dysfunction, arrhythmias, and respiratory derangements. The regulation and transport of calcium, phosphate, and magnesium is essential to maintain homeostatic biologic and cellular functioning. In the text that follows, we describe regulatory hormonal influences and transport of these ions.

TABLE 10.7 The Pineal Gland

Hormone(s) Synthesized	Hormone Class	Specific Hormone Function(s)
Melatonin	Amine	Helps to control circadian rhythm and regulate certain reproductive hormones

Calcium. Calcium is the most abundant ion in the human body. Calcium ions are essential for maintenance and control of many biologic processes, including cell-to-cell communication, cell aggregation and division, coagulation, neuromuscular excitability, cardiomyocyte depolarization, membrane integrity and permeability, and enzymatic synthesis and secretion (Blaine et al., 2015; O'Callaghan & Roth, 2022).

Nearly all calcium (99%) is found in the bones and teeth. The remaining 1% of calcium is found in the ECF and the soft tissues. Total body calcium levels rapidly rise during the final trimester of fetal development and then drop shortly after birth. After birth, total body calcium is found in three distinct forms: (a) "free" or ionized (50%); (b) bound to albumin and globulins (40%); or (c) bound to bicarbonate, phosphate, or citrate (10%). *Free (ionized) calcium is the active form of calcium* and can cross the plasma membrane; therefore, a low ionized calcium level is associated with the symptoms of hypocalcemia observed in newborns (O'Callaghan & Roth, 2022).

Postnatal calcium concentrations are regulated by PTH secretion, 1,25-$(OH)_2D$ (active vitamin D_3), and CT. Both PTH and vitamin D_3 work to promote calcium absorption, whereas CT works to increase calcium excretion. PTH promotes calcium resorption in the bone and renal system and within the intestine by way of facilitating 1,25-$(OH)_2D$-mediated intestinal absorption of calcium. Similarly, vitamin D stimulates the absorption of calcium (and phosphorus) from the bone, intestine, and kidney. As vitamin D can only be obtained through exposure to sunlight and enterally through the ingestion of infant formulas or vitamin supplements, the influence of vitamin D on calcium homeostasis is considered a "long-loop" (time-consuming) process, which often does not reach an influential status for the first few weeks of life (O'Callaghan & Roth, 2022). Conversely, CT acts to facilitate calcium homeostasis through *inhibition*. CT works to prevent hypercalcemic states by inhibiting calcium (and phosphorus) release from bone as well as facilitating renal excretion of calcium (and phosphorus; Abrams & Tiosano, 2025). Both CT and PTH are considered faster-acting "short loops" once PTH maturation is complete.

The neonate must quickly adapt to extrauterine life and the cessation of a calcium supply from the pregnant patient. Unfortunately for the newborn, the parathyroid response to evolving hypocalcemia is diminished in the first days after birth. As such, ionized calcium concentrations fall over the first 24 to 48 hours of life. In term infants, the ionized calcium nadir is approximately 4.9 mg/dL (1.2 mmol/L), which will rebound over the next 4 to 6 days of life and reach childhood levels by the end of postnatal week one (Abrams & Tiosano, 2025; Loughead et al., 1988; O'Callaghan & Roth, 2022). Of infants born prematurely, those weighing less than 1.5 kg at birth tend to experience a lower ionized calcium nadir.

Parathyroid immaturity, or the transient hypoparathyroid state observed after birth, is not fully understood, yet it contributes significantly to the risk for hypocalcemia in premature and term newborns. Factors understood to contribute to a stunted parathyroid response include method of delivery, decreased enteral calcium intake during the first days of life, and the functional immaturity of the GI and renal systems. Higher PTH values are reported in the umbilical cords of infants born by elective cesarean section, compared to those delivered by elective cesarean *with* trial of labor, emergent cesarean, and spontaneous vaginal delivery (O'Callaghan & Roth, 2022). It is understood that both breastfed and bottle-fed newborns slowly increase ingested enteral volumes, which leads to a steady increase in exogenous calcium intake over the first week of life. Similarly, intestinal absorption of essential nutrients steadily increases over the first 2 to 4 weeks of life (O'Callaghan & Roth, 2022), concurrent with increasing enteral feeding volumes. As the majority of calcium is absorbed in the small intestine, delayed intestinal maturity contributes to the observed decrease and slow restoration of calcium levels to normal values after birth. In addition, the renal system undergoes a process of functional maturation after birth, reaching competency by the second week of life. Once mature, virtually all filtered calcium is reabsorbed within the proximal tubules, with additional reabsorption occurring later in the distal convoluted tubules (Blaine et al., 2015; O'Callaghan & Roth, 2022).

Premature infants, infants of diabetic mothers, and those who suffer perinatal asphyxia are at a higher risk for early-onset calcium dysregulation. These risk factors and their mechanism of action in facilitating a hypocalcemic state are provided in **Table 10.8**. Osteopenia of prematurity (OoP) is one of the most common comorbidities associated with prolonged calcium dysregulation.

Clinical Application. Parathyroid activity offers the most significant influence upon calcium homeostasis. When the parathyroid glands sense hypocalcemia, several compensatory mechanisms are activated. PTH is synthesized and this hormone

TABLE 10.8 Factors Associated With Early-Onset Postnatal Hypocalcemia (1–4 Days of Age)

Factor	Mechanism
IUGR	Decreased placental calcium transfer
Maternal diabetes	Maternal renal loss of magnesium with glycosuria results in fetal hypomagnesemia and inability to produce sufficient PTH
	Fetal macrosomia may encourage premature delivery and resultant decreased PTH activity
Prematurity	Early termination of placental calcium transfer
	Inadequate calcium intake enterally or intravenously
	Urinary calcium loss secondary to immature renal function
Birth asphyxia	Inadequate calcium intake enterally or intravenously
	Renal failure, acute tubular necrosis
Immunodeficiency disorder	22q11.2 deletion (DiGeorge syndrome) is associated with underdeveloped or absent parathyroid gland development and function
Hyperphosphatemia	Increased phosphorus load (e.g., inappropriate enteral intake, high phosphorus, cow's milk)
Vitamin D deficiency	Low production of PTH secondary to hypomagnesemia triggered by insufficient vitamin D
Medications	Diuretics, aminoglycosides (e.g., gentamicin) increase urinary losses of calcium

Note: Infants born via elective cesarean *with* trial of labor, emergent cesarean, and by spontaneous vaginal delivery risk postnatal hypocalcemia. IUGR infants who succumb to any of the risk factors listed are considered at-risk for hypocalcemia.

IUGR, intrauterine growth restriction; PTH, parathyroid hormone.

Sources: Abrams, S. A., & Tiosano, D. (2025). Disorders of calcium, phosphorus and magnesium metabolism in the neonate. In R. J. Martin & A. A. Fanaroff (Eds.), *Fanaroff and Martin's neonatal-perinatal medicine, 2-volume set: Diseases of the fetus and infant* (12th ed., pp. 1697–1727). Elsevier; Molina, P. E. (2023). *Endocrine physiology* (6th ed.). McGraw-Hill Medical; Pfaff, D. W., & Joëls, M. (Eds.). (2016). *Hormones, brain and behavior* (3rd ed.). Elsevier/Academic Press.

frees calcium (and phosphorus) from the bone and permits entry into the bloodstream. PTH also triggers the synthesis of calcitriol (biologically active form of vitamin D), which summons calcium transporters to accumulate at the lumen of the small intestine and allow for increased GI calcium absorption. The kidneys also reabsorb calcium from the tubules (to reduce urinary losses) in exchange for allowing increased urinary excretion of phosphorus. Newborns who present with hypocalcemia shortly after birth may be experiencing this imbalance due to prematurity, IUGR, hypomagnesemia, asphyxia in the perinatal period, maternal drug influences, respiratory alkalosis, or more rare causes including DiGeorge syndrome (22q11). Remember that the majority of calcium crosses the placenta in the third trimester!

Newborns weighing more than 1.5 kg at birth should demonstrate ionized (physiologically active) calcium levels greater than 1.1 mmol/L (or greater than 4.4 mg/dL). Newborns weighing less than 1.5 kg at birth should demonstrate ionized calcium levels greater than 1 mmol/L (or greater than 4 mg/dL). Levels that are below these thresholds constitute hypocalcemia that may require further evaluation and treatment, particularly if infants are symptomatic. Common symptoms include an exaggerated startle reflex, jitters, myoclonic jerks, prolonged QTc on an ECG monitor, or seizures. Treatment initially involves the administration of IV calcium gluconate at 100 to 200 mg/kg/dose and may also include the administration of magnesium sulfate (if hypomagnesemia precipitates hypocalcemia) or vitamin D supplementation.

Phosphorus. Second to calcium, phosphorus is the most abundant mineral in the human body. Like calcium, nearly all phosphorus (85%) is found in the bones and teeth. The remaining 15% of phosphorus is found in

ECF and soft tissues. Total body phosphorus exists as (a) "free" or ionized (85%); (b) bound to albumin (11%); and (c) bound to sodium, calcium, or magnesium (5%–15%; Molina, 2023; O'Callaghan & Roth, 2022). Serum phosphorus concentrations vary, altered by factors, including gender, age, acidity, or alkalinity, and as influenced by other circulating hormones (O'Callaghan & Roth, 2022).

Phosphorus load is regulated by renal, skeletal, and intestinal transport mechanisms. In situations in which phosphorus load is decreased (hypophosphatemia), several mechanisms are activated to restore homeostasis in a manner that does not disrupt calcium concentrations. First, renal tubular reabsorption of phosphorus occurs. During this time frame, calcium and phosphorus are mobilized from the bone. In addition, 1,25-$(OH)_2$D is synthesized by the kidneys and released into the intestinal tract to promote increased absorption of calcium and phosphorus. The reverse of this cascade of events is elicited in the face of hyperphosphatemia (O'Callaghan & Roth, 2022).

Similar to calcium, total body phosphorus levels rapidly increase during the final trimester of fetal development and then drop over the first 48 hours after birth. Beginning around the second day of life, and as PTH and calcium levels begin to increase, an increase in plasma phosphorus is observed. It is likely that transient postnatal renal immaturity, which typically spans the first 1 to 2 postnatal days (see Chapter 8), spares newborns of renal phosphorus losses and facilitates the progressive increase in phosphorus load. Concurrently, as postnatal gluconeogenesis is established, circulating phosphorus levels increase; phosphorus is liberated from amino acids with this metabolic pathway.

Life-span implications associated with phosphorus dysregulation include parathyroid cell hyperplasia and phosphorus depletion syndrome. Both extremes are regarded as preventable, rare diseases of the neonate. Careful management of fluid and electrolyte status, and the provision of enteral and parenteral nutrition, is indicated among critically ill neonates who require a prolonged birth hospitalization.

Magnesium. Magnesium is an abundant intracellular cation whose serum concentrations influence calcium homeostasis. Nearly all magnesium (99%) is stored in the bone, muscle, and soft tissues. A small percentage (1%) of magnesium can be found in the ECF. Similar to both calcium and phosphorus, magnesium exists as three fractions: (a) "free" or ionized (55%–70%); (b) bound to albumin (20%–30%); and (c) bound to bicarbonate, phosphate, or citrate (5%–15%); due to differences in measurement methods, ranges for each fraction of magnesium vary considerably across the literature (O'Callaghan & Roth, 2022). Magnesium is essential to bone and teeth development, and influences cardiovascular smooth muscle contractility, neuromuscular excitability, and transmission (e.g., twitches, cramps, muscle spasms), as well as many enzyme reactions (often involving ATP; Blaine et al., 2015; Long & Romani, 2014; O'Callaghan & Roth, 2022).

Total body magnesium levels are tightly regulated by intestinal, renal, and bone transport mechanisms. Intestinal transport involves the active transport of magnesium across the ileum, with passive absorption occurring throughout the small intestine. Fecal excretion is a major determinant of overall magnesium retention, explaining why the neonate exposed to birth parent magnesium will have high serum levels until stooling begins, which is often delayed due to dysmotility from magnesium effects. Renal transport of magnesium involves filtration and reabsorption. Approximately 70% of total circulating (absorbed) serum magnesium is transported and filtered through the glomerulus. Nearly all (96%) of this filtered magnesium is reabsorbed within the proximal tubule, ascending loop of Henle, and distal convoluted tubule. As such, and under normal circumstances, little magnesium is lost to the urine. Magnesium transport and absorption within the bone are dynamic; however, transport mechanisms are currently poorly understood (Blaine et al., 2015; Long & Romani, 2014; O'Callaghan & Roth, 2022).

Life-span implications associated with magnesium dysregulation include fetal magnesium toxicity (rickets) secondary to maternal magnesium tocolysis leading to inhibition of PTH secretion and hypocalcemia.

Clinical Application. The ileum is responsible for absorption of many nutrients, including magnesium. In situations involving ileal resection (e.g., from complications of NEC) nutrient malabsorption can occur. Affected infants may require prolonged hyperalimentation that includes magnesium and micronutrient supplementation.

Glucose Homeostasis. Glucose is delivered to the fetus transplacentally. In contrast, glucose is produced within the liver after birth and delivered to target tissues by way of the systemic circulation. The demand for circulating glucose is highest during the newborn period. Therefore, it is of no surprise that newborns produce glucose at a rate that is two- to three-fold higher than children and adults, mainly because the brain is a substantial consumer of glucose and the newborn's brain-to-body weight is very disproportionate (favoring increased cerebral glucose consumption).

Glucose Metabolic Pathways. Four major metabolic pathways control glucose production, either through the synthesis of glucose from precursors for release into the bloodstream, synthesis of glycogen for storage in the liver or muscle cells, or the synthesis of pyruvate (Table 10.9; and Figure 10.11). These energy-generating carbohydrate-mediated metabolic pathways are essential "core knowledge" for the APRN. Among newborns, functional operation of two particular pathways, glycogenolysis and gluconeogenesis, are necessary within the first hours after birth in order to maintain necessary basal glucose utilization (4–6 mg/kg/minute; Beardsall et al., 2022; Wernimont & Norris, 2022).

TABLE 10.9 The Four Major Carbohydrate Metabolic Pathways

Metabolic Pathway	Major Function
Glycogenesis	Synthesis of glycogen
Glycogenolysis	Breakdown of glycogen to glucose
Glycolysis	Breakdown of glucose to pyruvate
Gluconeogenesis	Synthesis of noncarbohydrate sources (pyruvate, lactate, amino acids) to glucose

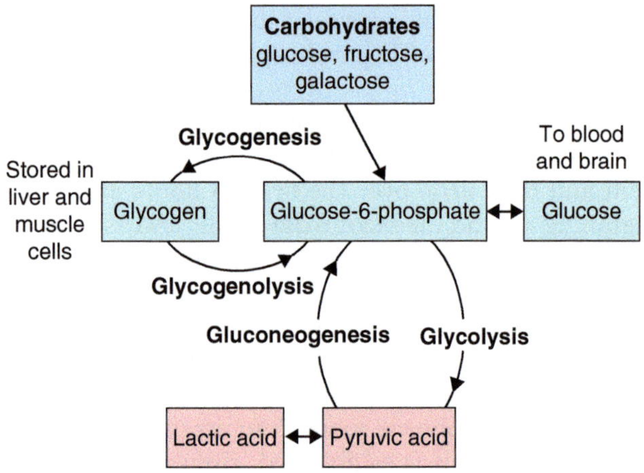

Figure 10.11 Summary of carbohydrate metabolism.

Glycogenesis. By definition, glycogenesis describes the biosynthesis of sugar into glycogen for storage and later use, which among fetuses occurs with glucose transport across the placenta, and in newborns occurs immediately after the ingestion of carbohydrate sources. Fetal glycogen accretion begins as early as week 9 of gestation (Beardsall et al., 2022). Thereafter, glycogen stores gradually increase across fetal development; at term, healthy, appropriate-for-gestational age (AGA) infants possess increased glycogen stores compared to adults. In some circumstances, the glycogen stores amassed during fetal development are sufficient to maintain euglycemia after birth. This is typically true among AGA infants and is helpful as the mother–infant dyad adjusts to oral enteral feeding regimens. Comparatively, premature, late preterm, and small-for-gestational age (SGA) infants typically possess insufficient (or virtually no) glycogen stores at birth. As a result, these infants are at increased risk for developing hypoglycemia after birth. APRNs and clinical nurses are responsible for ensuring the prompt and consistent provision of appropriate exogenous carbohydrates (by way of breast milk, formula, or a combination of both) in these situations, as this is the primary mechanism by which glucose can reach the systemic circulation and cerebral glucose uptake can occur (Beardsall et al., 2022).

Glycogenesis occurs primarily within the hepatocyte, and to a lesser degree within muscle cells. Key hormones, namely insulin (diminishes hepatic glucose production), glucagon, cortisol, and epinephrine (stimulates hepatic glucose production), modulate this process (Nelson & Cox, 2021; Wernimont & Norris, 2022). The stepwise biochemical process involved with the synthesis of glycogen is presented in Figure 10.12. More simply, let's review the steps that are required for glucose molecules to enter the liver and be stored as glycogen. Glucose molecules require special transporters, namely GLUT2 transporters, to enter hepatocytes. As the glucose molecule enters the hepatocyte, the enzyme glucokinase (or glucose kinase, found in the liver) catalyzes the phosphorlyation of glucose into glucose-6-phosphate. Next, the enzyme phosphoglucomutase converts glucose-6-phosphate into glucose-1-phosphate. The glucose-1-phosphate reacts with uridine trisphosphate (UTP) to form uridine diphosphate (UDP)-glucose. Ultimately, UDP-glucose interacts with the enzyme glycogenin, and a glycogen chain is formed. This process can also occur within the muscle tissue, with the primary difference being that glucose molecules require the enzyme hexokinase (or hexose kinase) to enter muscle cells. The remaining steps mimic what has been previously described.

Glycogenolysis. Recall that glycogen is the stored form of glucose, and under normal circumstances is mobilized from either hepatic or muscle cells when blood glucose levels fall. This process of converting stored glycogen into glucose is termed glycogenolysis. More specific, the glycogen stores are converted into glucose-1-phosphate (in muscle cells) and glucose (in hepatocytes). Glucose-1-phosphate offers a source of energy for muscle contraction, while glucose helps fuel the body and the developing brain. The same hormones that regulate glycogenesis also modulate glycogenolysis (Wernimont & Norris, 2022).

When blood glucose levels fall into a hypoglycemic range (a precise threshold has not been agreed upon by experts to date), the pancreas secretes glucagon. Glucagon travels to the liver, where it binds to hepatic receptors and initiates an increase in cAMP levels. The cAMP

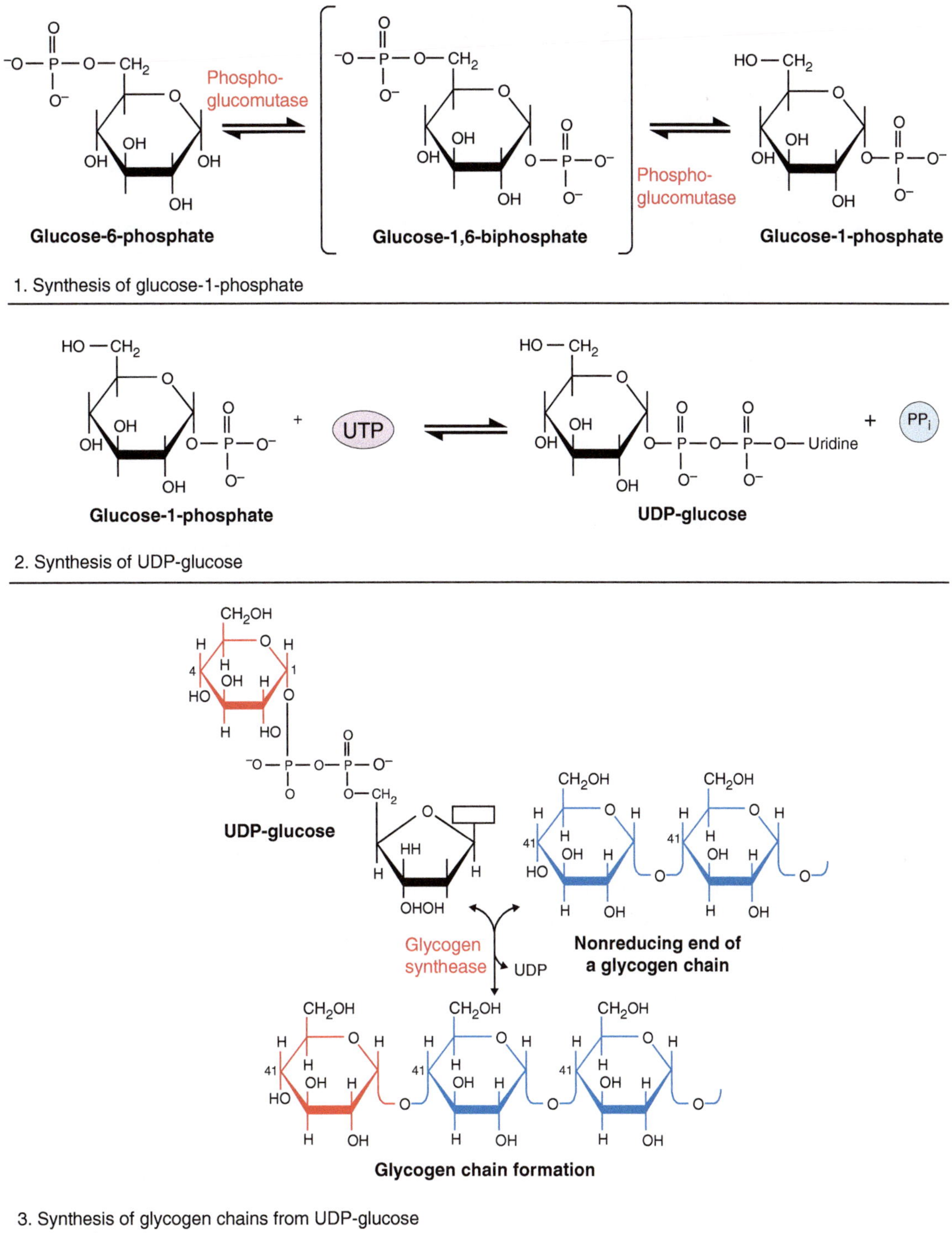

Figure 10.12 Glycogenesis pathway.
ADP, adenosine monophosphate; ATP, adenosine triphosphate; PP$_1$, protein phosphatase 1; UDP, uridine 5'-diphosphate; UTP, uridine 5'-triphosphate.

stimulates a phosphorylation cascade, activating *glycogen phosphorylase* and other enzymes. The glycogen phosphorylase enzyme begins by acting directly on glycogen polymers. It targets the alpha 1,4 glycosidic bonds and splits them apart. In doing so, the phosphate molecule (formerly a part of the glycogen *phosphor*ylase enzyme) attaches to five of the glucose molecules, forming glucose-1-phosphate. At the same time, a complementary debranching enzyme cleaves one glucose molecule from the polymer chain. Some glucose-1-phosphate molecules are diverted to muscle cells for optimized muscle contractility while others are converted (reversibly) to glucose-6-phosphate (by the enzyme phosphoglucomutase). Next, glucose-6-phosphate interacts with the enzyme glucose-6-phosphatase and is converted into glucose. The glucose molecules are released into the bloodstream to be utilized by target tissues (**Figure 10.13**; Nelson & Cox, 2021).

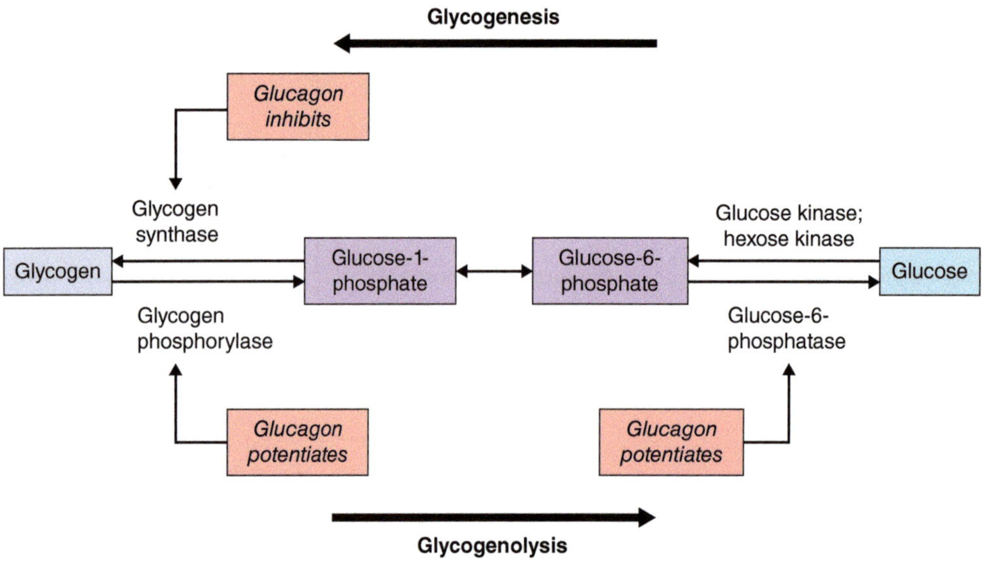

Figure 10.13 Glycogenesis and glycogenolysis.

Note: The influence of glucagon on the inhibition of glycogenolysis and potentiation of glycogenesis (formation of glycogen) is included to help learners recognize the physiologic function of glucagon and potential indication for the administration of exogenous glucagon in hypoglycemic neonates.

Image Credit: Amy J. Jnah.

Glycogenolysis can occur during fetal development or within the intrapartum period. Circumstances associated with intrauterine glycogenolysis include situations where the fetus is exposed to a prolonged delay in umbilical glucose uptake (e.g., placental insufficiency, abruption, perinatal asphyxia). That said, glycogenolysis primarily begins after birth. Among newborns with available glycogen stores, glycogenolysis provides a rapid source of glucose during the first 10 to 12 hours of postnatal life, until all glycogen stores have been utilized. Glycogenolysis may be initiated during periods of hypoglycemia or accelerated glucose uptake, as is the case with hypoxic-ischemic encephalopathy and during seizures (Garg & Devaskar, 2025). It is possible for an infant to exhibit glycogenolysis outside of the newborn period, once adequate enteral or parenteral nutrition is offered, and glycogen stores are replenished for later mobilization.

Clinical Application. Glycogen is stored in the liver and muscles. When hypoglycemia is present, glycogen stores can be a source to be tapped into in order to address the low blood sugar. However, in the SGA infant, glycogen stores are limited and may not be able to meet the demands. Glycolysis will take over as an emergency next step. To prevent hypoglycemia in these at-risk infants, providing exogenous glucose as soon as possible with feedings at least every 2 to 3 hours is a key factor. Despite early feedings, parenteral support may still be needed. The release of glucagon is impaired in the infant of a diabetic mother (IDM) as a result of long-term exposure to high blood sugars in utero. This exposure causes the fetal pancreas to adapt by increasing insulin production and decreasing glucagon production. With clamping of the cord at delivery, this continuous supply of glucose from the mother stops, and due to the inability of the neonate to begin suppressing insulin production and releasing glucagon, hypoglycemia is commonly seen.

Glycolysis. Glycolysis, an anaerobic process, is believed to be the oldest and most widely understood carbohydrate metabolic pathway. By definition, glycolysis involves the extraction of energy from glucose. To accomplish this, circulating glucose molecules are oxidized, split into two equal parts, and converted into pyruvate (a ketoacid). In addition, energy, primarily in the form of ATP, is cleaved and stored for later use. In order to best appreciate the complexity of chemical reactions involved in the production of pyruvate, the glycolytic pathway is summarized as a series of 10 specific chemical reactions as shown in Figure 10.14.

Gluconeogenesis. Gluconeogenesis can provide newborns with a source of glucose for cerebral and tissue consumption, but requires the use of noncarbohydrate sources, including lactate, glycerol, pyruvate, and amino acids. It is modulated by hormonal changes, including a reduction in the plasma insulin concentration and increased circulating concentrations of glucagon, catecholamines, GH, TSH, and other hormones including cortisol (Nelson & Cox, 2021; Thureen & Hay, 2006). Similar to glycogenolysis, gluconeogenesis is potentiated after the

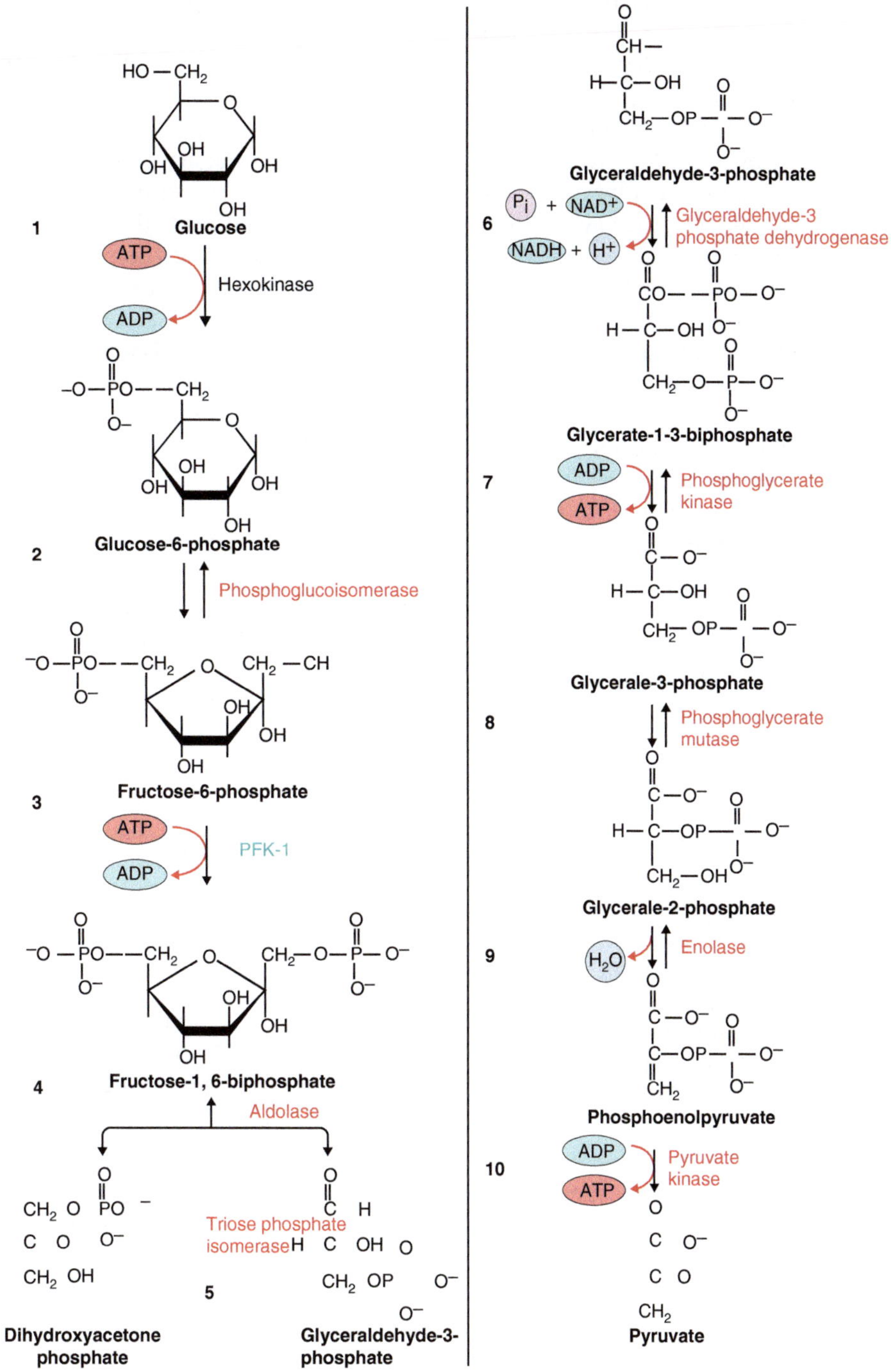

Figure 10.14 The glycolytic pathway.

Note: The glycolytic pathway steps are as follows: (1) synthesis of glucose-6-phosphate; (2) conversion of glucose-6-phosphate to fructose-6-phosphate; (3) phosphorylation of fructose-6-phosphate; (4) cleavage of fructose-1,6-biphosphate; (5) conversion of glyceraldehyde-3-phosphate and dihydroxyacetone phosphate; (6) oxidation of glyceraldehyde-3-phosphate; (7) phosphoryl group transfer; (8) conversion of 3-phosphoglycerate and 2-phosphoglycerate; (9) dehydration of 2-phosphoglycerate; (10) synthesis of pyruvate.

ADP, adenosine diphosphate; ATP, adenosine triphosphate; NAD+, nicotinamide adenine dinucleotide in oxidized form; NADH, nicotinamide adenine dinucleotide in reduced form; PKF-1, phosphofructokinase-1.

normal surge in glucagon occurs after birth. However, there are numerous enzymes necessary for the completion of this pathway and these enzymes only *begin* to emerge between 4 to 6 hours *after* birth. Therefore, this pathway cannot mitigate early postnatal hypoglycemia that occurs within the first few hours after birth (**Figure 10.15**).

The first step in gluconeogenesis involves the conversion of pyruvate to phosphoenolpyruvic acid (PEP). The second step is the conversion of fructose-1,6 biphosphate to fructose-6-phosphate with the use of the enzyme fructose-1,6-phosphatase. The conversion of fructose-6-phosphate to glucose-6-phosphate is modulated by the enzyme phosphoglucoisomerase. The final operational step in gluconeogenesis involves the interaction of glucose-6-phosphate with the enzyme glucose-6-phosphatase and production of glucose for use as an energy source throughout the body and, in particular, within the brain (Baynes, 2023; Nelson & Cox, 2021; Thureen & Hay, 2006).

Fetal Glucose Metabolism. Under normal conditions, the fetus does not independently produce glucose. Transplacental glucose, amino acids, free fatty acids, ketones, and glycerol are easily funneled from mother to fetus and glucose is obtained through a process of oxidation. The fetus is never directly exposed to periods of fasting and therefore does not develop associated compensatory mechanisms.

The fetus does demonstrate some competency with insulin secretion and regulation in response to the maternal glucose load; however, the function of insulin in utero differs from its postnatal function in that it is primarily synthesized to promote fetal growth and development. That said, insulin secretion *is* responsive to fetal glucose concentrations, but fetal glucose concentrations are controlled by the mother. Maternal hyperglycemia, which occurs with diabetes, can elicit fetal hyperglycemia and a compensatory increase in fetal insulin secretion. Conversely, maternal hypoglycemia can elicit fetal hypoglycemia and fetal suppression of insulin synthesis. Prolonged fetal exposure to uncontrolled maternal hyperglycemia can lead to persistent (excessive) glycogenesis. Manifestations include macrosomia and hypertrophic cardiomyopathy, which will be addressed later in this chapter (Krawczyk et al., 2022).

During the third trimester, fetal glycogen production and storage are increased (and abnormally upregulated in cases of uncontrolled maternal diabetes), with suppression of glycogenolysis. Cortisol and circulating insulin levels rise, which suppresses lipolysis and allows for subcutaneous energy storage. These subcutaneous storage sites, when established in adequate amounts, will become easily accessible sites for glucose mobilization in the hours immediately after birth (Tas et al., 2020; Wernimont & Norris, 2022). After birth, glucose concentrations are controlled by enteral or IV carbohydrate intake, glycogenolysis, and gluconeogenesis.

Postnatal Glucose Metabolism. The neonate's ability to independently produce glucose after the cessation of the transplacental lifeline is one of the most critical events involved in the "transition to extrauterine life" (**Figure 10.16**). Recall that both maternal and fetal glucose concentrations rise during labor (as glucose crosses the placenta). Once the umbilical cord is clamped and reduced, the newborn's glucose concentration decreases, and the plasma glucose nadir occurs within approximately 1 to 3 hours after birth (Sen et al., 2025). Among healthy, AGA, term newborns, a glucose nadir of 25 to 30 mg/dL may be observed over the first few hours of life with a range of 25 mg/dL to 110 mg/dL (Sen et al., 2025). During this time frame, three critical compensatory mechanisms should be activated in the newborn: (a) increased catecholamine and glucagon secretion, (b) "resetting" of insulin synthesis at higher glucose concentrations, and (c) the onset of glycogenolysis followed by gluconeogenesis (Adamkin, 2017; Poindexter & Martin, 2025; Tas et al., 2020). Importantly, hepatic enzymes must be present for glycogenolysis. Exogenous glucose precursors (enteral carbohydrates or IV dextrose) must be provided continuously or every 2 to 3 hours, as tolerated, to maintain adequate circulating glucose levels. Next, adequate stores of glycogen, free fatty acids, glycerol, amino acids, and lactate must be present within 3 to 4 hours of birth for gluconeogenesis to occur. Subsequently, over the following 48 to 72 hours after birth, the newborn's metabolic and endocrine system "resets" the threshold for insulin synthesis such that a higher glucose concentration (compared to in utero levels) must be reached before insulin is produced. By 72 hours of life, glucose concentrations in healthy, term, AGA newborns should range between 60 to 100 mg/dL (mean glucose 59+11 mg/dL within 48 hours of birth and 83+14 mg/dL after 72 hours of life; Sen et al., 2025).

Cerebral Glucose Utilization and Metabolism. All organs use glucose; however, the brain relies almost exclusively on glucose as its source for energy metabolism. Furthermore, cerebral glycogen stores are low, and for that reason, glucose delivery to the brain is an ongoing process that must be tightly regulated to maintain homeostasis. For infants, this is particularly important, as cerebral glucose requirements are increased compared to adults and alternative energy sources (lactate, ketone bodies) are limited. Cerebral glucose consumption accounts for a significant proportion of total glucose consumption in newborns. Given that the brain is disproportionately large in newborns, and there is likewise an increased brain-to-body ratio, a higher rate of glucose production occurs in newborns compared to older infants and children. Clearly, the brain is the primary driver for hepatic glucose production (Kalhan & Parimi, 2000, Sen et al., 2025).

Glucose is the largest contributor to ATP production, accounting for 72% to 84% of total cerebral ATP over the first 5 postnatal days (Sen et al., 2025). Once

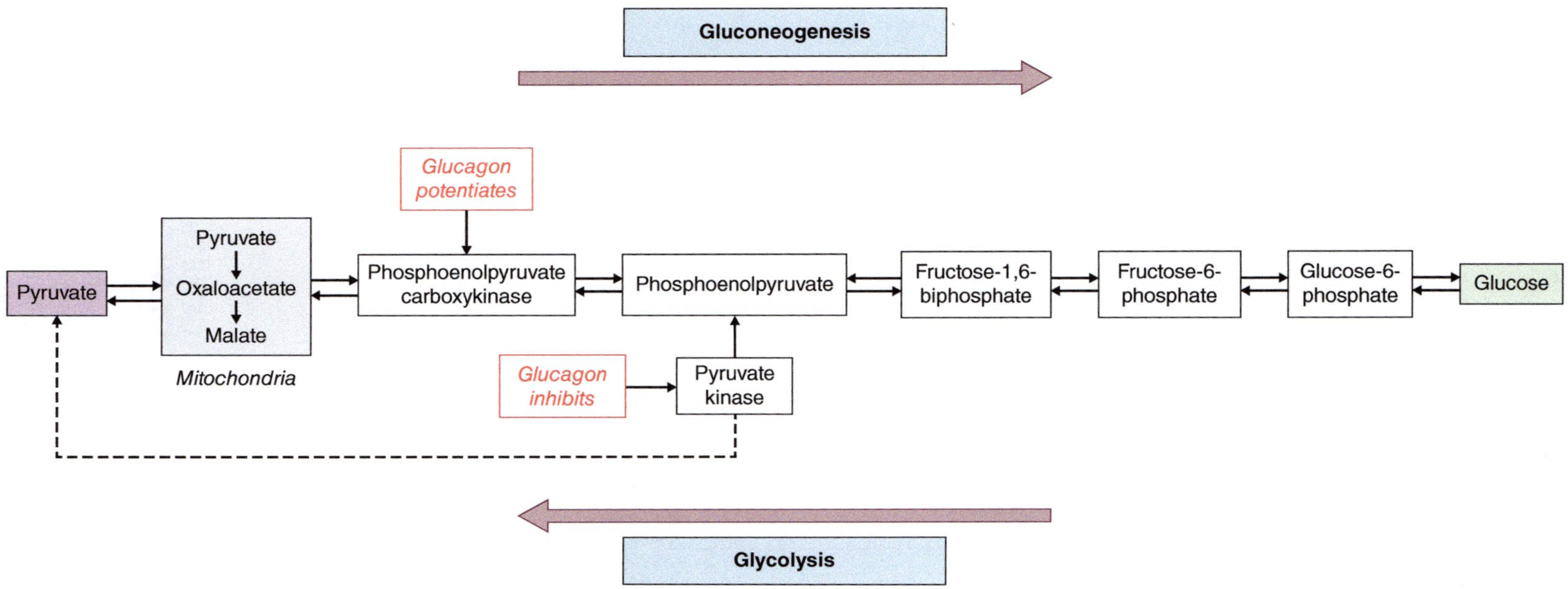

Figure 10.15 Gluconeogenesis and glycolysis pathways.

Note: This is a simplified depiction of both pathways. Several additional enzymes, including fructose-2,6-bisphosphatase, phosphofructokinase-1, and 6-phosphofructo-2-kinase, participate in the conversion of fructose to glucose. Glucagon exerts a potentiating effect on several of these enzymes in the gluconeogenesis pathway.

Image Credit: Amy J. Jnah.

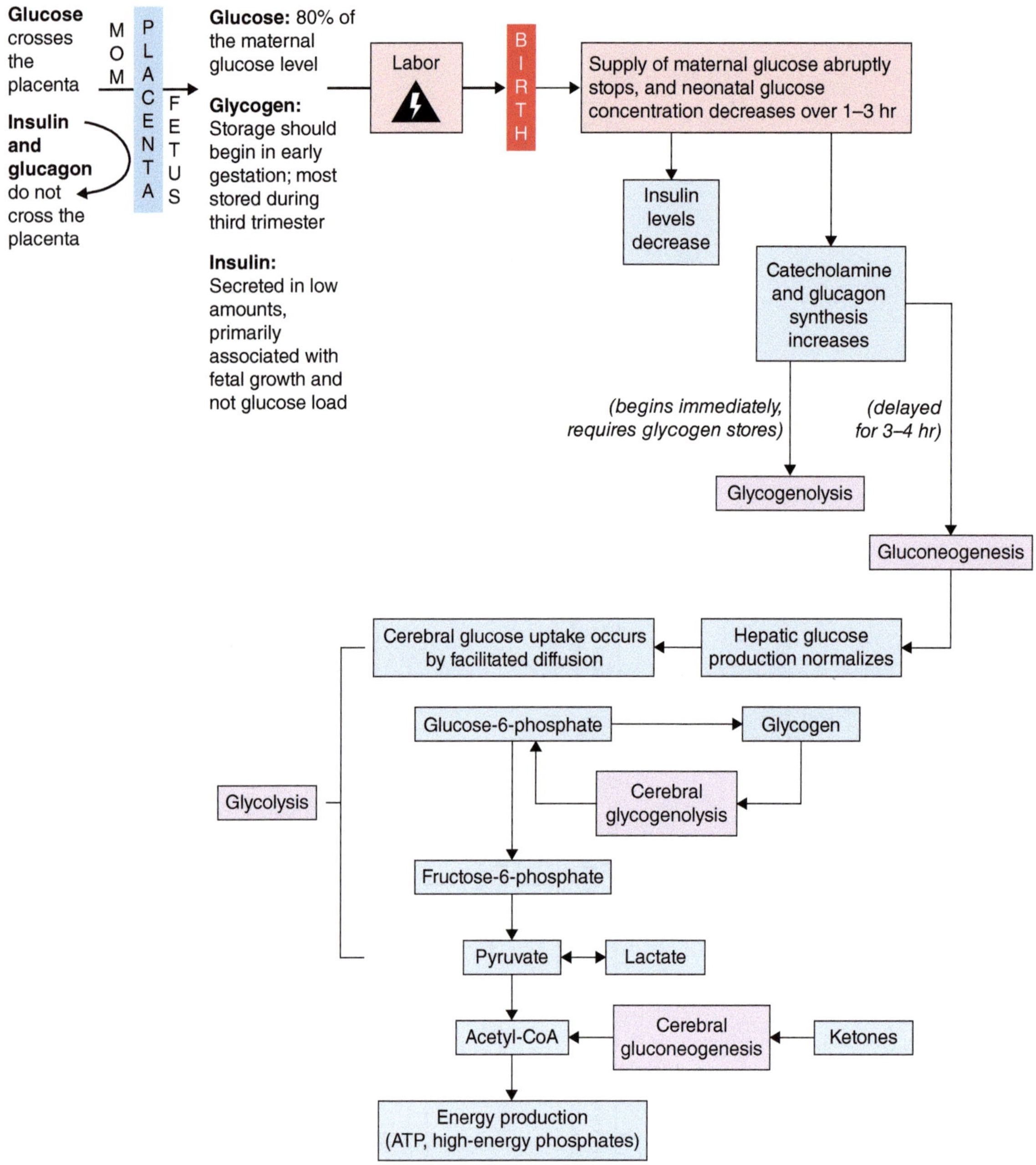

Figure 10.16 Normal postnatal glucose metabolism.

Note: The triangular alert icon provided at "birth" is intended to remind readers that traumatic events which occur in the intrapartum period and/or at the time of delivery of the infant can reduce or deplete energy stores in the fetus and exacerbate the postnatal glucose nadir as well as risk a severe reduction in glucose availability for cerebral uptake.

ATP, adenosine triphosphate.

Image Credit: Oksana Kasko and Amy J. Jnah.

glucose is available in the circulation, cerebral glucose uptake occurs by simple diffusion (active transport) with the use of GLUT transporters. Once glucose molecules enter the brain, each molecule of glucose can be oxidized to yield 38 molecules of ATP. Of note, preterm newborns are uniquely susceptible to reduced cerebral glucose uptake, as they often have 33% to 50% fewer GLUT transporters compared to term counterparts (Sen et al., 2025).

GENETIC INFLUENCES: INBORN ERRORS OF METABOLISM

Under normal circumstances, metabolic reactions occur within the body as a means to break down nutrients, such as amino acids, or to create energy, such as glucose. Inborn errors of metabolism (IEMs) occur secondary to genetic mutations that block normal metabolic pathways and cause disordered cellular functioning. The end result is an accumulation of toxic precursors (metabolites) or a deficiency of end-product production. IEMs are commonly classified by the pattern of inheritance, enzyme involvement, and clinical manifestations. These genetically influenced metabolic disorders commonly affect amino acid, carbohydrate, and lipid metabolisms, as well as other degradation pathways. Three common metabolic disorders are presented here, as is a list of the most commonly screened IEMs (Table 10.10).

TABLE 10.10 Newborn Screening Disorders Recommended Uniform Screening Panel

Metabolic Disorder (Type)	Screening Inborn Error of Metabolism
Organic acid	3-Hydroxy-3-methyglutaric aciduria
	3-Methylcrotonyl-CoA carboxylase deficiency
	ß-Ketothiolase deficiency
	Glutaric acidemia type I
	Holocarboxylase synthase deficiency
	Isovaleric acidemia
	Methylmalonic acidemia (cobalamin disorders)
	Methylmalonic acidemia (methylmalonyl-CoA mutase)
	Propionic acidemia
Fatty acid oxidation	Carnitine uptake defect/carnitine transport defect
	Long-chain L-3 hydroxyacyl-CoA dehydrogenase deficiency
	Medium-chain acyl-CoA dehydrogenase deficiency
	Trifunctional protein deficiency
	Very long-chain acyl-CoA dehydrogenase deficiency
Amino acid	Argininosuccinic aciduria
	Citrullinemia, type I
	Classic phenylketonuria
	Homocystinuria
	Maple syrup urine disease
	Tyrosinemia, type I
Endocrine	Congenital adrenal hyperplasia
	Primary congenital hypothyroidism
Hemoglobinopathies	S, ß-thalassemia
	S,C disease
	S,S disease (Sickle cell anemia)

(continued)

TABLE 10.10 Newborn Screening Disorders Recommended Uniform Screening Panel *(continued)*

Metabolic Disorder (Type)	Screening Inborn Error of Metabolism
Miscellaneous	Biotinidase deficiency
	Classic galactosemia
	Critical congenital heart disease
	Cystic fibrosis
	Glycogen storage disease type II (Pompe)
	Guanidinoacetate methyltransferase deficiency
	Hearing loss
	Infantile Krabbe disease
	Mucopolysaccharidosis type I and II
	Severe combined immunodeficiencies
	Spinal muscular atrophy
	X-linked adrenoleukodystrophy

Note: This list is non-exhaustive. Disorders provided in this table are commonly included in mandatory newborn screening tests across U.S. states. Clinicians are encouraged to consult their state laboratory and maintain awareness of inborn errors of metabolism screened in the state in which they practice.
Source: Advisory Committee on Heritable Disorders in Newborns and Children. (2024). *Recommended uniform screening panel.* https://www.hrsa.gov/advisory-committees/heritable-disorders/rusp/index.html

Disorders of Branched-Chain Amino Acid Metabolism

Recall that branched-chain ketoacids (BCKAs) are derived from the branched-chain amino acids (BCAAs) leucine, isoleucine, and valine. These are important precursors for gluconeogenesis, energy production, and the synthesis of cholesterol and fatty acids. BCAAs are commonly found in infant formulas and certain table foods (soy products, meats, fish, dairy products, and legumes). Once ingested, enzyme complexes facilitate the metabolism of valine, isoleucine, and leucine (**Figure 10.17**). The first step in the metabolic process involves transamination (transfer of one amino group to another) of BCAAs into BCKAs; this is facilitated by the enzyme branched-chain amino transferase (BCAT). The second step involves oxidative decarboxylation by way of the enzyme branched-chain ketoacid dehydrogenase (BCKDH). Disorders of BCAA metabolism often involve gene mutations that disrupt normal enzyme function. The most common BCAA disorder is maple syrup urine disease (MSUD).

Maple Syrup Urine Disease. MSUD is classified as an autosomal recessive disease and considered the most common disorder of BCKA metabolism. It is most often caused by mutations in the *BCKDHA, BCKDHB*, and *DBT* genes. Globally, classic type MSUD is diagnosed in one of every 185,000 newborns, and within the United States, MSUD is often diagnosed in the Mennonite population located within Lancaster County, Pennsylvania. An estimated one of every 176 newborns in Lancaster, Pennsylvania, is affected by MSUD (Kabbany & Murray, 2024). Five phenotypes of MSUD are reported in the literature (**Table 10.11**).

MSUD involves a disruption or dysfunction of enzyme complexes, commonly at step 2 (oxidative carboxylation). This results in toxic accumulation of both BCAA and BCKA, and failed synthesis of glutamate. Glutamate is a central nervous system (CNS) neurotransmitter, serving a key role in cognition, memory, and learning (Berry et al., 2025; Blackburn et al., 2017). Clinical manifestations of classic and intermediate MSUD present in the neonatal period, with the maple syrup urine odor noted as the most common manifestation of the disease process. Other clinical manifestations include irritability, feeding difficulties, CNS disturbances, and lethargy. Metabolic acidosis with an elevated anion gap can develop (Kabbany & Murray, 2024).

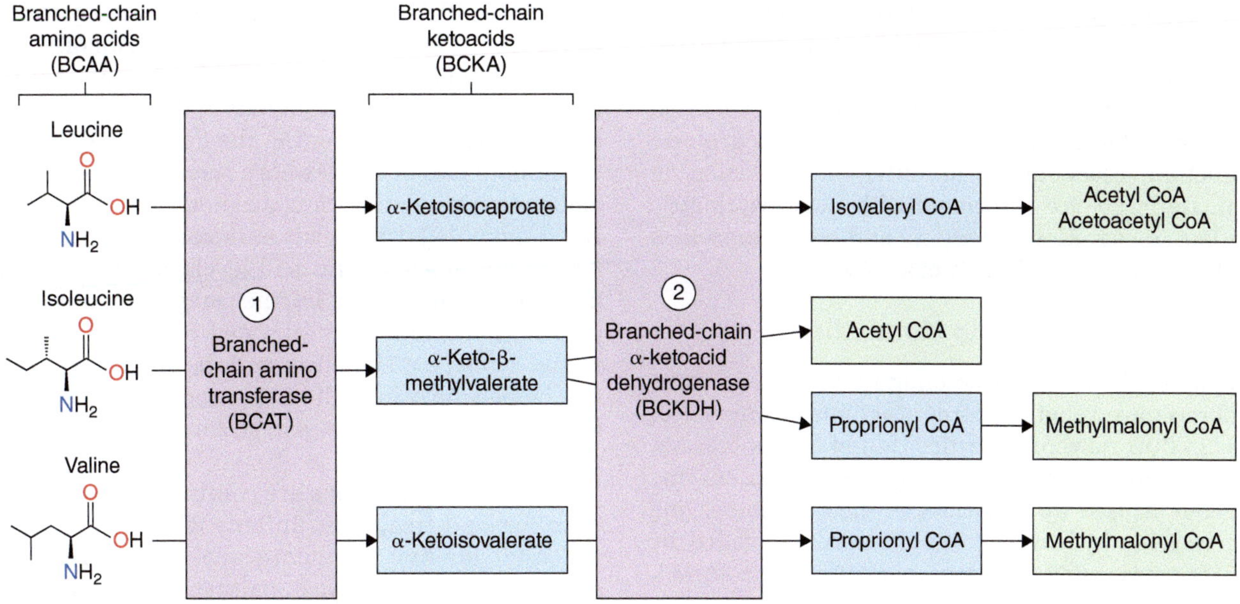

Figure 10.17 Branched-chain amino acid metabolism.
Note: (1) step 1 (transamination) in the degradation of branched-chain amino acids (BCAA). (2) step 2 in the degradation of branched-chain ketoacids (BCKA).
Image Credit: Amy J. Jnah.

TABLE 10.11 Five Phenotypes of Maple Syrup Urine Disease

MSUD Type	Gene Involvement	Onset of Symptoms	Common Clinical Manifestations
Classic	*BCKDHA, BCKDHB, DBT*	Neonatal period	*Neonatal period:* Maple syrup urine fragrance, irritability, feeding difficulties, lethargy, periodic apnea, opisthotonus *Infancy:* Nausea, anorexia, dystonia, ataxia *Childhood and beyond:* Cognitive impairment, sleep and mood disturbances, focal dystonia, ataxia
Intermediate type 1	*BCKDHA, BCKDHB, DBT*	Varies across the life span	*Neonatal period:* Maple syrup urine fragrance *Infancy and beyond:* Feeding difficulties, poor linear growth, developmental delay
Intermediate type 2	*BCKDHA, BCKDHB, DBT*	Varies across the life span	Stress-mediated encephalopathy
Thiamine-responsive	*DBT*	Varies across the life span	Same as intermediate manifestations
E3-deficient	*DLD*	Neonatal period or beyond	*Neurologic:* Hypotonia, lethargy, seizures, spasticity, emesis, hepatomegaly, poor linear growth/failure to thrive, developmental delays *Hepatic:* Nausea, emesis, hepatomegaly, hepatic encephalopathy

BCKDHA, branched chain keto acid dehydrogenase E1, alpha polypeptide; BCKDHB, branched chain keto acid dehydrogenase E1 subunit beta; DBT, dihydrolipoamide branched chain transacylase E2; DLD, dihydrolipoamide dehydrogenase; MSUD, maple sugar urine disease.
Source: Adapted from Blackburn, P. R., Gass, J. M., Vairo, F. P. E., Farnham, K. M., Atwal, H. K., Macklin, S., Klee, E. W., & Atwal, P. S. (2017). Maple syrup urine disease: Mechanisms and management. *The Application of Clinical Genetics, 10*, 57–66. https://doi.org/10.2147/TACG.S125962

Life-span implications of MSUD are directly related to elevated leucine levels and low circulating glutamate. Persistently elevated leucine levels are associated with altered water homeostasis within subcortical grey matter, encephalopathic syndrome, and associated neurologic dysfunction (Blackburn et al., 2017). Low circulating glutamate levels are associated with neuropsychiatric disorders of cognition, attention, and mood as well as cognitive impairment (Muelly et al., 2013).

Disorders of Amino Acid Metabolism

Phenylketonuria. Phenylketonuria (PKU) is an autosomal recessive genetic disorder that affects one out of every 25,000 newborns in the United States (Cleary, 2015; Merritt & Gallagher, 2024). PKU is an enzyme deficiency, caused by mutations in the hepatic enzyme phenylalanine hydroxylase (PAH), normally coded by the *PAH* gene located on chromosome 12 (Figure 10.18). PKU is detected on the newborn metabolic screening test as an abnormal ratio of phenylalanine (abnormally elevated) to tyrosine (abnormally decreased; Cleary, 2015; Merritt & Gallagher, 2024).

Phenylalanine is an essential amino acid. Under normal conditions, phenylalanine is hepatically metabolized by the PAH enzyme to tyrosine. Tyrosine is another essential amino acid that participates in the production of hormones, including thyroid hormones, epinephrine, and norepinephrine, as well as dopamine and melanin.

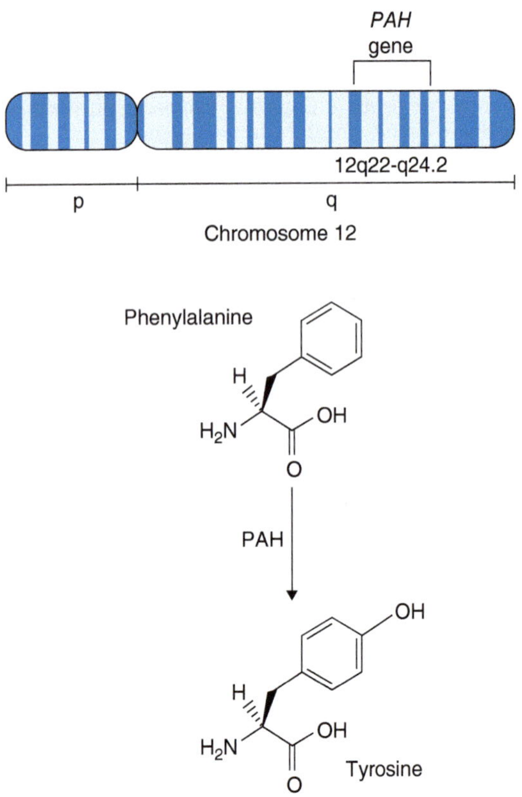

Figure 10.18 Genetic and molecular structure of PKU. PAH, phenylalanine hydroxylase; PKU, phenylketonuria.

In cases of PKU, the PAH enzyme deficiency impedes the ability to metabolize phenylalanine. Abnormally elevated levels of phenylalanine and low tyrosine levels are observed. Clinical manifestations of PKU are not evident at birth and rarely present in the first month of life because state-mandated newborn screening tests have facilitated early identification, diagnosis, and intervention. If left untreated, PKU leads to increased urinary phenyl ketone and phenylacetic acid levels, altering the smell of urine ("mousey odor"). Other manifestations include pale skin and blue eyes (elevated phenylalanine levels reduce tyrosine metabolism and the subsequent formation of melanin, which alters skin and eye pigmentation), low-circulating T_4 levels, and seizures (Merritt & Gallagher, 2024).

Life-span implications are contingent on early identification and treatment. Infants who remain undiagnosed for the first 3 or more weeks of life risk severe and irreversible cognitive impairment. A favorable long-term prognosis is offered to infants identified within the first week of life who are provided a medical diet supplemented with artificial amino acids. Females of childbearing age must undergo strict monitoring, as conception that occurs concurrent with a period of hyperphenylalanemia has been associated with maternal PKU syndrome, resulting in fetal growth restriction, microcephaly, congenital heart defects (CHDs), and other malformations (Cleary, 2015; Merritt & Gallagher, 2024).

Disorders of Hyperammonemia

The metabolism of amino acids, by way of the Krebs cycle, leads to the formation of ammonia, which is then converted to ammonium (a toxic molecule). Under normal circumstances, ammonium is subsequently hepatically (and to a smaller extent, renally) reduced to urea, a less toxic molecule (Figure 10.19). Urea is then transported via the circulation to the nephron, where it is eliminated in the urine. Alternatively, ammonium can interact with the enzyme glutamine synthetase, which is found within astrocytes in the brain, and convert glutamate into glutamine. Glutamine is an osmotically active molecule and can diffuse out of the brain. However, excessive accumulation of glutamine, which can occur with inborn errors of ammonia metabolism, can create an unfavorable osmotic shift and influx of water into the brain, risking cerebral edema, followed by ischemia and oligodendroglial and neuronal death. IEMs associated with a pathologic accumulation of ammonia include propionic acidemia (PA; an organic acidemia), methylmalonic acidemia (MMA; an organic acidemia), medium-chain Acyl-CoA dehydrogenase deficiency (MCADD; fatty acid oxidation defect), and mitochondrial disorders. Other conditions that can precipitate an abnormal accumulation of ammonia include prematurity (transient hyperammonemia) and perinatal asphyxia.

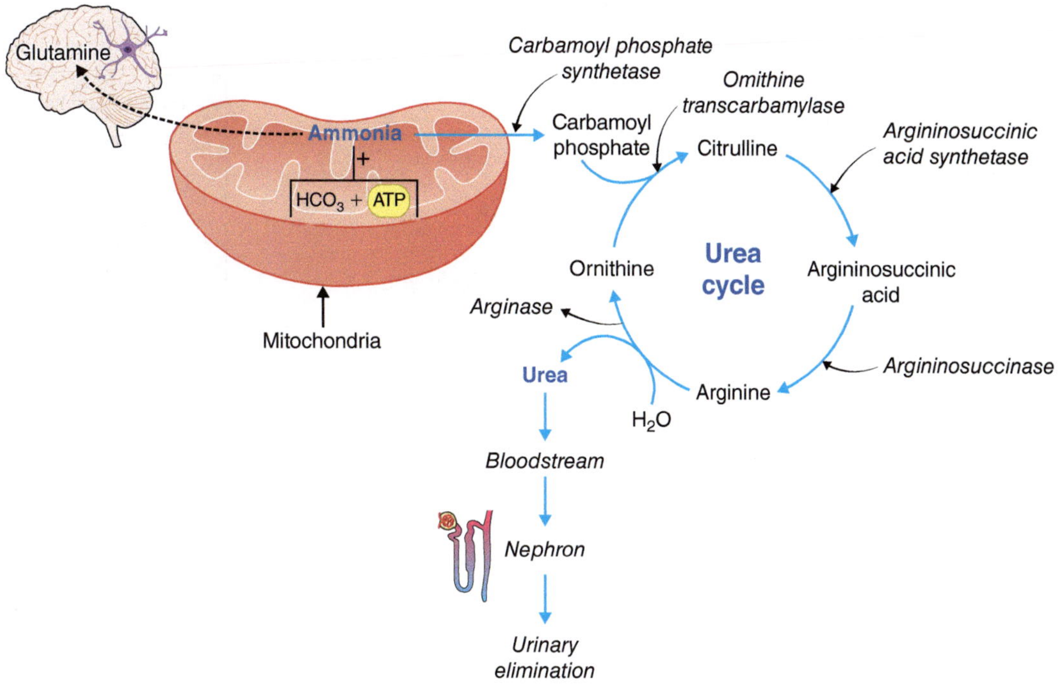

Figure 10.19 Pathways for ammonia metabolism.

Note: Solid arrows depict the principal method of ammonia biosynthesis, via the urea cycle (Krebs cycle), which results in the formation of urea for nitrogen removal from the body. Dotted arrows depict the alternative pathway of ammonia metabolism within the brain, at the level of astrocytes, which leads to the formation of glutamine. The overlying image of the brain includes the rendering of a single astrocyte, to enhance visual learning.

Image Credit: Amy J. Jnah.

Disorders of Organic Acid Metabolism

Organic acids are compounds that contain carboxylic acid. Disorders of organic acid metabolism occur due to an abnormal breakdown of amino acids and can manifest as an aciduria (accumulation of organic acids in the urine) and/or acidemia (accumulation of organic acids in the blood). In contrast to other IEMs, organic acidemias are rare, affecting between one in 20,000 to 250,000 newborns globally, per annum (National Organization for Rare Disorders [NORD], 2020). Both MMA and PA are the most commonly diagnosed organic acidemias in neonates and are the focus of this discussion.

IV or enterally administered lipids and proteins must be metabolized. Under normal circumstances, the catabolism of these lipids and fats, namely cholesterol, valine, odd-chain fatty acids, methionine, isoleucine, and threonine (cleverly memorized as "C-VOMIT" by scores of students!), proceeds in a stepwise fashion and results in the formation of succinyl CoA (**Figure 10.20**). Succinyl CoA participates in the Krebs cycle (or citric acid cycle), which leads to the production of energy in the form of high-energy phosphates. In situations where enzyme deficiencies present and organic acids cannot be metabolized to succinyl CoA, metabolic acidosis and hyperammonemia may develop.

PA is associated with *PCCA* or *PCCB* gene mutations. This causes a deficiency of the propionyl-CoA carboxylase enzyme and interrupts the normal process of catabolism of proteins and lipids. A deficiency of succinyl CoA develops with secondary inhibition of the urea cycle. This leads to metabolic acidosis and hyperammonemia. Other symptoms include seizures, tachypnea, hyperglycinemia, neutropenia, anemia, and/or thrombocytopenia (Berry et al., 2025). Long-term complications include metabolic encephalopathy, cardiomyopathy or arrythmias, movement disorders secondary to injury to the basal ganglia, and optic atrophy.

MMA is associated with *MMUT*, *MMAA*, or *MMAB* gene mutations. This causes a deficiency of the methylmalonyl-CoA mutase enzyme (most common), or the cobalamin A or cobalamin B enzymes. A deficiency of succinyl CoA develops with secondary inhibition of the urea cycle. As with PA, symptoms of MMA include metabolic acidosis and hyperammonemia, as well as seizures, tachypnea, hyperglycinemia, neutropenia, anemia, and/or thrombocytopenia (Berry et al., 2025). Long-term complications include metabolic encephalopathy, renal disease, hearing loss (acute or evolving), and movement disorders.

Clinical Application. Neonatal clinicians are encouraged to investigate the IEMs that are assessed on the state newborn metabolic

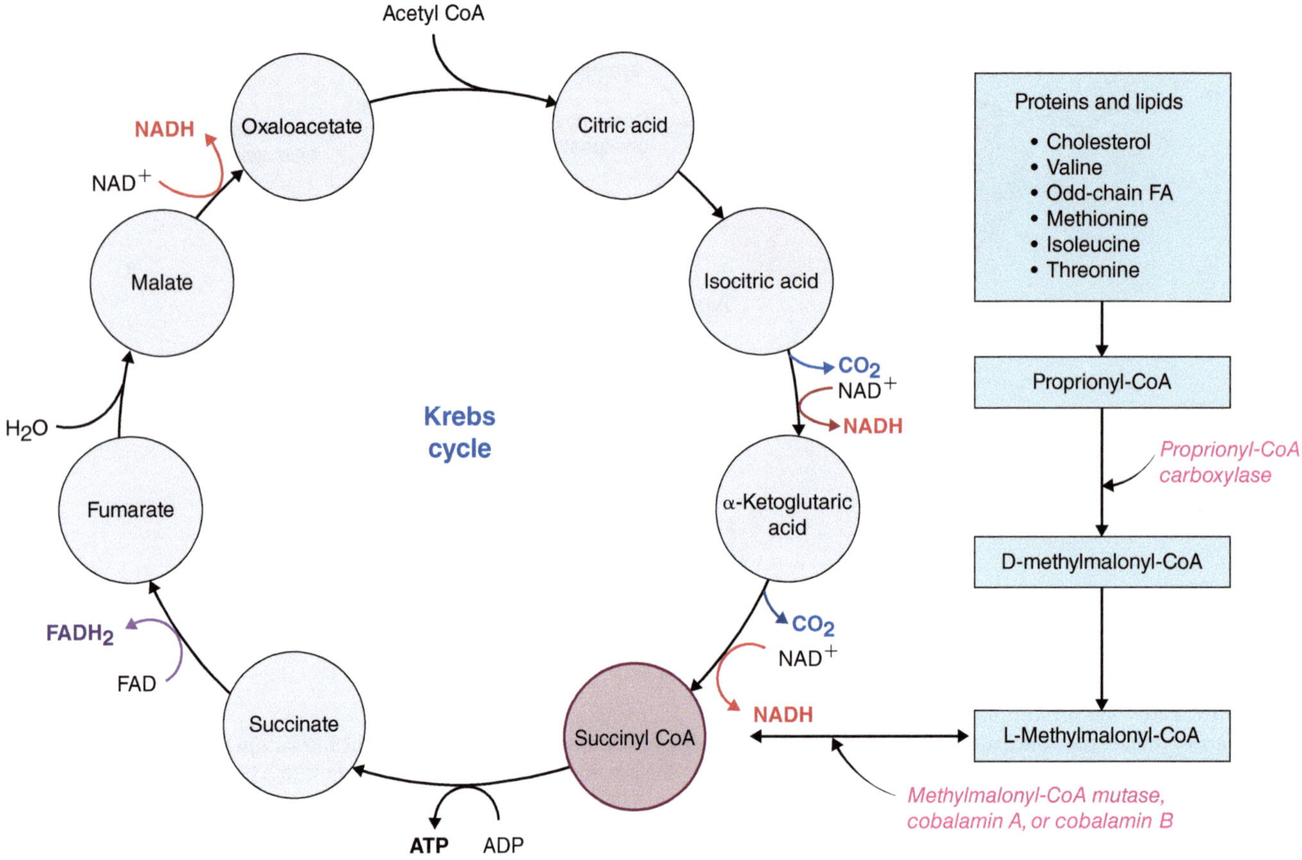

Figure 10.20 The metabolism of proteins and lipids with entry into the Krebs cycle.
ADP, adenosine diphosphate; ATP, adenosine triphosphate; CO2, carbon dioxide; FA, fatty acid; FAD, flavin adenine dinucleotide; FADH, reduced form of flavin adenine dinucleotide; NAD, nicotinamide-adenine; NADH, nicotinamide-adenine dinucleotide.
Image Credit: Amy J. Jnah.

screening test in the state in which they practice. In cases of MMA, the newborn screen may be returned with a positive result for "C4-DC" (methylmalonylcarnitine). A pediatric endocrinology consult is indicated, as further testing (2-methylcitrate, methylmalonic acid, 3-hydroxypropionate) will be indicated.

Disorders of Fatty Acid Metabolism

Free fatty acids are found in human milk and commercial formulas. These fatty acids comprise a substantial energy reserve within the body and provide significant energy to vital organs including the myocardium, skeletal muscle, and liver. Fatty acid oxidation leads to the production of energy, including ATP and ketones, which can be used during periods of fasting as a source of energy for the brain and peripheral tissues (Figure 10.21). This is particularly helpful for newborns with limited glycogen stores at birth.

Medium-Chain Acyl-CoA Dehydrogenase Deficiency. MCADD is the *most common* autosomal recessive inherited disorder of fatty acid oxidation. This disorder is associated with mutations at the *ACADM* and affects approximately one in every 50,000 liveborn infants globally (NORD, 2023). Only medium-chain fatty acids (C6-C12) are implicated with this disease.

Medium-chain acyl-CoA dehydrogenase (MCAD) is an enzyme that catalyzes the first step in β-oxidation of medium-chain fatty acids. With MCADD, the deficient MCAD enzyme complement decreases β-oxidation of medium-chain acyl-CoA molecules. The result is a toxic accumulation of medium-chain acyl-CoA within the mitochondria and inadequate formation of adequate high-energy phosphates. As the medium-chain acyl-CoA accumulates within the mitochondria, the toxic accumulation damages the inner mitochondrial membrane, allowing the molecules to escape the mitochondrial membrane. Some acyl-CoA molecules will enter the cytosol layer of the mitochondria, then the endoplasmic reticulum, and be converted into dicarboxylic acid which can enter the systemic circulation and be excreted

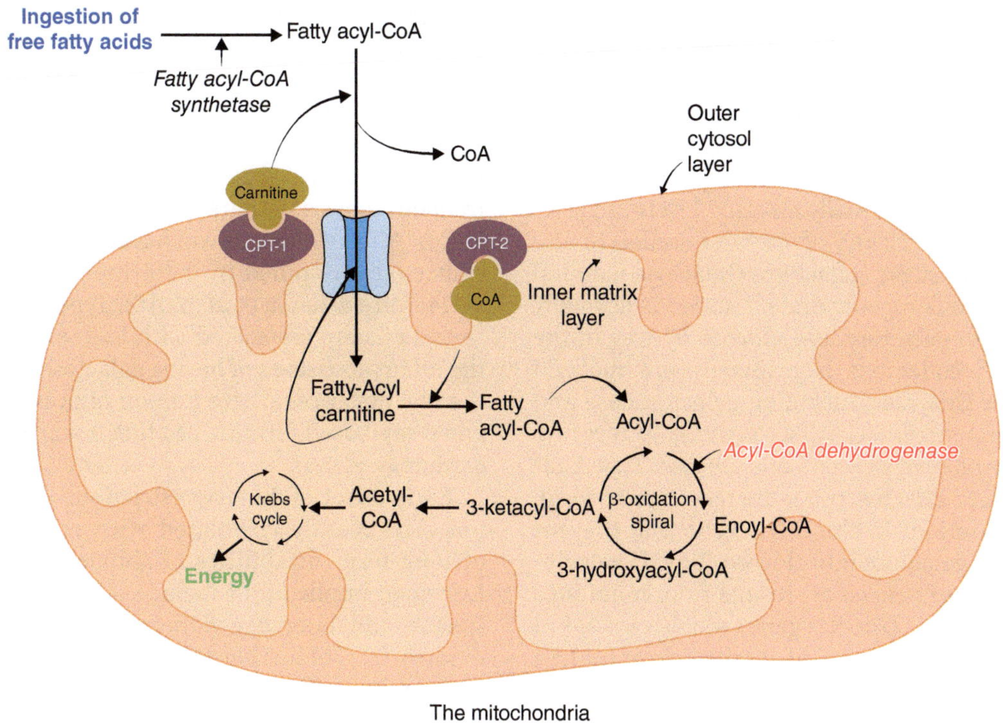

Figure 10.21 Basic overview of fatty acid oxidation.

Note: This image offers a broad overview of fatty acid oxidation of all types (short, medium, long-chain). Once cellular uptake has occurred, the enzyme fatty acyl-CoA synthetase converts the free fatty acid to fatty acyl-CoA. Next, the outer mitochondrial layer (cytosol) synthesizes the enzyme carnitine palmitoyltransferase I (CPT-1), which allows for binding of carnitine and dislodgement of CoA, producing fatty-acyl carnitine. Now, the molecule can enter the mitochondria. Upon entry, several additional reactions occur which lead to the production of acyl-CoA by carnitine palmitoyltransferase II (CPT-II), and then beta oxidation. Three enzymes participate in beta oxidation: acyl-CoA dehydrogenase, 3-hydroxyacyl CoA dehydrogenase, and e-ketoacyl CoA thiolase. Ultimately, acetyl-CoA is formed and can enter the Krebs cycle in order to produce high-energy phosphates.

Image Credit: Amy J. Jnah.

in the urine. Other molecules will enter the mitochondrial membrane and interact with the enzyme carnitine palmitoyltransferase I (CPT-1) in order to bind with carnitine, forming fatty acyl-CoA carnitine. This newly formed fatty acyl-CoA carnitine will enter the cytoplasm and then the systemic circulation.

Common observable manifestations include hypotonia, feeding intolerance, and respiratory distress. Metabolic symptoms include acidosis, hypoketotic hypoglycemia, hyperammonemia, and dicarboxylic aciduria. Further testing will show an abnormally high level of acylcarnitine and abnormally low proportion of free carnitine. The mortality risk is 45% in undiagnosed newborns, necessitating proper monitoring during the birth hospitalization and proper outpatient pediatric care coordination with diligent monitoring for the newborn metabolic screening test result (Berry et al., 2025).

Clinical Application. Newborn metabolic screening tests involve the performance of tandem mass spectrometry. As neonatal nurses are all too familiar, filter paper is used to collect drops of blood from the infant. Ideally, this test is performed after a newborn has been challenged with enteral nutrition, as the pathology of many inborn errors of metabolism will evolve only after exposure to human milk or commercial formula. In the case of MCADD, this fatty oxidation disorder leads to abnormally high blood acylcarnitine levels, and this can be detected by the state newborn screening lab. A “abnormal” or “critical” acylcarnitine result should prompt clinicians to pursue additional confirmatory diagnostic testing. In addition, it is crucial to evaluate for hypoglycemia, establish euglycemia, avoid periods of fasting, and consider the use of a high-carbohydrate and low-fat enteral diet.

Disorders of Carbohydrate Metabolism

Galactosemia. Galactosemia is an autosomal recessive inherited disorder caused by mutations in the *GALT*,

GALK1, and *GALE* genes. Three types of galactosemia are reported in the literature. Type I galactosemia occurs in one of every 30,000 to 60,000 newborns, type II is estimated to occur in less than one out of every 100,000 newborns, and type III galactosemia is extremely rare (Kabbany & Murray, 2024).

Galactosemia, or abnormally elevated levels of galactose, results from a deficiency of enzymes needed to metabolize the simple sugar, galactose. Galactose is found within lactose, a milk carbohydrate. Lactose is normally broken down into galactose and glucose by way of the lactase enzyme. Galactose is primarily metabolized within the liver. Enzymes, including galactokinase and Gal-1-P uridyl transferase (GALT), convert galactose into galactose 1-phosphate and eventually glucose. Type I galactosemia (classic galactosemia), the most severe form, results from mutations in the *GALT* gene that prevent the conversion of galactose into glucose. Type II galactosemia (galactokinase deficiency) results from mutations in the galactokinase 1 (*GALK1*) gene, which stunts, but does not completely eradicate, the production of GALK1 enzymes necessary for processing of galactose. Type III galactosemia results from mutations in the *GALE* gene responsible for providing instructions for making the enzyme UDP-galactose 4-epimerase, which is the final step in galactose metabolism (**Figure 10.22**; Berry, 2021).

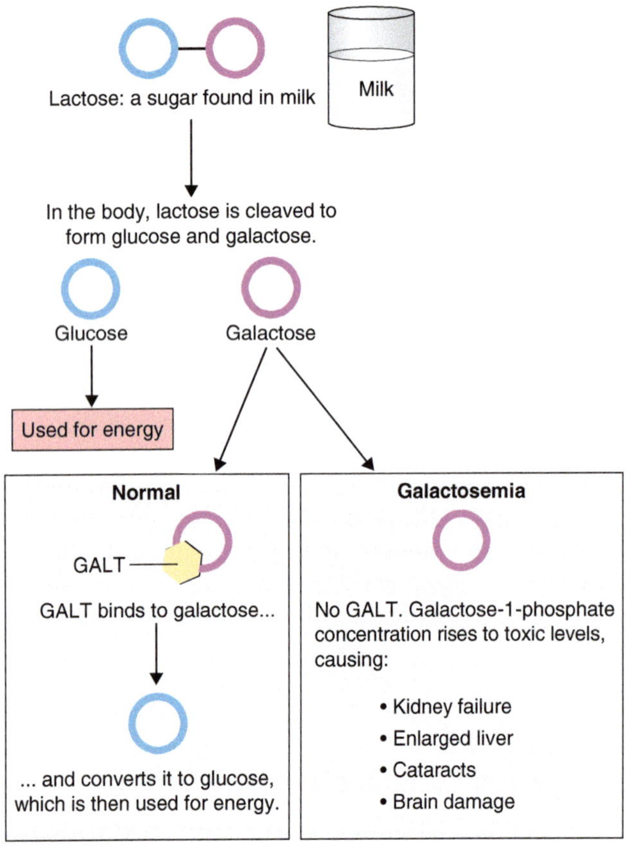

Figure 10.22 Normal lactose metabolism versus galactosemia. GALT, galactose-1-phosphate uridyl transferase.

Clinical manifestations vary depending on the affected gene mutation. Most newborns are typically well appearing after birth, and can remain so for the first 10 to 14 days of life. Thereafter, classic clinical manifestations of type I galactosemia include *Escherichia coli* bacteremia, hyperbilirubinemia, hepatomegaly, poor growth, frequent emesis, lethargy, and cataracts or cloudy optic lenses. Affected infants will have a positive reducing substance (sugar spilled in the urine; Kabbany & Murray, 2024; Varela-Lema et al., 2016). Type II and type III galactosemia are associated with less severe symptoms. In the infant suspected of having galactosemia, this is one of the few instances where human milk is contraindicated and a soy-based formula product is warranted (Kabbany & Murray, 2024).

Early onset of dietary restrictions and compliance is not significantly correlated with reduced observance of long-term disabilities (Kabbany & Murray, 2024). Life-span implications include intellectual impairment, speech and language deficits, apraxia/dyspraxia and dysarthria, motor disorders, and transient cataracts. Females with galactosemia may develop primary ovarian insufficiency. In addition, adolescents with galactosemia are at a higher risk for altered social function, often reporting difficulty coping with the disease process and maintaining compliance with the prescribed medical diet (Varela-Lema et al., 2016).

Clinical Application. Cataracts are an abnormal physical exam finding often noticed as a clinician is performing a red reflex examination. Any newborn with cataracts should be evaluated by a pediatric ophthalmologist and considered at-risk for galactosemia. This IEM is a standard part of mandatory state newborn metabolic screening tests and can be easily detected in newborns who did not receive a packed red blood cell transfusion prior to obtaining the newborn screening sample. Clinicians can always call the state laboratory and request an expedited turnaround time for results.

Endocrine Disorders

Congenital Hypothyroidism. In the majority of cases, CH is a sporadic occurrence; when inherited, it is an autosomal recessive pattern of inheritance. The incidence of CH in the United States is estimated at one of every 2,500 to 3,000 newborns, with the global incidence of CH on the rise due to the widespread adoption of rigorous newborn screening requirements and increased survivability of extremely premature infants (Kim et al., 2024; Sahai, 2024). Premature infants and infants of Hispanic or Asian descent are among those at a heightened risk for CH; females are twice as likely to be affected compared to male infants (Kim et al., 2024).

Two types of CH are known. Thyroid dysgenesis is the most common type of CH (85%) and involves the absence, hypoplastic development, or abnormal positioning of the gland. The exact cause of thyroid dysgenesis is unknown; however, the *PAX8*, *TSHR*, and *NKX2-5* genes are implicated with this genetic disorder and interrupt the normal genesis of the thyroid gland during fetal development (Kuhn-Riordon et al., 2022). Thyroid dyshormonogenesis is the second type of CH and involves a normal or enlarged thyroid gland (goiter) and associated decreased or absent synthesis of thyroid hormone. This inborn error of thyroid hormone biosynthesis occurs in up to 10% to 15% of all cases of CH. The *DUOX2*, *SLC5A5*, thyroglobulin (*TG*), and *TPO* genes undergo aberrant mutations, stunting or blocking the synthesis of thyroid hormone. The result is abnormally low-circulating thyroid hormone levels, which may be permanent and require lifelong hormone replacement, or transient with recovery to normal hormone synthesis within the first few years of life (**Figure 10.23**; Kim et al., 2024; Wassner & Brown, 2015).

The clinical presentation of CH may be nondescript and subtle. Common clinical manifestations of CH during the neonatal period and into infancy include large-for-gestational-age (LGA) status, a hoarse cry, decreased activity, fatigue with increased sleep interval, feeding difficulties, irregular stooling patterns, and prolonged physiologic hyperbilirubinemia lasting in excess of 3 weeks. Physical features that should increase the index of suspicion for CH include hypotonia, enlarged fontanelles (due to a lack of thyroid hormone production and resultant decreased bone maturation), facial edema, macroglossia, and the presence of abdominal distention with a coexisting umbilical hernia. CH can be associated with trisomy 21; midline defects, including cleft palate, cardiac and genitourinary malformations; and liver hemangiomas (Kim et al., 2024; Wassner, 2017).

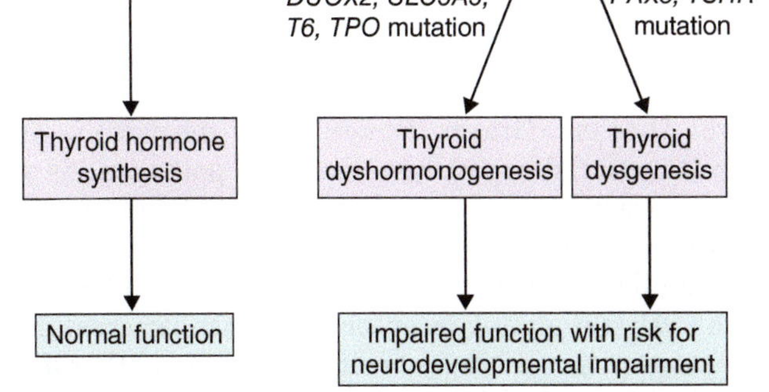

Figure 10.23 Normal thyroid function versus congenital hypothyroidism.
TPO, thyroperoxidase.

It is particularly important for practicing clinicians to appreciate the significance of performing a second metabolic screening test after the first month of life among premature infants, low birthweight infants, or critically ill infants, as TSH synthesis may be delayed until the third week of postnatal life, thereby providing a false negative result on the initial newborn screen (Kim et al., 2024; Sahai, 2024).

Life-span implications are primarily focused on neurodevelopmental delays. CH is the leading cause for cognitive impairment within the United States and on a global level. IQ and timing of diagnosis with subsequent treatment are inversely related; earlier identification is advantageous to affected infants and families.

NOTEWORTHY DISEASES IN THE XX PREGNANT PATIENT THAT INFLUENCE FETAL METABOLIC AND ENDOCRINE DEVELOPMENT AND FUNCTION

The maternal endocrine system undergoes significant changes prenatally to support the pregnancy and the developing fetus. Alterations in these changes lead to complications that can be experienced by the fetus and/or XX pregnant patient (Frise & Williamson, 2013). Myriad acute, chronic, and pregnancy-induced health issues can implicate fetal endocrine development as several hormones, minerals, and proteins are known to cross the placenta (**Table 10.12**). Disruptions in placental phosphate transfer observed with preeclampsia, chorioamnionitis, and placental infections increase the risk for IUGR and the acquisition of rickets. Thyroid disorders and diabetes in XX pregnant patients are two additional common disease states that can negatively affect the developing metabolic and endocrine system. Both disease processes are discussed in this section of the chapter. Additional disorders that affect the developing fetal endocrine system are summarized in **Table 10.13**.

Thyroid Disease

The developing fetus relies heavily on maternal production of thyroid hormones during the first few months of pregnancy, as these hormones are crucial for normal

TABLE 10.12 Hormones That Cross the Placenta and Influence the Developing Fetus

Organ	Physiologic Influence
Adrenal	*Glucocorticoids*: Increased deoxycorticosterone, CBG, ACTH, and free cortisol leading to physiologic hypercortisolism *Mineralocorticoids*: Stimulation of the RAA system leading to increased plasma volume
Pancreas	Diabetogenic state due to placental-hormone-inducing insulin resistance Maternal pancreatic dysfunction induces GDM
Parathyroid	Ionized calcium values are normal; intestinal calcium absorption increases; calcium is transferred to the fetus
Pituitary	*Anterior*: Proliferation of prolactin-producing cells; increased GH *Posterior*: Increased oxytocin and AVP; decreased serum sodium causes decreased osmolality requiring adjustment of osmoreceptors for thirst sensation and release of ADH
Thyroid	Increased TBG leading to higher levels of T_3/T_4 Relative iodine deficiency due to transplacental transfer to the fetus

ACTH, adrenocorticotropic hormone; ADH, antidiuretic hormone; AVP, arginine vasopressin; CBG, corticosteroid binding globulin; GDM, gestational diabetes mellitus; RAA, renin–angiotensin–aldosterone; TBG, thyroxine binding globulin; T_3, triiodothyronine; T_4, thyroxine.
Source: Data from Soma-Pillary, P., Nelson-Piercy, C., Tolppanen, H., & Mebazaa, A. (2016). Physiological changes in pregnancy. *Cardiovascular Journal of Africa, 27*(2), 89–94. https://doi.org/10.5830/CVJA-2016-021

brain development. Thyroid hormones can cross the placenta, and as such fetal growth and development can be negatively implicated by maternal thyroid disease. Thyroid disease is the second most common disease during pregnancy (Singh & Sandhu, 2023).

Hypothyroidism. Hypothyroidism involves the underproduction of circulating thyroid hormone. This disorder can develop prior to or during pregnancy. Hypothyroidism is a relatively common problem among pregnant patients of reproductive age, with a reported incidence ranging from 3% to 5% combined for overt and subclinical hypothyroidism (Abadi et al., 2023; Singh & Sandhu, 2023). Risk factors for pregnant patients include nutrient deficiencies and food sensitivities, adrenal dysfunction, and bacterial and viral infections.

Hashimoto Thyroiditis. With Hashimoto thyroiditis, antithyroid antibodies cross the placenta, causing decreased fetal circulating TSH and elevated T_4 levels. Significant fetal and maternal mortality risks are associated with persistently abnormal circulating thyroid hormone levels, including spontaneous abortion, intrauterine fetal demise, IUGR, fetal malformations, and maternal morbidity and mortality risks. Fetal manifestations to maternally acquired Hashimoto thyroiditis include arrhythmias and decreased cardiac output secondary to prolonged TSH suppression. Both manifestations require emergent delivery (Singh & Sandhu, 2023; Tudosa et al., 2010).

Early establishment of maternal euthyroid status significantly reduces the risks for immediate and long-term maternal and fetal/neonatal complications. With proper medical management, it is possible to carry a fetus to term without severe complications (Tudosa et al., 2010). Postnatal manifestations of maternal Hashimoto thyroiditis include congenital anomalies, acidosis, tachycardia, pulmonary hypertension, reduced cardiac output, and the onset of a congenital hypothyroid state. Lifespan implications associated with poorly controlled maternal thyroid hormone levels include low IQ and impaired psychomotor development (Kim et al., 2024).

Hyperthyroidism. Hyperthyroidism involves overproduction of circulating thyroid hormone. This disorder can develop prior to or during pregnancy. The incidence of maternal hyperthyroidism during pregnancy is 0.1% to 0.4%, although the incidence of transient disease states is 1.5% to 2.5% (Singh & Sandhu, 2023; van der Kaay et al., 2016). XX pregnant patients incur a fourfold higher risk for developing hyperthyroid disease as compared to men.

Graves Disease. Graves disease is the most common cause of maternal hyperthyroidism. The pathogenesis of Graves disease involves autoimmunity to TSH receptors. Antibodies bind to the TSH receptors, activating them and stimulating overproduction of thyroid hormone. These TSH-stimulating receptor antibodies can cross the placenta, and as such may facilitate fetal hyperthyroidism (after 20 weeks of gestation).

Generally speaking, medically managed hyperthyroidism does not complicate pregnancy. Fetal manifestations of poorly controlled maternal thyroid hormone

TABLE 10.13 Endocrine Disorders in Pregnant Patients That Influence the Developing Fetus

Organ	Abnormality	Effect(s) on Pregnancy
Adrenal	Cushing syndrome	Hypercortisolemia: weight gain, fatigue, glucose intolerance, hypertension
	Conn syndrome (primary hyperaldosteronism)	Hypokalemia, hypertension, proteinuria, placental abruption, preterm delivery
	Adrenal insufficiency	N&V, weight loss, hyperpigmentation, weakness, hyponatremia, hypoglycemia
	Congenital adrenal hyperplasia	Virilization, salt wasting, adult hirsutism, menstrual irregularity, subfertility, PIH, GDM
	Pheochromocytoma	Hypertension, placental insufficiency, placental abruption
Parathyroid	Hyperparathyroidism	Hypertension, preeclampsia, maternal mortality secondary to pancreatitis, maternal and fetal mortality secondary to hypercalcemic crisis
Pituitary	Prolactinoma	Reduced GRH: Infertility Maternal visual disturbances
	Acromegaly	PIH, GDM
	Pituitary insufficiency	Miscarriage; stillbirth
	Lymphocytic hypophysitis	ACTH deficiency
	Diabetes insipidus	Worsening of symptoms secondary to increased placental production of vasopressin
Thyroid	Hypothyroidism	Lethargy, weight gain, constipation, cold intolerance, bradycardia, amenorrhea, infertility, miscarriage, anemia, preeclampsia, LBW infant
	Hyperthyroidism	Infertility, miscarriage, preterm delivery, fetal growth restriction, fetal hyperthyroidism, goiter

ACTH, adrenocorticotropic hormone; GDM, gestational diabetes mellitus; GRH, gonadotropin-releasing hormone; LBW, low birthweight; N&V, nausea and vomiting; PIH, pregnancy-induced hypertension.

Source: Adapted from Frise, C. J., & Williamson, C. (2013). Endocrine disease in pregnancy. *Clinical Medicine: The Journal of the Royal College of Physicians, 13*(2), 176–181. https://doi.org/10.7861/clinmedicine.13-2-176

levels include tachycardia, heart failure with nonimmune hydrops, IUGR, preterm birth, and advanced skeletal maturation and craniosynostosis (van der Kaay et al., 2016). Thyroid storm, a life-threatening complication of hyperthyroidism, is rarely reported yet is associated with maternal fever, dehydration, diarrhea, cardiac dysrhythmias, shock, and maternal and fetal death (Kim et al., 2024).

Diabetes Mellitus

Diabetes is a metabolic disease resulting from defects in insulin secretion and/or insulin action that causes a hyperglycemic state. The World Health Organization (WHO) offers three major classifications for diabetes: type 1, type 2, and gestational diabetes. Other rarer forms of diabetes are reported and involve impaired glucose tolerance and fasting hyperglycemia (WHO, 2023).

Gestational diabetes mellitus (GDM), or glucose intolerance during pregnancy, affects up to 14% of all pregnancies in the United States; globally, approximately 20.9 million pregnancies are impacted (Melchior et al., 2017; Ornoy et al., 2015; Vambergue & Fajardy, 2011). Onset of GDM typically occurs in the second trimester. The etiology for GDM is rather poorly understood, yet it is accepted that GDM primarily occurs as a result of deficient pancreatic ß-cell responses to hyperglycemia, which promotes increased insulin resistance and decreased insulin sensitivity (Daher, 2015). The increased accumulation of adipose tissue among pregnant patients with GDM may also be associated with increased circulating inflammatory mediators (C-reactive protein, IL-6, and TNF-a), which may contribute to the pathogenesis of GDM.

Prolonged hyperglycemia has a significant impact on fetal well-being and the health of the pregnant patient. Consequences to the pregnant woman include cardiovascular disease and dysfunction as well as organ failure. Fetal sequela includes macrosomia; microsomia; defects of the cardiovascular, vascular, renal, GI, and neurologic systems; and death (Weiner et al., 2025).

COMMON PROBLEMS WITH IMPLICATIONS ACROSS THE LIFE SPAN

Many problems associated with the metabolic and endocrine system are genetically inherited (see the section "Genetic Influences: Inborn Errors of Metabolism"). The syndrome of inappropriate antidiuretic hormone (SIADH), AI, and OoP are three commonly *acquired* problems that affect normal metabolic and endocrine function.

Hypoglycemia

It is imperative that neonatal APRNs identify newborns at risk for an impaired metabolic transition to extrauterine life as well as quickly identify newborns who are presenting with clinical symptoms of hypoglycemia. Conditions that favor the development of hypoglycemia are summarized in Table 10.14.

TABLE 10.14 Risk Factors for Hypoglycemia and Associated Disorders

Risk Factor	Common Associations
Insufficient glycogen stores	• IUGR • Prematurity
Decreased glucose availability	• IUGR • Prematurity • Systemic hypotension
Decreased alternative energy sources (lactate, ketones)	• Absent or decreased gluconeogenesis • IUGR • Prematurity
Decreased cortisol, growth hormone	• Hypopituitarism
Decreased fatty acid oxidation	• Medium chain acyl-CoA dehydrogenase deficiency
Impaired galactose metabolism	• Galactosemia
Impaired glucose-6-phosphatate function	• Glycogen storage diseases
Impaired fructose-1-phosphate metabolism	• Hereditary fructose intolerance
Increased systemic glucose consumption	• Hypothermia • Infection • Respiratory distress
Increased cerebral glucose consumption	• Hypoxia ischemia • Seizure disorder
Increased insulin synthesis	• Beckwith-Wiedemann syndrome • Congenital hyperinsulinism • IDM • Turner syndrome

GH, growth hormone; IDM, infants born of diabetic mothers; IUGR, intrauterine growth restriction.

Source: Adapted from Rozance, P. J., & Wright, C. J. (2021). The neonate. In M. B. Landon, H. L. Galan, E. R. M. Jauniaux, D. A. Driscoll, V. Berghella, W. A. Grobman, S. J. Kilpatrick, & A. G. Cahill (Ed.), *Obstetrics: Normal and problem pregnancies* (8th ed., pp. 430–458). Elsevier.

Cerebral Responses to Hypoglycemia. A state of hypoglycemia, particularly when glucose concentrations fall below 30 mg/dL, elicits cerebral compensatory responses. First, the brain attempts to compensate for the abrupt loss of circulating glucose by increasing cerebral blood flow. The theory is rather simple: increasing blood flow is an attempt to quickly usher as much remaining glucose as possible to neurons, using as many available capillaries as possible. This compensatory response is short-lived, as it does not restore a normal glucose infusion rate to the brain. In addition, cerebral glycogenolysis may be initiated in an attempt to generate energy, if glycogen stores are available. Glycogenolysis involves the biochemical conversion of glycogen to glucose and will be described in the following section of this chapter (Box 10.2).

Next, alternative energy sources may be utilized, as available, to provide the brain with a compensatory source of chemical energy, in the form of ATP, for brain metabolism. These alternative sources include lactate and pyruvate, hepatic-generated ketone bodies, amino acids, and free fatty acids (Harris et al., 2021). Lactate is available in the immediate postnatal period and can provide upwards of 25% of necessary ATP, making it the second-largest source of energy for the brain. Under normal physiologic conditions, lactate enters neurons and is utilized as an energy source. During episodes of hypoglycemia or hypoxia, increased lactate uptake from the circulation and into the brain occurs, and lactation

BOX 10.2 Early Cerebral Responses to Hypoglycemia

↑ Cerebral blood flow
↑ Cerebral glycogenolysis
↑ Cerebral lactate production

is oxidized to pyruvate and used as energy. In contrast to glucose, lactate, and pyruvate, ketone bodies are not an effective source of ATP during episodes of early postnatal hypoglycemia and throughout the first 48 hours of life; overall, ketones contribute only 7% of the total ATP for brain metabolism (Stanley et al., 1979). In fact, most newborns present with *hypo*ketotic hypoglycemia in the newborn period. Afterward, ketones can be converted to acetyl-CoA and then to ATP for brain metabolism. Finally, amino acids and free fatty acids can be used as alternative energy sources in the brain, but at the expense of degradation of structural aspects of brain tissue and rising ammonia levels (as amino acids are catabolized). Recall that phospholipids (which form the membrane of neurons, glia, and other cells) must be degraded in order to produce free fatty acids (Hawkes et al., 2022; Sen et al., 2025).

Should hypoglycemia become severe or persistent, cerebral glucose metabolism will become severely diminished, as will the production of high-energy phosphates. The metabolism of alternative energy sources is significantly upregulated. For example, amino acid catabolism leads to a 10- to 15-fold increase in cerebral ammonia levels (Sen et al., 2025). These compensatory responses are not sufficient to curb the decline in high-energy phosphates and give way to a series of additional and deleterious effects. Once energy levels drop to the level that neurons can no longer maintain ion gradients, the Na+/K+ pump fails, and abnormal ion movements trigger the Na+/Ca++ exchanger pathway. The result is an abnormal extracellular accumulation of potassium and intracellular accumulation of sodium and calcium. The intracellular accumulation of calcium precipitates the abnormal accumulation of glutamate and aspartate (excitatory amino acid neurotransmitters) and accumulation of reactive oxygen and nitrogen species. In aggregate, these events lead to excitotoxic neuronal damage and apoptosis (Sen et al., 2025; Box 10.3).

Clinical Application. There remains no consensus between the American Academy of Pediatrics (AAP) and the Pediatric Endocrine Society (PES) on a glucose concentration threshold that requires intervention by neonatal clinicians. The AAP defines "operational thresholds," or

BOX 10.3 Cerebral Responses to Severe or Prolonged Hypoglycemia

↑↑ Alternative energy source metabolism
↑ Extracellular accumulation of K+
↑ Intracellular accumulation of Na+ and Ca++
↑ Accumulation of excitatory amino acid neurotransmitters (glutamate, aspartate)
↑ Excitotoxic neuronal damage and apoptosis

glucose concentrations that warrant treatment consideration (less than 40 mg/dL within the first 4 hours of life and less than 45 mg/dL within the first 24 hours of life). The PES defines normative glucose concentrations for healthy newborns (greater than 50 mg/dL within the first 48 hours of life and greater than 60 mg/dL after 48 hours of life) and newborns diagnosed with a metabolic or endocrine disorder (greater than 70 mg/dL at all times). Given how crucial adequate cerebral glucose uptake is for brain health and development, neonatal clinicians should dutifully ensure that at-risk newborns and symptomatic newborns are properly screened for hypoglycemia, and treatment is promptly initiated.

Special Populations: The Late-Preterm and Small-for-Gestational-Age Infant. *Late-preterm infants* are defined as those born between 34 and 36 6/7 weeks of gestation. *SGA* infants are defined as infants who weigh less than 2,500 grams and fall below the 10th percentile for their stated gestational age. Both of these special populations incur an increased risk for hypoglycemia within the first few days of life because they often lack adequate glycogen stores, the primary source of glucose in the first 6 hours of postnatal life, as well as triglyceride stores and a delayed maturation of enzymes necessary for gluconeogenesis. In addition, decreased glucose production in the liver, limited fat stores and ketogenesis, and the inability to oxidize free fatty acids and triglycerides and hyperinsulinism are often present (Edmundson & Jnah, 2024; Werny et al., 2024).

Clinical Application. Neonatal clinicians should screen all newborns for risk factors for hypoglycemia. Among SGA newborns, the initiation of enteral feedings within the first hour of life (in infants deemed eligible for enteral nutrition) and use of point-of-care glucose screenings shortly after birth (usually beginning at 1 hour of life) is essential to maintain adequate cerebral glucose uptake. Judicious use of glucose gel, supplemental use of donor breast milk or commercial formula among breastfed newborns, reduced intervals between feedings to shorten the fasting window, and/or increased enteral caloric intake with the use of higher-calorie commercial formulas are often very helpful in establishing and maintaining euglycemia.

Special Populations: The Infant of a Diabetic Mother. An IDM is defined as a newborn whose birthing parent has been diagnosed with diabetes before (type 1 or 2 diabetes) or during (gestational diabetes) pregnancy. The incidence of diabetes during pregnancy continues to rise, with over 21 million pregnancies affected by diabetes in 2021; of that total, 19.7% were classified as type 1 or 2 and 80.3% were diagnosed as gestational diabetes (Magliano et al., 2021).

Given that glucose easily diffuses across the placenta, the fetal glucose concentration will mimic the maternal concentration. Fetal hyperglycemia that develops early into pregnancy has been linked to increased oxidative stress, the production of reactive oxygen species, and an increased risk for diabetic embryopathy (Suhonen et al., 2000). A persistently high glucose load induces a compensatory increased synthesis of insulin (hyperinsulinemia) with upregulated glycogenesis and oxidative stress. The fetal metabolic rate increases, as does oxygen consumption, which leads to a chronic state of hypoxemia (due to oxygen offloading from tissue metabolic demand). This is evidenced by increased erythropoietin production and hematopoiesis, and postnatal polycythemia (hematocrit greater than 65%) and hyperbilirubinemia. Hyperinsulinemia is associated with hypertrophy and hyperplasia of pancreatic beta cells, which influences the growth of insulin-dependent organs and is associated with organomegaly. Of note, glycogen can be stored in the myocardial tissues and precipitate hypertrophic cardiomyopathy, which can progress to heart failure secondary to ongoing oxidative stress. Hyperinsulinism is also associated with suppressed cortisol production, which discourages surfactant synthesis and can manifest as postnatal respiratory distress syndrome. Additionally, hyperinsulinemia is associated with increased accretion of body fat, LGA status at birth, and macrosomia (Garg & Devaskar, 2025; Weiner et al., 2025). Approximately 5% to 27% of IDMs go on to develop hypoglycemia in the immediate newborn period, which can remain problematic for the first 3 to 7 days of life (Lord & DeLeón-Crutchlow, 2025). The subsequent downregulation of insulin synthesis occurs slowly, usually over the first 3 to 7 days of life, before reaching adult levels (Kansra, 2023; Lord & DeLeón-Crutchlow, 2025; Werny et al., 2024).

Life Span Implications of Neonatal Hypoglycemia. There remains no consensus between the AAP and the PES on a glucose concentration threshold that requires intervention by neonatal clinicians (Adamkin, 2017; Tas et al., 2020; Thornton et al., 2015). The AAP defines "operational thresholds," or glucose concentrations that warrant treatment consideration (less than 40 mg/dL within the first 4 hours of life and less than 45 mg/dL within the first 24 hours of life). The PES defines normative glucose concentrations for healthy newborns (greater than 50 mg/dL within the first 48 hours of life and greater than 60 mg/dL after 48 hours of life) and those diagnosed with a metabolic or endocrine disorder (greater than 70 mg/dL at all times).

Given that the glucose is the primary metabolic fuel for the brain, and AAP recommendations may not be inclusive of the operational threshold at which clinicians should be considering treatment to preserve neuronal health, investigators have attempted to define the minimum glucose concentration necessary to elicit the postnatal "reset" of insulin synthesis and maintain adequate cerebral glucose utilization (Edmundson & Jnah, 2024). It is certainly indisputable that persistent hypoglycemia should be avoided, and ample methods are available (e.g., glucose gel, higher calorie commercial formulas, supplemental donor breast milk, reduced intervals between oral feeding times, dextrose-containing IV fluids) to prevent and treat hypoglycemia in the neonatal period. What remains to be agreed upon is a pathologic glucose nadir and hypoglycemia exposure time frame that must be avoided to protect brain health and long-term cognition during childhood and possibly beyond.

Pyrds and colleagues (1990) and Powers and colleagues (1998) both reported that glucose concentrations less than 54 mg/dL are associated with reduced glucose transport to the brain and reduced glucose availability and utilization. Lucas et al. (1988) reported that in at-risk preterm infants, glucose concentrations less than 47 mg/dL on at least one occasion were associated with reduced math performance and motor disability through age 8. Tin and colleagues (2012) reported that a glucose level of less than 46 mg/dL within the first 24 hours of life is associated with a 3.7-fold increased risk for brain injury visible on MRI and 4.8-fold increased odds of lower motor, cognitive, and language scores at 1 year of age (Tam et al., 2012). J. R. Kaiser et al. (2015) reported that transient hypoglycemia (glucose concentrations less than 45 mg/dL) in at-risk newborns between 25 and 42 weeks of gestation were associated with a 50% reduction in passing fourth-grade literacy and math tests and continued academic deficits through age 8. McKinlay and colleagues (2017) identified that in at-risk newborns with a gestational age greater than 35 weeks, a single episode of severe hypoglycemia less than 36 mg/dL or three or more episodes of moderate hypoglycemia (less than 47 mg/dL) were associated with reduced executive function and reduced visual motor scores until age 9. Wickström and colleagues (2018) published outcomes of a recent study of 1,396 infants and reported a 2- to 3-fold higher risk for adverse neurodevelopmental (motor or cognitive) impairment with hypoglycemia (serum glucose less than 40 mg/dL) in the neonatal period. Clearly, this issue remains contentious and further investigation is indicated to safely define hypoglycemia and ensure that quality and safety remain at the forefront of clinical medicine. In the meantime, clinicians must use the proper growth charts to plot newborns and complete a risk assessment for hypoglycemia associated with SGA, AGA, or LGA status; proactively initiate point-of-care glucose screening for at-risk infants (e.g., premature, growth restricted, subject to perinatal hypoxia-ischemia, IDM, exclusively breastfed infant with suspected deficient milk transfer, rapid weight loss after birth), and *intervene*.

Syndrome of Inappropriate Antidiuretic Hormone

SIADH is the most frequent cause of euvolemic hyponatremia; it involves the inappropriate secretion of ADH in the presence of euvolemia. Hyponatremia affects approximately 25% of hospitalized children (Reid-Adam, 2013). Risk factors for SIADH are associated with neurologic, pulmonary, and other conditions (Table 10.15). In addition, genetic mutations triggering SIADH have been reported (Verbalis et al., 2013).

In the blood, solutes suspended in plasma constitute the density of the solution, also known as *serum osmolality*. The normal serum osmolality is 275 mOsm/L to 290 mOsm/L (Wright et al., 2024). The major contributor to the serum solute load is sodium, which contributes approximately 280 mOsm/L of the total value. The normal range for serum sodium is 135 to 145 mEq/L. When values fall below this range, hyponatremia is present. *Hypo*natremia may occur from a low sodium intake, body losses such as sweating or diarrhea, the inability of the renal tubule to reabsorb sodium from the filtrate, or an overabundance of free water that results in a dilutional state. *Hyper*natremia results from high amounts of sodium intake, poor intake of free water, or losses of body water as seen with renal or GI abnormalities.

ADH, also known as *vasopressin*, is a polypeptide hormone produced by the hypothalamus and stored in and released from the posterior pituitary gland. ADH controls water conservation; a paucity of ADH permits water removal to maintain the normal serum osmolality. In normal conditions, triggers for ADH release include hypovolemia, hypotension, angiotensin II, and an increase in serum osmolality (Michalopulos & Quigley, 2024). Hypovolemia stimulates baroreceptors in the major vessels, namely the aorta and carotid arteries, as well as within the left atrium. This activates the renin-angiotensin-aldosterone cascade, which leads to vasoconstriction. Simultaneously, when osmoreceptors in the brain detect a rising serum osmolality, signals are transmitted to the posterior pituitary to release ADH, which conserves body water. These mechanisms serve to maintain homeostasis by providing an adequate vascular volume at normal pressure and control serum osmolality within a normal range. On release from the posterior pituitary, ADH is transported via the vascular system to the renal tubule (Grimberg & Kutikov, 2022). ADH binds with receptors on principal cells of the collecting ducts of the renal tubule. Principal cells then place aquaporins, small apertures that allow water to move by diffusion from the filtrate out toward the high solute milieu surrounding the renal tubule, in the renal medulla portion of the kidney. This salvaging of water permits an increase in vascular volume and pressure and helps reestablish a normal range of serum osmolality.

In abnormal conditions, vasopressin (ADH) is released in excess. This is SIADH. This abnormality leads to water retention and, subsequently, to dilution of electrolytes, particularly sodium since it is the most abundant extracellular electrolyte. SIADH thereby manifests as oliguria, free water retention, decreased serum sodium concentration and osmolality, increased urine concentration, and weight gain with edema. It is essential that the APRN recognize that despite the low serum sodium concentrations, total body sodium concentrations are normal. The increase in total body water (edema with weight gain) causes the dilutional hyponatremic state; therefore, treatment is aimed at cause as well as fluid and sodium restriction (Wright et al., 2024).

Life-span implications of SIADH are correlated with early identification, management, and treatment. Delayed recognition of decreasing serum osmolality can increase the risk for cerebral edema and herniation. Alternatively, overzealous correction of hyponatremia can precipitate severe and long-term neurologic dysfunction.

Acquired Adrenal Insufficiency

Adrenal insufficiency (AI) can be an inherited steroidogenesis defect (congenital adrenal hyperplasia or congenital adrenal hypoplasia; see Chapter 11); a result of an injury to the hypothalamus or pituitary gland during fetal development (central adrenal insufficiency aka *ACTH* or *CRH deficiency*); a result of a hemorrhage within the adrenal gland, hypothalamus, or pituitary; or an acquired insufficiency. The acquired form of AI typically manifests during the postnatal period, often as a result of prolonged, supraphysiologic corticosteroid therapy. In addition, an immature HPA axis may be a root cause for AI, in particular among infants born at less than or equal to 30 weeks' gestation (Auron & Raissouni, 2015; Quintos & Boney, 2010; Witt, 1999). Precursors for acute AI are summarized in Table 10.16.

In cases of HPA axis immaturity, premature infants exposed to internal or environmental stressors exhibit normal to elevated ACTH synthesis and secretion with

TABLE 10.15 Common Risk Factors for SIADH

Body System	Risk Factor
CNS	Cerebral trauma
	Maternal renal loss of magnesium with glycosuria[a]
	Fetal macrosomia[a]
	Hypothermia
	Pain/stress
	Encephalitis
	Hydrocephalus
	Intraventricular hemorrhage
Cardiovascular	Early termination of placental calcium transfer
	Acute blood loss
	Urinary calcium loss secondary to immature renal function
	Patent ductus arteriosus[a]
	Inadequate calcium intake enterally or IV
Pulmonary	Hypoxia/asphyxia
	Acidosis
	Atelectasis
	Air leak syndrome (in particular pneumothorax)
Endocrine	Adrenal insufficiency
	Hyperlipidemia
	Hypothyroidism
	Improper enteral formula, high phosphorus, or cow's milk (seven times the phosphorus of breast milk)
	Low production of PTH secondary to hypomagnesemia triggered by insufficient circulating vitamin D
Immune	Infection (meningitis, respiratory syncytial virus, pneumonia)
	22q11.2 deletion (DiGeorge syndrome)
Other	Diuretic use (e.g., furosemide)

[a]Maternal renal loss of magnesium with glycosuria causes fetal hypomagnesemia and the inability to synthesize sufficient PTH. Fetal macrosomia may lead to premature birth and delivery complications. Surgical ligation of patent ductus arteriosus may increase the risk for onset of SIADH. Diuretic use is associated with natriuresis. The administration of any drug with tubular toxicity risks increases the likelihood for development of SIADH.

CNS, central nervous system; PTH, parathyroid hormone; SIADH, syndrome of inappropriate secretion of ADH.

Sources: Kim, Y.-J., Lee, J. A., Oh, S., Choi, C. W., Kim, E.-K., Kim, H.-S., Kim, B. I., & Choi, J.-H. (2015). Risk factors for late-onset hyponatremia and its influence on neonatal outcomes in preterm infants. *Journal of Korean Medical Science, 30*(4), 456–462. https://doi.org/10.3346/jkms.2015.30.4.456; Soto-Rivera, C. L., Breault, D. T., & Majzoub, J. A. (2025). Other abnormalities of arginine vasopressin metabolism and action. In R. M. Kliegman & J. W. St Geme III (Eds.), *Nelson textbook of pediatrics* (22nd ed., pp. 3375–3378.e1). Elsevier Inc; Wright, C. J., Posencheg, M. A., & Seri, I. (2024). Fluid, electrolyte, and acid-base balance. In C. A. Gleason & T. Sawyer (Eds.), *Avery's diseases of the newborn* (11th ed., pp. 231–252). Elsevier.

TABLE 10.16 Common Stressors (Precursors) for Acute Adrenal Insufficiency

Body System	Risk Factor
CNS	Hypoxia
	Immature HPA axis
Pulmonary	Prolonged, supraphysiologic corticosteroid replacement therapy with or without abrupt cessation
Endocrine	ACTH unresponsiveness
	Congenital adrenal hyperplasia
	Adrenal hypoplasia
	Adrenal hemorrhage
Immune	Sepsis
Other	Gestational age of 30 weeks or less, low birthweight, prolonged maternal steroid administration

Note: All risk factors noted in the table affect serum cortisol concentrations during the first few weeks of life. Congenital adrenal hyperplasia may be of the 21-hydroxylase, 11-hydroxylase, 3-β-hydroxylase, 17-hydroxylase, or lipoid type. Adrenal hemorrhage may occur secondary to birth injury, asphyxia, sepsis, or disseminated intravascular coagulation. Sepsis may occur secondary to fungal or viral etiologies.
ACTH, adrenocorticotropic hormone; CNS, central nervous system; HPA, hypothalamic–pituitary–adrenal axis.
Source: Adapted from Witt, C. L. (1999). Adrenal insufficiency in the term and preterm neonate. *Neonatal Network, 18*(5), 21–28. https://doi.org/10.1891/0730-0832.18.5.21

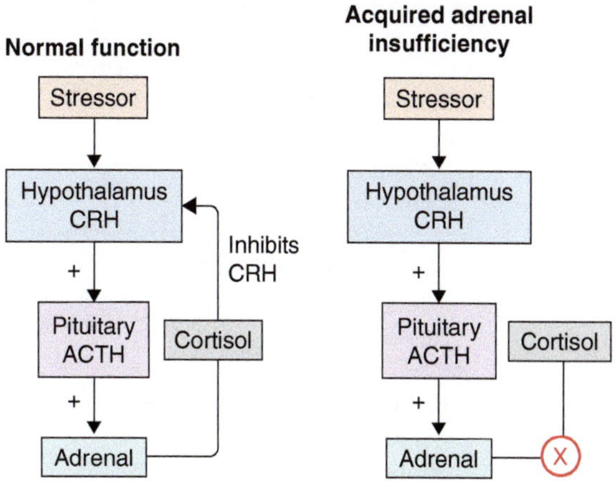

Figure 10.24 Normal adrenal feedback loop as compared to acquired adrenal insufficiency. The image depicts normal function compared to the interrupted feedback loop noted with acquired adrenal sufficiency.
ACTH, adrenocorticotropic hormone; CRH, corticotropin-releasing hormone.

suboptimal cortisol synthesis and secretion. Etiologies include an immature neurologic response to stress, adrenal immaturity to ACTH stimulation, and reduced enzymatic precursors necessary for cortisol synthesis and secretion. Of note, one particulary important precursor is 3-β-hydroxysteroid dehydrogenase (3-β-HSD). 3-β-HSD is essential for the biosynthesis of many hormonal steroids, including glucocorticoids and mineralocorticoids; the maturation of this enzyme is dependent on increasing gestational age (Kusuda et al., 2025). Specific to AI, decreased levels of this enzymatic precursor are associated with a reduced ability to synthesize cortisol. Low cortisol levels are detected by the hypothalamus, which secretes CRH to the pituitary, which thereby secretes ACTH. ACTH levels continue to rise relative to low cortisol; however, the adrenal gland fails to synthesize and secrete cortisol (Figure 10.24).

In cases of prolonged exposure to corticosteroids, an abnormal suppression of endogenous corticosteroid (ACTH) production is observed during the fight-or-flight response to an internal or environmental stressor. Decreased ACTH secretion occurs, which suppresses the HPA axis and causes insufficient cortisol synthesis and resultant hypotension refractory to volume or vasopressors (Auron & Raissouni, 2015; Quintos & Boney, 2010).

The early clinical presentation may be ill-defined during early manifestations of the disease process. Poor feeding and emesis are common. Biochemical indicators include hyponatremia, hyperkalemia, hypoglycemia, and ketonuria (Auron & Raissouni, 2015). AI is considered a life-threatening condition associated with a high risk for mortality when left untreated. Among medically managed infants, life-span implications are associated with complications of corticosteroid therapy. Neurodevelopmental and GI consequences, including lower mental developmental index (MDI) and Bayley infant developmental scores, in addition to spontaneous intestinal perforation, have been reported (Holmstrom & Jnah, 2021; Quintos & Boney, 2010).

Osteopenia of Prematurity

OoP (rickets of prematurity) is an acquired metabolic bone disease characterized by deficient bone mineralization and subsequent loss of bone mass. The precise incidence of OoP is rarely quantified in the literature, due to variability in screening and diagnostic methods. It is widely accepted that OoP is inversely proportional to gestational age and birthweight, with infants weighing less than 1,500 g at birth at the highest risk for acquisition of the disease process. A prevalence of OoP among male newborns is reported. Risk factors for OoP are summarized in Table 10.17 (Abrams & Tiosano, 2025).

Bone mineralization peaks during the third trimester; it is estimated that 80% of all calcium and phosphate ac-

TABLE 10.17 Common Risk Factors for Osteopenia of Prematurity

Body System	Risk Factor
CNS	Cerebral pathology
	Neuromuscular disorders
Pulmonary	Acidosis
	Bronchopulmonary dysplasia
Gastrointestinal	Short gut syndrome
	Cholestatic jaundice
	Unsupplemented human-milk feedings
	Prolonged parenteral nutrition therapy
Immune	Sepsis
	Enterocolitis
Endocrine	Vitamin D deficiency
Other	Placental insufficiency,[a] prematurity (birthweight less than 1,500 g, less than 34 weeks' gestation), male gender, prolonged periods of immobility, poor prenatal nutrition (maternal), methylxanthine administration, corticosteroid administration, loop diuretic administration

[a]Chronic damage to the placenta (e.g., preeclampsia) is positively associated with intrauterine growth retardation and an increased risk for osteopenia of prematurity.
CNS, central nervous system.
Source: Abrams, S. A., & Tiosano, D. (2025). Disorders of calcium, phosphorus, and magnesium metabolism in the neonate. In R. J. Martin & A. A. Fanaroff (Eds.), *Fanaroff and Martin's neonatal-perinatal medicine, 2-volume set: Diseases of the fetus and infant* (12th ed., pp. 1697–1727). Elsevier; Poindexter, B. B., & Martin, C. R. (2025). Nutritional support for preterm infant. In R. J. Martin & A. A. Fanaroff (Eds.), *Fanaroff and Martin's neonatal-perinatal medicine, 2-volume set: Diseases of the fetus and infant* (12th ed., pp. 720–738). Elsevier.

cumulation occurs at this time (Hodges, 2023). During this time, the fetal skeleton requires ample transfer of calcium, phosphorus, vitamin D, and protein. In fact, third trimester circulating calcium and phosphorus levels are approximately 20% higher in the fetus than the pregnant woman, as each of these minerals (and protein) cross the placenta. Fetuses delivered at less than 34 weeks' gestation are devoid of a full opportunity for phosphate and calcium accretion, and therefore are at higher risk for OoP (Rayannavar & Calabria, 2020; Rehman & Narchi, 2015).

Postnatally, premature infants are devoid of placentally supplied minerals (calcium and phosphate) necessary for optimal bone growth and development. Shortly after removal of the placental blood supply, the premature infant's parathyroid gland detects low-circulating calcium levels and synthesizes and secretes PTH. The secretion of PTH increases extracellular calcium concentrations, inhibits bone mineralization, and encourages osteoclast formation, which seeks to strip calcium from bones. During this time frame, the bones then undergo structural modifications, including widening of the internal cavity with rapid increases in bone length (Abrams & Tiosano, 2025; Rayannavar & Calabria, 2020). The chronic inhibition of bone mineralization over time increases the vulnerability to bone injury (rickets).

Clinical Application. Alkaline phosphatase is an enzyme involved in bone formation. In preterm infants, levels greater than 600 IU/L are suspicious for OoP; levels greater than 800 IU/L are associated with likely OoP. Keep in mind that elevations of alkaline phosphatase can also be related to the liver and intestines, so if unclear on etiology, consider doing a fractionated level. Other serum levels to consider if concerned about OoP are phosphorus, which is significantly low ranging from less than 1.1 to 1.5 mmol/L. Calcium levels are not as helpful as they may be normal, elevated, or even low.

Consequences of OoP include mechanical fractures to the ribs and long bones. A longer birth hospitalization is common among infants with OoP. In addition, comorbidities, including periventricular leukomalacia, intraventricular hemorrhage, retinopathy of prematurity, persistent patent ductus arteriosus, and spontaneous intestinal perforation, have been reported. Life-span implications, in addition to the aforementioned neurodevelopmental consequences, include poor growth in infancy and throughout childhood (Moreira et al., 2014).

CONCLUSION

The metabolic and endocrine system is a network of organs, complex by way of its multiorgan involvement and innervation. The endocrine system functions to achieve and maintain homeostasis by responding and adapting to both internal and external events by way of the synthesis of hormones that coordinate and control responses within cells, tissues, or organs within the body. Any failure in normal anatomic or functional development of these organ systems can result in developmental errors affecting growth, metabolism, fluid, and electrolyte balance; response to stress; reproduction; and influence on the immune system. Several problems associated with the metabolic and endocrine system are genetically inherited (IEM). New tests have expanded newborn metabolic screening to assess the newly born infant for 60 core and secondary conditions. Early detection permits treatment interventions decreasing morbidity and mortality.

LEARNING TOOLS AND RESOURCES

CourseConnect

To access self-assessment questions and interactive, competency-based learning activities for this chapter, visit www.springerpub.com/courseconnect. See inside front cover and tear-out card for CourseConnect details.

Podcast

This podcast is available online by visiting www.springerpub.com/courseconnect. See inside front cover and tear-out card for CourseConnect details.

Neonatal Dehydration and Hypoglycemia
Christie del Castillo-Hegyi

Discussion Prompts

1. It is recommended that a second newborn screen be obtained when a baby is receiving adequate protein intake (~100 mL/kg/day) and when the baby is 2 to 4 weeks postbirth. Discuss the rationale for these two parameters.
2. Insulin inhibits lipolysis and release of free fatty acids from adipose cells. Discuss the purpose for this action.
3. IDM are at an increased risk for hypoglycemia. Discuss the factors that predispose the IDM infant to glucose dysregulation.

MIND MAP

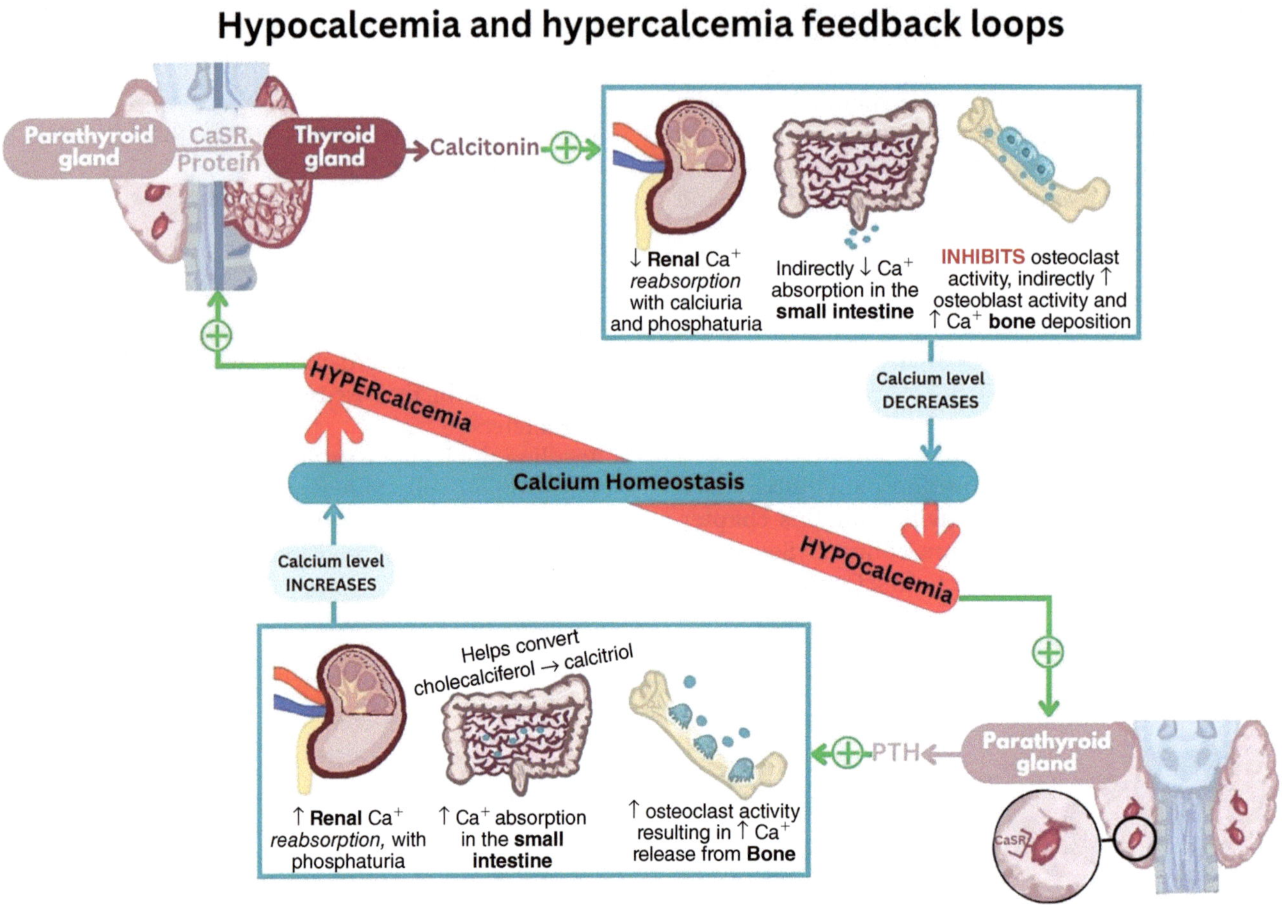

Note: This mind map reflects a former neonatal nurse practitioner student's interpretation of a concept addressed in this chapter. Readers should regard the mind maps woven throughout this textbook as examples of multisensory study tools that can be developed to aid conceptual understanding. Readers are encouraged to develop their own unique mind maps in consultation with academic faculty or clinical preceptors.
Image Credit: Kerri Rassa, MSN, NNP, RNC-NIC, C-ELBW.

TIMELINE OF ORGAN DEVELOPMENT

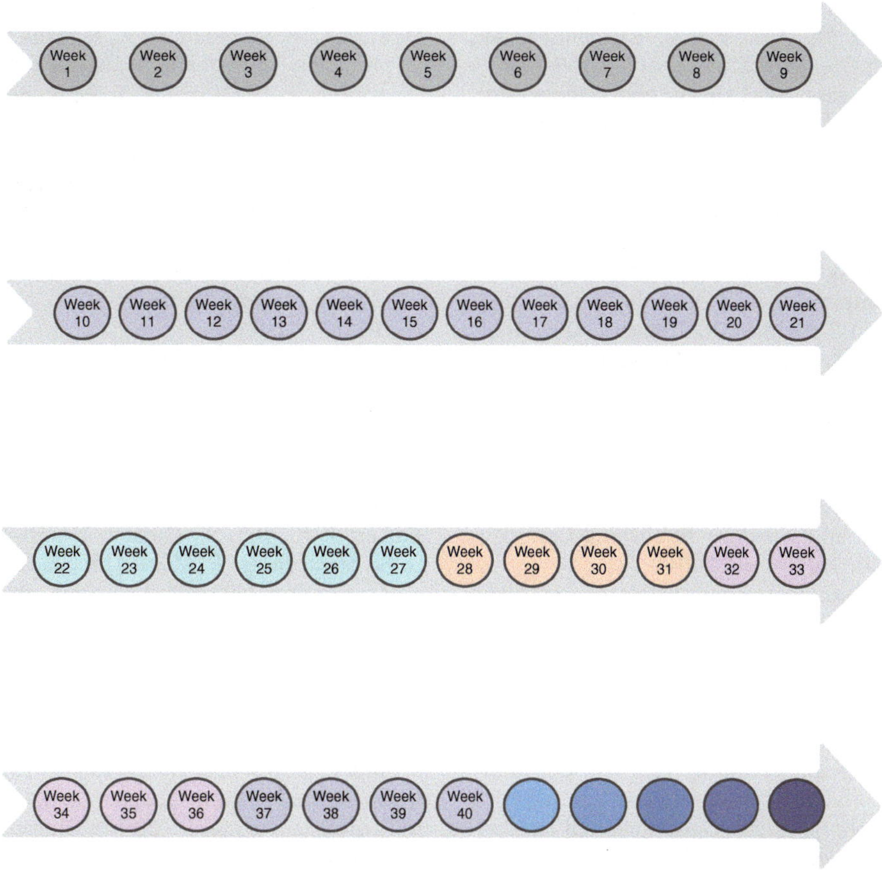

Note: Placement of common problems is meant to offer visual/conceptual perspective on the timing of onset of these commonly reported malformations. Variation exists across the literature.	***Legend:*** <22 – 27 6/7 weeks = extremely preterm 28 – 31 6/7 weeks = very preterm 32 – 36 6/7 weeks = late/moderate preterm 37 – 40 weeks = term

Note: Readers should annotate the blank timeline during studying, self-directed learning, and creation of feedback loops with mentors. To access the blank and completed timelines visit www.springerpub.com/courseconnect. See inside front cover and tear-out card for CourseConnect details.

REFERENCES

Abadi, K. K., Jama, A. H., Legesse, A. Y., & Gebremichael, A. K. (2023). Prevalence of hypothyroidism in pregnancy and its association with adverse pregnancy outcomes among pregnant women in a general hospital: A cross sectional study. *International Journal of Women's Health, 15*, 1481–1490. https://doi.org/10.2147/IJWH.S429611

Abrams, S. A., & Tiosano, D. (2025). Disorders of calcium, phosphorus and magnesium metabolism in the neonate. In R. J. Martin & A. A. Fanaroff (Eds.), *Fanaroff and Martin's neonatal-perinatal medicine, 2-volume set: Diseases of the fetus and infant* (12th ed., pp. 1697–1727). Elsevier.

Adamkin, D. H. (2017). Neonatal hypoglycemia. *Seminars in Fetal & Neonatal Medicine, 22*(1), 36–41. https://doi.org/10.1016/j.siny.2016.08.007

American Association of Endocrine Surgeons. (2024a). *Parathyroid gland.* http://endocrinediseases.org/parathyroid

American Association of Endocrine Surgeons. (2024b). *Thyroid gland.* http://endocrinediseases.org/thyroid

Auron, M., & Raissouni, N. (2015). Adrenal insufficiency. *Pediatrics in Review, 36*(3), 92–103. https://doi.org/10.1542/pir.36-3-92

Baynes, J. W. (2023). Biosynthesis and storage of carbohydrates. In J. W. Baynes & M. H. Dominiczak (Eds.), *Medical biochemistry* (6th ed., pp. 153–170). Saunders.

Beardsall, K., Ogilvy-Stuart, A., & Win, M. S. (2022). Role of glucoregulatory hormones in hepatic glucose metabolism during the perinatal period. In R. A. Polin, H. S. Abrams, D. H. Rowtich, & W. E. Benitz (Eds.), *Fetal and neonatal physiology* (6th ed., pp. 382–392.e2). Elsevier.

Berry, G. T. (2021). *Classic galactosemia and clinical variant galactosemia.* https://www.ncbi.nlm.nih.gov/books/NBK1518/

Berry, G., Demirbas, D., & Volpe, J. J. (2025). Amino acids. In J. J. Volpe & M. B. Inder (Eds.), *Volpe's neurology of the newborn* (7th ed., pp. 912–939). Elsevier.

Bilezikian, J. P., Marcus, R., Levine, M. A., Marcocci, C., Silverberg, S. J., & Potts, J. T., Jr. (Eds.). (2015). *The parathyroids: Basic and clinical concepts* (3rd ed.). Academic Press.

Blackburn, P. R., Gass, J. M., Vairo, F. P. E., Farnham, K. M., Atwal, H. K., Macklin, S., Klee, E. W., & Atwal, P. S. (2017). Maple syrup urine disease: Mechanisms and management. *The Application of Clinical Genetics,* 10, 57–66. https://doi.org/10.2147/TACG.S125962

Blaine, J., Chonchol, M., & Levi, M. (2015). Renal control of calcium, phosphate, and magnesium homeostasis. *Clinical Journal of the American Society of Nephrology, 10*(7), 1257–1272. https://doi.org/10.2215/CJN.09750913

Christ-Crain, M., Thompson, C. J., & Verbalis, J. G. (2025). Posterior pituitary. In S. Melmed, R. J. Ancus, A. B. Goldfine, C. J. Rosen, & P. A. Kopp (Eds.), *Williams textbook of endocrinology* (15th ed., pp. 296–323.e9). Elsevier.

Cleary, M. A. (2015). Phenylketonuria. *Paediatrics and Child Health, 25*(3), 108–112. https://doi.org/10.1016/j.paed.2014.10.00

Cowett, R. M. (Ed.). (2012). *Principles of perinatal–neonatal metabolism* (2nd ed.). Springer Publishing Company. https://doi.org/10/1007/978-1-4612-1642-1

Daher, S. (2015). Exploring the pathophysiology of gestational diabetes: Many questions still unanswered. *Placenta, 36*(4), 476. https://doi.org/10.1016/j.placenta.2015.01.405

Dingeldien, M. (2025). Development of the neonatal gastrointestinal tract. In R. J. Martin & A. A. Fanaroff (Eds.), *Fanaroff and Martin's neonatal–perinatal medicine, 2-volume set: Diseases of the fetus and infant* (12th ed., pp. 1598–1604). Elsevier.

Divall, S. A., & Merjaneh, L. (2024). Developmental endocrinology. In C. A. Gleason & T. Sawyer (Eds.), *Avery's diseases of the newborn* (11th ed., pp. 1173–1181). Elsevier.

Edmundson, K., & Jnah, A. J. (2024). Neonatal hypoglycemia. *Neonatal Network, 43*(3), 156–164. https://doi.org/10.1891/NN-2023-0068

Fechner, P. Y. (2024). Disorders of the adrenal gland. In C. A. Gleason & T. Sawyer (Eds.), *Avery's diseases of the newborn* (11th ed., pp. 1201–1214). Elsevier.

Felsenfeld, A. J., & Levine, B. S. (2015). Calcitonin, the forgotten hormone: Does it deserve to be forgotten? *Clinical Kidney Journal, 8*(2), 180–187. https://doi.org/10.1093/ckj/sfv011

Ferber, S. G., Als, H., McAnulty, G., Peretz, H., & Zisapel, N. (2011). Melatonin and mental capacities in newborn infants. *Journal of Pediatrics, 159*(1), 99–103.e1. https://doi.org/10.1016/j.jpeds.2010.12.032

Frise, C. J., & Williamson, C. (2013). Endocrine disease in pregnancy. *Clinical Medicine: The Journal of the Royal College of Physicians, 13*(2), 176–181. https://doi.org/10.7861/clinmedicine.13-2-176

Garg, M., & Devaskar, S. U. (2025). Disorders of carbohydrate metabolism in the neonate. In R. J. Martin & A. A. Fanaroff (Eds.), *Fanaroff and Martin's neonatal–perinatal medicine, 2-volume set: Diseases of the fetus and infant* (12th ed., pp. 1672–1696). Elsevier.

Grimberg, A., & Kutikov, J. K. (2022). Hypothalamus: Neuroendometabolic center. In R. A. Polin, H. S. Abrams, D. H. Rowtich, & W. E. Benitz (Eds.), *Fetal and neonatal physiology* (6th ed., pp. 1495–1504.e2). Elsevier.

Harris, D. L., Weston, P. J., & Harding, J. E. (2021). Alternative cerebral fuels in the first five days in healthy term infants: The glucose in well babies (GLOW) study. *The Journal of Pediatrics,* 231, 81–86. https://doi.org/10.1016/j.jpeds.2020.12.063

Hawkes, C. P., Stanescu, D. E., & Stanley, C. A. (2022). Pathophysiology of neonatal hypoglycemia. In R. A. Polin, H. S. Abrams, D. H. Rowtich, & W. E. Benitz (Eds.), *Fetal and neonatal physiology* (6th ed., pp. 1624–1633.e2). Elsevier.

Hodges, B. S. (2023). Metabolic bone disease of prematurity. In Pediatric Nutrition Practice Group, B. S. Hodges, M. Johnson, & S. M. Barr (Eds), *Pocket guide to neonatal nutrition* (3rd ed., pp. 249–255). Academy of Nutrition and Dietetics.

Holmstrom, L. E., & Jnah, A. J. (2021). Relative adrenal insufficiency. *Neonatal Network, 40*(6), 369–376. https://doi.org/10.1891/11-T-703

Holt, E. H., Lupsa, B., Lee, G. S., Bassyouni, H., Peery, H. E., 1946, & Goodman, H. M. (2021). *Goodman's basic medical endocrinology* (5th ed.). Elsevier.

Kabbany, M. N., & Murray, K. F. (2024). Disorders of the liver. In C. A. Gleason & T. Sawyer (Eds.), *Avery's diseases of the newborn* (11th ed., pp. 940–955). Elsevier.

Kaiser, J. R., Bai, S., Gibson, N., Holland, G., Lin, T. M., Swearingen, C. J., Mehl, J. K., & ElHassan, N. O. (2015). Association between transient newborn hypoglycemia and fourth-grade achievement test proficiency: A population-based study. *JAMA Pediatrics, 169*(10), 913–921. https://doi.org/10.1001/jamapediatrics.2015.1631

Kaiser, S. A., & Ho, K. K. Y. (2025). Pituitary physiology and diagnostic evaluation. In S. Melmed, R. J. Ancus, A. B. Goldfine, C. J. Rosen, & P. A. Kopp (Eds.), *Williams textbook of endocrinology* (15th ed., pp. 802–844.e15). Elsevier.

Kalhan, S., & Parimi, P. (2000). Gluconeogenesis in the fetus and neonate. *Seminars in Perinatology, 24*(2), 94–106. https://doi.org/10.1053/sp.2000.6360

Kansra, A. R. (2023). Hypoglycemia. In R. Kliegman, H. Roth, B. J. Bordini, & D. Basel (Eds.), *Nelson pediatric symptom-based diagnosis: Common diseases and their mimics* (2nd ed., pp. 1091–1105). Elsevier.

Katugampola, H., El-Khairi, R., & Dattani, M. T. (2025). Endocrinology of fetal development. In S. Melmed, R. J. Ancus, A. B. Goldfine, C. J. Rosen, & P. A. Kopp (Eds.), *Williams textbook of endocrinology* (15th ed., pp. 802–844.e15). Elsevier.

Khetan, S. K. (2014). *Endocrine disruptors in the environment* (pp. 29–50). John Wiley & Sons.

Kim, G., Nandi-Munshi, D., & DiBlasi, C. C. (2024). Disorders of the thyroid gland. In C. A. Gleason & T. Sawyer (Eds.), *Avery's diseases of the newborn* (11th ed., pp. 1238–1253). Elsevier.

Koutcherov, Y., Mai, J. K., Ashwell, K. W. S., & Paxinos, G. (2002). Organization of human hypothalamus in fetal development. *Journal of Comparative Neurology, 446*(4), 301–324. https://doi.org/10.1002/cne.10175

Krawczyk, S., Urbanska, K., Biel, N., Bielak, M. J., Tarkowska, A., Piekarski, R., Prokurat, A. I., Pacholska, M., & Ben-Skowronek, I. (2022). Congenital hyperinsulinaemic hypoglycaemia–A review and case presentation. *Journal of Clinical Medicine, 11*(20), 6020. https://doi.org/10.3390/jcm11206020

Kuhn-Riordon, K., Lee, Y. K., & Styne, D. M. (2022). Endocrine factors affecting neonatal growth. In R. A. Polin, H. S. Abrams, D. H. Rowtich, & W. E. Benitz (Eds.), *Fetal and neonatal physiology* (6th ed., pp. 224–241.e5). Elsevier.

Kusuda, S., Masumoto, K., & Nakanishi, H. (2025). Care of periviable micropreemies: The Japanese perspective. In R. J. Martin & A. A. Fanaroff (Eds.), *Fanaroff and Martin's neonatal-perinatal medicine, 2-volume set: Diseases of the fetus and infant* (12th ed., pp. 1697–1727). Elsevier.

Lechan, R. M. (2025). Neuroendocrinology. In S. Melmed, R. J. Ancus, A. B. Goldfine, C. J. Rosen, & P. A. Kopp (Eds.), *Williams textbook of endocrinology* (15th ed., pp. 93–166.e.20). Elsevier.

Long, S., & Romani, A. M. (2014). Role of cellular magnesium in human diseases. *Austin Journal of Nutrition and Food Sciences, 2*(10), 1051. http://austinpublishinggroup.com/nutrition-food-sciences/fulltext/ajnfs-v2-id1051.php

Lord, K., & DeLeón-Crutchlow, D. D. (2025). Hypoglycemia. In R. M. Kliegman & J. W. St Geme (Eds.), *Nelson textbook of pediatrics* (22nd ed., pp. 980–981). Elsevier.

Loughead, J. L., Mimouni, F., & Tsang, R. C. (1988). Serum ionized calcium concentrations in normal neonates. *American Journal of Diseases of Children, 142*(5), 516–518. https://doi.org/10.1001/archpedi.1988.02150050054030

Lucas, A., Morley, R., & Cole, T. J. (1988). Adverse neurodevelopmental outcome of moderate neonatal hypoglycaemia. *British Medical Journal, 297*(6659), 1304–1308. https://doi.org/10.1136/bmj.297.6659.1304

Macchi, M. M., & Bruce, J. N. (2004). Human pineal physiology and functional significance of melatonin. *Frontiers in Neuroendocrinology, 25*(3), 177–195. https://doi.org/10.1016/j.yfrne.2004.08.001

Magliano, D. J., Boyko, E. J., & IDF Diabetes Atlas 10th edition scientific committee. (2021). *IDF diabetes atlas* (10th ed.). International Diabetes Federation.

McKinlay, C. J. D., Alsweiler, J. M., Anstice, N. S., Burakevych, N., Chakraborty, A., Chase, J. G., Gamble, G. D., Harris, D. L., Jacobs, R. J., Jiang, Y., Paudel, N., San Diego, R. J., Thompson, B., Wouldes, T. A., Harding, J. E., & Children With Hypoglycemia and Their Later Development (CHYLD) Study Team. (2017). Association of neonatal glycemia with neurodevelopmental outcomes at 4.5 years. *JAMA Pediatrics, 171*(10), 972–983. https://doi.org/10.1001/jamapediatrics.2017.1579

Melchior, H., Kurch-Bek, D., & Mund, M. (2017). The prevalence of gestational diabetes: Aopulation-based analysis of a nationwide screening program. *Deutsches Ärzteblatt International, 114*(24), 412–418. https://doi.org/10.3238/arztebl.2017.0412

Melmed, S. (Ed.). (2022). *The pituitary* (5th ed.). Elsevier/Academic Press.

Melmed, S., Auchus, R. J., Goldfine, A. B., Rosen, C. J., & Kopp, P. A. (Eds.). (2025). *Williams textbook of endocrinology* (15th ed.). Elsevier.

Merritt, J. L., & Gallagher, R. C. (2024). Inborn errors of carbohydrate, ammonia, amino acid, and organic acid metabolism. In C. A. Gleason & T. Sawyer (Eds.), *Avery's diseases of the newborn* (11th ed., pp. 363–385). Elsevier, Inc.

Michalopulos, M. G., & Quigley, R. (2024). Pathophysiology and management of hyponatremia and hypernatremia in the neonate. In J. Lorenz, M. G. Baum, & K. G. Brennan (Eds.), *Neonatology questions and controversies: Renal, fluid and electrolyte disorders* (4th ed., pp. 74–95). Elsevier, Inc.

Molina, P. E. (2023). *Endocrine physiology* (6th ed.). McGraw-Hill Medical.

Moreira, A., Swischuk, L., Malloy, M., Mudd, D., Blanco, C., & Geary, C. (2014). Parathyroid hormone as a marker for metabolic bone disease of prematurity. *Journal of Perinatology: Official Journal of the California Perinatal Association, 34*(10), 787–791. https://doi.org/10.1038/jp.2014.97

Muelly, E. R., Moore, G. J., Bunce, S. C., Mack, J., Bigler, D. C., Morton, D. H., & Strauss, K. A. (2013). Biochemical correlates of neuropsychiatric illness in maple syrup urine disease. *Journal of Clinical Investigation, 123*(4), 1809–1820. https://doi.org/10.1172/JCI67217

National Organization for Rare Disorders. (2020). *Propionic academia*. https://rarediseases.org/rare-diseases/propionic-acidemia

National Organization for Rare Disorders. (2023). *Medium chain acyl CoA dehydrogenase deficiency*. https://rarediseases.org/rare-diseases/medium-chain-acyl-coa-dehydrogenase-deficiency

Nelson, D. L., &, Cox, M. M. (2021). *Lehninger principles of biochemistry* (8th ed.). W. H. Freeman.

O'Callaghan, K. M., & Roth, D. E. (2022). Fetal and neonatal calcium, phosphorus, and magnesium homeostasis. In R. A. Polin, H. S. Abrams, D. H. Rowtich, & W. E. Benitz (Eds.), *Fetal and neonatal physiology* (6th ed., pp. 265–281). Elsevier.

Ornoy, A., Reece, E. A., Pavlinkova, G., Kappen, C., & Miller, R. K. (2015). Effect of maternal diabetes on the embryo, fetus, and children: Congenital anomalies, genetic and epigenetic changes and developmental outcomes. *Birth Defects Research Part C: Embryo Today: Reviews, 105*(1), 53–72. https://doi.org/10.1002/bdrc.21090

Persaud, T. V. N., & Torchia, M. G. (2025). Alimentary system. In T. V. N. Persaud & T. G. Torchia (Eds.), *Before we are born* (11th ed.), 125–146. Elsevier, Inc.

Pfaff, D. W., & Joëls, M. (Eds.). (2016). *Hormones, brain, and behavior* (3rd ed.). Elsevier/Academic Press.

Poindexter, B. B., & Martin, C. R. (2025). Nutritional support for preterm infant. In R. J. Martin & A. A. Fanaroff (Eds.), *Fanaroff and Martin's neonatal-perinatal medicine, 2-volume set: Diseases of the fetus and infant* (12th ed., pp. 720–738). Elsevier.

Polin, R. A., Abman, S. H., Rowitch, D. H., & Benitz, W. E. (Eds.). (2022). *Fetal and neonatal physiology* (6th ed.). Elsevier.

Powers, W. J., Rosenbaum, J. L., Dence, C. S., Markham, J., & Videen, T. O. (1998). Cerebral glucose transport and metabolism in preterm human infants. *Journal of Cerebral Blood Flow and Metabolism, 18*(6), 632–638. https://doi.org/10.1097/00004647-199806000-00005

Quintos, J. B., & Boney, C. M. (2010). Transient adrenal insufficiency in the premature newborn. *Current Opinions in Endocrinology, Diabetes, and Obesity, 17*(1), 8–12. https://doi.org/10.1097/MED.0b013e32833363cc

Rayannavar, A., & Calabria, A. C. (2020). Screening for metabolic bone disease of prematurity. *Seminars in Fetal and Neonatal Medicine, 25*(1), 101086. https://doi.org/10.1016/j.siny.2020.101086

Rehman, M. U., & Narchi, H. (2015). Metabolic bone disease in the preterm infant: Current state and future directions. *World Journal of Methodology, 5*(3), 115–121. https://doi.org/10.5662/wjm.v5.i3.115

Reid-Adam, J. (2013). Hyponatremia. *Pediatrics in Review, 34*(9), 417–419. https://doi.org/10.1542/pir.34-9-417

Sahai, I. (2024). Newborn screening. In C. A. Gleason & T. Sawyer (Eds.), *Avery's diseases of the newborn* (11th ed., pp. 199–215). Elsevier

Salvatore, D., Schoenmakers, N., Coehn, R., & Kopp, P. A. (2025). Thyroid pathophysiology and diagnostic evaluation. In S. Melmed, R. J. Ancus, A. B. Goldfine, C. J. Rosen, & P. A. Kopp (Eds.), *Williams textbook of endocrinology* (15th ed., pp. 325–356). Elsevier.

Sen, S., Harding, J., Inder, T. E., & Volpe, J. J. (2025). Glucose. In J. J. Volpe & M. B. Inder (Eds.), *Volpe's neurology of the newborn* (7th ed., pp. 849–877). Elsevier.

Singh, S., & Sandhu, S. (2023). *Thyroid disease and pregnancy*. Stat Pearls. https://www.ncbi.nlm.nih.gov/books/NBK538485

Stanley, C. A., Anday, E. K., Baker, L., & Delivoria-Papadopolous, M. (1979). Metabolic fuel and hormone responses to fasting in newborn infants. *Pediatrics, 64*(5), 613–619. http://pediatrics.aappublications.org/content/64/5/613?download=true

Suhonen, L., Hiilesmaa, V., & K. Teramo, K. (2000). Glycaemic control during early pregnancy and fetal malformations in women with type I diabetes mellitus. *Diabetologia, 43*, 79–82. https://doi.org/10.1007/s001250050010

Tam, E. W. Y., Haeusslein, L. A., Bonifacio, S. L., Glass, H. C., Rogers, E. E., Jeremy, R. J., Barkovich, A. J., & Ferriero, D. M. (2012). Hypoglycemia is associated with increased risk for brain injury and adverse neurodevelopmental outcome in neonates at risk for encephalopathy. *Journal of Pediatrics, 161*(1), 88–93. https://doi.org/10.1016/j.jpeds.2011.12.047

Tas, E., Garibaldi, L., & Muzumdar, R. (2020). Glucose homeostasis in newborns: An endocrinology perspective. *NeoReviews, 21*(1), e14–e29. https://doi.org/10.1542/neo.21-1-e14

Thornton, P. S., Stanley, C. A., Leon, D. D. D., Harris, D., Haymond, M. W., Hussain, K., Levitsky, L. L., Murad, M. H., Rozance, P. J., Simmons, R. A., Sperling, M. A., Weinstein, D. A., White, N. H., Wolfsdorf, J. I., & Pediatric Endocrine Society. (2015). Recommendations from the Pediatric Endocrine Society for evaluation and management of persistent hypoglycemia in neonates, infants, and children. *Journal of Pediatrics, 167*(2), 238–245. https://doi.org/10.1016/j.jpeds.2015.03.057

Thureen, P. J., & Hay, W. W. (2006). *Neonatal nutrition and metabolism* (2nd ed.). Cambridge University Press.

Tin, W., Brunskill, G., Kelly, T., & Fritz, S. (2012). 15-year follow-up of recurrent "hypoglycemia" in preterm infants. *Pediatrics, 130*(6), e1497–e1503. https://doi.org/10.1542/peds.2012-0776

Tudosa, R., Vartej, P., Horhoianu, I., Ghica, C., Mateescu, S., & Dumitrache, I. (2010). Maternal and fetal complications of the hypothyroidism-related pregnancy. *Mœdica, 5*(2), 116–123. https://www.ncbi.nlm.nih.gov/pmc/articles/PMC3150006

Vambergue, A., & Fajardy, I. (2011). Consequences of gestational and pregestational diabetes on placental function and birth weight. *World Journal of Diabetes, 2*(11), 196–203. https://doi.org/10.4239/wjd.v2.i11.196

van der Kaay, D. C., Wasserman, J. D., & Palmert, M. R. (2016). Management of neonates born to mothers with Graves' disease. *Pediatrics, 137*(4), e20151878. https://doi.org/10.1542/peds.2015-1878

Varela-Lema, L., Paz-Valinas, L., Atienza-Merino, G., Zubizarreta-Alberdi, R., Villares, R. V., & López-García, M. (2016). Appropriateness of newborn screening for classic galactosaemia: Asystematic review. *Journal of Inherited Metabolic Disease, 39*(5), 633–649. https://doi.org/10.1007/s10545-016-9936-y

Verbalis, J. G., Goldsmith, S. R., Greenberg, A., Korzelius, C., Schrier, R. W., Sterns, R. H., & Thompson, C. J. (2013). Diagnosis, evaluation, and treatment of hyponatremia: Expert panel recommendations. *American Journal of Medicine, 126*(10, Suppl. 1), S1–S42. https://doi.org/10.1016/j.amjmed.2013.07.006

Wassner, A. J. (2017). Congenital hypothyroidism. *Clinics in Perinatology, 45*(1), 1–18. https://doi.org/10.1016/j.clp.2017.10.004

Wassner, A. J., & Brown, R. S. (2015). Congenital hypothyroidism: Recent advances. *Current Opinion in Endocrinology, Diabetes, and Obesity, 22*(5), 407–412. https://doi.org/10.1097/MED.0000000000000181

Watterberg, K. (2006). Fetal adrenal development: Implications for lung development and postnatal disease. *Neoreviews (Elk Grove Village, Ill.), 7*(3), e135. https://doi.org/10.1542/neo.7-3-e135

Weiner, M. R., Gurevich, P., Shinwell, E. S., & Yogev, Y. (2025). Pregnancy complicated by diabetes mellitus. In R. J. Martin & A. A. Fanaroff (Eds.), *Fanaroff and Martin's neonatal-perinatal medicine, 2-volume set: Diseases of the fetus and infant* (12th ed., pp. 307–317). Elsevier.

Wernimont, S. A., & Norris, A. W. (2022). Glucose metabolism in the fetus and newborn, and methods for its investigation. In R. A. Polin, H. S. Abrams, D. H. Rowtich, & W. E. Benitz (Eds.), *Fetal and neonatal physiology* (6th ed., pp. 358–368.e3). Elsevier.

Werny, D., Huang, A., Tenney, J., & Pihoker, C. (2024). Neonatal hypoglycemia and hyperglycemia. In C. A. Gleason & T. Sawyer (Eds.), *Avery's diseases of the newborn* (11th ed., pp. 1254–1268). Elsevier.

Wickström, R., Skiöld, B., Petersson, G., Stephansson, O., & Altman, M. (2018). Moderate neonatal hypoglycemia and adverse neurological development at 2–6 years of age. *European Journal of Epidemiology, 33*(10), 1011–1020. https://doi.org/10.1007/s10654-018-0425-5

Witt, C. L. (1999). Adrenal insufficiency in the term and preterm neonate. *Neonatal Network, 18*(5), 21–28. https://doi.org/10.1891/0730-0832.18.5.21

World Health Organization. (2023, April). *Diabetes fact sheet*. http://www.who.int/mediacentre/factsheets/fs312/en/

Wright, C. J., Posencheg, M. A., & Seri, I. (2024). Fluid, electrolyte, and acid-base balance. In C. A. Gleason & T. Sawyer (Eds.), *Avery's diseases of the newborn* (11th ed., pp. 231–252). Elsevier.

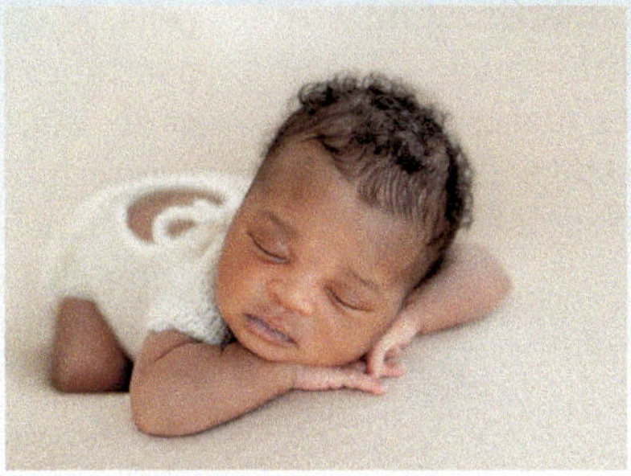
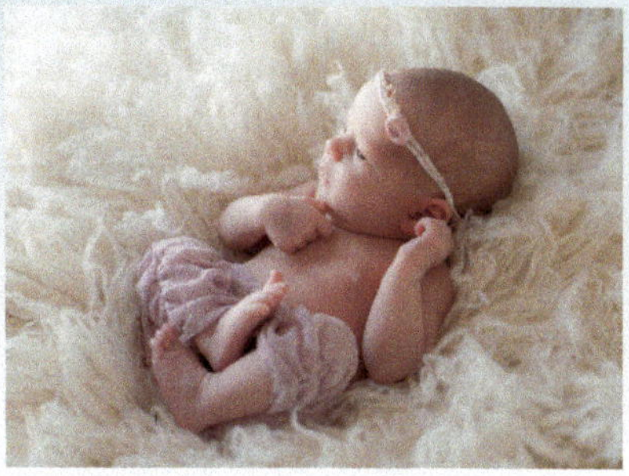

11

THE REPRODUCTIVE SYSTEM

Amy Williford and Amy J. Jnah

LEARNING OBJECTIVES

After completing this chapter, the reader should be able to:

- Understand normal reproductive system development.
- Analyze the physiologic function of the fetal and neonatal reproductive system.
- Discuss common inherited disorders and their effect on fetal and neonatal reproductive system development and function.
- Identify health issues in XX pregnant patients that have a potential impact on fetal and postnatal reproductive system development and function.
- Evaluate common disorders that affect the reproductive system and their implications across the life span.

INTRODUCTION

The development of the reproductive system is a complex process. Differentiation of sex progresses through discrete stages in a sequence from genetic to gonadal, hormonal, phenotypic, and psychologic development (Makiyan, 2016). Fertilization determines the genetic sex. Over the next 14 weeks, through the integrated action of genetic codes, hormones, and the nervous system, sexual differentiation occurs as the human moves from zygote to embryo to fetus. The observable physical properties of a fetus (phenotype) also include physical and psychologic development over time. Adverse events from fertilization through fetal development can result in abnormalities in genetic makeup, sexual differentiation, and external genitalia. This chapter discusses normal physiologic development with an emphasis on hormones that contribute to sexual differentiation and development of internal and external genitalia. Also included is an overview of disorders of sexual development.

TIMELINE OF ORGAN DEVELOPMENT

Gonads are reproductive glands that produce mature germ cells, either male or female, and carry a haploid chromosome set capable of initiating formation of a new individual. Fetal development of gonads begins in an undifferentiated state and progresses to development of specialized male or female organ systems capable of differentiated functions as a direct result of exposure to sex hormones. This development includes formation of the gonads, genital ducts, and external genitals from undifferentiated primordial structures within the embryo into adapted structures that meet the functional needs of the two sexes.

In the male fetus, gonads differentiate into testes and the duct system becomes the efferent ductules of the testes, the duct of the epididymis, the ductus deferens, the seminal vesicles, and the largest portion of the urethra. External genitalia become specialized to form the penis and scrotum. In the female fetus, gonads differentiate into the ovaries and the duct system becomes the fallopian tubes, uterus, and the upper third of the vagina. External genitalia become specialized to form the clitoris, labia majora and minora, vulva, and mons pubis.

This developmental process begins at fertilization with the determination of genetic sex as either male (XY) or female (XX). This differentiation of sex marks the end of the sex-indifferent or undifferentiated stage. In total, fetal and gonadal development progress through four phases:

- sex indifferent or bipotential gonad
- differentiation of gonadal sex
- differentiation of somatic sex
- differentiation of neuroendocrine sex

DEVELOPMENTAL PHYSIOLOGY

The Sex-Indifferent, Bipotential Gonad

Regardless of chromosomal sex as female (46 XX) or male (46 XY), the embryo and early fetus are sex-indifferent and have the potential to develop into either sex. For both sexes, gonadal development begins in an undifferentiated state. During week 4 of gestation, irrespective of sex, primordial germ cells arise from the mesonephros to form the genital ridge, the somatic precursor of gonads (Thompson & Wherrett, 2025). The genital ridge forms next to the developing kidney. Fetal sex determination is directed by the interaction of genes and primarily transcription factors. Transcription-factor genes that are essential for human genital ridge development and gonadogenesis include Wilms tumor 1 (*WT1*), homeobox genes, and steroidogenic factor 1 (*SF1*; M. Lee, 2022). Early gonads arise in pairs on day 10.5 of gestation, from the ventromedial surface of the intermediate mesoderm (Garcia-Alonso et al., 2022). They align on either side of the embryo and line the coelomic cavity between the limb buds during the first half of development (Wilhelm, Hiramatsu, et al., 2007). This development is triggered by the *SRY* gene.

***SRY* Gene.** The *SRY* gene is located on the short arm of the Y chromosome and is the testis-determining factor. The gene produces sex-determining region Y protein, a transcription factor that binds to a specific region of DNA and helps control activity of specific genes. It results in the production of hormones that guide male sexual differentiation and development. If there is absence or dysfunction of the *SRY* gene, ovaries develop (Hryhorczuk et al., 2022).

SRY encodes the transcription factor that is a member of the high-mobility group (HMG)-box family of DNA-binding proteins. *SRY* binds to *SF1* and together they bind to a specific region of the *SOX9* enhancer and activate the *SOX9* gene that is expressed in Sertoli cells (Kashimada & Koopman, 2010). The expression, timing, and pattern of *SRY* begins at day 41 of gestation and reaches its peak at day 44 of gestation, then decreases to low levels up until week 18 of gestation (Hanley et al., 2000).

***SOX9* Gene.** Both *SRY* and *SOX9* support cell lineage precursors with differentiation of these cells into Sertoli cells. *SOX9* expression starts at day 41 of gestation and continues to approximately 18 weeks of gestation (Hanley et al., 2000). The protein encoded by the *SOX9* gene is a transcription factor that binds to DNA and activates other genes, including blocking the gene pathway leading to the differentiation of ovarian cells (Thompson & Wherrett, 2025). There are two other essential products of *SOX9* upregulation. These products are prostaglandin D2 (PGD2) and fibroblast growth factor 9 (FGF9). PGD2 recruits cells of the supporting cell lineage in order to ensure enough Sertoli cells are provided for normal testis development (Ellis, 2022). In contrast, FGF9 promotes reproduction of Sertoli cell precursors (Brennan & Capel, 2004).

***DAX1* Gene.** The *DAX1* gene is another gene required for sex determination. *DAX1* is located on the X chromosome and is upregulated by *WT1* and *SF1*. This gene is ultimately necessary for the proper development and function of future hormone-producing tissues. *DAX1* expression occurs prior to *SRY* and remains in Sertoli cells throughout the sex determination period (Hanley et al., 2000). *DAX1* is expressed in both ovarian and testicular tissue, but downregulates the effectiveness of *SRY*. Overexpression of *DAX1* in XY individuals may result in sex reversal (Blecher & Erickson, 2007). A summary is presented in Table 11.1.

Differentiation of Gonadal Sex

The bipotential gonad, or genital ridge (urogenital ridge), proliferates from coelomic epithelium. The external genitalia for both sexes are derived from the urogenital sinus, genital tubercle, genital swellings, and genital folds. The differentiation of the genital ridge into the testis, with the formation of Sertoli cells, occurs in the presence of the Y chromosome. *SRY* is detected in the genital ridge soon after its formation. The primordial germ cells, which originate in the epiblast, migrate through the primitive streak to the posterior body wall of the yolk sac and then move into the mesenchyme of the genital ridge. The epithelium of the genital ridge proliferates and the cells enter the underlying mesenchyme. Under the influence of *SOX9*, primitive sex cords develop in the genital ridge and become enlarged and more defined. The cords are embedded within the surface of the coelomic epithelium. The indifferent gonad now consists of an external cortex and an internal medulla and resides in the Wolffian body.

When differentiation of the sex cords occurs, they are separated from the germinal epithelium. The tunica vaginalis is the outer layer that surrounds the testis and the tunica albuginea, a dense layer of connective tissue, divides the testis cords from the epithelium surface. The tunica albuginea ultimately attaches to the rete testis. The tunica albuginea thickens at the posterior margin of the testis and forms the mediastinum testis, which is a mass of fibrous tissue that is continuous externally with the tunica albuginea. The outer portion of the sex cords becomes the seminiferous tubules. The spaces between the seminiferous tubules are occupied by highly vascularized

TABLE 11.1 Developmental Physiology: Bipotential Gonad

Primordial germ cells form the genital ridge	Pronephros: Anterior region
	Mesonephros: Central region
	Metanephros: Posterior region
SRY gene	Located on the short arm of the Y chromosome
	Determines testis formation
SOX9 gene	Blocks differentiation of ovarian cells
	Precursor of prostaglandin D2
	Precursor of fibroblast growth factor 9
DAX1 gene	Located on the X chromosome
	Upregulated by *WT1* and *SF1*
	Remains in Sertoli cells through sex determination
	Expressed in ovarian and testicular tissue
	Overexpression can result in sex reversal

SF1, steroidogenic factor; *WT1*; Wilms tumor 1.

connective tissue containing fibroblasts, macrophages, and Leydig cells. Each seminiferous tubule forms a loop and connects to the rete testes. Fetal Leydig cells begin developing shortly after the differentiation of the testis cords with production of testosterone to impact sexual differentiation of the genital ducts and external genitalia.

Testis Differentiation

Peritubular Myoid Cells. Peritubular myoid cells are thought to migrate from the mesonephros and form a single layer of flattened cells that surround the Sertoli cells. Their main functions include providing structural support of the forming testis cords (M. Lee, 2022), in conjunction with Sertoli cells, and stimulating movement of mature sperm through the seminiferous tubules to the seminal vesicles. Peritubular myoid cells may represent the only cell type in the testis for which no corresponding cell type has been identified in the ovary (Wilhelm, Palmer, et al., 2007).

Leydig Cells. Development of Leydig cells in humans occurs during embryonic and fetal development, as well as during puberty. Leydig cell androgen production begins in embryonic life and is critical for intrauterine masculinization of the male fetus genital tract and brain, and continues until birth, at which time it decreases. The second increase of Leydig cells occurs at 2 months of age and then the cells remain dormant until the third surge occurs, when adult Leydig cells arise at puberty (S. Griswold & Behringer, 2009).

Fetal Leydig cells are thought to originate in the mesonephric or coelomic epithelium and develop outside the testicular cord in the testes. From week 8 of gestation, the Leydig cells (also known as *interstitial cells*) secrete testosterone. A rapid rise in production is noted between weeks 10 and 15 of gestation, when the cells comprise more than 50% of the volume of the fetal testis (Thompson & Wherrett, 2025).

The function of the Leydig cells is to respond to the luteinizing hormone (LH) secreted from the pituitary gland. The LH, which is released from the hypothalamus via the gonadotropin-releasing hormone (GnRH), is responsible for stimulating testosterone production from the Leydig cells in the testes. This acts as a negative feedback on the pituitary to suppress or modulate further LH secretion. The LH binds to the cell surface receptors on the Leydig cells, activating the synthesis and secretion of androgens: testosterone, androstenedione, and dehydroepiandrosterone. Some testosterone is converted into dihydrotestosterone (DHT), which influences the development of the penis, scrotum, and prostate.

Sertoli Cells. During week 7 of gestation, Sertoli cells (sustentacular cells) differentiate in the testis and organize to form the testis cords, surrounding the incoming germ cells in the center of the cords and expressing *SOX9* (Estermann & Smith, 2020). The cords form loops in the mesenchymal region of the developing testis and are connected to the rete testis located in the hilum of the testicle.

Sertoli cells are the supporting cells for germ cells. These cells are important in establishing testis vasculature and inducing differentiation of peritubular myoid cells and fetal Leydig cells. The function of the Sertoli cells is controlled by the follicle-stimulating hormone (FSH) via the hypothalamus, which secretes GnRH. FSH stimulates the Sertoli cells to produce androgen-binding protein (ABG) and the anti-Müllerian hormone (AMH). ABG is a protein that binds to testosterone and keeps it concentrated within the seminiferous tubules so that spermatogenesis can progress. AMH is a glycoprotein and is responsible for the regression of Müllerian ducts in male fetuses; it is the first hormone secreted by the Sertoli cells (Thompson & Wherrett, 2025).

Blood–Testis Barrier. The specialized junctions of the Sertoli cells create a barrier separating the testes from the normal circulation and testicular tubules. The barrier restricts fluids from entering or exiting the lumen (Mital et al., 2011). The blood-testis barrier only allows secretion from Sertoli cells to enter the lumen of the seminiferous tubules and support spermatogenesis (M. Lee, 2022). The primary function of this barrier is to provide an environment for germ cell development and maturation. A summary is provided in **Table 11.2** and **Figure 11.1**.

TABLE 11.2 Developmental Physiology: Testis Differentiation

Peritubular myoid cells	Migrate from the mesonephros
	Form a single layer surrounding the Sertoli cells
	Provide structural support for formation of testis cords
	Contribute to movement of mature sperm cells through seminiferous tubules
	May be the only cells in the testis lacking a corresponding cell type in the ovaries
Leydig cells	Originate in the mesonephros
	Begin in embryonic stage
	In utero androgen production essential for masculinization
	Key to fetal genital tract development
	Key to fetal brain development
	Increase in second month; more than half the volume of testis
	Respond to LH secreted by the pituitary and stimulate testosterone production
	Secrete testosterone between weeks 10–15
	Activate synthesis and secretion of androgens
	A portion is converted to dihydrotestosterone and influences development of penis, scrotum, and prostate
	Third surge in adulthood
Sertoli cells	Differentiate in week 7 within the testis
	Form the testis cords in the mesenchymal region
	Express *SOX9*
	Cords form loops
	Act as support for germ cells
	Key to formation of testis vasculature
	Induce differentiation of peritubular myoid cells and fetal Leydig cells
	Function controlled by FSH and GnRH
	Produce ABG, which binds to testosterone and retains it in the seminiferous tubules
	Produce AMH responsible for regression of Müllerian ducts
Blood–testis barrier	Junction of Sertoli cells
	Forms barrier between systemic circulation and that of the testis
	Provides environment for germ cell development and maturation

ABG, androgen-binding hormone; AMH, anti-Müllerian hormone; FSH, follicle-stimulating hormone; GnRH, gonadotropin-releasing hormone; LH, luteinizing hormone.

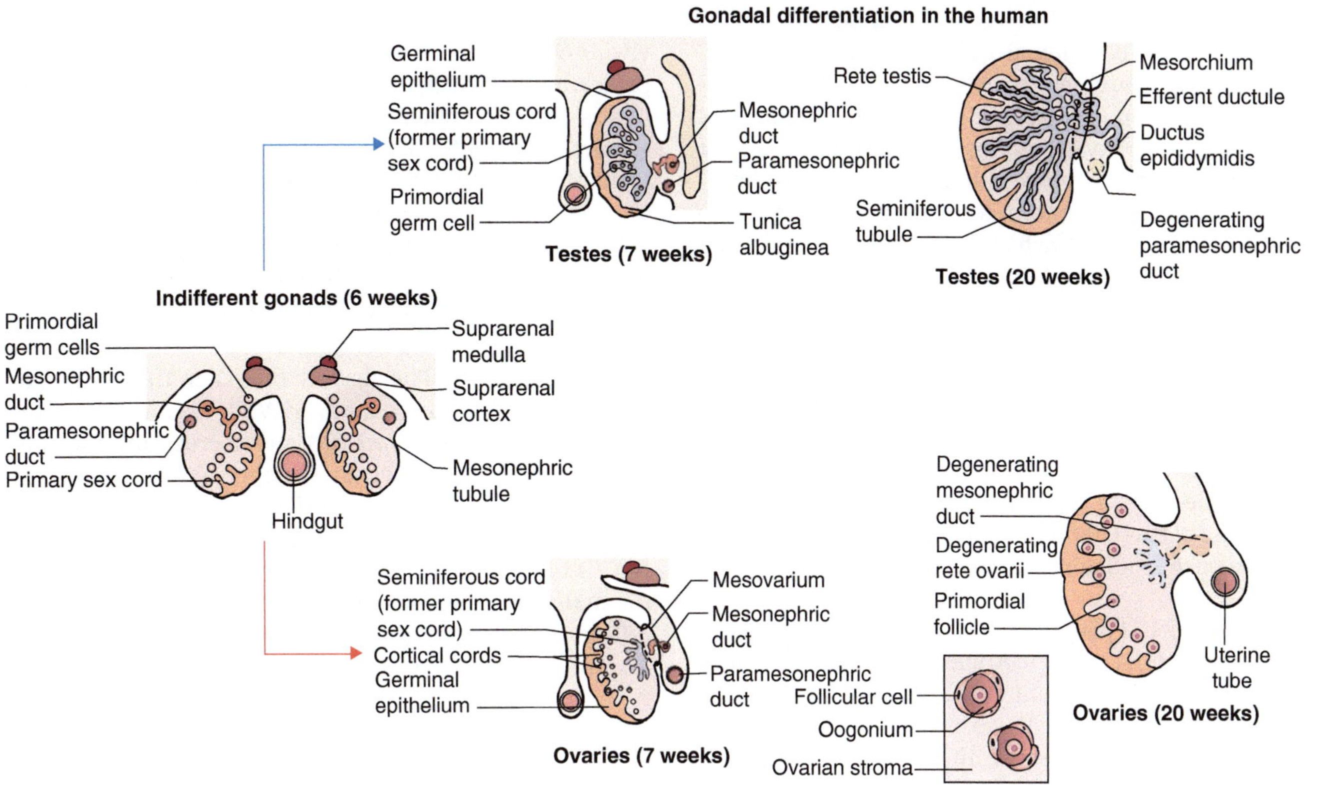

Figure 11.1 Overview of gonadal development.

Development of the Ovary

The development of the ovary occurs more slowly than the development of the testis. Ovarian development is very complex and not well understood. The common belief that females are the "default sex" has been challenged since the early 2000s with the discovery of genes that stimulate ovary development and prevent testicular development (Ainsworth, 2015; Ellis, 2022).

The primordial germ cells arise from the yolk sac and migrate through the primitive gut to incorporate into the extracellular matrix of the dorsal mesentery and then cluster on the outer half of the genital ridge. If the primordial germ cells do not migrate, streak gonads (gonadal dysgenesis) develop; in these circumstances, the ovary is replaced by functionless tissue. In embryos with the XX sex chromosome, the cortex differentiates into an ovary and the medulla regresses. The primary sex cords, which are in the medullary region of the ovary, develop from the gonadal ridge but are not prominent in the female gonad and develop from the mesonephros into the rete ovarii, which eventually degenerates and disappears.

After the primordial germ cells reach the ovary, they proliferate in vast number through mitosis from 7 weeks through month 5 of gestation (Thompson & Wherrett, 2025). These are called *oogonia* (primordial female sex cells). Research indicates that this occurs under the influence of retinoic acid (Childs et al., 2011; M. Griswold et al., 2012; Le Bouffant et al., 2010). During this time the oogonia divide, forming germ-cell nests. These nests are partitioned into ovigerous cords that are open to the surface of the ovary. Ovigerous cords consist of a cluster of primordial germ cells surrounded by somatic cells (Nef et al., 2005). No oogonia form postnatally and many of them degenerate before birth through apoptosis.

The first stage of folliculogenesis occurs during week 10 of gestation, when the oogonia undergo meiosis, enlarge, and develop into oocytes. During this same time frame, somatic cells develop into the follicular epithelial granulosa cells (Maheshwari & Fowler, 2008). Granulosa cells can have specific names depending on their location within the follicle. They may derive from the mesonephros (primitive sex cords), the coelomic epithelium (the secondary sex cords), or from ovarian mesenchyme.

One oocyte is surrounded by a single layer of flat pregranulosa cells, which become primordial follicles (Thompson & Wherrett, 2025). Primordial follicles contain the germinal vesicle oocytes, which are actually oocyte nuclei at this stage of development (Virant-Klun, 2015). Primordial follicles are found on the edge of the cortex and medulla as well as in the internal cortex (Maheshwari & Fowler, 2008). It is estimated that the ovaries contain approximately 5 to 7 million primordial follicles. The majority of primordial follicles undergo atresia (meaning a natural process of degeneration and resorption of follicles) mediated by programmed cell death or apoptosis (Markström et al., 2002). Atresia occurs at every stage of follicular development which ultimately leaves 300,000 to 2.5 million oocytes within the ovaries of newborn females (Mamsen et al., 2022).

The tunica albuginea, which forms at the corticomedullary junction of the ovary, contains the majority of oocytes. The majority of oocytes degenerate across fetal development and the entire volume of oocytes is determined at birth. The primordial follicles enter the diplotene stage of prophase 1, which lasts until puberty (onset of ovulation; Figure 11.2).

The molecular regulation of early ovarian development is not well understood. There are several genes that are directly linked to ovarian development, and research by Nef and colleagues (2005) indicate that gene expression in ovarian development is detected as early as postcoital day 11.5 of gestation (Nef et al., 2005). At least 1,000 female-specific genes have been identified, but for the purpose of this chapter, we discuss four gene markers that have been studied in humans.

***DAX1* Gene.** *DAX1* plays a complex role in the downregulation of the AMH, leading to Müllerian duct development and internal female differentiation. Elevated levels of this hormone are associated with sex reversal in XY chromosomes in mouse models; this is thought to be repression of transcription factor *SOX9* (Lalli et al., 1998). The loss of *DAX1* function is associated with X-linked congenital adrenal hypoplasia (Suntharalingham et al., 2015).

***FOXL2*.** *FOXL2* is a female-specific marker of the Forkhead box transcription factor (FOX) family and has been evolutionarily conserved. This marker is expressed in the supporting cells of the XX gonad as early as day 12.5 of gestation. *FOXL2* is vital for the development and maintenance of the ovaries (Thompson & Wherrett, 2025). In vivo, *FOXL2* represses testis differentiation through repression of the *SOX9* cis-regulatory sequence of TESCO (testis-specific enhancer core element). Cis-regulatory sequences of TESCO are areas of noncoding DNA important to the understanding of gene regulatory mechanisms. The majority of research, done in mice, has demonstrated that deletion of *FOXL2* causes ovarian dysgenesis and infertility; therefore, it may be a primary female-determining gene (Dupont et al., 2000).

***WNT4* and *FST1*.** The absence of *SRY* in the XX gonad releases *WNT4* expression. *WNT4* also upregulates *DAX1*, which antagonizes *SF1* and thereby inhibits steroidogenic enzymes. Recent evidence has demonstrated that the signaling pathway of *WNT4* may be a multigene signaling pathway. *FST1* (follistatin) acts downstream of *WNT4* to impede the formation of the coelomic vessel in the male gonad and also maintains survival of the germ cells in the cortical region of the ovary (Yao et al., 2004). A summary is presented in Table 11.3.

Sexual Duct Systems

Although gonads are sex determined at the end of week 7 of gestation, reproductive ducts are still indifferent (Figure 11.3; Torchia & Persaud, 2025). Male (Wolffian) external genitalia originate from the mesonephric ducts, whereas female (Müllerian) external genitalia originate from the paramesonephric ducts. The mesonephric tubules grow into the gonadal ridge and are connected to the mesonephric duct. The paramesonephric duct invaginates into the coelomic epithelium. By the end of week 8 of gesta-

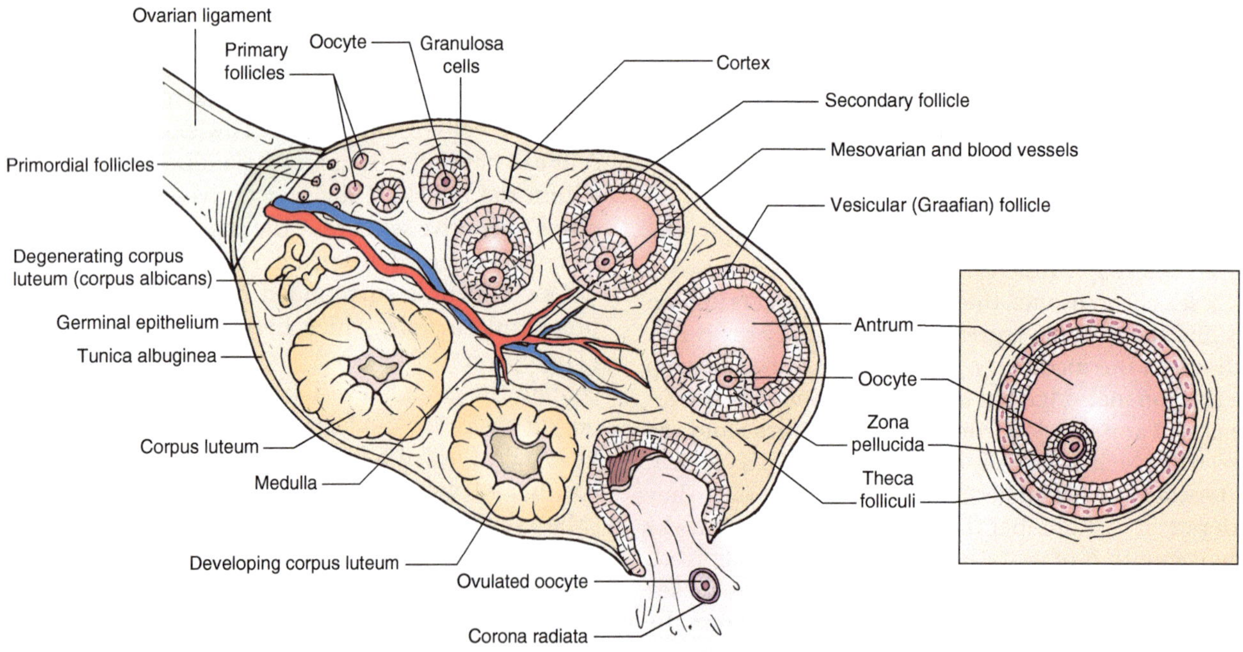

Figure 11.2 Oogenesis in the ovary.

TABLE 11.3 Developmental Physiology: Ovarian Development

Oogenesis	Primordial germ cell arises from the yolk sac to cluster on the outer half of the genital ridge.
	Primary sex cords in the medullary region arise from the gonadal ridge.
	Cells proliferate under the influence of retinoic acid to form oogonia.
	Oogonia divide to form germ cells.
	Germ cells cluster into nests.
	Nests partition to form ovigerous cells that are surrounded by somatic cells.
	Five to seven million primordial follicles form and situate at the inner cortex, the outer edge of the cortex, and medulla.
	Most follicles will die by apoptosis.
	Atresia occurs at every stage of development.
	Tunica albuginea, containing the majority of oocytes, forms.
DAX1 gene	Complex role in downregulation of anti-Müllerian hormone
	Contributes to Müllerian duct formation
	Contributes to female differentiation
	Elevated levels associated with sex reversal in XY mouse models
	Loss associated with X-linked congenital adrenal hypoplasia
FOXL2 gene	Forkhead box transcription factor
	Female-specific marker
	Expressed as early as day 12 postcoitus
	Represses testis differentiation by suppressing *SOX9*
WNT4	Expressed in the absence of *SRY* in the XX gonad
	Upregulates *DAX1*
	Antagonizes *SFI*
FST1	Acts downstream to *WNT4* to impede formation of coelomic vessel in male gonads
	Maintains survival of germ cells in the ovary

FST, follistatin; SF1, steroidogenic factor 1.

tion, the embryo has an undifferentiated gonadal primordium and two embryonic duct systems (Sobel et al., 2004).

Differentiation of the Male Duct System. After the gonads have differentiated into testes, the secretion of testicular hormones is required to develop the sexual duct system in the male. The Müllerian-inhibiting substance (MIH) belongs to the transforming growth factor-β (TGFβ) superfamily. MIH is expressed in Sertoli cells and causes regression of the Müllerian (paramesonephric) ducts by week 9 of gestation. In the Leydig cells, the LH initiates the production of pregnenolone, which is converted to Dhea (dehydroepiandrosterone) and then to testosterone. This promotes development of the

Wolffian (mesonephric) ducts. The Wolffian ducts then differentiate to form the ductus deferens and urethra as well as the male accessory sex glands: the seminal vesicle, prostate, and bulbourethral gland (Cowper's gland). The formation of the accessory sex glands in the male depends on androgenic stimulation (Figure 11.4).

Differentiation of the Female Duct System. Two mesenchymal projections border the cloacal membrane laterally; these are the paired primordia of the genital tubercle. The cloacal fold surrounds the cloacal membrane and prolongs the genital tubercle; on either side of the cloacal folds are the genital swellings. The cloacal membrane divides into the urogenital membrane anteriorly and the anal membrane posteriorly. During week 9 of gestation, the urogenital membrane dissipates and the phallic segment of the urogenital sinus opens to the exterior.

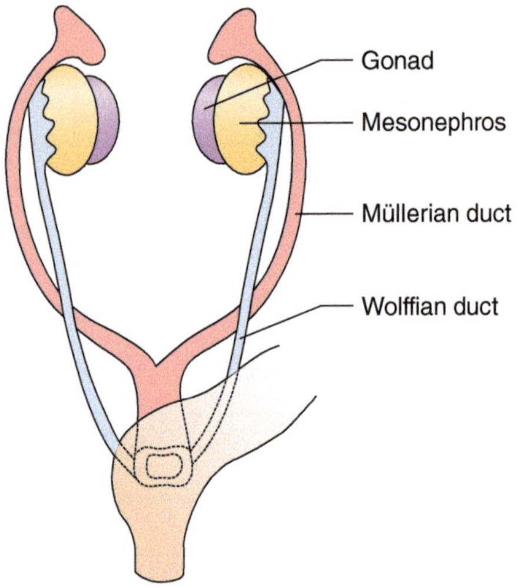

Figure 11.3 Indifferent reproductive duct system (predifferentiation).

The Müllerian ducts develop laterally to the Wolffian ducts. In the absence of male hormones, the Wolffian ducts degenerate and the Müllerian ducts are retained and differentiate into the Fallopian tubes (oviducts), uterus, and vagina. The caudal end of the Müllerian ducts form the Müllerian tubercle at the dorsal wall of the urogenital sinus. The Müllerian tubercle is destroyed and becomes the vaginal plate. By weeks 16 to 18 of gestation, the central core breaks down to form the vaginal lumen. The upper two thirds of the vagina is formed by the Müllerian tubercle, whereas the lower third of the vagina is formed by the urogenital sinus. See Figure 11.5.

The role of steroids in female development has not been determined. The ovary does not produce steroids during embryogenesis and the female reproductive tract is independent of gonadal secretions. A summary is presented in Table 11.4.

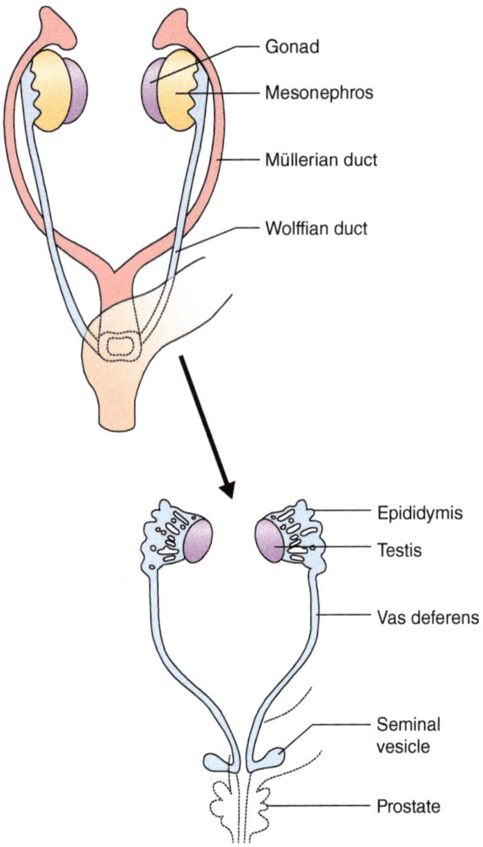

Figure 11.4 Differentiation of the male duct system.

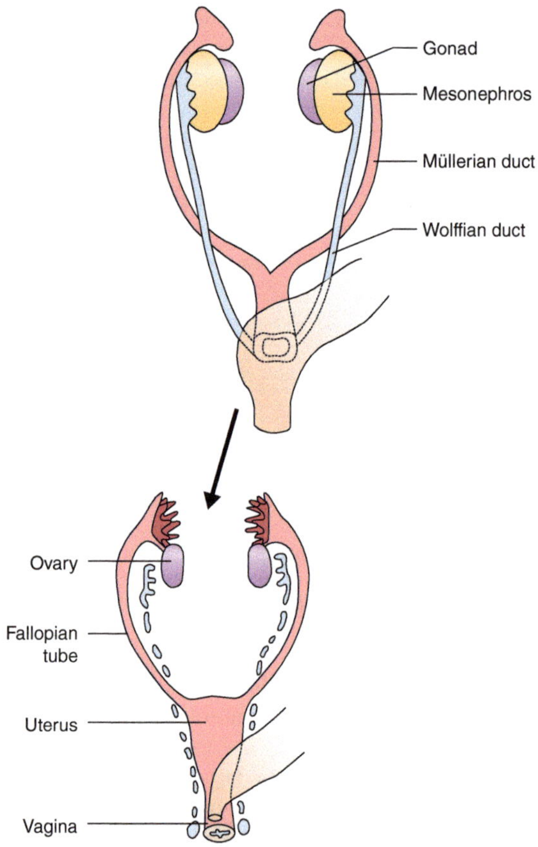

Figure 11.5 Differentiation of the female duct system.

TABLE 11.4 Developmental Physiology: Duct Systems

Male	Gonads differentiate into testis.
	Testosterone signals development of male duct system.
	Müllerian-inhibiting hormone is expressed from Sertoli cells.
	MIH leads to regression of Müllerian ducts by week 9.
	LH in Leydig cells produces pregnenolone.
	Pregnenolone converts first to DHEA and then to testosterone.
	Testosterone promotes development of Wolffian ducts.
	Wolffian ducts form the ductus deferens, urethra, and male sex glands.
	Seminal vesicle, prostate, and bulbourethral glands develop dependent on stimulation by androgen.
Female	Two mesenchymal projections border the cloacal membrane.
	Cloacal fold extends the genital tubercle.
	Cloacal membrane forms urogenital membrane anteriorly.
	Cloacal membrane forms anal membrane posteriorly.
	Phallic segment opens to the urogenital sinus at week 9.
	Müllerian duct develops lateral to the Wolffian.
	Wolffian duct degenerates in the absence of male hormones.
	Müllerian ducts differentiate into fallopian tubes.
	Caudal end of Müllerian duct forms dorsal wall of urogenital sinus.
	Müllerian tubercle degenerates to form vaginal plate.
	Central core breaks down at weeks 16–18 to form vagina.
	Upper vagina formed by Müllerian tubercle and lower formed from sinus.

DHEA, dehydroepiandrosterone; LH, luteinizing hormone; MIH, Müllerian-inhibiting hormone.

Clinical Application. A cloacal malformation is a complex anomaly which exclusively affects females. It is characterized by failure of the genitourinary, gastrointestinal, and gynecologic tracts to separate properly during fetal development. Since separation does not occur as it should, the urinary tract, vagina, and rectum are fused and present as one tract. The most severe form of this anomaly is termed a cloacal exstrophy, which also involves the abdominal wall such that the bladder and a portion of the intestinal tract are situated outside of the abdomen. Cloacal exstrophy, or "OEIS syndrome," can be confused with a disorder of sex development (DSD). Therefore, a thorough exam using proper technique is necessary for prompt diagnosis. The APRN must distinguish between clitoral hypertrophy that appears phallus-like versus the redundant labial skin folds and abnormal single perineal orifice of a cloacal anomaly. This is vital to properly direct the appropriate diagnostic workup and management.

Development of External Genitalia

Although the sex of the embryo is genetically determined at fertilization, the morphologic characteristics of normal male and female external genitalia remain undifferentiated until week 7 of development. If the sexual determination of the zygote is male, masculinization occurs through physical growth and fusion. The development of the external genitalia cannot be accomplished without DHT, an essential androgenic hormone. It is derived from testosterone via the action of the enzyme 5-alpha-reductase (Sajjad, 2010). Without DHT present, the external genitalia will be female.

Male External Genitalia. Inguinal-canal development provides the testes with the ability to migrate to the labioscrotal swellings. The gubernaculum starts to develop during week 6 of gestation and is the primary structure in testicular descent. This process is regulated by insulinlike 3 (Inls-3), which is secreted by the Leydig cells (Nation et al., 2009). The gubernaculum, attached to the caudal end of the testis, descends on each side from the lower poles of the gonads and migrates from the abdominal wall to the internal inguinal ring (Favorito et al., 2014), where it innervates the cremaster muscle and then migrates across the pubic region to the scrotum (Hughes & Acerini, 2008). Migration occurs as the abdominal cavity and the pelvic region enlarge.

The processus vaginalis, an invagination of the peritoneum, develops ventral to the gubernaculum and pushes through the lower abdominal wall using the path formed by the gubernaculum. The processus vaginalis carries layers of the abdominal wall, which covers the testes and spermatic cord. The mesonephric duct develops into the epididymis. At 26 to 36 weeks of gestation, the epididymis enters the processus vaginalis prior to the testis. The epididymis and testis descend into the scrotum and fuse with the posterior layers of the scrotum to prevent the testis from rotating. At 37 to 40 weeks of gestation, the processus vaginalis closes, preventing communication between the peritoneum and the inguinal canal or scrotum.

During this phase of sexual development, the genital tubercle elongates to form a phallus, which pulls the urethral folds forward to form the lateral walls of the urethral groove, resulting in the penile portion of the male urethra. The growth of the phallus is dependent on DHT and testosterone. At the base of the urethral groove, ectoderm grows toward the penile urethra. Originating in the endoderm, the epithelial lining of the groove forms the urethral plate. The two urethral folds close over the urethral plate, which does not reach the glans. Ectoderm cells from the tip of the glans penetrate inward and form an epithelial cord known as the *glandular epithelial plate*. When this plate splits, it forms the glandular urethra on the ventral part of the glans. The movement of the urethral opening to the tip of the glans forming the external urethral meatus occurs as a result of the closing of the groove in the glans. The labioscrotal folds fuse at midline to form the scrotal raphe (Thompson & Wherrett, 2025).

Clinical Application. The APRN must complete a detailed physical examination, which includes a genitourinary assessment. Two penile defects that can affect male newborns are hypospadias and epispadias. Hypospadias is one of the most common congenital defects of the male external genitalia (1:250 males are born with it), increasing the likelihood of finding this on the routine physical exam. It develops when the urethral groove fails to properly close between weeks 7 and 14 of gestation. Failed closure causes the urethral meatus to assume an abnormal position along the ventral (underside) shaft of the penis rather than at the tip of the glans (normal position). Hypospadias is often an isolated finding, but other genital anomalies may occur concomitantly, such as chordee (curvature of the penis), hydrocele, meatal stenosis, cryptorchidism (undescended teste[s]), and inguinal hernia. Circumcision is typically deferred and pediatric urology follow-up is arranged. Surgical repair, which requires general anesthesia and typically takes 1 to 2 hours, customarily occurs between 6 and 18 months of age.

Epispadias is a rare abnormality of the external genitalia (1:117,000 males are born with it) and may occur when the urethral tube fails to fully form. This leaves the urethral plate exposed on the dorsum (topside) of the male phallus. Even less common, this can present in females (1 in 484,000 females are born with it) as a bifid clitoris with a widely open and exposed urethral meatus and an abnormal or absent mons pubis. Epispadias often occurs as part of a constellation of malformations, most often with bladder exstrophy. Like with hypospadias, circumcision is deferred and pediatric urology follow-up is arranged. Surgical repair may be indicated with moderate or severe cases, and may require both urology and orthopedic involvement.

Female External Genitalia. Without androgen influence on the development of external female genitalia, the genital tubercle remains small and differentiates into the body and glans of the clitoris. The urogenital sinus remains open with the urethra opening anteriorly and the vagina posteriorly, within the vestibular portion of the urogenital sinus. The majority of the labioscrotal swelling remains unfused and becomes the labia majora. The labioscrotal folds fuse anteriorly to form the mons pubis and posteriorly to form the posterior labial commissure. The urethral folds fuse posteriorly to form the frenulum of the labia minora. The urethral folds that do not fuse become the labia minora. The accessory glands of female genitalia include the Skene or lesser vestibular glands and the urethral glands. All arise from the urogenital sinus. The Bartholin glands (greater vestibular glands) are located on the right and left side of the vaginal vestibule. A summary is presented in Table 11.5 and Figure 11.6.

TABLE 11.5 Developmental Physiology: External Genitalia

Male testis	Inguinal canal provides path for testis migration.
	Gubernaculum provides structure for testicular descent and development begins in week 6.
	INLS-3 secreted by Leydig cells; regulates descent.
	Gubernaculum migrates from abdominal wall to inguinal ring.
	Gubernaculum then innervates the cremaster muscle and scrotum.
	Processus vaginalis follows the path of the gubernaculum, carrying layers of the abdominal wall to cover the testis and spermatic cord.
	Epididymis enters the processus vaginalis and then joins the testes to descend into and fuse with the walls of the scrotum at week 26.
	Processus vaginalis closes at weeks 37–40.
Male phallus	Genital tubercle elongates to form phallus.
	Urethra is pulled forward to form lateral walls of urethral groove.
	DHT and testosterone influence formation of the phallus.
	Ectoderm grows from the base toward the penile urethra.
	Endothelial lining originates in the endoderm and forms the epithelial lining of the urethral plate.
	Ectoderm cells from the glans move inward to form the epithelial cord and plate.
	Plate splits to form the urethra and ventral glans.
	Opening of the urethra moves to the tip of the glans, forming the urinary meatus and closing the groove of the glans.
	Labiosacral fold fuses at midline.
Female external genitalia	Absence of androgen leads to small genital tubercle, which differentiates into the body and glans of the clitoris.
	Labia minora urethral folds become one.
	Labiosacral folds become labia majora.
	Labiosacral folds join anteriorly to form mons pubis.
	Labiosacral folds join posteriorly to form labial commissure.
	Skene, lesser vestibular, urethral, and Bartholin's glans form.

DHT, dihydrotestosterone; INLS-3, insulinlike substance.

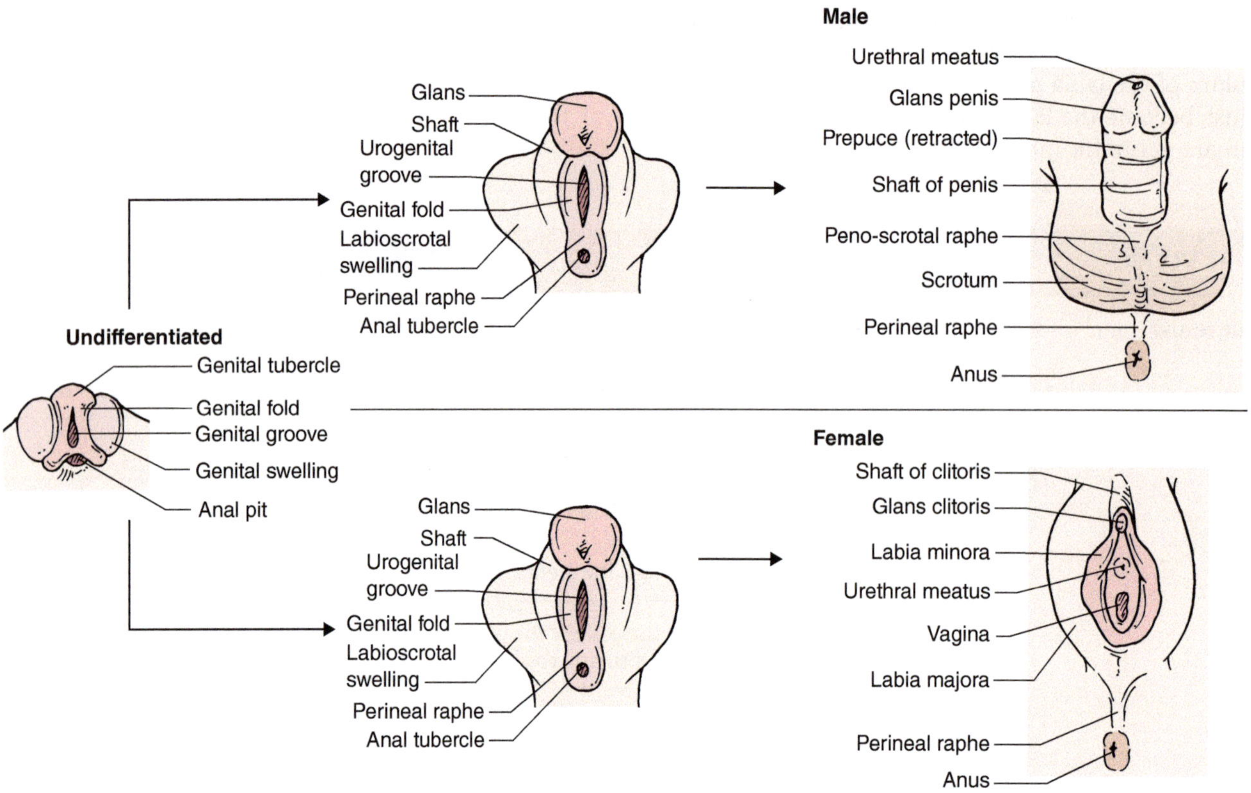

Figure 11.6 Development of male and female external genitalia.

COMMON PROBLEMS WITH IMPLICATIONS ACROSS THE LIFE SPAN

Variations in development of gonads and sex that present at birth impose lifelong implications. In 2005, an international consensus group on intersex disorders proposed the term *disorders of sex development* to describe the conditions. Subsequently, advocates proposed *sex development* as a more fitting label, because it accommodates identity rather than exclusively medical criteria. Both can be referred to as *DSD*, which comprise a variety of patterns of atypical development (Meyer-Bahlburg, 2017). This set of disorders consists of a variety of conditions characterized by complex interactions between multiple organ systems and psychologic development that affect individuals in varying degrees and have long-lasting impact (Van Batavia & Kolon, 2016). These DSDs can be classified by karyotype (47XXY, 45XO/46XY, 46XX/46XY, and a few other variations), phenotype, or gonadal histology (Figure 11.7; Hughes et al., 2006).

For the purpose of linking genetic, gonadal, and somatic sex development to interconnected body systems, a few of the more prevalent intersex conditions are highlighted in the final section of this chapter. These conditions are Turner syndrome (TS), Klinefelter syndrome (KS), complete androgen insensitivity syndrome (CAIS), and congenital adrenal hyperplasia (CAH).

Differences of Sex Development

Differences of sex development (or sometimes called "disorders of sexual differentiation" [DSD]) refers to a set of atypical patterns of development involving both internal and external genitalia. Labeled in the past as *ambiguous genitalia* or *intersex*, these conditions lead to questions about gender assignment and long-term management. Such variations occur once in every 1,500 to 2,000 births in the United States (Davis & Preves, 2017; Sax, 2002). The root cause of DSD is dysfunctional androgen activity, commonly androgen insensitivity syndrome, or AIS. Individuals with AIS will develop testicular dysgenesis and exhibit either female external genitalia or DSD as a result of incomplete masculinization. In some cases, gonads will develop ovotesticular gonads composed of both ovarian tissue and testicles joined together end to end via the primordial tubular and ductal structures. A summary is presented in Table 11.6.

Turner Syndrome (Female)

TS is characterized by a single X chromosome and found in one of 2,500 to 5,000 female births (Kikkeri & Nagalli, 2023; Thompson & Wherrett, 2025). Among the most common forms of aneuploidy, individuals with TS have short stature, sexual infantilism, and a variety of malformations, including webbing of the neck, widening between nipples, a low hairline on the neck, brown nevi

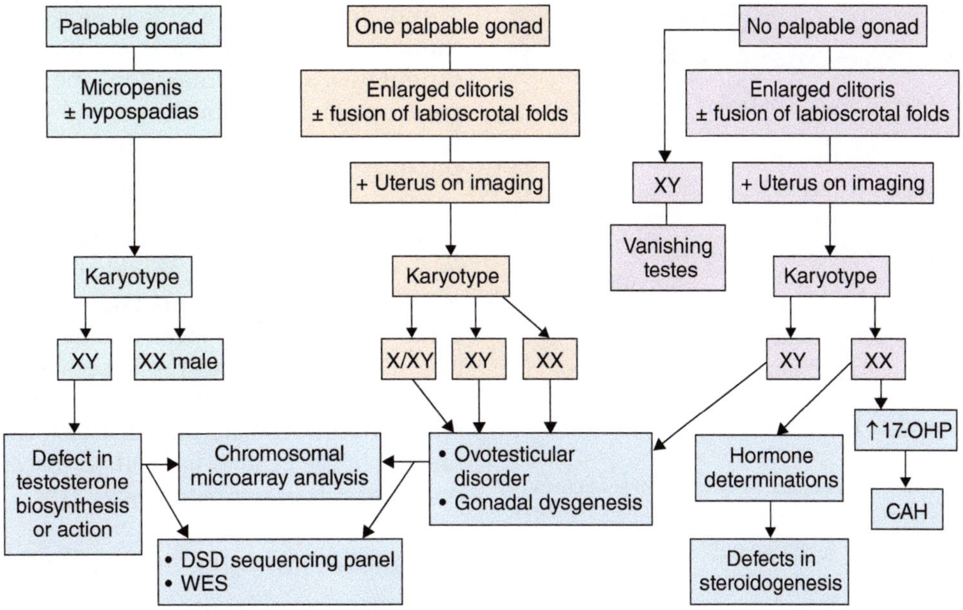

Figure 11.7 Infant with differences of sex development (DSD). This decision tree offers a practical approach to the diagnosis and determination of the pathogenesis of DSD.

CAH, congenital adrenal hyperplasia; WES, whole exome sequencing.

Source: Yatsenko, S. A., & Witchel, S. F. (2017). Genetic approach to ambiguous genitalia and disorders of sex development: What clinicians need to know. *Seminars in Perinatology, 41*, 232–243. https://doi.org/10.1053/j.semperi.2017.03.016

TABLE 11.6 Differences of Sex Development

Incidence	One in every 1,500–2,000 live births in the United States
Etiology	Androgen dysfunction or insensitivity
Impact	Testicular dysgenesis and incomplete masculinization
Presentation	Either female or ambiguous external genitalia

on the skin, elbow deformities, short metacarpals, small fingernails, and lymphedema in hands and feet (Oliveira et al., 2009). Individuals with TS may also present with a shield-shaped chest, horseshoe-shaped kidney, and coarctation of the aorta (Pennington et al., 1985). Undifferentiated gonads are a hallmark of the disorder. Both external and internal genitals are female, but the breasts are small and underdeveloped, as are the uterus and ovaries; primary amenorrhea is common (Oliveira et al., 2009).

Approximately 99% of all embryos with the pure 45X karyotype die in utero. However, mosaicism is higher among live-born fetuses with TS than among aborted fetuses and is considered necessary for survival and the source of variability in presentation (Hassold et al., 1988; Held et al., 1992). Risk for gonadal tumors results from abnormal gonadogenesis (Verp & Simpson, 1987). Gonadoblastoma is one such tumor, which despite its benign presentation can transform into more invasive tumors. For this reason, careful monitoring is required.

Individuals with TS also face increased risk for catastrophic aortic dissection. Among 85 reported cases, more than half of the dissections presented in XX pregnant patients below the age of 30. No additional risk factors were identified in 21% of the cases. Congenital heart disease was reported in 69% of the cases, and among these 54% were hypertensive, although blood pressure measurements were unavailable (Carlson & Silberbach, 2007; Thompson & Wherrett, 2025). A summary is presented in Table 11.7.

Klinefelter Syndrome (Male)

KS, also known as *47,XXY* or simply *XXY*, is characterized by hypergonadotropic hypogonadism. The most common sex-chromosome–linked DSD in males, KS presents as often as one in 500 to 1,000 live births (Butler et al., 2023; National Organization for Rare Disorders [NORD], 2024). However, many times KS is not recognized until later in life or sometimes not at all, or may be found incidentally with antenatal testing (Butler et al., 2023). It is often diagnosed after identifying developmental or speech delays. Individuals with KS face greater risk for all-cause mortality (40%) as well as cardiovascular risk, present with subclinical cardiovascular abnormalities, and perform poorly during exercise stress testing (Salzano et al., 2016). In addition to issues with cognitive development, individuals with KS have a higher prevalence of metabolic syndrome, insulin resistance, and type 2 diabetes (Salzano et al., 2016).

Individuals with KS are trapped in a cycle of hypogonadism, increasing body fat, failing carbohydrate metabolism, insulin resistance, suppressed testosterone production, and progressive hypogonadism. In theory,

TABLE 11.7 Turner Syndrome (Female)

Incidence	One in every 2,500–5,000 live female births
Etiology	Single X chromosome
Impact	99% of embryos die in utero
	Mosaicism common in live-born fetus may be necessary for survival
Long-term outcomes	Gonadal tumors may develop (benign and/or invasive)
	Congenital heart disease in 69% of cases
	Essential hypertension
	Risk for aortic dissection
Presentation	Short stature
	Sexual infantilism
	Webbing of neck
	Widening between nipples
	Hairline low on neck
	Brown nevi
	Elbow deformities
	Short metacarpals
	Small fingernails
	Lymphedema in hands and feet
	Shield-shaped chest
	Horseshoe-shaped kidney
	Coarctation of the aorta
	Undifferentiated gonads
	Female internal and external gonads; underdeveloped breasts, uterus, and ovaries
	Primary amenorrhea

supplemental testosterone can break the cycle and may reduce levels of C-reactive protein associated with persistent inflammation. However, robust data are not yet available to support this practice (Salzano et al., 2016).

Individuals with KS face increased risk for both thromboembolic and stasis events. Mesenteric venous thrombosis, arterial infarction, and ischemic injury are more common than in the general population adjusted for age (Campbell & Price, 1981; Campbell et al., 1980; Rouffy et al., 1973).

The cardiovascular function is also altered by the hypogonadism of KS. Shortened QTC intervals are common. It is interesting to note that the alteration is more pronounced in KS patients taking testosterone replacements as compared to those who do not (Jørgensen et al., 2015). This introduces the hypothesis that individuals with KS may be protected against the cardiovascular danger of low testosterone identified across males more broadly in the general population (Salzano et al., 2016). A summary is presented in Table 11.8.

Complete Androgen Insensitivity Syndrome

CAIS refers to a condition in which affected individuals are nonresponsive to male sex hormones (androgens). Androgen insensitivity syndrome is differentiated ac-

TABLE 11.8 Klinefelter Syndrome (Male)

Incidence	One in 660 live births
Etiology	47,XXY
Impact	Hypergonadotropic hypogonadism
Presentation and long-term outcomes	Increased risk for mortality from all causes (40%)
	Subclinical cardiovascular abnormalities
	Issues with cognitive development
	Metabolic syndrome
	Insulin resistance
	Persistent inflammatory processes
	Increasing body fat
	Failing carbohydrate metabolism
	Suppressed testosterone production
	Progressive hypogonadism
	Thromboembolic events
	Vascular stasis
	Arterial infarction and ischemic injury

TABLE 11.9 Complete Androgen Insensitivity (Male)

Incidence	2 to 5 per 100,000 live births
Etiology	Unresponsive to male sex hormones
Impact	No masculinization of male genitalia
Presentation	Genetic males present with female external phenotype
	Sparse axillary and pubic hair
	Breasts may develop
	Primary amenorrhea in individuals thought to be female

cording to the degree of genital masculinization. CAIS is only significant when it occurs in genetic males and is reported among two to five of every 100,000 individuals (Hughes & Deeb, 2006; Singh & Ilyayeva, 2023). Due to the unresponsiveness to male hormones, there is no masculinization of male genitalia. Genetic male individuals affected by CAIS will have female external phenotypic development despite the presence of a Y chromosome; they may have a separate urethral and vaginal orifice. Individuals may have sparse axilla and pubic hair. Breast development may occur due to conversion of excessive testosterone to estrogen. Females have primary amenorrhea and are diagnosed with CAIS during puberty. A summary is presented in Table 11.9.

Congenital Adrenal Hyperplasia

CAH is a group of autosomal recessive genetic disorders with varying phenotypic presentations. This defect results from a deficiency in reduced activity of one of the five crucial enzymes required for cortisol and aldosterone biosynthesis (from cholesterol) in the adrenal cortex. In approximately 95% of cases of CAH, the genetic defect affects the enzyme 21-hydroxylase (21-OH), which is a cytochrome P450 enzyme. The gene for 21-OH is found on chromosome 6 and is known as *CYP21A2* (Online Mendelian Inheritance in Man, 2018). Classic CAH is the most common cause of DSD in the newborn, affecting one in 14,000 to 20,000 newborns (Burdea & Mendez, 2023; Thompson & Wher-

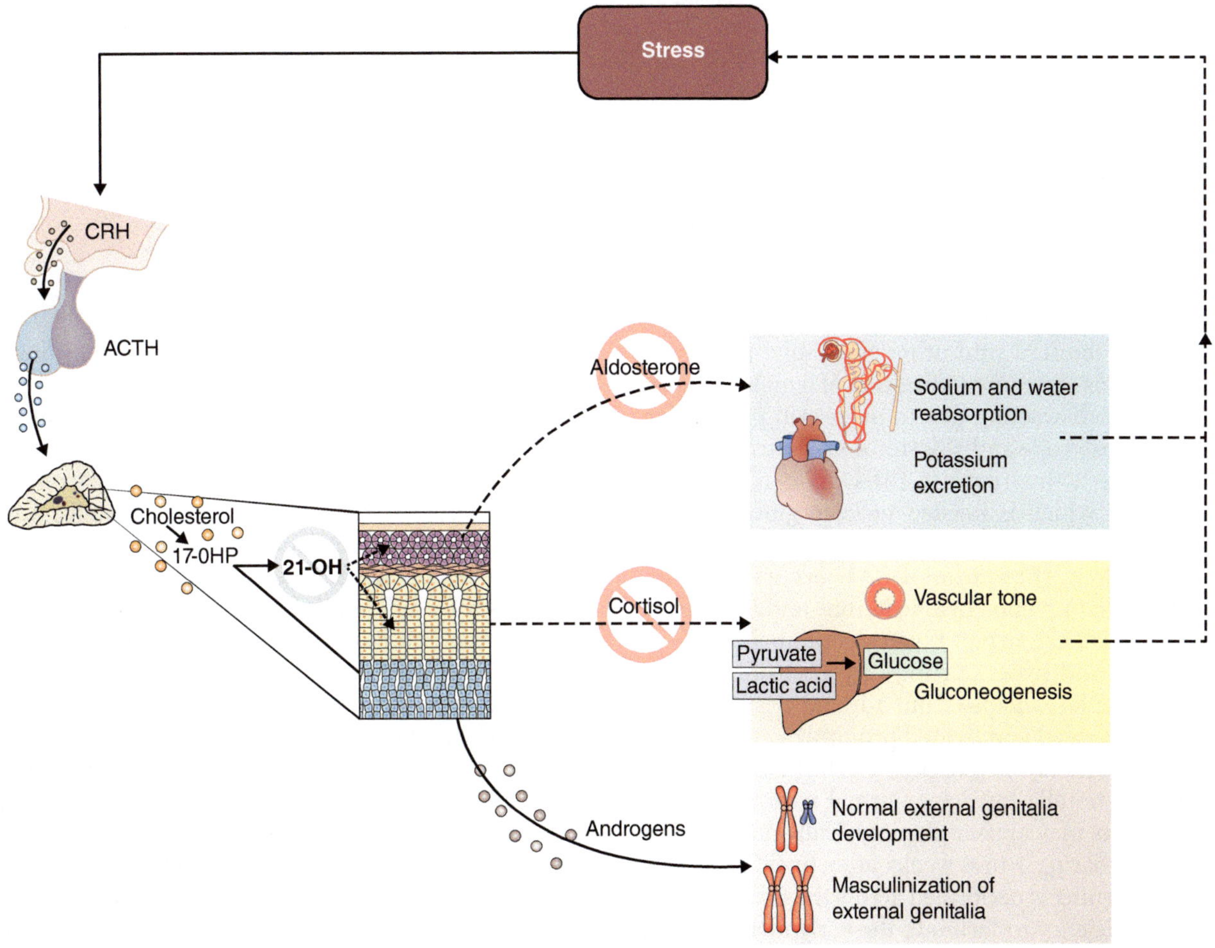

Figure 11.8 Pathophysiology of congenital adrenal hyperplasia.
ACTH, adrenocorticotropic hormone; CRH, corticotropin-releasing hormone.

TABLE 11.10 Congenital Adrenal Hyperplasia

Incidence	One in every 12,000–15,000 live births
Etiology	Autosomal recessive disease; gene is found on chromosome 6 (CYP21A2)
Impact	Virilization of female genitalia with incorrect sexual assignment
	Periods of adrenal crisis
Long-term outcomes	Decreased fertility in XX pregnant patients
	Short stature
	Severe acne
	Early puberty changes, as early as 3–4 years of age
Presentation	*Classic CAH (salt-wasting):* vomiting, diarrhea, dehydration, low blood pressure, weight loss, hyponatremia, poor feeding, metabolic acidosis
	Classic CAH (simple virilizing form): DSD, fused labia, enlarged clitoris, adrenal crisis
	Nonclassic CAH: variable symptoms with milder effects • *Males and females*: rapid growth during childhood, early puberty, hirsutism, severe acne • *Males only*: small testicles, enlarged penis, early facial hair • *Females only*: irregular menses, infertility, behavior becomes masculinized

CAH, congenital adrenal hyperplasia; DSD, disorder of sex development.

rett, 2025). Nonclassic disease is reported among one in 1,000 individuals (Burdea & Mendez, 2023).

The basic pathophysiology of this condition, specific to the reproductive system, involves the decrease of cortisol synthesis resulting in hyperplasia of the adrenal cortex due to (a) continuous stimulation by adrenocorticotropic hormone (ACTH) and (b) an overproduction of androgens that are shunted into other metabolic pathways. These androgens can cause virilization of female genitalia (and possible salt-wasting due to decreased production of deoxycorticosterone and aldosterone; Figure 11.8).

The enzyme 21-hydroxylase (21-OH) is required to make cortisol, which is needed to keep glucose levels normal. Newborns with CAH may present with hypoglycemia. The salt-wasting form of CAH occurs when infants do not produce enough aldosterone and lose excess salt and water to the urine. Electrolyte imbalance (i.e., hyponatremia and hyperkalemia), hypotension, shock, and cardiovascular collapse from adrenal crisis may result if not recognized and treated promptly.

Female infants may be recognized at birth due to atypical external genitalia but have normal internal genitalia. Male infants may appear phenotypically normal with symptoms appearing 1 to 4 weeks after birth. Newborn metabolic screening is performed across the United States for 21-OH deficiency to facilitate the early identification of infants at risk for developing life-threatening adrenal crisis. In addition, early identification prevents affected female infants with DSD from receiving an incorrect sex assignment (Levine, 2000). A summary is presented in Table 11.10.

CONCLUSION

Sex hormones, which are primarily androgens, are produced in small amounts; this process begins during early embryonic development and extends across the life span. The formation of the accessory sex glands in the male depends on androgenic stimulation. Females rely on androgen secretion for normal development of genitalia. An error in genetic, gonadal, ductal, or genital development, as a result of dysfunctional androgen activity, may result in a disorder of sexual differentiation. TS involves normal ovarian differentiation until the early fetal period of development, when degeneration and atresia of the primordial ovarian follicles occurs. These infants exhibit normal Müllerian duct development, absent Wolffian ducts, and phenotypically female external genitalia with bilateral streak gonads. Many affected infants manifest with impaired lymphatic drainage and cardiac anomalies. KS typically manifests during puberty with persistently small testes and impaired spermatogenesis. CAH is a group of autosomal recessive disorders that occurs as the result of impaired cortisol synthesis, most often due to 21-hydroxylase deficiency, an enzyme responsible for the conversion of cholesterol to cortisol and aldosterone. CAH is the most common cause for DSD among females, and, depending on its severity, females may manifest with a simple virilizing form of CAH or a more severe salt-wasting form of the disease. Clinically, term males with bilateral impalpable gonads and infants who present with ambiguous genitalia must be considered positive for CAH until proven otherwise. An understanding of normal sexual differentiation and the more common disorders of sexual differentiation that may manifest during the birth hospitalization or early childhood is essential. Clinicians must remain vigilant and prioritize the early identification, diagnosis, and treatment of these disorders, and, in some cases, offer timely counseling and psychosocial support for family members.

LEARNING TOOLS AND RESOURCES

CourseConnect

To access self-assessment questions and interactive, competency-based learning activities for this chapter, visit www.springerpub.com/courseconnect. See inside front cover and tear-out card for CourseConnect details.

Podcast

This podcast is available online by visiting www.springerpub.com/courseconnect. See inside front cover and tear-out card for CourseConnect details.

Congenital Adrenal Hyperplasia/ 21-Hydroxylase Deficiency
Andrea N. Trembath

Discussion Prompts

1. Contrast the concepts of development and differentiation.
2. What is meant by the bipotential gonad?
3. Describe the function of estrogen and progesterone.
4. Explain the differences between the sexes with respect to ductal system differentiation.
5. When is the sex of the embryo genetically determined?

MIND MAP

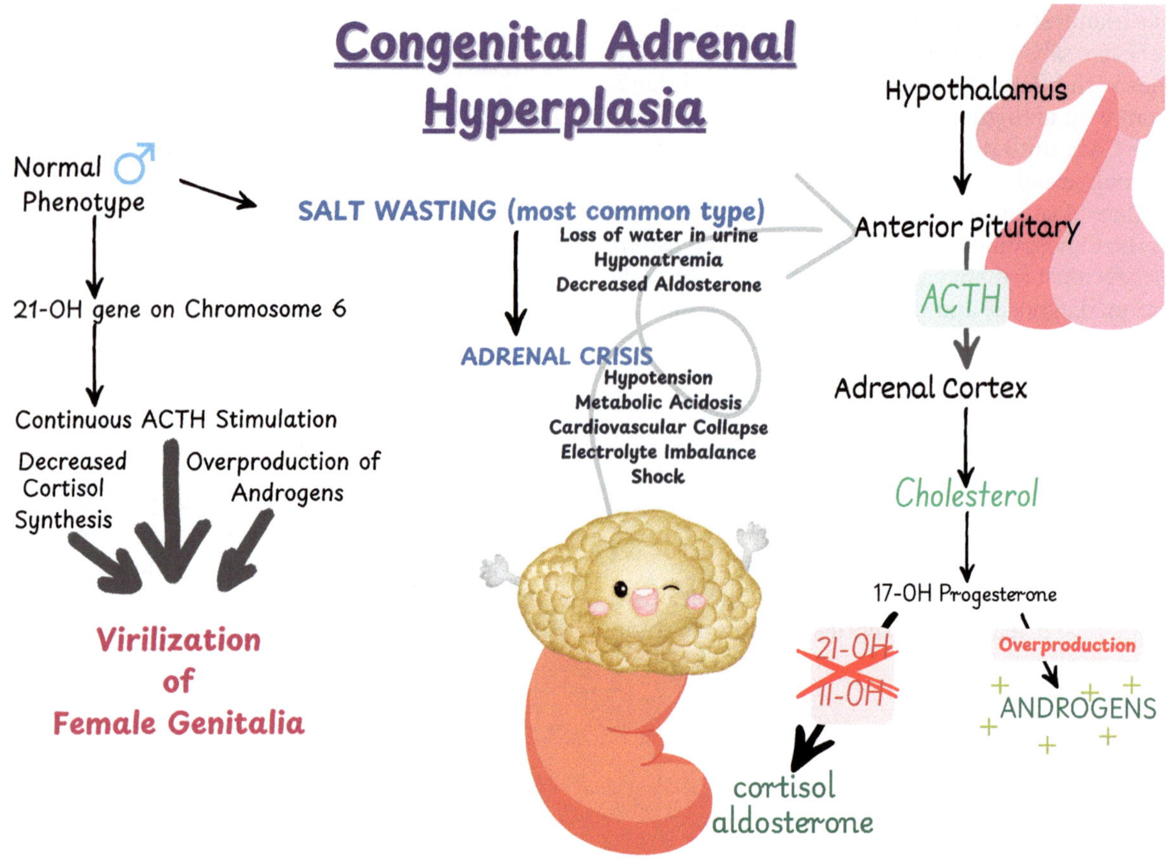

Note: This mind map reflects one student's interpretation of a portion of one or more concepts addressed in this chapter. Readers should regard the mind maps woven throughout this textbook as examples of multisensory study tools that can be developed to encourage conceptual understanding. Readers are encouraged to develop their own unique mind maps in consultation with academic faculty or clinical preceptors.

Image Credit: Courtney McDaniel, BSN, RNC-NIC.

TIMELINE OF ORGAN DEVELOPMENT

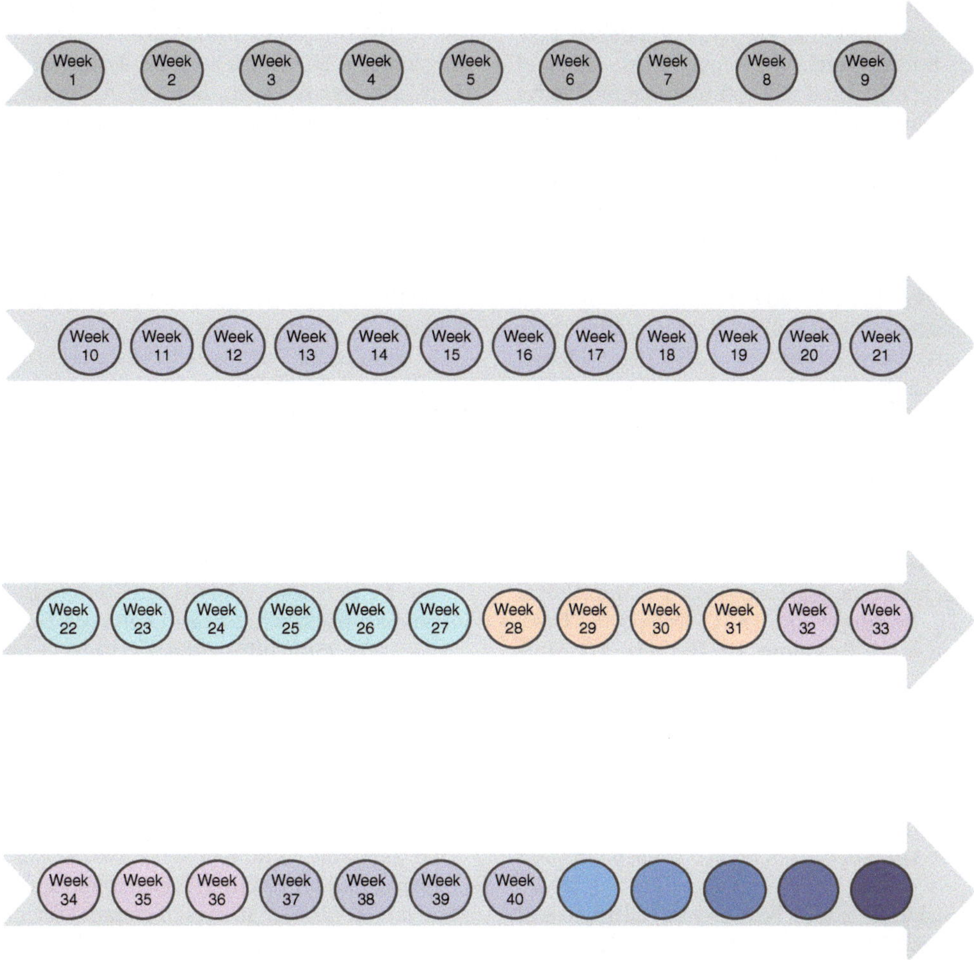

Note: Placement of common problems is meant to offer visual/conceptual perspective on the timing of onset of these commonly reported malformations. Variation exists across the literature.	***Legend*:** <22–27 6/7 weeks = extremely preterm 28–31 6/7 weeks = very preterm 32–36 6/7 weeks = late/moderate preterm 37–40 weeks = term

Note: Readers should annotate the blank timeline during studying, self-directed learning, and creation of feedback loops with mentors.

REFERENCES

Ainsworth, C. (2015). Sex redefined. *Nature*, 518, 288–291. https://doi.org/10.1038/518288a

Blecher, S., & Erickson, R. (2007). Genetics of sexual development: A new paradigm. *American Journal of Medical Genetics: Part A, 143A*(24), 3054–3068. https://doi.org/10.1002/ajmg.a.32037

Brennan, J., & Capel, B. (2004). One tissue, two fates: Molecular genetic events that underlie testis versus ovary development. *Nature Reviews Genetics, 5*, 509–521. https://doi.org/10.1038/nrg1381

Burdea, L., & Mendez, M. D. (2023, July 31). 21-hydroxylase deficiency. In *StatPearls*. StatPearls Publishing. https://www.ncbi.nlm.nih.gov/books/NBK493164

Butler, G., Srirangalingam, U., Faithfull, J., Sangster, P., Senniappan, S., & Mitchell, R. (2023). Klinefelter syndrome: Going beyond the diagnosis. *Archives of Disease in Childhood, 108*(3), 166–171. https://doi.org/10.1136/archdischild-2020-320831

Campbell, W. A., Newton, M. S., & Price W. H. (1980). Hypostatic leg ulceration and Klinefelter's syndrome. *Journal of Mental Deficiency Research, 24*, 115–117. https://doi.org/10.1111/j.1365-2788.1980.tb00064.x

Campbell, W. A., & Price, W. H. (1981). Venous thromboembolic disease in Klinefelter's syndrome. *Clinical Genetics, 19*, 275–280. https://doi.org/10.1111/j.1399-0004.1981.tb00709.x

Carlson, M., & Silberback, M. (2007). Dissection of the aorta in Turner syndrome: Two new cases and review of 85 cases in the literature. *Journal of Medical Genetics, 44*, 745–749. https://doi.org/10.1136/jmg.2007.052019

Childs, A., Cowan, G., Kinnell, A., Anderson, R., & Saunders, P. (2011). Retinoic acid signaling and the control of meiotic entry in the human fetal gonad. *PLoS One, 6(6)*, e20249. https://doi.org/10.1371/journal.pone.0020249

Davis, G., & Preves, S. (2017). Intersex and the social construction of sex. *Contexts, 16*(1), 80. https://doi.org/10.1177/1536504217696082

Dupont, S., Krust, A., Gansmuller, A., Dierich, P., Chambon, P., & Mark, M. (2000). Effect of single and compound knockouts of estrogen receptor μ (ERμ) and (ER) on mouse reproductive phenotypes. *Development, 127*(19), 4277–4291. http://dev.biologists.org/content/develop/127/19/4277.full.pdf

Ellis, P. (2022). Genetics of sex determination and differentiation. In R. Polin, S. H. Abman, D. H. Rowitch, & W. Benitz (Eds.), *Fetal and neonatal physiology* (6th ed., pp. 1555–1566). Elsevier.

Estermann, M. A., & Smith, C. A. (2020). Applying single-cell analysis to gonadogenesis and DSDs (disorders/differences of sex development). *International Journal of Molecular Sciences, 21*(18), 6614. https://doi.org/10.3390/ijms21186614

Favorito, L., Costa, S., Julio-Junior, H., & Sampaio, F. (2014). The importance of the gubernaculum in testicular migration during the human fetal period. *International Brazilian Journal of Urology, 40*(6), 722–729. https://doi.org/10.1590/S1677-5538.IBJU.2014.06.02

Garcia-Alonso, L., Lorenzi, V., Mazzeo, C. I., Alves-Lopes, J., Roberts, K., Sancho-Serra, C., Engelbert, J., Marečková, M., Gruhn, W. H., Botting, R. A., Li, T., Crespo, B., Dongen, S. V., Kiselev, V. Y., Prigmore, E., Herbert, M., Moffett, A., Chédotal, A., Bayraktar, O. A., . . . Vento-Tormo, R. (2022). Single-cell roadmap of human gonadal development. *Nature, 607*(7919), 540-4,547A-547W. https://doi.org/10.1038/s41586-022-04918-4

Griswold, M., Hogarth, C., Bowles, J., & Koopman, P. (2012). Initiating meiosis: The case for retinoic acid. *Biology of Reproduction, 86*(2), 1–7. https://doi.org/10.1095/biolreprod.111.096610

Griswold, S., & Behringer, R. (2009). Fetal Leydig cell origin and development. *Sexual Development, 3*(1), 1–15. https://doi.org/10.1159/000200077

Hanley, N., Hagan, D., Clement-Jones, M., Ball, S., Strachan, T., Salas-Cortés, L., McElreavey, K., Lindsay, S., Robson, S., Bullen, P., Ostrer, H., & Wilson, D. (2000). *SRY, SOX9* and DAX1 expression patterns during human sex determination and gonadal development. *Mechanisms of Development, 91*(1–2), 403–407. https://doi.org/10.1016/S0925-4773(99)00307-X

Hassold, T., Benham, F., & Leppert, M. (1988). Cytogenetic and molecular analysis of sex-chromosome monosomy. *American Journal of Human Genetics, 42*(4), 534–541.

Held, K. R., Kerber, S., Kaminsky, E., Singh, S., Goetz, P., Seemanova, E., & Goedde, H. W. (1992). Mosaicism in 45, X Turner syndrome: Does survival in early pregnancy depend on the presence of two sex chromosomes? *Human Genetics, 88*(3), 288–294. https://doi.org/10.1007/BF00197261

Hryhorczuk, A. L., Phelps, A. S., Yu, R. N., & Chow, J. S. (2022). The radiologist's role in assessing differences of sex development. *Pediatric Radiology, 52*(4), 752–764. https://doi.org/10.1007/s00247-021-05147-z

Hughes, I., & Acerini, C. (2008). Factors controlling testis descent. *European Journal of Endocrinology, 159*(Suppl. 1), s75–s82. https://doi.org/10.1530/EJE-08-0458

Hughes, I., & Deeb, A. (2006). Androgen resistance. *Best Practices and Research Clinical Endocrinology and Metabolism, 4*, 577–598. https://doi.org/10.1016/j.beem.2006.11.003

Hughes, I. A., Houk, C., Ahmed, S. F., & Lee, P. A. (2006). Consensus statement on management of intersex disorders. *Archives of Diseases in Children, 91*(7), 554–563. https://doi.org/10.1136/adc.2006.098319

Jørgensen, I. N., Skakkebæk, A., Andersen, N. H., Pedersen, L. N., Hougaard, D. M., Bojesen, A., Trolle, C., & Gravholt, C. H. (2015). Short QTc interval in males with Klinefelter syndrome—Influence of CAG repeat length, body composition, and testosterone replacement therapy. *Pacing and Clinical Electrophysiology, 38*, 472–482. https://doi.org/10.1111/pace.12580

Kashimada, K., & Koopman, P. (2010). SRY: The master switch in mammalian sex determination. *Development, 137*, 3921–3930. https://doi.org/10.1242/dev.048983

Kikkeri, N., & Nagalli, S. (2023, August 8). Turner syndrome. In *StatPearls*. StatPearls Publishing. https://www.ncbi.nlm.nih.gov/books/NBK554621

Lalli, E., Melner, M. H., Stocco, D. M., & Sassone-Corsi, P. (1998). DAX-1 blocks steroid production at multiple levels. *Endocrinology, 139*(10), 4237–4243. https://doi.org/10.1210/endo.139.10.6217

Le Bouffant, R., Guerquin, M., Duquenne, C., Frydman, N., Coffigny, H., Rouiller-Fabre, V., Frydman, R., Habert, R., & Livera, G. (2010). Meiosis initiation in the human ovary requires intrinsic retinoic acid synthesis. *Human Reproduction, 25*, 2579–2590. https://doi.org/10.1093/humrep/deq195

Lee, M. (2022). Testicular development and descent. In R. Polin, S. H. Abman, D. H. Rowitch, & W. Benitz (Eds.), *Fetal and neonatal physiology* (6th ed., pp. 1574–1581). Elsevier.

Levine, L. (2000). Congenital adrenal hyperplasia. *Pediatrics in Review, 21*(5), 159–170. https://doi.org/10.1542/pir.21-5-159

Maheshwari, A., & Fowler, P. A. (2008). Primordial follicular assembly in humans-revisited. *Zygote, 16*(4), 285–296. https://doi.org/10.1017/S0967199408004802

Makiyan, Z. (2016). Studies of gonadal sex differentiation. *Organogenesis, 12*(1), 42–51. https://doi.org/10.1080/15476278.2016.1145318

Mamsen, L. S., Andersen, C. Y., Childs, A. J., & Anderson, R. A. (2022). Differentiation of the ovary. In R. Polin, S. H. Abman, D. H. Rowitch, & W. Benitz (Eds.), *Fetal and neonatal physiology* (6th ed., pp. 1566–1574). Elsevier.

Markström, E., Svensson, E., Shao, R., Svanberg, B., & Billig, H. (2002). Survival factors regulating ovarian apoptosis-dependence on follicle differentiation. *Reproduction, 123*(1), 23–30. https://rep.bioscientifica.com/view/journals/rep/123/1/23.xml?rskey=x2TV2d&result=1

Meyer-Bahlburg, H. F. L. (2017). Intersex care development: Current priorities. *LGBT Health, 4*(2), 77–80. https://doi.org/10.1089/lgbt.2017.0021

Mital, P., Hinton, B., & Dufour, J. (2011). The blood–testis and blood–epididymis barriers are more than just their tight junctions. *Biology of Reproduction, 84*, 851–858. https://doi.org/10.1095/biolreprod.110.087452

Nation, T., Balic, A., Southwell, B., Newgreen, D., & Hutson, J. (2009). The hormonal control of testicular descent. *Pediatric Endocrinology Review, 7*(1), 22–31.

National Organization of Rare Disorders. (2024). *47, XXY (Klinefelter syndrome)*. https://rarediseases.org/rare-diseases/47-xxy-klinefelter-syndrome

Nef, S., Schaad, O., Stallings, N. R., Cederroth, C. R., Pitetti, J.-L., Schaer, G., Malki, S., Dubois-Dauphin, M., Boizet-Bonhoure, B., Descombes, P., Parker, K. L., & Vassalli, J.-D.

(2005). Gene expression during sex determination reveals a robust female genetic program at the onset of ovarian development. *Developmental Biology, 287*(2), 361–377. https://doi.org/10.1016/j.ydbio.2005.09.008

Oliveira, R. M., Verreschi, I., Lipay, M. V., Eça, L., Guedes, A., & Bianco, B. (2009). Y chromosome in Turner syndrome: Review of the literature. *Sao Paulo Medical Journal, 127*(6), 1–11. https://doi.org/10.1590/S1516-31802009000600010

Online Mendelian Inheritance in Man. (2018). *#201910 adrenal hyperplasia, congenital, due to 21-hydroxylase deficiency.* http://www.omim.org/entry/201910

Pennington, B. F., Heaton, R. K., Karzmark, P., Pendleton, M. G., Lehman, R., & Shucard, D. W. (1985). The neuropsychological phenotype in Turner syndrome. *Cortex, 21*, 391–404. https://doi.org/10.1016/S0010-9452(85)80004-6

Rouffy, J., Pestel, M., Cortot, A., Sikorav, H., Michaux, A., & Julien, R. (1973). Klinefelter's syndrome, endogenous hypertriglyceridemia, and arteriopathy of the lower limbs. Apropos of a case. *Annales de Médecine Interne, 124*, 201–206.

Sajjad, Y. (2010). Development of the genital ducts and external genitalia in the early human embryo. *Journal of Obstetrics and Gynaecology Research, 6*(5), 929–937. https://doi.org/10.1111/j.1447-0756.2010.01272.x

Salzano, A., Acropinto, M., Marra, A., Bobbio, E., Esposito, D., Accardo, G., Giallauria, F., Bossone, E., Vigorito, C., Lenzi, A., Pasquali, D., Isidori, A. M., & Cittadini, A. (2016). Klinefelter syndrome, cardiovascular system, and thromboembolic disease: Review of the literature and clinical perspectives. *European Journal of Endocrinology, 175*(1), R27–R40. https://doi.org/10.1530/EJE-15-1025

Sax, L. (2002). How common is intersex? A response to Anne Fausto-Sterling. *Journal of Sex Research, 39*(3), 174–178. https://doi.org/10.1080/00224490209552139

Singh, S., & Ilyayeva, S. (2023, February 23). Androgen insensitivity syndrome. In *StatPearls*. StatPearls Publishing. https://ghr.nlm.nih.gov/condition/androgen-insensitivity-syndrome

Sobel, V., Zhu, Y., & Imperato-McGinley, J. (2004). Fetal hormones and sexual differentiation. *Obstetrical and Gynecological Clinics of North America, 31*, 837–856. https://doi.org/10.1016/j.ogc.2004.08.005

Suntharalingham, J., Buonocore, F., Duncan, J., & Achermann, J. (2015). DAX-1 (NR0B1) and steroidogenic factor-1 (SF-1, NR5A1) in human disease. *Best Practices and Research Clinical Endocrinology and Metabolism, 29*(4), 607–619. https://doi.org/10.1016/j.beem.2015.07.004

Thompson, S., & Wherrett, D. K. (2025). Disorders of sex development. In R. J. Martin & A. A. Fanaroff (Eds.), *Fanaroff & Martin's neonatal–perinatal medicine, 2-volume set: Diseases of the fetus and infant* (12th ed., pp. 1750–1789). Elsevier.

Torchia, M. G., & Persaud, T. V. N. (2025). *The developing human: Clinically oriented embryology* (12th ed.). Elsevier.

Van Batavia, J. P., & Kolon, T. F. (2016). Fertility in disorders of sex development: A review. *Journal of Pediatric Urology, 12*(6), 418–425. https://doi.org/10.1016/j.jpurol.2016.09.015

Verp, M. S., & Simpson, J. L. (1987). Abnormal sexual differentiation and neoplasia. *Cancer Genetics & Cytogenetics, 25*(2), 191–218. https://doi.org/10.1016/0165-4608(87)90180-4

Virant-Klun, I. (2015). Postnatal oogenesis in humans: A review of recent findings. *Stem Cells and Cloning: Advances in Application, 8*, 49–60. https://doi.org/10.2147/SCCAA.S32650

Wilhelm, D., Hiramatsu, R., Mizusaki, H., Widjaja, L., Combes, A., Kanai, Y., & Koopman, P. (2007). SOX9 regulates prostaglandin D synthase gene transcription *in vivo* to ensure testis development. *Journal of Biological Chemistry, 282*(14), 10553–10560. https://doi.org/10.1074/jbc.M609578200

Wilhelm, D., Palmer, S., & Koopman, P. (2007). Sex determination and gonadal development in mammals. *Physiological Review, 87*, 1–28. https://doi.org/10.1152/physrev.00009.2006

Yao, H., Matzuk, M., Jorgez, C., Menke, D., Page, D., Swain, A., & Capel, B. (2004). *Follistatin* operates downstream of *Wnt4* in mammalian ovary organogenesis. *Developmental Dynamics, 230*(2), 210–215. https://doi.org/10.1002/dvdy.20042

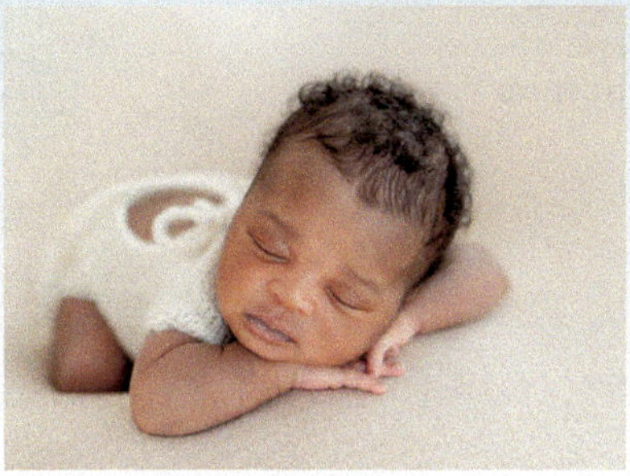 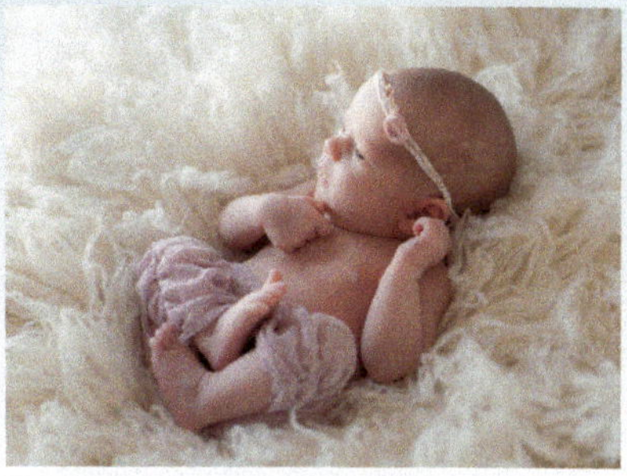

12

THE SKIN

Colleen R. Moss, Jennifer Fitzgerald, and Amy J. Jnah

LEARNING OBJECTIVES

After completing this chapter, the reader should be able to:

- Understand normal skin development.
- Analyze the physiologic function of the fetal and neonatal skin.
- Discuss common inherited disorders and their effect on fetal and neonatal skin development and function.
- Identify health issues in XX pregnant patients that have a potential impact on fetal and postnatal skin development and function.
- Evaluate common disorders that affect the skin and their implications across the life span.

INTRODUCTION

The skin, or integumentary system, is the largest organ in the body. It modulates multiple functions, including protection, sensation, metabolic functions, and thermoregulation. It does so by forming a physical barrier to the environment, harmful microorganisms, ultraviolet radiation, toxic agents, and mechanical injuries. The skin functions as a conduit for sensation and a metabolic organ that allows or limits the transmission of passage of water, electrolytes, and various substances as well as energy stored as fat and the synthesis of vitamin D. The skin is critical to thermoregulatory homeostasis and impacts the maintenance of euthermia through an intricate process of capillary dilatation and restriction, as well as the regulation of moisture. This chapter reviews embryologic development, lists the primary functions, explores the anatomic layers and their physiologic functions, discusses genetic influences, and outlines common neonatal skin problems.

TIMELINE OF ORGAN DEVELOPMENT

The skin is embryologically derived from two separate origins. The epidermis, or the superficial layer, originates from the ectoderm, whereas the deeper layer, known as the *dermis*, arises from the mesenchyme (Sadler, 2023). The following is an overview of embryologic development of the skin and its derivatives. It is important to remember that studying the details of skin-layer–specific maturation with the use of visual aids may create the false perception of spaciousness. Rather, we encourage students and clinicians to be mindful of the fact that the five major layers of the skin are tightly connected and account for, on average, 0.9 mm (premature infants) to 1.2 mm (term infants) of depth (Bolender, 2022).

Epidermis

Embryonic Period. The epidermis arises from the embryonic ectoderm (neural crest; Figure 12.1). During week 4 of gestation, a single layer of ectodermal cells appears. Between weeks 4 and 6 of gestation, these cells stratify into peridermal (outermost) and basal (innermost) layers (Bolender, 2022; Carlson, 2024; Persaud & Torchia, 2025. The periderm protects the developing epidermis from amniotic fluid and manages glucose uptake. The periderm thereby begins a cyclic process of cellular generation, keratinization, and exfoliation. Simultaneously, the lower basal layer begins synthesizing skin cells (Persaud & Torchia, 2025). Around week 4, the sebaceous glands begin to form, and mammary ridges begin to appear. Melanocytes start appearing in the basal layer from weeks 5 to 8 of gestation. The ectodermal cells begin to form ridges around week 6 and, by week 8, epidermal mammary ridges begin to disappear.

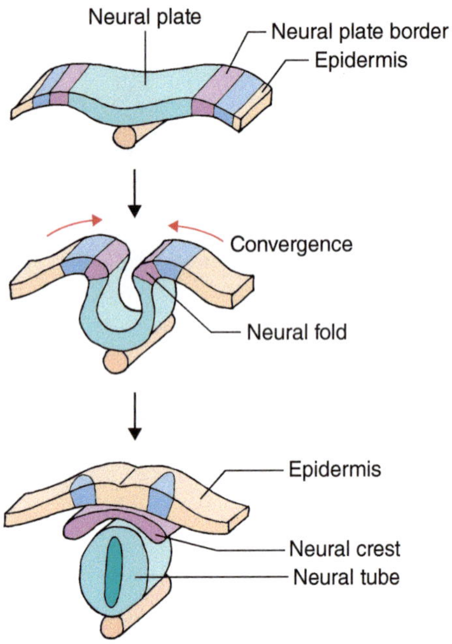

Figure 12.1 Origin of the epidermis.

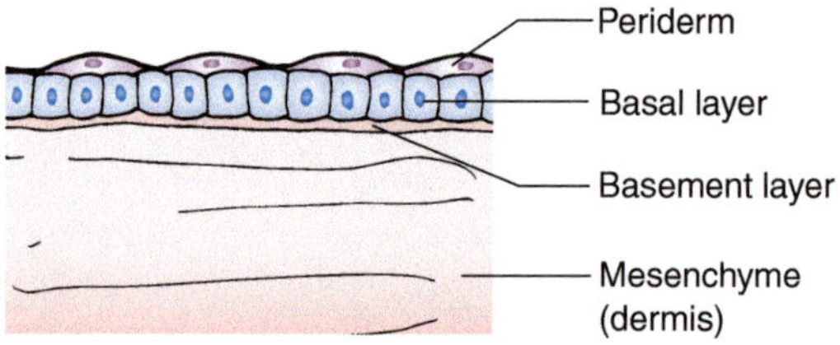

Figure 12.2 Early layers of the epidermis.

Fetal Period. The early fetal period is marked by epidermal differentiation into a three-layered structure, which begins between weeks 8 and 11 of gestation. Proliferation and maturation of basal layer keratinocytes proliferate to form the spinous cell layer between the basal layer and the periderm (Figure 12.2). The lowest basal layer (stratum germinativum) increases production of cells and assumes the role of germinal matrix for cellular synthesis. The rapid synthesis and upward migration of new skin cells exceeds the turnover rate of normally expiring peridermal cells and gives rise to an intermediate skin layer (Bolognia et al., 2025). Periderm, spinous cells (two layers), basal cells, desmosomes, hair follicles, and mesenchymal cells of the hair bulb appear between weeks 12 and 16 of gestation. There are six to eight basal layers for each periderm layer, and the upper spinous cells flatten from weeks 14 to 17 of gestation (Visscher & Narendran, 2014).

Basal layer cellular proliferation also projects in a downward direction, toward the deeper mesenchyme (dermis). This gives rise to epidermal ridges, or invaginations, that resemble U-shaped curves. By week 15 of gestation, these ridges give rise to touch pads and grooves at the hands and feet (Persaud & Torchia, 2025). These grooves develop curves and whorls by week 35 of gestation, bestowing a unique fingerprint to the infant; abnormal matriculation of the pads and grooves are commonly observed among individuals with trisomy 21 (Persaud & Torchia, 2025).

By week 16 to 23 of gestation, the five epidermal layers are evident (Table 12.1). These layers are both thick and thin, uniquely equipped with a complement of follicles, arrector muscles, sebaceous glands, and sweat glands (Table 12.2; Persaud & Torchia, 2025; Sadler, 2023). Polygon-shaped cells, composed of keratin, appear in the interfollicular regions and hair follicles. At 18 to 19 weeks of gestation, the stratum corneum (SC) can be seen around the hair follicle. By week 21, it can be seen along the hair canal. This demonstrates the important role of the hair follicle in epidermal barrier development. The terminally differentiated outermost layer, or SC, can be seen at week 23, but may be only a few layers thick. Periderm is no longer observed around week 23. By week 26, the epidermis is fully keratinized, composed of (a) one basal layer, (b) two to three spinous layers, (c) a granular layer containing keratohyalin granules, and (d) five to six layers of SC. The interfollicular epidermis cornifies programmatically from head (initially, week 23) to toe and dorsal–ventral (week 25, abdomen) across the developing infant (Visscher & Narendran, 2014). Cornification of the appendages and trunk usually begins between weeks 24 and 26 of gestation and continues throughout gestation. The time for complete maturation of the neonatal epidermal barrier, to achieve structure and function comparable to adults, is currently unknown (Visscher & Narendran, 2014).

Dermis and Hypodermis

Embryonic Period. The origin of the dermis is shared between the neural crest and mesoderm (Carlson, 2024). Dermal mesenchyme that comprise the face and scalp arise from the neural crest. Dermal mesenchyme of the back arises from the embryonic somite. In addition, the dermal mesenchyme associated with the appendages and trunk (ventral) arise from the lateral plate mesoderm. No rationale for this phenomenon exists. Primitive dermal cells can be seen during the latter end of the embryonic period of development (week 8 of gestation); however, they are not active until the early fetal period of development (Figure 12.3).

Fetal Period. Proliferation commences early into the fetal period, as the dermis subdivides into its two primary layers, the (a) dermal papillae and (b) reticular layer. Although the previously described epidermal cells invade the topmost layer of the dermis, creating epidermal ridges,

TABLE 12.1 The Epidermis

Epidermal Sublayer	Composition and Function
Corneum (outermost layer)	*Composition*: On average, 16 layers composed of nonviable cells known as corneocytes consisting of water-retaining keratin proteins and a highly structured cell envelope to provide strength. *Function*: Barrier to external agents and transepidermal water loss; contains antimicrobial proteins
Granulosum and lucidum	*Composition*: Consists of 3–5 cell layers with the lucidum present only in skin of palms and soles; keratinocytes at this stage contain keratohyalin granules *Function*: Keratohyalin granule proteins aggregate keratin proteins and move the cells toward the stratum corneum
Spinosum	*Composition*: 8–10 layers of keratinocytes with tonofibrils and Langerhans cells *Function*: Formation of keratinocytes begins here; keratins are synthesized; intermediate filaments that form to strengthen cells and connect to desmosomes; initiates cell-mediated immune response
Basal (deepest layer)	*Composition*: Single germinal cell layer of proliferating and stem keratinocytes and melanocytes (pigment cells) *Function*: Melanocytes produce melanin pigmentation to protect the living cells from solar radiation damage

Note: This information is based on normal adult skin values. Comparable data for premature and full-term infant skin is currently incomplete.
Sources: Carlson, B. M. (2024). *Human embryology and developmental biology* (7th ed., pp. 1154–1194). Elsevier/Saunders; Leung, A., Balaji, S., & Keswani, S. G. (2013). Biology and function of fetal and pediatric skin. *Facial Plastic Surgery Clinics of North America, 21*(1), 1–6. https://doi.org/10.1016/j.fsc.2012.10.001; Persaud & Torchia. (2025). Integumentary system. *The developing human: Clinically oriented embryology* (12th ed., pp. 415–431). Elsevier.

TABLE 12.2 Features of Epidermal Skin Thickness

	Thick Skin Layer (Hands, Feet)	Thin Skin Layer (All Areas Except Hands and Feet)
Follicles	No	Yes
Arrector muscles	No	Yes
Sebaceous glands	No	Yes
Sweat glands	Yes	Yes

Source: Persaud, T. V. N. & Torchia, M. G. (2025). *The developing human: Clinically oriented embryology* (12th ed., pp. 415–431). Elsevier.

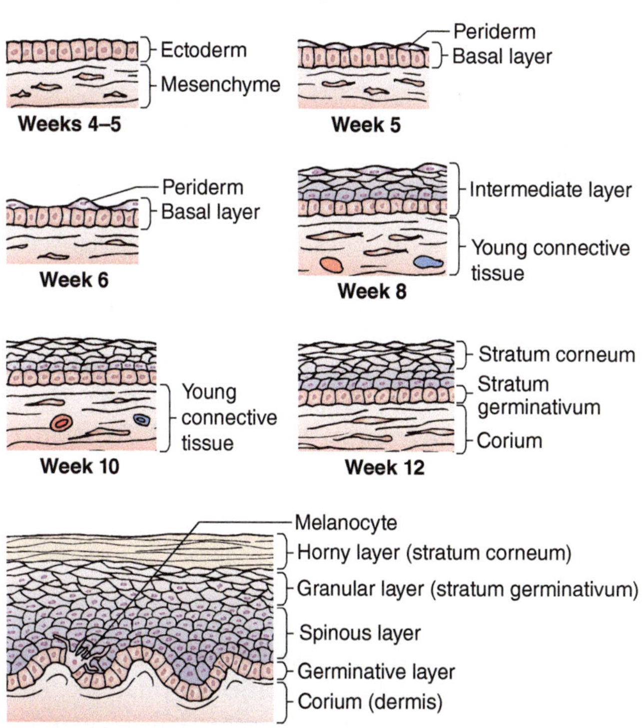

Figure 12.3 Stages of histogenesis of the skin.

the dermis reciprocates by developing rounded, finger-like extensions (papillae) that project upward and into the epidermal ridges. This marks the genesis of the *dermal papillae* (papillary layer), the most superficial layer of the dermis. Papillae permit the proliferation of primitive blood vessels and the matriculation of afferent sensory nerves. This process of vascular proliferation directs the differentiation of primitive capillaries into arterioles and arteries, whereas others become veins (Table 12.3). The *reticular layer*, which lies below the papillary layer, thereby begins to form. Collagen fibers arranged in parallel ranks and lymphatic meshes, which drain into larger lymphatic vessels, comprise this layer of the dermis.

TABLE 12.3 The Dermis and Hypodermis

Dermal Sublayer	Composition and Function	Visual Depiction
Papillary	*Composition:* Vasculature and afferent nerves *Function:* Renders vascular and sensory (afferent) nervous innervation	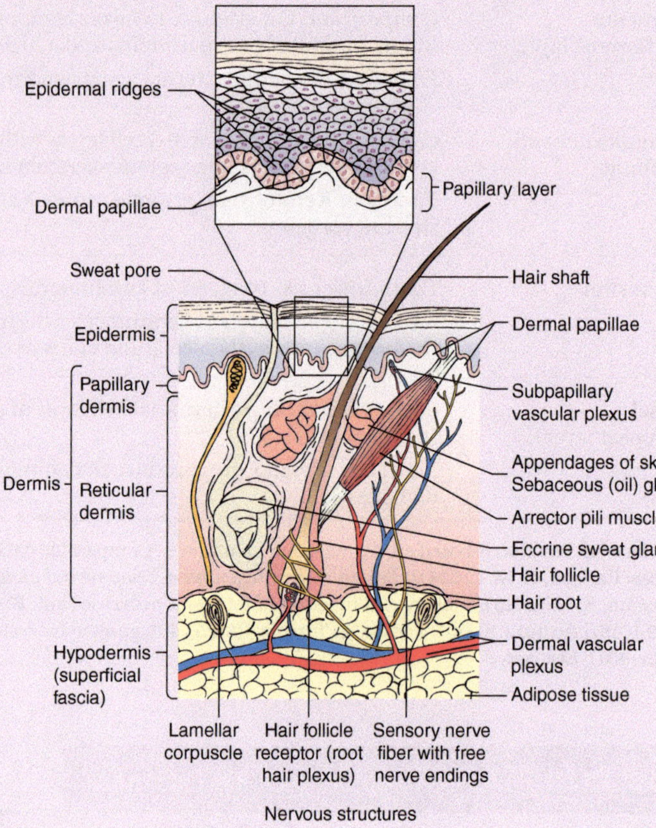
Reticular	*Composition:* Collagen fibers, lymphatic meshes *Function:* Contains loosely organized collagen fibers	
Hypodermis	*Location:* Innermost layer of the skin *Composition:* Fibroblasts, adipose cells and collagen fibers, and macrophages *Function:* Insulation and shock absorption; renders vascular and sensory (afferent) nervous innervation	

Source: Vandergriff, T. W. (2025). Anatomy and pathophysiology. In J. Bolognia, J. V. Schaffer, & L. Cerroni (Eds.), *Dermatology* (5th ed., pp. 47–57). Elsevier.

Evidence of the hypodermis can be seen between weeks 7 and 9 of gestation, as distinct from the dermis. Fibroblasts, adipose cells, and macrophages comprise this layer of the skin and have been observed using electron microscopes beginning with week 22 of gestation (Bolognia et al., 2025; Schoenwolf et al., 2021). From this period through birth, the dermis shifts from a well-hydrated and cellular-dense structure to a thicker, more fibrous structure (Bolognia et al., 2025).

Hair

Embryonic Period. Hair is derived from the surface ectoderm (Carlson, 2024). In fact, dermal-to-epidermal signaling is responsible for follicle formation. The dermis modulates a process of epidermal thickening, which forms hair placode cells within the basal layer of the epidermis. These placodes are observed by the end of week 11 of gestation and participate in the formation of the dermal papillary layer (Bolender, 2022). The placodes interact with genes, including sonic hedgehog (*SHH*), wingless type (*WNT*), bone morphogenic proteins (*BMPs*), and fibroblast growth factor (*FGF*), which signals further downward movement and differentiation. This movement pushes the placodes deeper while carving a canal for the future expression of hairs.

Fetal Period. By week 12 of gestation, the keratinocytes of the placode reach the dermis and the germinal matrix and hair formation is established. Peripheral cells along the hair shaft take on a cuboidal shape and give rise to the epithelial hair sheath. This hair sheath bulges, allowing innervation of arrector pili muscles and sebaceous glands (Chu & Loomis, 2022). By week 14 of gestation, the base of the follicle is properly situated within the papillary layer. The hair canal is fully formed by week 21 of gestation (Bolender, 2022). The proliferation of hair begins as cells are pushed upward by the arrector muscles, keratinized, and expressed. In fact, contraction of the arrector muscles elicits the "goose bump" response (Persaud & Torchia, 2025).

Hair first appears on the surface of the fetus, in particular along the regions of the eyebrow and upper lip. The majority of body hair is visible by week 20 of gestation. Over time, several cycles of hair proliferation and shedding occur during intrauterine development; hair that is shed can be found within the amniotic fluid (Bolender, 2022; Persaud & Torchia, 2025). The first fine and downy hair that appears along the embryo's body, and is particularly abundant among premature infants, is termed *lanugo* (Table 12.4; Sadler, 2023). Lanugo appears around 24 weeks of gestation and is abundant over the upper back and shoulders by 28 weeks of gestation. By term, lanugo has worn away, as the back is mostly bald (Ballard et al., 1991).

Clinical Application. Consider the Ballard examination with focus on skin maturity. The neonatal advanced practice nurse (APRN) evaluates the amount of lanugo covering the newborn's back, shoulders, and lumbo-sacral region. Thinning of the lanugo first appears over the lower back and is typically absent in term and postterm infants. The APRN describes the lanugo as sparse, abundant, thinning, or bald areas. Of note, infants of diabetic mothers typically have abundant lanugo on the pinnae and upper back at term.

Nails

The nails are derived from the surface ectoderm (Carlson, 2024). The fingernails are first to develop, beginning during early fetal development (weeks 9 and 10 of gestation) as thickenings in the epidermal layer (Bolender, 2022; Persaud & Torchia, 2025). The toenails follow in a similar fashion and begin matriculating within 4 weeks of the fingernails (Persaud & Torchia, 2025). Nails reach the fingertips by 32 weeks of gestation and the distal edges of the toes by week 36 of gestation (Persaud & Torchia, 2025; Sadler, 2023).

Glands

The glands (sebaceous, sweat, apocrine, mammary, lacrimal, and salivary) are derived from the surface ectoderm (Carlson, 2024). The skin contains several types of glands, including sebaceous, sweat, and mammary glands. Each has a distinct developmental timeline, location, and function.

Sebaceous Glands. Sebaceous glands are found only where hair grows and are directly connected to the hair's sheath. These are, at first, solid, hemispherical protuberances on the posterior surfaces of the hair pegs. The sebaceous glands are formed from the epidermal cells and begin to develop between weeks 13

TABLE 12.4 The Hair and Glands

Hair and Glands	Primary Function
Epidermis	The *epidermis* is the outermost layer of the skin.
Sweat pore	The *sweat pore* is an opening through which sweat emerges on the surface of the skin (not functional in neonates).
Hair follicle Hair sheath Hair shaft	Each hair is made of a hair shaft, hair sheath, and root. The *hair shaft* contains the keratinized fibers that appear as a single hair. The *hair sheath* surrounds the hair shaft and connects to the sebaceous glands. The body's hair serves to protect the skin.
Duct of eccrine gland	The *duct of the eccrine gland* is a conduit through which sweat rises from the eccrine gland to the surface of the skin (not fully functional in neonates).
Arrector pili	Connected to each hair is a tiny muscle known as the *arrector pili* muscle that contracts in response to cool temperatures or emotions, such as fear, causing the hair to stand on end.
Sebaceous glands	The *sebaceous glands* are attached to each hair and secrete an oily sebum. This lipid-based substance functions to provide an epidermal permeability barrier as well as structure and differentiation, signal skin-specific hormones, transport antioxidants to the skin's surface, and offer protection from ultraviolet radiation.
Dermal papillae (hair root)	The *hair root*, or *dermal papilla*, is fed by tiny blood vessels and is responsible for thermoregulation.
Eccrine gland	The *eccrine glands* are found over a majority of the body and are secretory glands that are under psychologic and thermal control through sympathetic (cholinergic) nerve fibers. Eccrine glands secrete sweat containing chloride, lactic acid, fatty acids, urea, glycoproteins, and mucopolysaccharides.

Source: Vandergriff, T. W. (2025). Anatomy and pathophysiology. In J. Bolognia, J. V. Schaffer, & L. Cerroni. (Eds.), *Dermatology* (5th ed., pp. 47–57). Elsevier.

and 14 of gestation (Niemann & Horsley, 2012). Sebaceous glands are well developed and generally large at term. Yet, after birth, the size rapidly diminishes, and only after puberty do they once again enlarge to become functional.

Sweat Glands. There are two primary types of sweat glands: eccrine and apocrine; each type of gland is located within the dermal layer. Eccrine glands reside over most of the body, with the exception of the lips and external ear canals and are derived as buds from the basal layer of the epidermis (Cui & Schlessinger, 2015). These glands begin to form between weeks 28 (palmoplantar region) and 35 (rest of body) of gestation (Cui & Schlessinger, 2015). Apocrine glands reside within the axillae and external genitalia (Sadler, 2023). These glands form during early adolescence, commensurate with the onset of puberty.

Mammary Glands. Mammary glands are adapted sweat glands that first appear during week 4 of gestation as bilateral buds of thickened epidermis (Persaud & Torchia, 2025). These buds are commonly referred to as *mammary ridges* or *crests*. By the end of week 5 of gestation, the mammary crests penetrate the underlying mesenchyme and form 16 to 24 sprouts, which give rise to the mammary buds. Mammary buds undergo a progressive process of canalization and form lactiferous ducts. By term, up to 20 lobes of breast tissue have formed, each affixed with one lactiferous duct (Javed & Lteif, 2013; Persaud & Torchia, 2025; Sadler, 2023). Further differentiation of the buds gives rise to the glands, located at the tips of each mammary bud. The glands are well established by week 24 of gestation and breast tissue is evident on physical examination (Javed & Lteif, 2013). Although the term neonate is affixed with lactiferous ducts at birth, the breasts are devoid of milk-releasing alveoli unless stimulated by hormones from the XX pregnant patient.

Nipples

Nipple formation also begins during late fetal development. The epidermis invaginates within the pectoral region at the fourth intercostal space on the chest region, forming a pit. Abnormal positioning yields supernumerary nipples, which are observed in 2% to 5% of newborns (Javed & Lteif, 2013). These pits give rise to each nipple, which often remain below the level of the epidermis for several weeks into postnatal life. During this time, connective tissue infiltrates the surrounding area and raises the nipple to a position above the level of the epidermis. During puberty, females will undergo progressive breast development, whereas male breasts remain in their primitive form across the life span (Persaud & Torchia, 2025).

DEVELOPMENTAL PHYSIOLOGY

The skin, or integumentary system, is the largest organ in the body. Known physiologic functions include barrier protection, thermoregulation, sensation, and metabolic functions. Through its anatomic construct and physiologic function, the skin resists infection and offers immunosurveillance, an acid mantle, antioxidant function, and protection from ultraviolet light (Visscher et al., 2015). We offer a discussion of the core functions of the skin, which serves as an expansion of core concepts discussed within Chapter 9.

Barrier Protection

The epidermal barrier forms as a result of a well-orchestrated progression that culminates in the formation of flattened, cornified keratinocytes. The keratinocytes are imbedded within a sophisticated bilayer lipid matrix, connected together by specialized structures called *desmosomes*. This outermost barrier provides protection from chemicals and irritants as well as physical dangers and mechanical trauma (Mancini & Lawley, 2015). At birth, this role becomes immediately crucial, as the fetus transitions from the hospitable environment provided by the womb to a cold, dry, and microorganism-filled atmosphere (Visscher & Narendran, 2022).

Skin barrier function is typically effective among infants born at or beyond 37 weeks of gestation, yet immature among infants born at less than 37 weeks of gestation. As with other organ systems, skin barrier function increases with advancing gestational age (GA). Well-developed skin is affixed with a thick epidermis and SC; these layers offer physical barrier function (Mancini & Lawley, 2015). In contrast, the skin of premature infants is affixed with fewer cornified layers, resulting in reduced barrier function, an increased risk for the penetration of exogenous materials and pathogens, transepidermal water loss (TEWL), and mechanical injuries (skin tears; Visscher et al., 2015). TEWL decreases with maturation of the SC, which among premature infants occurs between 2 to 9 weeks postnatal age; complete acid mantle formation may require additional months. Time required for epidermal maturation among infants less than 28 weeks GA is unknown (Visscher & Narendran, 2014).

Thermoregulation

The skin also participates in postnatal thermoregulation, a function that was unnecessary before birth and largely performed by the placenta. Maintaining optimal body core temperature (37°C or 98°F–99°F), or thermoregulation, involves balancing heat loss and production. The majority of thermoreceptors are located at the face, neck, and shoulder region; activation elicits a thermoregulatory response that involves increased caloric expenditures.

Thermoregulatory function is modulated through a complex series of neurogenic, myogenic, and metabolic processes; collectively, these processes regulate vasomotor tone within the dermis. Neurogenic and myogenic processes trigger the constriction or expansion of blood vessels. This controls blood flow and determines whether heat is dispelled or conserved.

Heat production, or *thermogenesis*, is modulated through oxidative metabolism as regulated by sympathetic nervous system modulation of nonshivering thermogenesis (NST), thyroid hormone synthesis, peripheral vasoconstriction, and muscle flexion. Oxidative metabolism involves the mobilization of glucose, fats, and proteins.

Recall that newborns have a high surface area-to-volume ratio compared to children and adults, and are more susceptible to heat loss, particularly in the immediate time frame after birth. Among infants who have accumulated brown fat (which is accrued between 26–30 weeks of gestation), NST leads to the production of heat without the use of muscle contractions associated with shivering. This is achieved through lipolysis of brown fat, a highly vascularized substance composed of mitochondria, lipid molecules, numerous capillaries, and innervated by sympathetic neurons. A sequence of events occurs to stimulate brown fat lipolysis. Norepinephrine is released in response to exposure to the colder extrauterine environment. This elicits vasoconstriction and an increase in the metabolic rate. The stimulation of sympathetic nervous system pathways encourages a surge in TSH, which leads to the release of thyroxine (T_4) and triiodothyronine (T_3). The release of T_3 into the circulation stimulates the upregulation of thermogenin, which acts directly upon brown fat to initiate chemical thermogenesis (fatty acid oxidation and uncoupling of ATP) and the resultant lipolysis of brown fat. When brown fat is metabolized, heat is produced and this warms the organs and bloodstream, leading to an increase in body temperature. Importantly, brown fat accounts for only 4% to 10% of total adipose tissue among term infants whose size is appropriate for GA (Mancini & Lawley, 2015). Premature infants possess even less brown fat and glycogen stores. In fact, brown adipose tissue is often not generated until 26 to 30 weeks of gestation. In addition, premature infants often cannot remain in a flexed position (to prevent heat loss through increased surface area exposure to colder temperatures), as well as reduced ability to mobilize existing brown adipose tissue. Neonatal APRNs should remain vigilant when attending the birth of growth-restricted newborns (term and preterm) and preterm infants born before 30 weeks of gestation and anticipate the need for supplemental heat sources (e.g., warmer pads) to establish euthermia.

Thermolysis refers to the loss of heat. Infants born at less than 38 weeks of gestation are at increased risk for heat loss. Heat loss can occur by way of (a) conduction, (b) convection, (c) radiation, and (d) evaporation (**Figure 12.4**). *Conduction* involves heat lost through direct contact with a cold surface, such as a cold blanket or neonatal scale. *Convection* involves heat lost from cooler air flowing over the body's surface, such as from an air-conditioning vent. *Radiation* is electromagnetic heat lost from heat radiating toward a cooler surface, which does not come into direct contact with the neonate's skin. Examples include a cold exterior window or the walls of an isolette. *Evaporation* is the final mechanism of heat loss and can be the result of bathing, birth, and sweating. Evaporation involves heat lost through wet skin.

Neurosensory Function

Skin contains both somatic sensory and sympathetic autonomic nerve fibers (**Figure 12.4**). These fibers function to innervate with arrector pili muscles, cutaneous blood vessels, and sweat glands. They serve as receptors for touch, pain, temperature, itch, and mechanical stimuli (Mancini & Lawley, 2015). Each stimulus provides the brain with afferent information that the brain translates into an efferent response. At the level of the skin, responses may include "goose bumps" or mottling. Thus, evidence of central nervous system maturation and responses to stimuli at the skin depend on sensory input received during the immediate postnatal period (Visscher & Narendran, 2022).

Glandular Function

As mentioned earlier, the skin contains glands, including apocrine, eccrine, mammary, and sebaceous glands. The apocrine glands are secretory glands found within the face, axilla, and pubic region. These glands open solely into hair follicles, develop during puberty, and are under thermal control by way of sympathetic (adrenergic) nerve fibers (Schaller & Plewig, 2025). Sweat, a by-product of the apocrine glands, is composed of lipids, proteins, and pheromones. Typically, once children reach puberty, the bacterial breakdown of sweat produces foul odors.

The eccrine glands are also sweat glands and are found throughout the body. The highest density of eccrine glands is noted in the palms of the hands and soles of the feet. Eccrine sweat glands are composed of a secretory coil and a duct (located in the lower dermis), as well as subcutaneous tissue. Components of eccrine sweat include water, sodium, chloride, potassium, urea, lactate, ammonia, antimicrobial peptides, cytokines, and immunoglobulins (Schaller & Plewig, 2025). *Eccrine glands* are innervated by the sympathetic nervous system. Pharmacologic stimulation or emotional or thermal stress stimulates the secretion of acetylcholine, which activates eccrine activity (Mancini & Lawley, 2015). Among neonates, eccrine activity manifests as thermal and emotional sweating. The core temperature required to induce neonatal sweating is

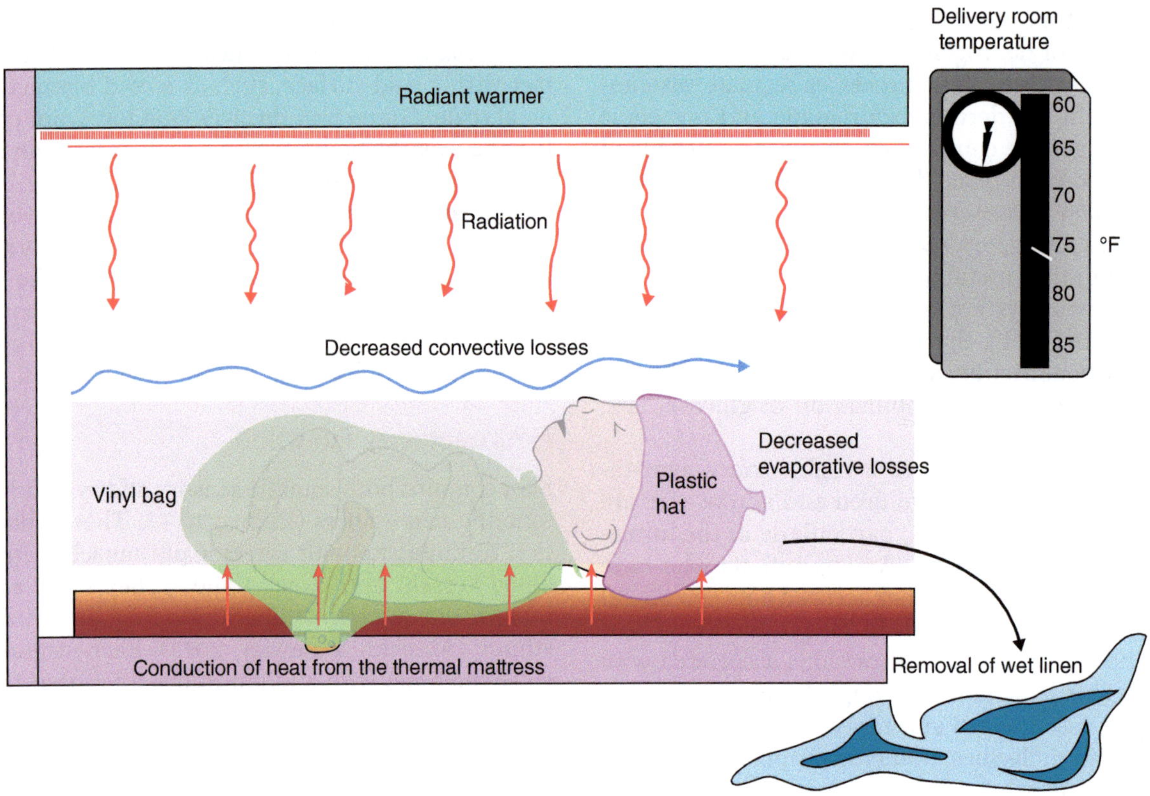

Figure 12.4 The four mechanisms of heat loss.
Source: Image courtesy of Dr. Satyan Lakshminrusimha. Reprinted with permission.

approximately 37.2°C/98.9°F (Mancini & Lawley, 2015). This is typically immature among premature neonates and is a process that matures over time among all neonates.

Mammary glands are found in the breast tissue. These glands should not exhibit secretory activity at birth, although transient galactorrhea (pseudolactation, or "witch's milk") has been observed in the neonatal period. This can develop from placental-transmitted estrogen, which can enlarge the fetal breast nodules; as levels in the newborn levels decline after birth, they elicit prolactin synthesis from the pituitary gland. As a result, a milky discharge from the newborn's nipples can be observed; this discharge is not pathologic, does not require treatment, and is self-limiting (Grabowski, 2022). Later during puberty, estrogen and progesterone levels rise and stimulate the lactiferous ducts to form alveoli and secretory cells primarily for future milk production (Sadler, 2023).

Sebaceous glands are numerous at birth. During fetal development, secretions from the sebaceous glands contribute to vernix formation. This early sebaceous gland activity is modulated by maternal hormonal (androgen) influences. After birth, hormone concentrations from the XX pregnant patient wane; however, residual hormonal influence may trigger continued sebaceous activity, which manifests as scalp flaking, or cradle cap. Once this transient phenomenon subsides, physiologic function of the sebaceous glands is not observed until puberty.

Vernix

During the last trimester, vernix caseosa, a whitish pastelike substance, begins to coat fetal skin from head to toe and back to front (Visscher et al., 2015). The cells in vernix may originate from the hair follicles, suggesting that vernix is "extruded" out through the hair shaft onto the skin surface initially around the hair and spreading over the entire surface as gestation progresses (Sadler, 2023). Vernix is primarily composed of sebaceous gland secretions and desquamated SC cells and provides physical protection from maceration by amniotic fluid and enzymes due to its hydrophobic lipids. Vernix also influences the antimicrobial function of the skin by (a) lowering the pH of the skin's surface, and (b) providing hydration and lipids for further formation of the cutaneous layers (Visscher et al., 2015). Each of these aforementioned functions is enhanced by allowing vernix to remain in place at least 6 hours after birth (Visscher et al., 2015). Clinicians are encouraged to delay the first postnatal bath, as appropriate.

Histologic Function

Although an investigation into cell-mediated skin function may seem like a daunting task, it is particularly significant for the neonatal clinician. Neonates, specifically premature neonates, depend on their skin for barrier protection against surface pathogens. In order to achieve this functional status, certain cells must matriculate into the epidermis.

Skin Coloration. Beginning with the second month of gestational development, primitive epidermal neural crest cells migrate from the dermis into the epidermis. This stimulates the synthesis of melanocytes. Under the influence of *WNT* signaling pathways, skin pigment granules are synthesized. These processes modulate melanin production and skin coloring, which is known to be influenced by ethnicity (Persaud & Torchia, 2025). Darker skin coloration is associated with earlier production of melanocytes and an increased number of pigment granules per cell (Carlson, 2024; Persaud & Torchia, 2025).

Immune Response. Toward the end of the first trimester, Langerhans cells migrate from the bone marrow to the stratum germinativum. These cells participate in cell-mediated immune responses to pathogens that persistently attempt to penetrate the skin barrier. The quantity of Langerhans cells increases across gestational development, with the most significant amount of proliferation noted during the third trimester. As such, infants born prematurely are often affixed with a significantly reduced number of Langerhans cells, which reduces the skin's ability to protect the body from antigens (Carlson, 2024).

GENETIC INFLUENCES

There are certain hereditary disorders that manifest with noteworthy dermatologic aberrations. Here, we review some common genetic disorders and their associated dermatologic findings.

Noonan Syndrome

Noonan syndrome is one of a group of related autosomal dominant inherited disorders, collectively known as the *RASopathies,* caused by a mutation in the genes of the RAS/MAPK pathway. In addition to Noonan syndrome, the RASopathies include cardiofaciocutaneous syndrome, Costello syndrome, neurofibromatosis 1, and Legius syndrome. Noonan syndrome affects one in every 1,000 to 2,500 births (National Institutes of Health [NIH], 2024b). Heterozygous mutations in the genes affect the *RAS/MAPK* (mitogen-activated protein kinase) signaling pathway, most commonly isolated at the *PTPN11* gene (75%). This disrupts normal cellular proliferation, differentiation, and migration (Bertola et al., 2014). Common skin-related manifestations include a deep groove at the philtrum, webbing of the skin of the neck, and a low posterior hairline. Abnormal synthesis and secretion of growth hormone may implicate the aforementioned manifestations, as well as stunt overall growth and development.

Neurofibromatosis (Type 1)

Neurofibromatosis type 1 (NF1) is the more common form of autosomal dominant neurofibromatosis, with an estimated incidence of one in every 3,000 to 4,000 individuals (NIH, 2020). Germline mutations in the *NF1* gene (involved in the RAS/MAPK pathway) overstimulate the RAS signaling activity, which alters normal keratinocyte differentiation (Peltonen et al., 2017). Therefore, although NF1 is commonly characterized by the growth of tumors on the nerves, this disease can also affect the skin. Common skin-related manifestations include cutaneous neurofibromas, café-au-lait lesions (infancy), freckles (childhood), and palpable neurofibromas (noncancerous tumors) that manifest under the skin; these tumors often present in adulthood.

Localized Hypotrichosis

Localized autosomal recessive hypotrichosis is characterized by sparse hair on the scalp beginning in infancy. The global incidence is unknown; however, an incidence of one in every 10,000 individuals is reported among Japanese infants, as this condition prevails among the Japanese population (NIH, 2018). Males and females are equally affected. Mutations in the *LIPH*, *LPAR6*, and *DSG4* genes alter the normal synthesis and proliferation of the hair and also may contribute to epidermal dysfunction. Common skin-related manifestations of hypotrichosis may include erythema, pruritis, or coarse, dry skin. At birth, scalp hair ranges from sparse and tightly curled whorls of hair to thin hair, which typically gradually decreases as the infant ages. A decreased complement of eyebrows, eyelashes, and axillary hair has also been reported (Basit et al., 2015).

Sturge–Weber Syndrome

Sturge–Weber syndrome is a congenital neurocutaneous disorder that affects one in every 20,000 to 50,000 individuals (National Organization for Rare Disorders [NORD], 2021). It commonly manifests during infancy as a triad of three classic features: (a) port-wine stains, usually located to the cutaneous distribution of the first branch of the trigeminal nerve, (b) a leptomeningeal venous malformation, and (c) glaucoma (Jnah et al., 2017). Life-span implications do not relate to the skin. Rather,

TABLE 12.5 Epidermolysis Bullosa: Inheritance Pattern, Level of Skin Cleavage, and Affected Proteins

	Inheritance Pattern	Level of Skin Cleavage	Percentage of Each Type
EB simplex	Autosomal dominant[a]	Intraepidermal (*basal and basal epidermis*)	Most common (70%)
Junctional EB	Autosomal recessive	Intralamina lucida (*basement membrane*)	(5%)
Dystrophic EB	Autosomal dominant *and* autosomal recessive	Sublamina densa (*dermis*)	(25%)
Kindler syndrome	Autosomal recessive	Multiple points	Rare (< 1%)

[a]Most forms of EB simplex are autosomal dominant, with the exception of suprabasilar types and forms with muscular dystrophy or pyloric atresia.
EB, epidermolysis bullosa.
Source: Dystrophic Epidermolysis Bullosa Research Association of America. (2025). *Understanding epidermolysis bullosa (EB).* https://www.debra.org/about-eb/eb-depth; Gonzalez, M. E. (2013). Evaluation and treatment of the newborn with epidermolysis bullosa. *Seminars in Perinatology, 37,* 32–39. https://doi.org/10.1053/j.semperi.2012.11.004

affected individuals may suffer visual disturbances (associated with choroidal hemangiomas), intellectual disabilities (secondary to seizures or leptomeningeal angiomas), and hemiparesis (NORD, 2021).

Epidermolysis Bullosa

Epidermolysis bullosa (EB) refers to a group of heterogeneous diseases that may affect the epidermis, dermal–epidermal junction, and dermis (Jnah et al., 2017; Persaud & Torchia, 2025). Current evidence suggests that EB affects one in every 50,000 individuals (NORD, 2024). The four major types of EB are (a) EB simplex (most common), (b) junctional EB, (c) dystrophic EB, and (d) Kindler syndrome (rarest; 250 cases worldwide); at least 39 subtypes have been reported (Table 12.5; Fine & Mellerio, *2025*). At present, 16 distinct structural genes representing more than 1,000 different mutations are linked etiologically to EB and affect at least 19 different structural proteins (Fine & Mellerio, *2025;* Narendran, 2025). The degree (severity) of gene mutation directly affects protein synthesis and disease severity.

In 2020, EB was reclassified based on genetics (Narendran, 2025). Ultra-rapid targeted genomic sequencing and whole genome sequencing are now utilized, as genetic testing is the new standard for diagnosis (Lucky et al., 2021). Clinical manifestations vary in the newborn period; however, *skin fragility and blistering are consistent findings across all types and subtypes of EB* (Figure 12.5). Nikolsky sign is a hallmark feature of the disorder. This sign is elicited when the examiner gently rubs or applies friction to the skin, eliciting a blister in response to the friction. EB simplex usually manifests with small and localized blisters without a history of trauma to the skin. Junctional and dystrophic EB, most notably the recessive forms, involve deeper blisters that may implicate a larger surface area (Jnah et al., 2017). Blisters are termed a *congenital localized absence of skin* (CLAS); the classic appearance is a red, shiny blister with clearly defined margins (Fine & Mellerio, 2025). Infants who do not manifest with intrauterine-acquired blisters will develop them in the postnatal period, often secondary to friction imposed during the birth process. Blisters are composed of serous or hemorrhagic fluid; many heal without scarring, yet the breach in the skin barrier increases the risk for nosocomial infection during the birth hospitalization and later bacterial infections. Other consequences of EB include TEWL and fluid and electrolyte imbalances.

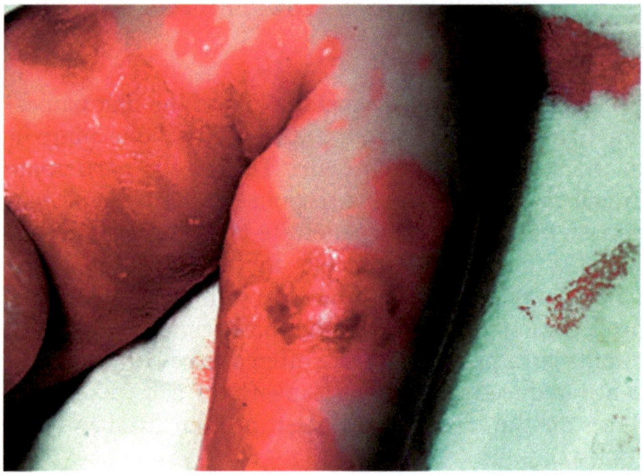

Figure 12.5 Denudation and erosion as a result of blistering in an infant with epidermolysis bullosa.
Source: Antaya, R. J., & Robinson, D. M. (2010). Blisters and pustules in the newborn. *Pediatric Annuals, 39,* 635–645. https://doi.org/10.3928/00904481-20100922-01

The care of EB extends across the life span and may involve rigorous and frequent dressing changes, rehospitalizations, recurrent infections, dehydration, or poor nutrition secondary to oral or esophageal blistering. Activity restrictions are common in order to reduce high-friction blistering. Affected children and adults are at risk for psychosocial disturbances due to disfigurement (Adni et al., 2012).

NOTEWORTHY DISEASES IN THE XX PREGNANT PATIENT THAT INFLUENCE FETAL SKIN DEVELOPMENT AND FUNCTION

The health of the XX pregnant patient can influence fetal skin development and function. In particular, maternal autoimmune disorders, infectious diseases, and nutritional deficits can implicate fetal and neonatal skin. We discuss the effect of maternal lupus infection and nutritional deficits on the developing skin. The effect of maternal viral infections, when acquired by the fetus or neonate, is presented later in this chapter.

Systemic Lupus Erythematosus

Mothers with anti-Ro/SSA and/or anti-La/SSB antibodies are at increased risk for giving birth to infants with neonatal lupus, an autoimmune disease that occurs in approximately 10% of infants whose mothers test positive for systemic lupus erythematosus (SLE). Common clinical manifestations of neonatal lupus include dermatologic, cardiac, and hepatic abnormalities (Bermas & Smith, 2024). Specific to the skin, cutaneous lesions may present at birth, but often appear within the first few weeks of life. Erythematous or polycystic plaques appear mainly on the scalp, neck, or face, but similar plaques may appear on the trunk or extremities. This dermatitis resembles the rash of subacute cutaneous lupus erythematosus rather than the malar rash of SLE. Periorbital erythema, referred to as *raccoon eye* or *owl eye*, is a very common characteristic (Figure 12.6). Bullous lesions may be seen on the soles of the feet. Besides the dermatologic signs, the most serious complication of neonatal lupus that all clinicians should be mindful of is complete heart block (Lun Hon & Leung, 2012). Children with neonatal lupus have an excellent long-term outcome when only skin lesions are present. The cutaneous lesions usually disappear by 6 months of age (Lun Hon & Leung, 2012).

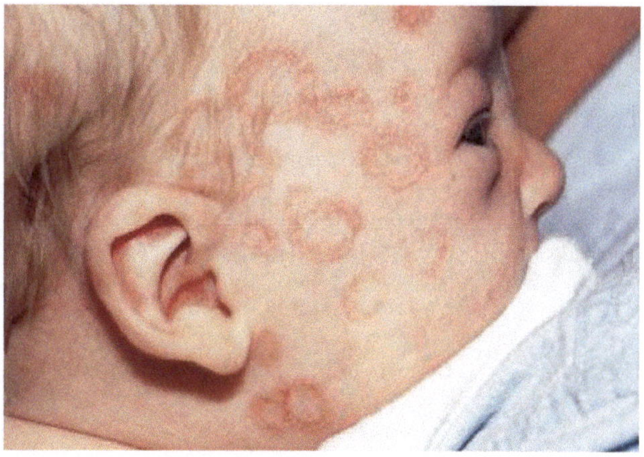

Figure 12.6 Cutaneous neonatal lupus erythematosus.
Note: "Racoon eye" appearance is noted over the right periorbital area. Customary erythematous annular plaques are seen over the glabella, along with central atrophy.
Source: Weston, W. L., Morelli, J. G., & Lee, L. A. (1999). The clinical spectrum of anti-Ro-positive cutaneous neonatal lupus erythematosus. *Journal of the American Academy of Dermatology, 40*(5 Pt 1), 675–681. https://doi.org/10.1016/s0190-9622(99)70146-5

Nutritional Deficits

Biotin Deficiency. Biotin deficiency is a rare nutritional disorder, more often observed in poorly developed countries. Biotin is a water-soluble vitamin, generally classified as a b-complex vitamin. Genetic disorders, such as biotinidase deficiency, multiple carboxylase deficiency, and holocarboxylase synthetase deficiency, can lead to inborn or late-onset forms of biotin deficiency (NORD, 2019). In all cases, dietary, genetic, or otherwise, supplementation with biotin is the primary method of treatment.

Pregnancy alters biotin catabolism and, despite a regular biotin intake, approximately 50% of pregnant patients in the United States are recognized as marginally biotin deficient (Zempleni et al., 2009). Signs and symptoms of neonatal biotin deficiency include red, patchy rashes near the mouth (erythematous periorofacial macular rash), fine and brittle hair, alopecia, anemia, birth defects, seborrheic dermatitis, and fungal infections. Fortunately, biotin supplements are readily available within the United States, and when prenatal care is pursued and continued throughout pregnancy, biotin deficiency is typically averted.

COMMON PROBLEMS WITH IMPLICATIONS ACROSS THE LIFE SPAN

The skin is a critical interface between the body and environment. This layer differentiates between "self" and "nonself." In fact, maternal–infant bonding is, in large part, a complex dynamic interaction between skin surfaces. Cutaneous characteristics are routinely used as determinants of GA. Pathologic processes visible on the skin surface range from general signs of systemic dysfunction to clinical evidence of specific diseases. Table 12.6 presents a list of common dermatology-specific terms and associated definitions. Readers should refer to this table while studying the

TABLE 12.6 Common Dermatological Terms

	Brief Description	Examples of Association(s)	Primary or Secondary
Cicatricial	Fibrous and contracted scar tissue	Congenital VZV	Primary
Crusted ulcerations	Crusted skin lesions composed of dried exudate (blood, pus, or other serous or serosanguinous fluid) found on the epidermal layer of the skin	Trauma, viral/infectious etiologies, genetic or congenital syndromes, or vascular or other malformations	Secondary
Erythema	Redness of the skin that can occur in one or more locations and cover a small to large volume of surface area of the skin	Erythema toxicum, periumbilical erythema (omphalitis or funusitis), erythema multiforme, and SSSS	Secondary
Exanthem	Widespread rash	Toxoplasmosis, HSV	Primary
Fissures	Linear breaches at the skin surface, resulting in an often painful separation of the epidermal layer	Keratodermas, eczema	Secondary
Scaling	Heaping of the stratum corneum with resultant shedding upon exfoliation	Ichthyosis, seborrheic dermatitis	Secondary
Scarring	Permanent, fibrotic alteration in skin integrity incurred as a result of trauma or tissue injury	Congenitally acquired infections, EB, infantile acne	Secondary

EB, epidermolysis bullosa; HSV, herpes simplex virus; SSSS, staphylococcal scalded skin syndrome; VZV, varicella zoster virus.
Source: Data from S. Bellini & M.J. Beaulieu (Eds.). (2016). *Neonatal advanced practice nursing: A case-based approach* (pp. 217–218). Springer Publishing.

common problems described in this final section of the chapter.

Transient Cutaneous Lesions

A number of benign and transient skin lesions are commonly observed in a normal newborn nursery population. It is important for the clinician to distinguish such transient lesions from cutaneous manifestations associated with life-threatening diseases. A precise description of primary and secondary skin cutaneous lesions forms the basis for understanding the skin pathology. Tables 12.7 and 12.8 describe the basic lesional morphology of infant skin with associated clinical exemplars.

Acrocyanosis. Acrocyanosis is one of the most common and typically transient cutaneous blood flow abnormalities; it is caused by reduced capillary reperfusion to the hands and feet. Reduced perfusion may be secondary to vasomotor immaturity, or caused by vasoconstriction secondary to cold temperatures (Maguiness & Garzon, 2015). Common clinical manifestations include a bluish color to the hands and feet. Because this phenomenon commonly self-resolves within 24 to 48 hours after birth and is not typically a primary or sole indicator of a congenital heart lesion, it is considered a benign finding (Jnah et al., 2017).

Sebaceous Gland Hyperplasia and Milia. These two conditions are presented in a side-by-side manner because they are easily confused in the clinical setting. Sebaceous gland hyperplasia is reported in approximately 20% to 40% of well-appearing newborns, with recent reports indicating occurrences of 89% (Haveri & Inamadar, 2014). The enlarged glands manifest secondary to increased sebum secretion at birth, likely due to an increased placental concentration of the androgen dehydroepiandrosterone (Brzezinski & Chiriac, 2015). Defining characteristics include yellow-white papules with swelling of the sebaceous glands (Figure 12.7). These papules are often clustered together into small groupings, often located on the nose or midface region (Lucky, 2015).

Clinical Application. Take a moment to look at Figure 12.7. Consider the appearance of the smaller and flatter papules of sebaceous gland hyperplasia located on the infant's nose. Contrast these lesions with milia, which are typically white and scattered across the infant's face.

TABLE 12.7 Primary Cutaneous Lesions

Type	Description	Clinical Examples
Abscess	Same as a pustule but >1 cm in size	Pyodermas
Bulla	Same as a vesicle but >1 cm in size	Sucking blisters EB Bullous impetigo
Nodule	A circumscribed, elevated, solid lesion with depth, up to 2 cm in size	Neuroblastoma
Macule	A circumscribed, flat lesion with color change, up to 1 cm in size; by definition, they are not palpable	Café-au-lait spots Capillary ectasias
Papule	A circumscribed, elevated, solid lesion, <1 cm in size; elevation may be accentuated with oblique lighting	Milia
Patch	Same as macule but >1 cm in size	Congenital dermal melanocytoses Nevus simplex
Plaque	A circumscribed, elevated, plateau-like, solid lesion, >1 cm in size	Nevus sebaceous
Pustule	A circumscribed, elevated lesion filled within purulent fluid, <1 cm in size	Neonatal pustular melanosis Erythema toxicum neonatorum Infantile acropustulosis
Tumor	Same as a nodule but >2 cm in size	Hemangioma Rhabdomyosarcoma
Vesicle	A circumscribed, elevated, fluid-filled lesion up to 1 cm in size	HSV Varicella zoster virus Miliaria crystalline
Wheal	A circumscribed, elevated, edematous, often evanescent lesion, caused by accumulation of fluid within the dermis	Urticaria Bite reactions Drug eruptions

EB, epidermolysis bullosa; HSV, herpes simplex virus.
Source: Adapted from Yan, A. C., Kim, H. J., & Honig P. J. (2015). Lesional morphology and assessment. In L. F. Eichenfield, I. J. Frieden, E. F. Mathes, & A. L. Zaenglein (Eds.), *Neonatal and infant dermatology* (3rd ed., pp. 24–35). Elsevier Saunders.

TABLE 12.8 Secondary Cutaneous Lesions

Type	Description	Clinical Examples
Atrophy	Localized diminution of skin. *Epidermal atrophy* results in a translucent epidermis with increased wrinkling, whereas *dermal atrophy* results in depression of the skin with retained skin markings. Use of topical steroids can result in epidermal atrophy, whereas intralesional steroids may result in dermal atrophy.	Aplasia cutis congenita Intrauterine scarring Focal dermal hypoplasia
Crust	Results from dried exudates overlying an impaired epidermis. Can be composed of serum, blood, or pus.	EB Impetigo
Erosion	Intraepithelial loss of epidermis; heals without scarring.	Herpes simplex

(continued)

TABLE 12.8 Secondary Cutaneous Lesions *(continued)*

Type	Description	Clinical Examples
Fissure	Linear, often painful break within the skin surface, as a result of excessive xerosis.	Inherited keratodermas Epidermolysis bullosa Eczema (hands, feet)
Lichenification	Thickening of the epidermis with exaggeration of normal skin markings caused by chronic scratching or rubbing.	Sucking blister Atopic dermatitis
Scale	Results from increased shedding or accumulation of stratum corneum as a result of abnormal keratinization and exfoliation. Can be subdivided further into pityriasiform (branny, delicate), psoriasiform (thick, white, and adherent), and ichthyosiform (fish scale–like).	Ichthyoses Postmaturity desquamation Seborrheic dermatitis
Scar	Permanent fibrotic skin changes that develop as a consequence of tissue injury. In utero scarring can occur as a result of certain infections or amniocentesis or postnatally from a variety of external factors.	Congenital varicella Aplasia cutis congenita
Ulcer	Full-thickness loss of the epidermis with damage into the dermis. Will heal with scarring.	Ulcerated hemangiomas Aplasia cutis congenita

Note: Lesions arise as characteristic modifications of primary lesions through environmental interaction (e.g., drying) or subject interaction (e.g., scratching).

Source: Adapted from Yan, A. C., Kim, H. J., & Honig P. J. (2015). Lesional morphology and assessment. In L. F. Eichenfield, I. J. Frieden, E. F. Mathes, & A. L. Zaenglein (Eds.), *Neonatal and infant dermatology* (3rd ed., pp. 24–35). Elsevier Saunders.

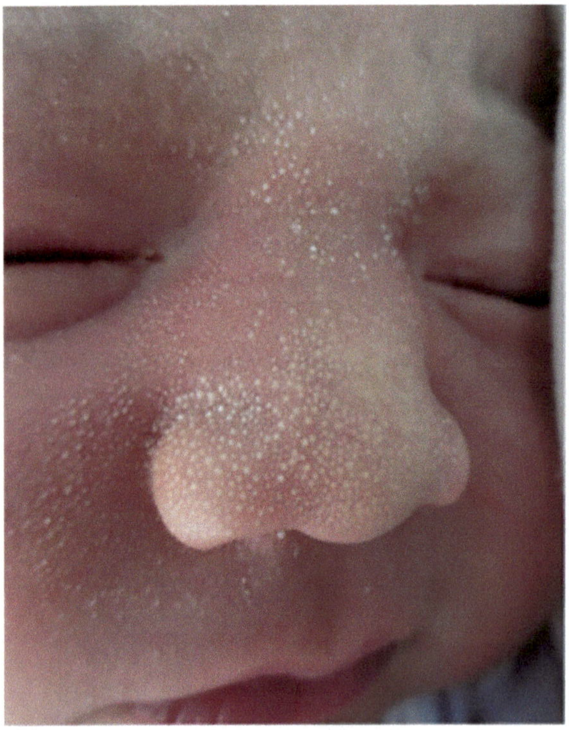

Figure 12.7 Sebaceous gland hyperplasia.

Source: De María, M. K., Borda, K. M., Arretche, V. N., Gugelmeier, N., Mombelli, R., de Los Santos, A. V., Acosta, M. A., Álvarez, M., Pose, G. L., Borbonet, D., & Martínez, M. A. (2021). Neonatal dermatologic findings in Uruguay: Epidemiology and predisposing factors. *Actas Dermo-Sifiliograficas, 112*(5), 414–424. https://doi.org/10.1016/j.ad.2020.11.019

On the contrary, milia are characterized as white cysts measuring approximately 1 mm in diameter. Milia is typically scattered over the cheeks, forehead, nose, and nasolabial folds. They may be few or numerous, but they frequently occur in clusters. Because all of these cysts exfoliate or involute spontaneously within the first few weeks of life, they are considered a benign finding.

Pigmentary Abnormalities

The melanocyte system of the newborn skin usually is not mature at birth. As a result, all babies, regardless of racial pigmentation, may look lighter than their parents at birth. Within the first few weeks, pigmentation becomes more evident because melanin production has been stimulated by exposure to the postnatal environment.

Albinism. Albinism (e.g., complete albinism, oculocutaneous albinism), which occurs in all races, has an incidence of one per 17,000 to 20,000 individuals in the United States; the phenotypic picture is caused by an autosomal recessive gene (NIH, 2024a). Several forms of this disorder have been delineated, including albinism type 1 and type 2 (Chan & Tay, 2015).

The biochemical defect responsible for oculocutaneous albinism type 1 is a deficiency of tyrosinase, the enzyme responsible for converting tyrosine to dopamine, an early step in the formulation of melanin. Structurally, the melanosomes appear to be normal. In oculocutaneous albinism type 2, however, mutations in the *OCA2* gene affect function of a melanosomal protein. Both conditions reduce melanin synthesis and yield reduced pigmentation.

Clinical manifestations include markedly reduced skin pigment, yellow or white hair, pink pupils, gray irises, photophobia, and cutaneous photosensitivity. Among African American infants, the skin may be tan, the hair may have a yellow or orange color, and freckles can appear upon exposure to light (Wright et al., 2015). Over the lifetime, reduced pigmentation and associated increased susceptibility to ultraviolet radiation can result in elastosis, actinic keratoses, and skin cancers including squamous cell carcinoma, basal cell carcinoma, and melanoma (Figure 12.8).

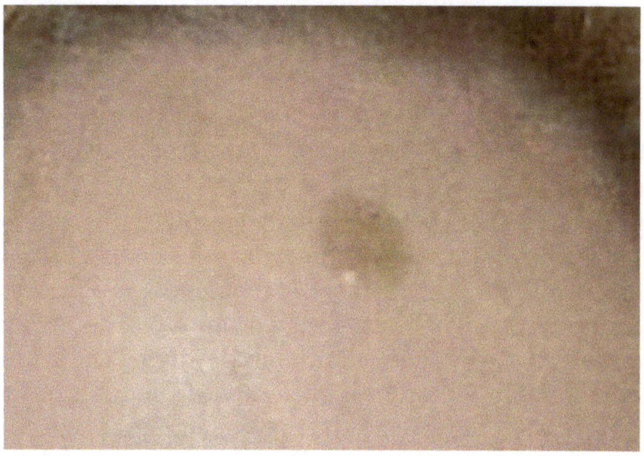

Figure 12.9 Café-au-lait macules.
Source: Bellini, S., & Beaulieu, M. J. (Eds.). (2017). *Neonatal advanced practice nursing: A case-based learning approach.* Springer Publishing Company.

Café-au-Lait Macules. Café-au-lait macules are flat, pigmented macules with distinct borders that may be present in the newborn infant. The macules are light brown in Caucasians and dark brown in African Americans (Simkin et al., 2023). Lesions are commonly seen on the trunk in older children, and over the buttocks in newborns (Price & Marghoob, 2015; Figure 12.9).

The pathogenesis involves an accumulation of melanin within the epidermis. Because the macules may be associated with several syndromes, including NF1, Leopard syndrome, Russell–Silver syndrome, and tuberous sclerosis (TS), a differential diagnosis is recommended based on size and number (single versus multiple; Taieb et al., 2014). *Lesions that are larger than 0.5 cm in diameter and more than six in number, especially when accompanied by "freckling" in the flexures, strongly suggest neurofibromatosis, a disorder characterized by mutations of the* NF1 *gene.* The *NF1* gene makes neurofibromin, a protein that regulates cell growth and prevents tumor formation. In neurofibromatosis, neurofibromin is deficient, thereby allowing tumors to grow along nerves in various locations. Patients with TS also may have café-au-lait spots that are identical in appearance to those of neurofibromatosis, but they are usually accompanied by white macules.

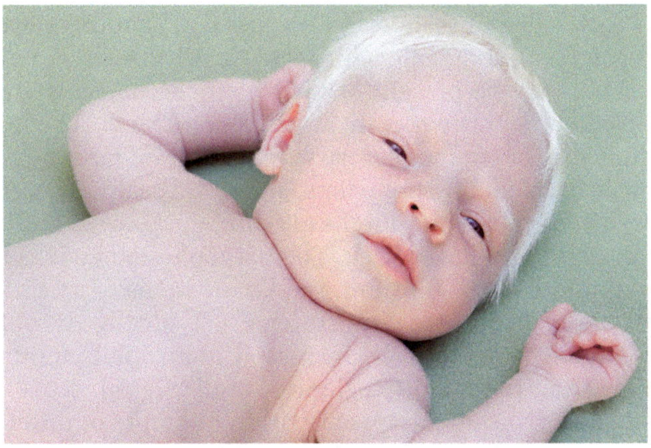

Figure 12.8 Albinism.
Source: Fernandes, F. (n.d.). Albino newborn. https://www.flickr.com/photos/felipefdesign/12135299916/

Clinical manifestations may include axillary freckles, which actually represent tiny café-au-lait macules. Café-au-lait spots are usually the first cutaneous lesions to appear in a patient with neurofibromatosis, but additional genetic and clinical investigations are required to establish a diagnosis. Café-au-lait macules may change size, and even increase over the first few years of life, but they do not spontaneously resolve. Because these skin lesions persist, they may be cosmetically problematic as the child ages. Lesions associated with neurofibromatosis incur additional life-span issues addressed in prior chapters of this textbook, which include neurologic or cognitive difficulties and/or tumor formation.

Congenital Melanocytic Nevi, Small to Intermediate. Congenital melanocytic (pigmented) nevi present at birth or within the first few months of life. Small nevi (smaller than 1.5 cm) are seen in 1% to 2% of newborns and intermediate nevi (1.5 to 20 cm) in 0.6% (Price & Marghoob, 2015). These skin lesions are believed to arise due to mutations in *Nras* and *Braf* genes. The mutations provoke an abnormal proliferation of cells with a melanocytic phenotype, which nest together in the epidermis; at least three melanocytic cells touch the dermis or other tissues (Roh et al., 2015). Clinical manifestations of small nevi are flat and light- to dark-brown lesions, often with variegated color or speckling and an accentuated epidermal surface ridge pattern. These lesions vary in site, size, and number, but most often are solitary. Melanocytic nevi may be malignant and should be monitored diligently from birth through adulthood (Figure 12.10).

Congenital Melanocytic Nevi, Large. The occurrence of large nevi is less than 0.02%. The giant (greater than 20 cm) nevus is associated with a lifetime risk for malignant transformation, and melanoma is estimated to occur in 6% to 8% of affected individuals (Price & Marghoob, 2015). The onset of melanoma in utero has been reported. These nevi may occupy 15% to 35% of the body surface, most commonly involving the trunk. The pigmentation often is variegated from light brown to black. The affected skin may be smooth, nodular, or leathery in consistency. Prominent hypertrichosis is often present. Almost invariably, numerous satellite nevi coexist elsewhere on the body. Leptomeningeal melanocytosis has been documented in some of these patients, and this complication may manifest as seizures. Because of the significant incidence of malignant transformation, the hideous deformity, and the intense pruritus that may accompany them, it is desirable, when feasible, to excise these lesions surgically as soon as possible.

Nevus Anemicus. Nevus anemicus is a congenital vascular anomaly that occurs in about 1% to 2% of individuals, and typically yields lesions that measure 5 to 10 cm in diameter (Kolb & Krishnamurthy, 2024). These lesions present as permanently pale, mottled lesions located on the trunk. The cause is believed to be secondary to a heightened response to the effects of catecholamines (adrenaline noradrenaline). For that reason, the nevus is best characterized as a pharmacologic abnormality, rather than an anatomic one. The lesions appear hypopigmented, but contain normal amounts of pigment. Pallor results from increased local reactivity to catecholamines, which provokes vasoconstriction and subsequent pallor. When rubbed, the lesion does not redden like the surrounding skin. These lesions do not spontaneously resolve and, therefore, may impose cosmetic issues over time.

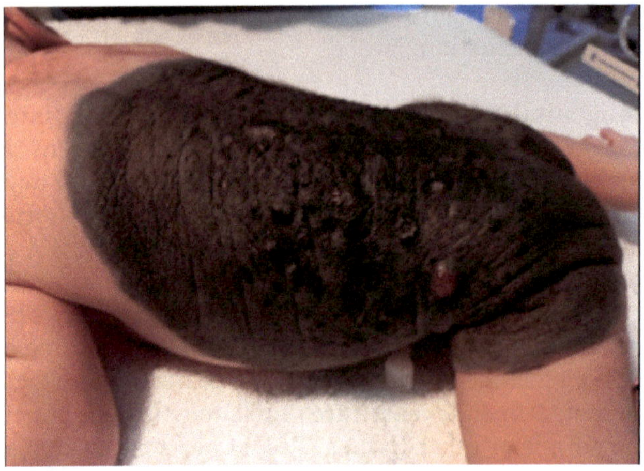

Figure 12.10 Congenital melanocytic nevi.
Source: Mumtaz Hashmi, H., Shamim, N., Kumar, V., & Idrees, S. (2021). Giant congenital melanocytic nevi in a Pakistani newborn. *Cureus, 13*(5), e15210. https://doi.org/10.7759/cureus.15210

Pigmentary Lesions

Erythema Toxicum. Erythema toxicum is a benign and self-limited inflammatory reaction that usually manifests within the first 24 to 72 hours of life; new lesions may appear until 2 to 3 weeks of age (Narendran, 2025). The disorder is more common among term than premature infants, which suggests that the inflammatory reaction requires mature skin. The pathogenesis involves skin reactions to elevated concentrations of IL-8, L11, eotaxin, and psoriasin, further supporting the inflammatory etiology for this type of transient lesion (Monteagudo et al., 2012). Lesions may be firm, 1 mm to 3 mm in diameter, pale yellow to white, and manifest as papules or pustules that sit on an erythematous base resembling flea bites. They may also manifest as erythematous macules as large as 3 cm in diameter. Individual lesions are fleeting, often lasting only a matter of hours. They may be found on any area of the body, but only rarely to the palms and soles. They are asymptomatic with no related systemic involvement. A microscopic examination of a Wright- or Giemsa-stained smear of the pustule contents will yield numerous eosinophils; Gram stains are negative for bacteria and cultures are sterile. Spontaneous resolution occurs in 6 days to 2 weeks (Figure 12.11).

Transient Neonatal Pustular Melanosis. Transient neonatal pustular melanosis is a distinctive eruption that consists of three types of lesions. First-stage lesions are small, superficial vesiculopustules with little or no surrounding erythema (Narendran, 2025). These rapidly progress to the second stage, which consists of collarettes of scale or scale crust surrounding a hyperpigmented macule (third stage). All three types of lesions may be present at birth, but the macules are observed more frequently at the time of birth. The lesions may be profuse or sparse and occur on most body surfaces, including the palms, soles, and scalp. Sites of predilection are the forehead, submental area, anterior neck, and lower back. The pathophysiology is not well understood. Cultures and Gram stains of smears prepared from intact pustules are typically devoid of organisms; however, increased neutrophil counts have been observed (Reginatto, Muller, et al., 2017). Pustules typically disappear within 48 hours of onset, whereas the hyperpigmented macules may persist for as long as 3 months. The disorder is benign and transient (Figure 12.12).

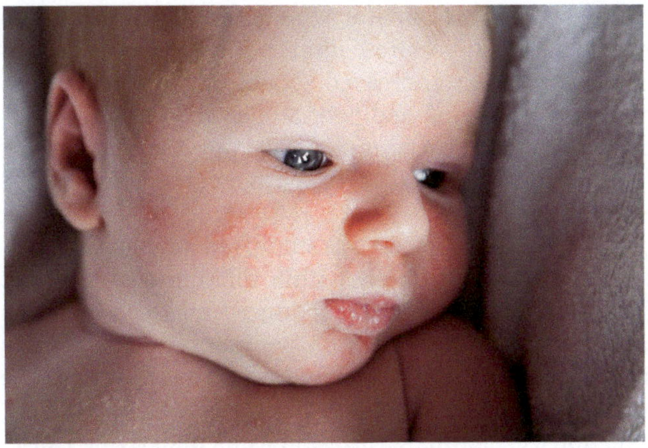

Figure 12.11 Erythema toxicum.
Source: © David Gee/Alamy Stock Photo.

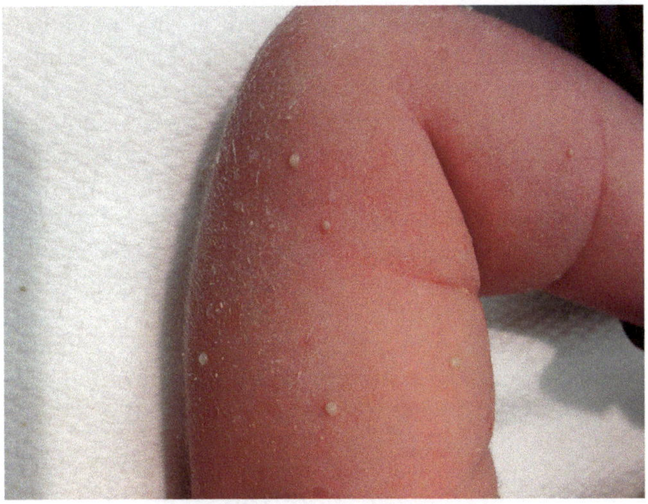

Figure 12.12 Transient neonatal pustular melanosis.
Source: Gzzz. (2014, January 31). *Transient neonatal pustular melanosis.* https://commons.wikimedia.org/wiki/File:Transient_Neonatal_Pustular_Melanosis_2.jpg

Clinical Application. Note the difference between the hyperpigmented macules identified with transient neonatal pustular melanosis and the hypopigmented lesions associated with TS. Infants affected with TS have white macules, also known as ash-leaf macules because they resemble the leaf of an ash tree, typically located on the trunk and buttocks (Narendran, 2025). Since these lesions are light in color, they may be challenging to identify in fair-skinned newborns. In this scenario, a Wood (ultraviolet) light may be used to illuminate these hypopigmented macules (Witt, 2024). It is important to identify these hypopigmented lesions because infants with TS have seizures and intellectual disabilities (Narendran, 2025).

Harlequin Color Change. Harlequin color change is a transient phenomenon observed in the immediate neonatal period, commonly noticed among low-birthweight infants. The pathophysiology is attributed to a temporary imbalance in the autonomic regulatory mechanism of the cutaneous vessels; there are no accompanying vital sign changes (Figure 12.13; Khemani et al., 2017). The dependent side of the body becomes intensely red, the upper side pales, and a sharp, vertical line of demarcation appears down the trunk (midline). The episodes can be observed during the first 3 weeks of life and are of no pathologic significance.

Miliaria. Miliaria is a skin eruption that results from eccrine sweat duct obstruction. This leads to sweat retention (Hölzle & Kligman, 1978; Narendran, 2025). Three clinical presentations are observed: (a) superficial thin-walled vesicles without inflammation (i.e., miliaria crystalline); (b) small, erythematous, grouped papules (i.e., miliaria rubra); and (c) nonerythematous pustules (i.e., miliaria pustulosis). The eruption most frequently develops in the intertriginous areas and over the face and scalp. It is exacerbated by exposure to a warm and humid environment. Rapid resolution occurs when the infant is placed in a cooler environment. A Wright-stained smear of vesicular lesions demonstrates only few squamous cells or lymphocytes. In a seminal controlled study, *Staphylococcus epidermidis* produced miliaria but *S. haemolyticus, S. hominis, S. cohnii, S. saprophyticus*, and *S. simulans* did not (Mowad et al., 1995). The condition resolves spontaneously (Figure 12.14).

Congenital Dermal Melanocytoses. The most frequently encountered pigmented lesion is the congenital dermal melanocytoses (previously called a “slate grey patch” or “Mongolian spot”), which occurs in 90% to 100% of African American and Asian infants, 50% in Hispanic infants, and less frequently (less than 10%) among Caucasian infants (Griswold & Srinivas, 2025; Gupta & Thappa, 2013). The pathophysiology relates

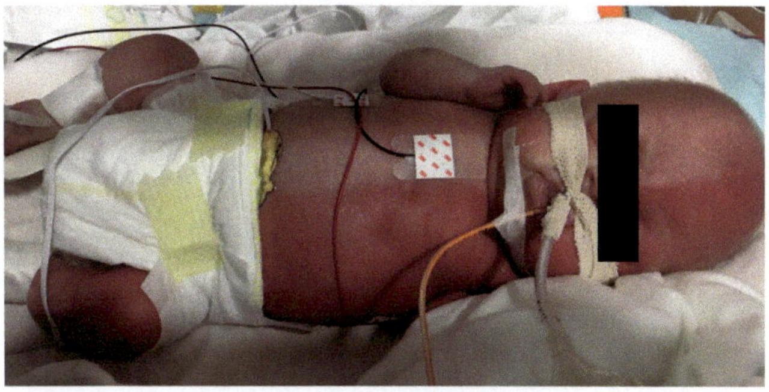

Figure 12.13 Harlequin color change.

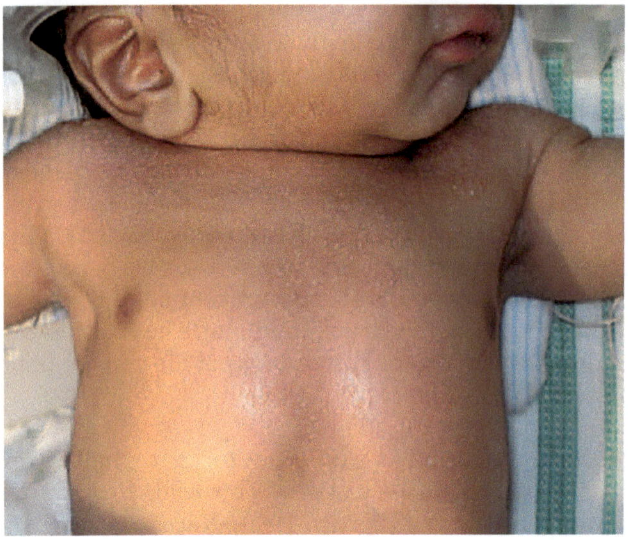

Figure 12.14 Miliaria.
Source: Babu, T. A., & Sharmila, V. (2012). Congenital miliaria crystallina in a term neonate born to a mother with chorioamnionitis. *Pediatric Dermatology, 29*(3), 306–307. https://doi.org/10.1111/j.1525-1470.2011.01435.x

to the excessive accumulation and delayed disappearance of melanocytes in varying numbers. Although most of these lesions are found in the lumbosacral area, they can occur at other sites. The pigmentation is macular and gray-blue, lacks a sharp border, and may span a diameter of 10 cm or more. Most of these lesions gradually disappear during the first few years of life, but aberrant lesions in unusual sites are more likely to persist. There is some indication that they are associated with metabolism disorders or neurocristopathies (**Figure 12.15**).

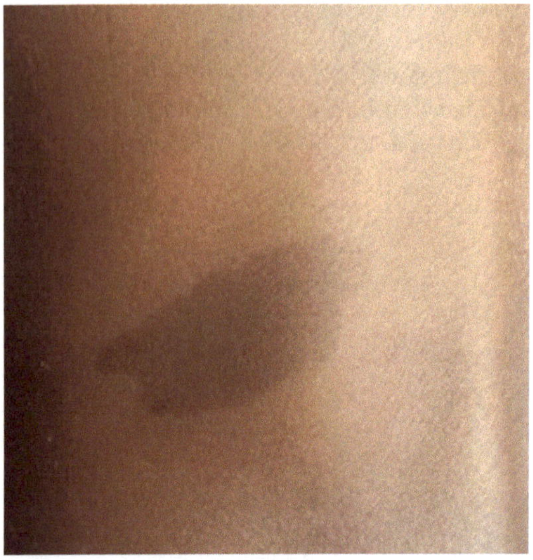

Figure 12.15 Congenital dermal melanocytosis.
Source: Image courtesy of Amy J. Jnah.

Neonatal Acne. Neonatal acne occurs in up to 20% of newborns, and is more common among males (Yeo & Ormerod, 2014). Increased sebaceous secretions, secondary to maternal and neonatal androgens, and colonization of the sebaceous glands by the yeast *Malassezia furfur* are implicated in its pathogenesis (Schachner et al., 2023).

Neonatal acne presents as small, red papules and pustules on the face, usually within the first weeks of life. Unlike in adolescence, comedones and cysts are usually absent. The lesions are asymptomatic and resolve spontaneously without scarring over several weeks. The clinical significance lies in differentiating this rash from infections, excluding virilization as its underlying cause, and potential implication of severe acne in adolescence.

Nevus Simplex (Salmon Patch). The nevus simplex (stork bite) is the most common neonatal cutaneous lesion, and is present in up to 80% of normal newborns (Kanada et al., 2012; Narendran, 2025). Stork bites manifest as a result of distended dermal capillaries and blanch when compressed. The lesions are transient and typically manifest within the first 72 hours of life (Reginatto, Devilla, et al., 2017). Clinicians will commonly note their central location and symmetric presentation; lesions typically appear at the nape of the neck, eyelids, and glabella. In a prospective study of affected infants, most of the facial lesions had faded by 1 year of age, but those on the neck were more persistent (Reginatto, Devilla, et al., 2017). Surveys of adults confirm the persistence of the nuchal lesions in approximately 25% of affected individuals (**Figure 12.16**).

Disorders of Cornification: The Scaly Baby

The most common and benign cause for excessive scaling is attributed to physiologic desquamation (normal term infants) and dysmaturity (postmature and small-for-gestational-age infants), neither of which have long-term sequelae. Less common causes include the congenital ichthyoses and the ectodermal dysplasias, both of which are chronic, heritable disorders (Craiglow, 2013; Foley et al., 2015). In the normal infant with accentuated physiologic scaling and the dysmature infant, desquamation is a transient phenomenon. The integument continues to serve its intended protective function. In contrast, the infant with congenital ichthyosis may exhibit impaired barrier function and incur a heightened risk for secondary infections.

Ichthyoses. *Ichthyosis* refers to a complex and often confusing plethora of conditions characterized by disorders of cornification with or without systemic symptoms (Foley et al., 2015; Narendran, 2025). Ichthyosis is a genetic disorder, characterized by mutations in the genes that produce keratin (i.e., *KRT1, KRT2*, or *KRT10*), which disrupt normal skin barrier formation (Vahlquist et al.,

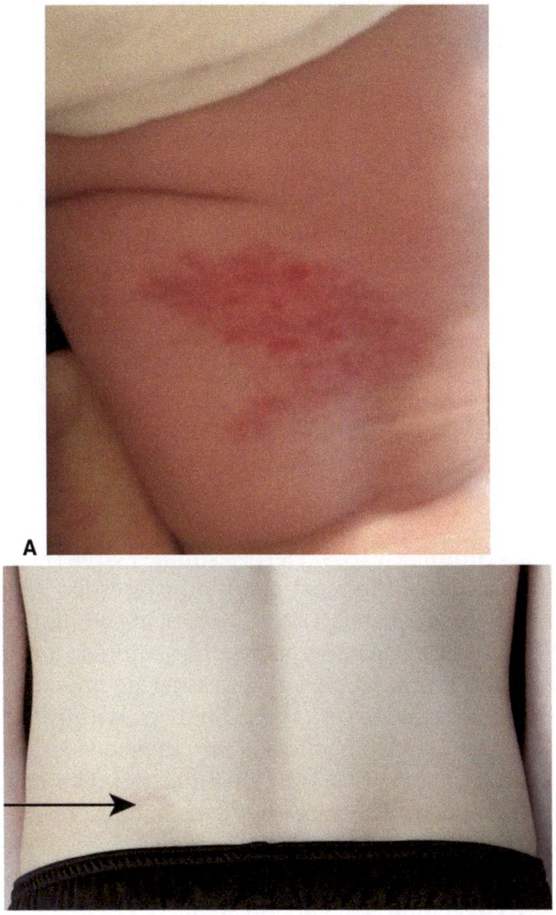

Figure 12.16 (**A**) Nevus simplex (salmon patch) on 2-month-old infant. (**B**) A faded salmon patch on a 13-year-old child.
Source: (**A**) Image courtesy of Elizabeth Carmac; (**B**) image courtesy of Amy J. Jnah.

2018). The major clinical phenotypes in the newborn of ichthyoses are enumerated in the "Genetic Influences" section of this chapter (**Figure 12.17**). Clinical manifestations during the neonatal period include isolated scaling, scaling with erythroderma, a collodion membrane, or thickened plates of harlequin ichthyosis. Although rare, early recognition is critical. Ichthyosis compromises the skin barrier, which increases the risk for secondary infection and increased penetration of irritants.

Infectious Etiologies

Candidiasis. Candidiasis is an infection caused by *Candida*, a species of yeast. The incidence of confirmed cases ranges from 2% to 26% in U.S. NICUs (Aliaga et al., 2014). Among extremely premature infants (smaller than 1,000 g), the incidence ranges from 4% to 8% and the mortality risk is 30% (Kelly et al., 2015). Fecal contamination is the usual source of the organism in *Candidal* dermatitis. *Candida* species are commensal organisms commonly found in the gastrointestinal and female genital tracts. Roughly 33% of healthcare workers in NICUs test positive for *Candida* on routine surveillance cultures, and up to 40% of XX pregnant patients are positive for *Candida* at the time of delivery (Filippidi et al., 2014).

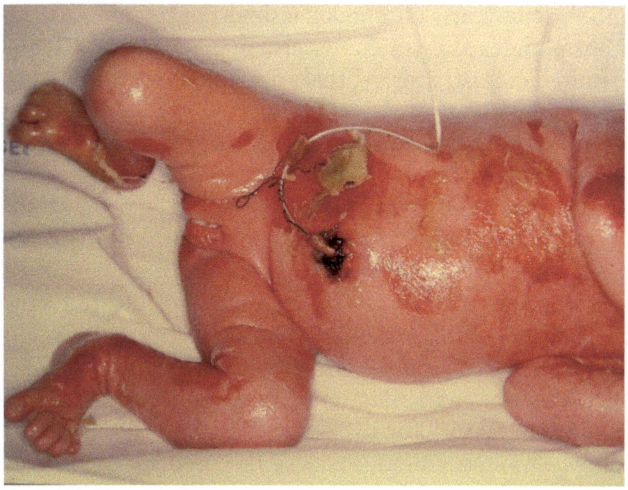

Figure 12.17 Ichthyoses.
Source: Waikato District Health Board/DermNet New Zealand.

Rarely, cutaneous candidiasis is congenitally acquired as a result of vertical (ascending) infection from a vaginal or cervical focus. Affected infants usually manifest with pustules to the palms and soles, and occasionally nail dystrophy. Candidiasis in the first 4 weeks of life is more common, usually benign, and typically localized to the oral cavity (thrush) or diaper area (**Figure 12.18**). The lesions of thrush are detectable as creamy-white patches of friable material on the buccal mucosa, gums, palate,

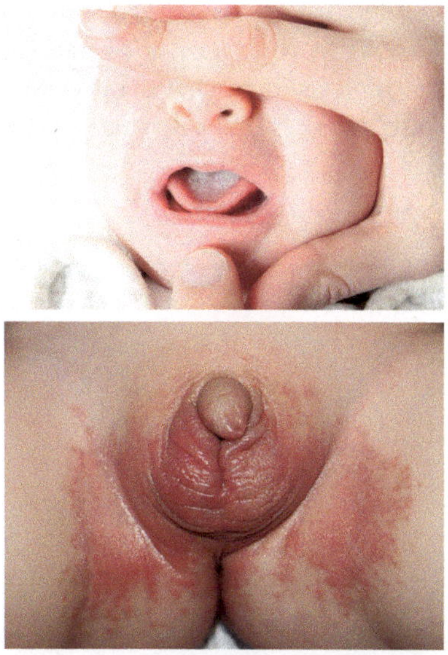

Figure 12.18 Candidiasis. (**A**) White, curdlike patch to the buccal mucosa, consistent with early stages of oral thrush. (**B**) Red, shiny rash with satellite lesions located within diaper region, consistent with *Candida* diaper rash.
Sources: (**A**) RioPatuca/Alamy Stock Photo; (**B**) Coughlin, C. C., Eichenfield, L. F., & Frieden, I. J. (2014). Diaper dermatitis: Clinical characteristics and differential diagnosis. *Pediatric Dermatology, 31*(Suppl 1), 19–24. https://doi.org/10.1111/pde.12500

and tongue. Early cutaneous lesions consist of erythematous papules and vesicopustules that become confluent, forming a moist, erosive, scaly dermatitis surrounded by satellite pustules.

In contrast to acquired cutaneous candidiasis, congenital candidiasis has lesions at nonflexural sites (Narendran, 2025). Distinctive yellow-white papules on the umbilical cord and placenta represent *Candida* granulomas. *C. albicans* may be demonstrable on histologic examination of these tissues and may be cultured from the amniotic fluid. Although *Candida* infection is usually localized to skin, infants who weigh less than 1,500 g are at risk for systemic infections (Shope et al., 2023). Additional risk factors for disseminated candidiasis include central-line placement, invasive mechanical ventilation, broad-spectrum antibiotic exposure, and the provision of intravenous parenteral nutrition.

Congenital Syphilis. Congenital syphilis occurs as a result of vertical transmission of *Treponema pallidum,* a spiral-shaped and coiled spirochete that invades the mucosa or skin during sexual intercourse. Sixty to ninety percent of infants with congenital syphilis are asymptomatic at birth. Clinical manifestations include erythematous vesicles or bullae atop a polished base (macule with erythematous halo); lesions located on the palms and soles are pathognomonic (Figure 12.19). Skin lesions may be accompanied by hepatosplenomegaly, periostitis of long bones, snuffles, and iritis. If undiagnosed, the symptoms persist or worsen. Diagnosis is confirmed through nontreponemal antibody titers (Church et al., 2023).

Clinical Application. Congenital syphilis cases have increased by 291% between 2015 and 2019 (Church et al., 2023). As many as 25% to 45% of untreated syphilis infections in XX pregnant patients result in spontaneous abortion or perinatal death. Symptoms associated with early congenital syphilis include low birthweight, maculopapular/vesicular skin rashes, hypercholesterolemia, hepatosplenomegaly, jaundice, anemia, thrombocytopenia, and purulent nasal discharge (rhinitis; Church et al., 2023). It is important for the APRN to remember that paired maternal and neonatal serum rapid plama reagin (RPR) testing is required to confirm the diagnosis. In addition, a lumbar puncture is required to evaluate the neonate for congenital syphilis.

Herpes Simplex Virus. Herpes simplex virus (HSV) infection is one of the most common causes for vesicular rashes in the neonatal period (Desai et al., 2025; Howard & Frieden, 2015). The virus may be acquired in utero or during the perinatal period. Intrauterine infection typically presents with vesicles at birth, or within the first 24 hours of life. An inconspicuous cutaneous lesion heralds the onset of severe systemic infection. The vesicular eruption may be widespread or even bullous, resembling EB (Figure 12.20). Vesicles may also present on the torso or buttocks, especially with a breech presentation. Rarely, congenital scars are present.

HSV infection acquired during the perinatal period is often limited to the skin, eyes, and mouth; disseminated infection is possible. Cutaneous lesions usually manifest during the second week of life, concurrent with or after nonspecific systemic signs and symptoms. Typically, the vesicles measure 1 mm to 3 mm in diameter and are usually noted on the scalp or face. Rarely, pustules, erosions, or oral ulcerations appear as isolated manifestations.

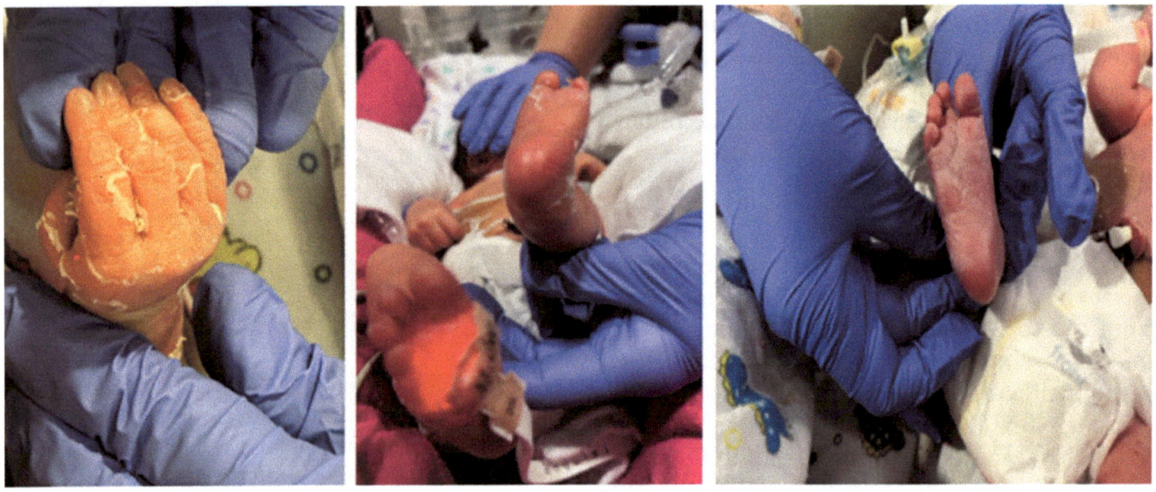

Figure 12.19 Congenital syphilis. Note the peeling vesiculobullous lesions on the hands and feet.
Source: Church, S., Willis, S., & Jnah, A. J. (2023). Congenital syphilis infection: A case study. *Neonatal Network, 42*(3), 156–164. https://doi.org/10.1891/NN-2022-0024

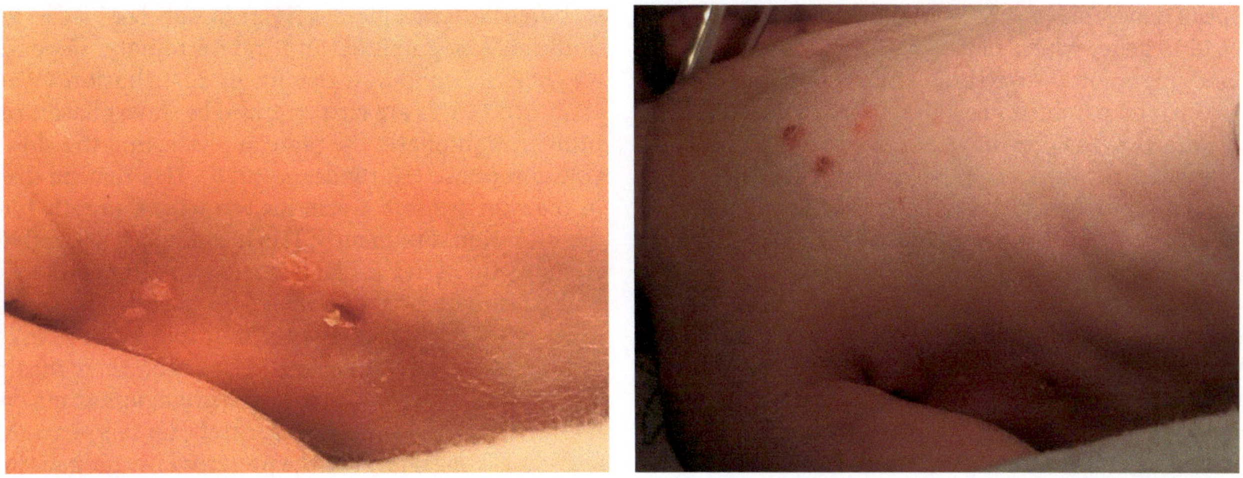

Figure 12.20 Herpes simplex virus.
Source: Bellini, S., & Beaulieu, M. J. (Eds.). (2017). *Neonatal advanced practice nursing: A case-based learning approach*. Springer Publishing Company.

Staphylococcal Infection and Impetigo. Superficial skin infections caused by *Staphylococcus aureus* are a concern because of the increase in community acquired *Methicillin-resistant Staphylococcus aureus* (*MRSA*). The *S. aureus* organism disrupts the host immune response by mechanisms that include isolation of host antibodies, the formation of a polysaccharide biofilm, and prevention of chemotaxis of leukocytes (Tong et al., 2015). Infections range from localized bullous impetigo to generalized cutaneous involvement with systemic illness. In contrast to congenital blistering diseases, which are often present at birth, skin infections with *S. aureus* usually develop after the first few days of life (Newnam, 2016). Lesions may be bullous, crusted, or pustular; typical lesions are small vesicles or pustules, or large, fragile bullae filled with clear, turbid, or purulent fluid. They rupture easily, leaving red, moist, denuded areas often with a superficial varnishlike crust (Figure 12.21; Nguyen et al., 2016). Although they may develop anywhere on the body, the blisters and pustules commonly occur on the diaper area, axillae, and periumbilical skin.

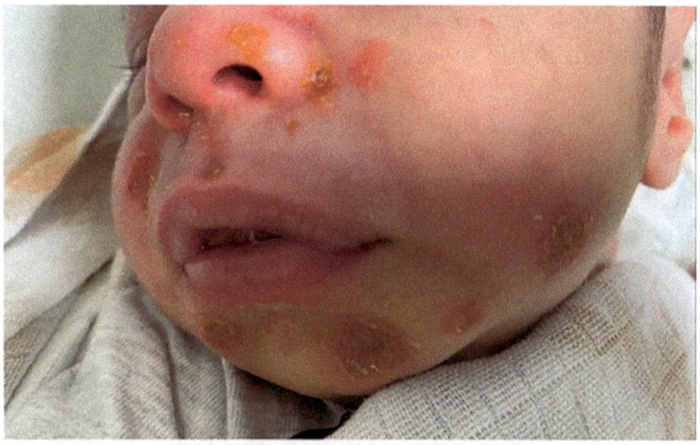

Figure 12.21 Infant with perioral impetigo, an acute contagious staphylococcal or streptococcal skin disease that presents as vesicles or pustules, and yellowish crusts.
Source: De Rose, D. U., Pugnaloni, F., Martini, L., Bersani, I., Ronchetti, M. P., Diociaiuti, A., El Hachem, M., Dotta, A., & Auriti, C. (2023). Staphylococcal infections and neonatal skin: Data from literature and suggestions for the clinical management from four challenging patients. *Antibiotics, 12*(4), 632. https://doi.org/10.3390/antibiotics12040632.

Staphylococcal Scalded Skin Syndrome. Staphylococcal scalded skin syndrome (*SSSS*) is a blistering skin disorder. Premature infants are at increased risk for SSSS due to a lack of maternal antitoxin antibodies. The infecting organism is *S. aureus*, usually a group 2 phage type, although other phage types occasionally have been incriminated. These organisms produce exotoxins (e.g., exfoliatin) that exert proteolytic activity on desmoglein-1, a molecule found within the desmosomes of keratinocytes responsible for the cutaneous manifestations (Hennigan & Riley, 2016; McKeown & Baker, 2022). The release of the endotoxins (epidermolytic toxin a and b) provokes widespread epidermal necrolysis with severe bullous eruptions. The bullous eruptions usually present between days 3 and 7 of life. Denudation and blister formation characteristically occur after gentle rubbing of the skin, which is referred to as *Nikolsky's sign*. Histologic examination of the skin shows a striking absence of inflammatory infiltrate. Infants are typically febrile, irritable, and exhibit marked cutaneous tenderness. Crusting around the mouth and eyes results in atypical facies. Conjunctivitis is common, along with hyperemia of the mucous membranes, but oral ulcerations do not occur.

Vascular Anomalies: Vascular Malformations and Vascular Tumors

Arteriovenous Malformations. Arteriovenous malformations (AVMs) are a more aggressive type of simple malformation. They are composed of malformed arteries, veins, and capillaries; direct arteriovenous communications result in arteriovenous shunting (Wassef et al., 2015). The incidence is estimated to be 0.001% within northern

European geographies. AVMs arise due to a mutation in the *RASA1* gene, which normally directs cell proliferation and migration (Weitz et al., 2015). Lesions are large, red, warm, and painful and exhibit pulsations, thrills, or a bruit. Rarely, AVMs present as ulcerated and bleeding lesions or with high output congestive cardiac failure. AVMs may remain quiescent through early childhood, and display sudden growth at puberty or following a local trauma. A high recurrence risk is reported (Richter & Suen, 2010).

Epidermal Nevi. Epidermal nevi occur among one to three of every 1,000 newborns (NIH, 2016). *RAS* gene mutations have been implicated in the formation of this skin lesion, which provoke overgrowth of keratinocytes (Hafner et al., 2012; Prendiville, 2015). Variations in size, clinical appearance, histologic characteristics, and evolution are reported. Lesions occurring in sites normally rich in sebaceous glands (e.g., scalp) may appear similar to sebaceous nevi, whereas others found in areas where the epidermis is thick (e.g., elbow) appear wartlike.

The most common type of epidermal nevus in the newborn infant is the sebaceous nevus, a hairless, papillomatous, yellow or pink, slightly elevated plaque on the scalp, forehead, or face (Prendiville, 2015). These lesions have a characteristic oval or lancet shape. Because a significant incidence of basal cell epitheliomas occurs in these lesions after puberty, they should be surgically removed.

Hemangiomas. Hemangiomas are the most common soft tissue tumors of infancy, occurring in up to 12% of infants (Narendran, 2025). These are benign vascular neoplasms that undergo rapid endothelial cell proliferation shortly after birth, stabilize, and then slowly involute with diminishing cellular activity and fibrous fatty deposition for up to 5 to 7 years (Shah et al., 2016).

Infantile hemangiomas (IHs) are subclassified as focal, multifocal, segmental, and indeterminate, depending on their morphology, extent, or distribution (Wassef et al., 2015). IHs are characterized by three phases: rapid proliferation phase, the plateau phase, and the slow involution phase (Narendran, 2025). IHs that lie deeper in the skin are soft, warm masses with a slightly bluish discoloration. Frequently, IHs have superficial and deep components. They range from a few millimeters to several centimeters in diameter and usually are solitary; up to 20% of infants display multiple lesions (**Figure 12.22**). Generally, superficial IHs reach their maximal size by 6 to 8 months, but deep hemangiomas may proliferate for 12 to 14 months or, rarely, up to 2 years. MRI and ultrasonography are the preferred imaging methods and should be considered when lesions are detected on the scalp, orbits, airways, or are found in groups of five or more.

Despite the benign nature of most cutaneous hemangiomas, a significant number cause functional compromise or permanent disfigurement. Approximately 65% of hemangiomas are on the head and neck. Even with treatment, half of hemangiomas located on the lip, eyelid, nose, cheek, or glabella require surgical treatment (Brennan et al., 2017). Nasal tip, lip, and parotid hemangiomas are notorious for slow involution, and very large superficial facial hemangiomas often leave disfiguring scarring. Ulceration, the most frequent complication, can be excruciatingly painful and carries the risk of infection, hemorrhage, and scarring. Occasionally, hemangiomas manifest as congenital ulcerations with only a very small rim of typical hemangioma, making the diagnosis difficult.

Periorbital hemangiomas and hemangiomas that involve the ear pose considerable risk to vision, hearing,

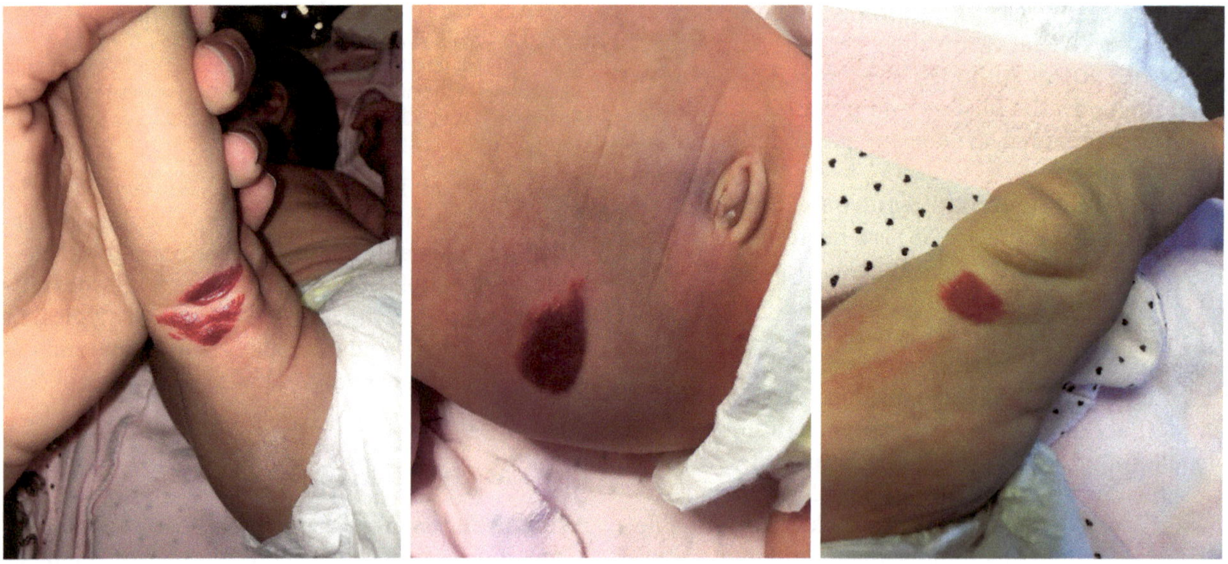

A B C

Figure 12.22 Images of a female newborn with five focal cutaneous hemangiomas (four shown here: [**A**] two lesions to the right leg, [**B**] lesion to the right abdomen, and [**C**] lesion to the left thigh). Further examination revealed normal thyroid function and an absence of associated hepatic hemangiomas.

and speech. Multiple cutaneous (i.e., diffuse hemangiomatosis) and large facial hemangiomas may be associated with visceral hemangiomas. Due to the potential for visceral hemangiomas, additional evaluations including ultrasounds and/or MRI may be warranted (Friedland et al., 2017; Reimer & Hoeger, 2016). Subglottic hemangiomas manifest with hoarseness and stridor, and progression to respiratory failure may be rapid. Approximately 50% of these infants have associated cutaneous hemangiomas. Any "noisy breathing" by an infant with a cutaneous hemangioma involving the chin, lips, mandibular region, and neck warrants direct visualization of the airway. Sixty percent of young infants with extensive facial hemangiomas in the "beard" distribution develop symptomatic airway hemangiomas.

The presence of an extensive cervicofacial hemangioma may indicate PHACE syndrome, where the hemangioma is associated with other anomalies; **P** = posterior fossa (possible abnormal structures in the brain, especially the cerebellum), **H** = hemangioma, **A** = arterial (possible brain artery abnormalities), **C** = cardiac (possible abnormalities of the great vessels of the heart), and **E** = eyes (possible eye anomalies). This syndrome has a marked female predominance (9:1) and is thought to represent a developmental field defect that occurs between weeks 8 and 10 of gestation. Lumbosacral hemangiomas may be markers for occult spinal dysraphism and anorectal and urogenital anomalies.

Congenital hemangiomas are relatively uncommon, present fully grown at birth, and either undergo rapid involution (RICH: rapidly involuting congenital hemangioma) or persist into adulthood (NICH: noninvoluting congenital hemangioma). Congenital hemangiomas that resolve rapidly often leave pronounced atrophic skin changes in their wake.

Most hemangiomas require "active nonintervention" coupled with a careful discussion of the natural history of the lesions and photographic documentation of involution (Maguiness & Garzon, 2015; Narendran, 2025; Tripathi et al., 2021). Up to 40% of children develop complications requiring intervention. Ulceration is the most common complication, but other problems include bleeding, airway or visual axis obstruction, cosmetic disfigurement, and high-output cardiac failure (Maguiness & Garzon, 2015; Narendran, 2025).

Kaposiform hemangioendothelioma (Kasabach–Merritt phenomenon), a complication of a rapidly enlarging vascular lesion, is characterized by hemolytic anemia, thrombocytopenia, and coagulopathy. These massive tumors are usually a deep red-blue color, firm, grow rapidly, have no sex predilection, tend to proliferate for a longer period (2–5 years), and have a different histologic pattern than other hemangiomas. Most patients with Kasabach–Merritt phenomenon manifest with proliferative vascular tumors, usually kaposiform hemangioendotheliomas or tufted angiomas (Maguiness & Garzon, 2015; Narendran, 2025). The Kasabach–Merritt phenomenon carries a significant mortality risk.

Lymphangiomas. Lymphangiomas are congenital hamartomatous malformations composed of dilated lymph channels that are lined by normal lymphatic endothelium (Maguiness & Garzon, 2015). Fetal skin and subcutaneous tissues are involved in this malformation that affects 1.1 to 5.3 of every 10,000 births (Ersoy et al., 2016). These malformations may be observed prenatally via ultrasound, may be superficial or deep, and are often associated with anomalies of the regional lymphatic vessels (Figure 12.23).

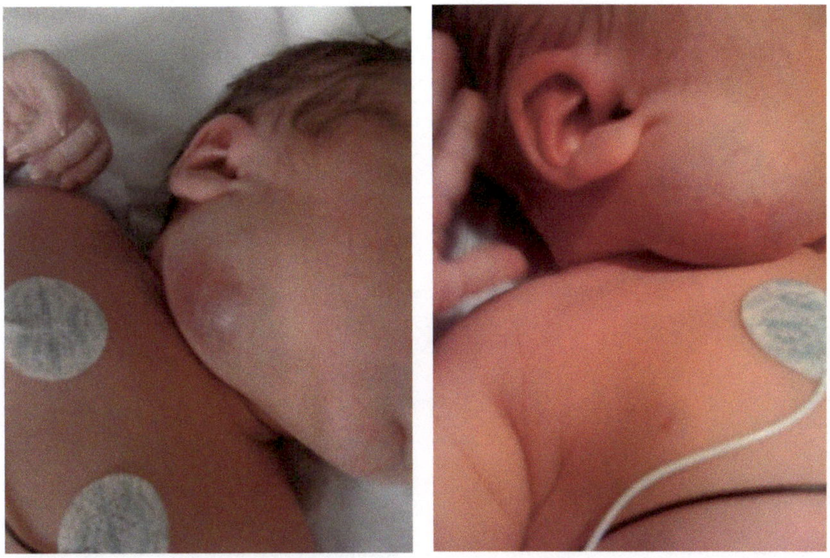

Figure 12.23 Lymphatic malformation ("cystic hygroma") present at birth.
Image Credit: Amy J. Jnah.

Milroy primary congenital lymphedema may present at birth and often affects the dorsal aspects of the feet. This autosomal dominant condition arises from a congenital dysgenesis of the lymphatic microvessels secondary to mutation in the *FLT4* (*VEGFR3*) gene. This condition is rarely associated with significant complications.

Simple and deep lymphangiomas, as well as cystic hygromas, may present at birth or during infancy. Simple lymphangiomas appear as solitary, skin-colored, dermal or subcutaneous nodules. After trauma, they may exude serous fluid. On occasion, these lesions have been associated with more extensive lymphatic involvement. Alternatively, deep lymphangiomas are more diffuse and consist of large, cystic dilations of lymphatics in the dermis, subcutaneous tissue, and intermuscular septa. Cystic hygroma is a benign, multilocular tumor usually found in the neck region. These tumors tend to increase in size.

Lymphangioma circumscriptum is probably the most common type of lymphangioma and may be present at birth or appear in early childhood. Areas of predilection are the oral mucosa, proximal limbs, and flexures. This malformation consists of clustered, small, thick-walled vesicles resembling frog spawn; it is often skin colored but may have a red or purple cast because of the presence of blood mixed with lymph in the vesicles.

Port-Wine Stain. Port-wine stains are capillary malformations that are almost always present at birth and should be considered permanent developmental defects (Maguiness & Garzon, 2015; Narendran, 2025). They occur in 0.3% of neonates (Elias et al., 2021). These lesions may span a few millimeters in diameter or cover extensive areas, but facial lesions are the most common (Figure 12.24). They do not proliferate after birth, but may appear to increase in size with the growth of the child. Port-wine stains are sharply demarcated and flat during infancy, but with time develop a pebbly or slightly thickened surface and frequently darken (Narendran, 2025). Most port-wine stains occur as isolated defects; occasionally, these lesions may be associated with ocular defects or certain vascular malformation syndromes.

Inflammatory Diseases of the Skin

Several inflammatory skin conditions may occur in the neonate. Irritant contact dermatitis and seborrheic dermatitis are the most frequently encountered (Cordoro & Schulman, 2015; Tom & Eichenfield, 2015). They may be difficult to distinguish because their clinical features have a significant degree of overlap.

Irritant Contact Dermatitis. Primary irritant contact dermatitis (as opposed to allergic contact dermatitis) is probably the most common exogenous cause for dermatitis in the newborn. Irritant contact dermatitis is generally a result of penetration of external agents, or iatrogenic causes, via a damaged or underdeveloped SC. External agents may disrupt the SC barrier by way of hydration or alteration of the lipid bilayer structure. Irritants penetrate into the epidermis, causing inflammation, cytokine release, and acceleration of barrier repair (Visscher et al., 2015). The distribution of the eruption varies somewhat, depending on the precipitating agent. The principal irritants in diaper dermatitis are fecal enzymes, skin maceration, friction, high pH, and prolonged contact with urine and feces (Figure 12.25; Atherton, 2016). Detergent bubble bath, antiseptic proprietary agents, and soap zealously used to clean the perianal area may cause acute eczematous diaper dermatitis, which may become generalized. Obtaining precise information about what has been applied to the skin and how it has been applied is imperative in making an accurate diagnosis.

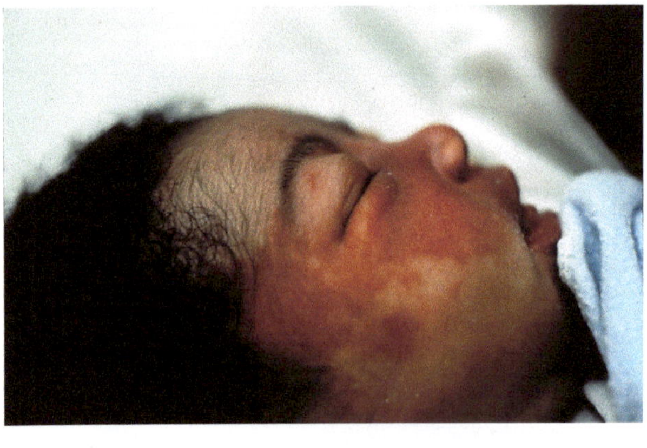

Figure 12.24 Port-wine nevus.
Source: Clark, D. A. (2000). *Atlas of neonatology*. Saunders.

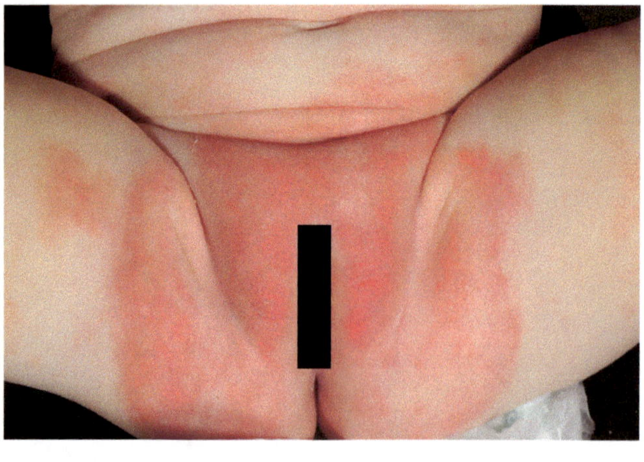

Figure 12.25 Irritant contact dermatitis.
Source: Fölster-Holst R. (2018). Differential diagnoses of diaper dermatitis. *Pediatric Dermatology, 35*(Suppl 1), s10–s18. https://doi.org/10.1111/pde.13484

Seborrheic Dermatitis. Seborrheic dermatitis affects as many as 10% of neonates. It typically occurs on the scalp but may develop on the face, neck, and in the diaper area (Cohen, 2017). Seborrheic dermatitis is characterized by greasy, nonpruritic scaling associated with patchy redness, fissuring, and occasional weeping, usually involving the scalp, ears, axillary, and perineal folds (Figure 12.26).

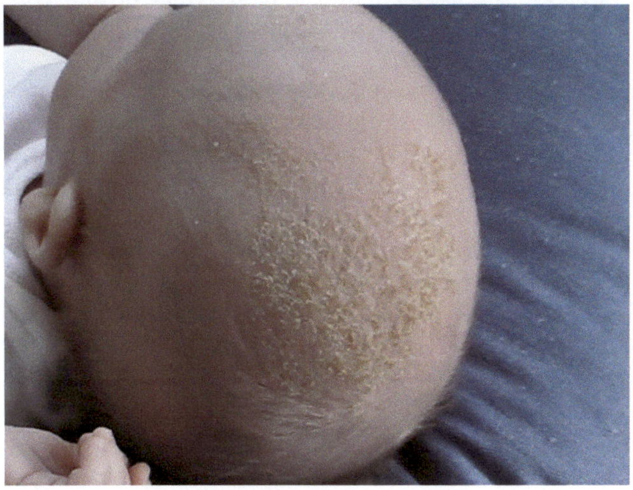

Figure 12.26 Infant with scales on the scalp, consistent with seborrheic dermatitis ("cradle cap").
Source: Starfoxy. (2005). *An infant with cradle cap.* https://commons.wikimedia.org/wiki/File:Baby_With_Cradle_Cap.jpg.

The yeast *Malassezia* is believed to contribute to the pathophysiology. There is controversy about whether seborrheic dermatitis is a distinct entity or presages the advent of atopic dermatitis. Some infants never progress beyond the seborrheic phase of the dermatitis, which in its classic form rarely is seen in the first month of life. Cradle cap is a minor variant of seborrheic dermatitis.

Other Skin Disorders

Sucking Blisters. Sucking blisters present in 0.4% of neonates (Aydin et al., 2013). They are benign, fluid-filled erosions on the skin surface secondary to in utero fetal sucking maneuvers. Episodic or short-term sucking produces a soft and fluid-filled blister, whereas chronic sucking may increase the likelihood for postnatal calluses (Figure 12.27). Asymmetric or irregular borders are common and, unlike infectious blisters, these are often limited to one blister in a specific location. As such, these blisters often present on the hands, lips, or inside the mouth (Bruckner & O'Regan, 2015).

CONCLUSION

The skin is the largest organ in the body and plays vital roles in protection, thermoregulation, and communication with the environment. Understanding its

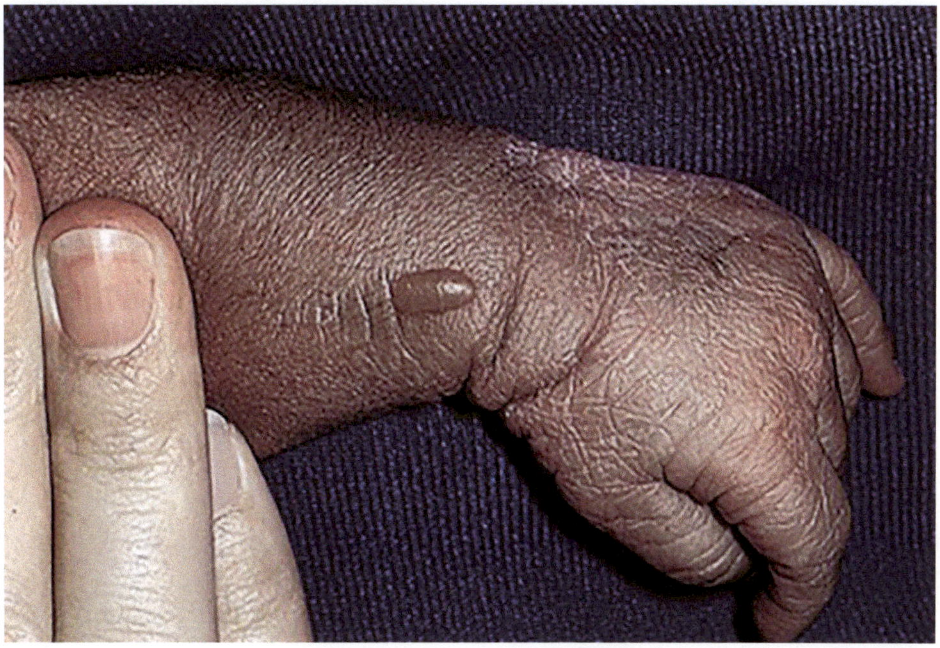

Figure 12.27 Evidence of sucking blister to left hand, which presented at birth.
Source: Lucky, A. W. (2015). *Transient benign cutaneous lesions in the newborn.* https://clinicalgate.com/transient-benign-cutaneous-lesions-in-the-newborn/

embryologic origins is important. Genetic and maternal influences should be explored. Finally, accurate visual diagnosis is key to uncovering neonatal skin conditions.

LEARNING TOOLS AND RESOURCES

CourseConnect

To access self-assessment questions and interactive, competency-based learning activities for this chapter, visit www.springerpub.com/courseconnect. See inside front cover and tear-out card for CourseConnect details.

Podcast

This podcast is available online by visiting www.springerpub.com/courseconnect. See inside front cover and tear-out card for CourseConnect details.

Neonatal Skin and Innate Immunity: Differences Between the Term and Preterm Infant

Rani Delaney, Lauren Fraser, Maryellen Lane, and Melissa Bauserman

Discussion Prompts

1. Discuss the purpose and derivatives of vernix. How might the presence or absence of vernix implicate newborn skin?
2. Identify and discuss the major issues for the premature infant as a result of underdeveloped skin.
3. What is the most common neonatal skin condition? Correlate the etiology with your understanding of the physiology of the skin.
4. Describe the difference between a vascular malformation and a vascular tumor in neonates.
5. Describe the causes and appearance of *Candida* infections.

MIND MAP

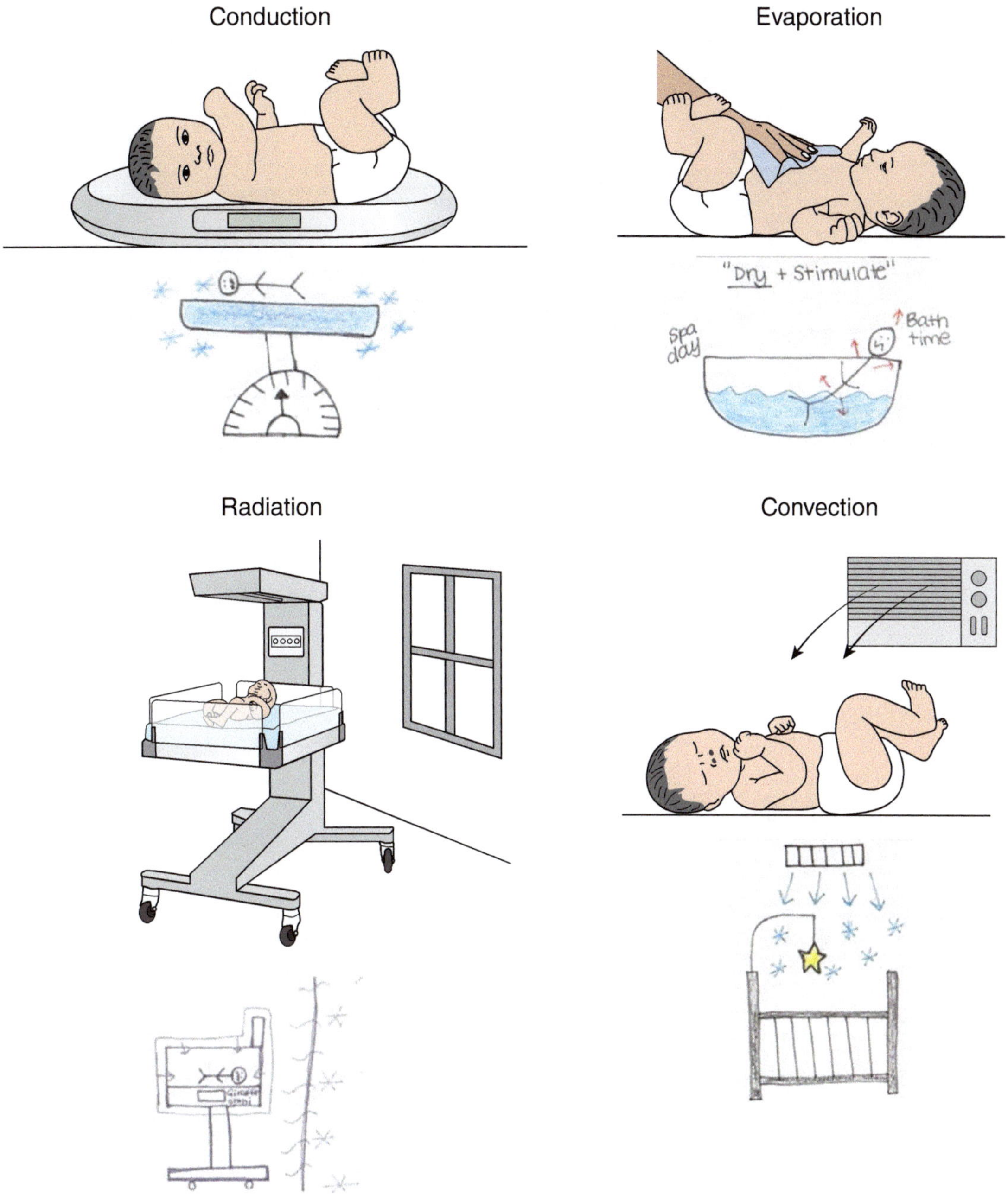

Note: This mind map reflects one neonatal nurse practitioner student's interpretation of a concept addressed in this chapter. Readers should regard the mind maps woven throughout this textbook as examples of multisensory study tools that can be developed to aid conceptual understanding. Readers are encouraged to develop their own unique mind maps in consultation with academic faculty or clinical preceptors.

Image Credit: Courtesy of Ellie Essick, BSN, RN.

TIMELINE OF ORGAN DEVELOPMENT

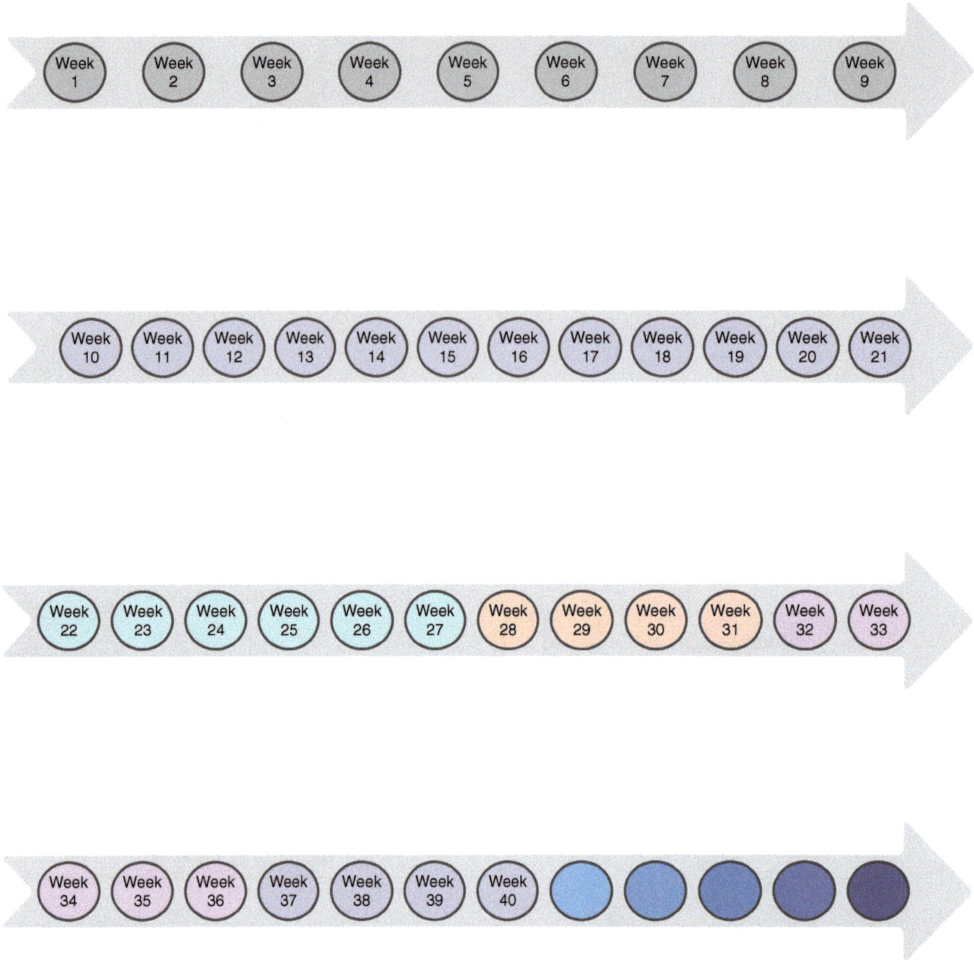

Note: Placement of common problems is meant to offer visual/conceptual perspective on the timing of onset of these commonly reported malformations. Variation exists across the literature.	***Legend:*** <22 – 27 6/7 weeks = extremely preterm 28 – 31 6/7 weeks = very preterm 32 – 36 6/7 weeks = late/moderate preterm 37 – 40 weeks = term

Note: Readers should annotate the blank timeline during studying, self-directed learning, and creation of feedback loops with mentors. To access the blank and completed timelines visit www.springerpub.com/courseconnect. See inside front cover and tear-out card for CourseConnect details.

REFERENCES

Adni, T., Martin, K., & Mudge, E. (2012). The psychosocial impact of chronic wounds on patients with severe epidermolysis bullosa. *Journal of Wound Care, 21*(11), 528–538. https://doi.org/10.12968/jowc.2012.21.11.528

Aliaga, S., Clark, R. H., Laughon, M., Walsh, T. J., Hope, W. W., Benjamin, D. K., Kaufman, D., Arrieta, A., Benjamin, D. K., Jr., & Smith, P. B. (2014). Changes in the incidence of candidiasis in neonatal intensive care units. *Pediatrics, 133*(2), 236–242. https://doi.org/10.1542/peds.2013-0671

Atherton, D. J. (2016). Understanding irritant napkin dermatitis. *International Journal of Dermatology, 55(1)*, 7–9. https://doi.org/10.1111/ijd.13334

Aydin, M., Hakan, N., Zenciroglu, A., & Demirol, H. A. (2013). A rare location of sucking blister in newborn: The lips. *European Journal of Pediatrics, 172*(10), 1423–1424. https://doi.org/10.1007/s00431-013-2055-y

Ballard, J. L., Khoury, J. C., Wedig, K., Wang, L., Eilers-Walsman, B. L., & Lipp, R. (1991). New Ballard score, expanded to include extremely premature infants. *The Journal of Pediatrics, 119*(3), 417–423. https://doi.org/10.1016/s0022-3476(05)82056-6

Basit, S., Khan, S., & Ahmad, W. (2015). Genetics of human isolated hereditary hair loss disorders: Genetics of hereditary hair loss disorders. *Clinical Genetics, 88*(3), 203–212. https://doi.org/10.1111/cge.12531

Bermas, B. L., & Smith, N. A. (2024). Pregnancy in women with systemic lupus erythematosus. In M. Ramirez Curtis (Ed.), *UpToDate*. Retrieved September 23, 2025, from https://www.uptodate.com/contents/pregnancy-in-women-with-systemic-lupus-erythematosus

Bertola, D. R., Yamamoto, G. L., Almeida, T. F., Buscarilli, M., Jorge, A. A. L., Malaquias, A. C., Kim, C. A., Takahashi, V. N., Passos-Bueno, M. R., & Pereira, A. C. (2014). Further evidence of the importance of RIT1 in Noonan syndrome.

American Journal of Medical Genetics Part A, 164(11), 2952–2957. https://doi.org/10.1002/ajmg.a.36722

Bolender, D. L. (2022). Basic embryology. In R. A. Polin, S. H. Abman, D. H. Rowitch, W. E. Benitz, & W. W. Fox (Eds.), *Fetal and neonatal physiology* (6th ed., pp. 23–38). Elsevier.

Bolognia, J., Schaffer, J. V., & Cerroni, L. (Eds.). (2025). *Dermatology* (5th ed.). Elsevier.

Brennan, T. E., Waner, M., & O. T. M. (2017). The tissue expander effect in early surgical management of select focal infantile hemangiomas. *JAMA Facial Plastic Surgery, 19*(4), 282–286. https://doi.org/10.1001/jamafacial.2016.1991

Bruckner, A. L., & O'Regan, G. M. (2015). Inherited and acquired blistering diseases. In L. F. Eichenfield, I. J. Frieden, E. F. Mathes, & A. L. Zaenglein (Eds.), *Neonatal and infant dermatology* (3rd ed., pp. 140–154). Elsevier Saunders.

Brzezinski, P., & Chiriac, A. (2015). Sebaceous hyperplasia in neonates and adults. *Our Dermatology Online, 6*(1), 107–108. https://doi.org/10.7241/ourd.20151.29

Carlson, B. M. (2024). Integumentary, skeletal, and muscular systems. In B. M. Carlson, *Human embryology and developmental biology* (5th ed., pp. 154–194). Elsevier Saunders.

Chan, Y., & Tay, Y. (2015). Hypopigmentation disorders. In L. F. Eichenfield, I. J. Frieden, E. F. Mathes, & A. L. Zaenglein (Eds.), *Neonatal and infant dermatology* (3rd ed., pp. 369–387). Elsevier Saunders.

Chu, D. H., & Loomis, C. A. (2022). Structure and development of the skin and cutaneous appendages. In R. A. Polin, S. H. Abman, D. H. Rowitch, W. E. Benitz, & W. W. Fox (Eds.), *Fetal and neonatal physiology* (6th ed., pp. 446–454). Elsevier.

Church, S., Willis, S., & Jnah, A. (2023). Congenital syphilis infection: A case study. *Neonatal Network, 42*(3), 156–164. https://doi.org/10.1891/NN-2022-0024

Cohen, B. (2017). Differential diagnosis of diaper dermatitis. *Clinical Pediatrics, 56*(5 Suppl), 16S–22S. https://doi.org/10.1177/0009922817706982

Cordoro, K., & Schulman, J. (2015). Papulosquamous & lichenoid disorders. In L. F. Eichenfield, I. J. Frieden, E. F. Mathes, & A. L. Zaenglein (Eds.), *Neonatal and infant dermatology* (3rd ed., pp. 233–244). Elsevier Saunders.

Craiglow, B. G. (2013). Ichthyosis in the newborn. *Seminars in Perinatology, 37*(1), 26–31. https://doi.org/10.1053/j.semperi.2012.11.001

Cui, C., & Schlessinger, D. (2015). Eccrine sweat gland development and sweat secretion. *Experimental Dermatology, 24*(9), 644–650. https://doi.org/10.1111/exd.12773

Desai, A. P., Lim, P. P. C., Ogundare, M. O., & Gonzalez, B. E. (2025). Viral infections in the neonate. In R. J. Martin & A. A. Fanaroff (Eds.), *Fanaroff and Martin's neonatal-perinatal medicine* (12th ed., pp. 917–978). Elsevier Saunders.

Elias, A. J., Hand, J. L., Tollefson, M. M., & Davis, D. M. R. (2021). The anatomic distribution of isolated and syndrome-associated port-wine stain. *Pediatric Dermatology, 38*(1), 77–82. https://doi.org/10.1111/pde.14392

Ersoy, A. O., Oztas, E., Saridogan, E., Ozler, S., & Danisman, N. (2016). An unusual origin of fetal lymphangioma filling right axilla. *Journal of Clinical and Diagnostic Research, 10*(3), QD09–QD11. https://doi.org/10.7860/JCDR/2016/18516.7513

Filippidi, A., Galanakis, E., Maraki, S., Galani, I., Drogari-Apiranthitou, M., Kalmanti, M., Mantadakis, E., & Samonis, G. (2014). The effect of maternal flora on *Candida* colonisation in the neonate. *Mycoses, 57*(1), 43–48. https://doi.org/10.1111/myc.12100

Fine, J.-D., & Mellerio, J. E. (2025). Epidermolysis bullosa. In J. L. Bolognia, J. V. Schaffer, & L. Cerroni (Eds.), *Dermatology* (5th ed., pp. 545–559). Elsevier Saunders.

Foley, C. C., Paller, A. S., & Irvine, A. D. (2015). Disorders of cornification (ichthyosis). In L. F. Eichenfield, I. J. Frieden, E. F. Mathes, & A. L. Zaenglein (Eds.), *Neonatal and infant dermatology* (3rd ed., pp. 281–302). Elsevier Saunders.

Friedland, R., Ben Amitai, D., & Zvulunovs, A. (2017). Screening for brain involvement in infants with multifocal cutaneous infantile hemangiomas. *Dermatology, 233*(6), 435–440. https://doi.org/10.1159/000484598

Grabowski, J. (2022). Disorders of the breast. In P. Mattei (Ed.), *Fundamentals of pediatric surgery*. Springer Publishing Company.

Griswold, K., & Srinivas, G. (2025). Examination of the newborn. In R. J. Martin & A. A. Fanaroff (Eds.), *Fanaroff and Martin's neonatal-perinatal medicine* (12th ed., pp. 453–474). Elsevier Saunders.

Gupta, D., & Thappa, D. M. (2013). Mongolian spots: How important are they? *World Journal of Clinical Cases, 1*(8), 230–232. https://doi.org/10.12998/wjcc.v1.i8.230

Hafner, C., Toll, A., Gantner, S., Mauerer, A., Lurkin, I., Acquadro, F., Fernández-Casado, A., Zwarthoff, E. C., Dietmaier, W., Baselga, E., Parera, E., Vicente, A., Casanova, A., Cigudosa, J., Mentzel, T., Pujol, R. M., Landthaler, M., & Real, F. X. (2012). Keratinocytic epidermal nevi are associated with mosaic *RAS* mutations. *Journal of Medical Genetics, 49*(4), 249–253. https://doi.org/10.1136/jmedgenet-2011-100637

Haveri, F. T. T. S., & Inamadar, A. C. (2014). A cross-sectional prospective study of cutaneous lesions in newborn. *ISRN Dermatology, 2014*, 1–8. https://doi.org/10.1155/2014/360590

Hennigan, K., & Riley, C. (2016). Staphylococcal scalded skin syndrome: A case review. *Neonatal Network, 35*(1), 8–12. https://doi.org/10.1891/0730-0832.35.1.8

Hölzle, E., & Kligman, A. M. (1978). The pathogenesis of miliaria rubra: Role of the resident microflora. *British Journal of Dermatology, 99*(2), 117–137. https://doi.org/10.1111/j.1365-2133.1978.tb01973.x

Howard, R., & Frieden, I. (2015). Vesicles, pustules, bullae, erosions, and ulceration. In L. F. Eichenfield, I. J. Frieden, E. F. Mathes, & A. L. Zaenglein (Eds.), *Neonatal and infant dermatology* (3rd ed., pp. 111–139). Elsevier Saunders.

Javed, A., & Lteif, A. (2013). Development of the human breast. *Seminars in Plastic Surgery, 27*(1), 5–12. https://doi.org/10.1055/s-0033-1343989

Jnah, A. J., Newberry, D., & Robertson, T. (2017). Dermatology cases. In S. Bellini & M. Beaulieu (Eds.), *Neonatal advanced practice nursing: A case-based learning approach* (pp. 213–254). Springer Publishing Company.

Kanada, K. N., Merin, M. R., Munden, A., & Friedlander, S. F. (2012). A prospective study of cutaneous findings in newborns in the United States: Correlation with race, ethnicity, and gestational status using updated classification and nomenclature. *Journal of Pediatrics, 161*(2), 240–245. https://doi.org/10.1016/j.jpeds.2012.02.052

Kelly, M. S., Benjamin, D. K., Jr., & Smith, P. B. (2015). The epidemiology and diagnosis of invasive candidiasis among premature infants. *Clinics in Perinatology, 42*(1), 105–117. https://doi.org/10.1016/j.clp.2014.10.008

Khemani, S., Ali, S. B., Karim, S., & Yezdan, M. A. (2017). Harlequin colour change. *Journal of the College of Physicians*

Surgeons Pakistan, 27(9), S127–S128. https://www.jcpsp.pk/archive/2017/SS_Sep2017/25.pdf

Kolb, L., & Krishnamurthy, K. (2024). *Nevus anemicus.* https://www.ncbi.nlm.nih.gov/books/NBK459139

Lucky, A. W. (2015). Transient benign cutaneous lesions of the newborn. In L. F. Eichenfield, I. J. Frieden, E. F. Mathes, & A. L. Zaenglein (Eds.), *Neonatal and infant dermatology* (3rd ed., pp. 65–76). Elsevier Saunders.

Lucky, A. W., Whalen, J., Rowe, S., Marathe, K. S., & Gorell, E. (2021). Diagnosis and care of the newborn with epidermolysis bullosa. *Neoreviews, 22*(7), e438–e451. https://doi.org/10.1542/neo.22-7-e438

Lun Hon, K., & Leung, A. K. C. (2012). Neonatal lupus erythematosus. *Autoimmune Diseases, 2012*, 1–6. https://doi.org/10.1155/2012/301274

Maguiness, S., & Garzon, M. (2015). Vascular malformations. In L. F. Eichenfield, I. J. Frieden, E. F. Mathes, & A. L. Zaenglein (Eds.), *Neonatal and infant dermatology* (3rd ed., pp. 352–368). Elsevier Saunders.

Mancini, A. J., & Lawley, L. P. (2015). Structure and function of newborn skin. In L. F. Eichenfield, I. J. Frieden, E. F. Mathes, & A. L. Zaenglein (Eds.), *Neonatal and infant dermatology* (3rd ed., pp. 14–23). Elsevier Saunders.

McKeown, K. E., & Baker, R. B. (2022). Staphylococcal scalded skin syndrome, identification, and wound care: A case report series. *Advances in Neonatal Care: Official Journal of the National Association of Neonatal Nurses, 22*(4), 325–332. https://doi.org/10.1097/ANC.0000000000000979

Monteagudo, B., Labandeira, J., Cabanillas, M., Acevedo, A., & Toribio, J. (2012). Prospective study of erythema toxicum neonatorum: Epidemiology and predisposing factors. *Pediatric Dermatology, 29*(2), 166–168. https://doi.org/10.1111/j.1525-1470.2011.01536.x

Mowad, C. M., McGinley, K. J., Foglia, A., & Leyden, J. J. (1995). The role of extracellular polysaccharide substance produced by *Staphylococcus epidermidis* in miliaria. *Journal of the American Academy of Dermatology, 33*(5), 729–733. https://doi.org/10.1016/0190-9622(95)91809-4

Narendran, V. (2025). The skin of the neonate. In R. J. Martin & A. A. Fanaroff (Eds.), *Fanaroff and Martin's neonatal-perinatal medicine: Diseases of the fetus and neonate* (12th ed., pp. 1992-2026). Elsevier.

National Institutes of Health. (2016). *Genetics home reference: Epidermal nevus.* https://medlineplus.gov/genetics/condition/epidermal-nevus/#frequency

National Institutes of Health. (2018). *Genetics home reference: Autosomal recessive hypotrichosis.* https://ghr.nlm.nih.gov/condition/autosomal-recessive-hypotrichosis#genes

National Institutes of Health. (2020). *Genetics home reference: Neurofibromatosis type 1.* https://ghr.nlm.nih.gov/condition/neurofibromatosis-type-1#statistics https://medlineplus.gov/genetics/condition/neurofibromatosis-type-1/#frequency

National Institutes of Health. (2024a). *Genetics home reference: Albinism.* https://www.ncbi.nlm.nih.gov/books/NBK519018

National Institutes of Health. (2024b). *Genetics home reference: Noonan syndrome.* https://www.ncbi.nlm.nih.gov/books/NBK532269

National Organization for Rare Disorders. (2019). *Biotinidase deficiency.* https://rarediseases.org/rare-diseases/biotinidase-deficiency/

National Organization for Rare Disorders. (2021). *Sturge-Weber syndrome.* https://rarediseases.org/rare-diseases/sturge-weber-syndrome

National Organization for Rare Disorders. (2024). *Epidermolysis bullosa.* https://rarediseases.org/rare-diseases/epidermolysis-bullosa

Newnam, K. M. (2016). Surveillance and isolation of methicillin-resistant *Staphylococcus aureus* colonization in the neonatal intensive care unit. *Advances in Neonatal Care, 16*(4), 298–307. https://doi.org/10.1097/ANC.0000000000000312

Nguyen, T. A., Wang, A. S., Eichenfield, L. F., & Barrio, V. (2016). "EB, or not EB?" Neonatal desquamative impetigo in a degloving pattern. *Pediatric Dermatology, 33*(2), e147–e148. https://doi.org/10.1111/pde.12766s

Niemann, C., & Horsley, V. (2012). Development and homeostasis of the sebaceous gland. *Seminars in Cell & Developmental Biology, 23*(8), 928–936. https://doi.org/10.1016/j.semcdb.2012.08.010

Peltonen, S., Kallionpää, R. A., & Peltonen, J. (2017). Neurofibromatosis type 1 (*NF1*) gene: Beyond café au lait spots and dermal neurofibromas. *Experimental Dermatology, 26*(7), 645–648. https://doi.org/10.1111/exd.13212

Persaud, T. V. N., & Torchia, M. G. (2025). *The developing human: Clinically oriented embryology* (12th ed., pp. 415–431). Elsevier.

Prendiville, J. (2015). Lumps, bumps, and hamartomas. In L. F. Eichenfield, I. J. Frieden, E. F. Mathes, & A. L. Zaenglein (Eds.), *Neonatal and infant dermatology* (3rd ed., pp. 422–442). Elsevier Saunders.

Price, H., & Marghoob, A. (2015). Disorders of hyperpigmentation and melanocytes. In L. F. Eichenfield, I. J. Frieden, E. F. Mathes, & A. L. Zaenglein (Eds.), *Neonatal and infant dermatology* (3rd ed., pp. 388–409). Elsevier Saunders.

Reginatto, F. P., DeVilla, D., Muller, F. M., Peruzzo, J., Peres, L. P., Steglich, R. B., & Cestari, T. F. (2017). Prevalence and characterization of neonatal skin disorders in the first 72 h of life. *Jornal de Pediatria, 93*(3), 238–245. https://doi.org/10.1016/j.jped.2016.06.010

Reginatto, F. P., Muller, F. M., Peruzzo, J., & Cestari, T. F. (2017). Epidemiology and predisposing factors for erythema toxicum neonatorum and transient neonatal pustular: A multicenter study. *Pediatric Dermatology, 34*(4), 422–426. https://doi.org/10.1111/pde.13179

Reimer, A., & Hoeger, P. H. (2016). Lesion morphology in multifocal infantile hemangiomas. *Pediatric Dermatology, 33*(6), 621–626. https://doi.org/10.1111/pde.12956

Richter, G. T., & Suen, J. Y. (2010). Clinical course of arteriovenous malformations of the head and neck: A case series. *Otolaryngology—Head and Neck Surgery, 142*(2), 184–190. https://doi.org/10.1016/j.otohns.2009.10.023

Roh, M. R., Eliades, P., Gupta, S., & Tsao, H. (2015). Genetics of melanocytic nevi. *Pigment Cell & Melanoma Research, 28*(6), 661–672. https://doi.org/10.1111/pcmr.12412

Sadler, T. W. (2023). *Langman's medical embryology* (15th ed.). Lippincott, Williams & Wilkins.

Schachner, L. A., Andriessen, A., Benjamin, L., Dones, M., Kircik, L., Pinera-Llano, A., & Hebert, A. A. (2023). The many faces of pediatric acne: A practical algorithm for treatment, maintenance therapy, and skincare recommendations for pediatric acne patients. *Journal of Drugs in Dermatology: JDD, 22*(6), 539–545. https://doi.org/10.36849/JDD.7440

Schaller, M., & Plewig, G. (2025). Structure and function of eccrine, apocrine, and sebaceous glands. In J. Bolognia, J. V. Schaffer, & L. Cerroni (Eds.), *Dermatology* (5th ed., pp. 586–591). Elsevier.

Schoenwolf, G. C., Bleyl, S. B., Brauer, P. R., & Francis-West, P. H. (2021). *Larsen's human embryology* (6th ed., pp. 150–165). Churchill Livingstone

Shah, S. D., Baselga, E., McCuaig, C., Pope, E., Coulie, J., Boon, L. M., Garzon, M. C., Haggstrom, A. N., Adams, D., Drolet, B. A., Newell, B. D., Powell, J., García-Romero, M. T., Chute, C., Roe, E., Siegel, D. H., Grimes, B., & Frieden, I. J. (2016). Rebound growth of infantile hemangiomas after propranolol therapy. *Pediatrics, 137*(4), e20151754. https://doi.org/10.1542/peds.2015-1754

Shope, C., Ritter, A., Karlin, S., Lee, L. W., & Cotton, C. H. (2023). Congenital cutaneous candidiasis in preterm infants. *NeoReviews, 24*(3), e175–e180. https://doi.org/10.1542/neo.24-3-e175

Simkin, D. J., Mavropoulous, J. C., & Cohen, B. A. (2023). Pigmentary disorders. In B. Cohen (Ed.), *Pediatric dermatology* (5th ed., pp. 157–159). Elsevier Saunders.

Taieb, A., Ezzedine, K., & Morice-Picard, F. (2014). Diagnosis of some common and uncommon hyperpigmentation disorders in children. *Dermatlogica Sinica, 32(4)*, 211–216. https://doi.org/10.1016/j.dsi.2014.08.001

Tom, W. L., & Eichenfield, L. F. (2015). Eczematous disorders. In L. F. Eichenfield, I. J. Frieden, E. F. Mathes, & A. L. Zaenglein (Eds.), *Neonatal and infant dermatology* (3rd ed., pp. 216–232). Elsevier Saunders.

Tong, S. Y. C., Davis, J. S., Eichenberger, E., Holland, T. L., Fowler, J., & Vance, G. (2015). *Staphylococcus aureus* infections: Epidemiology, pathophysiology, clinical manifestations, and management. *Clinical Microbiology Reviews, 28*(3), 603–661. https://doi.org/10.1128/CMR.00134-14

Tripathi, R., Mazmudar, R. S., Knusel, K. D., Ezaldein, H. H., Belazarian, L. T., Bordeaux, J. S., & Scott, J. F. (2021). Impact of congenital cutaneous hemangiomas on newborn care in the United States. *Archives of Dermatological Research, 313*(8), 641–651. https://doi.org/10.1007/s00403-020-02147-1

Vahlquist, A., Fischer, J., & Törmä, H. (2018). Inherited nonsyndromic ichthyoses: An update on pathophysiology, diagnosis and treatment. *American Journal of Clinical Dermatology, 19*(1), 51–66. https://doi.org/10.1007/s40257-017-0313-x

Visscher, M. O., Adam, R., Brink, S., & Odio, M. (2015). Newborn infant skin: Physiology, development and care. *Clinics in Dermatology, 33*(3), 271–280. https://doi.org/10.1016/j.clindermatol.2014.12.003

Visscher, M. O., & Narendran, V. (2014). The ontogeny of skin. *Advances in Wound Care, 3*(4), 291–303. https://doi.org/10.1089/wound.2013.0467

Visscher, M. O., & Narendran, V. (2022). Physiologic development of the skin. In R. A. Polin, S. H. Abman, D. H. Rowitch, W. E. Benitz, & W. W. Fox (Eds.), *Fetal and neonatal physiology* (6th ed., pp. 454–472). Elsevier.

Wassef, M., Blei, F., Adams, D., Alomari, A., Baselga, E., Berenstein, A., Burrows, P., Frieden, I. J., Garzon, M. C., Lopez-Gutierrez, J. C., Lord, D. J., Mitchel, S., Powell, J., Prendiville, J., Vikkula, M., & on behalf of the ISSVA Board and Scientific Committee. (2015). Vascular anomalies classification: Recommendations from the International Society for the Study of Vascular Anomalies. *Pediatrics, 136*(1), e203–e214. https://doi.org/10.1542/peds.2014-3673

Weitz, N. A., Lauren, C. T., Behr, G. G., Wu, J. K., Kandel, J. J., Meyers, P. M., Sultan, S., Anyane-Yeboa, K., Morel, K. D., & Garzon, M. C. (2015). Clinical spectrum of capillary malformation–arteriovenous malformation syndrome presenting to a pediatric dermatology practice: A retrospective study. *Pediatric Dermatology, 32*(1), 76–84. https://doi.org/10.1111/pde.12384

Witt, C. (2024). Skin assessment. In C. A. Witt & C. M. Wallman (Eds.), *Tappero & Honeyfield's physical assessment of the newborn* (7th ed., pp. 59–74). Springer Publishing Company.

Wright, C. Y., Norval, M., & Hertle, R. W. (2015). Oculocutaneous albinism in Sub-Saharan Africa: Adverse sun-associated health effects and photoprotection. *Photochemistry and Photobiology, 91*(1), 27–32. https://doi.org/10.1111/php.12359

Yeo, L., & Ormerod, A. D. (2014). Treatment of acne in children. *American Journal of Clinical Dermatology, 15*(2), 77–86. https://doi.org/10.1007/s40257-013-0057-1

Zempleni, J., Wijeratne, S. S. K., & Hassan, Y. I. (2009). Biotin. *BioFactors, 35*(1), 36–46. https://doi.org/10.1002/biof.8

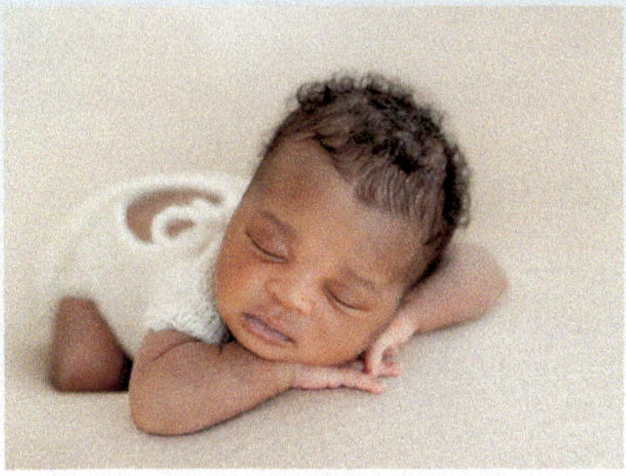

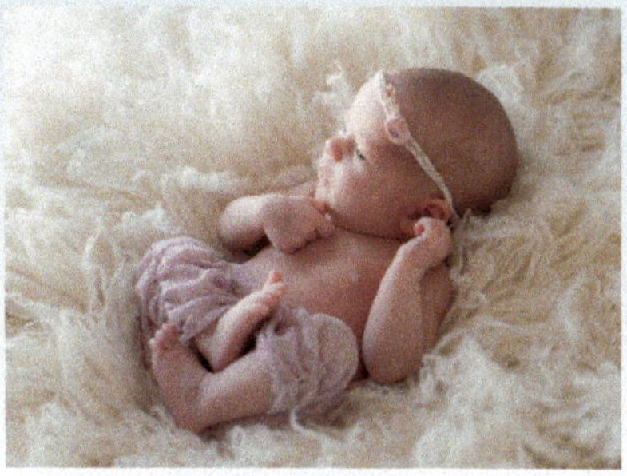

13 THE EYES

Jennifer Fitzgerald, Colleen R. Moss, and Amy J. Jnah

LEARNING OBJECTIVES

After completing this chapter, the reader should be able to:

- Understand normal ocular development.
- Analyze the physiologic function of the fetal and neonatal ocular system.
- Discuss common inherited disorders and their effect on fetal and neonatal ocular system development and function.
- Identify health conditions in XX pregnant patients that have a potential impact on fetal and postnatal ocular system development and function.
- Evaluate common disorders that affect the ocular system and their implications across the life span.

INTRODUCTION

The human eyes allow us to see the world as we know it. The human fetus can detect light as early as 16 weeks of gestation. Term infants exhibit farsightedness at birth with eye function developing rapidly over the first 6 months of life. At term, the eye is 70% of its adult size, and by age 3, the cornea and eyeball measure 95% of adult diameter (Diniz et al., 2025; Örge & Selem, 2025). Full ocular maturity, both in size and visual acuity, is achieved by 7 years of age. Maturation of the eyes can be affected by abnormal visual conditions early in life, prematurity, and poor nutrition, among others. The development of the human eye may also be affected by various genetic conditions, infectious diseases, and maternal substance abuse. Furthermore, retinopathy of prematurity (ROP) represents the leading cause of blindness in developed countries. In this chapter, we review the embryology, developmental physiology, and genetic and maternal health influences on the human eyes. In addition, a relevant discussion of common eye problems, including ROP, and the potential implications of these problems across the life span is presented.

TIMELINE OF ORGAN DEVELOPMENT

Eye development involves a complex and interconnected morphologic differentiation and maturation. Most primitive eye structures arise at the same time, during the early embryonic period, while the fetal and postnatal periods primarily involve structural and functional maturation. Note that as you progress through this section of the chapter, our use of plurality accounts for the bilateral development of structures which comprise each individual eye.

Eye structures arise from the neuroectoderm, surface ectoderm, mesoderm, and neural crest cells beginning during week 3 of gestation (Table 13.1; Persaud & Torchia, 2025). During this time, the neural folds approximate and fuse, which creates the forebrain. During the process of folding and fusion, optic sulci (grooves) protrude at the cranial end of the neural folds and give rise to the optic vesicles (primitive eyes). These primitive optic vesicles undergo two concurrent and critical processes, invagina-

TABLE 13.1 Summary of Embryologic Origins of Eye Structures

Mesoderm	Neural Crest Cells	Ectoderm	
		Neural	Surface
Extraocular muscle cells Vascular endothelia Schlemm's canal endothelium	Corneal endothelium Trabecular meshwork Stroma: iris Stroma: cornea Stroma: ciliary bodies Choroid Sclera Episclera Ciliary muscle Perivascular connective tissue and smooth muscle cells Meninges of optic nerve Orbital cartilage and bone Connective tissue of extrinsic ocular muscles Secondary vitreous Zonules	Neural retina Epithelium: retinal pigment Epithelium: ciliary body Epithelium: posterior iris Pupillary muscles	Lens Corneal epithelium Conjunctival epithelium Caruncle Eyelid epidermis Eyelid cilia Epithelium of adnexal glands Epithelium of nasolacrimal duct Lacrimal gland

Sources: From Persaud, T. V. N., & Torchia, M. G. (2025). *The developing human* (12th ed.). Elsevier; Schoenwolf, G. C., Bleyl, S. B., Brauer, P. R., & Francis-West, P. H. (2021). *Larsen's human embryology* (6th ed.). Churchill Livingstone.

tion and stimulation of the surface ectoderm, which ultimately give rise to the major structures and vasculature of the eye (**Figure 13.1**; Schoenwolf et al., 2021).

Invagination

The process of invagination (folding inward) begins during week 6 of gestation. The distal ends of the optic vesicles increase in size and invaginate, giving rise to the primitive optic cups (future retina and iris) and optic stalks. Fissures, or grooves, develop on the ventral sides of both structures, which give rise to the optic discs and the primitive vascular supply. The outer mesenchyme surrounding the optic cups differentiates into the choroid (vascular layer which lies between the retina and sclera) and scleral (opaque, fibrous outer layer of the eye) layers.

Primitive vascular supply to the retina is established by week 15 to 16 of gestation. This primitive vascular supply includes the hyaloid artery and vein (future central retinal artery and vein). The hyaloid artery will nourish the retina and lens during early development, while the hyaloid vein offers venous outflow (**Figure 13.2**). Later, the choroid will supply the outer retina, whereas the ophthalmic artery and its branches, including the central retinal artery and long posterior and anterior ciliary arteries, will supply the inner retina. These vessels are derivatives of the internal carotid artery (a portion of the circle of Willis), which receives its arterial supply from the right and left brachiocephalic arteries, which are branches of the ascending aorta. The central retinal vein will modulate venous outflow to the superior, then inferior ophthalmic vein, which then drains into the internal jugular vein and superior vena cava, and finally into the right atrium.

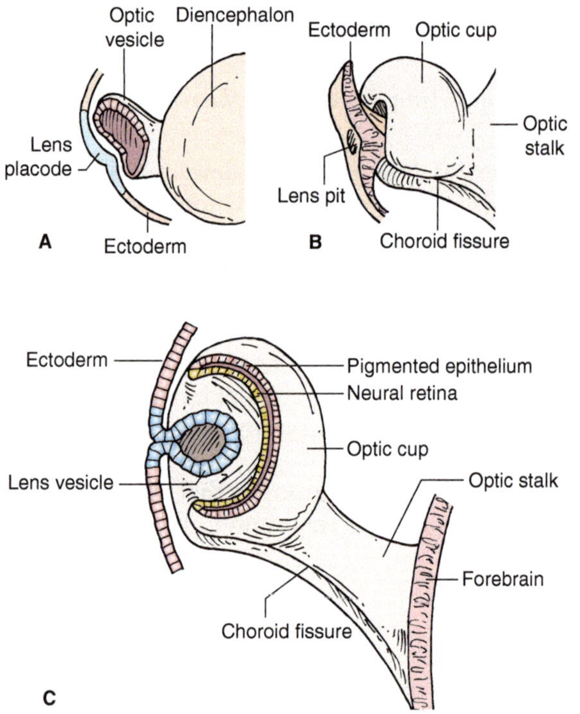

Figure 13.1 Early eye formation from initial protrusions (**A**) to invagination of optic cups with connection (**B**) to developing forebrain (**C**). The time for movement from image A to C is 7 to 10 days between weeks 4 and 5.

Formation of the Retina

During week 5 of gestation, the walls of the optic cup give rise to each retina. This primordial retina begins as a two-layered structure, transiently separated by an in-

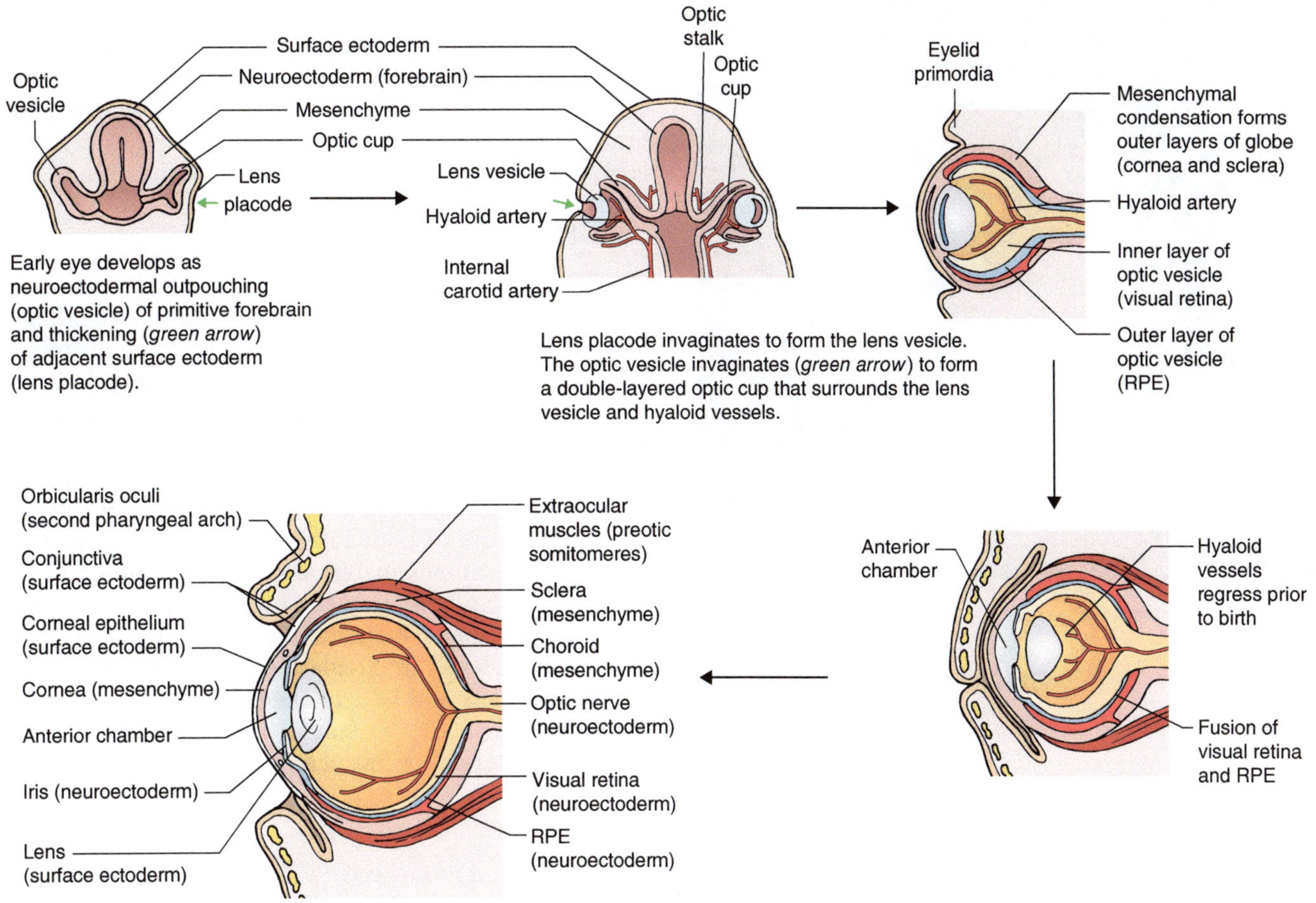

Figure 13.2 The eye and adnexa.
RPE, retinal pigment epithelium.

traretinal space. The outermost layer is the pigmented layer (not to be confused with the pigmented layer of the iris which dictates eye coloration), while the inner layer is the neural retina. As morphologic development continues, the two retinal layers fuse, and the intraretinal space is obliterated. The neural retina continues to differentiate and develop a neuroepithelium. The cells within the neuroepithelium give rise to the photoreceptors (rods and cones) and neurons (retinal ganglion cells). Ganglion cells thereby grow toward the optic stalk (optic nerve). Photoreceptor cells, which are primarily responsible for the process of light transduction, begin their differentiation during week 25 of gestation (Schoenwolf et al., 2021).

The processes of vasculogenesis (the differentiation of precursor cells into the primitive vascular network) and angiogenesis (growth of new capillaries) support the growth and differentiation of the retina (Hughes et al., 2000). Prior to week 15, a rudimentary vascular supply is apparent. By week 25 of gestation, angiogenesis increases, and vascular density in the incipient fovea (a small depression in the retina where acuity is highest) is notably increased (Figure 13.3; Hughes et al., 2000). Vascularization progresses from the central to peripheral retina and is complete by 36 to 40 weeks of gestation (Chan-Ling et al., 2018).

Formation of the Iris

The iris, which arises and develops between weeks 4 and 7 of gestation, forms from the outer wall of the optic cup. Over time, the iris evolves into a covering over the lens of the eye. Two major layers comprise the iris: the pigmented epithelium (outermost layer) and stroma (supporting tissue). The muscles of the iris function to control light entering through the pupil and therefore influence the image quality delivered to the retina. Definitive iris coloration is not established until 6 to 10 months of postnatal life and depends upon distribution of melanin. Genetic inheritance patterns influence melanin distribution. Genes located on chromosome 15, in particular the *OCA2* and *HERC2* genes, modulate the synthesis and expression of P protein, which influence the production of melanin. Similar to skin tone, the amount of melanin located in the pigmented epithelium or stroma influences eye coloration (Table 13.2; Persaud & Torchia, 2025). Reduced production of P protein results in lighter (blue) colored eyes, whereas an increased quantity of melanin throughout the stroma is associated with darker (brown) colored eyes. While it is uncommon for brown-eyed parents to have blue-eyed children, it is not impossible (Persaud & Torchia, 2025). Therefore,

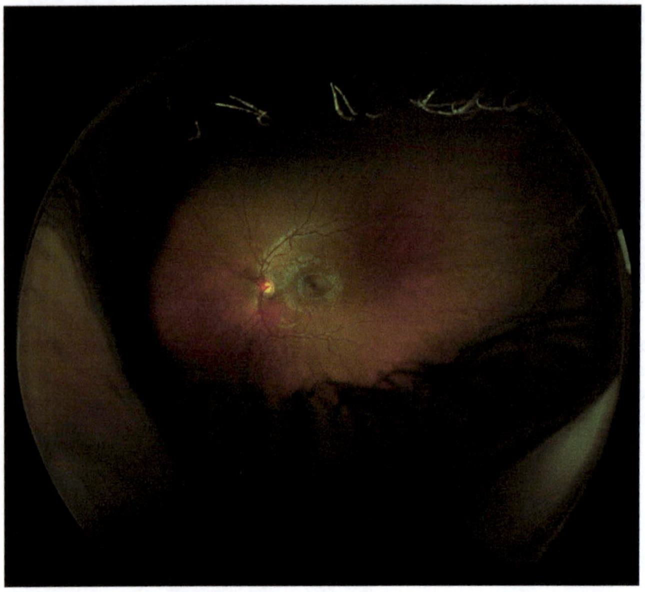

Figure 13.3 Retinal scan.

TABLE 13.2 Eye Coloration

Eye Color	Melanin Pigmentation
Albino	Minimal to none
Blue	Low
Green/hazel	Moderate
Dark brown	High

Source: From Persaud, T. V. N., & Torchia, M. G. (2025). *The developing human* (12th ed.). Elsevier.

neonatal APRNs should exercise caution when opining on definitive eye coloration, as genetic variations can give rise to unexpected results.

Formation of the Optic Nerve

As previously discussed, during week 4 of gestation, the distal ends of the optic vesicles increase in size and invaginate, giving rise to the primitive optic cups and optic stalks. The optic stalks exist as hollow tubules and arise from the fusion of retinal fissures (grooves). The tubules are progressively infiltrated by retinal ganglion cells from the neural retina (innermost layer). By week 8 of gestation, axons extend off the ganglion cells and extend through the optic stalk, connecting the neural retina to the brain. These ganglion clog and permanently obliterate the hollow interior of the optic stalk, thereby converting it to the optic nerve. The optic nerve becomes covered within three layers of myelin. The outermost layer arises from the dura mater and is fibrous in construct. The middle layer originates from the arachnoid mater and is relatively thin when compared to the outer layer. Last, the interior layer originates from the pia mater and is a densely vascular layer, which provides blood supply to the optic nerve from the ophthalmic artery (main blood supply), a branch of the internal carotid artery. The first branch of the ophthalmic artery is the central artery and vein, which are the main blood supply for the retina.

Lens Formation

Optic vesicles also induce the formation of the lens placodes (primitive lens of each eye). The surface ectoderm undergoes a process of folding and separation, forming hollow lens vesicles (lens placodes). These primitive lenses fold inward, forming pits (lens pits). Over time, these lens pits fuse together and form the lens vesicles. The lens vesicles give rise to the eye's lens and the cornea. Maternal infections, such as rubella, or the development of inborn errors of metabolism can derange lens formation. For example, maternal rubella infection during weeks 4 and 7 of gestation can predispose the developing eyes to cataracts. Postnatally, untreated galactosemia leads to high levels of circulating galactose, which can damage the lens and lead to cataract formation; treatment of the inborn error of metabolism facilitates resolution of the cataracts (Persaud & Torchia, 2025).

Clinical Application. The neonatal APRN should become skilled at performance of the noninvasive red reflex test. The red reflex can be elicited beginning with week 30 of gestation. When shining the ophthalmoscope at the newborn's eye, the reflex should be round and symmetric and present as a red, reddish-yellow, or light gray coloration. Abnormal colorations include a white reflex (leukocoria) and blue coloration (associated with osteogenesis imperfecta). The exam should be repeated at discharge to home, in the outpatient setting at every well-baby visit through the first year of life, and then periodically throughout childhood. Identification of potential pathologic conditions warranting immediate referral, evaluation, and treatment by a pediatric ophthalmologist can enable preservation of vision in up to 75% of pediatric cases of blindness. Common diagnoses that can be detected with this relatively simple assessment include congenital cataracts, glaucoma, retinoblastoma, and osteogenesis imperfecta, resulting from infectious, genetic, or metabolic disorders.

Cornea, Ciliary Bodies, Iris, and Pupil

By week 8 of gestation, the stromal layer of the developing cornea appears between the two corneal layers. The cornea evolves into the transparent covering of the iris, pupil, and anterior chamber of the eye. Ciliary bodies and muscles arise during this time. Ciliary bodies are highly vascularized structures that synthesize and secrete aqueous humor, a watery and transparent fluid primarily composed of amino acids and glucose. The aqueous humor travels from the ciliary epithelium to the anterior chamber of the eye to nourish the cornea, iris, and mature lens, as well as maintain homeostatic intraocular pressures. Any disruption to this pathway can lead to the development of congenital glaucoma.

The lens of the eye is essentially suspended by the ciliary muscle, which modulates focusing of the lens (Figure 13.4). Parasympathetic and sympathetic neurons innervate the ciliary muscle during early embryogenesis. Once mature, parasympathetic stimulation causes constriction, and sympathetic stimulation causes relaxation of the ciliary muscle.

Support Structures

Eyelids. By week 6 of gestation, the surface ectoderm and mesenchyme fold to create the primitive eyelids and conjunctival sac, a space between the corneas and eyelids. The lids thereby remain fused until months 5 to 7 of gestation. Failure of the eyelids to separate, ankyloblepharon, may present as partial or complete fusion and may be associated with other facial anomalies (Dallalzadeh et al., 2023).

Nasolacrimal Glands. Nasolacrimal glands arise from within the conjunctival sacs and undergo a progressive maturational process until approximately week 6 of postnatal life (Schoenwolf et al., 2021). The lacrimal gland is located behind the lateral aspect of the upper eyelid and, when mature, functions to lubricate, cleanse, and protect the eye (Figure 13.5; Dallalzadeh et al., 2023; Persaud & Torchia, 2025). Small ducts carry tear fluid into the conjunctiva and then medially across the surface of the cornea. Tears thereby enter the lacrimal punctum (superior and inferior) and drain into the nasal cavity via the nasolacrimal duct and nasolacrimal canal (Dallalzadeh et al., 2023; Persaud & Torchia, 2025; Schoenwolf et al., 2021).

Eyelashes. A double row of eyelashes is usually present by 28 to 32 weeks of gestation. The eyelashes cover the edge of the eyelids along with associated sebaceous glands. Medially, the eyelashes end at the lacrimal punctum and serve as a sensing mechanism to protect the eye from debris and damage (Gosling et al., 2016).

Ocular Orbit. The bony walls of the orbit separate its contents from the cranial fossa, ethmoidal air cells, nasal cavity, maxillary sinus, temporal fossa, and lateral surface of the face (Figure 13.6; Gosling et al., 2016). The orbit contains the eye globe, extraocular muscles, fat, vasculature, cranial nerves (CNs), and lacrimal gland (Gosling et al., 2016). The fascia bulbi (or vagina bulbi) is the fascial sheath that allows for eye movement. The bulbi are attached to the eye at the corneal edge by suspensory ligaments (Gosling et al., 2016). The sclera is a tough structure that supports the inner structures of the eye (Schoenwolf et al., 2021). The six muscles (four recti, two obliques) that control eye movement, and the levator palpebrae superioris (which elevates the eyelid), pierce the fascia to connect to the eye. These muscles

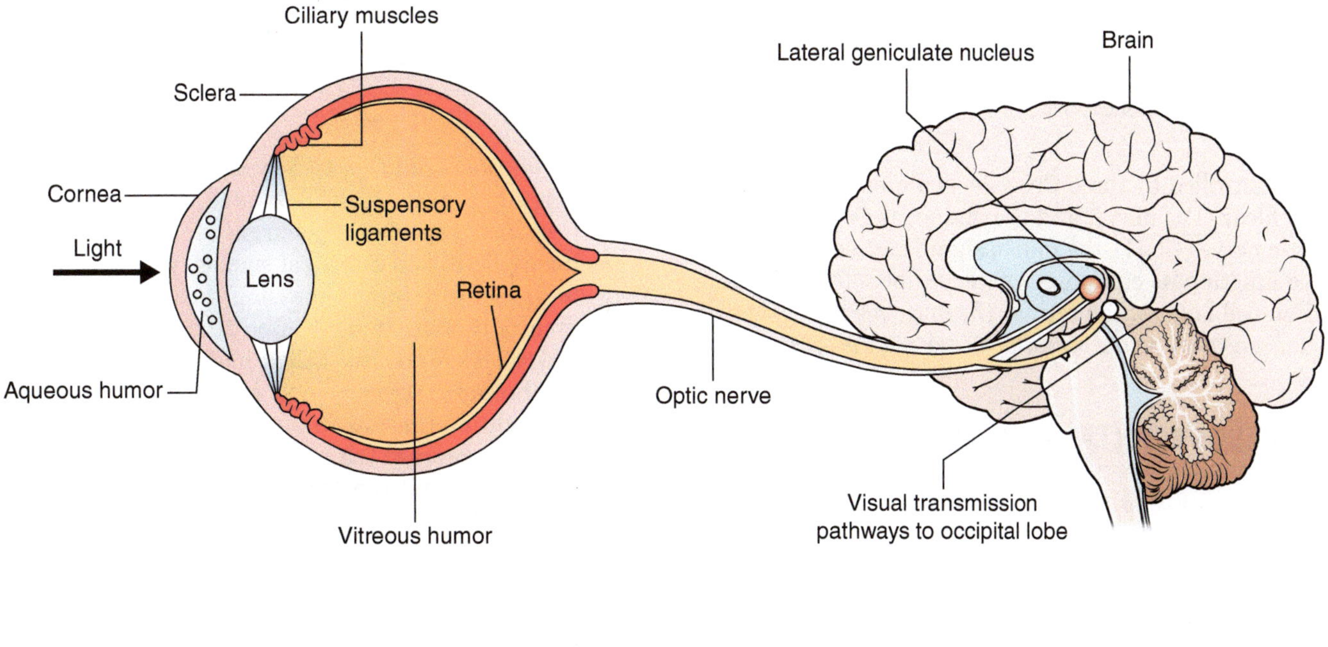

Figure 13.4 The visual pathway.
Image Credit: Layla Williford.

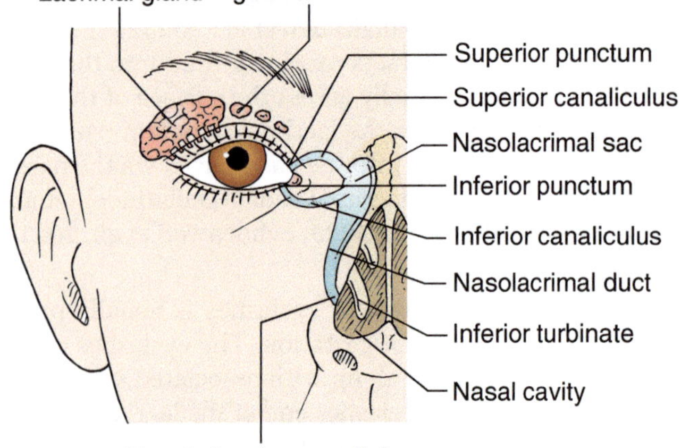

Figure 13.5 The nasolacrimal gland.

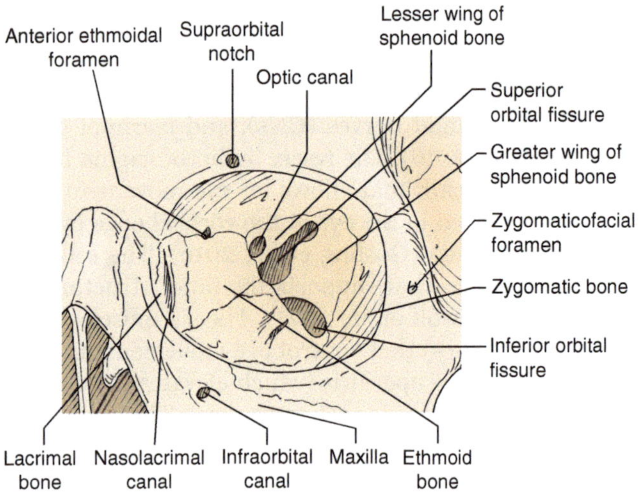

Figure 13.6 Anatomy of the orbit (left eye).
Source: Adapted from Gosling, J. A., Harris, P. F., Humpherson, J. R., Whitmore, I., & Willan, P. L. T. (2016). *Human anatomy: Color atlas and textbook* (6th ed.). Elsevier.

are controlled by three CNs: the oculomotor (III) nerve, trochlear (IV) nerve, and the abducens (VI) nerve. The optic nerve (CNII), the fourth significant nerve affecting eye function, is composed of nerve fibers from the ganglion cell layer of the retina. *The optic nerve conveys visual sensation to the occipital cortex via the optic chasm.*

DEVELOPMENTAL PHYSIOLOGY

Sensory Innervation to the Eye

Recall that the eyes are innervated by several CNs, and each modulates a specific process. Cranial nerve II (optic nerve) transmits visual information, whereas CNs III, IV, VI, and VII (facial nerve) modulate ocular motor function. Cranial nerve V (trigeminal nerve) holds the unique role of transmitting sensory information from the eye to the cranial structures and is the focus of this section of the chapter.

As you may recall from Chapter 3, neurons within the cerebral cortex and other areas of the brain work collaboratively (in circuits). The neurons transmit information received via afferent (input) pathways and orchestrate responses via efferent (motor output) pathways. Afferent pathways are either somatic or visceral and, as such, involve the CNs. This is particularly important when considering organs, such as the eyes, because they are richly innervated with somatic (sensory) nerve fibers. Sensory nerve receptors, located at the tips of second-order nerve fibers, are in abundance at the cornea, iris, sclera, and conjunctiva. Therefore, these structures are particularly sensitive to pain, temperature, and touch. It is interesting to note that the cornea consists of more sensory nerve fibers than other tissues of the body.

Three types of sensory receptors innervate the eye. *Mechanoreceptors* sense mechanical irritants (ocular contact with foreign bodies or other mechanical forces) and modulate a localized pain response. *Polymodal receptors* also sense mechanical irritants, as well as chemical and thermal (heat) irritants, and perpetuate the pain response even after the acute injury phase has passed (Guerrero-Moreno et al., 2020). *Cold receptors* sense reductions in corneal surface temperature.

The introduction of any mechanical, thermal, or chemical stimuli (irritant) to the corneal surface activates the corresponding second-order neuron. Nerve impulses (often pain impulses) travel along afferent pathways and to the central nervous system (**Figure 13.7**). Once the sensory input has been processed within the brain, an efferent motor or autonomic response is returned from the brain to the eye in the form of motor and autonomic responses. Typical responses include blinking and tearing; both seek to protect the eye as well as raise ocular surface temperature.

Retinal Function: The Rods and Cones

The human eye contains two types of photoreceptor cells, rods and cones, which are located in the neural retina. These highly specialized neurons are responsible for transducing light into electrical signals, which, in turn, provide the sensory input for vision throughout the diurnal cycle of illumination (Wensel, 2025; Werner & Chalupa, 2014). This process, called *phototransduction*, is achieved through a series of biochemical processes stimulated by light and results in decreased ongoing release of neurotransmitters at the synapse. In essence, light enters the eye, comes into contact with rhodopsin (a photosensitive chemical contained in rods), and, as a result of chemical reactions, sends electrical impulses to the brain where it is interpreted as light (Diniz et al., 2025; Purves et al., 2018; Wensel, 2025).

There are approximately 6.5 million cones in the human eye. Three main types of cones are observed: S-cones ("blue cones"), M-cones ("green cones"), and

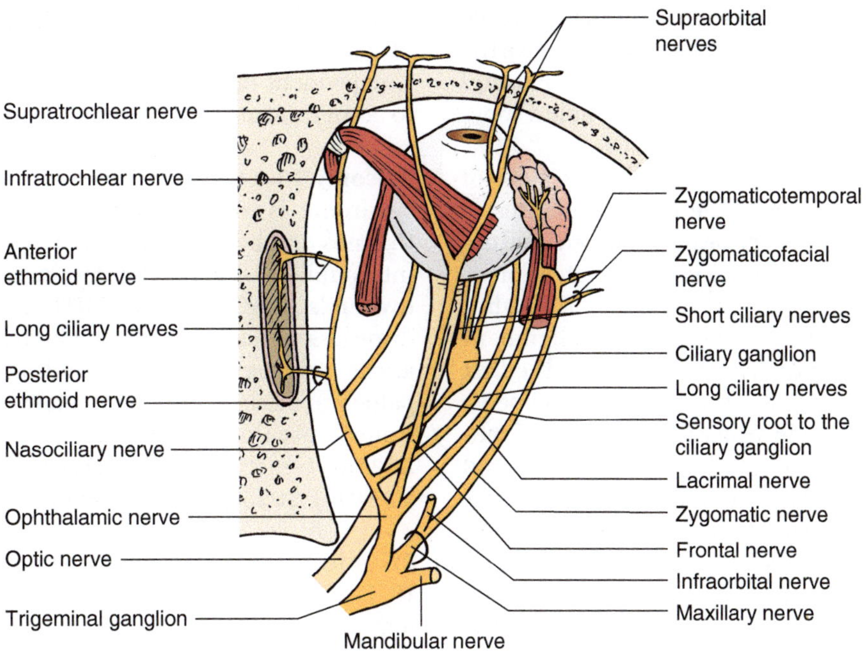

Figure 13.7 Trigeminal nerve branches with the ocular orbit.

L-cones ("red cones"). A high concentration of cones is found in the macula, providing sharp, detailed vision (Purves et al., 2018; Wu, 2025). Cones are responsible for photopic vision (vision in well-lit conditions), color vision, and detail. As such, cones function best in bright illumination and are relatively unresponsive in low light (MacLeish & Makino, 2025; Purves et al., 2018).

There are approximately 120 million rods in the human eye. Rods are responsible for scotopic vision (vision in dim light) and do not differentiate colors. Rhodopsin enables vision in low-light conditions. Rods have a limited sensitivity over a narrow range of light intensities; the benefit of this is a decreased metabolic demand (Lamb & Kefalov, 2025; Werner & Chalupa, 2014).

Adaptation to Light

Light itself is integral to functional maturation of synaptic function within the inner retina (Werner & Chalupa, 2014). Light adaptation is the ability of the visual system to adjust between light and dark. This ability matures quickly among infants born after 35 weeks' gestation but is functionally immature among infants 30 to 35 weeks' gestation and absent among infants younger than 30 weeks' gestation (Ikeda et al., 2015; Lamb & Kefalov, 2025).

Rods are primarily responsible for visual adaptation (image-forming systems and pupillary reflex) in dimly lit areas. Cones remain responsible for visual adaptation in well-lit areas. The combined effort of both systems, in low lighting, is termed mesopic vision and is evident among infants greater than 35 weeks' gestation (Lamb & Kefalov, 2025; Werner & Chalupa, 2014). The pupillary (blink-to-light) reflex is mediated by these photoreceptor cells (rods and cones) and implicated by pupillary size. Reduced ocular and corneal diameter, which is commonly noted among infants younger than 38 weeks' gestation, corresponds with reduced pupillary size. In fact, infants born at less than 30 weeks of gestation typically exhibit no blink-to-light reflex and only primitive image-forming systems, due to pupillary and retinal immaturity (Ikeda et al., 2015).

Visual Milestones

The fetus is able to detect light as early as 16 weeks of gestation (Örge & Selem, 2025). By week 26, the fetal eye is affixed with most histologic features of the mature eye; visual milestones are evident beginning with week 30 of gestation.

The first visual milestone to appear is the pupillary light reflex. This reflex is noted at 30 weeks of gestation and involves a reduction in pupillary diameter with lid closure in response to light stimulation (Örge & Selem, 2025). The preterm neonate is able to focus and track objects and has a preference for patterns by 33 to 34 weeks of gestation. Vestibular rotations, or the doll's eye maneuver, in which the eyes deviate to the opposite direction when the head is quickly rotated from side to side are well developed at 34 weeks of gestation.

At term, infants are farsighted (objects nearby are blurry) and have the ability to respond to light (Persaud & Torchia, 2025). The visual field is typically limited to approximately 8 to 10 inches, with estimated visual acuity of 20/400 (Lam & Suh, 2022). Patterned stimuli are preferred over uniform brightness (Norcia, 2025; Oatts et al., 2024). This is likely due to the functional immaturity of vision processing centers in the brain, which improve over time. Visual fixation, conjugate horizontal gaze, and optokinetic nystagmus are also well developed at birth

(Örge & Selem, 2025). Visual fixation is the maintenance of visual gaze on a single location. The ability to move the eyes together horizontally refers to *conjugate horizontal gaze*. Optokinetic nystagmus is the ability to follow moving objects while keeping the head still.

Preterm and term infants are born into a state of functional immaturity; as such, the first few months of postnatal life are regarded as a critical period for visual development. The blink response to a visual threat, color vision (the ability to discern different wavelengths of light), stereopsis (depth perception), and ocular alignment (normal eye alignment) rapidly develop during the first 6 months of life (Norcia, 2025). Additional developments in the first 6 months include visual following, accommodation, conjugate vertical gaze, fusional convergence, and differentiation of fovea and iris stromal (the front fibrovascular layer of the iris) pigmentation (Örge & Selem, 2025). *Visual following* involves the ability to control where eyes are aimed, whereas *accommodation* refers to the ability to maintain clear focus as the distance of an object varies. The ability to move the eyes together vertically refers to *conjugate vertical gaze*. *Fusional convergence* is the ability of the two eyes to perceive one single image.

The eye is considered to be mature, both in size and visual acuity, by 7 years of age. Color perception and accommodation, as well as visual acuity, are considered equal to that of the adult eye by this time. As a result, APRNs must recognize the importance of early identification and treatment of ocular disorders as a critical means to optimize eye health across the life span.

GENETIC INFLUENCES

There are a number of genetic conditions that are accompanied by ocular abnormalities. Conditions, such as trisomy 13, 18, and 21, as well as Turner syndrome, are more common, whereas others are quite rare. Additional inherited disorders affecting the ocular system are provided in Table 13.3.

Chromosomal Abnormalities

Trisomy 21. Trisomy 21, or Down syndrome, is the most common inherited disorder and is slightly more common in males than females. This syndrome affects a total of one in 700 births, with an increased incidence of one in 50 to 300 births reported among pregnant women over the age of 35 (Jones et al., 2022; National Institutes of Health [NIH], 2020a). There are a number of ocular findings common to trisomy 21. Epicanthal folds, an extra layer of skin that covers the inner canthus (corner) of the eye, are a classic feature of this disorder. Palpebral fissures, the opening between the eyelids from the medial to lateral canthus, are upturned. Other findings include refractive errors, usually myopia (70%), lens opacities (59%), nystagmus (35%), strabismus (45%), blepharitis, glaucoma, Brushfield spots (speckling or nodules on the iris), and adult-onset cataracts (30%–60%; American Academy of Ophthalmology [AAO], 2023b; Jones et al., 2022; Örge & Selem, 2025). Long-term visual outcome is dependent on the degree of myopia, ability of the eye to accommodate, and the impact of cataracts.

Trisomy 13. Ocular involvement in trisomy 13, Patau syndrome, is common, with anophthalmos or microphthalmos and hyper/hypotelorism (widened or shortened interpupillary distance) noted in more than 80% of individuals (AAO, 2024m; NIH, 2021). Additional eye disorders seen in individuals with trisomy 13 include cataracts, colobomas of the iris and retina, short/upslanted palpebral fissures, persistent fetal vasculature, persistent tunica vasculosa lentis, and retinal dysplasia (AAO, 2024m; Genetic and Rare Diseases Information Center [GARD], 2025e; Örge & Selem, 2025).

Trisomy 18. Of the trisomy genetic abnormalities, trisomy 18, Edwards syndrome, is the second most common. Ocular abnormalities noted in individuals with trisomy 18 include epicanthal folds, hypertelorism, and short palpebral fissures with limitations in eyelid opening (blepharophimosis). Occasionally, glaucoma, cataracts, coloboma of the iris, cyclopia, and microphthalmia may accompany this diagnosis (GARD, 2025f; Örge & Selem, 2025).

Turner Syndrome. As the result of a spontaneous error, girls with Turner syndrome have an absent (or abnormal) set of genes on the short arm of one X chromosome (GARD, 2025g). The global incidence is one in every 2,500 females (Jones et al., 2022; NIH, 2023a). The karyotype in Turner syndrome is usually 45 X; however, affected individuals who have a mosaic form of the syndrome (XX/X; XY/X) or are missing genetic material on the X chromosome experience variable expression of typical findings (Jones et al., 2022). Ocular findings are present in 35% of cases of Turner syndrome and include ptosis, strabismus, epicanthal folds, amblyopia, and myopia (GARD, 2025g). Visual impairment will depend on the severity of the refractive error.

Craniofacial Syndromes

Craniosynostosis. Craniosynostosis involves the premature fusion of one or more of the cranial sutures. Craniosynostosis affects approximately one in 2,000 to 2,500 live births with up to 75% of cases occurring in nonsyndromic individuals (Kajdic et al., 2018). Ocular findings include hypertelorism, amblyopia (reduced vision in the affected eye) related to strabismus, anisometropia (in which eyes have unequal refractive power), ametropia (nearsightedness or farsightedness), astigmatism (blurred vision caused by irregular shaped cornea or lens), and optic neuropathy secondary to damage to the optic nerve from increased intracranial pressure or anomalies in the development of the orbit (AAO, 2024c). Small orbits increase the risk for globe subluxation and drying, as well as ulcerations of the cornea (keratopathy) resulting from exposure (AAO, 2024c; Örge & Selem,

TABLE 13.3 Other Inherited Disorders of the Eyes

Disorder	Incidence	Inheritance Pattern	Developmental Impact
Apert syndrome	1/65,000	Autosomal dominant	Associated with craniosynostosis; exophthalmos (proptosis): bulging or protrusion of the optic globe; hypertelorism
Congenital stromal corneal dystrophy	<1/1,000,000	Autosomal dominant	Opacity of the cornea associated with moderate to severe visual loss
Crouzon syndrome	1.6/100,000	Autosomal dominant	Associated with craniosynostosis; hypertelorism, proptosis, ptosis, and strabismus
Focal dermal hypoplasia	<1/1,000,000	X-linked dominant	Coloboma of the iris or retina, corneal clouding, hypertelorism, micro/anophthalmia, ptosis, strabismus
Fraser syndrome	1/200,000	Autosomal recessive	Blindness, cryptophthalmos (abnormalities in eyelid development), hypertelorism, lacrimal duct abnormalities, micro/anophthalmia
Marfan syndrome	1/5,000–10,000	Autosomal dominant	Cataracts, glaucoma, lens dislocation (ectopia lentis), myopia, retinal detachment
Moebius syndrome	~1/50,000	Autosomal dominant	Blepharitis, CN VII palsy impacting eyelid closure, corneal clouding, eye muscle paralysis, ptosis, strabismus
Ocular albinism	1 male/ 20,000 births	X-linked recessive	Astigmatism, decreased iris and retinal pigmentation, foveal hypoplasia, nystagmus, photophobia, strabismus
Renal coloboma syndrome	Unknown	Autosomal dominant	Myopia, optic nerve dysplasia, retinal coloboma
Zellweger syndrome	Unknown	Autosomal recessive	Corneal opacity or cataracts, epicanthal folds, retinal defects, up-slanted palpebral fissures, vision loss

Note: Incidence reflects knowledge known at the time of publication. A more comprehensive list is provided by the National Institutes of Health, Genetic and Rare Diseases Information Center (https://rarediseases.info.nih.gov or https://rarediseases.org/rare-diseases).

Sources: Genetic and Rare Diseases Information Center. (2025). *Apert syndrome*. https://rarediseases.info.nih.gov/diseases/5833 /apert-syndrome; Genetic and Rare Diseases Information Center. (2025). *Congenital stromal corneal dystrophy*. https://rarediseases.info.nih.gov/diseases/16943 /congenital-stromal-cornealdystrophy; Genetic and Rare Diseases Information Center. (2025). *Crouzon syndrome*. https://rarediseases.info.nih .gov/diseases/6206/crouzon-syndrome; Genetic and Rare Diseases Information Center. (2025). *Focal dermal hypoplasia*. https://rarediseases .info.nih.gov/diseases/6457/focal-dermal-hypoplasia; Genetic and Rare Diseases Information Center. (2025). *Fraser syndrome*. https://rarediseases .info.nih.gov/diseases/6465/fraser-syndrome; Genetic and Rare Diseases Information Center. (2025). *Neonatal Marfan syndrome*. https:// rarediseases.info.nih.gov/diseases/21128/neonatal-marfan-syndrome; Genetic and Rare Diseases Information Center. (2025). *Ocular albinism, type 1*. https://rarediseases.info.nih.gov/diseases/8471/x-linked-recessive-ocular-albinism; Genetic and Rare Diseases Information Center. (2025). *Oromandibular-limb hypogenesis spectrum*. https://rarediseases.info.nih.gov/diseases/8549/moebius-syndrome; Genetic and Rare Diseases Information Center. (2025). *Renal coloboma syndrome*. https://rarediseases.info.nih.gov/diseases/4106/renal-coloboma-syndrome; Genetic and Rare Diseases Information Center. (2025). *Zellweger spectrum syndrome*. https://rarediseases.info.nih.gov/diseases/7917/zellweger-syndrome.

CN, cranial nerve.

2025). The impact of craniosynostosis on long-term visual outcome is dependent on the underlying cause of the disorder as well as the severity of cranial malformation.

Oculo-Auriculo-Vertebral Spectrum (Hemifacial Microsomia). Underdevelopment of the lower portion of the face is sometimes referred to as first and second brachial arch syndrome, lateral facial dysplasia, or facio-auriculo-vertebral sequence, and includes both hemifacial microsomia and Goldenhar syndrome diagnoses. The etiology is unknown and usually occurs with no family history, although it is estimated to occur in an estimated one in 3,000 to 5,000 births (Jones et al., 2022). Ocular findings include coloboma of the upper eyelid or iris, vertical displacement of the orbit, and less frequently anopthalmia (missing eye) or microphthalmia (AAO, 2024e; Örge & Selem, 2025). Other findings include minor fissure abnormalities and orbital lipodermoids, a collection of adipose tissue found on the cornea, conjunctiva, and sclera (AAO, 2024e).

Gene Mutations

11p Abnormalities. WAGR syndrome (**W**ilms tumor, **A**niridia, **G**enitourinary abnormalities, and a **R**ange of developmental delays) results from a deletion on the short arm of chromosome 11 (Örge & Selem, 2025). This syndrome is rare, occurring in one in 500,000 to 1 million individuals (NIH, 2023b). Most cases result from a de novo mutation, although, rarely, a family history is present. Aniridia (absence of the colored part of the iris) occurs in 80% to 99% of cases. Other ocular abnormalities include aplasia or hypoplasia of the iris and nystagmus (GARD, 2025i). Life-span implications include cataract formation, glaucoma, and corneal opacification (Moosajee et al., 2018).

Syndromes

Pierre Robin Sequence. Pierre Robin sequence (PRS) is characterized by micro/retrognathia, glossoptosis, cleft palate, and airway obstruction (GARD, 2025d). The reported prevalence of this disorder ranges from one in 2,000 to 3,000 live births; isolated PRS accounts for up to 40% of cases (GARD, 2025d, NIH, 2016). Of infants diagnosed with PRS, approximately 10% also have Stickler syndrome (Örge & Selem, 2025). Stickler syndrome is an inherited disorder that involves mutations in the *COL2A1* and *COL11A1* genes. These genes normally modulate the formation of collagen and the vitreous humor within the eyes. Ocular manifestations include congenital high myopia (eyeball is very long from front to back), nearsightedness, cataracts, and glaucoma; an increased risk for retinal tears or detachment is reported (AAO, 2023a). Visual outcomes are dependent on treatment of refractive errors and management of retinal detachment.

Waardenburg Syndrome. Waardenburg syndrome (WS) is a group of genetic disorders that result in congenital sensorineural hearing loss, as well as the loss of eye, hair, and skin pigmentation (GARD, 2025h; Waardenburg, 1951). There is an estimated prevalence of one in every 40,000 individuals, and the syndrome is classified into four different subtypes (NIH, 2022d). Mutations in the *WS1*, *WS4*, or *PAX3* genes disrupt melanocyte development and lead to abnormal eye pigmentation (different colored eyes), as well as abnormal skin and hair pigmentation. Other ocular findings include dystopia canthorum, a lateral displacement of the inner canthum of the eyes (GARD, 2025h). Vision is usually normal in WS.

Cornelia de Lange Syndrome. Cornelia de Lange syndrome (CdLS) is a genetic condition resulting from mutations in the *Nipbl* (65%), *SMC1A*, *SMC3*, *HDAC8*, or *RAD21* (5%) genes. Experts estimate that CdLS affects one in every 10,000 to 30,000 newborns (NIH, 2022a). Most cases are de novo mutations; however, both autosomal dominant and x-linked inheritance patterns have been described (GARD, 2025b). Ocular findings include long eyelashes and a brushed-on appearance to the arch of the eyebrows (NIH, 2022a). In addition, myopia, blepharitis (inflammation of the eyelids at the base of the eyelashes), nasolacrimal duct obstruction, and ptosis can occur (GARD, 2025b).

CHARGE Syndrome. CHARGE is an acronym for **C**oloboma of the retina, **H**eart abnormalities, **A**tresia of the choanae, **R**estricted growth and mental development, **G**enital hypoplasia or anomalies, and **E**ar anomalies (Jones et al., 2022). CHARGE occurs in one in 8,500 to 10,000 newborns (NIH, 2017) and, in more than 50% of cases, is the result of mutations in the *CHD7* gene. Most cases of CHARGE result from de novo mutations; some are autosomal dominant disorders. Ocular findings include coloboma of the eyelid, iris, or retina; anophthalmia or microphthalmia; nystagmus; optic nerve atrophy; ptosis; and strabismus (GARD, 2025a). Facial palsies associated with CHARGE syndrome may result in corneal scarring due to drying of the cornea from the inability to close the eyelids. Retinal detachment has also been reported (GARD, 2025a).

Neurocutaneous Disorders (Phakomatoses)

Neurofibromatosis Type 1. Neurofibromatosis type 1 (NF1) is an autosomal dominant disorder reported to affect one in 3,000 to 4,000 people (NIH, 2020b; Örge & Selem, 2025). In neonates, the presence of *six or more café-au-lait patches* should raise the index of suspicion for NF1. Ocular findings include pigmented iris hamartomas (Lisch nodules), which do not impact vision. Additional findings of retinal hamartomas and optic nerve gliomas may impact vision. Symptoms of optic glioma include optic atrophy and vision loss, pain, and bulging of the eye. Life-span implications include the risk for cataract formation as early as the teenage years (GARD, 2025c).

Sturge–Weber Syndrome. Sturge–Weber syndrome (SWS), a neurocutaneous disorder occurring in one in every 20,000 to 50,000 births, is characterized by port-wine stains of the upper trigeminal region of the face and underlying vascular malformations of the eye and leptomeninges (Greene et al., 2009; NIH, 2018). SWS is caused by a spontaneous mutation in the *GNAQ* gene (NIH, 2018). Glaucoma and vascular malformations of the conjunctiva, choroid, retina, and sclera occur in SWS. However, glaucoma is the most common finding with intraocular pressure elevating to a high enough level that the eye may appear as a bulging and enlarged globe (buphthalmos; Jones et al., 2022; NIH, 2018). According to a seminal study of adults with SWS, the onset of glaucoma ranges from birth to 41 years of age (Sujansky & Conradi, 1995).

Tuberous Sclerosis Complex. Tuberous sclerosis complex (TSC) is a multisystem genetic disorder occurring in one in 6,000 individuals (NIH, 2022c). TSC has an autosomal dominant pattern of inheritance and affects males and females equally. Mutations in the *TSC1* or *TSC2* genes provoke the pathogenesis of *TSC* and clinical manifestations, such as ash-leaf shaped (depigmented) macules (NIH, 2022c). The presence of three or more of these macules is highly associated with TSC and should prompt the clinician to obtain further imaging of the heart, eyes, kidneys/abdomen, and brain. Retinal tumors occur in up to 53% of patients with tuberous sclerosis. These small gray-white infiltrating tumors are classified as astrocytic hamartomas and are usually slow growing and benign. Retinal detachment leading to blindness and vitreous seeding has been reported (Cruess & Sharma, 2018).

X-Linked Disorders

Norrie Disease. Norrie disease, an X-linked, recessive disorder, results from a mutation on the *NDP* gene on chromosome Xp11.4. The incidence is unknown. Norrie disease involves incomplete retinal vascularization, retinal dysgenesis, and incomplete regression of primary hyaloid structures. Bilateral retinal detachment is common and may be present at birth; the detachment manifests as a white pupil. Infantile symptoms include leukocoria (white pupillary reflex), iris atrophy, retrolental fibroplasia (excessive fibrous tissue behind the lens of the eye), vitreous hemorrhage, dysplastic retinae, retinal folds, and retinal detachments. The disease may progress to cataract, glaucoma, retinal schisis, and/or atrophy of the globe (Örge & Selem, 2025). Males affected by Norrie are considered legally blind and have no light perception.

Recessive Disorders

Leber Congenital Amaurosis. Leber congenital amaurosis (LCA) occurs in two to three per 100,000 newborns, and accounts for 10% to 18% of congenital blindness (NIH, 2022b). LCA is an autosomal recessive condition due to a mutation in the *Ckbi* gene. LCA presents with poor vision (hyperopia or farsightedness), mainly attributed to poor light perception, nystagmus, and poor papillary reactions. Children with this condition often rub their eyes excessively, which is known as *blindism behavior*. Nystagmus presents after a few months, and severe visual impairment develops during infancy (Örge & Selem, 2025).

NOTEWORTHY DISEASES IN THE XX PREGNANT PATIENT THAT INFLUENCE FETAL OCULAR DEVELOPMENT AND FUNCTION

Intrauterine Infections

The eyes can be affected by any of the STORCH (**S**yphilis, **T**oxoplasmosis, **O**ther agents, **R**ubella, **C**ytomegalovirus [CMV], and **H**erpes simplex) infections (Örge & Selem, 2025; Stokes & Melvin, 2024). These infections can be transmitted via the placenta or via contact in the birth canal and represent a preventable cause of childhood blindness. Infections occurring in the first 2 to 8 weeks of fetal life, during organogenesis, are concerning for the impact on the development of the eyes. The most common ocular manifestation of congenital or prenatal infection is chorioretinal scarring (Table 13.4; Örge & Selem, 2025). The sequelae of prenatal infections can result from teratogenesis in the form of cell death, cell growth alteration, or chromosomal damage.

Syphilis. Maternal syphilis cases are rising worldwide across all races and ethnicities. Cases of maternal syph-

TABLE 13.4 Common Ocular Findings Associated With Congenital Infections

Congenital Infection	Percent (%) of ocular findings at birth	Transmission	Ocular Findings
Syphilis	10%	Transplacental, vertical, postnatal	Chorioretinitis ("salt & pepper" pseudoretinitis), glaucoma, uveitis, keratitis
Toxoplasmosis	75%	Transplacental	Retinitis, retinal scarring, inflammation of the choroid and vitrius
Rubella	50% of CRS	Transplacental, postnatal	Cataracts, glaucoma, chorioretinitis ("salt and pepper" pseudoretinitis)
Cytomegalovirus	Less than 10%	Transplacental, postnatal	Cataracts; chorioretinitis; optic nerve atrophy, microphthalmos, strabismus
Herpes simplex virus		Transplacental, vertical, postnatal	Vesicular lesions, conjunctivitis, cataracts

ilis have nearly tripled in the United States, with an increase of 222% from 2016 to 2022 (Centers for Disease Control and Prevention [CDC], 2024b). Rates are higher in underdeveloped nations and within racial and ethnic groups with greater disparities and barriers that lead to decreasing access to prenatal care, limiting screening and treatment for syphilis. Most cases of congenital syphilis are transmitted vertically during the prenatal period but can also occur perinatally and postnatally. The likelihood of vertical transmission increases with advancing gestational age and with early maternal stages of syphilis rather than late latent infections. Approximately 33% of infants are asymptomatic at birth but develop signs and symptoms later in life (Maldonado et al., 2025).

Neonatal ocular manifestations of congenital syphilis are rare and include chorioretinitis, eyelid skin rash, orbital and intraocular inflammation, interstitial keratitis, CN involvement, "salt and pepper" fundus, uveitis, glaucoma, cataract, and central visual pathway involvement, including optic nerve atrophy and pupillomotor disturbances (Maldonado et al., 2025; Örge & Selem, 2025). Chancres of the eyelid are rare. Keratitis is seen in untreated children over 5 years old who present with acute photophobia, lacrimation, corneal edema, and iritis.

Toxoplasmosis. The fetus is susceptible to infection with *Toxoplasma gondii* throughout gestation, during the first trimester (15% chance of transmission), second trimester (30% chance of transmission), and up until the last few weeks of pregnancy (60% chance of transmission; Michaels et al., 2024). Perinatal infections occurring at earlier gestational ages are generally more severe, and greater than 80% of affected premature infants develop either learning or visual disabilities (Michaels et al., 2024). Approximately one in 1,000 women will seroconvert during pregnancy with fetal transmission risk of 40% (Michaels et al., 2024). A delay of 8 weeks between maternal seroconversion and initiation of treatment has been identified as a risk factor for retinochoroiditis in the first 2 years of life in infants treated for congenital toxoplasmosis (Kieffer et al., 2008). In a 10-year follow-up study of children with congenital toxoplasmosis in France, 30% had at least one ocular manifestation, with approximately 20% demonstrating vision loss (Wallon et al., 2014).

Neonatal and recurrent ophthalmologic findings are seen with congenital toxoplasmosis. *Chorioretinitis is the most common presenting manifestation at birth* and can present with leukocoria (Khazaeni, 2017; Maldonado et al., 2025). Neonatal and recurring manifestations include necrotizing chorioretinitis and associated retinal vasculitis resulting in chorioretinal scars that may occur anywhere on the retina but are more common in the macula (Khazaeni, 2017; Örge & Selem, 2025). Recurrent infection can result in worsening visual outcomes. Inflammation in the tissues caused by cysts results in the damage seen. Associated pathologies can be thought of in terms of what part of the eye is impacted. The anterior portion of the eye includes such pathologies as cataract, glaucoma, microphthalmia, microcornea, nystagmus, and strabismus. The pathologies seen in the posterior portion of the eye include optic nerve atrophy, retinal detachment, retinitis, and vitritis; these frequently contribute to impaired visual function (Khazaeni, 2017; Maldonado et al., 2025). Visual loss is a problem noted in long-term survivors and is impacted by the location and number of chorioretinal scars, with those occurring in the macula leading to significant visual impairment (Khazaeni, 2017).

Human Immunodeficiency Virus. Transmission of HIV can occur prenatally, perinatally, or postnatally through breastfeeding. In the United States, perinatal HIV transmission rates have decreased to 2% or less due to universal HIV testing, antiretroviral treatment during pregnancy, and avoidance of breastfeeding in HIV-positive mothers. Without intervention, the vertical transmission rate is estimated at 25% to 30%. Infants with congenital HIV are often asymptomatic at birth; if present, symptoms are generally nonspecific and subtle (Maldonado et al., 2025).

Ocular findings, mainly chorioretinitis, are generally associated with concurrent infections, including herpes simplex virus (HSV), CMV, and toxoplasmosis (Maldonado et al., 2025; Michaels et al., 2024). Loss of vision is low unless complicated by a concurrent infection.

Congenital Rubella Syndrome. Congenital rubella syndrome has declined since the implementation of routine vaccination for rubella in 1969. Ocular insults related to congenital rubella syndrome are dependent on the timing of maternal infection. The incidence of associated congenital defects is highest in the first 11 weeks of gestation (70%), lower between weeks 12 and 20 (30%) of gestation, and nonexistent thereafter (Maldonado et al., 2025; Stokes & Melvin, 2024). Exposure during the first 2 months of gestation is associated with cataracts and glaucoma, as maximum blood supply to the lens occurs between 2 and 11 weeks of gestation, whereas retinopathy is associated with exposure during the first 5 months (Stokes & Melvin, 2024).

Common ocular findings in congenital rubella syndrome include microphthalmia, corneal haze, cataract, glaucoma, uveitis, and pigmentary ("salt and pepper") retinopathy, or chorioretinitis (Khazaeni, 2017; Örge & Selem, 2025; Stokes & Melvin, 2024). Cataracts and retinopathy are the two most common ocular manifestations of congenital rubella and are often bilateral. Cataracts occur in approximately 30% of cases and are associated with the greatest risk for visual loss if not treated with surgery and lens replacement within the first few months of life (Khazaeni, 2017; Örge & Selem, 2025). Visual impairment is not generally associated with retinopathy unless neovascularization develops (Örge & Selem, 2025). Other reported ophthalmologic associations include dacryostenosis, edema to the cornea, keratoconus, iris hypoplasia, iris coloboma, anisocoria, posterior synechiae, persistent pupillary membrane, mesodermal dysgenesis, optic atrophy, nystagmus, and strabismus (Michaels et al., 2024).

Cytomegalovirus. CMV transmission can occur transplacentally, via the birth canal, or postnatally through breast milk or transfusion of CMV-positive blood. CMV is the most common congenital viral infection, occurring in 0.2% to 2.2% of all newborns, with incidence higher in underdeveloped nations (Khazaeni, 2017; Maldonado et al., 2025; Stokes & Melvin, 2024). Primary maternal CMV infection carries a 24% to 75% risk for fetal infection, whereas transplacental infection is associated with a 24% risk for fetal infection during the first trimester (Choodinatha et al., 2023). The relative risk increases with advancing trimesters of pregnancy; recurrent infections are less likely to affect the fetus and are reported in 1% to 2.2% of cases (Choodinatha et al., 2023). Symptomatic infection may be more likely in those exposed in the first half of pregnancy.

In general, infants are rarely symptomatic at birth; however, congenital CMV illnesses may be severe and lead to significant long-term developmental delays. Ocular involvement can be seen in up to 40% of symptomatic infants and includes chorioretinitis, keratitis, cataract, conjunctivitis, microphthalmos, strabismus, cortical blindness, anterior chamber malformations with glaucoma, retinal necrosis and calcification, blindness, optic disc malformations, and optic atrophy (Khazaeni, 2017; Örge & Selem, 2025; Stokes & Melvin, 2024). Chorioretinitis is the most common finding, present in 10% to 21% of symptomatic patients, and is evidenced by chorioretinal scars. Cortical visual impairment and optic atrophy are the most common etiology for common visual impairment in symptomatic patients. Asymptomatic patients rarely have visual impairments.

Herpes Simplex Virus. Congenital HSV can be acquired in utero, intrapartum, or postnatally. Passage through the birth canal is the most common method of acquisition of congenital HSV (86% of cases), with type 2 most commonly responsible (Örge & Selem, 2025). Intrauterine infection is rare and estimated at one in 100,000 births or three of every 100 infected infants (Maldonado et al., 2025).

Congenital infection with HSV is associated with blepharoconjunctivitis, keratitis, iritis, chorioretinitis with vitritis, corneal dendrites and ulcers, cataracts, optic atrophy, and bilateral macular scars without other ocular signs (Maldonado et al., 2025; Örge & Selem, 2025). Lid, conjunctival, and corneal lesions may occur with acute ocular involvement. The timing of conjunctivitis onset is usually 0 to 14 days of age, but retinitis may not be noted until over 1 month of age. Late ocular sequelae of congenital HSV infection include cortical blindness, cortical visual loss, squint, chorioretinal scars, optic atrophy, corneal scarring, and cataracts. Keratoconjunctivitis may lead to chorioretinitis, cataracts, and retinal detachment.

Ocular Manifestations of Maternal Substance Abuse

The fetal eyes are not immune to the effects of maternal substance abuse. Substances, such as alcohol, cocaine, and tobacco, have all been associated with teratogenic effects on the developing eyes.

Fetal Alcohol Syndrome. The incidence of fetal alcohol syndrome (FAS) ranges between 0.3 to nine per every 1,000 children in the United States (CDC, 2024a). The exact mechanism for the teratogenic effects of alcohol on the embryogenic eye are not known but may be related to the effects of ethyl alcohol or acetaldehyde, its metabolite. The type of insult may determine the timing of exposure, with insults to the optic nerve beginning at week 6 of gestation through birth and retinal vascularization beginning after week 16 of gestation. Environmental factors, genetics, timing of exposure, and dose may all play a part in and help explain the variation in the ophthalmologic expression of FAS (AAO, 2024d).

Ocular findings associated with FAS include blepharophimosis, epicanthal folds, microphthalmia, ptosis, telecanthus, cataracts, refractive errors, optic nerve hypoplasia (ONH), persistent fetal vasculature, strabismus, nystagmus, amblyopia, and anterior segment abnormalities (AAO, 2024d). Studies report approximately 25% to 48% of infants manifest with accompanying ONH; these estimates may be falsely inflated due to limited sample sizes (AAO, 2024d).

Cocaine. Cocaine use is often associated with polysubstance abuse, and it is therefore difficult to tease out the effects of cocaine alone. Ocular manifestations associated with prenatal exposure to cocaine have not changed over the past several decades and include optic nerve abnormalities/atrophy, delayed visual maturation, and prolonged eyelid edema (Good et al., 1992; Peragallo et al., 2013). In a study of 55 children prenatally exposed to cocaine, strabismus was significantly higher in the cocaine-exposed group in comparison to 100 controls when comparing full-birthweight infants ($p < 0.05$). However, these differences did not persist in low-birthweight infants. ROP, although rare, was also associated with prenatal cocaine exposure in the same study (Peragallo et al., 2013).

Tobacco. Prepregnancy smoking rates range from 2.6% to 32.9% within the United States. Smoking at any time during pregnancy is reported among 8.4% of pregnant women, and third-trimester smoking is reported in approximately 10.9% of pregnant women (Curtin & Matthews, 2016).

Prenatal exposure to cigarette smoking is a risk factor for the esotropia and exotropia type of strabismus, refractive errors, and ROP. The ROP association is significant for progression to Stages 3 or 4 disease (see the section "Retinopathy of Prematurity" later in the chapter). This is likely secondary to fetal retinal and intraocular muscle sensitivity. A dose-dependent relationship between smoking and ocular disturbances in infancy and childhood has been reported; however, further research is indicated (Fernandes et al., 2015).

COMMON PROBLEMS WITH IMPLICATIONS ACROSS THE LIFE SPAN

Early detection and treatment of congenital eye disorders is critical to optimize vision development. Although congenital eye disorders can be isolated, they are often part of a broader genetic syndrome and frequently accompany brain malformations. The timing of embryonic insult determines the type of eye abnormalities; disruption of the optic field occurs in the earliest embryonic stage, and includes anophthalmia, whereas abnormalities of various components of the eye occur in later embryonic stages and include microphthalmia (Figure 13.8) and coloboma (Schoenwolf et al., 2021). Microphthalmia is the underdevelopment of one or both eyes and is defined as 2 standard deviations (SD) below the mean for age. Several common ocular problems are discussed in this section of the chapter.

Congenital Dacryostenosis

Congenital dacryostenosis involves narrowing or obstruction of the nasolacrimal duct (Figure 13.9). This defect affects up to 20% of newborns (Örge & Selem, 2025; Zitelli et al., 2023). The obstruction causes a stagnant pool of tears in the lacrimal sac that leads to chronic

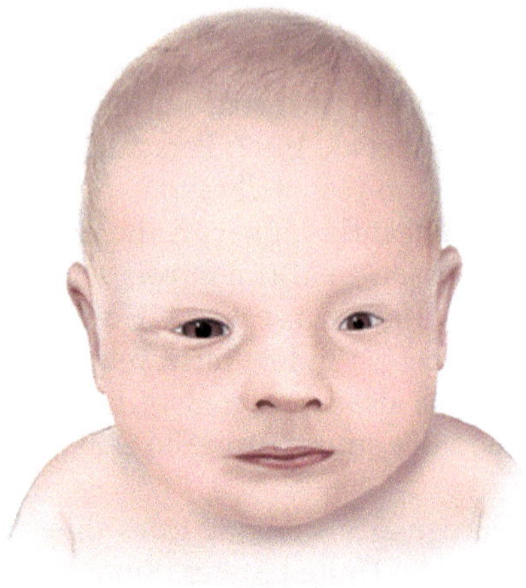

Figure 13.8 Microphthalmia of the left eye.

Source: Centers for Disease Control and Prevention. (2024). *Anophthalmia/microphthalmia*. https://www.cdc.gov/birth-defects/about/anophthalmia-microphthalmia.html?CDC_AAref_Val=https://www.cdc.gov/ncbddd/birthdefects/anophthalmia-microphthalmia.html

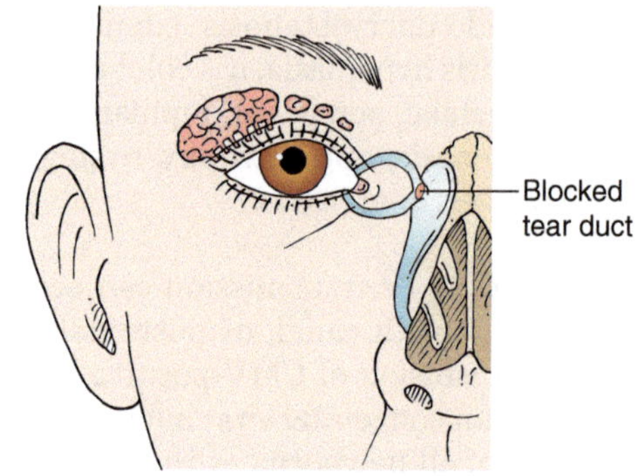

Figure 13.9 Congenital dacryostenosis.

or recurrent inflammation, or dacryocystitis. In a recent study, massage of the lacrimal duct resulted in resolution of the blockage in more than 85% of cases, with 70% of those cases resolving within 6 months (Nanda & Sarkar, 2022). No common long-term complications are reported.

Primary Congenital Glaucoma

Congenital glaucoma is a primary cause for blindness in children, accounting for up to 5% of all cases (AAO, 2024i). This condition involves uncontrolled increased ocular pressure. The incidence of congenital glaucoma is one in 10,000 to 20,000 infants. A male prevalence is observed, as males account for approximately 65% of all cases of congenital glaucoma.

Three subtypes of primary congenital glaucoma affect children: congenital glaucoma (the focus of this discussion), infantile glaucoma (1–3 years of age at onset), and juvenile glaucoma (4 years to adulthood; AAO, 2024i). Most cases are a result of spontaneous mutation; however, some reports suggest an autosomal recessive or polygenic inheritance pattern accounting for onset of the disease process. Secondary glaucoma is the result of a spontaneous mutation or a manifestation of a genetic disorder such as SWS. Lastly, acquired glaucoma occurs in an otherwise healthy eye due to pharmacologic treatment, trauma, surgery, or inflammation.

The pathogenesis of congenital glaucoma involves an obstruction to aqueous flow that increases intraocular pressure. The obstruction may occur secondary to trabeculodysgenesis, or angle maldevelopment. The iris abnormally inserts into the surface of the trabeculum in two possible ways: (a) flat insertion at or anterior to the scleral spur, or (b) concave insertion with the plane of the iris posterior to the scleral spur. Alternatively, the pathogenesis may involve uncontrolled ocular pressure secondary to drainage abnormalities (Figure 13.10).

Common clinical manifestations include a cloudy cornea and progressive myopia. A corneal diameter of greater than 12 mm (enlarged cornea) with corneal haze, tearing, blepharospasm, and photophobia should raise suspicion for congenital glaucoma (AAO, 2024i; Örge & Selem, 2025). An enlarged eye should raise concern

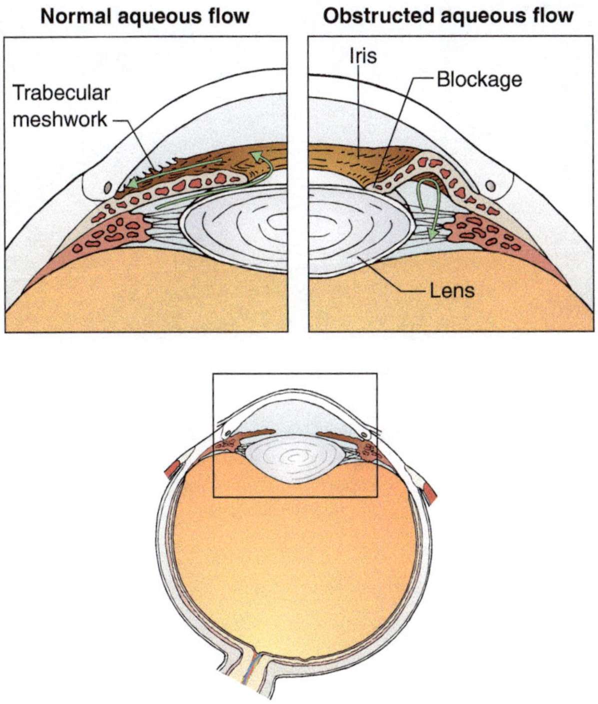

Figure 13.10 Normal and abnormal iris insertion with congenital glaucoma.

for later infantile glaucoma, which needs to be treated quickly to preserve visual development.

Life-span implications are primarily associated with untreated glaucoma. Photophobia with loss of vision may occur due to stretching of the eye from increased intraocular pressure. The age at onset and time to diagnosis will affect visual outcome (Örge & Selem, 2025). Delayed diagnosis after 1 year of age is associated with poor visual acuity across the life span.

Colobomas

Colobomas are among the most common congenital abnormalities of the eyelid and/or structures of the eye, occurring in approximately one in every 10,000 newborns. A coloboma is a defect in closure of the structure and can occur in the eyelid or structures of the eye, including the iris, lens, retina, or optic nerve, and is associated with microphthalmia (AAO, 2024b).

Eyelid colobomas range from partial-thickness to full-thickness defects. The extent of the defect can range from a small notch on the lid border to involvement of the entire length of the lid. The pathogenesis of eyelid colobomas involves failed closure of the optic fissure. Eyelid colobomas often involve the upper eyelid and are the result of defects during eyelid fusion or reseparation (AAO, 2024b). The etiology is unknown but may be a result of adhesion failure of lid folds resulting in lack of growth or the effect of amniotic bands; epigenetic influences; or environmental factors, including alcohol consumption during pregnancy (Örge & Selem, 2025). Eyelid colobomas may prevent complete lid closure and manifest with exposure of the cornea. This leads to thickening, opacification, infection, ulceration, and/or perforation of the exposed cornea.

Colobomas involving the lower aspect of the iris create a "keyhole" appearance of the pupil (Figure 13.11). Coloboma defects involving the pupil typically do not derange vision; however, visual difficulties, including refractive errors and light sensitivity, occur when colobomas involve the retina, optic nerve, or macula (Örge & Selem, 2025).

Lens Abnormalities

Congenital Cataracts. Similar to congenital glaucoma, congenital cataracts are a major cause for blindness during the childhood years, accounting for 5% to 20% of childhood blindness worldwide (Heidar & Tropathi, 2025; Örge & Selem, 2025). The incidence of congenital cataracts is one in every 250 children; however, the rate of cataracts that impact vision is estimated at three to four per 10,000 live births (Heidar & Tropathi, 2025). Cataracts can have a hereditary, chromosomal, metabolic, traumatic, or infectious etiology and range in size from a small dot to complete lens opacity. The majority of congenital cataracts result from either genetic abnormalities or are isolated disorders (Örge & Selem, 2025).

Congenital cataracts involve an opacity or abnormality within the structure of the lens that clouds its appearance. Clinical manifestations of cataracts are dependent on the timing during organogenesis. Insults occurring early in embryogenesis result in opacification in the center of the lens (Figure 13.12). Insults occurring later in fetal development cause the emergence of ringlike opacifications surrounded by central and peripheral clear zones. Alternatively, recent damage results in peripheral opacifications near the surface of the lens. Congenital or infantile cataracts may be subtle and likewise overlooked. In these cases, diagnosis is rendered secondary to abnormal loss of visual function or white pupillary reflex. Presenting symptoms include absent red reflex, nystagmus, and inability to fix and follow.

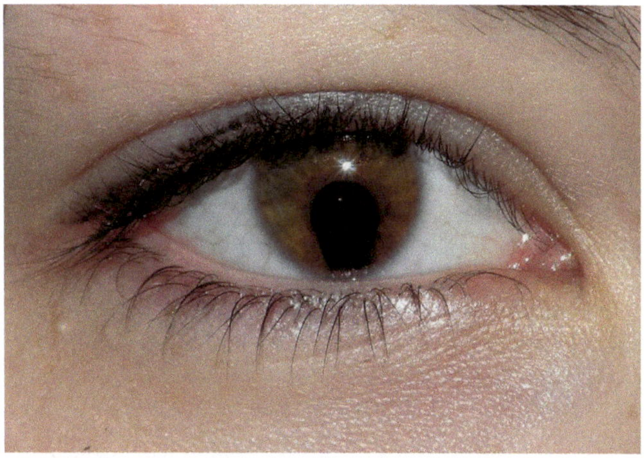

Figure 13.11 "Keyhole" appearance with coloboma.
Source: Jmarchn. (2016). *Coloboma of the iris.* https://commons.wikimedia.org/wiki/File:Coloboma_of_the_iris.JPG

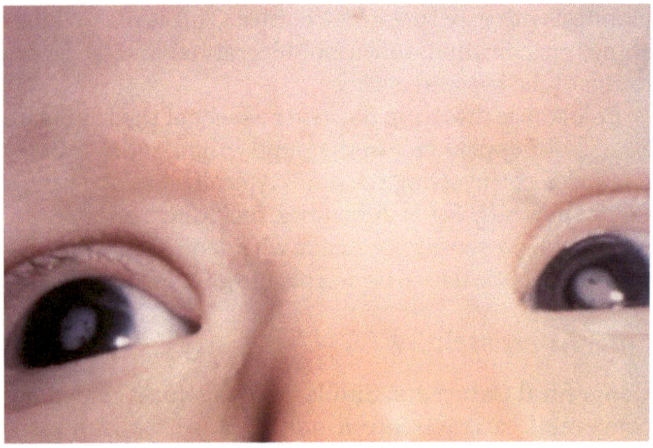

Figure 13.12 Congenital cataracts. This photograph illustrates leukocoria (white discoloration of the pupil) secondary to congenital cataracts in a child's eyes secondary to congenital rubella syndrome.
Source: Centers for Disease Control and Prevention. (1976). *Public health image library, ID #4284*. https://phil.cdc.gov/Details.aspx?pid=4284

Prognosis for vision is poorer when only one eye is involved due to the increased risk for amblyopia. Management of congenital cataracts is challenging in the neonate and young infant due to the increased risk of postoperative complications (Heidar & Tripathi, 2025). Some very small cataracts can be managed with close follow-up and medical management, while those children with evidence of vision impairment (amblyopia) should have prompt surgical intervention (Heidar & Tripathi, 2025).

Optic Nerve Hypoplasia

ONH, the most common congenital disc anomaly, involves an abnormally small, underdeveloped optic nerve with decreased nerve axons (Figure 13.13). ONH has been reported to occur in approximately 11 per 100,000 children under 18, and experts posit that this once rare disease is on the rise (AAO, 2024h).There are a number of genetic mutations impacting transcription factors that have been discovered in connection with ONH. ONH may present as an isolated defect impacting one or both eyes or may occur in association with other intracranial anomalies. When associated with other intracranial anomalies (absent septum pellucidum, agenesis of the corpus callosum, or in conjunction with deficient pituitary hormones) the APRN should be concerned for septo-optic dysplasia (AAO, 2024h). When associated with other intracranial anomalies, there is an increased risk for neurodevelopmental deficits.

The pathogenesis of ONH is thought to involve a vascular interruption of the anterior cerebral artery during embryonic and fetal development between weeks 6 and 16 of gestation (AAO, 2024h). Risk factors noted to have some impact on the development of ONH are summarized in Table 13.5.

Clinical manifestations are usually subtle in the newborn period and through early childhood. Unless other

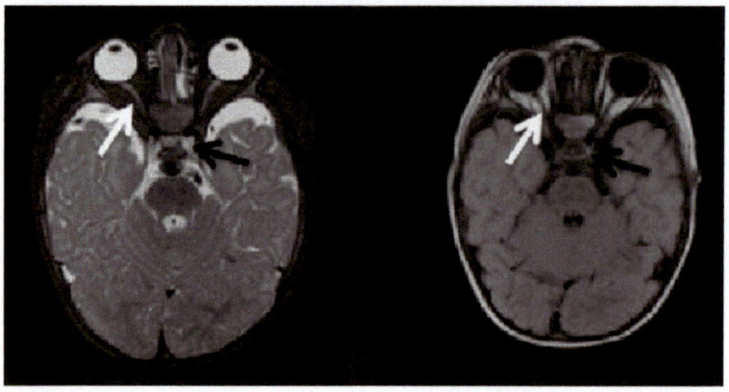

Figure 13.13 Optic nerve hypoplasia. Arrows denote optic nerve fiber thinning.
Source: Pensiero, S., Cecchini, P., Michieletto, P., Pelizzo, G., Madonia, M., & Parentin, F. (2011). Congenital aplasia of the optic chiasm and esophageal atresia: A case report. *Journal of Medical Case Reports, 5*, 335. https://doi.org/10.1186/1752-1947-5-335

TABLE 13.5 Common Risk Factors for Optic Nerve Hypoplasia

Maternal	Fetal
• Addictive behaviors (smoking, recreational drugs, alcohol) • Anemia • CMV infection • Depression • Gestational diabetes • Metabolic disorder • Young primigravida	• Low birthweight • Intrauterine growth restriction • Prematurity • Twin–twin transfusion syndrome

Note: Metabolic conditions may include hypothyroidism, hypocortisolism, panhypopituitarism, diabetes insipidus, and hyperprolactinemia.
Source: Data from Kaur, S., Jain, S., Sodhi, H. B. S., Rastogi, A., & Kamlesh. (2013). Optic nerve hypoplasia. *Oman Journal of Ophthalmology, 6*(2), 77–82. https://doi.org/10.4103/0974-620X.116622
CMV, cytomegalovirus.

hypothalamic dysfunction is noted during early childhood, the defect is typically identified in early childhood with the onset of routine clinical ophthalmic examinations. This defect manifests with a gray or pale optic nerve head. In addition, the optic disc may be bordered by a yellowish, mottled parapapillary halo surrounded by an increase or decrease in pigmentation. An altered pupillary light reflex may be evident. Visual acuity may be decreased (Kaur et al., 2013).

Prognosis ranges from 20/20 vision to no light perception; visual-evoked responses range from normal to fully extinguished. ONH is associated with astigmatism, nystagmus, amblyopia, and visual field and associated nerve fiber bundle defects (AAO, 2024h; Örge & Selem, 2025).

Retinoblastoma

Retinoblastoma is the most common intraocular tumor in children, accounting for 6% of all pediatric cancers seen in children under 5 years of age. It occurs at a rate of approximately 11.6 per million live births (AAO, 2024j). These neoplasms arise within the developing retina as a result of a mutation in both alleles of the *RB1*, or retinoblastoma tumor suppressor gene, on chromosome 13 (AAO, 2024j). The majority (60%) of cases are nonhereditary and unilateral. The remainder of retinoblastomas are inherited or a result of gene mutation and typically affect both eyes. Retinoblastomas will be categorized as either a germline (inherited from a mutation in either the sperm or egg) or somatic mutation (AAO, 2024j). Retinoblastoma usually presents in children younger than 5 years of age with leukocoria or strabismus.

The pathogenesis of retinoblastoma involves tumor formation near the photoreceptors and subsequent extension into the vitreous cavity of the eye. The tumor manifests as a fleshlike, heterogeneous structure that rapidly proliferates and fills the posterior chamber of the eye (**Figure 13.14**). The tumor often invades the choroid, providing ample vascular supply and margin for expansion. Metastasis into the sclera and orbit, ciliary body and lymph nodes, or optic nerve and intracranial cavity has been reported.

Clinical manifestations during infancy are often noticed by way of photographs. Parents or caregivers may observe leukocoria, or a white-colored reflection from the retina. Other clinical manifestations include strabismus and glaucoma, which present with advanced cases of retinoblastoma secondary to tumor size and increased intraocular pressure (AAO, 2024j). On average, children with bilateral disease present 9 months earlier than those with unilateral disease. Life-span implications are contingent on the type and severity of retinoblastoma; cases that involve metastasis into intracranial structures are associated with high mortality (AAO, 2024j).

Rhabdomyosarcoma

Rhabdomyosarcoma (RMS), a soft-tissue sarcoma, is the most common orbit malignancy in children. The mean age of onset is 6 to 8 years, although a subset of cases has been noted in infants within the first few months of age and is known as infantile and congenital RMS (Yan et al., 2023). Most cases of RMS are not familial, but rather are the result of sporadic mutations and epigenetic influences causing hypermethylation of genes tasked with coding proteins for skeletal muscle development.

RMS has two subtypes: the more common embryonal type that is less aggressive and the less common but more aggressive alveolar type (Yan et al., 2023). Common ocular manifestations of RMS include proptosis, globe displacement, swelling of the eyelid and conjunctiva, ptosis, and diplopia. Ocular tumors, including but not limited to RMS, often demonstrate rapid proliferation causing bulging and displacement of the affected eye (**Figure 13.15**). Hemorrhage, pain, and excessive tearing may also be present (AAO, 2024l). Life-span implications of embryonal RMS involve age of onset and metastasis to the lungs. Failure-free survival, or the length of time a treated infant or child survives without disease progression, is dependent on the cell type of the tumor, with the more common embryonal cell type having a greater than 90% 5-year survival, unless diagnosed within the first year of life. Infants diagnosed in the first year of life have nearly a 50% chance of death (AAO, 2024l).

Neuroblastoma

Neuroblastoma is a common solid tumor found in infants and children and arises from neural crest cells. It is the most common cancer in children; approximately 7% of all pediatric cancers are attributed to neuroblastoma. Risk factors include autosomal dominant inheritance as well as Turner syndrome; Noonan syndrome; neuro-cardio-facial syndromes, including Costello syndrome; and overgrowth disorders such as Beckwith–Weidemann syndrome (Orkin et al., 2015). Epigenetic factors may implicate the formation of a neuroblastoma, as deficient methylation has been associated with the onset of non-Wilms tumors.

The pathogenesis of neuroblastoma is poorly understood. However, similar to other ocular tumors, neuroblastomas are thought to arise secondary to epigenetic influences, causing abnormal proliferation of embryonal cells. Tumors present as small, blue-colored, dense cellular masses. Tumors may appear anywhere that involves

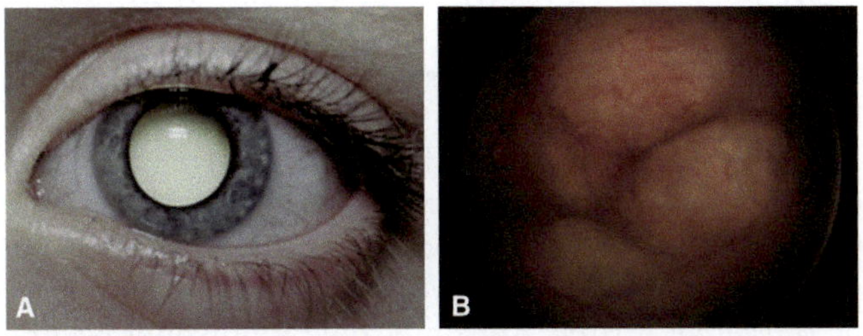

Figure 13.14 Retinoblastoma. Gross appearance of leukocoria (**A**) with an enucleated eye; (**B**) maximally dilated pupil shows large retinoblastoma filling the posterior chamber, vitreous seeds, and retinal detachment.

Source: Rodriguez-Galindo, C., Orbach, D. B., & VanderVeen, D. (2015). Retinoblastoma. *Pediatric Clinics of North America, 62*(1), 201–223. https://doi.org/10.1016/j.pcl.2014.09.014

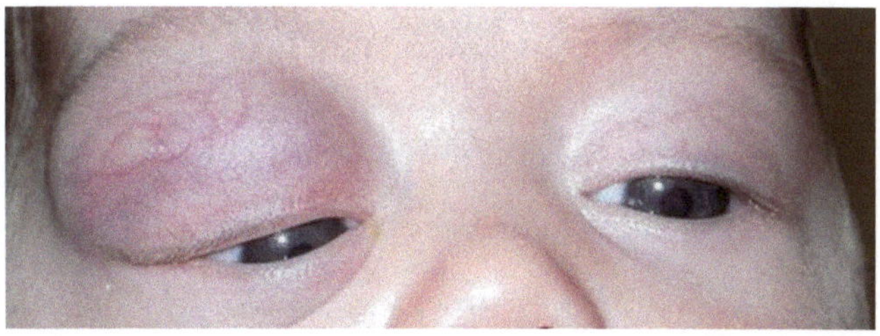

Figure 13.15 Orbital mass in small child (rhabdomyosarcoma is most common).

Source: Goddard, K. (Ed.). (2008). Ophthalmology for the oncologist. *Pediatric Oncology Education Materials.* http://www.pedsoncologyeducation.com/OpthalmologyProptosis.asp

sympathetic innervation, including the orbit, neck, chest, pelvis, and abdomen. Similar to RMS, orbital symptoms include bulging of the eye and bruising around the eyes (AAO, 2024f). A 5-year survival rate of 50% is reported for those diagnosed with the metastatic form of the disease (Orkin et al., 2015).

Strabismus

Strabismus, a neuromuscular abnormality, presents as the misalignment of gaze and is a result of abnormal extraocular muscles or their innervation and is the most common pathology impacting pediatric visual development (Lam & Suh, 2022; Schoenwolf et al., 2021). Strabismus can occur as horizontal deviations, esodeviations, exodeviations, or, rarely, vertical deviations which impair the ability of both eyes to focus on the same target (Table 13.6). Strabismus can be either concomitant, with deviation the same regardless of gaze position, or incomitant, with variable deviation as gaze is shifted up, down, or to the side (Örge & Selem, 2025).

The most common infantile forms of concomitant strabismus include congenital exotropia, early intermittent exotropia, congenital/infantile esotropia, early accommodative esotropia, and sensory esotropia. Accommodative esotropia occurs secondary to exaggerated accommodative efforts, whereas sensory strabismus is due to vision loss in one or both eyes (Örge & Selem, 2025).

Impaired globe movements secondary to muscle restriction or weakness result in noncomitant strabismus. Etiologies for noncomitant strabismus include fractures, orbital tumors, CN palsies, and congenital myasthenia gravis (Örge & Selem, 2025).

Two situations occur that can confuse the diagnosis of strabismus. Pseudostrabismus can present as esotropia and exotropia. A large nasal bridge and prominent epicanthal folds can create the appearance of pseudoesotropia. In addition, immaturity of foveal fixation and binocularity and the establishment of firm control of eye movement can also create a small misalignment of one or both eyes (Örge & Selem, 2025).

Pseudostrabismus is self-limiting and presents no long-term visual deficits. True strabismus requires early corrective surgery (within 4–6 months) after correction of refractive errors and any associated amblyopia in order to improve binocular cooperation (Örge & Selem, 2025).

TABLE 13.6 Strabismus Eye Positions

Type	Eye Position
Esotropia	Affected eye turns inward
Exotropia	Affected eye turns outward
Hypertropia	Affected eye deviates upward
Hypotropia	Affected eye deviates downward

Nystagmus

Nystagmus, involuntary eye movements, usually present as rapid, rhythmic, and repetitious movements. Congenital nystagmus is noted at birth, while acquired nystagmus presents after 6 months of age. Congenital nystagmus is the result of motor defects (infantile idiopathic nystagmus), as well as abnormal eye or brain development (AAO, 2024g). Acquired nystagmus affects 17 of every 10,000 live births (AAO, 2024g). Risk factors for acquired nystagmus include medications, stroke, brain injuries, and vestibular impairment. Sensory abnormalities and diseases, including albinism, achromatopsia, ONH, aniridia, and congenital cataracts, are often responsible for nystagmus presenting in infants at 3 to 4 months of age (Örge & Selem, 2025).

The pathogenesis of nystagmus is not well understood. Clinical manifestations include periods of slow and rapid eye movements. Essentially, infants are unable to hold a gaze; slow eye movements evolve into rapid fluttering movements away from an initial focal point. The fluttering movements permit refocusing of the eye to the focal point. Life-span implications are significant and include visual degeneration, psychosocial dysfunction secondary to altered self-image, and driving limitations among older adolescents.

Amblyopia

Often called *lazy eye*, amblyopia is the reduction in vision from abnormal visual development during infancy and early childhood. For at least the past decade, amblyopia has been regarded as the most common cause of monocular vision loss in children and young adults (AAO, 2024a). The incidence is estimated at 1% to 5%, with approximately 12 million children affected by uncorrected amblyopia (World Health Organization, 2023). Risk factors include prematurity, low birthweight, visual deprivation through early childhood, family history of amblyopia, and strabismus.

Amblyopia likely results secondary to strabismus (ocular misalignment is the most common risk factor), anisometropia (uncorrected refractive errors between both eyes), opacities (cataracts), or visual deprivation (often caused by eyelid drooping; AAO, 2024a). More specifically, refractive amblyopia results from two types of refractive errors: Anisometropic amblyopia occurs when there is an unequal refractive error that prevents the normal fusing of an image seen by each eye; more commonly, bilateral hyperopia (farsightedness) also causes refractive amblyopia. Deprivation amblyopia results from blocked visual axis information received by the retina during a critical period of eye development.

The most notable clinical manifestation in young children is eye rubbing observed secondary to abnormal processing of visual images, secondary to loss of visual acuity. On exam, the cornea, lens, retina, and optic disc appear normal.

Early childhood life-span implications include difficulty with participation in athletics, psychosocial dysfunction secondary to teasing from peers, and altered depth perception. Although the incidence is reported to be less than 2%, vision loss in the affected eye can significantly impair visual acuity.

Blindness

Loss of vision in the neonatal population can result from a number of causes, including congenital abnormalities affecting the optic nerve or brain, genetic syndromes, trauma, infection, hypoxia, and ROP. In developed countries, cortical visual impairment and optic nerve abnormalities are the most common causes of severe visual impairment. ROP, glaucoma, cataracts, and injury are the most common preventable causes of blindness in developed countries secondary to advances made in long-term survival of extremely premature neonates.

Neonatal Conjunctivitis

Ophthalmia neonatorum, conjunctivitis occurring in the first month of life, is most commonly the result of infection with *Staphylococcus aureus*, *Staphylococcus epidermidis*, *Streptococcus pneumoniae*, or *Moraxella catarrhalis* (Richards & Guzman-Cottrill, 2010). Infections caused by *Chlamydia trachomatis*, *Neisseria gonorrhea*, or HSV can be acquired through the birth canal. Table 13.7 provides a summary of common causes of conjunctivitis presenting in the neonatal period along with symptoms, outcomes, and treatment options.

Viral Conjunctivitis. Viral conjunctivitis is less common in the neonatal population compared to older children. The most common cause of this self-limiting condition is adenovirus.

Ocular Trauma

Eye-related birth injuries are more common with operative deliveries and include orbital fracture and corneal lacerations. Subconjunctival and retinal hemorrhages are common with precipitous or vacuum-assisted de-

TABLE 13.7 Causes of Neonatal Conjunctivitis

Organism	Presentation Timeline	Symptoms	Outcomes	Treatment
Chemical (following silver nitrate or antibiotic ointment)	First 24 hours	Clear, thin watery discharge; redness	Good, no impact to vision	None
Neisseria gonorrhea	2–4 days	Purulent discharge—copious; marked eyelid and conjunctival edema	Good with early recognition and treatment; if unrecognized and treatment delayed, may lead to corneal ulceration and perforation	IV antibiotics, topical irrigation, topical antibiotics if corneal ulceration present
Chlamydia trachomatis	5–14 days (occurs in 30%–40% of neonates born to untreated mothers)	Edema and redness of conjunctiva; copious discharge—initially thin/watery before progressing to purulent Associated with pneumonia if left untreated	Good with early recognition and treatment	Oral erythromycin or azithromycin
Herpes simplex virus (HSV)	6–14 days	Unilateral or bilateral serous discharge; vesicles or skin sloughing noted on eyelid	Depends on type: skin, eye, mouth (SEM) disease has best long-term outcome	Acyclovir IV for 2–3 weeks depending on type followed by oral suppression for 6 months

Note: For additional treatment recommendations refer to Jnah & McPherson's *Fetal and Neonatal Pharmacology for Advanced Practice Nurse* (2024).
Source: Oatts, J. T., De Alba Campomanes, A. G., & Binenbaum, G. (2024). Eye and vision disorders. In C. A. Gleason & T. Sawyer (Eds.), *Avery's diseases of the newborn* (11th ed., p. 1399). Elsevier.

livery, or in the presence of a tight nuchal cord. Owing to the protective bony prominence surrounding the eye, traumatic eye injury is relatively uncommon in neonates. Retinal hemorrhages increase the risk of visual impairment if the optic nerve is involved (Örge & Selem, 2025). A focal globular hemorrhage at the posterior pole of the eye, as well as severe retinal hemorrhage, is associated with shaken baby syndrome (Örge & Selem, 2025). Severe hemorrhage may involve the covering (sheath) of the optic nerve. Shaken baby syndrome should be considered among infants who present with the aforementioned findings.

Retinopathy of Prematurity

ROP, first reported in 1942 and labeled *retrolental fibroplasia (RLF)*, was the consequence of supplemental oxygen use. Oxygen therapy inhibited normal retinal vascular proliferation among premature infants, leading to retinal detachment, and, in some cases, blindness (Terry, 1942). In the 1950s, as awareness of causative factors for ROP increased, the supplemental use of oxygen became more restrictive; this practice extends into modern times. Although the judicious use of oxygen has led to a decrease in the incidence of ROP, an optimum saturation range remains unknown. Efforts to narrow the oxygenation saturation (SaO_2) range endorsed by the American Academy of Pediatrics (AAP; 90%–95%), so as to reduce ROP and avoid a consequential increase in mortality, have been subject to debate and ongoing discussion as the likely target range is dynamic and influenced by patient-specific pathophysiology (Cummings et al., 2016).

The incidence of ROP is highest among premature infants born at less than 28 weeks of gestation. The incidence has increased due to increased survival of infants at lower gestational ages. This is balanced somewhat by the proliferation of neonatal intensive care. In the United States, for infants weighing less than 1,250 grams at birth, 68% are noted to have ROP of any stage with approximately 40% of those with ROP progressing to treatment thresholds (Kim et al., 2018). ROP remains the leading cause of blindness in developed countries.

The primary risk factors for ROP include prematurity, low birthweight, and postnatal oxygen exposure. The use of supplemental oxygen increases oxidative injury from damaging reactive oxygen species (ROS). Premature infants have fewer antioxidants (low levels of vitamin E) to counteract the ROS; the result is endothelial cell damage, apoptosis, and capillary constriction. Infants born at earlier than 33 weeks of gestation exhibit decreased circulating growth factors, which contribute to an increased risk for ROP. Hyperglycemia and insulin use have also been implicated in the incidence of ROP. Secondary risk factors in the development of ROP include hyperoxia, apnea, sepsis, blood transfusions, antioxidant deficiency, and patent ductus arteriosus (Shah et al., 2016). According to the AAO, the primary risk factors that warrant routine screening in the NICU include those listed in Box 13.1.

BOX 13.1 Common Risk Factors for Retinopathy of Prematurity

- Prematurity
- Supplemental use of oxygen
- Prolonged mechanical ventilation
- Low birthweight
- Hyperglycemia and insulin use
- Apnea
- Sepsis
- Blood transfusions
- Antioxidant deficiency
- Patent ductus arteriosus

Blood vessels that supply the retina begin to develop at the optic disc at 15 to 16 weeks of gestation; this process is stimulated by the release of vascular endothelial growth factor (VEGF) and insulin growth factor (IGF-1). The retinal vasculature moves in a predictable pattern from the optic nerve to the periphery; at 36 and 40 weeks of gestation, the vessels reach the nasal and temporal edge of the retina, respectively. In utero, VEGF controls the proliferation of the retinal vasculature as well as its regression. However, premature birth, and exposure to relative hyperoxia, halts the proliferation of the retinal vasculature and the normal, physiologic expression of VEGF (Sun et al., 2025). This predisposes the premature infant to abnormal retinal development.

Phase-1 ROP. The development of ROP is explained as a series of two sequential phases. Phase-1 ROP encompasses the cessation of normal growth of blood vessels, which occurs at birth. As a result, VEGF and IGF-1 levels drop. Concurrent with the onset of phase 1, and in the immediate window after birth, is a brief and possibly subtle period of postnatal hypoxia as the infant adjusts to extrauterine life. This elicits significant upregulation of VEGF with a slower increase in IGF-1 concentrations. Subsequently, and throughout the early postnatal period, any exposure to physiologic stressors, including illness, stress, or persistent fluctuations in oxygen levels, can encourage additional abnormal downregulation and upregulation of VEGF concentrations. Abnormally high saturation levels (in comparison to normal intrauterine paO_2 less than 50 mmHg) downregulate VEGF and favor vasoobliteration, whereas periods of hypoxia upregulate VEGF and encourage abnormal vasoproliferation (Sun et al., 2025).

Phase-2 ROP. Phase-2 ROP involves one of two possible pathways: spontaneous regression of ROP, or progression to pathologic proliferative retinopathy (neovascularization). Spontaneous regression involves the return of VEGF levels to normal, physiologic concentrations. This facilitates normal, progressive retinal vascularization and marks the resolution of ROP.

Alternatively, pathologic proliferation is modulated by markedly elevated increases in factors, including VEGF, erythropoietin (EPO), IGF-1, and long-chain polyunsaturated fatty acids (LCPUFA; Eldweik & Mantagos, 2016). Recall that VEGF and EPO are oxygen-regulated angiogenic growth factors. IGF-1 is essential for normal growth of blood vessels (among other tissues), and omega LCPUFA is crucial for retinal development (AAO, 2024k). The end result is a retina that is metabolically active, yet poorly vascularized. Neovascularization provides poor oxygenation to the retina, leading to disease progression and the potential for retinal detachment and blindness.

Classification of ROP. ROP is classified according to the International Classification of Retinopathy of Prematurity (ICROP) by zone, extent of disease severity, and stage. ROP begins with the cessation of normal retinal neuronal and vascular development. Vessel growth may become pathologic and result in neovascularization (pathologic vessel growth) of the retina.

ROP zone, or location, of the disease is distinguished by dividing the retina into three concentric areas centered on the optic disc. The more posterior the disease occurs, the more severe the disease. There are three zones used to describe the location of progressive vascular development. Zone 1 is the most posterior zone; it is defined by a circle around the optic nerve head. Zone 1 represents the most immature vascularization; as such, zone 1 is considered the area of most concern and is associated with increased disease severity. Zone 2 consists of a concentric circle around zone 1 and is twice the radius of zone 1. Zone 2 extends to the ora serrata nasally. Zone 3 encompasses the remaining crescent-shaped retina and extends to the temporal side (Table 13.8; AAO, 2024k).

The extent of disease is expressed as clock hours of retinal involvement. The clock hours are separated into 30-degree segments. For APRNs, the temporal side of the right eye corresponds with 9 o'clock, whereas the temporal side of the left eye corresponds with 3 o'clock.

Furthermore, ROP is divided into five stages (Table 13.9). Stages 1 to 3 describe increasing degrees of abnormal blood vessel growth. Stage 1 consists of a flat demarcation line at the junction of the vascular and avascular retina. Stage 2 involves a slightly elevated ridge of fibrovascular tissue. In stage 3, the vessels grow into the vitreous humor (clear jelly that fills the eyeball) and may be severe enough to cause partial (stage 4) or complete (stage 5) retinal detachment (AAO, 2024k). *Plus disease* describes venous dilation and arterial tortuosity that increase the risk for retinal detachment (AAO, 2024k; Oatts et al., 2024). Plus disease is evidence of active and progressive disease. Per the most recent ICROP recommendations, aggressive ROP (A-ROP) is an additional classification used to describe a more severe retinopathy that progresses rapidly without following the typical disease progression stages (Chiang et al., 2021). A-ROP involves a very marked neovascularization in addition to plus disease and can progress very quickly to stage 5 ROP and blindness (AAO, 2024k; Oatts et al., 2024).

ROP regresses spontaneously in over 90% of cases; the remaining cases require treatment to avoid negative sequelae. Stage 1 or stage 2 ROP is considered mild and is likely to resolve spontaneously. Even with spontaneous regression of mild ROP, neural deficits are possible and include loss of photoreceptor function (Chan-Ling et al., 2018). Premature infants with stage 1 or stage 2 ROP have only a slightly increased risk for optical conditions, including myopia/hyperopia, strabismus, and amblyopia, in comparison to their full-term counterparts. The onset of ROP in zone 2 is more likely to resolve spontaneously and achieve good prognosis (Chan-Ling et al., 2018).

ROP requiring treatment, such as stages 3, 4, and 5 ROP, carry a poor prognosis; when untreated, retinal detachment leads to blindness. There are now two therapies most often used in the treatment of ROP: anti-VEGF intraocular injections and laser ablation surgery. Infants who have required treatment for ROP have increased risk for adverse visual outcomes including strabismus, amblyopia, refractive errors (myopia and anisometropia), and optic atrophy. Strabismus is likely to occur in

TABLE 13.8 Zones of Retinopathy of Prematurity

Zones	Visual Depiction
Zone 1: Twice the radius from optic nerve to macula (fovea centralis) *Zone 2:* Nasal edge of Zone 1 to temporal equator *Zone 3:* Residual crescent anterior to Zone 2	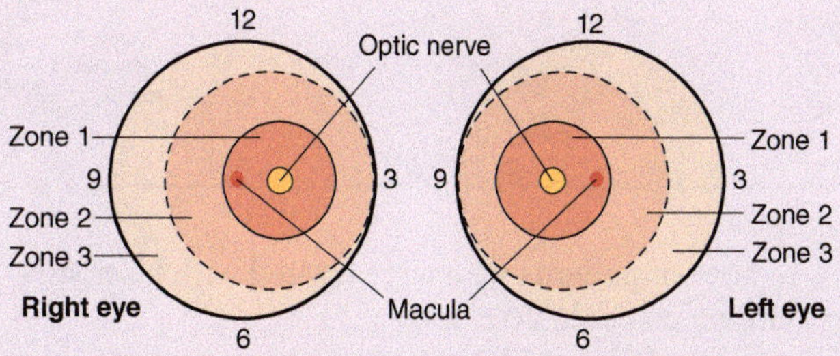

TABLE 13.9 Stages of Retinopathy of Prematurity

Stage	Definition	Visual Depiction	Life-Span Implications
1	Line of demarcation separates avascular and vascularized portions of the retina	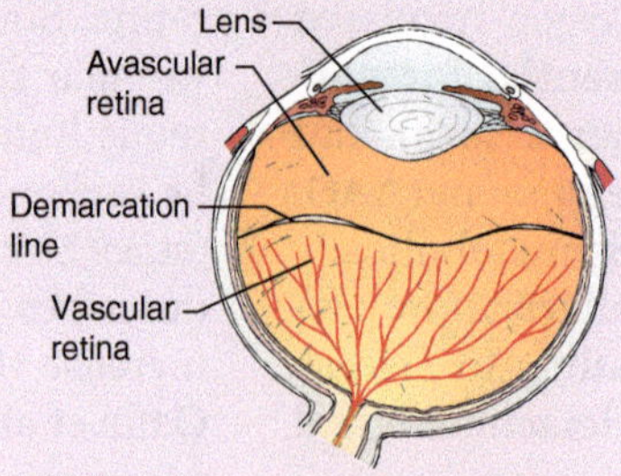	Likely to resolve spontaneously, loss of photoreceptor cell function possible, slightly increased risk for myopia/hyperopia, strabismus, and amblyopia
2	The line of demarcation develops into fibrous ridge of tissue, often with small tufts of new blood vessels	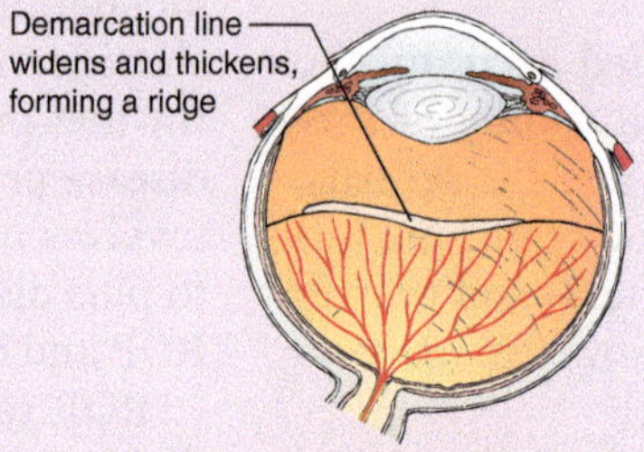	Likely to resolve spontaneously, loss of photoreceptor cell function possible, slightly increased risk for myopia/hyperopia, strabismus, and amblyopia
3	Ridge of blood vessel development extends, demonstrating extraretinal fibrovascular proliferation beyond the retina and into the vitreous humor	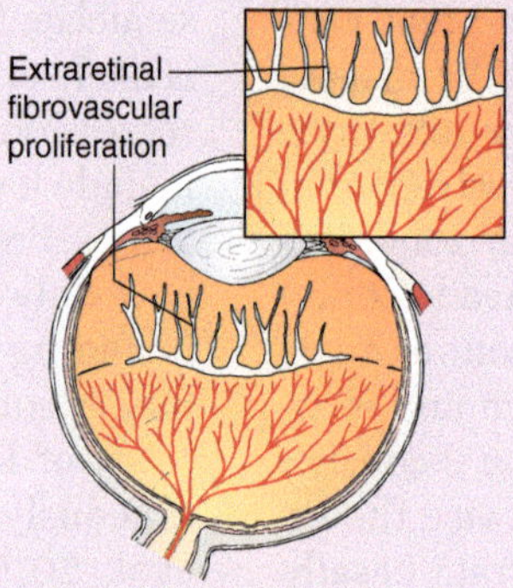	May be severe enough to cause partial (stage 4) or complete (stage 5) retinal detachment and blindness
4	Partial retinal detachment	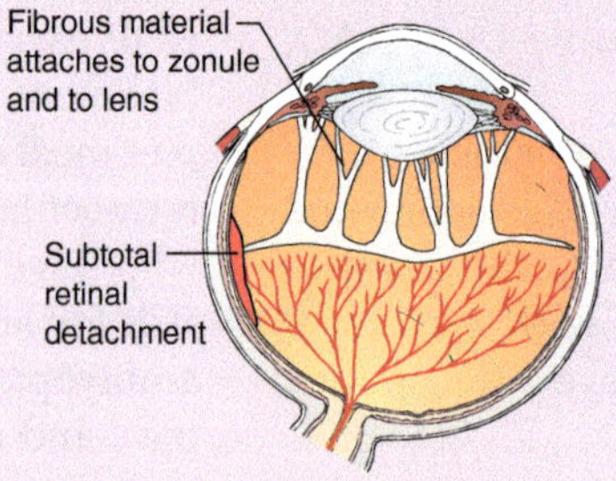	Poor prognosis; when untreated can progress to total retinal detachment, retinal detachment leads to blindness.
5	Total retinal detachment	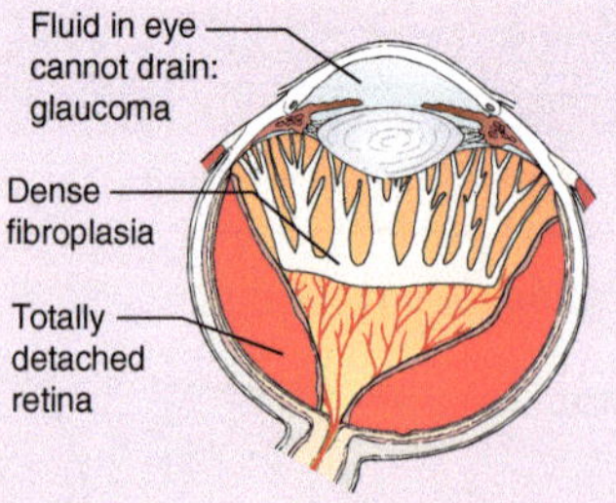	Poor prognosis; when untreated, retinal detachment leads to blindness.

30% to 40% of patients who were treated with laser surgery (Gundlach et al., 2022).

The role of the APRN in determining screening and identifying those neonates most at risk can not be understated. Table 13.10 provides the most recent screening recommendations for premature neonates based on the policy statement from the AAP, AAO, and the American Association for Pediatric Ophthalmology and Strabismus (AAPOS). All neonates born at a gestational age of 30 weeks or less and size of less than or equal to 1,500 grams should be screened for ROP. Additional risk factors for infants between 1,500 and 2,000 grams and greater than 30 weeks' gestation may prompt screening and include hypotension requiring vasopressor support, or oxygen requirement for a prolonged period or without saturation monitoring. Follow-up exams should be based on the presence and severity of ROP findings with more frequent follow-up eye exams occurring for neonates with any ROP in zone 1, stage 3 ROP (presence of stage 3 ROP in zone 1 requires treatment), or if A-ROP is suspected.

Preterm infants who do not develop ROP by 42 weeks postmenstrual age are at low risk for the development of ROP (Fierson et al., 2018). Infants discharged prior to resolution of ROP risk require parental education and agreement to continue to follow all regularly scheduled eye appointments. The anticipatory guidance provided to parents should contain information on the significant risk of blindness if ROP advances to retinal detachment, not to scare caregivers, but to clearly communicate the potential adverse sequelae of advanced stages of ROP.

TABLE 13.10 ROP Screening Recommendations

	Age at First Exam	
Gestational Age at Birth	Postmenstrual Age (Weeks)	Chronologic Age (Weeks)
22 weeks	31	9
23 weeks	31	8
24 weeks	31	7
25 weeks	31	6
26 weeks	31	5
27 weeks	31	4
28 weeks	32	4
29 weeks	33	4
30 weeks	34	4
>30 weeks with high risk factors		4

ROP, retinopathy of prematury.

Source: Fierson, W. M., American Academy of Pediatrics Section on Ophthalmology, American Academy of Ophthalmology, American Association for Pediatric Ophthalmology and Strabismus, & American Association of Certified Orthoptists. (2018). Screening examination of premature infants for retinopathy of prematurity. *Pediatrics, 142*(6), e20183061. https://doi.org/10.1542/peds.2018-3061

CONCLUSION

Embryologic development of the eye begins at 4 weeks of gestation. Sensory innervation of the eye is mediated by several CNs to allow a response, usually blinking or tearing, to pain and temperature. Sensory input—the transduction of light into electrical signals—is provided by the photoreceptor cells (rods and cones). The development of visual milestones begins at 16 weeks of gestation and continues on throughout early childhood. Factors, such as abnormal visual conditions, prematurity, and poor nutrition, can affect the physiologic maturation of the eyes. Genetic aberrations, intrauterine infections, and maternal substance abuse all have associated ocular sequelae, whereas ROP remains a leading cause of blindness in developing nations worldwide. The prompt identification and treatment of common eye problems is essential to optimize visual development.

LEARNING TOOLS AND RESOURCES

CourseConnect

To access self-assessment questions and interactive, competency-based learning activities for this chapter, visit www.springerpub.com/courseconnect. See inside front cover and tear-out card for CourseConnect details.

Podcast

This podcast is available online by visiting www.springerpub.com/courseconnect. See inside front cover and tear-out card for CourseConnect details.

#1—Visual Input; #2—Retinopathy of Prematurity; #3—The Red Reflux

Desi M. Newberry, Debbie Fraser,
Sofia Aliaga, Bill Diehl-Jones, and Amy J. Jnah

Discussion Prompts

1. Review the timeline of visual milestones in the premature and term neonate. What milestones should you expect for each gestational age?
2. What are the most common causes of conjunctivitis? Differentiate the most common causes based on symptoms and timing of symptoms.
3. Discuss the timing of ROP development in relation to screening recommendations. Why do we screen when we do? Which zone/stage combination is most concerning?

MIND MAP

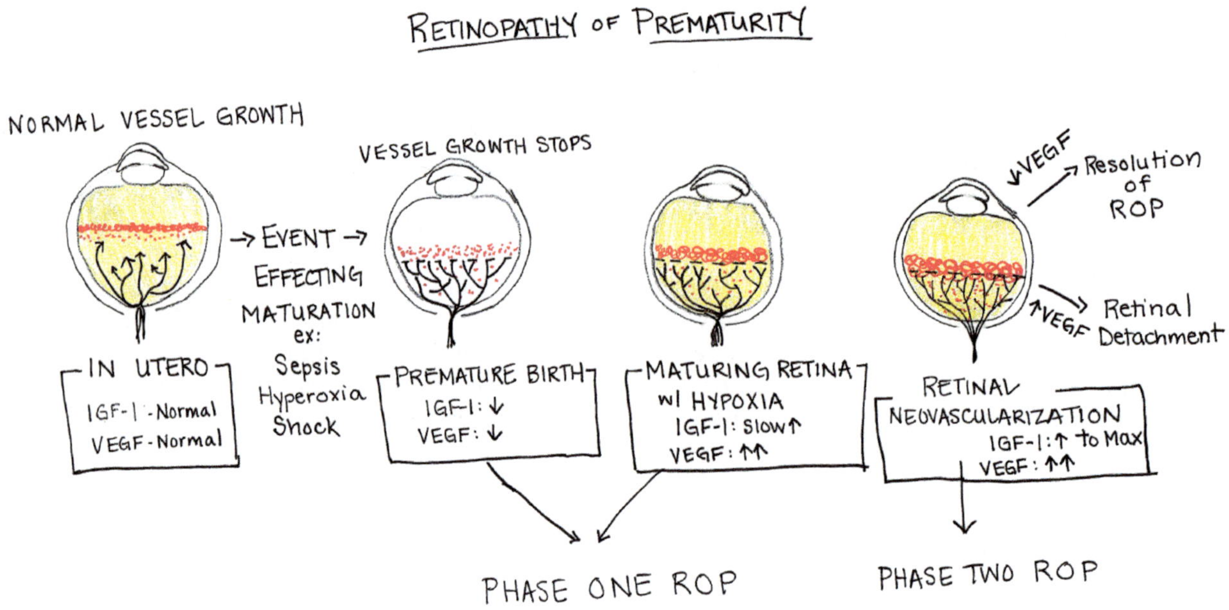

Note: This mind map reflects one student's interpretation of a portion of one or more concepts addressed in this chapter. Readers should regard the mind maps woven throughout this textbook as examples of multisensory study tools that can be developed to encourage conceptual understanding. Readers are encouraged to develop their own unique mind maps in consultation with academic faculty or clinical preceptors.
Image credit: Nicole Harvey, MSN, APRN, NNP-BC.

TIMELINE OF ORGAN DEVELOPMENT

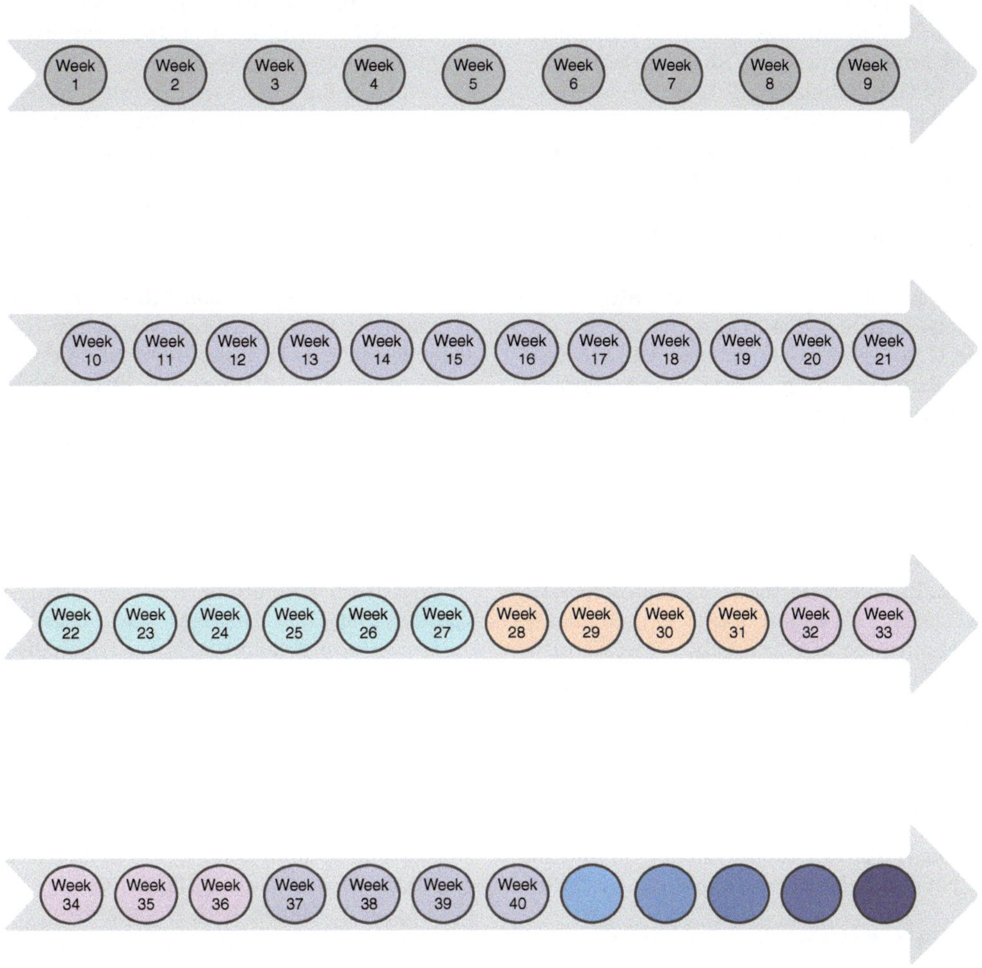

Note: Placement of common problems is meant to offer visual/ conceptual perspective on the timing of onset of these commonly reported malformations. Variation exists across the literature.	***Legend:*** <22 – 27 6/7 weeks = extremely preterm 28 – 31 6/7 weeks = very preterm 32 – 36 6/7 weeks = late/moderate preterm 37 – 40 weeks = term

Note: Readers should annotate the blank timeline during studying, self-directed learning, and creation of feedback loops with mentors. To access the blank and completed timelines visit www.springerpub.com/courseconnect. See inside front cover and tear-out card for CourseConnect details.

REFERENCES

American Academy of Ophthalmology. (2023a). *Stickler syndrome.* EyeWiki. https://eyewiki.org/Stickler_Syndrome

American Academy of Ophthalmology. (2023b). *Trisomy 21.* EyeWiki. https://eyewiki.org/Trisomy_21/Down_Syndrome

American Academy of Ophthalmology. (2024a). *Amblyopia.* EyeWiki. https://eyewiki.org/Amblyopia

American Academy of Ophthalmology. (2024b). *Coloboma.* EyeWiki. https://eyewiki.org/Coloboma

American Academy of Ophthalmology. (2024c). *Craniosynostosis syndromes.* EyeWiki. https://eyewiki.org/Cranio synostosis_Syndromes

American Academy of Ophthalmology. (2024d). *Fetal alcohol.* EyeWiki. https://eyewiki.org/Fetal_Alcohol

American Academy of Ophthalmology. (2024e). *Goldenhar syndrome.* EyeWiki. https://eyewiki.org/Goldenhar_Syndrome

American Academy of Ophthalmology. (2024f). *Neuroblastoma.* EyeWiki. https://eyewiki.aao.org/Neuroblastoma

American Academy of Ophthalmology. (2024g). *Nystagmus.* EyeWiki. https://eyewiki.aao.org/Nystagmus

American Academy of Ophthalmology. (2024h). *Optic nerve hypoplasia.* EyeWiki. https://eyewiki.aao.org/Optic_Nerve_Hypoplasia

American Academy of Ophthalmology. (2024i). *Primary congenital glaucoma.* EyeWiki. https://eyewiki.aao.org/Primary_Congenital_Glaucoma

American Academy of Ophthalmology. (2024j). *Retinoblastoma.* EyeWiki. https://eyewiki.aao.org/Retinoblastoma

American Academy of Ophthalmology. (2024k). *Retinopathy of prematurity*. EyeWiki. https://eyewiki.aao.org/Retinopathy_of_Prematurity

American Academy of Ophthalmology. (2024l). *Rhabdomyosarcoma*. EyeWiki. https://eyewiki.org/Rhabdomyosarcoma

American Academy of Ophthalmology. (2024m). *Trisomy 13*. EyeWiki. https://eyewiki.org/Trisomy_13

Centers for Disease Control and Prevention. (2024a). *Fetal alcohol spectrum disorders (FASDs)*. https://www.cdc.gov/fasd/index.html

Centers for Disease Control and Prevention. (2024b). *Trends and characteristics in maternal syphilis rates during pregnancy: United States, 2016–2022*. https://cdc.gov/nchs/products/databriefs/db496.htm

Chan-Ling, T., Gole, G. A., Quinn, G. E., Adamson, S. J., & Darlow, B. A. (2018). Pathophysiology, screening and treatment of ROP: A multidisciplinary perspective. *Progress in Retinal and Eye Research, 62*, 77–119. https://doi.org/10.1016/j.preteyeres.2017.09.002

Chiang, M. F., Quinn, G. E., Fielder, A. R., Ostmo, S. R., Paul Chan, R. V., Berrocal, A., Binenbaum, G., Blair, M., Peter Campbell, J., Capone, A., Jr, Chen, Y., Dai, S., Ells, A., Fleck, B. W., Good, W. V., Elizabeth Hartnett, M., Holmstrom, G., Kusaka, S., Kychenthal, A., Lepore, D., ... Zin, A. (2021). International classification of retinopathy of prematurity, third edition. *Ophthalmology, 128*(10), e51–e68. https://doi.org/10.1016/j.ophtha.2021.05.031

Choodinatha, H. K., Jeon, M. R., Choi, B. Y., Lee, K.-N., Kim, H. J., & Park, J. Y. (2023). Cytomegalovirus infection during pregnancy. *Obstetrics & Gynecology Science, 66*(6), 463–476. https://doi.org/10.5468/ogs.23117

Cruess, A., & Sharma, S. (2018). Tuberous sclerosis and the eye. In A. Schachat (Ed.), *Ryan's retina* (6th ed., pp. 2438–2445). Elsevier.

Cummings, J. J., Polin, R. A., & Committee on Fetus and Newborn. (2016). Oxygen targeting in extremely low birth weight infants. *Pediatrics (Evanston), 138*(6). https://doi.org/10.1542/peds.2016-2904

Curtin, S. C., & Matthews, T. J. (2016). Smoking prevalence and cessation before and during pregnancy: Data from the birth certificate, 2014. *National Vital Statistics Reports, 65*(1), 1–13. https://www.cdc.gov/nchs/data/nvsr/nvsr65/nvsr65_01.pdf

Eldweik, L., & Mantagos, I. S. (2016). Role of VEGF inhibition in the treatment of retinopathy of prematurity. *Seminars in Ophthalmology, 31*(1-2), 163-168. https://doi.org/10.3109/08820538.2015.1114847

Dallalzadeh, L. O., Robillard, E. G., Goodyear, K., & Khitri, M. R. (2023). Eyelid, orbital, and lacrimal disorders in the neonate. *NeoReviews, 24*(10), e616–e625.

Diniz, D., Taguchi, F., & Schor, P. (2025). Optics. In L. A. Levin, P. L. Kaufman, & M. E. Hartnett (Eds.), *Adler's physiology of the eye* (12th ed., pp. 1a–26). Elsevier.

Fernandes, M., Yang, X., Li, J. Y., & Cheikh Ismail, L. (2015). Smoking during pregnancy and vision difficulties in children: A systematic review. *Acta Ophthalmologica, 93*(3), 213–223. https://doi.org/10.1111/aos.12627

Fierson, W. M., American Academy of Pediatrics Section on Ophthalmology, American Academy of Ophthalmology, American Association for Pediatric Ophthalmology and Strabismus, & American Association of Certified Orthoptists. (2018). Screening examination of premature infants for retinopathy of prematurity. *Pediatrics, 142*(6), e20183061. https://doi.org/10.1542/peds.2018-3061

Genetic and Rare Diseases Information Center. (2025a). *CHARGE syndrome*. https://rarediseases.info.nih.gov/diseases/29/charge-syndrome

Genetic and Rare Diseases Information Center. (2025b). *Cornelia de Lange syndrome*. https://rarediseases.info.nih.gov/diseases/10109/cornelia-de-lange-syndrome

Genetic and Rare Diseases Information Center. (2025c). *Neurofibromatosis*. https://rarediseases.info.nih.gov/diseases/10420/neurofibromatosis

Genetic and Rare Diseases Information Center. (2025d). *Isolated Pierre-Robin syndrome*. https://rarediseases.info.nih.gov/diseases/4347/pierre-robin-sequence

Genetic and Rare Diseases Information Center. (2025d). *Complete trisomy 13 syndrome*. https://rarediseases.info.nih.gov/diseases/7341/trisomy-13

Genetic and Rare Diseases Information Center. (2025f). *Trisomy 18*. https://rarediseases.info.nih.gov/diseases/6321/trisomy-18

Genetic and Rare Diseases Information Center. (2025g). *Turner syndrome*. https://rarediseases.info.nih.gov/diseases/7831/turner-syndrome

Genetic and Rare Diseases Information Center. (2025h). *Waardenburg syndrome*. https://rarediseases.info.nih.gov/diseases/5525/waardenburg-syndrome

Genetic and Rare Diseases Information Center. (2025i). *11p partial monosomy syndrome*. https://rarediseases.info.nih.gov/diseases/5528/wagr-syndrome

Good, W. V., Ferriero, D. M., Golabi, M., & Kobori, J. A. (1992). Abnormalities of the visual system in infants exposed to cocaine. *Ophthalmology, 99*(3), 341–346. https://doi.org/10.1016/S0161-6420(92)31967-0

Gosling, J. A., Harris, P. F., Humpherson, J. R., Whitmore, I., & Willan, P. L. T. (2016). *Human anatomy: Color atlas and textbook* (6th ed.). Elsevier.

Greene, A. K., Taber, S. F., Ball, K. L., Padwa, B. L., & Mulliken, J. B. (2009). Sturge–Weber syndrome: Soft-tissue and skeletal overgrowth. *Journal of Craniofacial Surgery, 20*, 617–621. https://doi.org/10.1097/SCS.0b013e318192988e

Guerrero-Moreno, A., Baudouin, C., Parsadaniantz, S. M., & Réaux-Le Goazigo, A. (2020). Morphological and functional changes of corneal nerves and their contribution to peripheral and central sensory abnormalities. *Frontiers in Cellular Neuroscience, 14*, 1–17. https://doi.org/10.3389/fncel.2020.610342

Gundlach, B. S., Kokhanov, A., Altendahl, M., Suh, S. Y., Fung, S., Demer, J., Pineles, S., Khitri, M., Chu, A., & Tsui, I. (2022). Real-world visual outcomes of laser and anti-VEGF treatments for retinopathy of prematurity. *American Journal of Ophthalmology, 238*, 86–96. https://doi.org/10.1016/j.ajo.2021.11.015

Heidar, K., & Tropathi, P. (2025). *Cataracts in children, congenital and acquired*. https://eyewiki.org/Cataracts_in_Children,_Congenital_and_Acquired

Hughes, S., Yang, H., & Chan-Ling, T. (2000). Vascularization of the human fetal retina: Roles of vasculogenesis and angiogenesis. *Investigative Ophthalmology & Visual Science, 41*(5), 1217–1228.

Ikeda, T., Ishikawa, H., Shimizu, K., Asakawa, K., & Goseki, T. (2015). Pupillary size and light reflex in premature infants.

Neuro-Ophthalmology, 39(4), 175–178. https://doi.org/10.3109/01658107.2015.1055363

Jones, K. L., Jones, M. C., & Del Campo, C. M. (2022). *Smith's recognizable patterns of human malformation* (8th ed.). Elsevier.

Kajdic, N., Spazzapan, P., & Velnar, T. (2018). Craniosynostosis: Recognition, clinical characteristics, and treatment. *Bosnian Journal of Basic Medical Sciences, 18*(2), 110–116. https://doi.org/10.17305/bjbms.2017.2083

Kaur, S., Jain, S., Sodhi, H. B. S., Rastogi, A., & Kamlesh. (2013). Optic nerve hypoplasia. *Oman Journal of Ophthalmology, 6*(2), 77–82. https://doi.org/10.4103/0974-620X.116622

Khazaeni, L. M. (2017). Ocular complications of congenital infections, *NeoReviews, 18*(2), e100–e104. https://doi.org/10.1542/neo.18-2-e100

Kieffer, F., Wallon, M., Garcia, P., Thulliez, P., Peyron, F., & Franck, J. (2008). Risk factors for retinochoroiditis during the first 2 years of life in infants with treated congenital toxoplasmosis. *Pedaitric Infectious Disease, 27*(1), 27–32. https://doi.org/10.1097/INF.0b013e318134286d

Kim, S. J., Port, A. D., Swan, R., Campbell, J. P., Chan, R. V. P., & Chiang, M. F. (2018). Retinopathy of prematurity: A review of risk factors and their clinical significance. *Survey of Ophthalmology, 63*, 618–637. https://doi.org/10.1016/j.survophthal.2018.04.002

Lam, M., & Suh, D. (2022). Screening, diagnosis, and treatment of pediatric ocular diseases. *Children, 9*(12), 1939. https://doi.org/10.3390/children9121939

Lamb, T. D., & Kefalov, V. J. (2025). Light adaptation in photoreceptors. In L. A. Levin, P. L. Kaufman, & M. E. Hartnett (Eds.), *Adler's physiology of the eye* (12th ed., pp. 451–463). Elsevier.

MacLeish, P. R., & Makino, C. L. (2025). Photoresponses of rods and cones. In L. A. Levin, P. L. Kaufman, & M. E. Hartnett (Eds.), *Adler's physiology of the eye* (12th ed., pp. 432–450). Elsevier.

Maldonado, Y., Nizet, V., Barnett, E. D., Edwards, K. M., & Malley, R. (2025). *Remington and Klein's infectious diseases of the fetus and newborn* (9th ed.). Elsevier Saunders

Michaels, M. G., Sánchez, P. J., & Lin, P. L. (2024). Congenital toxoplasmosis, syphilis, malaria, and tuberculosis. In C. A. Gleason & T. Sawyer (Eds.), *Avery's diseases of the newborn* (11th ed.). Elsevier.

Moosajee, M., Hingorani, M., & Moore, A. T. (2018). *PAX6*-related aniridia. In M. P. Adam, J. Feldman, G. M. Mirzaa, R. A. Pagon, S. E. Wallace, & A. Amemiya (Eds.), *GeneReviews* (pp. 487–511). University of Washington. https://www.ncbi.nlm.nih.gov/books/NBK1360

Nanda, D., & Sarkar, M. (2022). Efficacy of lacrimal sac massage in management of congenital nasolacrimal duct obstruction in infants: An observational study of 853 cases from a single institute of eastern Asia. *Middle East African Journal of Ophthalmology, 29*(4), 216–219. https://doi.org/10.4103/meajo.meajo_122_23

National Institutes of Health. (2016). *Pierre Robin sequence*. Medline Plus. https://medlineplus.gov/genetics/condition/isolated-pierre-robin-sequence/#statistics

National Institutes of Health. (2017). *CHARGE syndrome*. Medline Plus. https://medlineplus.gov/genetics/condition/charge-syndrome

National Institutes of Health. (2018). *Sturge-Weber syndrome*. Medline Plus. https://medlineplus.gov/genetics/condition/sturge-weber-syndrome/#statistics

National Institutes of Health. (2020a). *Down syndrome*. Medline Plus. https://medlineplus.gov/genetics/condition/down-syndrome/#statistics

National Institutes of Health. (2020b). *Neurofibromatosis type 1*. Medline Plus. https://medlineplus.gov/genetics/condition/neurofibromatosis-type-1/#statistics

National Institutes of Health. (2021). *Trisomy 13*. Medline Plus. https://medlineplus.gov/genetics/condition/trisomy-13

National Institutes of Health. (2022a). *Cornelia de Lange syndrome*. Medline Plus. https://medlineplus.gov/genetics/condition/cornelia-de-lange-syndrome/#inheritance

National Institutes of Health. (2022b). *Leber congenital amaurosis*. Medline Plus. https://medlineplus.gov/genetics/condition/leber-congenital-amaurosis

National Institutes of Health. (2022c). *Tuberous sclerosis complex*. Medline Plus. https://medlineplus.gov/genetics/condition/tuberous-sclerosis-complex

National Institutes of Health. (2022d). *Waardenburg syndrome*. Medline Plus. https://medlineplus.gov/genetics/condition/waardenburg-syndrome/#statistics

National Institutes of Health. (2023a). *Turner syndrome*. Medline Plus. https://medlineplus.gov/genetics/condition/turner-syndrome/#statistics

National Institutes of Health. (2023b). *WAGR syndrome*. Medline Plus. https://medlineplus.gov/genetics/condition/wagr-syndrome

Norcia, A. M. (2025). Development of vision in infancy. In L. A. Levin, P. L. Kaufman, & M. E. Hartnett (Eds.), *Adler's physiology of the eye* (12th ed., pp. 735–747). Elsevier.

Oatts, J. T., De Alba Campomanes, A. G., & Binenbaum, G. (2024). Eye and vision disorders. In C. A. Gleason & T. Sawyer (Eds.), *Avery's diseases of the newborn* (11th ed., pp. 1391–1413). Elsevier.

Örge, F. H., & Selem, Z. M. (2025). Examination and common problems of the neonatal eye. In R. J. Martin & A. A. Fanaroff (Eds.), *Fanaroff and Martin's neonatal–perinatal medicine* (12th ed., pp. 2028–2063). Saunders/Elsevier.

Orkin, S. H., Nathan, D. G., Ginsburg, D., Look, A. T., Fisher, D. E., & Lux, S. (Eds.). (2015). *Nathan and Oski's hematology and oncology of infancy and childhood* (8th ed.). Saunders.

Peragallo, J., Biousse, V., & Newman, N. J. (2013). Ocular manifestations of drug and alcohol abuse. *Current Opinion in Ophthalmology, 24*(6), 566–573. https://doi.org/10.1097/ICU.0b013e3283654db2

Persaud, T. V. N., & Torchia, M. G. (2025). *The developing human* (12th ed.). Elsevier.

Purves, D., Augustine, G. J., Fitzpatrick, D., Hall, W. C., LaMantia, A.-S., Mooney, R. D., Platt, M. L., & White, L. E. (Eds.). (2018). *Neuroscience* (6th ed.). Sinauer Associates.

Richards, A., & Guzman-Cottrill, J. A. (2010). Conjunctivitis. *Pediatrics in Review, 31*(5), 196–208. https://doi.org/10.1542/pir.31-5-196

Schoenwolf, G. C., Bleyl, S. B., Brauer, P. R., & Francis-West, P. H. (2021). *Larsen's human embryology* (6th ed.). Churchill Livingstone.

Shah, P. K., Prabhu, V., Karandikar, S. S., Ranjan, R., Narendran, V., & Kalpana, N. (2016). Retinopathy of prematurity: Past, present and future. *World Journal of Clinical Pediatrics, 5*(1), 35–46. https://doi.org/10.5409/wjcp.v5.i1.35

Stokes, C., & Melvin, A. J. (2024). Viral infections of the fetus and newborn. In C. A. Gleason & T. Sawyer (Eds.), *Avery's diseases of the newborn* (11th ed., pp. 450–486). Elsevier.

Sujansky, E., & Conradi, S. (1995). Outcome of Sturge–Weber syndrome in 52 adults. *American Journal of Medical Genetics Part A, 57*(1), 35–45. https://doi.org/10.1002/ajmg.1320570110

Sun, Y., Hellström, A., & Smith, L. E. H. (2025). Retinopathy of prematurity. In R. J. Martin, A. A. Fanaroff, & M. C. Walsh (Eds.), *Fanaroff and Martin's neonatal–perinatal medicine: Diseases of the fetus and infant* (12th ed., pp. 6944–6975). Saunders/Elsevier.

Terry, T. L. (1942). Fibroblastic overgrowth of persistent tunica vasculosa lentis in infants born prematurely: II. Report of cases—Clinical aspects. *Transactions of the American Ophthalmological Society, 40*, 262–284. https://www.ncbi.nlm.nih.gov/pmc/articles/PMC1315050/pdf/taos00059-0283.pdf

Waardenburg, P. J. (1951). A new syndrome combining developmental anomalies of the eyelids, eyebrows and nose root with pigmentary anomalies of the iris and head hair and with congenital deafness. *American Journal of Human Genetics, 3*(3), 195–253. https://www.ncbi.nlm.nih.gov/pmc/articles/PMC1716407/pdf/ajhg00426-0007.pdf

Wallon, M., Garweg, J. G., Abrahamowicz, M., Cornu, C., Vinault, S., Quantin, C., Bonithon-Kopp, C., Picot, S., Peyron, F., & Binquet, C. (2014). Ophthalmic outcomes of congenital toxoplasmosis followed until adolescence. *Pediatrics, 133*(3), e601–e608. https://doi.org/10.1542/peds.2013-2153

Wensel, T. G. (2025). Biochemical cascade of phototransduction. In L. A. Levin, S. F. P. L. Kaufman, & M. E. Hartnett (Eds.), *Adler's physiology of the eye* (12th ed., pp. 414a–431). Elsevier.

Werner, J. S., & Chalupa, L. M. (Eds.). (2014). *The new visual neurosciences*. MIT Press.

World Health Organization. (2023). *Blindness and vision impairment*. https://www.who.int/news-room/fact-sheets/detail/blindness-and-visual-impairment

Wu, S. M. (2025). Signal processing in the outer retina. In L. A. Levin, P. L. Kaufman, & M. E. Hartnett (Eds.), *Adler's physiology of the eye* (12th ed., pp. 480-494). Elsevier.

Yan, A. P., Venkatramani, R., Bradley, J. A., Lautz, T. B., Urla, C. I., Merks, J. H. M., & Oberoi, S. (2023). Clinical characteristics, treatment considerations, and outcomes of infants with rhabdomyosarcoma. *Cancers, 15*(8), 2296–2311. https://doi.org/10.3390/cancers15082296

Zitelli, B. J., McIntire, S., Nowalk, A. J., & Garrison, J. (Eds.). (2023). *Zitelli and Davis' atlas of pediatric physical diagnosis* (8th ed.). Saunders/Elsevier.

III

TRANSITION TO EXTRAUTERINE LIFE

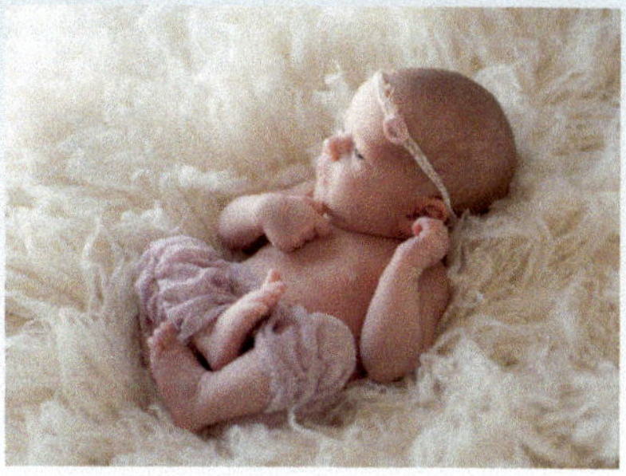

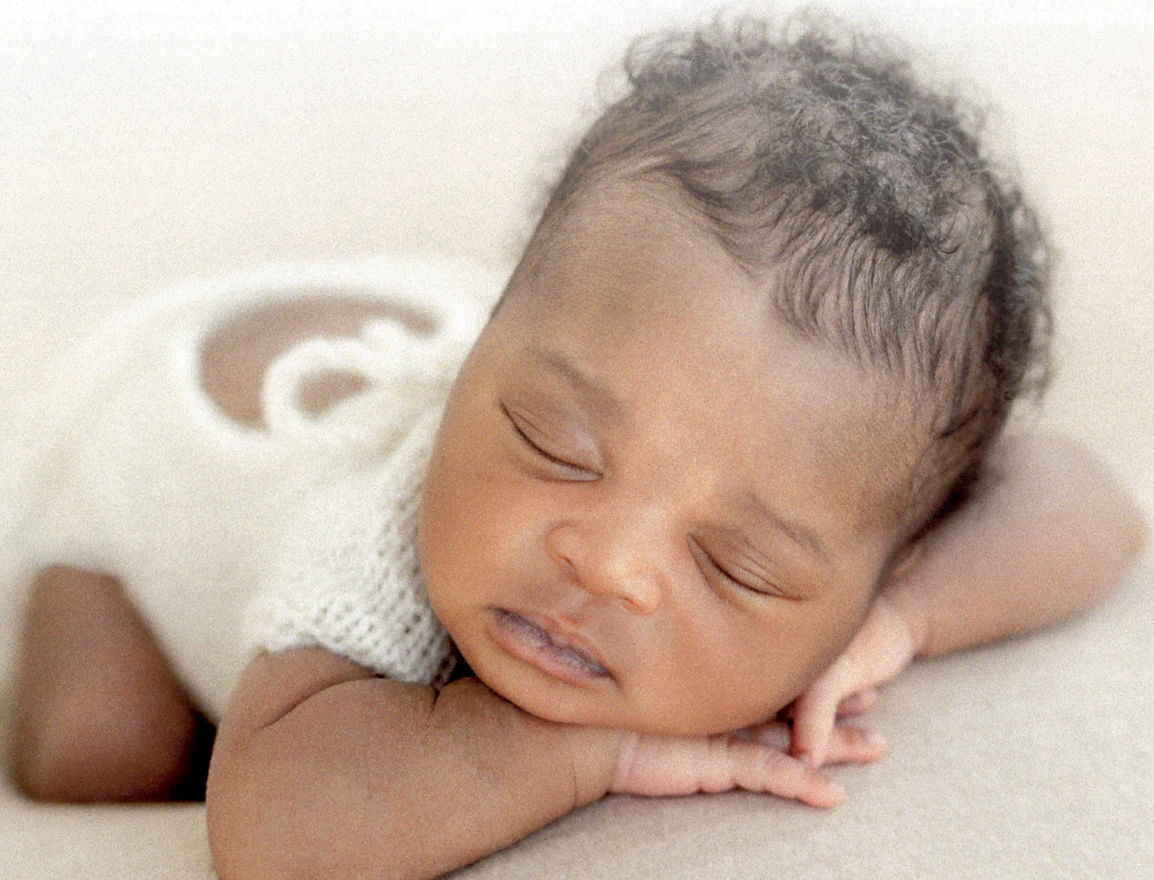

14

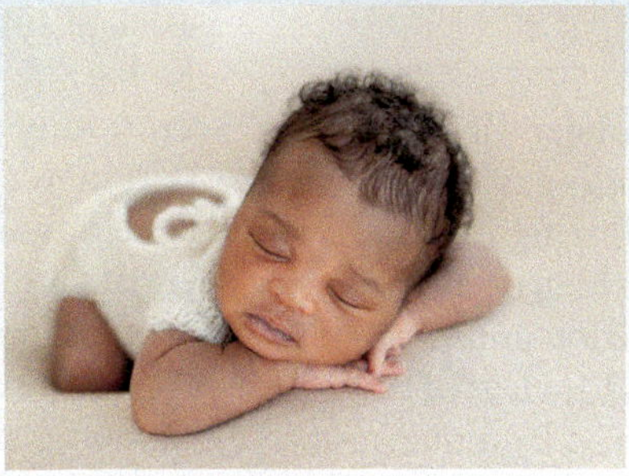

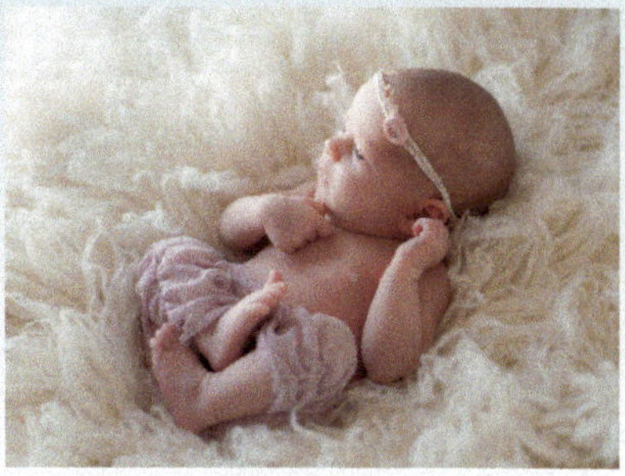

THE BIOLOGY OF BIRTH, PERIPARTUM RISKS, AND HYPOXIC-ISCHEMIC INJURY IN THE TERM NEWBORN

Amy J. Jnah and Jennifer Fitzgerald

LEARNING OBJECTIVES

After completing this chapter, the reader should be able to:

- Review the role of cardiovascular development in overall fetal growth and development.
- Review the cardiorespiratory transition from intrauterine to extrauterine life.
- Identify factors that influence the neonate's transition to extrauterine life.
- Analyze indications for and implications of an emergent cesarean delivery.
- Analyze indications for and implications of an operative vaginal delivery.
- Recognize common contraindications for spontaneous and operative vaginal deliveries.
- Differentiate among risk factors, pathophysiology, clinical findings, and long-term effects of common pathologies that arise during the peripartum period and affect the fetus and neonate.
- Identify appropriate means to assess for common birth injuries in neonates.

INTRODUCTION

The transition from placenta-dependent to postnatal life is a complex and vulnerable period for all newborns. All organ systems must quickly adjust to postnatal life; however, the establishment of placenta-independent cardiovascular and respiratory function is the most immediate and necessary adaptation, and contingent upon the first postnatal breath. Extrauterine adaptation is influenced by epigenetic, genetic, chronic maternal health, prenatal, and intrapartum-related complications, as well as the gestational age of the fetus at the time of delivery. In fact, a fetus subject to acute or prolonged interruptions in uterine blood flow is at increased risk for a pathologic transition to extrauterine life and neurologic morbidity. In addition, the delivery method may implicate the transition to extrauterine life, and in some circumstances injure the fetus. Neonatal APRNs are expected to recognize maternal, fetal, and intrapartum risk factors that increase the likelihood for an altered transition to extrauterine life. These risk assessments help ensure that proper personnel are immediately available during and after the birth process, to reduce the high burden of neonatal mortality and morbidity.

THE BIOLOGY OF BIRTH

Placental and fetal circulation have been described in prior chapters to establish understanding of the genesis of fetal blood flow and its function during intrauterine development; however, use of a spiral curriculum is essential to promote knowledge acquisition and retention. Therefore, we present an abbreviated review of normal placental and fetal circulation, followed by a discussion of the biology of labor, circulatory transition to extrauterine life, and common factors that may compromise fetal blood flow, oxygenation, and an otherwise healthy transition to life outside the womb.

Review of the Placental and Fetal Circulations

Although the heart technically marks the starting point for fetal circulation, beginning a review with oxygen uptake and flow at the placenta is often ideal for student learners (**Figure 14.1**). Recall from Chapter 2 that freshly oxygenated blood travels down the spiral arteries and enters the uterus at the intervillous space. Oxygen and nutrients are transferred from the maternal side of the placenta into capillaries within chorionic villi on the fetal side of the placenta. These capillaries converge to form the umbilical vein, which delivers the highest amount of oxygen molecules (70%–80% saturation) to the fetal circulation and overall provides approximately 40% of total fetal cardiac output (Goldsmith, 2025; M. K. Park & Salamat, 2021). While this blood oxygen saturation is considerably lower than acceptable postnatal parameters, it does not compromise fetal growth and development. The fetus compensates by increasing renal erythropoietin production (which increases blood cell production and mean cell volume), utilizing hemoglobin F (which increases placental oxygen uptake and carrying capacity) and maintaining a lower energy expenditure and rate of oxygen consumption than that of newborns (Brown et al., 2024).

Recall from Chapters 4 and 5 that fetal circulation relies upon the patency of four critical shunts: (a) the placenta, (b) ductus venosus, (c) foramen ovale, and (d) ductus arteriosus to function as a circuit. Once blood flow from the umbilical vein reaches the liver, it splits. A lesser proportion of this well-oxygenated blood flow enters the hepatic circulation. A greater proportion of this well-oxygenated blood flow enters the ductus venosus and preferentially streams across the foramen ovale, into the left atrium and left ventricle, and finally out to the brain and peripheral tissues by way of the aorta (Brown et al., 2024; M. K. Park & Salamat, 2021).

In addition, deoxygenated blood returning to the heart from the systemic circulation, by way of the inferior vena cava, superior vena cava, and the coronary system, is deposited into the right atrium. This blood preferentially streams into the right ventricle and pulmonary artery. From there, the majority of blood flow shunts across the

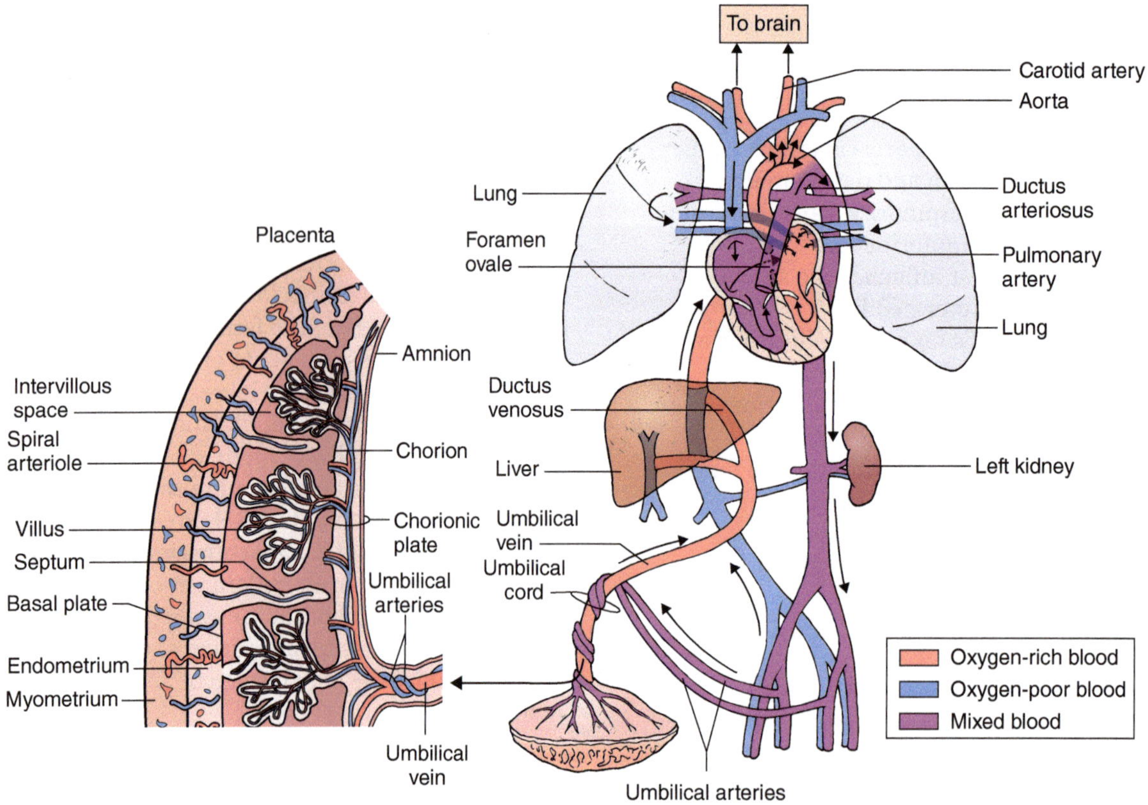

Figure 14.1 Anatomy of maternal-fetal circulatory pathway.

ductus arteriosus and into the descending aorta, in order to perfuse the lower body organs and extremities (Figure 14.2). Around 10% of fetal blood flows through the right or left pulmonary artery to the lungs, providing nutrients to the developing lung tissue.

Placental and Fetal Circulation During Labor

Human labor integrates a complex set of changes within the uterus and fetal membranes that occur over a period of days to weeks. Changes include an increase in prostaglandin synthesis, an increased uptake of oxytocin receptors, fetal influence on placental steroid hormone production, and secretion of multiple hormones that stimulate prostaglandin synthesis. The interplay of these physiologic and hormonal changes is termed a *parturition cascade.*

Labor can alter normal placental and fetal blood flow. The onset of labor and subsequent contractions of the uterine wall compresses the myometrium and the umbilical vessels. During normal labor, intrauterine pressures do not compromise gas exchange within the placenta and do not endanger the fetus. However, changes in placental resistance can reduce placental blood flow and favor hypoxemia and/or ischemia. Recall that flow within the umbilical circuit is determined by cardiac force (blood pressure and kinetic energy) as well as vascular resistance (geometry and viscosity; Mir & Rosenfeld, 2021). Blood flow to the fetus is temporarily decreased with uterine contractions, with the time in between contractions utilized as a "recovery period" for the fetus as transplacental gas exchange normalizes. As labor progresses and contractions continue, the cumulative effect of contraction-induced temporary interruptions in gas exchange can manifest in the fetus as hypercapnia and hypoxia with mild/transient metabolic acidosis. However, in cases that prohibit a normal recovery period, involve altered vascular resistance and decreased blood flow, or feature a perinatal sentinel event, the fetus may be subject to pathologic hypoxia–ischemia and show an intolerance of labor; expedited delivery will be necessary (Goldsmith, 2025).

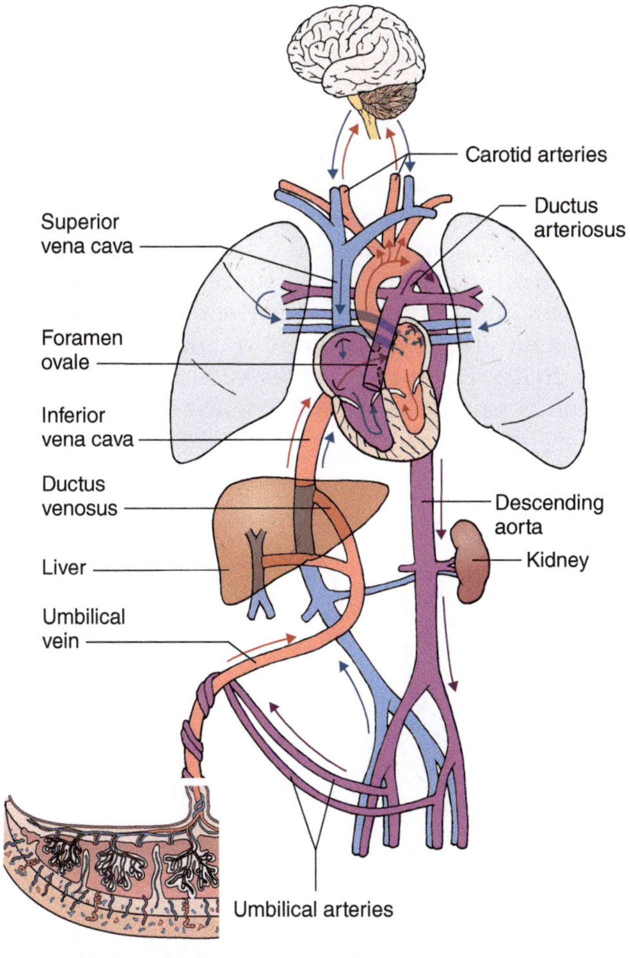

Figure 14.2 Directional blood flow within fetal circulation.

Review: Cardiovascular and Pulmonary Transition to Postnatal Life

The most critical step in accomplishing the pulmonary transition from intrauterine to extrauterine life is the conversion of the lung from a fluid-filled to air-filled organ capable of gas exchange. With the onset of labor, the tissues change from fluid production to fluid absorption, using active transport to draw fluid into the interstitium and allow for air to fill the lungs. The first breath, typically elicited with routine drying and stimulation (which activates peripheral and central chemoreceptors), induces forced expansion of the lungs and increases the partial pressure of oxygen (PaO_2). These changes accelerate the normal reabsorption of fetal lung fluid. In term newborns, all fluid is typically cleared from the lungs within the first 5 breaths (spontaneous or assisted; Goldsmith, 2025).

Clamping of the umbilical cord also activates peripheral and central chemoreceptors and elicits an increase in systemic vascular resistance (SVR). As this occurs, left atrial pressure increases and exceeds right atrial pressure. This change in pressure elicits functional closure of both the foramen ovale and ductus arteriosus.

Clinical Application. Recent data suggest that spontaneously breathing term newborns exhibit one to three unique breaths immediately after birth. These breaths are characterized by short inhalations with high inspiratory pressure, short inspiratory time, and extended expiratory time (with high expiratory pressure). This respiratory pattern helps to force any remaining fetal lung fluid into the interstitium. When resuscitating a term, apneic newborn who requires positive pressure ventilation, it is important to provide adequate inflating pressure with the first few breaths to open the lungs and establish functional residual capacity. The clinician providing positive pressure ventilation must confirm chest wall movement and execute corrective ventilation steps in a timely manner to facilitate the transition to extrauterine life.

NOTEWORTHY DISEASES IN THE PREGNANT PATIENT AND KNOWN EFFECTS UPON THE INTRAPARTUM PERIOD

Placenta Previa

Placenta previa, a condition of abnormal placentation in which the internal cervical os is completely or nearly covered by placental tissue, is often characterized by its classic symptom of painless vaginal bleeding. The incidence is estimated at 5.2 per 1,000 live births (Jenabi et al., 2022). Risk factors for placenta previa include prior cesarean delivery, assisted reproductive technology (e.g., in vitro pregnancy), prior abortion, male fetus, smoking, advanced maternal age, and multiple-gestation pregnancy (Cresswell et al., 2013; Francois & Foley, 2017; Jenabi et al., 2022; Oyelese & Smulian, 2006; Walfisch & Sheiner, 2016).

Placenta previa can be classified as complete or marginal (**Figure 14.3**). Complete placenta previa is diagnosed when the internal opening of the cervix or internal cervical os is entirely covered by the placenta. However, in cases in which the placenta does not cover the cervical os but is attached within 2 to 3 cm from the opening, the condition is categorized as marginal placenta previa. The pathogenesis relates to thinning of the uterine wall that normally occurs during the third trimester. Typically, placental implantation will take place in the fundus, as opposed to implantation occurring in the lower segment, as seen with placenta previa. When this occurs, thinning continues at the site of implantation, causing interruption in placental attachment as the uterus prepares for labor. As a result, hemorrhage may occur and persist from the inability of the thin-walled uterus to constrict bleeding vessels. This may create a cycle of bleeding that stimulates uterine contractions, which are followed by continued bleeding. As labor progresses and causes cervical change in the form of dilation and effacement, the potential for hemorrhage increases from continued separation of the placenta from the uterine wall (Oyelese & Smulian, 2006; Walfisch & Sheiner, 2016).

Placenta previa is associated with a higher risk for preterm delivery, emergency delivery, and/or the use of general anesthesia. Adverse neonatal outcomes that have been reported in the literature include hypoglycemia, NICU admission, hyperbilirubinemia requiring phototherapy, respiratory distress syndrome, and exposure to mechanical ventilation (Levin et al., 2021).

Abruptio Placentae/Placental Abruption

Abruptio placentae, a condition of abnormal placentation, occurs when separation of the placenta takes place prior to childbirth (**Figure 14.4**). The incidence of abruptio placentae is approximately 1% worldwide, but the mortality risk is 10% (Bączkowska et al., 2022). This condition, also known as *placental abruption*, involves separation of a normally implanted placenta from the uterus and typically takes place in the third trimester of pregnancy, but may be diagnosed any time after 20 weeks of gestation. The separation of the placenta from the uterine wall often occurs as a result of bleeding, which has great potential to develop into a life-threatening hemorrhage. Risk factors include a prior history of placental abruption (10-fold to 93-fold recurrence risk), hypertensive disorders of pregnancy, underweight, advanced age at conception, adolescent pregnancy, illicit drug use, concurrent polyhydramnios or placenta previa, and uterine trauma (Bączkowska et al., 2022). Hallmark manifestations include sharp abdominal pain (70% of cases), uterine contractions,

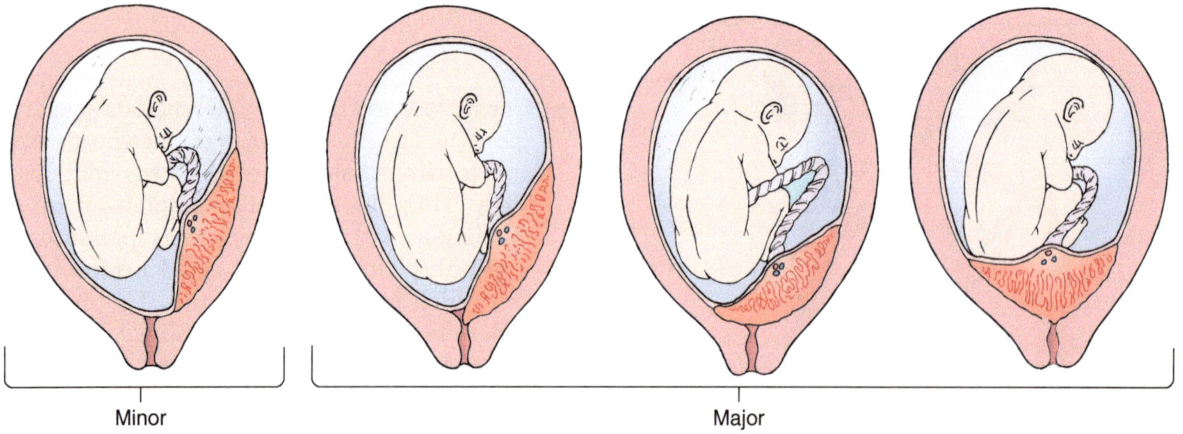

Figure 14.3 Placenta previa. Classification into "major" and "minor" placenta previa depends on the distance of the placenta from the internal os. It is also important to note whether the placenta is anterior or posterior, as cesarean section is more difficult through an anterior placenta.

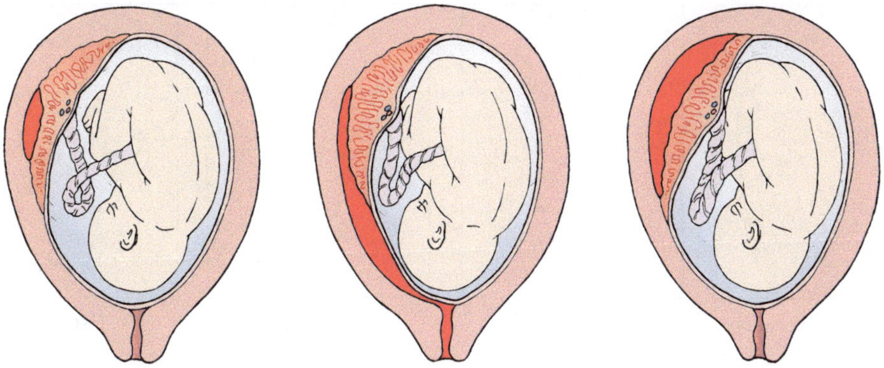

Figure 14.4 Abruptio placentae.

tenderness, fetal heart rate (FHR) abnormalities (75% of cases), and vaginal bleeding (35%–80% of cases; Hiersch et al., 2017).

The pathogenesis involves rupture of maternal or fetal–placental vessels located in the decidua basalis. The accumulation of blood from hemorrhage acts to separate layers of the decidua from the maternal side of the placenta. Further separation may ensue from the formation of a decidual hematoma. As a result, placental tissue in the detached area is destroyed and unable to facilitate gas exchange, provide nutrients, or eliminate waste, each of which may contribute to fetal compromise (Ananth et al., 2016; Tikkanen et al., 2013).

Fetal and neonatal risks include preterm birth, small for gestational age status, hypoxia–ischemia, and death. The risk for poor fetal outcomes is inversely proportional to gestational age at birth (Bączkowska et al., 2022).

Placenta Accreta Spectrum

Placenta accreta spectrum disorders are conditions involving an abnormal degree of invasion of trophoblasts of the placenta into the uterine myometrium (American College of Obstetricians and Gynecologists [ACOG], 2021). The incidence of this spectrum has increased in recent years, occurring in nearly one in 272 births, due to the overall increase in cesarean delivery, which is a significant risk factor for development of the condition (ACOG, 2021).

Three possible presentations can arise: placenta accreta, increta, or percreta (**Figure 14.5**). Placenta accreta involves a superficial invasion of trophoblast cells into the myometrium. Placenta percreta involves a deep invasion of trophoblast cells into the myometrium. Placenta increta involves a deep invasion of trophoblast cells into the myometrium with involvement of adjacent structures. The most significant risk factors for any of these presentations is prior cesarean delivery, placenta previa, advanced age at conception, multiparity, prior obstetric surgery or curettage, and Asherman syndrome (ACOG, 2021).

Neonatal providers should be cognizant of fetal risks associated with placenta accreta spectrum, with the most severe being uterine rupture and hemorrhage. Hemorrhage that occurs as a result of conditions related to abnormal placentation has a great potential to alter uteroplacental circulation, thus reducing fetal oxygen supply. This gives rise to a nonreassuring fetal heart rate (FHR) pattern, which is identified by way of cardiotocography (electronic fetal monitoring). When maternal and/or fetal compromise arise from conditions causing obstetric hemorrhage, emergent cesarean delivery may be carried out in an effort to optimize birth outcomes (ACOG, 2021).

Chorioamnionitis ("Triple I")

Intraamniotic infection, *chorioamnionitis*, or *Triple I* are terms used to describe an infectious process affecting approximately 2% to 5% of all pregnancies that leads to inflammation of any of the following: the placenta, decidua, amniotic fluid, fetal membranes, or fetus (ACOG, 2022a). The term "Triple I" more recently originated from the National Institute of Child Health and Human Development (NICHD) as the more appropriate term for this disease because it can be associated with intrauterine inflammation and a confirmed infection, or intrauterine inflammation with no confirmed microorganism (Jain et al., 2022). When microorganisms (aerobic or anaerobic) are involved, they typically originate from the vaginal canal and translocate in an ascending manner into the amniotic cavity (ACOG, 2022a). Pathogens thereby enter the intrauterine space and invade the gestational membranes (maternal decidua and fetal chorion and amnion). This invokes a proinflammatory response that disrupts normal placental transfer of nutrients and other placental barriers that should protect the fetus (Greenberg et al., 2014). In aggregate, this facilitates weakening and invasion of the maternal decidua, followed by invasion of the fetal chorion and amnionic cavity (Anders et al., 2017).

The ACOG (2022a) separates the clinical manifestations of Triple I into three possible diagnostic categories: isolated maternal fever, suspected Triple I, and confirmed Triple I. *Isolated maternal fever* is defined as one (single) maternal oral temperature greater than 39°C or abnormal temperatures greater than 38°C for longer than 30 minutes. *Suspected Triple I* is defined as maternal

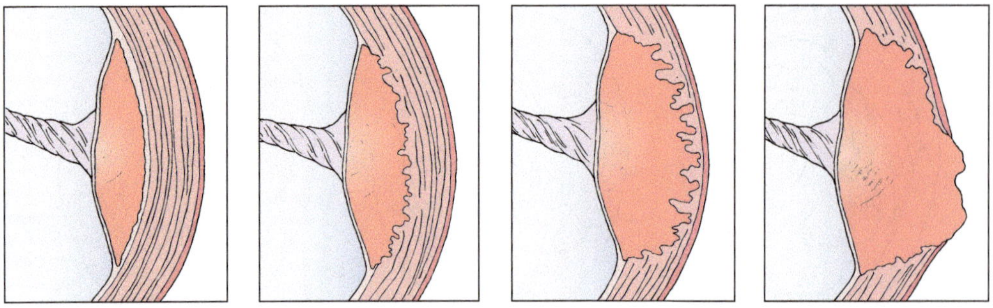

Figure 14.5 Placenta accreta, increta, and percreta.

fever and one or more of the following findings: leukocytosis, purulent cervical drainage, or fetal tachycardia. *Confirmed Triple I* is defined as a positive amniotic fluid test result or positive placental pathology report. Common pathogens associated with Triple I include *Mycoplasma, Ureaplasma*, Group B *Streptococcus* (GBS), *Toxoplasma gondii, Listeria monocytogenes, Treponema pallidum*, parvovirus, HIV, varicella zoster virus, rubella, cytomegalovirus, herpes virus 1 and 2, Zika virus, and *plasmodium* (Jain et al., 2022). Of note, neonatal sepsis risk models consider maternal GBS colonization and peak intrapartum maternal temperature significant factors for predicting early onset sepsis risk among term and premature neonates. It is common for neonatal providers to learn of chorioamnionitis (Triple I) at the time they arrive to prepare for the resuscitation of a newborn. Consistent use of the Neonatal Resuscitation Program (NRP) "4 pre-birth questions" will help ensure full transparency. Neonatal providers should clarify the type of antibiotic regimen provided, particularly in cases of suspected GBS infection.

The neonatal morbidity and mortality risk is 2- to 3.5-fold higher with cases of Triple I. Complications observed shortly after birth include intraventricular hemorrhage (IVH), meningitis, necrotizing enterocolitis, sepsis and septic shock, pneumonia, and death. Later complications include cerebral white matter damage and retinopathy of prematurity. Life-span implications include chronic asthma, chronic obstructive pulmonary disease, cerebral palsy, and associated developmental delays, as well as hearing impairment and schizophrenia/autism phenotypes (Jain et al., 2022).

Obstetric Hemorrhage

Obstetric hemorrhage may be defined as excessive uterine or vaginal bleeding that exceeds 1,000 mL, which occurs during the antepartum or postpartum period (ACOG, 2022b). Obstetric hemorrhage that happens in the postpartum period is one of the leading causes of morbidity and mortality in XX pregnant patients throughout the world, accounting for 11% of all pregnancy-related deaths in the United States (ACOG, 2022b). Risk factors for hemorrhage and the need for a blood transfusion include a classical cesarean incision, preeclampsia, prolonged labor, and chorioamnionitis (Triple I; Table 14.1; Association of Women's Health, Obstetric and Neonatal Nurses, 2019; Salcido et al., 2023). Other causes of postpartum hemorrhage that exclusively affect the pregnant patient (and not the fetus or newborn) in the postpartum period are not included in this review.

Recall that significant hemodynamic changes occur during pregnancy, the first of these being an increase in the pregnant patient's plasma volume. XX pregnant patients also increase their red blood cell (RBC) mass by an expected 20% to 30%. The maternal cardiac output increases by 30% to 50% to manage the increased volume and increased baseline heart rate. Concurrently, SVR falls. Finally, fibrinogen and the majority of procoagulant blood factors, most notably factors VII, VIII, X, and von Willebrand factor, increase during pregnancy. Under normal circumstances, suppression of clot busting and a state of hypercoagulability arise. Although these systemic changes are vital for maternal hemodynamic stability during pregnancy, the combination also facilitates a rapid decompensation during an obstetric hemorrhage (Francois & Foley, 2017; Key et al., 2017).

When a maternal hemorrhage occurs, the body's arterial and venous compartments vasoconstrict, but can only compensate with up to 20% of total volume loss. With massive hemorrhage, cardiovascular collapse occurs, as cardiac output falls due to decreased preload, leading to poor end-organ perfusion. Shock and acidosis thereby ensue and, if left uncorrected, will result in maternal, and possibly fetal, demise (Francois & Foley, 2017). The long-term effects to the liveborn neonate subject to an obstetric hemorrhage are dictated by its etiology and severity.

THE FETAL HEART RATE

A normal FHR is defined as 110 bpm to 160 bpm with beat-to-beat variability ranging between 6 and 25 bpm (ACOG, 2017; Gutvirtz et al., 2022). In order for the FHR to vary, normal parasympathetic input from the cortex, diencephalon, and brainstem toward the medulla and then to the vagus nerve must be present. Therefore, *normal beat-to-beat variability is the single most significant indicator of fetal well-being.* Conditions that favor a loss of beat-to-beat variability include premature gestation; fetal exposure to drugs including narcotics, analgesics,

TABLE 14.1 Obstetric Hemorrhage Risk Assessment

Prenatal Risk Factors
- Clinically significant bleeding disorder
- Prepregnancy BMI >50
- Suspected placenta accreta, previa, increta, percreta
- Other risk factors (e.g., refusal of blood transfusion)

Antepartum Risk Factors
- Placenta accreta
- Placenta previa
- Prior classical cesarean section
- Prior myomectomy

Intrapartum Risk Factors

Low Intrapartum Risk	Medium Intrapartum Risk	High Intrapartum Risk
• ≤4 prior vaginal births	• >4 prior vaginal births	• Active bleeding > bloody show
• No history of hemorrhage	• Chorioamnionitis (Triple I)	• Hematocrit <30%
• No known bleeding disorder	• Estimated fetal weight >4 kg	• History of >1 hemorrhage
• No previous uterine incision	• Family history of hemorrhage[a]	• Known coagulopathy
• Singleton pregnancy	• Fetal demise	• Low-lying placenta
	• History of prior hemorrhage	• Placenta accreta
	• Induction of labor	• Placenta percreta
	• Intraamniotic (Triple I) infection	• Placenta previa
	• Morbid obesity (BMI >50)	• Platelet count <100,000/mcL
	• Polyhydramnios	
	• Preeclampsia	
	• Prior cesarean birth	
	• Prior uterine incision	
	• Prolonged labor	

[a]Family history is limited to a first-degree relative with a history of hemorrhage.
BMI, body mass index.
Source: Adapted from Association of Women's Health, Obstetric and Neonatal Nurses. (2019). *Safe motherhood initiative.* https://www.acog.org/community/districts-and-sections/district-ii/programs-and-resources/safe-motherhood-initiative/obstetric-hemorrhage

benzodiazepines, and sedatives; and congenital neurologic defects (e.g., anencephaly). Furthermore, *when beat-to-beat variability is accompanied by variable or late FHR decelerations, the neonatal clinician should suspect that the fetus is suffering from worsening acidosis and hypoxic injury in utero.* This should prompt neonatal teams to prepare for a potential advanced resuscitation.

Recall that increases in the FHR above baseline are considered *accelerations* and decreases in the FHR below baseline are *decelerations*. The presence of accelerations is customarily reassuring. However, decelerations can be problematic. These are further classified as either early, variable, or late decelerations. While neonatal providers will not interpret fetal monitoring strips and diagnose FHR changes, it is important to understand the customary proximate cause for the various types of decelerations. Early decelerations are associated with benign compression of the fetal head during a contraction, which increases intracranial pressure (briefly), widens the pulse pressure, and causes short-term bradycardia (also known as the "Cushing reflex"). A noteworthy biochemical indicator of early decelerations is isolated respiratory acidosis on cord blood gas analysis. Variable decelerations are associated with umbilical cord compression (e.g., true knot, nuchal, prolapse). The mechanism for the bradycardic event involves the following sequence: umbilical cord compression induces a state of increased peripheral resistance and fetal hypertension, which activates stretch-sensitive baroreceptors. Baroreceptor activation stimulates the cardioinhibitory center causing a vagally mediated response (bradycardia). Late decelerations are most often associated with placental insufficiency and are associated with fetal hypoxia, acidosis, and hypotension. This type of deceleration occurs 30 to 60 seconds after a contraction has finished and is vagally mediated. Tissue oxygen deprivation elicits the onset of anaerobic glycolysis and the slow accumulation of organic acids (e.g., lactate, ketone bodies; Jia et al., 2023).

Obstetric experts use a three-tiered system to describe the features of the FHR, both baseline (rate and beat-to-beat variability) and periodic (accelerations and decelerations), as these features inform fetal acid–base status (Box 14.1). It is important that neonatal clinicians remain familiar with this tiered system as the information should be used to prepare for neonatal resuscitation and stabilization after birth. Category I FHR is defined as a normal baseline FHR with normal variability; this is indicative of normal fetal acid-base balance (ACOG, 2017; Zullo et al., 2023). Category II findings are characterized as FHR tracings that are not by definition able to be classified as category I or III. Tracings may include bradycardia, tachycardia, minimal or absent variability, variable decelerations, or late decelerations occurring with moderate FHR variability. Although this categorization should be closely evaluated, additional surveillance and/or monitoring tools should be implemented to further evaluate fetal health and determine the need for prompt delivery (ACOG, 2017). Category III FHR monitoring tracings are determinant of abnormal fetal acid–base status and require prompt intervention. Examples of compromising fetal patterns include absent FHR variability occurring with persistent bradycardia, as well as late or variable decelerations (ACOG, 2014, 2017; Zullo et al., 2023).

DELIVERY METHODS

The ACOG and the Society for Maternal-Fetal Medicine (SMFM) have long discouraged nonindicated delivery before 39 weeks of gestation. The reason for this long-standing principle is that the neonatal risks of late-preterm (34 0/7–36 6/7 weeks of gestation) and early-term (37 0/7–38 6/7 weeks of gestation) births are well established (ACOG, 2017). Delivery methods include planned vaginal delivery, operative vaginal delivery, elective cesarean delivery without labor, cesarean delivery with trial of labor, and emergency cesarean delivery. FHR patterns described in the prior section of this chapter can inform the type of delivery method.

Vaginal Delivery

Vaginal deliveries, including planned and operative vaginal deliveries, account for approximately 67.9% of all deliveries within the United States (Osterman et al., 2024). Planned vaginal births are associated with fewer postpartum risks, including a lower incidence of postpartum hem-

BOX 14.1 The Three-Tier Fetal Heart Rate Classification System

Category 1

Tracings are strongly predictive of normal fetal acid–base status with FHR 110 to 160 bpm; may be monitored in a routine manner and no specific action is required. The tracing includes:

- absent early, variable, or late decelerations
- moderate beat-to-beat variability
- presence or absence of accelerations

Category 2

Tracings are not predictive of abnormal fetal acid–base status; tracings require evaluation and continued surveillance and reevaluation, taking into account the entire associated clinical circumstances. The tracing may include any of the following:

- absence of beat-to-beat variability with bradycardia
- absent, minimal, or significant FHR variability
- accelerations may be absent
- intermittent, recurrent, or prolonged decelerations
- recurrent late decelerations
- tachycardia
- variable decelerations with slow recovery to baseline

Category 3

Tracings are associated with abnormal fetal acid–base status at the time of observation. Category III FHR tracings require prompt evaluation. If a category III tracing does not resolve with conservative intervention measures, delivery should be undertaken. The tracing will include absent beat-to-beat variability and:

- bradycardia
- recurrent variable and/or late decelerations
- sinusoidal FHR pattern

FHR, fetal heart rate.

orrhage, blood transfusions, procedural complications, infection, and anesthesia-related complications (ACOG, 2017). Neonatal benefits include earlier onset of breastfeeding, with reductions in rates of iatrogenic prematurity, hypothermia, hypoglycemia, retained fetal lung fluid, and other causes for respiratory distress during the immediate postnatal period. Finally, the mother–neonate dyad often benefits from earlier initiation of breastfeeding practices and incurs a shorter length of stay (ACOG, 2017). Contraindications to a planned vaginal delivery may include, but are not limited to, multiple gestation; fetal malposition; maternal disease states, such as obesity and diabetes mellitus; or other safety issues. One particular mechanical complication that precludes a vaginal birth is umbilical cord prolapse, which may present at any time during the intrapartum period and warrants a cesarean delivery.

Operative Vaginal Delivery

Operative vaginal deliveries involve the use of obstetric instruments to expedite delivery in cases of maternal or fetal compromise. The current incidence in the United States is 3.3% (ACOG, 2020). Indications for operative vaginal delivery include a prolonged second stage of labor, suspicion for fetal compromise (immediate or potential), or to shorten the second stage of labor for the benefit of the pregnant patient (ACOG, 2020). Forceps-assisted delivery has fallen out of favor in exchange for vacuum assistance.

The risk for birth trauma is 3-fold higher with vacuum extraction and 4-fold higher with forceps extraction, with 60% to 90% of all cases of subgaleal hemorrhage associated with vacuum extraction (Kong & To, 2024). Other neonatal complications include *late* decelerations (from head compression when forceps assist is utilized), bruising, lacerations, external ocular trauma, cephalohematoma, and brachial plexus injury. Rare, life-threatening complications include subgaleal hemorrhage, intracranial hemorrhage, and IVH. In rare instances, death may occur (ACOG, 2020).

Cesarean Delivery

Between 2015 and 2022, 32% of all births involved cesarean deliveries (Centers for Disease Control and Prevention, 2024). This is a decline from 2009, when the rate was 60%, yet remains substantially higher than 5% in 1960 (Martin et al., 2013). Common medical indications for cesarean birth include arrest of labor, nonreassuring fetal status, malpresentation, placental abruption or previa, severe preeclampsia, and chorioamnionitis. Socioeconomic inequities are reported in the literature, with a higher percentage of cesarean births occurring in Black, Latinx, and Asian patients (Manns-James et al., 2024).

When conditions compromise maternal or fetal well-being during childbirth, the decision must be made by healthcare providers to determine the urgency of delivery. Intrapartum cesarean delivery classified as emergent should be carried out immediately if presenting conditions pose life-threatening risks to the mother or fetus (Veltman, 2017). Recommendations endorsed by the ACOG (2017) and the American Academy of Pediatrics (AAP) state, "Historically, the consensus has been that hospitals need to have the capability of beginning a cesarean delivery within 30 minutes of the decision to operate. However, the scientific evidence to support this threshold is lacking. The decision-to-incision interval should be based on the timing that best incorporates maternal and fetal risks and benefits [...] it is reasonable to tailor the time to delivery to local circumstances and logistics" (Bank et al., 2023, p. S1111).

DELIVERY COMPLICATIONS AND BIRTH-RELATED INJURIES

A *birth-related injury* can be defined as an event that causes injury to the fetus during the birth process. Birth injuries run a spectrum from mild and self-limiting to so severe they result in the death of the neonate. They are classified by location or etiology. The risk for birth-related injury increases with fetal prematurity, macrosomia, and with fetal malpresentation (e.g., breech, transverse, face, brow positioning) or with shoulder dystocia. Maternal conditions that increase the risk of birth-related injuries are a contracted pelvis, cephalopelvic disproportion, and prolonged or precipitous labor. Instruments, such as fetal scalp electrodes, forceps, and vacuum extractors, are also associated with an increase in birth-related injuries. A comprehensive list of common birth injuries with associated risk factors is presented in Table 14.2. Next, we explore hypoxic–ischemic encephalopathy (HIE), a significant injury and proximate cause for neurologic morbidity in newborns.

Hypoxic–Ischemic Encephalopathy in the Term Neonate

Birth asphyxia results when an interruption in the supply of oxygen from the mother to the developing fetus occurs. Nearly 1 million newborns worldwide die from asphyxia, which most commonly occurs during the perinatal period (World Health Organization, 2024). Among those newborns who survive the birth process, hypoxic–ischemic injury, which manifests as abnormal neurologic behavior in the neonate following a period of perinatal hypoxia–ischemia, may be diagnosed. This form of abnormal neurologic behavior has been classically termed *hypoxic–ischemic encephalopathy*. More recently, the terms include perinatal hypoxia–ischemia, asphyxia neonatorum, and *neonatal encephalopathy* (NE). The global incidence of NE is approximately 1.5 per every 1,000 liveborn infants (J. Park et al., 2023).

Common risk factors for HIE are summarized in Table 14.3. Of note, the two most common intrapartum events associated with hypoxic–ischemic insults

TABLE 14.2 Common Birth Injuries With Associated Risk Factors

Birth Injury	Risk Factors	Incidence
Injuries to the Head and Neck		
Extracranial hemorrhages		
Caput succedaneum	Prolonged labor, primiparous mothers, vacuum-assisted delivery, large baby, small maternal pelvis	Common
Cephalohematoma	Prolonged labor, primiparous mothers, forceps- or vacuum-assisted delivery, large baby, small maternal pelvis	Common
Lacerations	Rupture of membranes prior to delivery, oligohydramnios or anhydramnios with cesarean birth, or in emergent situations	Common
Subgaleal hemorrhage	Prolonged labor, primiparous mothers, forceps, vacuum-assisted delivery with traction applied, large baby, small maternal pelvis	Uncommon
Intracerebellar hemorrhage	Preterm, difficult delivery	Uncommon
Subdural hemorrhage	Prolonged labor, forceps, vacuum-assisted delivery	Uncommon
Subarachnoid hemorrhage	Prolonged labor, forceps, vacuum-assisted delivery	Common
Skull fracture	Prolonged labor, primiparous mothers, difficult labor, vacuum extraction, forceps	Common
Facial palsy	Fetal position, prolonged labor, forceps, large baby, small maternal pelvis, increased pressure from maternal sacral promontory	Common
Vocal cord paralysis	Fetal malpresentation, breech, large baby, small maternal pelvis	Rare
Injuries to the Shoulders, Chest, and Other Bones		
Clavicular fracture	Large baby, small maternal pelvis, shoulder dystocia, breech	Common
Brachial plexus injuries	Fetal malpresentation, breech, increased traction on presenting part during delivery, large baby, small maternal pelvis	
Erb palsy		Common
Klumpke palsy		Rare
Erb–Duchenne–Klumpke Paralysis		Uncommon
Phrenic nerve paralysis	Fetal malpresentation, breech, increased traction on presenting part during delivery, large baby, small maternal pelvis	Uncommon
Humerus fracture	Fetal malpresentation, breech, large baby, small maternal pelvis	Rare
Femur fracture	Breech	Rare
Injuries to the Abdomen		
Rupture of the liver	Breech, large baby, small maternal pelvis	Rare
Rupture of the spleen	Breech, large baby, small maternal pelvis	Rare
Rupture of the adrenal glands	Breech, large baby, small maternal pelvis	Rare

TABLE 14.3 Risk Factors for Hypoxic–Ischemic Injury

Risks for Hypoxia	Risks for Ischemia
• Impaired placental gas exchange (e.g., maternal diabetes, preeclampsia) • Perinatal sentinel event (e.g., placental abruption, uterine rupture, cord prolapse, rotational maneuvers) • Persistence of fetal circulation after birth (e.g., PPHN, CCHD) • Postnatal respiratory disease or failed establishment of spontaneous breathing at birth	• Cardiovascular dysfunction (e.g., persistent right-to-left shunting across ductus arteriosus) • Failed cerebral autoregulation • Cardiovascular dysfunction (e.g., persistent left-to-right shunting across ductus arteriosus) • Sepsis

Note: Diabetes and preeclampsia are the two maternal diseases most significantly associated with a higher risk for HIE and need for body cooling. CCHD, congenital cyanotic heart disease; HIE, hypoxic–ischemic encephalopathy; PPHN, persistent pulmonary hypertension in the newborn
Source: Mrelashvili, A., Ferriero, D., Inder, T. E., & Volpe, J. J. (2025). Hypoxic-ischemic injury in the term infant: Clinical-neurological features, diagnosis, imaging, management, and prognosis. In J. J. Volpe & T. E. Inder (Eds.). *Volpe's neurology of the newborn* (7th ed., pp. 643–696). Elsevier.

are acute circulatory events (placental abruption, cord prolapse, prolonged labor with transverse arrest, complicated forceps extraction, and rotational maneuvers; Mrelashvili et al., 2025). Less common are antepartum events including uterine hemorrhage, maternal trauma, or maternal hypotension; these events are responsible for fewer than 20% of all cases of NE. However, antepartum complications such as those mentioned, as well as maternal diabetes and preeclampsia, increase the risk for hypoxia–ischemia once labor begins. Therefore, neonatal clinicians must remain vigilant and inquire about antepartum events and maternal diagnoses, particularly when a newborn presents with signs of neurologic depression. Diabetes is associated with placental vascular disease (insufficiency), and when combined with preeclampsia increases the likelihood for NE requiring therapeutic hypothermia by 3-fold to 5-fold (Mrelashvili et al., 2025). Many affected infants will be growth restricted (less than 5th percentile), which correlates with placental insufficiency, maternal diabetes, and/or preeclampsia. The least common causes for NE are postpartum events, namely severe pulmonary hypertension in the newborn, recurrent and severe apneic events, and congenital heart disease; these events account for 5% to 50% of all cases of NE (Mrelashvili et al., 2025).

Terms and Definitions. *Hypoxia* denotes a partial loss of oxygen supply to the tissues (e.g., brain) or circulation. *Ischemia* denotes a reduction or complete cessation of blood flow to a particular region of the body (e.g., brain). Hypoxia and ischemia can both result from the larger problem of perinatal asphyxia. *Asphyxia*, the Greek word for *suffocation*, denotes the condition in which the supply of oxygen through the placenta and/or umbilical cord is interrupted.

Pathophysiology. With NE, blood flow and oxygen deprivation caused by any of the aforementioned risk factors (see Table 14.3) provokes a state of myocardial dysfunction and systemic hypotension in the fetus or newborn experiencing an asphyxial event. A state of cerebral ischemia emerges. The neuron is most vulnerable to ischemia, followed by oligodendrocyte, microglia, and astrocyte (Figure 14.6; Pierson & Volpe, 2025). A series of three major phases of energy failure and injury ensue once the primary ischemic insult (e.g., perinatal sentinel event) to the brain ceases. We discuss these phases of energy failure in this section of the chapter.

Primary and Latent Energy Failure. The primary phase of energy failure and associated neuronal changes begin within 5 to 30 minutes after the primary insult ceases (Box 14.2). The newborn, having been subject to a period of hypoxemia, can develop myocardial dysfunction. This precipitates a loss of cerebral autoregulatory capacity; the brain will enter into a pressure-passive state. The anterior, middle, and posterior cerebral arteries (which originate from the circle of Willis) do not effectively autoregulate during the hypotensive state and blood flow through these vessels to critical regions of the brain, the watershed region (parasagittal region), is deficient. This induces a state of cerebral hypoxia–ischemia and consequent brain injury.

The ischemia induced by the primary insult induces a rapid demand for energy metabolites (e.g., adenosine triphosphate, ATP) in the brain. ATP is depleted quickly and a state of anaerobic glycogenolysis and consequential metabolic (lactic) acidosis occurs. Recall that glycogenolysis involves glycogen metabolism and the formation of glucose molecules, which are then metabolized into lactate. The state of metabolic acidosis is associated with a destructive influx of hydrogen ions, sodium, chloride, water, and calcium into the neuronal cells (Groenendaal & DeVries, 2025). Increased potassium efflux occurs due to hydrogen influx, and anoxic depolarization at the neuron is observed. Free radicals and nitric oxide are formed, which in aggregate lead to oxidative stress and cytotoxic edema with resultant cellular necrosis. Throughout this time frame, glutamate, an excitatory neurotransmitter accumulates in the extracellular spaces. Neuronal necrosis occurs, and as cells rupture, inflammatory mediators

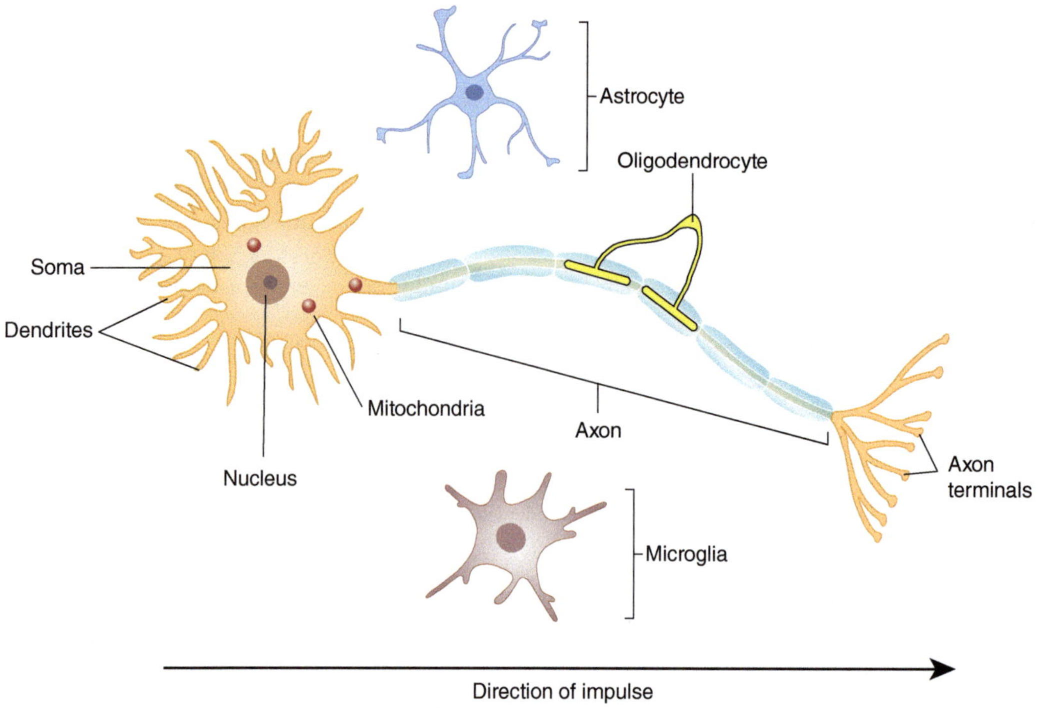

Figure 14.6 Basic anatomy of the neuron, oligodendrocyte, and astrocyte.
Note: Oligodendrocytes participate in the myelination of neurons. Microglia are immune cells found in the brain that assist with neuronal development and the formation of synapses. They are also activated when neurons are damaged. Astrocytes assist with the formation of neurons and synapses, help control the permeability of the blood-brain barrier, and help maintain normal extracellular ion levels in the brain. Astrocytes are activated by microglia.
Image Credit: Amy J. Jnah.

BOX 14.2 Primary Energy Failure: Sequence of Pathologic Events

1. Energy stores are depleted (glucose, ATP)
2. Loss of membrane potentials (anoxic depolarization)
3. Cellular edema begins
4. Oxidative stress begins
5. Glutamate accumulation and neuronal excitotoxicity occurs
6. Neuronal necrosis (primary cell death) occurs

ATP, adenosine triphosphate.

BOX 14.3 Latent Energy Failure: Sequence of Pathologic Events

1. Brief cessation of oxidative stress with restoration of oxidative metabolism
2. Cellular edema slows
3. Glutamate accumulation ceases
4. Reperfusion injury occurs
5. Oxidative stress resumes
6. Astrocytes release toxins
7. Mitochondrial membrane becomes more permeable, permitting leakage of pro-apoptotic proteins (e.g., cytochrome C, caspase-8)
8. Epileptiform changes observed on EEG
9. Connexin channels open
10. Neuroinflammation begins

EEG, electroencephalogram.

(interleukin [IL]-1, IL-6, and tumor necrosis factor alpha [TNFa]) are sequestered. These factors are responsible for early damage to the white matter (Pierson & Volpe, 2025).

The *latent phase of energy failure* begins next and extends through approximately the sixth hour after the primary insult ceased. Early into the latent phase, conditions begin to favor reperfusion. Oxidative metabolism resumes, cellular edema slows, and excess glutamate accumulation briefly ceases (Box 14.3). Astrocytes initially buffer the extracellular glutamate and potassium, participate in glycogenolysis for energy production, and help maintain the integrity of the blood-brain-barrier. Unfortunately, energy stores are again quickly depleted and oxidative stress with lactic acidosis reemerges. Next, astrogliosis (excess accumulation of astrocytes) develops and elicits pathologic extrinsic signaling which leads to the activation of cell death receptors, increased mitochondrial membrane permeability with the formation of openings (pores) in the mitochondria, the influx of calcium into the cells, leakage of proteins (e.g., cytochrome

C, capsases) from the mitochondria which favor cell death (apoptosis), and the opening of connexin-43 channels. Of note, in times of ischemia, connexin-43 channels that are found mostly on astrocytes can pathologically alter the cell membrane potential, releasing unregulated amounts of ATP or glutamate into the extracellular space. Neuroinflammation subsequently begins (Pierson & Volpe, 2025).

Clinical Application. Given the deleterious effects of excessive extracellular glutamate, and pathologic changes that can occur within the first 6 hours after a hypoxic-ischemic event ceases, it is imperative that infants who meet criteria for whole body cooling begin this therapy within the first 6 hours of life. Neonatal clinicians who staff smaller, rural hospitals should initiate transfer of care within the first hour of life, to allow adequate time for coordination of care by the accepting facility and the initiation of cooling within the allotted time frame. In addition, when a clinician cannot definitively discern why a baby is presenting with signs of neonatal encephalopathy, a lumbar puncture should be done. Early-onset meningitis presents similar to neonatal encephalopathy.

Secondary Energy Failure. During the *secondary phase of energy failure*, which can span up to approximately 72 hours after the initial insult ended, oxidative metabolism continues to fail, and cellular edema and inflammation continue (Box 14.4). In addition, a state of microgliosis develops in addition to worsening astrogliosis. Microglia are immune cells found in the central nervous system that normally assist with neuronal development and the formation of oligodendrocytes, myelin, and synapses, as well as the activation of astrocytes. Microglia are activated in times of neuronal injury and cases of neonatal encephalopathy, during which a state of microgliosis (overaccumulation of microglia) occurs (Figure 14.7). This results in the recruitment of proinflammatory mediators along with excessive phagocytosis, and the overactivation of astrocytes. Seizure activity often accompanies these changes and is a nefarious indicator of significant white (and grey) matter injury. Ultimately, selective, programmed cell death occurs, most often affecting the watershed (parasagittal) region and cerebral white matter (Pierson & Volpe, 2025).

BOX 14.4 Secondary Energy Failure: Sequence of Pathologic Events

1. Mitochondrial collapse
2. Cellular edema and neuroinflammation worsens
3. Poor cerebrovascular autoregulation develops
4. Seizures can manifest
5. Programmed cell death occurs

Tertiary Energy Failure. The tertiary phase of energy failure involves a continuum of neuroinflammation, gliosis, reduced oligodendrocyte maturation, and the potential for continued seizure activity (Box 14.5). The exact duration of this phase is unknown, but experts posit that it can span weeks to months. During phagocytosis, glial cells consume the lipid component of myelin sheaths from apoptotic neurons, which causes them to take on a "white" and foamy appearance. They are then appropriately labeled as "foamy macrophages." The foamy macrophages continue to consume debris left over from cell necrosis and a glial mat (scar tissue) forms in its place while a state of chronic neuroinflammation persists. In severe cases, extensive neuronal apoptosis may leave behind large cavities, most notably at the cortex. In fact, severe cases of NE are associated with 8% to 20% cell loss at the cortex (Gonzalez et al., 2025). The cumulative effect of these pathologic changes includes impaired formation and maturation of neurons along with faulty synaptogenesis. In addition, there is a loss of production of trophic factors that normally assist with neurogenesis and physiologic repair of damaged neurons across the life span (Pierson & Volpe, 2025).

Postnatal Clinical Manifestations. The timing, degree, and duration of impaired cerebral perfusion and hypoxia impact the severity of brain injury in term newborns and the clinical manifestations evident at birth (Table 14.4). Term neonates are depressed at birth and display clinical symptoms consistent with neurologic injury. These infants typically require advanced neonatal resuscitation, including chest compressions, thereby resulting in low Apgar scores. When an umbilical arterial cord gas pH is less than 7.00 and/or the base deficit is greater than 12 mmol/L in combination with signs of clinical illness (abnormal FHR pattern, Apgar score less than 5 at 10 minutes, respiratory dysfunction necessitating intubation), the likelihood for neurologic disease increases (Mrelashvili et al., 2025).

Therefore, three factors should increase the index of suspicion for hypoxic–ischemic injury: (a) fetal distress, (b) low Apgar scoring or the need for advanced neonatal resuscitation, and (c) manifestations of neurologic injury within the first 24 hours of life (Mrelashvili et al., 2025). The peripartum neurologic presentation is categorized by severity (mild, moderate, and severe), commonly measured using the modified Sarnat staging system (Table 14.5). Other scoring systems are available, including the Thompson scale, Score of the Ibero-American Society of Neonatology (SIBEN) scale, and the NICHD scale. The SIBEN and NICHD scales are limited to use within the first 6 hours of life and are useful for research (randomization) purposes. Although an exploration into each scoring method is

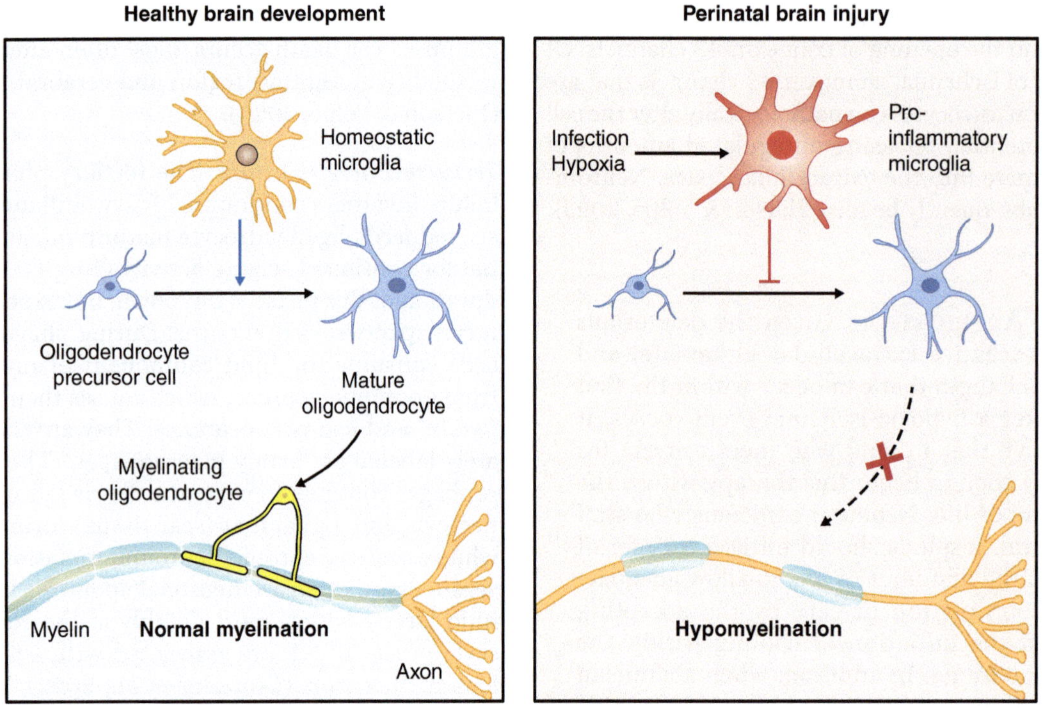

Figure 14.7 Microglia and the developing brain.

Note: During healthy brain development, microglia modulate the formation and maturation of oligodendrocytes. However, with perinatal brain injury, proinflammatory activation inhibits the maturation of oligodendrocytes. Over time, this leads to neuronal hypomyelination, which is associated with cognitive, sensory, and motor deficits.

Image Credit: Amy J. Jnah.

BOX 14.5 Tertiary Energy Failure: Sequence of Pathologic Events

1. Impaired neuronal maturation
2. Faulty synaptogenesis
3. Chronic neuroinflammation
4. Loss of trophic production of factors including erythropoietin and IGF-1

IGF, insulin-like growth factor.

TABLE 14.4 Clinical Features of Neonatal Encephalopathy

Mild to Moderate	Severe
• Decreased spontaneous activity • Disturbed respiratory function • Hyperalert or irritable • Hypotonia with distal hypertonia • Seizures	• Hypotonia exceeding hypertonia • Intact oculomotor response • Intact pupillary response • Respiratory dysfunction • Seizures • Stupor or coma

Source: Adapted from Mrelashvili, A., Ferriero, D., Inder, T. E., & Volpe, J. J. (2025). Hypoxic-ischemic injury in the term infant: Clinical-neurological features, diagnosis, imaging, management, and prognosis. In J. J. Volpe, & T. E. Inder (Eds.), *Volpe's neurology of the newborn* (7th ed., pp. 643–696). Elsevier.

beyond the scope of this textbook, we encourage clinicians who indirectly or directly participate in research initiatives to take time to compare and contrast the study-specific scoring tool with available alternatives.

It is common for affected neonates to manifest with neurologic impairment paired with at least one other indicator of major organ dysfunction. Therefore, cardiovascular, liver, and kidney dysfunction are commonly observed among affected neonates. Impaired myocardial contractility leads to a significant reduction in cardiac output, hypotension, and impairment of blood flow to other organs. Transient elevation in liver enzymes and impaired coagulation is to be expected; both are considered transient, reversible problems. Disseminated intravascular coagulation (DIC) is well recognized and is related to the low levels of factor XIII and alterations to the thrombin–antithrombin complexes and soluble fibrin monomer complexes (Groenendaal & DeVries, 2025). In addition, the majority of neonates who experience hypoxic–ischemic injury will develop acute renal failure, due to decreased renal perfusion. Careful maintenance of fluid balance with daily measurement of serum and urine electrolytes, as well as daily weights, is required (Groenendaal & DeVries, 2025).

TABLE 14.5 Clinical Staging of Hypoxic–Ischemic Encephalopathy

	Stage 1 (Mild)	Stage 2 (Moderate)	Stage 3 (Severe)
Level of consciousness	Hyperalert	Lethargic	Stupor or coma
Pupils	Dilated	Constricted	Variable, unequal
Breathing	Spontaneous	Periodic	Apnea
Heart rate	Tachycardia	Bradycardia	Lack of HR variability
Seizures	None	Present-infrequent	Present-frequent
Spontaneous activity	Normal	Decreased	Absent
Muscle Tone	Normal	Hypotonia	Flaccid
Posture	Mild distal flexion	Marked distal flexion	Decerebrate
Suck	Weak	Weak or absent	Absent
Moro	Strong	Weak	Absent

HR, heart rate.
Source: Adapted from Mrelashvili, A., Ferriero, D., Inder, T. E., & Volpe, J. J. (2025). Hypoxic-ischemic injury in the term infant: Clinical-neurological features, diagnosis, imaging, management, and prognosis. In J. J. Volpe & T. E. Inder (Eds.), *Volpe's neurology of the newborn* (7th ed., pp. 643–696). Elsevier.

Neuropathologic Manifestations of Neonatal Encephalopathy. Although neuropathologic features of hypoxic–ischemic injury vary with gestational age, certain patterns of injury can be identified after the tertiary phase of NE has completed. These patterns include selective neuronal necrosis, parasagittal injury, and cerebral white matter injury. We review the anatomic locus for each pattern of injury in this section of the chapter.

Selective Neuronal Necrosis. Selective neuronal necrosis, the most common neuropathologic finding, refers to necrosis of *neurons* at select, characteristic locations and in a widespread manner. The severity of the hypoxic–ischemic insult and gestational age of the neonate can affect the distribution of injury. The common locations associated with selective neuronal necrosis include the cerebellum, brainstem, thalamus, basal ganglia, hippocampus, and cortex (Figure 14.8). Keeping these loci in mind, three patterns of distribution are reported: deep nuclear-brainstem injury, cerebral-deep nuclear injury, and diffuse injury. Deep nuclear-brainstem is associated with severe yet abrupt hypoxia–ischemia and involves selective neuronal necrosis within the cerebellum, brainstem, thalamus, and basal ganglia. Cerebral-deep nuclear injury is associated with moderate to severe and prolonged hypoxia–ischemia and involves selective neuronal necrosis within the thalamus, basal ganglia, hippocampus, and cortex. Diffuse injury is associated with severe and prolonged hypoxia–ischemia and causes selective neuronal necrosis within the brainstem, thalamus, basal ganglia, hippocampus, and cortex. Severe diffuse disease is known to implicate the calcarine cortex, or vision center (Pierson & Volpe, 2025).

Parasagittal Cerebral Injury. Recall that the cerebral cortex sits atop the cerebrum, and subcortical white matter is contained within the cerebrum. Major cerebral arteries (middle cerebral artery, anterior and posterior cerebral arteries) that comprise part of the circle of Willis innervate the cortex and subcortical white matter at an area known as the parasagittal watershed region ("watershed" referring to an outflow point where blood from the circle of Willis enters the brain). Parasagittal cerebral injury, or a *watershed infarct*, occurs when perfusion to major cerebral arteries is interrupted and neurons within the cortex and the adjacent subcortical white matter are devoid of blood flow and oxygen. This injury manifests on both hemispheres of the brain (Figure 14.9). The injury is usually symmetrical although small differences in the extent of injury between the hemispheres may exist. Nearly 40% to 60% of term infants with NE manifest with this pattern of injury (Pierson & Volpe, 2025).

Cerebral White Matter Injury. White matter injury is a common finding associated with NE, as it also is with preterm infants who suffer IVH. This makes the neuropathology of both injuries extremely similar. The posterior white matter of the brain is customarily more profoundly affected by hypoxia–ischemia than anterior and central white matter. The damage to white matter

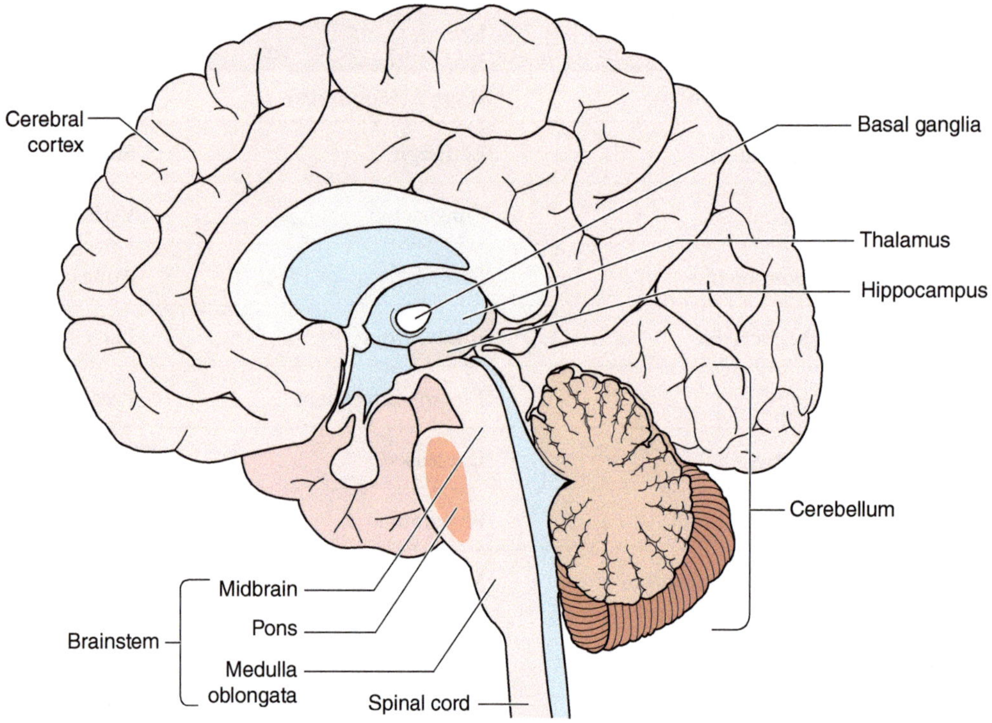

Figure 14.8 Locations associated with selective neuronal necrosis.
Image Credit: Amy J. Jnah.

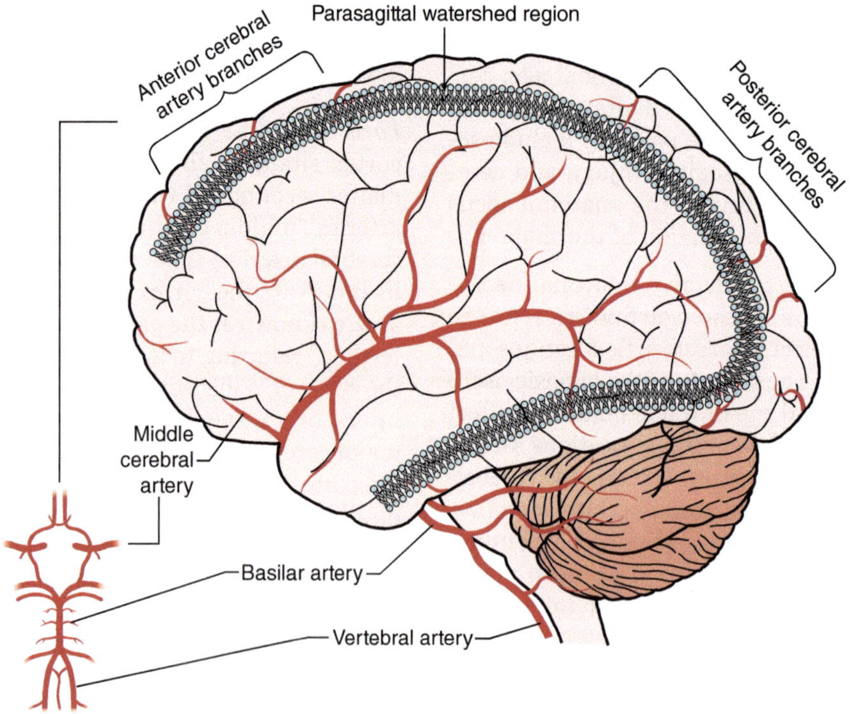

Figure 14.9 Border zones of major cerebral arteries implicated with watershed injury.
Note: The gray shaded region denotes the watershed region.
Image Credit: Amy J. Jnah.

crosses a spectrum of severity from "focal necrotic/cystic" (most severe) to "nonnecrotic/noncystic" (least severe) disease. Focal necrotic/cystic disease involves the formation of large focal necrotic lesions that evolve to cysts. Less severe are *focal necrotic/noncystic* lesions that do not evolve into cysts, but rather scar tissue. In contrast, nonnecrotic/noncystic disease involves the formation of tiny lesions or cysts that tend to be diffusely spread throughout the white matter but are difficult to identify with neuroimaging (Back & Volpe, 2025).

Life-Span Implications. Cognitive impairment with or without cerebral palsy, seizure disorders, a notable weakening and/or spasticity of all extremities, visual impairments, and death are reported among affected neonates. In fact, the presence of seizures increases the risk for neurologic sequelae by as much as 40-fold. Clinicians must also recognize that mild injury may lead to no long-term consequences, whereas those with moderate to severe hypoxic–ischemic injury have exhibited long-term neurodevelopmental and cognitive deficits (Mrelashvili et al., 2025). The aforementioned Sarnat and Thompson scales, in conjunction with MRI findings, offer clinicians the ability to discuss prognostics with family members.

CONCLUSION

Multiple intricate angiogenic factors must align to build a functional circulatory system, and this involves coordination of both maternal and fetal components. The fetal heart begins to beat during early embryologic development, and subsequent vascular development is crucial for other organ placement and formation. Maternal health prior to and in the early stages of pregnancy significantly impacts fetal development. The transition from fetal to neonatal circulation is a crucial time for the newborn and can be heavily influenced again by maternal health and also by mode of delivery. Delays or complications in delivery impact the cardiopulmonary transition and result in neonatal injury and disease. Birth injuries can also occur as a result of the mode of delivery and carry long-term neurologic, orthopedic, and dermatologic implications. Should a worst-case scenario arise, the neonatal APRN requires a strong communication skill set in order to communicate with the family in an empathetic manner.

LEARNING TOOLS AND RESOURCES

CourseConnect

To access self-assessment questions and interactive, competency-based learning activities for this chapter, visit www.springerpub.com/courseconnect. See inside front cover and tear-out card for CourseConnect details.

Podcast

This podcast is available online by visiting www.springerpub.com/courseconnect. See inside front cover and tear-out card for CourseConnect details.

Transition to Extrauterine Life
Janice L. Wilson and Jennifer Fitzgerald

Discussion Prompts

1. Discuss how economic investment in comprehensive maternal healthcare could prevent elevated costs associated with maternal disease states and neonatal morbidities, including prematurity.
2. Discuss how indications of fetal health status should or should not impact the decision to proceed with vaginal versus operative delivery.
3. You are performing a newborn exam on a 3.9-kg, 2-hour-old neonate. In your assessment you find the right arm is not flexed and there is an absent Moro reflex on the right side; the left side shows a normal expected response. Discuss the possible etiology for this finding, what other assessments will need to be made, possible long-term outcomes, and the conversation that will occur with the parents.
4. You are counseling a family that is attempting to lay blame for their 4-hour-old neonate having experienced a hypoxic–ischemic injury during a forceps-assisted delivery that failed and required an emergency cesarean section. The parents are convinced that their child will have permanent, long-term brain damage and claim they asked for the cesarean early in the birth process and were denied. How do you answer their challenges and concerns?

REFERENCES

American College of Obstetricians and Gynecologists. (2017). ACOG practice bulletin No. 106: Intrapartum fetal heart rate monitoring: Nomenclature, interpretation, and general management principles. *Obstetrics and Gynecology, 114*(1), 192–202. https://doi.org/10.1097/AOG.0b013e3181aef106

American College of Obstetricians and Gynecologists. (2020). Operative vaginal birth: ACOG practice bulletin, Number 219. *Obstetrics and Gynecology, 135*(4), e149–e159. https://doi.org/10.1097/AOG.0000000000003764

American College of Obstetricians and Gynecologists. (2021). *Placenta accreta spectrum.* https://www.acog.org/clinical/clinical-guidance/obstetric-care-consensus/articles/2018/12/placenta-accreta-spectrum

American College of Obstetricians and Gynecologists. (2022a). *Committee Opinion No. 712: Intrapartum management of intraamniotic infection.* https://www.acog.org/clinical/clinical-guidance/committee-opinion/articles/2017/08/intrapartum-management-of-intraamniotic-infection

American College of Obstetricians and Gynecologists. (2022b). *Committee Opinion No. 794: Quantitative blood loss in obstetric hemorrhage*. https://www.acog.org/clinical/clinical-guidance/committee-opinion/articles/2019/12/quantitative-blood-loss-in-obstetric-hemorrhage

Ananth, C. V., Lavery, J. A., Vintzileos, A. M., Skupski, D. W., Varner, M., Saade, G., Biggio, J., Williams, M. A., Wapner, R. J., & Wright, J. D. (2016). Severe placental abruption: Clinical definition and associations with maternal complications. *American Journal of Obstetrics and Gynecology, 214*(2), 272.e1–272.e9. https://doi.org/10.1016/j.ajog.2015.09.069

Anders, A. P., Gaddy, J. A., Doster, R. S., & Aronoff, D. M. (2017). Current concepts in maternal–fetal immunology: Recognition and response to microbial pathogens by decidual stromal cells. *American Journal of Reproductive Immunology, 77*(3), e12623. https://doi.org/10.1111/aji.12623

Association of Women's Health, Obstetric and Neonatal Nurses. (2019). *Safe motherhood initiative*. https://www.acog.org/community/districts-and-sections/district-ii/programs-and-resources/safe-motherhood-initiative/obstetric-hemorrhage

Back, S. A., & Volpe, J. J. (2025). Encephalopathy of prematurity: Pathophysiology. In J. J. Volpe & T. E. Inder (Eds.), *Volpe's neurology of the newborn* (7th ed., pp. 523–546). Elsevier.

Bączkowska, M., Kosińska-Kaczyńska, K., Zgliczyńska, M., Brawura-Biskupski-Samaha, R., Rebizant, B., & Ciebiera, M. (2022). Epidemiology, risk factors, and perinatal outcomes of placental abruption-detailed annual data and clinical perspectives from Polish tertiary center. *International Journal of Environmental Research and Public Health, 19*(9), 5148. https://doi.org/10.3390/ijerph19095148

Bank, T. C., Macones, G., & Sciscione, A. (2023). The "30-minute rule" for expedited delivery: Fact or fiction? *American Journal of Obstetrics and Gynecology, 228*(5), S1110–S1116. https://doi.org/10.1016/j.ajog.2022.06.015

Brown, D. W., Freed, M. D., & Mayer, J. E. (2024). Fetal and transitional circulation. In E. P. Walsh, J. E. Mayer Jr., S. A. Teele, & D. W. Brown (Eds.), *Nadas' pediatric cardiology* (pp. 49–54). https://doi.org/10.1016/B978-1-4557-0599-3.00013-2

Centers for Disease Control and Prevention. (2024). *Births—Method of delivery*. https://www.cdc.gov/nchs/fastats/delivery.htm

Cresswell, J. A., Ronsmans, C., Calvert, C., & Filippi, V. (2013). Prevalence of placenta praevia by world region: A systematic review and meta-analysis. *Tropical Medicine & International Health, 18*(6), 712–724. https://doi.org/10.1111/tmi.12100

Francois, K., & Foley, M. (2017). Antepartum and postpartum hemorrhage. In S. G. Gabbee, J. R. Niebyl, J. L. Simpson, M. B. Landon, H. L. Galan, E. R. M. Jauniaux, D. A. Driscoll, V. Berghella, & W. A. Grobman (Eds.), *Obstetrics: Normal and problem pregnancies* (7th ed., pp. 395–424). Elsevier.

Goldsmith, J. (2025). Overview and initial management of delivery room resuscitation. In R. J. Martin & A. A. Fanaroff (Eds.), *Fanaroff and Martin's neonatal-perinatal medicine: Diseases of the fetus and infant* (12th ed., pp. 530-544). Elsevier.

Gonzalez, F. F., Ferriero, D. M., & Volpe, J. J. (2025). Hypoxic-ischemic injury in the term infant: Pathophysiology. In J. J. Volpe & T. E. Inder (Eds.), *Volpe's neurology of the newborn* (7th ed., pp. 632–646). Elsevier.

Greenberg, J., Narendran, V., Schibler, K., Warner, B., & Haberman, B. (2014). Neonatal morbidities of prenatal and perinatal origin. In R. Creasy, R. Resnik, J. Iams, C. Lockwood, T. Moore, & M. Greene (Eds.), *Creasy and Resnik's maternal–fetal medicine: Principles and practice* (7th ed., pp. 1215–1239). Elsevier.

Groenendaal, F., & DeVries, L. (2025). Hypoxic–ischemic encephalopathy. In A. A. Fanaroff & R. J. Martin (Eds.), *Fanaroff and Martin's neonatal–perinatal medicine: Diseases of the fetus and infant* (11th ed., pp. 1059–1084). Elsevier.

Gutvirtz, G., Pariente, G., Wainstock, T., & Sheiner, E. (2022). Intrapartum fetal heart rate monitoring and offspring long-term neurological health. *American Journal of Obstetrics and Gynecology, 226*(1), S731–S731. https://doi.org/10.1016/j.ajog.2021.11.1204

Hiersch, L., Shinar, S., Melamed, N., Aviram, A., Hadar, E., Yogev, Y., & Ashwal, E. (2017). Recurrent placenta-mediated complications in women with three consecutive deliveries. *Obstetrics and Gynecology, 129*, 416–421. https://doi.org/10.1097/AOG.0000000000001890

Jain, V. G., Willis, K. A., Jobe, A., & Ambalavanan, N. (2022). Chorioamnionitis and neonatal outcomes. *Pediatric Research, 91*(2), 289–296. https://doi.org/10.1038/s41390-021-01633-0

Jenabi, E., Salimi, Z., Bashirian, S., Khazaei, S., & Ayubi, E. (2022). The risk factors associated with placenta previa: An umbrella review. *Placenta, 117*, 21–27. https://doi.org/10.1016/j.placenta.2021.10.009

Jia, Y., Ghi, T., Pereira, S., Gracia Perez-Bonfils, A., & Chandraharan, E. (2023). Pathophysiological interpretation of fetal heart rate tracings in clinical practice. *American Journal of Obstetrics and Gynecology, 228*(6), 622–644. https://doi.org/10.1016/j.ajog.2022.05.023

Key, N., Makris, M., & Lillicrap, D. (Eds.). (2017). *Practical hemostasis and thrombosis* (3rd ed.). John Wiley.

Kong, C. W., & To, W. W. K. (2024). Precision of vacuum cup placement and its association with subgaleal hemorrhage and associated morbidity in term neonates. *Archives of Gynecology and Obstetrics, 309*(4), 1411–1419. https://doi.org/10.1007/s00404-023-07018-4

Levin, G., Rottenstreich, A., Ilan, H., Cahan, T., Tsur, A., & Meyer, R. (2021). Predictors of adverse neonatal outcome in pregnancies complicated by placenta previa. *Placenta, 104*, 119–123. https://doi.org/10.1016/j.placenta.2020.12.005

Manns-James, L., Vines, S., Alliman, J., Hoehn-Velasco, L., Stapleton, S., Wright, J., & Jolles, D. (2024). Race, ethnicity, and indications for primary cesarean birth: Associations within a national birth center registry. *Birth, 51*(2), 353–362. https://doi.org/10.1111/birt.12791

Martin, J. A., Hamilton, B. E., Osterman, M. J. K., Curtin, S. C., & Mathews, T. J. (2013). *Births: Final data for 2012*. https://www.cdc.gov/nchs/data/nvsr/nvsr62/nvsr62_09.pdf

Mir, I. N., & Rosenfeld, C. R. (2021). Regulation of placental circulation. In R. Polin, S. H. Abman, D. H. Rowitch, & W. Benitz (Eds.), *Fetal and neonatal physiology* (6th ed., pp. 80-88). Elsevier.

Mrelashvili, A., Ferriero, D., Inder, T. E., & Volpe, J. J. (2025). Hypoxic-ischemic injury in the term infant: Clinical-neurological features, diagnosis, imaging, management, and prognosis. In J. J. Volpe & T. E. Inder (Eds.), *Volpe's neurology of the newborn* (7th ed., pp. 643–696). Elsevier.

Osterman, M. J. K., Hamilton, B. E., Martin, J. A., Driscoll, A. K., & Valenzuela, C. P. (2024). *Births: Final data for 2022.* https://www.cdc.gov/nchs/data/nvsr/nvsr73/nvsr73-02.pdf

Oyelese, Y., & Smulian, J. C. (2006). Placenta previa, placenta accreta, and vasa previa. *Obstetrics and Gynecology, 107*(4), 927–941. https://doi.org/10.1097/01.AOG.0000207559.15715.98

Park, J., Park, S. H., Kim, C., Yoon, S. J., Lim, J. H., Han, J. H., Shin, J. E., Eun, H. S., Park, M. S., & Lee, S. M. (2023). Growth and developmental outcomes of infants with hypoxic ischemic encephalopathy. *Scientific Reports, 13*(1), 23100. https://doi.org/10.1038/s41598-023-50187-0

Park, M. K., & Salamat, M. (2021). Fetal and perinatal circulation. In M. K. Park & M. Salamat (Eds.), *Park's pediatric cardiology for practitioners* (7th ed., pp. 92–95). Elsevier.

Pierson, C. R., & Volpe, J. J. (2025). Hypoxic-ischemic encephalopathy in the term infant: Neuropathology. In J. J. Volpe & T. E. Inder (Eds.), *Volpe's neurology of the newborn* (7th ed., pp. 619–631). Elsevier.

Salcido, C., Shahidi, S. A., Poeltler, D. M., Gollin, Y., Johnston, L. A., & Katheria, A. C. (2023). Maternal bleeding complications and neonatal outcomes following early versus delayed umbilical cord clamping in cesarean deliveries for very low birthweight infants. *Journal of Perinatology, 43*(1), 39–43. https://doi.org/10.1038/s41372-022-01558-4

Tikkanen, M., Luukkaala, T., Gissler, M., Ritvanen, A., Ylikorkala, O., Paavonen, J., Nuutila, M., Andersson, S., & Metsäranta, M. (2013). Decreasing perinatal mortality in placental abruption. *Acta Obstetricia et Gynecologica Scandinavica, 92*(3), 298–305. https://doi.org/10.1111/aogs.12030

Veltman, L. (2017). The "6 A's": A risk manager's guide to emergency cesarean delivery. *Journal of Healthcare Risk Management, 36*(4), 19–24. https://doi.org/10.1002/jhrm.21269

Walfisch, A., & Sheiner, E. (2016). Placenta previa and immediate outcome of the term offspring. *Archives of Gynecology and Obstetrics, 294*(4), 739–744. https://doi.org/10.1007/s00404-016-4044-7

World Health Organization. (2024). *Perinatal asphyxia.* https://www.who.int/teams/maternal-newborn-child-adolescent-health-and-ageing/newborn-health/perinatal-asphyxia

Zullo, F., Di Mascio, D., Raghuraman, N., Wagner, S., Brunelli, R., Giancotti, A., Mendez-Figueroa, H., Cahill, A. G., Gupta, M., Berghella, V., Blackwell, S. C., & Chauhan, S. P. (2023). Three-tiered fetal heart rate interpretation system and adverse neonatal and maternal outcomes: A systematic review and meta-analysis. *American Journal of Obstetrics and Gynecology, 229*(4), 377–387. https://doi.org/10.1016/j.ajog.2023.04.008

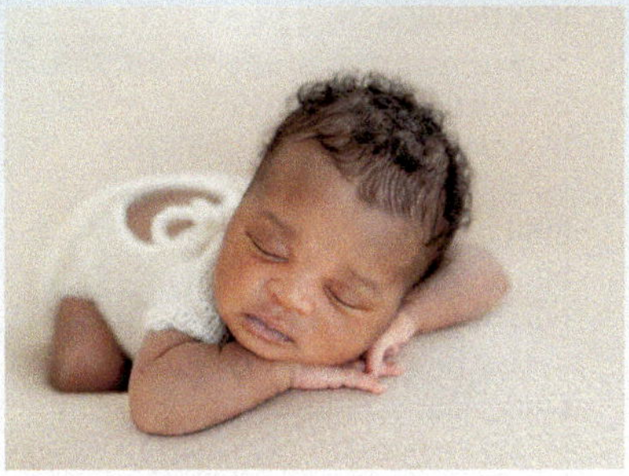
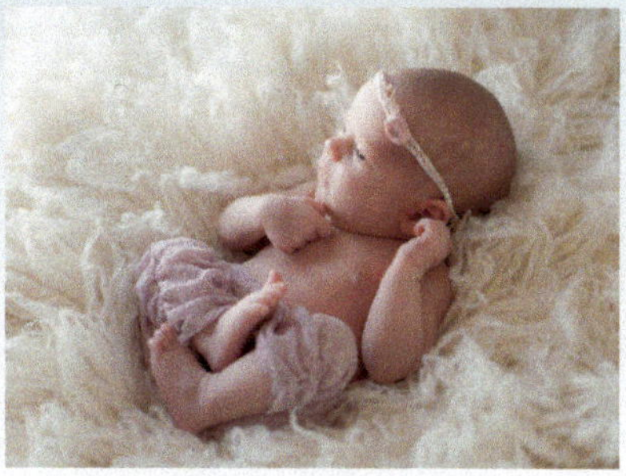

INDEX